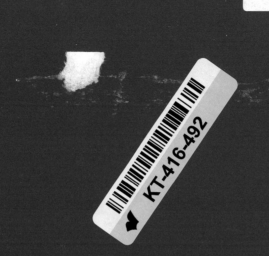

Companion to Psychiatric Studies

Edited by

Eve C. Johnstone MD FRCP(Glasgow and Edinburgh) FRCPsych
Professor of Psychiatry and Head of the Department of Psychiatry, University of Edinburgh, UK

C.P.L. Freeman MB ChB MPhil FRCPsych
Consultant Psychotherapist, Royal Edinburgh Hospital; Senior Lecturer, Department of Psychiatry, University of Edinburgh, UK

A.K. Zealley MB ChB FRCP(Edinburgh) FRCPsych DPM
Consultant Psychiatrist, Royal Edinburgh Hospital; Honorary Senior Lecturer, Department of Psychiatry, University of Edinburgh, UK

SIXTH EDITION

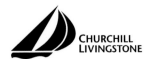

EDINBURGH LONDON NEW YORK SAN FRANCISCO SYDNEY TORONTO 1998

CHURCHILL LIVINGSTONE
A division of Harcourt Brace and Company Limited

Churchill Livingstone, 1-3 Baxter's Place, Leith Walk,
Edinburgh EH1 3AF

Distributed in the United States of America by Churchill
Livingstone Inc., 650 Avenue of the Americas, New York,
N.Y. 10011, and by associated companies, branches and
representatives throughout the world.

First edition 1973
Second edition 1978
Third edition 1983
Fourth edition 1988
Fifth edition 1993
Sixth edition 1998

ISBN 0443 057826

British Library of Cataloguing in Publication Data
A catalogue record for this book is available from the British
Library.

Library of Congress Cataloging in Publication Data
A catalog record for this book is available from the Library of
Congress.

Medical knowledge is constantly changing. As information
becomes available, changes in treatment, procedures,
equipment and the use of drugs become necessary. The
author and publisher have, as far as it is possible, taken care
to ensure that the information given in the text is accurate and
up-to-date. However, readers are strongly advised to confirm
that the information, especially with regard to drug usage,
complies with current legislation and standard of practice.

For Churchill Livingstone:

Publisher: Michael Parkinson
Project editor: Barbara Simmons
Copy-editor: Rosaline Crum
Project controller: Nancy Arnott
Design direction: Erik Bigland

Produced by Addison Wesley Longman China Limited, Hong Kong
CTPS/01

Preface

The first edition of this textbook was published in 1973, and since then a new edition has been published every five years, this being the sixth. Like its predecessors, this volume attempts to incorporate the advances and changes in psychiatric knowledge and practice over the last five years, retain the important elements from previous editions and remove any material which is no longer been up-to-date or relevant. A number of chapters have been coalesced so that, for example, measurement, statistics and research design are now dealt with together.

Since the last edition, many authors have moved on and much new material has been included by the authors of this volume. Some new chapters have been added, for example 'Psychiatric disorders specific to women' by Dr Rachel Jenkins and Professor Jan Scott, and 'Legal and ethical aspects of psychiatry' by Dr Stephen Potts. Sincere thanks are due to all of the authors and those who helped them to prepare their chapters, but it is a pleasure to acknowledge the particular contribution of the late Professor William Parry-Jones, who, when he was already suffering from his rapid final illness, sent in a neat, well-nigh perfect manuscript, exactly on time.

This book is intended as a general textbook for all postgraduate students of psychiatry. Although it is hoped that it will be useful for candidates for both parts of the Membership of the Royal College of Psychiatrists examination, it is meant to serve a wider audience. It is hoped that it will be valuable to others involved in the study of mental disorders, such as clinical psychologists, neuroscientists and psychiatric nurses, and that psychiatrists who have not had to sit an examination for many years will find it a useful source for updating information and reference.

Most, although not all, of the authors, work or have worked in Edinburgh. The book is, however, not intended merely for a local or indeed a UK-wide readership. Issues are addressed from a broader perspective and it is intended to be a relevant text for psychiatrists and others throughout the English-speaking world.

The editors of the previous editions of this book have, in the prefaces, expressed the view that so many advances have taken place over the last five years that a new edition is necessary. Perhaps the latest advances always seems more exciting than those viewed from a distant perspective, but the developments in neuroimaging, psychopharmacology, genetics and neuropsychology that have lately taken place do seem to have brought about great changes in the way that we think about mental disorders. Not all changes are ever for the better, and the last five years have certainly seen increasing concern about the delivery of mental health. These issues too are covered in this edition. In psychiatry, it is very much the case that as some things change, so too do others remain the same. Recent advances in the understanding of the functioning of the nervous system have not been paralleled by improvements in the outcome of treatment to the extent that we might have wished, and it is hoped that issues relating to the burden of disease have not been overlooked here.

Throughout, where the male pronoun is used, this also refers to the female unless otherwise indicated.

Edinburgh 1998

E.C.J
C.P.F.
A.K.Z.

Contributors

Gordon W. Arbuthnott BSc PhD
Honorary Professor, Centre for Neuroscience and
Preclinical Veterinary Sciences, University of Edinburgh

John Bancroft MD FRCP FRCP(Edin) FRCPsych
Director, The Kinsey Institute of Research in Sex,
Gender and Reproduction, Indiana University, USA

Douglas Blackwood PhD FRCP FRCPsych
Reader in Psychiatry, University of Edinburgh,
Edinburgh, UK

Tom M. Brown MB MPhil MRCP MRCPsych
Consultant Psychiatrist, St John's Hospital at Howden,
Livingston, UK

Malcolm Bruce MB ChB MRCPsych PhD
Consultant Psychiatrist in Addiction, Royal Edinburgh
Hospital, Edinburgh, UK

Jonathan T. O. Cavanagh MB ChB MRCPsych MPhil
Research Fellow in Psychiatry, University of
Edinburgh, Edinburgh, UK

Derek Chiswick MB ChB MPhil FRCPsych
Consultant Forensic Psychiatrist, Edinburgh
Healthcare NHS Trust; Honorary Senior Lecturer in
Psychiatry, University of Edinburgh, UK

David G. Cunningham Owens MD(Hons) FRCP FRCPsych
Reader in Psychiatry and Honorary Consultant
Psychiatrist, University Department of Psychiatry,
Royal Edinburgh Hospital, Edinburgh, UK

Ian J. Deary BSc PhD MB ChB MRCPsych FRCP(Edin)
Professor of Differential Psychology, Department of
Psychology, University of Edinburgh, Edinburgh, UK

John C. Duffy BSc MSc CStat
Senior Lecturer, Department of Mathematics and
Statistics, University of Edinburgh, on secondment to
the Scottish Office as Research Manager, Chief
Scientist Office, Scottish Office Department of Health,
Edinburgh

Klaus Peter Ebmeier MD MRCPsych
Professor of Psychiatry, University of Edinburgh, Royal
Edinburgh Hospital, Edinburgh, UK

Christopher P.L. Freeman MB ChB MPhil FRCPsych
Consultant Psychotherapist, Royal Edinburgh
Hospital; Senior Lecturer, Department of Psychiatry,
University of Edinburgh, UK

Linda Gask MB ChB MSc PhD FRCPsych
Senior Lecturer in Community Psychiatry, University
of Manchester; Honorary Consultant Psychiatrist,
Royal Preston Hospital, Preston, UK

John R. Geddes MD MRCPsych
Senior Clinical Research Fellow, University of Oxford,
Warneford Hospital, Oxford, UK

Guy Goodwin MA DPhil FRCPsych FRCP(Edin)
W A Handley Professor of Psychiatry, University
Department of Psychiatry, Warneford Hospital,
Oxford

Peter Hoare DM FRCPsych
Senior Lecturer, University of Edinburgh; Honorary
Consultant Psychiatrist, Royal Edinburgh Hospital,
Edinburgh, UK

Alan Jacques BSc MB BCh FRCPsych
Medical Commissioner, Mental Welfare Commission
for Scotland, Edinburgh, UK

Rachel Jenkins MA MB BCh MRCPsych MD
Director of WHO Collaborating Centre for Mental
Health Research and Training, Institute of Psychiatry;
Honorary Senior Lecturer, Institute of Psychiatry,
London, UK

Eve C. Johnstone MD FRCP(Glasgow and Edinburgh) FRCPsych
Professor of Psychiatry and Head of the Department of
Psychiatry, University of Edinburgh, UK

Stephen M. Lawrie MD MB ChB MPhil MRCPsych
Lecturer in Psychiatry, University of Edinburgh, UK

Glyn Lewis PhD MRCPsych
Professor of Community and Epidemiological
Psychiatry, University of Wales College of Medicine,
Cardiff, UK

George Masterton BSc MD FRCPsych
Consultant Psychiatrist, Royal Infirmary of Edinburgh,
Edinburgh, UK

Diana P. Morrison MB ChB MRCPsych MD MFPM
Consultant Psychiatrist (General Adult Psychiatry),
Royal Edinburgh Hospital, Edinburgh, UK

Walter J. Muir BSc (Hons) MB ChB MRCPsych
Senior Lecturer in the Psychiatry of Learning
Disability, Department of Psychiatry, University of
Edinburgh; Honorary Consultant Psychiatrist,
Edinburgh Healthcare NHS Trust

William Parry-Jones MA MD FRCP(Glas) FRCPsych DPM
Late Professor of Child and Adolescent Psychiatry,
University of Glasgow, Royal Hospital for Sick
Children, Glasgow, UK

David F. Peck BA DAP(Clin) FBPsS
Area Clinical Psychologist, Highland Communities
NHS Trust, Craig Phadrig Hospital, Inverness, UK

Stephen G. Potts MA BM BCh MRCPsych
Consultant in Liaison Psychology, Department of
Psychological Medicine, Royal Infirmary of Edinburgh,
UK

Michael J. Power BSc DPhil MSc
Professor of Clinical Psychology, Department of
Psychiatry, University of Edinburgh; Clinical
Psychologist, Royal Edinburgh Hospital, UK

Ian C. Reid MB ChB BMed Biol PhD MRCPsych
Head of Psychiatry Department, University of
Dundee, Dundee, UK

Bruce Ritson MD FRCP FRCPsych
Senior Lecturer and Consultant, University
Department of Psychiatry, Royal Edinburgh Hospital,
Edinburgh, UK

Allan I.F. Scott BSc MPhil MD MBA MRCPsych
Consultant Psychiatrist and Honorary Senior Lecturer,
Royal Edinburgh Hospital, Edinburgh, UK

Jan Scott MB BS MD FRCPsych
Professor of Community Psychiatry, University
Department of Psychiatry, Royal Victoria Hospital,
Newcastle-upon-Tyne, UK

Michael Sharpe MA MB BChir MRCP MRCPsych
Senior Lecturer in Psychological Medicine, University
of Edinburgh, UK

Lindsay D.G. Thomson MB ChB MPhil MRCPsych
Senior Lecturer in Forensic Psychiatry, University of
Edinburgh; Honorary Consultant Forensic
Psychiatrist, The State Hospital, Carstairs, UK

Kirstie Woodburn MA BM BCh MRCPsych MD
Senior Registrar in Old Age Psychiatry, Royal
Edinburgh Hospital, Edinburgh, UK

Andrew K. Zealley MB ChB FRCP(Edinburgh) FRCPsych DPM
Consultant Psychiatrist, Royal Edinburgh Hospital;
Honorary Senior Lecturer, Department of Psychiatry,
University of Edinburgh, UK

Contents

1

Psychiatry – its history and boundaries

Eve C. Johnstone

HISTORY

Introduction and early aspects

Psychiatry may be defined as the branch of medicine concerned with mental disorders (Walton et al 1994), these being divided into three broad classes: severe learning difficulty, personality disorder and mental illness. These categories are not, of course, mutually exclusive and, as will be discussed, their boundaries are matters of debate.

Mental disorders have a long history. Early Egyptian papyri contain references to mental disturbances – in about 1500 BC it was written of senility that 'the heart grows heavy and remembers not yesterday', and cases of mental disorder (affecting, for example, Saul, David and Nebuchadnezzar) are recorded in the Old Testament. Mental disorders receive extensive discussion in Ancient Greek medical texts and the writers, for example Hippocrates writing in the 4th century BC (Jones 1972) and Aretaeus writing in about AD 150 (Adams 1856), appeared to regard mental illnesses as having bodily causes and as requiring medical treatment. Phrenitis, mania, melancholia and paranoia were the core categories of Greek psychiatry (Roccatagliata 1973), and it would appear that for the Greeks phrenitis was a disturbance of thought, mood and action associated with physical disease (Sakai 1991). The concept of melancholia described by Aretaeus has obvious similarities to our current concepts of severe depressive illness, and the link between morbid depression and morbid elevation of mood was clearly appreciated at that time:

> And yet in certain of these cases there is mere anger and grief and sad dejection of mind... those affected with melancholy are not every one of them affected according to one particular form but they are either suspicious of poisoning or flee to the desert from misanthropy or turn superstitious or contract a hatred of life. Or if at any time a relaxation takes place, in most cases hilarity

supervenes. The patients are dull or stern, dejected or unreasonbly torpid... they also become peevish, dispirited and start up from a disturbed sleep.

None the less, while it is possible and perhaps appealing to link such descriptions over gaps of centuries, it is important to recognise that the conceptual framework within which psychopathological descriptions have been set has changed greatly over the years. The meanings ascribed to terms used for describing diagnostic concepts and behaviours may vary considerably from time to time so that the assumption that terms such as 'mania', 'melancholia' and 'hypochondria' mean the same now as they did even two centuries ago may not be justified and the nature of the parallel with more ancient times is appropriately the focus of the work of professional historians (Berrios & Porter 1995).

Whether or not the syndromes that were described in the ancient world closely resemble those which we see now, it is evident that mental disorders have been studied since Graeco-Roman times. The work ascribed to Hippocrates (4th century BC) was followed by that of Celsus, Aretaeus and Galen, writing in the 1st and 2nd centuries AD. The heritage of ancient times was developed by Arab scientists, notably Avicenna, the Persian physician who in the 11th century developed Galen's ideas in his *Canon of Medicine*. Greek, Roman, Arab and Byzantine texts spread into the Western world from the 11th century and the work of Galen was developed in the 12th century by Trotula of Salerno (1940).

The Middle Ages to the modern era

Universities in which medical subjects were taught were set up throughout Europe in the 13th century and a degree of development of these ideas continued. None the less, ideas that mental disorder was a spiritual rather than a medical problem were prominent throughout the Middle Ages, it being considered that the mentally ill were possessed by the Devil or were practitioners of witchcraft (Sprenger & Kramer 1486). Although these views were prominent, ideas of a medical kind were used against them, for example by Weyer (1564).

Lunacy legislation in England dates from 1320, when it was enacted during the reign of Edward II that the property of lunatics should be vested in the Crown (Henderson & Batchelor 1962). Bethlem, the first hospital in the British Isles to care for the insane, was funded in 1247 as a priory of the Order of the Star of Bethlem, and it is recorded that in 1403 six lunatics were confined there. In 1546, at the time of the dissolution of the monasteries, Henry VIII granted St Bartholomew's Hospital and Bethlem to the laity.

Sydenham's work, published in the late 17th century (1696), was a turning point on the road towards modern psychiatry, as well as to modern medicine as a whole. In the ancient world symptoms and signs, e.g. fever, asthma, rashes, joint pains, were themselves regarded as diseases to be studied separately, and it was really only with Sydenham's work that the idea of disease as a syndrome or constellation of symptoms having a characteristic prognosis became established. This laid the foundation for rational diagnosis and classification of disease.

As far as psychiatry in Britain was concerned, the unfortunate recurrent mental disorder suffered by King George III in the 18th century had the benefit of arousing much public interest and controversy. He was cared for by Francis Willis, a clergyman who had a reputation for dealing with such cases, derived from his experience in the management of a private mental home. The controversies provoked by the differences of opinion between Willis and other physicians called upon to treat the King led to the decision by the House of Lords to appoint a committee to institute a detailed enquiry. This provided consideration not only of the treatment of the King's illness but also of the care of the mentally ill throughout the century (Henderson & Batchelor 1962). The modern era of the treatment of mental disorder dates from this time, i.e. the end of the 18th century. The first phase of this may be described as the period of humane reform.

The modern era – the 18th century to the present day

The period of humane reform

In 1794 Philippe Pinel commenced work at the Bicetre Hospital in Paris, a hospital for male patients suffering from mental disorders in which physical restraints were widely used. He wrote extensively on psychiatric subjects (1801, 1806) and popularised methods of treatment involving non-restraint. His pupil, Jean Etienne Dominique Esquirol, wrote a textbook of psy-

chiatry (1838) and developed a lecture course on the subject.

At the same time as these reforms were taking place in France, the so-called moral treatment of the insane began in Britain in the Retreat at York, opened by the Quaker William Tuke in 1796. The regime of 'moral treatment' at the Retreat was regarded as successful and similar programmes of care were put into practice in the new lunatic asylums that were being built in the first half of the 19th century and were replacing the private madhouse, which had until then provided care for the mentally disordered. The principal elements of moral treatment appeared to be kindness, an ordered regime with regular occupation, religious observance, wholesome food and an avoidance of passion and excess.

In Scotland in 1792 Dr Andrew Duncan, who was Professor of Medicine at the University of Edinburgh, sponsored an appeal for funds to establish the Royal Edinburgh Mental Hospital, which was opened in 1813. In Germany the modern era began with Fricke, who in Brunswick in 1793 put humane medical treatment into practice and greatly reduced mechanical restraint.

The reforms begun in England by Tuke were followed by the introduction in 1808 of a bill into Parliament for the purpose of providing 'better care and maintenance of lunatics being paupers or criminals in England'. A series of amendments of the Act in 1811, 1815, 1819 and 1824 was followed by the establishment in 1845 of the Lunacy Commission, which later (1913) became organised as the Board of Control. The powers of this Board were dissolved in England at the time of the introduction of the Mental Health Act, 1959 but were resurrected in 1983 in the form of the Mental Welfare Commission.

The development of academic psychiatry

European academic psychiatry began in France with the work of Pinel, who published his *Traité de la Manie* in 1801. This work was developed by Esquirol, whose series of lectures on psychological medicine formed the model for the course of nine systematic lectures in psychiatry set up in Edinburgh in 1823 by Sir Alexander Morison. It was in Germany, however, that psychiatry first became established as a subject for academic study in universities. In 1811, Heinroth was appointed to the first Chair of 'Mental Therapy' in Leipzig, and this was renamed the Chair of Psychiatry in 1828. Griesinger was appointed first Professor of Psychiatry and Neurology in Berlin in 1865 and developed a department for the study of mental disorders. This work involved clinical and pathophysiological research based upon the hypothesis that 'mental illness is a somatic illness of the brain' (Griesinger 1861). This oft-quoted statement is an oversimplification of Griesinger's views on pathogenesis but it is an illustration of a point of view that has been central to the difficulties in defining the boundaries to psychiatry, which will shortly be discussed. Further Chairs of Psychiatry were established in Gottingen (1866), Heidelberg (1871), Leipzig (1882) and Bonn (1882), although in Britain no such post was developed until the Chair of Psychiatry in Edinburgh was set up in 1919.

With the development of these academic departments the study of psychiatric disorder began to flourish in Germany. The first important theme was the natural course of mental disorders studied by Kahlbaum and Kraepelin. It was largely upon the basis of these outcome studies that Kraepelin developed his comprehensive classification of mental illness which is the foundation of the schemes now in use throughout the world, such as ICD-10 Classification of Mental and Behavioural Disorders (WHO 1992). Kraepelin was Professor of Psychiatry in Heidelberg and later in Munich and wrote nine editions of his *Lehrbuch der Psychiatrie*, published between 1883 and 1927. In the first three editions of his book he was concerned to move away from the earlier 19th century nosological concepts, which he criticised as unreliable from a clinical and especially prognostic point of view (Hoff 1995). The term 'dementia praecox', the disorder with which he is most closely associated, was not used in these editions; it was in the fourth to eighth editions of *Lehrbuch der Psychiatrie* (1893–1915) that Kraepelin created a nosological system and finalised his concept of natural disease entities. In the fifth (1896) and sixth (1899) editions he developed the concept of dementia praecox and the separation of dementia praecox with a poor prognosis and manic–depressive illness with a good, or at least a better, prognosis. In defining dementia praecox he had drawn together hebephrenia as described by Hecker (1871), catatonia as described by Kahlbaum (1874) and his own dementia paranoides, regarding them as manifestations of the same disorder which typically had its onset in early adult life and had a poor outcome.

A further major theme concerned the relationship of mental disorder to brain pathology. Griesinger's ideas had stimulated this area of work but it was greatly encouraged by the progress that was being made in identifying pathological lesions in neurological disorders. The disorder, which came to be known as 'general paralysis of the insane', was a particular focus for study. This condition had been described by Bayle (1822) under the title 'arachnitis chronique'. This was the first example in psychiatry of a demonstrable morbid entity which presented itself as a sequential process unfold-

ing into successive clinical syndromes. Three clinical types were recognised: manic-ambitious, melancholic, hypochondriac and dementia. The unitary view, i.e. that all three represented stages of a single disease, the order of their appearance depending upon the progress of the brain lesions, received widespread but not universal support. Neuropathological approaches to dementia were also successful. Marcé described cortical atrophy, enlarged ventricles and softening of the brain in 1863. In 1881 Wernicke published a description of the encephalopathy which was named after him, and Alzheimer in 1907 reported neurofibrillary tangles, plaques and other changes in a 51-year-old woman with cognitive impairment and psychotic features. Neuropathological work was also conducted on patients where replicable findings were less easy to demonstrate. For example, with regard to dementia praecox, Alzheimer (1897, 1913), Wernicke (1900) and Klippel & Lhermitte (1909) described changes such as 'lacunae', pyknotic neuronal atrophy, focal demyelination and metachromatic bodies. Histological techniques were in their infancy at this time and progress was limited. This work was, however, the forerunner of the imaging studies of the brain in psychiatric disorder that have been conducted since the introduction of pneumoencephalography by Dandy in 1919, and which have led to the advances associated with the development of non-invasive neuroimaging and modern quantitative and molecular neuropathology.

A further theme of early research concerned hereditary issues. This developed from the work of Morel (1860), who proposed what came to be known as the theory of degeneration. He had suggested an aetiological rather than symptomatic classification and put forward six groups: hereditary (four classes), by intoxication (alcoholism, pellagra, etc.), neuroses, idiopathic, sympathetic and dementia. Although hereditary taint had been mentioned in relation to insanity before this time, it was highlighted by Morel's work. His degeneration theory involved the idea that mental illness affecting one generation could be passed on to the next, in ever worsening degree. Two mechanisms were thought to be involved: transmission and degradation of the tainted seed (Berrios & Beer 1995). As the hereditary taint was thought not only to be behavioural but also physical, stigmata of degeneration, such as deformed teeth, ears, head, etc., were assessed (Talbot 1898). The notion that behaviours such as alcohol abuse and masturbation could promote degeneration was included in the general theory. These ideas influenced the views of Sir Thomas Clouston (1890), who in addition put forward the concept of developmental insanity and considered that the results of his investigations of palatal structure in adolescent insanity (which he saw as being part of

Kraepelin's disease entity of dementia praecox) demonstrated that this disorder represented a form of developmental defect of ectodermal tissue (Clouston 1891). The moral and religious overtones of the degeneration theory seemed increasingly inappropriate by the end of the 19th century and these ideas encouraged a pessimistic approach to treatment and generally negative attitudes towards the mentally ill. On the positive side, the emphasis upon the hereditary aspect of mental disorders has pointed the way to the genetic studies which are now such a promising avenue forward in unravelling the basis of psychiatric disorders (Craddock & Owen 1996). Similarly, the neurodevelopmental ideas put forward by Clouston (1891) have resurfaced after 100 years, although of course in a somewhat altered form (Murray & Lewis 1987, Weinberger 1995). None the less, it was partly as a reaction to the pessimistic and unsympathetic view of the mentally ill put forward by the degeneration theories that an increasing interest in psychological causes of mental disorder developed from the end of the 19th century.

Psychoanalytic theories

Sigmund Freud, working in Vienna, began his career in neurological research and visited Charcot in Paris with a view to learning about the use of hypnotism in cases of hysteria. He began to use hypnosis in such cases but developed the alternative method of free association, in which patients were encouraged to speak about what was in their mind. Although initially intended as a treatment, Freud went on to try to use this technique to develop an understanding of the psychological causes of these disorders. He proceeded to develop his own theories, which included ideas that were already to some extent current, such as the importance of childhood experience on the behaviour of adults and the part played by the unconscious and irrational parts of the mind in influencing behaviour, and he gave emphasis to sexual motives as determinants of symptomatology. These theories have had a great influence on the development of literature in the 20th century, and as far as psychiatry is concerned have had importance in highlighting the role of psychological factors in the causation and management of mental disorder, but Freud's psychoanalytic theories are not now considered to have provided a satisfactory explanation for most psychiatric conditions. They are not put forward in terms of scientific hypotheses which can be confirmed or refuted and are thus difficult to reconcile with the ideas of evidence-based medicine. Other prominent figures in this field were Jung and E. Bleuler, both of whom departed from the psychoanalytic movement after some years. The French psychiatrist Pierre Janet was also concerned

with psychological causes of mental disorder. He shared with Freud concepts of the unconscious mind and of mental forces but saw recent rather than childhood experiences as important in the causation of neurotic illness.

The effects of the First World War

Interest in the idea that exposure to untoward events could cause nervous symptoms developed during the second half of the 19th century in relation to compensation claims following railway accidents. There was controversy between those who held that the complaints had a physical cause (Erichsen 1866, Oppenheim 1889) and those who considered that the symptoms resulted from the effects upon the mind. It was against this background that cases of 'shell shock' began to be diagnosed during the First World War. The British Army in France suffered 157 cases of 'shock' or 'shell shock' between the outbreak of the war and December 1914, among 520 cases of functional nervous disease (Macpherson et al 1923). The problem became very much more common, the peak incidence being 16,138 from July to December 1916, following the Battle of the Somme (War Office, 1922). Mott (1916) considered that there was a pathological basis for 'shell shock' in terms of minute haemorrhages in the nervous system, but it seemed improbable that such explanations could be present in all cases, as they did not all arise in circumstances close to the scene of combat, where exploding shells or carbon monoxide could have caused such effects. Functional explanations were put forward and this raised the unhappy issue of possible malingering (War Office, 1922). From the point of view of the military authorities the distinction between intentional and unintentional symptoms was of 'vital importance' (Myers 1915). Cowardice and desertion continued to be capital offences in the British Army during the First World War. The numbers affected by 'shell shock' in the latter part of 1916 meant that a clear distinction between neuropathologically and emotionally based disorders was not tenable, and that the Battle of the Somme could be considered as marking the point where the moral order represented by the dichotomy of courage and cowardice had to make way for a scientific and medical order represented by the idea of neurosis (Brown 1995). From 1917 the term 'shell shock' was replaced for official purposes by the label 'Not yet diagnosed – nervous' and front line triage stations were established so that doctors were integrated more closely into the early stages of the management of affected individuals. It was accepted that in some cases symptoms persisted, so that in 1921 65 000 men in Britain were drawing war pensions for neurasthenia and related conditions (Macpherson et al 1923) and in 1939 120 000 such pensions were still being drawn (Ahrenfeldt 1958). These circumstances led to a recognition of psychological illness and to the acceptance in the general public, as well as among military and medical authorities, that overwhelming stress could produce such illness, even in soldiers whose bravery had been recognised by military decorations. Indeed, psychological explanations of war neuroses had become so much accepted that they were used as a paradigm for neurosis in general in popular work (Riggs 1922).

The 1920s to the present day

After the First World War there was an expansion of psychiatric facilities and broadening of their scope. The Maudsley Hospital, with its emphasis on teaching, research and early treatment, was opened. Academic Departments of Psychiatry began to develop outpatient clinics for the treatment of milder disorders, and child guidance clinics were set up. The 1930s saw the introduction of new forms of physical treatment. Sakel had introduced insulin coma treatment for the management of drug addiction, but later promoted its use in schizophrenia (Sakel 1938). By 1950 it was regarded as the best available treatment for that condition (Sakel 1952), but its effects were later shown to be nonspecific (Ackner et al 1957). Convulsive treatment was introduced by Cerletti & Bini (Bini, 1938). Initially this was recommended for schizophrenia upon a theoretic basis which was later shown to be mistaken, but experience showed that its most striking effects were in severe depressive illness, for which it is still used. Psychosurgery was introduced in 1935 by Moniz. There is evidence of benefit from leucotomy – the most commonly used form of psychosurgery (Birley 1964) – but randomised placebo-controlled trials have never proved possible and it is rarely used now.

Lithium salts were introduced into psychiatric practice by Cade in 1949. The value of this treatment was not at first appreciated, but in recent decades lithium has come into increasingly widespread use. Chlorpromazine was synthesised in France in 1950 and initially used as a sedative and to induce hypothermia; it was introduced into psychiatric practice by Delay & Deniker in 1952.

Monamine oxidase inhibitor antidepressants in the form of iproniazid were introduced in 1957 (Loomer et al 1957), the effects of this antituberculous drug as a 'psychic energiser' having been observed by astute clinicians. In a similar fashion the antidepressant effect of the tricyclic imipramine, which was being assessed as a tranquilliser, was noted by Kuhn in 1958. All of these physical treatments were thus introduced on an empirical, indeed serendipitous, basis. The effects of these advances have, however, been far reaching. In clinical terms the benefits for patients of the introduction of effective antipsychotic, antidepressant and mood stabilising drugs have been enormous. In addition, the fact that methods of treatment which have measurable modes of action in physiological terms have effects upon psychiatric illnesses may be taken as evidence that these disorders do have a basis in physiological dysfunction. It is clearly possible that understanding of the mode of action of an effective treatment will give information about the biological basis of the condition that it relieves. Much research in this area has been conducted over the past 40 years and well-accepted theories of the pathogenesis of both schizophrenia and depressive illness initially relied heavily upon the known pharmacological actions of effective treatment for these disorders (Schildkraut & Kety 1967, Snyder et al 1974).

After the introduction of the National Health Service in Britain in 1948 a comprehensive system of general practice was introduced. This, together with the development of effective drug treatments, allowed many milder cases of psychiatric disorder to be managed entirely in general practice. Less restrictive regimes for patients with serious mental disorders were introduced, and there was a greater emphasis on social rehabilitation. Psychiatric practice in Britain was much influenced by Sir Aubrey Lewis in London and Sir David Henderson in Edinburgh, both of whom (like other distinguished psychiatrists of their generation) had been taught by Adolph Meyer, who emphasised the need for an eclectic approach, combining social, physical and psychological aspects.

In the United States this wide-ranging approach was less popular and psychoanalytic practice was heavily emphasised until the 1970s, although in the last two decades, as in Europe, this has become one approach among many.

The advances of the last 20 years are largely dealt with in the individual chapters. In Britain, however, major themes have been the effects of closure of the mental hospitals (first proposed by Tooth & Brooke in 1961 but gaining in momentum through the 1980s) and the move to community care, the increased importance given to the randomised placebo-controlled trial and the value of evidence-based medicine, and the possibilities for the investigation of the biological basis of psychiatric disorders arising from recent technical advances, particularly in neuroimaging and in molecular genetics (Johnstone 1996).

Of necessity, this has been a very much abbreviated account of how psychiatric thinking and practice have developed over the centuries. It is evident, however, that issues about the nature of mental disorders – those conditions where management is the province of psychiatrists – have repeatedly been raised, and it is a good deal less clear that they have ever been satisfactorily resolved. Questions arise as to what is really meant by mental disorder and what are the boundaries of psychiatric practice.

THE NATURE OF MENTAL DISORDER AND THE BOUNDARIES OF PSYCHIATRIC PRACTICE

As noted above, mental disorder is conventionally divided into three categories: mental illness, severe learning disability and personality disorder. The matter of what constitutes 'illness' or 'disease' is not quite as clear as it might at first appear (Kendell 1975). It was really only with Sydenham's work in the 17th century that the idea of disease as a syndrome or constellation of symptoms having a characteristic prognosis became established (Sydenham 1696). With the increasing popularity of postmortem examination in the 19th century, disease became defined by pathological findings rather than by the clinical picture, and later technological development has allowed diseases to be defined in bacteriological, biochemical and molecular biological terms. Although in the mid-19th century Griesinger had put forward the idea that 'mental illness is a somatic illness of the brain', psychiatry has had great difficulty in moving into these realms. The principal model of disease in psychiatry remains the syndrome model, i.e. a cluster of symptoms and signs which are associated with a characteristic course over time. The development of morbid anatomy and histology in the 19th century, and later advances in physiology and biochemistry, showed that many diseases initially defined as syndromes were in fact associated with identifiable lesions. This led to the view that the demonstration of such an identifiable lesion was the defining characteristic of disease. There are many problems with this clear-cut and initially appealing view. As far as much of psychiatry is concerned, at least until very recently, there was the very considerable drawback that no physical basis has been defined for most of the major syndromes.

This lack of a demonstrable physical basis has been a major difficulty for some earlier categorisations. As far as shell shock was concerned, it was evident that the haemorrhages in the nervous system, thought to be responsible for the symptoms in some cases (Mott 1916), were unlikely to be present in all those affected. This was one of the factors leading to the replacement of the diagnostic label and to the acceptance of a psychological cause for the symptoms. Neurasthenia was widely diagnosed in the United States and Europe during the 19th century (Beard 1880, Dubois 1909) and initially simple organic models of both aetiology and treatment were put forward. When these could not be sustained the diagnosis fell into disuse (Wessely 1995). For some psychiatrists, however, the lack of a demonstrable physical basis for the disorders with which they were concerned did not seem to be as much a problem as their views might have led one to expect. Kraepelin (1896), who defined dementia praecox – later known as schizophrenia – on the basis of the characteristic course and outcome of a cluster of symptoms and signs, stated that this was a disorder in which if 'every detail' were known a specific anatomical pathology with a specific aetiology would be found. Schneider (1950) saw no difficulty in accepting the idea that the word 'illness' should only be used in situations in which 'some actual change' or 'defective structure' was present in the body. In this context, he stated that he did not regard either neurotic states or personality disorders as illness but simply as 'abnormal varieties of sane mental life'. He still, however, considered schizophrenia and manic–depressive psychosis as illness, along with dementias and delirious states, on the basis of the assumption that in time they would prove to have an 'underlying morbid physical condition'.

This rather uncertain position, of believing on the basis of inadequate evidence that diseases which were in fact defined on a syndromal basis would later be demonstrated to be definable on a pathological basis, was maintained by most biological psychiatrists (in which grouping I would include myself) for many years, but it is becoming possible to move on to firmer ground. As Weinberger (1995) has written, '20 years ago the principal challenge in schizophrenia research was to gather objective scientific evidence that would implicate the brain. This challenge no longer exists.' This is equally true of other mental disorders, and indeed of mental functioning generally, although psychiatrists have probably been rather slow to appreciate this. The fact is that advances have taken place which allow us to see how the brain works in health as well as in disease.

For a good many years now there has been evidence of a cerebral substrate for mental phenomena. It is, for example, well established that stimulating electrodes within the brain of conscious subjects can evoke sensory experiences, emotions or vivid memories that have the subjective characteristics of familiar mental phenomena and come and go as the stimulating electrode is switched off. We know that lesions in specific areas of the brain will produce predictable changes in the subject's ability to speak, to understand the speech of others, to remember past events, to recognise familiar people or objects, to hear, see, taste or smell. For some time functional brain imaging has allowed us to see increased regional blood flow, oxygen consumption or glucose utilisation in relation to roughly localised activities, so that there would be increased left hemisphere activity when a verbal problem is attempted and right hemisphere activity when the task is spatial.

In the last 5 years, however, technical advances in functional neuroimaging – PET (positron emission tomography), SPET (single photon emission tomography) and FMRI (functional magnetic resonance imaging) – have meant that it is now possible to delineate the pattern of cerebral activity associated with specific neuropsychological tests or mental acts both in the well and in those affected by mental disorders (for example, Liddle 1996, McGuire et al 1996). In addition, complex analyses allow the relative amounts of activation in different parts of the brain in response to specific tasks to be assessed and to be compared in health and disease (Friston & Frith 1995). This means that the long years of trying to decide whether disorders defined on a syndromal basis are actually associated with a demonstrable physical basis in the brain can pass into history. If the very act of silently reading words can be shown to have a physiological basis, concern about the meaning in terms of brain pathology of altered regional blood flow in people with auditory verbal hallucinations becomes less pressing.

It is true that these advances have raised some uncertainties – that, as is said in the section on unsolved problems in the guide to ICD-10 (WHO 1994), we no longer know what to call 'organic'. Now that we have a demonstrable basis in brain physiology for the activities of the mind, we need not concern ourselves whether or not 'some actual change' or 'defective structure' underlies the conditions that we seek to treat. The mind–body distinction can become a thing of the past once the activities of the mind have been shown to be measurable by bodily change. This does not, of course, mean that it is ever going to be thought useful (even if it were affordable) for there to be a PET scanner in every hospital. It is never going to be helpful to measure the regional cerebral blood flow in response to provocative neuropsychological tests in every patient. It is the fact that functions of the mind can be shown to be measurable in the activity of the brain that is important. In the light of this, it becomes clear that psychiatric illnesses do not differ in any fundamental way from other illnesses – for example, cardiovascular illnesses where symptoms such as chest pain or breathlessness are measurable in terms of disordered cardiovascular physiology.

This view does not in any way imply that psychological or social factors are not important in psychiatric disorders. We know that they are. Now that we have the possibility of measuring physiological correlates of mental function, the opportunity of investigating the mechanism by which psychological and social factors have their effects as precipitants, modifiers or treatments of disease becomes available. Indeed, in general it is important to move on from the position of defining physiological or structural abnormality in psychiatric syndromes. It has been very rewarding to demonstrate these abnormalities (Ch. 16) but the important challenge now is to explore the mechanisms whereby these findings, be they physiological, structural or indeed molecular, produced the clinical features of the disorders that we seek to treat.

Much of this may seem a digression from the question of the boundaries of psychiatry, but as there has in the past been so much discussion about whether or not brain lesions of some kind underlie certain psychiatric disorders, it is important to make the point that it is probably no longer relevant to try to define psychiatric disorders in these terms. Psychiatric disorders are essentially those conditions in which the symptoms refer to mental functions, i.e. to emotion, to cognition, to perception, and they are perhaps most simply defined as those conditions which are conventionally referred to psychiatrists for diagnosis and treatment. They comprise the various conditions included in the psychiatric classifications described in Chapter 10 but of course these are very much a matter of convention, dependent upon custom and practice. It is clear that psychoses such as bipolar illness, schizophrenia, deliria and dementias are central to psychiatric practice, as are neurotic conditions such as panic disorder, anxiety states and obsessive compulsive disorder, but eating disorders, substance abuse and alcohol dependence fit less clearly within such a framework.

At the time at which it was first described (Gull 1874), anorexia nervosa was treated by physicians and certainly it could well have come within the province of endocrinologists or gynaecologists, but conventionally it does not. A case could be made for suggesting that alcohol problems could be treated by gastroenterologists but, although patients of this kind have considerable input from general medical services (Persson & Magnusson 1987), clinics for those with alcohol problems are generally run by psychiatrists. Similar arbitrary limits divide the practice of neurologists and psychiatrists in relation to progressive central nervous system disorders like Huntington's chorea, Parkinson's disease and the Steele–Richardson syndrome, and in relation to less severe disorders the division between the work of psychiatrists and that of general practitioners is very much a matter of individual clinicians and the circumstances of their services. In some places psychiatrists may advise on the management of people who are suffering from adjustment reactions, i.e. personal difficulties due to life circumstances which have caused emotional stress. In other areas such individuals would be managed by general practitioners, if indeed they sought medical help at all, and the work of psychiatrists would be confined to those with more clear-cut symptomatology.

Mental disorders include personality disorders and severe learning disability, as well as mental illnesses. Personality disorders represent an enduring pattern of inner experience and behaviour in the absence of mental illness which arises in adolescence and continues into adulthood. They represent deviations from the way in which the average individual in a given culture perceives, thinks, feels and particularly relates to others (WHO 1992). A wide range of subdivisions of personality disorder is described; for example DSM-IV (APA 1994) lists 10 main types, including paranoid, schizoid, histrionic, antisocial, etc. Personality disorders are frequently but not always associated with various degrees of subjective distress or impaired performance. It is obvious that the point at which a deviation in thinking, feeling or relating to others differs sufficiently from that of the average person in the same culture to allow a diagnosis of personality disorder is arbitrary. If there is no subjective distress or impaired performance, the individual concerned will not come to the attention of the medical or psychiatric services. Difficulties over the point at which the diagnosis of personality disorder should be made most often arise in relation to antisocial personality disorder, where issues of responsibility for antisocial acts may be discussed in judicial circumstances.

Severe learning difficulties are evident from childhood and are characterised by limited intelligence and restricted development of other aspects of psychological functioning. Although psychiatrists are often involved in the planning of services for those with learning disability, by no means all affected individuals require any form of psychiatric treatment. While learning disability (especially when severe) may result from some specific genetic anomaly (e.g. Down syndrome, fragile X syndrome), or environmental insult (e.g. perinatal damage), such identifiable lesions are not demonstrated or even postulated in a substantial percentage of affected individuals, and again the point at which deviation from the average is sufficient to allow this diagnosis is an arbitrary one.

It is obvious that subdivisions of the learning disabled population can be made on the basis of the presence or absence of an identifiable genetic or environmental lesion. Experience of similar divisions in relation to mental illness has not necessarily led to progress (see above) but, as far as learning disability is concerned, modern genetic approaches may allow research to proceed along more useful lines (Flint & Wilkie, 1996). The fact that genes play some part in determining intelligence quotient (IQ) is not seriously disputed. Chromosomal mapping of loci that determine genetic variability in multifactorial conditions is now possible (Davies et al 1994), and attempts to map the loci determining quantitative variation, (quantitative trait loci QTL) in IQ have already begun (Plomin et al 1994). It is possible that a combination of QTL mapping and other molecular biological techniques will identify the many genes that are responsible for learning disability (Flint & Wilkie 1996). Psychiatrists are, of course, only peripherally involved in such work, their main responsibility towards the severely learning disabled being in the treatment of the mental illness to which these individuals have an excessive liability (for example, Turner 1989).

The Future

Although the importance of advanced techniques in genetics and neuroimaging in moving our understanding of psychiatry on to a firm biological basis has been emphasised in this chapter, this enhanced understanding should not be considered as diminishing the importance of psychological or social factors in psychiatric practice. Indeed, recent advances may allow us to see how matters such as life events in the precipitation of depressive illness, or cognitive behaviour therapy (CBT) in the relief of panic disorder, exert their effects. While the most important future developments in treatment and prevention of psychiatric disorders are likely to be derived from the biological sciences, there is no reason why psychological and social interventions should not continue to play a major role. The various disorders resulting from substance abuse provide an illustration of this point. It is likely that the means by which alcohol and other psychoactive substances produce intoxication dependence and tissue damage will come to be understood at a cellular and molecular level in the foreseeable future. Such knowledge could lead to new methods of detecting, reducing and possibly reversing intoxication dependence and tissue damage, and of identifying high-risk individuals. Such advances would not mean that it would no longer be important to understand the social forces and psychological pressures that lead people into careers of abuse and dependence, or that political, social and economic measures may not continue to be the most effective means of combating drug misuse on a national scale. However detailed our understanding of underlying neuronal mechanisms becomes, and however potent the resulting pharmacological and other physical therapies may be, the understanding and treatment of psychiatric disorders is always going to require a rounded appreciation of the social setting in which they develop and an empathic understanding of the patient's inner feelings.

REFERENCES

Ackner B, Hartris A, Oldham A T 1957 Insulin treatment of schizophrenia: a controlled study. Lancet i: 607–611

Adams F (ed) 1856 The extant works of Aretaeus the Cappadocian. Sydenham Society, London

Alzheimer A 1897 Beitrage zur pathologischen Anatomie der Hirnrinde und zur anatomischen Grundlage der Psychosen. Monatsschrift für Psychiatrie und Neurologie 2: 82–120

Alzheimer A 1907 Uber eine eigenartige Erkrankung der Hirnrinde. Allgemeine Zeitschrift für Psychiatrie und Psychisch-Gerichtlich Medizine 64: 146–148

Alzheimer A 1913 Beitrage zur pathologischen Anatomie der Dementia Praecox. Allgemeine Zeitschrift für Psychiatrie 70: 810–812

APA 1994 Diagnostic and statistical manual of mental disorders, 4th edn. American Psychiatric Association, Washington, DC

Bayle A L J 1822 Recherches sur les maladies mentales. Medical thesis

Beard G 1880 A practical treatise on nervous exhaustion (neurasthenia). William Wood, New York

Berrios G E, Bear D 1995 Unitary psychosis concept. In: Berrios G, Porter R (eds) History of clinical psychiatry. Athlone Press, London

Berrios G, Porter R (eds) 1995 Introduction. In: A history of clinical psychiatry. Athlone Press, London

Bini L 1938 Experimental researches on epileptic attacks induced by the electric current. American Journal of Psychiatry 94 (suppl 172)

Birley J L T 1964 Modified leucotomy: a review of 106 cases. British Journal of Psychiatry 110: 211–221

Brown E M 1995 Post-traumatic stress disorder and shell shock. In: Berrios G, Porter R (eds) A history of clinical psychiatry. Athlone Press, London

Cade J F J 1949 Lithium salts in the treatment of psychotic excitement. Medical Journal of Australia 2: 349–352

Clouston T S 1890 Clinical lectures on mental diseases, 6th edn. Churchill, London

Clouston T S 1891 The neuroses of development being the Morison Lectures of 1890. Oliver & Boyd, Edinburgh

Craddock N, Owen M 1996 Modern molecular genetic approaches to psychiatric disease. In: Biological psychiatry. British Medical Bulletin 52(3): 434–452

Dandy W E 1919 Roentgenography of the brain after injection of air into the cerebral ventricles. American Journal of Roentgenography 6: 26

Davies J L, Kawaguchi Y, Bennett S T et al 1994 A genome-wide search for human type I diabetes susceptibility genes. Nature 371: 130–136

Delay J, Deniker P 1952 Le traitment des psychoses par une méthode neuroleptique derivé de l'hibernotherapie. In: Cossa P (ed) Congrès de médecine aliénistes et neurologistes de France. Masson, Paris

Dubois P 1909 The psychic treatment of nervous disorders, 6th edn. Jelliffe S E, White W (trans). Funk & Wagnalls, New York

Erichsen J E 1866 On railway and other injuries of the nervous system. Lea, Philadelphia

Esquirol J E D 1838 Des maladies mentales. Baillière, Paris

Flint J, Wilkie A O M 1996 The genetics of mental retardation. In: Biological psychiatry. British Medical Bulletin 52(3): 453–464

Friston K J, Frith C D 1995 Schizophrenia: a disconnection syndrome. Clinical Neurosciences 3: 88–97

Griesinger W 1861 Die Pathologie und Therapie der psychischen Krankheiten. 1st edn 1845. Krabbe, Stuttgart

Gull W W 1874 Anorexia nervosa (apepsia hysteric, anorexia hysterica). Transactions of the Clinical Society of London 7: 22–28

Hecker E 1871 Die Hebephrenie. Ein Beitrag zur klinischen Psychiatrie. Archiv für Pathologische, Anatomie und Physiologie und für Klinische Medizin 52: 394–429

Henderson D, Batchelor I R C 1962 Henderson & Gillespie's textbook of psychiatry. Oxford University Press, London

Hoff P 1995 Kraepelin. In: Berrios G, Porter R (eds) A history of clinical psychiatry. Athlone Press, London

Johnstone E C 1996 Concluding summary. In: Biological psychiatry. British Medical Bulletin 52(2): 656–662

Jones W H S (trans) 1972 (reprint) Works of Hippocrates. Loeb Classical Library. Heinemann, London, vol I

Kahlbaum K L 1874 Die Katatonie onder das Spannungirresein. Eine klinische Form psychischer Krankheit. Hirschwald, Berlin

Kendell R E 1975 The role of diagnosis in psychiatry. Blackwell, Oxford

Klippel M, Lhermitte J 1909 Un cas de démence précoce à type catatonique avec autopsie. Revue Neurologique 17: 157–158

Kraepelin E 1883–1927 Lehrbuch der Psychiatrie, nine editions. Abel, Leipzig (1883, 1887, 1889, 1893); Barth, Leipzig (1896, 1899 2 vols, 1903/1904 2 vols, 1909/1910/1913/1915 4 vols, 1927 2 vols)

Kuhn R 1958 The treatment of depressive states with G 22355 (imipramine hydrochloride). American Journal of Psychiatry 115: 459–464

Liddle P F 1996 Functional imaging – schizophrenia. In: Biological psychiatry. British Medical Bulletin 52(3): 486–494

Loomer H P, Saunders L C, Kline N S 1957 A clinical and pharmacological evaluation of iproniazid as a psychic energizer. Psychiatric research. Reports of the American Psychiatric Association 8: 129–141

McGuire P K, Silbersway D A, Murray R M, David A S, Frackowiak R S, Frith C D 1996 Functional anatomy of inner speech and auditory verbal imagery. Psychological Medicine 26: 29–38

Macpherson W G, Herringham W P, Elliott T R, Balfour A 1923 History of the great war medical services. Diseases of war. HMSO, London, vol 11

Marcé L V 1863 Recherches cliniques et anatomo-pathologiques sur la démence senile et sur les différences qui la separent de la paralysie générale. Gazette Médicale de Paris 34: 433–435

Morel B A 1860 Traité des maladies mentales. Masson, Paris

Mott F W 1916 Special discussion on shell shock without visible signs of injury. Proceedings of the Royal Society of Medicine part III (suppl 9): 1–44

Murray R M, Lewis S W 1987 Is schizophrenia a neurodevelopmental disorder? British Medical Journal 295: 681–682

Myers C S 1915 A contribution to the study of shell shock. Lancet i: 316–320

Oppenheim H 1889 Die traumatischen Neurosen. Hirschwald, Berlin. See Oppenheim H 1911 Textbook of nervous diseases for physicians and students. Bruce A T N (trans). Foulis, London

Persson J, Magnusson P H 1987 Prevalence of excessive or problem drinkers among patients attending somatic outpatient clinics: a study of alcohol related to medical care. British Medical Journal 295: 467–472

Plomin R, McClearn G E, Smith D L et al 1994 DNA markers associated with high versus low IQ. The IQ quantitative trait loci (QTL) project. Behavioural Genetics 24: 107–118

Pinel P 1801 Traité medico philosophique sur L'alienation mentale ou la manie, 1st edn. Caille & Ravier, Paris

Pinel P 1806 A treatise on insanity. Davis D D (trans). Cadell & Davies, Sheffield

Riggs A F 1922 Just nerves. Houghton Mifflin, Boston

Roccatagliata G 1973 Storia della psichiatria antica. Ulrico Hoepli, Milan. Simon B (trans) 1978 Mind and madness in Ancient Greece. Cornell University Press, London

Sakai A 1991 Phrenitis: inflammation of the mind and body. History of Psychiatry 2: 193–206

Sakel M 1938 The pharmacological shock treatment of schizophrenia. Nervous and mental diseases monograph series no 62. Nervous & Mental Disease Publication Company, New York

Sakel M 1952 Insulinotherapy and shock therapies. International Congress on Psychiatry 1950 4: 163

Schildkraut J J, Kety S S 1967 Biogenic amines and emotion. Science 56: 21–30

Schneider K 1950 Die psychopathischen Personlichkeiten. Hamilton M W (trans) 1958 9th edn. Cassell, London

Snyder S H, Banerjee S P, Yamamura H I, Greenberg D 1974 Drugs, neurotransmitters and schizophrenia. Science 184: 1243–1253

Sprenger J, Kramer H 1486 Malleus maleficarium – the hammer of witchcraft, second part, question two, chapter V, Prescribed remedies for those who are obsessed owing to some spell. Summers M (trans) 1968. Folio Society, London

Sydenham I 1696 The whole works of that excellent physician Dr Thomas Sydenham. Pechy J (trans). Richard Wellington & Edward Castle, London

Talbot E S 1898 Degeneracy: its causes, signs and results. Walter Scott, London

Tooth G C, Brooke E M 1961 Trends in the mental hospital population and their effect on future planning. Lancet i: 710–713

Trotula of Salerno 1940 De passionibus mulierum. Ward Ritchie Press, Los Angeles

Turner T H 1989 Schizophrenia and mental handicap: an historical review, with implications for further research. Psychological Medicine 19: 301–314

Walton J, Barondess J A, Lock S (eds) 1994 Oxford medical companion. Oxford University Press, Oxford

War Office 1922 Report of the War Office committee on enquiry into 'shell shock'. HMSO, London

Weinberger D R 1995 From neuropathology to neurodevelopment. Lancet 346: 552–557

Wernicke C 1881 Lehrbuch der Gehirnkrankheiten für Arzte und Studierende I. Fischer, Berlin

Wernicke C 1900 Grundiss de Psychiatrie. Barth, Leipzig

Wessely S 1995 Neurasthenia and fatigue syndrome In: Berrios G, Porter R (eds) A history of clinical psychiatry. Athlone Press, London

Weyer J 1564 De praestigiis daemonium (On the trickery of demons). Cited in Trillat E 1995 Conversion disorder and hysteria. In: Berrios G, Porter R (eds) A history of clinical psychiatry. Athlone Press, London, pp 433–450

WHO 1992 The ICD-10 classification of mental and behavioural disorders: clinical description diagnostic guidelines (CDDG). World Health Organization, Geneva

WHO 1994 Cooper J E (ed) Pocket guide to the ICD-10 classification of mental and behavioural disorders. Churchill Livingstone, Edinburgh

2
Functional neuroanatomy

K. P. Ebmeier   I. C. Reid

INTRODUCTION

Neuroanatomy analyses the structure of the nervous system. The three-dimensional organisation of the central nervous system (descriptive anatomy) and its development during the individual's lifespan (developmental anatomy) provide the substrate for its function. Functional neuroanatomy needs to combine such structural knowledge with behavioural data. It puts anatomy into the context of the living organism, by asking not only 'How?', but also 'Why?' and 'To what purpose?' This chapter cannot give a systematic overview as it would be provided by an anatomy atlas or a standard undergraduate textbook. We will rather try to focus on aspects of functional anatomy that are of relevance to the psychiatrist. We will use the more detailed discussion of a limited number of topics to illustrate important principles of the organisation of the central nervous system (CNS). For an introduction, we will discuss the research methods employed to link the anatomical substrate with behaviour. This will hopefully allow the reader to see the inherent limitations of established 'knowledge'. The second part of the chapter will deal with the visual system, which is the most important sensory system in most humans. It will serve to illustrate the principles of neuronal organisation to achieve complex information processing. The third part will deal with the important frontosubcortical circuits underlying movement, cognition and affect. The emphasis is here on the circular nature of connections which lead to the interaction of such diverse structures as the basal ganglia, the cerebellum and the frontal cortex. Part four deals with the limbic system, which is generally thought to be associated with motivations and emotions. The close interconnection of cognitive function, such as memory, with emotion, autonomic responses and automatic behavioural sequences will be demonstrated by pointing to the common anatomical substrates for these functions. The final section of the chapter will use a hybrid approach to anatomy, combin-

ing the pharmacology of transmitter substances with the anatomical distribution of these transmitter systems throughout the CNS in order to localise function. It should be apparent by now that we are concerned with the investigation of brain–behaviour relationships, an exciting, fast growing area that in our mind represents the essence of psychological medicine. It is just over 100 years ago that Fritsch and Hitzig, and a little later Herrick and Tite, electrically stimulated the brains of animals to demonstrate movements, much to the amazement of their peers. Today the assumption that CNS function is specifically localised is a commonly held belief that receives further growing support by new methods of investigation such as functional magnetic resonance imaging (MRI) and transcranial magnetic stimulation.

THE METHODS OF FUNCTIONAL NEUROANATOMY

In order to relate CNS structure with function, clear and objective methods have to be developed to identify both the anatomical substrate and the functional correlate. The first task has been tackled in a variety of ways, using macroscopic anatomy, histology, pharmacology and neurochemistry. One system that is still valid after 90 years is Brodmann's classification of cortical areas according to the architecture of their cell layers. Primary sensory cortex, for example, receives large inputs from the thalamus, which end in layer 4, so that this layer is disproportionately thick. In primary motor cortex, layer 4 is relatively underdeveloped. Cortical architecture thus reflects functional variety, and Brodmann's system is still widely used, for example by researchers employing functional neuroimaging methods (Fig. 2.1). Behavioural measures are generally more subjective, more difficult to quantify and to elicit in a reliable way. We are talking here of animal behaviour, reward driven learning or the performance of neuropsy-

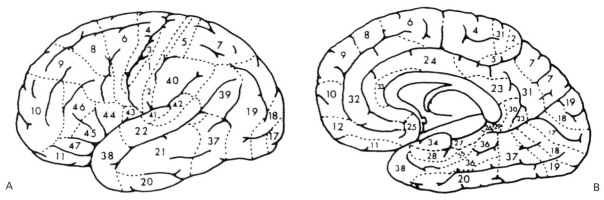

Fig. 2.1 The cytoarchitectural map of the cerebral cortex after Brodmann. **A** lateral surface; **B** medial surface.

chological tests in humans. The localisation of function in humans has for a long time only been possible by examining patients with focal CNS lesions. The characterisation of such lesions was only possible post mortem. Recent advances in in vivo imaging methods have made it possible to pinpoint the site of such lesions within the millimetre range. Nevertheless, lesion studies have a number of limitations that make firm conclusion about brain–behaviour relationships difficult. The CNS is characterised by a high degree of connectivity. Any lesion is likely to affect function in remote areas, which can seriously limit the localising power of any clinical observations. Discrete subcortical lesions, for example, can result in widespread cortical underactivity and be associated with clinical depression or dementia (Grasso et al 1994, Tatemichi et al 1995). The natural history of lesions can further exaggerate (post-traumatic oedema) or reduce (plasticity) the impact of a focal disturbance at different times. Using a purely logical approach, focal lesions may identify structures necessary for a specific function, but these structures need not be sufficient for the performance of the function, in fact they may only constitute a small link in the causal chain. The concepts of dissociation and double dissociation are often used to support specific brain–behaviour relationships between certain localised lesions and psychological impairments. A dissociation between two types of psychological deficits is said to exist if one is associated with a particular lesion, but the other is not. A double dissociation is then found if two separate psychological deficits are each associated with their own specific lesion sites, and are not affected by lesions at the other site. A more fine-grained method of localisation was used by Penfield & Rasmussen (1950), who used electrodes to stimulate the cortex of epileptic patients undergoing neurosurgery for the treatment of their illness. Their research resulted in the famous

homunculi for the primary motor and sensory cortices (Fig. 2.2). While direct electrical stimulation gives meaningful results over primary sensorimotor cortex, the effects of stimulation over association or limbic cortex are more difficult to interpret. A further drawback of this method is that the subjects examined are of necessity epileptic patients, whose brain disease may have already resulted in functional changes. Finally, even contemporary criticism was based on the possibility of current spread to related pathways (Phillips et al 1984). As a major advance on intracranial stimulation, for the last 10 years it has been possible to stimulate superficial cortex, using strong magnetic fields generated by a coil held over the head. This allows us to examine healthy volunteers (or indeed any patient group) and map primary sensorimotor function over the pre- and postcentral gyri with a spatial resolution of several millimetres. Such studies can, for example, track changes in the size of responsive neuronal areas in motor cortex with learning, and thus give a first-hand demonstration of neuronal plasticity. During the repeat performance of a complex serial reaction time task in one study, subjects performed faster with time (implicit learning), with motor cortical output maps for the muscles involved in the task covering an increasingly larger area. Once subjects became aware of the 'rules' of the task (explicit learning), motor output maps shrank to the original size (Pascual-Leone et al 1994).

The new methods of functional neuroimaging have revolutionised the investigation of brain–behaviour correlations (Ch. 15). Three strategies have been employed to quantify this relationship. Experiments can be designed in a modular manner, for example a verbal memory task is compared with a control task that contains all components, such as sensory input and motor response, except the memory task itself. The principle of this approach is that by subtracting the two brain

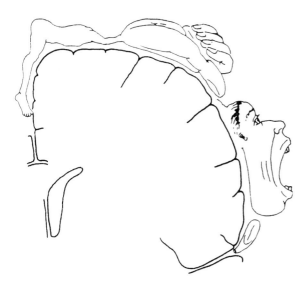

Fig. 2.2 The motor homunculus. (After Penfield & Rasmussen 1954.)

activity states it is possible to isolate the anatomical substrate linked with memory function. Studies using this paradigm have generated a number of intriguing findings, such as deactivations of certain brain regions during tasks and reciprocal changes between certain regions (e.g. frontal and temporal cortex). A more sophisticated approach uses factorial designs, such as different drug treatments (or placebo) crossed with several different activation tasks, so that interactions between task and treatment can be observed. A further interesting example of such a factorial design involves the effect of time on cerebellar activation during a finger apposition task. During this task, which is used by pianists or guitarists as a finger exercise, all fingers of one hand have to touch the thumb of the same hand in succession. In untrained subjects, motor learning takes place over repeated trials. It is, in fact, the interaction between task and repeat performance that demonstrates the effect of learning. Such an effect can be observed in the cerebellum, i.e. with increasing practice the cerebellar activation becomes less pronounced. This may be caused by long-term depression, which has been observed in animals during motor learning and may involve synapses on apical dendrites of Purkinje cells in the neocerebellar cortex (Friston 1994). If the behaviour under study is quantifiable, a parametric design can be employed that correlates, for example, performance measures during a task, or psychiatric symptom scores with brain activity. This assumes a linear relationship between symptoms or performance and

brain activity, although all or nothing (modular), or other non-linear relationships can be modelled in principle. In addition to factorial and parametric designs, it is possible to examine the correlation between the activity of different brain areas during several activation procedures. Such inter-regional correlations can be interpreted as evidence of coordinated activity in functional neuronal networks. An example for this approach is given by Friston (1994). Principal components analysis of brain activity during a sequence of 12 alternating word generation and word shadowing tasks produced two main components. The first accounted for the experimentally introduced variability in brain activity (71% of the variability over the time of the experiment) and involved increases in anterior cingulate, left dorsolateral prefrontal cortex, Broca's area, thalamus and cerebellum, with decreases in both temporal lobes and posterior cingulate. The second component reflected change over time (maybe attentional change) and mainly involved anterior cingulate activity. Time series of scans with changing task conditions, therefore, provide a most powerful tool to unravel the cooperation of remote structures in the brain for achieving the tasks. Functional MRI, which can be repeated many times over, is likely to be the standard method used in such studies in the future.

The methods described so far have in common the fact that they can be applied to human subjects. Animal studies, particularly in other mammals, have provided and still do provide essential information on functional neuroanatomy that cannot be generated from human studies. Amongst the most informative approaches in neuroscience have been in vivo recording techniques. Electrodes are implanted very precisely into an area of interest and spontaneous (single cell) neuronal activity during animal behaviour can be recorded. The spatial resolution of this method combined with postmortem confirmation of the electrode location is higher than any imaging mode has achieved so far, and information in the time domain is naturally superior. Recording, rather than stimulation, techniques avoid the problem of current spread (see above). Single cell recording in frontal cortex can, for example, identify neurones that fire during a delay after presentation of a stimulus which has to be compared with other stimuli later on. This method can therefore identify the 'neuronal working memory trace'. Some neurones fire depending on the spatial localisation of the stimulus, others depending on its shape or colour (Goldman-Racic 1995). Local neurotransmitter concentrations can be measured with an implanted probe that is equally able to deliver pharmacologically active agents to a small region in the brain. Mechanical, chemical and thermal lesioning and ablation techniques have played an important part in identifying the functional roles of different brain regions. In contrast to clinical studies, the size and location of the lesion can be rigorously controlled, so that many of the limitations discussed earlier can be circumvented. Kainic acid is used as a non-specific neurotoxin to create localised lesions. For some transmitter systems very specific toxins that are taken up only into one type of neurone and destroy it selectively, are available. An example is 1-methyl-4-phenyl-1,2,3,6-tetrahydropyridine (MPTP), a specific toxin of the nigrostriatal dopaminergic system, that has been used as a model of Parkinson's disease. Post mortem, many methods are now available to explore the functional role of brain structures and systems. Brain slice preparations are used for electrophysiological and pharmacological experiments. Neurones belonging to specific transmitter systems can be tracked in their projections by certain neurochemical reactions, such as fluorescence of catecholaminergic and serotoninergic neurones. Immunohistochemistry provides in vitro markers for neurotransmitters, enzymes and other proteins; in situ hybridisation allows for the localisation of specific mRNA. Axon transsection in vivo results in anterograde (Wallerian) degeneration; post mortem their course can be followed, for example using myelin staining. Locally applied markers, such as amino acids, fluorescent dyes or neurotoxins, are taken up into the axon and are transported in anterograde (proline/leucine) or retrograde (pseudorabies virus) directions. Some markers also bridge the synaptic cleft and allow for the tracing of projections beyond the original neurone (Cooper et al 1996). Receptor distributions can be mapped by radioactively labelled receptor ligands. After labelling, the brain is sectioned in a micro-tome, thin sections are apposed to sensitive film, and maps of radioactivity patterns are generated which can be compared with the histology of the original brain slice (Fig. 2.3). Similar to positron emission tomography (PET) and single photon emission computerised tomography (SPECT), cerebral blood flow and metabolism can be measured and mapped by autoradiographic methods, which allow for the localisation of specific pharmacological effects. The most recent addition to the armamentarium of the functional anatomist is the generation of transgenic animals with specific localised abnormalities in brain proteins, such as receptors. At the time of writing, ('knockout') mice have been created which miss the gene for the R1 subunit of the N-methyl-D-aspartate receptor specifically in CA1 pyramidal neurones of the hippocampus. These mice appear to show abnormalities in spatial memory (Morris & Morris 1997, Wilson & Tonegawa 1997). Functional neuroanatomy is thus increasingly based on a large variety of complex analytic methods which need to be integrated with clinical observation in order to achieve a balanced appreciation of brain function. It is self-evident that this chapter cannot be comprehensive: it reflects the clinical and scientific bias of the authors. We hope, however, that our subjective selection will give the reader an appreciation of the principles involved in functional neuronal organisation and transmit some of the excitement of modern neuroscience.

PRINCIPLES OF FUNCTIONAL NEURAL ORGANISATION

This section considers the functional anatomy of infor-

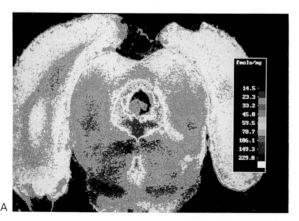
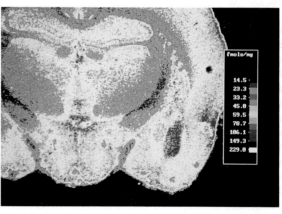

Fig. 2.3 Autoradiography of paroxetine binding sites in the rat brain. High transporter binding in (**a**) central raphe and (**b**) hippocampus. Reproduced with kind permission by Dr Judith K. McQueen, MRC Brain Metabolism Unit and Dr John Sharkey, Fujisawa Institute of Neuroscience.)

mation processing in the brain, using sensory systems in general and the visual system in particular as examples. We begin with a brief overview of the cortex and the general functional properties of sensory systems, and then turn in more detail to visual processing. Functionally relevant anatomical features are described, but the emphasis here is on how cellular arrangements process information, rather than detailed discussion of structural anatomy. Some basic knowledge of neuroanatomy is assumed, but it is not essential in order to follow the principles embodied in the aspects of neural processing described below. Structural anatomical detail can be found in relevant undergraduate textbooks. Although much of the information which follows has been derived from the study of the brains of cats and monkeys, it is likely that the principles described apply also in the human brain.

The cortex

The cerebral hemispheres consist of two large, thin, wrinkled sheets of cell bodies and their associated dendritic processes (cortex – grey matter) overlying myelinated (white matter) tracts. The hemispheres are connected by a white matter tract, the corpus callosum. The wrinkles in the cortical sheet – sulci and gyri – indicate the extensive folding necessary to contain the remarkable processing power of the cortex within the limited confines of the skull. The gyral and sulcal pattern provides the basis of the division of the cortex into anatomical lobes, which in turn show some degree of functional specialisation. Folded under the neocortex and within the temporal lobe are important grey matter structures, such as the hippocampus and amygdala, which will be discussed later when considering the limbic system.

Focusing in on the cortex, the cortical sheet is seen to have a laminar structure, consisting of six layers, numbered (top to bottom) from 1 to 6 – essentially a stack of six sheets (laminae), on average 2 mm thick, with layer 1 below the pial meningeal covering, and layer 6 above the white matter tracts. The layers are made distinct by their variable composition of different cell types and cell processes, and the relative proportions of cells and processes. The thickness and composition of individual laminae varies across the cortical sheet, and provides the basis for a more detailed 'cytoarchitectural' classification of cortical divisions proposed by Brodmann, mentioned above (Fig. 2.4). Though Brodmann's classification is still used, insight into the functional and anatomical complexity of the microstructure of the cortex has led to a more fine-grained subclassification – as we shall see later when

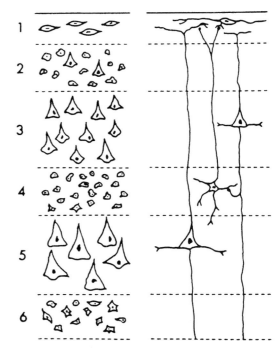

Fig. 2.4 Cellular layers in the neocortex. The right of the figure shows the connections between pyramidal and stellate cells.

considering the structure and function of the visual cortex.

Superimposed over this laminar (horizontal) organisation of the cortex are vertical aggregations of cylinders or columns of cells with rich interconnections which share functional properties. These properties vary with the overall function of the cortical areas that the columns inhabit, and are determined by the input that they receive and process. It may help to imagine the columns as many regularly spaced buildings arranged into many city blocks (individual cortical areas), which in turn make up an entire city (the cortex). Each building has six floors – each representing one of the six laminae – though the floors must be numbered in reverse to follow cortical convention, such that the bottom floor is the sixth floor, and the top floor is the first floor. As described earlier, the lamina vary in size depending on the function of the cortical area in which they are located: the fourth floor (layer 4, which receives input) in a sensory area (or city block) will be larger than the fourth floors of buildings in a motor output 'district', where floor 5 (layer 5 – concerned with output) is bigger.

Sensory systems

All sensory systems follow a similar general plan. In

functional terms, sensory receptors in each system transduce the energy of stimuli (mechanical, thermal, chemical or electromagnetic) into electrochemical energy and, by means of a variety of neural coding strategies, detect the modality, intensity, duration and location of stimuli. Sensory systems conduct, transform and integrate neural impulses actively in a variety of ways to allow us to perceive our environment. In order to achieve this, sensory systems are organised in a hierarchical, parallel and topographic fashion. They are hierarchical in the sense that successive stages extract increasingly complex features from the sensory environment; their parallel nature ensures that different kinds of information are processed separately; and their topographic organisation reflects the spatial relationship of stimuli from adjacent parts of the sensory field and their ability to affect each other. Neurones belonging to a particular sensory system, therefore, respond specifically to more or less complex stimuli, to particular aspects of sensory events, and to a specific locality within the sensory field – depending on their position within the chains of information processing. In the visual system there are cells which respond only to points of light from a highly restricted portion of the visual field, no matter what gestalt this point belongs to. In contrast, other cells respond to complex stimuli, such as faces, located anywhere in the visual field. These are manifestations of the hierarchical and topographical aspects of processing. Parallel processing, on the other hand, segregates information about movement from information about colour and shape. Thus the visual system makes a neurological distinction between 'where' something is as opposed to 'what' it is (Macko et al 1982). It is important to remember that cells within sensory systems have a 'projective field', as well as a receptive field. This determines how information received is subsequently transformed.

The visual system: complex information processing

Visual processing begins in the retina

The receptor organ of the visual system is the retina. Light is absorbed and transduced into electrochemical energy by photoreceptor cells – the rods and cones. Information collected by these receptors passes into a network of four further types of retinal cell: horizontal cells, bipolar cells, amacrine cells and ganglion cells. The cells are arranged such that final retinal output is from the ganglion cells, modified by the precise, regular network of connections between the various cell types. In this way, the network confers specific receptive field

properties to the ganglion cells (Tessier-Lavigne 1991). Ganglion cells have circular receptive fields, with a central circular portion surrounded by a concentric outer area which operates as 'antagonistic surround'. This means that stimuli in the centre of the receptive field have the opposite effect to stimuli falling within the more peripheral area of the receptive field of any individual cell. The 'effect' of a stimulus is to alter the firing rate of a ganglion cell. There are 'on-centre' cells and 'off-centre' ganglion cells. Cells with an 'on-centre' field fire more vigorously when a point of light falls on the central portion of the field, and less vigorously when the antagonistic, surrounding area is illuminated. 'Off-centre' cells have the opposite property: increased firing is encouraged by a stimulus within the outer portion, while firing is dampened down when the central portion of the field is activated. If illumination falls evenly across the receptive fields of either cell type, there is very little change in firing rate. The receptive fields of ganglion cells are therefore interested in contrasts and movement in their small portions of the visual field: even at this very early stage in visual processing, active computational processes are abstracting features of the electromagnetic environment by segregating information into parallel ('on-centre' and 'off-centre') streams.

A further, parallel division of information also occurs at this level. There are two types of ganglion cell, each type including cells with 'on-centre' fields and with 'off-centre' fields. One type, called M cells (magnocellular – large cells), respond mainly to rapid changes in the visual field and are primarily interested in movement. The other type, P cells (parvocellular – small cells), are more numerous and respond more to contrast changes and wavelength in their portions of the visual field. In some of these cells, the centre and 'antagonistic surround' areas of their receptive fields are responsive in an oppositional way to different wavelengths of light (such as red versus green light) – so called 'single-opponent' cells – in addition to the presence or absence of light: these cells are interested in colour. Other P cells are more interested in achromatic contrast and thus fine detail.

Leaving the retina

Information from the retina projects to a variety of brain areas: to the pretectal area in the midbrain, where pupillary reflexes are controlled; to the superior colliculus to provide information for the control of eye muscles; and to the lateral geniculate nuclei – the thalamic relay of the visual perception system. Retinal ganglion cell axons form the optic nerves, which course through the optic chiasm to become the optic tracts and terminate in the lateral geniculate nucleus (LGN). A further set of parallel information streams must be considered at this point: visual information is coming, of course, from each of two eyes. The nasal halves of each retinal projection decussate in the optic chiasm, the temporal halves do not. The left half of each retina (the left visual 'hemifield') projects to the left LGN; the right half of each retina (right 'hemifield') to the right LGN. Therefore, each nucleus receives input from both eyes.

In general, sensory systems project along a chain of neurones from their receptor sheet through peripheral sensory nerves to the spinal cord, via a relay in the thalamus, and then to their individual 'primary' sensory cortex and beyond. The olfactory system, however, has no thalamic relay, and the visual system has no 'peripheral' nerve – the optic nerve strictly speaking is a central neuronal pathway heading for the thalamus.

The thalamus is an egg-shaped structure which constitutes the largest part of the diencephalon. It acts as a gateway to the cortex for sensory information – its output to the cortex can be modified by the reticular activating system in the brainstem, for example. In view of its massive, widespread projection to (and back projection from) the cortex, the thalamus exerts considerable influence on cortical processing: it has been described as a 'brain within the brain'. The thalamus is divided up into several regions in terms of the cortical areas to which it projects. The parts of the thalamus concerned with visual information are the left and right lateral geniculate nuclei.

The lateral geniculate nucleus

The lateral geniculate nucleus has six layers, receiving highly ordered ganglion cell projections. The most ventral two layers have larger cells than the more rostral four layers. Each of the ventral, large cell layers are contacted by projections from the retinal ganglion M cells – one layer from M cells responding to stimuli activating the right eye's retinal contribution to the hemifield, the other responding to the left eye contribution. The four smaller cell layers receive P cell input, alternately segregated into left and right eye projections, two layers for each eye. Pathways carrying P cell (colour, detail) information remain separate from, but run parallel to, M cell (movement, flicker) projections. Information from the left and right eyes within a hemifield is similarly segregated, again illustrating the parallel nature of neural processing. Relationships between elements of the visual field are preserved at this level, following the principle of topographic organisation. Cells responding to adjacent portions of the visual field in the retina project to adjacent cells in the LGN. The LGN is said to possess a 'retinotopic' map, or rather several retinotopic maps, layer by layer. The receptive fields of the LGN

cells are therefore similar to those observed in the corresponding retinal ganglion cells – circular, with a central portion and an antagonistic surround – and they too respond best to points of light falling on the retina. There are few collateral connections or cross-talk between cells within the LGN; the information they obtain from the retina therefore appears to pass on to visual cortex with little modification. In this sense, the LGN may seem to act as a rather 'dumb', though highly ordered, relay. However, more than 80% of synaptic contacts within the LGN come not from the retinal ganglion cells but from cortical back-projections, and from the reticular formation in the brainstem. Higher order processing can therefore exert a profound influence on the LGN's activities, as can different arousal states. The details of these back-projections, and indeed cortical back-projections in general, are poorly understood. We therefore have to await new insights into such arrangements before a fuller understanding of LGN function becomes available.

Visual cortex: 'V1'

The first stage of cortical processing takes place in the striate cortex surrounding the calcarine sulcus of the occipital lobe and extending over the occipital pole at the back of the brain. Much of the visual cortex is hidden from view because it is folded into the depths of the calcarine sulcus. Again, it is more helpful to think of the visual cortex unfolded and laid out as a sheet. The striate cortex is so named because of its prominent striations or stripes of myelinated axons running parallel to the cortical sheet in layer 4. Brodmann classified striate cortex as area 17, and contiguous 'extrastriate' visual areas as 18 and 19. More detailed analysis and understanding of visual cortical areas has led to further subdivisions. At least 20 distinct cortical areas have been identified, with still more having partial visual properties. They are designated by number (striate cortex is now area V1), or by anatomical designation and number (such as area MT – middle temporal area, V5 – located on the posterior edge of the superior temporal sulcus). Not all visual areas will be described here, but the structure and function of important examples will be considered.

V1 is relatively thin, six-layered cortex. From a vertical perspective, taking each lamina in turn, layer 1 (the outermost layer, nearest the pial surface) contains many cell processes, such as the apical dendrites from cells in lower layers, but few cell bodies. Some input from other cortical areas arrives here. Layers 2 and 3 contain many pyramidal cells, which project to cells in other cortical areas. Layer 4 has spiny, stellate cells and few pyramidal cells. This is the main input layer of V1, where axons from cells in the LGN terminate. The cells here contact cells in other layers of V1, principally in layers 2 and 3. Layers 5 and 6 have many pyramidal cells. Cells in layer 5 receive some of their input from layer 3 and project beyond the cortex. Cells in layer 6 both receive input from and project back to, the thalamus, in addition to receiving input from layer 5. It also sends a (negative) feedback loop to layer 4. To return to our city block analogy, the foregoing describes activities on the six floors of one of the buildings. To grossly simplify, the fourth floor receives information from the LGN, passes it up to floors 2 and 3 (remember that the floors are numbered in reverse!). From there it is sent out to other city blocks and districts (other cortical areas) and also down to the fifth floor. From the fifth floor some information is then sent to the sixth floor, and some right out of the city to 'other lands' (to non-cortical areas, such as the spinal cord). The sixth floor sends inhibitory signals back to the fourth (input) floor – in this case, completing a negative feedback loop (Lund 1988). While this analogy does little justice to the complexity of cortical processing (and is somewhat inaccurate, as it does not take account of the fact that there is enormous information transfer amongst layers between vertical elements – between floors in different buildings – and that cells in lower layers have dendrites in upper layers and are thus influenced by inputs to other floors), it is intended to convey the idea that complicated but orderly integration of information is going on.

Input to V1 from the LGN

As noted in the preceding section, projections from the LGN terminate principally in layer 4 of V1. The M (magnocellular – concerned with flicker and movement) and P (parvocellular – concerned with fine contrast detail and colour) cell projections terminate, however, in different sublaminae of layer 4, preserving parallel but segregated information streams. Topographic mapping is also maintained, but the map is transformed, or distorted, such that there is increased representation of cells responding to stimuli closer to the centre of gaze. The receptive fields of the cells directly receiving input from the LGN in layer 4 are, of course, otherwise similar to the LGN cells themselves: circular, and responding to points of light. However, presumably as a consequence of the complex integration within V1 described above, cells above and below layer 4 have very different receptive field properties altogether.

Orientation columns

These cells do not respond preferentially to points of light, but to linear stimuli – bars or lines of light excite the cells. Furthermore, individual cells respond to bars with specific orientations: some cells to vertical bars, some to horizontal bars, some to transverse bars. These response characteristics are similar to those encountered earlier, in that the receptive field consists of an area which when 'stimulated' enhances cell activity, and a surrounding area which inhibits it – except that rather than concentric circles, the central area consists of a linear strip with a particular orientation. It is believed that the integration of overlapping, circular centre/surround fields in layer 4 generates these new, higher order receptive fields. Indeed, there are cells which respond individually to each orientation around the central axis of a bar stimulus through 360°. Moving horizontally across the V1 cortex, cells are found which respond to an orderly progression of bar orientations. The first cell may respond to a vertical bar. The next cell to a bar tipped 15° from vertical. The next cell to a bar 30° from vertical – and so on, until, over a distance of about 1 mm, we reach cells again responding to vertical bars. From a vertical perspective, cells one above the other tend to respond to the same orientation – while moving horizontally, the next 'column' of cells all respond to a slightly different orientation (for example, Hubel and Wiesel 1979).

Returning to our analogy, it is as if we were walking down a street in a cortical city, passing buildings (columns of cells), each specialising in dealing with different orientations of bars of light. Each floor (layer) within any one building deals with the same orientation, but the next building along deals with the next 15° rotation of the bar, and the next building a further rotation and so on. By the time we reach the end of the street (a distance of about a millimetre), we will have passed one building for each orientation – right around the clock. The first building of the next block we meet starts again at the first orientation we encountered, and the orderly progression continues. Each vertical column of cells (building) dealing with one orientation is known as an 'orientation' column, and the entire block with each orientation represented is considered to be part of a 'hypercolumn' (see below). All the cells which contribute to the same part of the retinal map (a whole city block) each have a different line orientation selectivity, so in essence every portion of the visual field has an element dedicated to every line orientation. Thus the next block, in which all the buildings are concerned with a different, adjacent part of the visual field, also has a full set of orderly arranged buildings dealing with each line orientation. The discovery of orientation columns – amongst other work – earned David Hubel and Torsten Wiesel the Nobel prize.

Within V1 there are cells with more complex receptive fields still – sensitive to linear stimuli throughout the visual field rather than in specific portions, or linear stimuli moving in a particular direction across the visual field, or to lines of particular length, and so on. Presumably these more complex fields are abstracted from integration of output from cells with simpler receptive field characteristics. Given that, as we have seen, fields tend to be responsive to changes in contrast and movement, it seems likely that the linear preoccupation of V1 cells is concerned with the detection of edges at different angles, and thus the construction of static and moving outlines in the visual field from short line segments with a variety of orientations.

Ocular dominance columns

What of the input from each eye? Remember that the left hemifield is conducted to the right hemisphere and the right hemifield to the left, such that each visual area has parallel input from each eye. The six layers of the LGN maintained separation of right and left eye contributions to hemifield input: the two ventral layers receiving M cell input, one for right, one for left; the four upper layers receiving P cell input, left and right eye information alternately. These left and right eye contributions are projected separately to another set of columns in V1– the ocular dominance columns. The ocular dominance columns thus contain vertical aggregations of cells which all tend to respond to stimuli falling on a small portion of the field of view of one eye, either right or left. The columns are arranged such that right eye and left eye responsive columns alternate as we move horizontally across the cortical sheet. It is likely that this arrangement plays an important role in stereoscopic vision (Hubel et al 1978).

The 'horizontal' route, which reveals the orderly left/right responsiveness alternation, is orthogonal to the orientation column axis that we encountered earlier. To make this clearer, we can employ again our city map analogy. Imagine that we have just walked one 'block', say east to west, past each of the 'buildings' responsible for each orientation of a strip of light (see above). If we turn 90°, and head north, we are now passing buildings alternately responsible for left eye input and right eye input. If we consider a complete 'block' as bounded east–west by a row of buildings comprising a complete set of line orientation columns, and bounded north–south by a left eye building and a right eye building, then our whole block contains the parallel distributed information for a single hemifield portion – a 'hypercolumn'. It is tempting to think of such units as individual cortical processing 'modules'. The principle of topographic mapping is sustained by finding that the next block in the city deals with an adjacent portion of the visual hemifield, and so on.

The features of this arrangement are not unique to the visual system. Auditory cortex, for example, has a topographic 'cochleotopic' map which receives ordered input, preserved through the many way stations from the cochlea, in terms of the sound frequency spectrum (analogous to the parallel processing of information from the visual field of the visual system). Each hemisphere also receives input from both ears, such that blocks in the 'auditory city' have a frequency dimension and a 'binaural' dimension: thus enabling the identification and localisation of sound.

Blobs and interblobs in V1

A further aspect of V1 structure must now be considered. Situated above and below layer 4 in the centre of the cortical visual 'blocks' are small peg-like regions called 'blobs' (the larger surrounding area of the block is sometimes described as the 'interblob' region). The blobs can be identified on the basis of their particular staining characteristics on histological examination. Cells within the blob regions are responsive to colour information, rather than the orientation of linear stimuli. They receive information initially generated by the 'single-opponent' P (parvocellular) cells described earlier when considering the retina. Information from the other P cells, which are concerned with fine (but colourless) contrast detail, eventually arrives in the interblob regions where cells do respond selectively to the orientation of stimuli. We can, therefore, distinguish two parallel pathways: the M (magnocellular) pathway originating with the M ganglion cells in the retina and concerned with detection of movement; and the P pathway, initiated by the P ganglion cells. The P pathway can be subdivided into a P-blob pathway, concerned with colour vision, and a P-interblob pathway concerned with detail and shape.

A parallel distributed system

Drawing these aspects of V1 together, we can see that this cortical area identifies line segments in the visual field, maintains and processes parallel pathways for colour, form and movement, and takes part in the ordering of information from both eyes for depth perception. Various elements across the visual field are, unsurprisingly, interconnected – such that cells concerned with a particular linear orientation (or a particular colour characteristic) from one part of the visual field talk to cells with similar colour or orientation interests, but with receptive fields serving a different part of the visual field.

Why does the cortex process information in this parallel, distributed way? There are certainly advantages to the arrangement. Multiple distributed modules might solve wiring problems: to mangle an analogy of Francis Crick's (1994), and give it a psychiatric flavour, the existence of distributed modules may be similar to the convenience to the population of many community resource centres – rather than having to travel some distance to a central asylum. (Crick thought more in terms of many convenience stores versus one large supermarket in a city). Distributed networking is also 'damage resistant'. Losing a single resource centre is not as catastrophic as losing the whole asylum. The mathematical neural network models beloved by theoretical neurobiologists demonstrate the principle of 'graceful degradation' in response to damage – just as small lesions to portions of V1 reduce visual acuity rather than causing complete blindness.

Extrastriate cortex: beyond V1

As noted above, there are many distinct cortical visual areas. In general, as we move in the direction of information flow, the size of individual cellular receptive fields increases, and the stimuli eliciting a response become more complex (Tanaka 1993). None the less, parallel information streams carrying specific kinds of information continue. The pathway originating in the M cells in the retina, initially responding to changes in contrast, and later orientation and movement in V1, projects via area V2 (part of Brodmann's area 18) to the middle temporal area – area MT (or V5, part of Brodmann's area 19). Here, more complex features are constructed, such as speed and direction of movement. Further projections terminate in parietal regions where a complex analysis of position and motion is carried out. It is in this sense that the visual system makes a neurological distinction between 'what' and 'where' – the M pathway terminating in parietal cortex is the 'where' pathway. The P pathway, arising from the parvocellular ganglion cells in the retina, and eventually dividing into blob (colour) and interblob (detail and form) streams in V1, projects via area V2 to area V4, where a great deal of colour processing occurs. Recordings from cells receiving information via the P-blob stream in area V4 do not simply respond to wavelength, but to perceived colour – which, despite invariant wavelength, can be changed by altering the background colour against which a coloured cue is placed. Cells in the P-interblob pathway are sensitive initially to edges, and ultimately to outlines and therefore shapes. Their projection from area V4 along with the P-blob stream to the inferotemporal visual area represents the end of the 'what' pathway. A small proportion of cells in this area respond uniquely to some very complex stimuli indeed, such as any orientation of a hand, anywhere in the visual field; or to faces. The 'what' and 'where' streams finally merge in the entorhinal and frontal cortices. Complex polysensory information is believed to be processed and constructed into memories in the hippocampus and the related entorhinal cortex (see limbic system, below); while the integration of 'what' and 'where' information may take place in the 'working memory' systems of the prefrontal cortex (Rao et al 1997).

Perception, attention and consciousness

Where, then, is visual awareness in this complex scheme? There is no 'homunculus' sitting inside the brain watching information about shape and colour and movement arriving on a monitor. Nor does the loss of the hippocampal system, where visual information eventually mingles, result in a loss of visual perception. Perhaps surprisingly, there is evidence that the mechanisms underlying visual awareness are, in fact, distributed throughout the visual system. Study of neural responses to visual illusions which make use of ambiguous stimuli have been used to show this. (The fact that visual illusions occur at all reveals the active, constructive nature of perceptual processing.) Consider the well known Necker cube illusion, where a two-dimensional drawing of a cube can appear at one moment to be viewed from above, while at another from below. The patterns of light being detected by the retina are not changing – some internal representation of the image is responsible for the perceived alteration in form. The effects of analogous illusions on the firing of neurones in the monkey visual pathway have provided clues as to where and how the illusion is represented. In an experiment conducted by Richard Andersen and his colleagues (Barinaga 1997), monkeys were presented with a computer-generated pattern of moving dots on a screen. The pattern is arranged such that the dots appear to form a rotating three-dimensional cylinder, and, as in the Necker cube illusion, it is sometimes viewed as rotating clockwise, sometimes anticlockwise – even though the pattern of dots and their movement has not changed. The monkeys were trained to indicate in which direction the cylinder appeared to them to move, while recordings were made from area MT where, as we have seen, there are cells which respond to direction of movement. Some 50% of the cells increased their firing rate only when the monkey indicated apparent movement in one particular direction, and firing was dampened down when the other direction of movement was perceived. Andersen and his colleagues interpreted this finding as indicating that the subset of MT neurones showing this activity reflect what the monkey perceives, rather the image falling on the retina. Similar experiments have shown that artificially stimulating neurones in area MT can bias monkeys' decisions about direction of movement in related visual tasks, suggesting that the MT neurones may themselves shape the perception – rather than simply passively conducting information.

Attentional processes appear to be important in directing these neural correlates of perceptual experience within the visual pathways. In an experiment designed to study neural responses in area V4 to the simultaneous presentation of variously coloured shapes, Robert Desimone and his colleagues trained monkeys to pay attention to individual shapes with a particular colour. As described earlier, V4 neurones respond to perceived colour. When the monkey attended to a red shape, red responsive neurones in V4 would fire vigorously. However, when attention was directed to a green shape, the red responsive neurone ceased responding, even though the red shape was still within the receptive field.

Analogous experiments have been conducted in humans. Steven Petersen and his colleagues (Corbetta et al 1990) used PET to measure changes in regional cerebral blood flow in subjects set the task of discriminating different attributes (shape, colour and velocity) of the same set of visual stimuli. When the subjects attended selectively to shape, brain activity was enhanced in the inferotemporal cortex (the 'what' pathway); when they attended to colour, activity was increased in an area likely to contain the human equivalent of V4; and when they attended to velocity, activity in a region analogous to MT was enhanced. These attention-directed variations occurred despite the fact that all three attributes of the stimulus set were within the visual field throughout.

How are these responses directed and coordinated? Speculation abounds. It has been suggested that frontal areas may be involved (Crick 1994). The experiments described above focus on the neural correlates of perception, visual awareness and consciously directed attention. Some neuroscientists believe that they are now taking the first steps towards understanding the biological basis of consciousness itself.

FRONTOSUBCORTICAL LOOPS – CONTROLLING MOVEMENT AND COGNITION

Frontal cortex does not only have an important role in the execution of movements, in cognition, social and motivated behaviour: it also appears to be implicated in psychiatric illness. Abnormalities in frontal lobe func-

tion have been described in the dementias, in depression and schizophrenia, and in obsessional disorder. The anatomical organisation of the frontal lobe and its functional implications are therefore of great interest to psychiatrists. As an important organisational principle, the parallel arrangement of neural loops connecting cortex with subcortical structures, such as striatum, pallidum and thalamus, has emerged over the last 15 years. These loops appear to be mutually exclusive, i.e. they connect clearly separated compartments in frontal cortex with similarly separate areas in basal ganglia (Alexander et al 1990). Of these, the 'motor circuit' has been characterised in most detail (Fig. 2.5). Before describing this circuit in greater detail a few more general observations on motor function are necessary to put the corticobasal ganglia–thalamic circuit into a wider functional context.

Motor function

Movement is essential for the expression of language, planned action, learning with practice and instinctive activity. Output from primary motor cortex (area 4) is a final common anatomical pathway for such behaviour. Area 4 projects to motor neurones in the anterior horn, directly and indirectly via spinal interneurones. There is also output to nuclei of the dorsal columns, the reticular formation, the pons and the inferior olive, the centromedian nucleus of the thalamus, and the putamen. Input to area 4 converges directly from other cortical areas, e.g. the parietal association cortex, or more indirectly from the basal ganglia and cerebellum via the thalamus. The motor function of the cerebellum has long been appreciated by the clinical effects of cerebellar lesions which result in disturbances of fine coordination, posture and walk, depending on the site of the lesion. The cerebellum receives input from vestibular, ascending sensory and descending pontine fibres. The pontine nuclei have input from the contralateral cerebral hemispheres, mainly primary motor (area 4), premotor (area 6), primary sensory (areas 1, 2, 3) and somatosensory association cortex (area 5). The cerebellum is thus equipped with a wealth of sensorimotor information. It projects via the dentate nucleus to the somatotopically organised ventral lateral thalamus and from there back to areas 4 and 6, closing the functional loop and enabling the cerebellum to act as a parallel processor to modulate movement and be involved in motor learning (see above). The ventrolateral portion of the dentate nucleus in fact projects to prefrontal association cortex and may be involved in cognitive processes (Martin 1996). A shorter loop courses from the dentate nucleus to the red nucleus, to the inferior olivary nucleus and via climbing fibres back to the cere-

Motor circuit

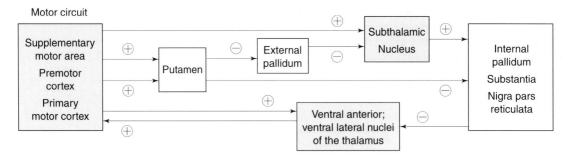

Fig. 2.5 The motor-circuit. (Modified from Alexander et al 1990 and Martin 1996.)

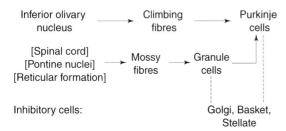

Fig. 2.6 Internal circuitry of the cerebellum. (After Martin 1996.)

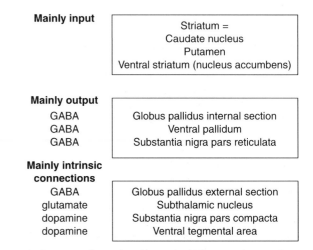

Fig. 2.7 Basal ganglia structures. (After Martin 1996.)

bellum. The internal circuitry of the cerebellum is relatively simple (Fig. 2.6). Granule cells are the only excitatory (glutamatergic) neurones in the cerebellum; all other cells are inhibitory, using γ-aminobutyric acid (GABA) or taurine (stellate cell) as a transmitter (Martin 1996). The output of Purkinje cells to the dentate nucleus is inhibitory as well. The detailed functional significance of this simple, relatively orderly arrangement of negative feedback is not yet clear, but its potential as a modulating circuit parallel to the neocortical motor centres is obvious.

The motor circuit

The terminology describing the basal ganglia is somewhat confusing. Figure 2.7 summarises the structures involved, grouped by their connection with input, output and internal structures. Putamen and pallidum are sometimes combined under the name lenticular nucleus. Similar to the cerebellum, the putamen receives motor input from area 4, but also from the supplementary motor cortex (medial area 6), the premotor cortex (lateral area 6), and sensory input from areas 1, 2, 3 and 5 (Fig. 2.5). This input is somatotopically organised, so that the leg zone lies dorsolateral, the orofacial zone ventromedial, and the arm zone in between. Neurones with GABA and substance P as transmitters project from putamen to the internal segment of the

globus pallidus, as well as to the pars reticulata of the substantia nigra, while neurones with GABA and enkephalin project to the external segment of the pallidum. There is thus a direct and an indirect pathway from putamen to thalamus. A short direct path leads via the internal segment of the pallidum or the substantia nigra back to the ventral lateral, ventral anterior and the centromedian nucleus of the thalamus (Fig. 2.5). An indirect pathway links the external segment of the globus pallidus with the subthalamic nucleus, hence the internal segment of the globus pallidus or substantia nigra and the thalamus. These two paths have opposite effects on the internal segment of the pallidum or the substantia nigra: excitatory glutamatergic input from cortex to putamen activates GABAergic cells in the putamen, which in turn inhibit GABAergic cells in the internal segment of the globus pallidus projecting to the thalamus. The net result is an activation of the thalamus (+−−), which itself has an activating input to cortex (and striatum). The indirect path involves inhibition of the external segment of the globus pallidus by GABAergic putamen cells; their output to the subthalamic nucleus is GABAergic too, whereas the output from the subthalamic nucleus to the internal segment of the globus pallidus or substantia nigra is excitatory. The net result is an inhibition of the thalamus $(+ - - + -)$. Moreover, there seems to be a differential effect of dopamine on striatal cells projecting to the external (GABA/enkephalin, inhibitory) and the internal (GABA/substance P, excitatory) globus pallidus. The depletion of dopaminergic input from the substantia nigra (pars compacta) to the striatum would, therefore, result in reduced thalamic excitation via the direct path and increased thalamic inhibition via the indirect path, both consistent with thalamic and consequently cortical underactivity. This additive effect explains the akinesia observed in parkinsonism. Recent results have qualified this simple model somewhat, in particular the straight linear connections within the indirect path are probably more complex than described (Chesselet & Delfs 1996, Feger 1997). Lesions of the subthalamic nucleus result in hemiballismus. A reduced excitatory input to the internal pallidum leads to decreased inhibition of the thalamus and consequent motor overactivity. Similarly, in Huntington's chorea there is a reduction of inhibitory enkephalinergic input from putamen to the external pallidum. This causes increased inhibition of the subthalamic nucleus by the external pallidum, reduced excitation of the internal pallidum by the subthalamic nucleus, and reduced inhibition of the thalamus by the internal pallidum, thus again causing increased movement. Finally, pallidotomy has been employed in the treatment of parkinsonism. Stereotactic lesions of the internal pallidum result in reduced thalamic inhibition and consequent reversal of the akinesia.

A similar circuit subserving oculomotor function exists but will not be discussed here in any detail. The corticobasal ganglia–thalamic circuits are described here in a simplified manner. A diversity of inputs to all stations of the circuits exists; there may also be links between the parallel loops.

The prefrontal circuit

The other parallel but mainly separate circuits linking dorsolateral prefrontal, orbitofrontal and anterior cingulate cortex with basal ganglia and thalamus (Figs 2.8 and 2.9) are not as well characterised as the motor circuit. The dorsolateral prefrontal cortex has long been implicated in cognitive function based on animal (Goldman-Racic 1995) and human studies (Petrides 1995, Stuss et al 1995). It receives input from a loop that includes the head of the caudate, the substantia nigra and the globus pallidus via the ventral anterior and medial dorsal nuclei of the thalamus. Both posterior parietal association cortex and premotor cortex project into this circuit via the head of the caudate. The most convincing interpretation of neuronal function in this circuit is that it subserves working memory. Working memory requires the active manipulation of a number of items within a memory store. Such a function is required during delayed matching-to-sample tasks: the subject has to select stimuli after evaluating their similarity in shape, colour or position with a previously presented sample. Similarly, self-ordering tasks require the retention and manipulation of a number of items, for example numbers. The word generation or verbal fluency task also requires the remembering of self-generated words in order to avoid repetition of the same word. There is now some evidence that spatial properties are processed separately from object properties in working memory. In non-human primates this may involve different regions within each hemisphere, whereas in humans the equivalent distinction between verbal and visuospatial properties likely maps on to different hemispheres. Closely associated with working memory are the concepts of the articulatory loop and the visuospatial scratch pad, where verbal and non-verbal information is held, and the central executive or supervisory attentional system, which is responsible for the manipulation of verbal and visuospatial information (Shallice 1982, Baddeley 1986). It has been suggested

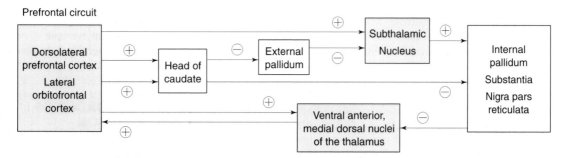

Fig. 2.8 Prefrontal circuit. (Modified from Alexander et al 1990 and Martin 1996.)

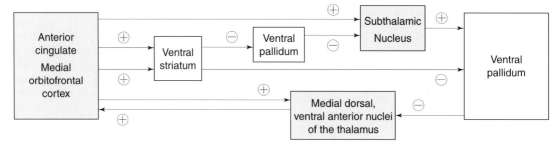

Fig. 2.9 Limbic circuit. (Modified from Alexander et al 1990 and Martin 1996.)

that these storage and processing functions of working memory in fact map on to different parts of the lateral prefrontal cortex (Goldman-Racic 1995), but there may also be a common area (area 46) that is involved in working memory of any type (Wickelgreen 1997).

So-called frontal dementias have been described in connection with a variety of illness processes, with an overactive, disinhibited presentation in association with orbitofrontal, and an apathetic presentation with dorsolateral prefrontal atrophy (Neary 1995). The basal ganglia are said to be invariably involved. In fact, primarily subcortical diseases, such as Huntington's disease, are occasionally associated with a 'subcortical' dementia of a frontal type. A similar explanation has been suggested for the cognitive abnormalities associated with severe depression, which often shows functional basal ganglia as well as prefrontal cortex underactivity. The hypofrontality associated with cognitive impairment in schizophrenia mainly affects the dorsolateral prefrontal cortex, possibly after an initial hyperactivity of this region (Ebmeier 1995, Wiesel et al 1987).

The limbic circuit

The limbic circuit receives cortical input from temporal lobe structures, such as the medial and lateral temporal lobes and the hippocampal formation. Anterior cingulate and medial orbitofrontal cortex are part of a circuit including the ventral striatum, the ventral pallidum and the medial dorsal and ventral anterior thalamic nuclei (Fig. 2.9). Baxter et al (1996) have advanced an argument implicating corticobasal ganglia–thalamic loops in obsessive–compulsive disorder. A relative increase in the neural tone of the direct path is said to result from medial orbitofrontal cortex input to the GABAergic cells of the ventral striatum (ventral medial head of caudate), which in turn inhibits GABAergic cells in the ventral pallidum that project to the dorsomedial nucleus of the thalamus. The end-result is an activation of the thalamus (+−−). The thalamus itself has reciprocal positive feedback with cortex (Fig. 2.9), so

that an escalating or at least driven circuit with associated inescapable compulsive behaviour may result. Compulsions to engage in stereotypical behaviour and obsessional ruminations thus may have a functional anatomical counterpart. The postulated relative increase in thalamic activity may be due to an imbalance between the direct (activating) and the indirect (inhibitory) paths. The model explains the excessive activation of orbitofrontal cortex, basal ganglia and thalamic nuclei found in symptomatic patients, as well as the observed correlations in activity between these regions. Both overactivity and correlations disappear with the resolution of symptoms. Based on this theory, internal capsulotomy, which interrupts the limbic circuit, has been employed in treatment-resistant obsessive–compulsive patients.

Similar increases in medial orbitofrontal and anterior cingulate cortex have been observed during short-term worsening of depressive symptoms, in particular vital symptoms, including anergia, and during pain syndromes (Ebert et al 1996).

The detailed anatomy of the prefrontal and limbic circuits remains to be determined. Although the principle of parallel circuits with somatotopic organisation throughout the circuit probably holds, the amount of cross-talk between the circuits is unknown. The above summary is, of course, incomplete without the multiple inputs from non-frontal structures, especially parietal and temporal association cortex and structures of the limbic system. The purpose of the simplified presentation has been to illustrate the principle of cortical–subcortical loops as an anatomical example of parallel processing within the brain, subserving behaviour, i.e. in the wider sense motor function.

THE LIMBIC SYSTEM: BORDER OF COGNITION AND EMOTION

The limbic system is essentially a collection of interconnected cortical and subcortical structures, described and defined in a variety of ways, and generally implicated in aspects of emotion, learning and memory (see limbic loop above). The concept of the limbic system can be confusing because both anatomical and functional considerations have determined its components over the years, and our understanding of brain and behaviour relationships has evolved over this time.

Historical background and conceptual overview

Paul Pierre Broca, a 19th century French surgeon and anthropologist (perhaps best known for describing the motor speech centre of the brain), first used the term 'limbic lobe' to delineate the tissues constituting the border (L. *limbus*, border) between neocortex and diencephalon. Although Broca himself regarded the limbic lobe as representing 'the seat of the lower faculties which predominate in the beast' and the extralimbic mass (neocortex) as 'the seat of superior faculties' – thus anticipat-

ing some later conceptualisations – neuroanatomists in the succeeding decades ascribed incorrectly a sensory (largely olfactory – hence rhinencephalon) role to the lobe. The early history of the limbic lobe is succinctly reviewed by Corsellis & Janota (1985).

The concept of a limbic system involved in emotional function developed later, from the speculations of James Papez (1937) and the subsequent theorising of Paul McLean (1949). On largely theoretical grounds, and drawing on the work of physiologist Walter Cannon, Papez proposed that a specific circuit (encompassing the hypothalamus, anterior thalamic nuclei, cingulate cortex and hippocampus) was responsible for the apprehension and expression of emotion. In the same year, Klüver & Bucy (1937) rediscovered the emotional effects of temporal lobe lesions which included limbic structures (originally described by Brown & Schafer (1888)). In the preceding year, Egas Moniz had begun treating pathological anxiety and agitation using the neurosurgical procedure of prefrontal leucotomy,

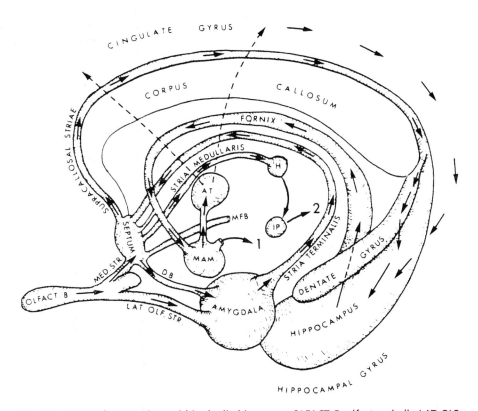

Fig. 2.10 Internal connections within the limbic system: OLFACT. B, olfactory bulb; LAT. OLF. STR., lateral olfactory stria; MED. STR., medial olfactory stria; AT, anterior nucleus of the thalamus; MFB, medial forebrain bundle; MAM, nucleus of the mamillary body (1, connection to midbrain reticular formation); DB, diagonal band of Broca; H, habenular nucleus; IP, interpeduncular nucleus (2, connection to midbrain reticular formation). (Modified from MacLean 1949.)

and it became increasingly appreciated that damage to frontal white matter had a marked effect on emotion and feeling – amongst other effects. In 1949, McLean extended the Papez circuit to include the prefrontal cortex, septum and amygdala and thus invented the original version of the limbic system (see Fig. 2.10). Reprising Broca's notions, McLean elaborated the concept of the limbic system as the visceral brain, the presumed source of basic emotions. It is easy to see the analogies being made in the minds of early investigators between the central tenets of Freudian psychoanalysis and non-cortical brain structure.

In 1957, Scoville and Milner reported that bilateral neurosurgical resection of the medial temporal lobes, including the hippocampus and amygdala, resulted in a severe impairment in memory function. Their now famous case (known in the literature as patient H.M.) had suffered from intractable temporal lobe epilepsy, and the lesions had been made in an effort – which was largely successful – to relieve the disorder. The role of limbic structures in memory function has been extensively studied in the years since. Further diencephalic structures, such as the mamillary bodies of the hypothalamus and the dorsomedial nucleus of the thalamus, earn their place in the limbic system both on grounds of anatomical considerations and the fact that they are implicated in the memory dysfunction which occurs in Korsakoff's syndrome.

Limbic structures thus play a role in memory and emotional function, and this overlap underscores the potential for confusion generated by the naive assumption that psychological concepts need to relate in any simple way to brain structure. Part of the problem in defining the limbic system is simply a reflection of the way in which research has developed: structures have come to be defined both in terms of crude gross anatomy (the original limbic lobe, for example) and in terms of function (such as those structures which when compromised or stimulated are observed to interfere with emotional behaviour, or memory function). These provisional approaches to classification do not map easily one to another. They are provisional in the sense that psychological constructs such as emotion, or memory, are subject to continuous conceptual refinement. Memory function, for example, is no longer considered a unitary entity and is at present better characterised as a series of dissociable subsystems, each of which may have its own structural substrate (see below). The same is true of emotion. Ultimately, the distinction between memory and emotion is likely to be modified: structural and functional concepts have mutually coevolved in the light of new findings, and continue so to do. The term 'limbic' therefore now fails to serve a variety of masters (not least the ingenious MCQ authors of the Royal College of Psychiatrists), but though there have been calls for its abolition, it has not yet been removed from office.

Here, the functional neuroanatomy of selected major limbic structures is described: the limbic cortex, the hippocampal formation (with a brief note regarding the role of the dorsomedial nucleus of the thalamus in memory function), the hypothalamus and the amygdaloid complex. The role of limbic structures in emotional and cognitive behaviour is the focus of each review.

Limbic cortex: cingulate and related prefrontal regions

The cingulate cortex (Brodmann areas 23, 24, 25 and 32) forms the superior arch of a ring of cortex on the medial surface of the temporal lobe, bounded above by the cingulate sulcus and below by the corpus callosum, over which it curves anteriorly, downwards and inward, merging into subgenual prefrontal cortex, and outward laterally into orbitofrontal cortex. The inferior half of the cortical ring is completed by pyriform, entorhinal and parahippocampal cortex (discussed below). This ring of cortex has been designated paralimbic (Pandya & Selzer, 1982): it differs from the primary sensory cortex or associational cortex encountered in our survey of the visual system in that it is older in evolutionary terms, and is composed largely of three rather than six layers. Paralimbic cortex receives higher order information from secondary associational sensory cortices (e.g. area V5 of the visual system), with which it is richly interconnected. The posterior portion of the cingulate cortex, for example, receives information from parietal association cortex, where visual and somatosensory information merge. Thalamic fibres, carrying pain-related information, project to the anterior portion of the cingulate. The anterior cingulate does not, however, play a part in the perception of pain per se, but rather appears to orchestrate the aversive emotional responses to painful stimuli. Surgical lesions here have been used in the treatment of chronic intractable pain – while pain is still perceived, its aversive qualities are abolished. It is likely that interconnections between anterior cingulate and other components of the limbic system, such as the hypothalamus and amygdala, confers this property of adding emotional tone to sensory stimuli.

The cingulate and its intimately associated prefrontal cortical areas (sometimes designated together as limbic association cortex) thus play an important role in emotional behaviour and have an interesting and controversial psychiatric history. It is said that an important spur to Moniz's development of prefrontal neurosurgery for mental disorder was the demonstration by Fulton & Jacobsen (Jacobsen, 1935) that previously aggressive chimpanzees were rendered passive and placid by bilateral frontal damage (see, for example, Damasio, 1994). Moniz reasoned that surgical destruction of frontal white matter pathways might attenuate the pathological anxiety and agitation experienced by some psychiatric patients, and set about developing his psychosurgical treatment, prefrontal leucotomy. Though the aim of early frontal lobe surgery was to reduce suffering without interfering with intellectual function, it became clear that gross frontal damage led not only to a marked reduction in emotional reactivity but also to alterations in personality, drive and social function. Subtle aspects of cognitive function are also perturbed, including deficits in planning, spatial and working memory, with a tendency to perseveration. This last deficit is revealed by the failure of some patients with frontal lesions to complete tasks requiring them to change strategies, such as the Wisconsin Card Sorting Test.

Refined lesion studies in animals, and neuropsychological studies of brain-injured patients, reveal that limbic cortex is functionally heterogeneous, responsible for a variety of cognitive and emotional functions. Damasio (1994) considers the anterior cingulate in particular as a 'fountainhead' region, where 'systems concerned with emotion/feeling, attention and working memory interact so intimately that they constitute the source for the energy of both external action (movement) and internal action (thought animation, reasoning)'.

Neuroimaging studies reveal functional and structural abnormalities in the frontal lobe generally in schizophrenia, which parallel neuropsychological deficits in tests of frontal lobe function (reviewed by Ebmeier 1995). More recent neuroimaging studies in affective disorder implicate functional changes in anterior cingulate activity. At the time of writing, Drevets and colleagues (Drevets et al 1997) have described both structural and functional abnormalities in anterior cingulate and associated prefrontal cortex in mood disorders. Using PET and MRI, they report both decreased activity and a reduction in cortical volume of the left subgenual prefrontal cortex (curving forward under the anterior edge of the corpus callosum) in depressed patients with a history of bipolar or unipolar affective disorder. While the structural abnormality does not change with the phase of the illness, a small group of bipolar patients studied during the manic phase showed increased cerebral metabolism in the same region, implying a mood-state-dependent change in activity in the affected area.

The hippocampal formation

The hippocampus and related structures are known collectively as the hippocampal formation (fancifully compared in shape to a seahorse = hippocampus). The structures are bilateral. The formation comprises the subiculum, hippocampus proper (sometimes called Ammon's horn – cornu Ammonis) and the dentate gyrus. Together, they represent a fold of three-layered evolutionarily ancient cortex which projects into the floor of the lateral ventricle in each hemisphere. The three layers are designated in terms of their cellular characteristics, with an inner polymorphic cell layer, a prominent pyramidal cell layer in the middle, and an outer molecular layer, consisting of fine nerve fibres and small neurones, which is continuous with the outermost layer of neocortex. The pyramidal cells of the hippocampus proper are replaced by smaller granule cells in the transition to the dentate gyrus. The formation is continuous with the six-layered entorhinal neocortex, the transition from six to three layers occurring at the subiculum. The entorhinal cortex merges with perirhinal cortex anteriorly and forms part of the parahippocampal gyrus posteriorly. These cortical areas merge laterally with the cortex of the inferior edge of the temporal lobe, and medially meet the subiculum and dentate gyrus where the fold of cortex turns in on itself.

The hippocampal formation and associated entorhinal cortex occupies an important nodal point in the processing of polysensory information. As a result, the structure has been very intensively investigated. The formation has reciprocal connections via the entorhinal cortex, with polysensory associational neocortical regions in the frontal, temporal and parietal lobes and the paralimbic cortex of the cingulate gyrus and prefrontal cortex (see above). Highly processed information is thus passed to entorhinal cortex, from there to the hippocampus proper, and then back to cortex. Information is passed around a circuit or loop within the hippocampus prior to projection back to cortical areas. This internal circuit starts in the dentate gyrus, where projections from the entorhinal cortex synapse on granule cells. These in turn project in series to subdivisions within the hippocampus, distinguished by their cytoarchitectural features. The granule cells of the dentate gyrus project to the pyramidal cells of area CA3 (cornu Ammonis), which themselves project in turn to pyramidal cells in area CA1. The axons of the CA1 cells then project to the subiculum, which projects back to the entorhinal cortex, completing the loop. This circuit (dentate–CA3–CA1–subiculum) is known as the trisynaptic loop. Damage to any component within the circuit essentially disables the entire loop. The hippocampus has a lamellar organisation, with the lamellae in transverse orientation to the long axis of the structure. Each lamella contains a complete hippocampal circuit loop, an arrangement which is exploited in the study of hippocampal function.

Individual living lamellar slices can be isolated after dissection of the hippocampus from experimental animals, and the trisynaptic loop examined electophysiologically in vitro.

Significant output from the hippocampus and subiculum is also carried via a structure known as the fornix. Axons arising from the pyramidal and polymorphic cell layers stream together on the ventricular surface of each hippocampus (forming the alveus), developing into increasingly substantial tracts (the fimbriae) as fibres accumulate together posteriorly. The fimbriae continue from each hippocampal formation as the crura of the fornix, merging together as the body of the fornix which loops up and anteriorly over the thalamus and underneath the corpus callosum, to curve down and largely (mainly subicular output) terminate in the mamillary bodies of the hypothalamus (see below). Though predominantly an output pathway, the fornix also carries cholinergic connections from the septal area back to the hippocampus. The fornix link between hippocampus and hypothalamus is a prominent component of Papez's original circuit.

Further inputs from locus coeruleus (noradrenergic system) and the raphe nuclei (serotonergic system) modulate hippocampal activity. The hippocampal formation also communicates extensively with the amygdala, with principal projections from the lateral and basal nuclei of the amygdala (both via entorhinal cortex and directly to the hippocampus proper). Reciprocal projections from the hippocampus back to the amygdala appear to be more rare, though the basal nucleus of the amygdala receives input from CA1, the subiculum and entorhinal cortex.

From a functional point of view, the hippocampus has been most extensively implicated in memory function. Though entorhinal cortex and other medial temporal lobe structures degenerate early and extensively in Alzheimer's disease, accounting for the prominent memory impairment which characterises the disorder, specific evidence for the role of the hippocampal formation in memory function comes from the neuropathology of a more rare and circumscribed disorder of memory, the amnesic syndrome. The syndrome is characterised by an anterograde memory impairment of varying severity (an inability to learn and remember new material), usually accompanied by a variable degree of retrograde amnesia (failure to recall events occurring prior to the onset of amnesia), in the setting of a clear sensorium with preserved intellectual and language function. In contrast to the anterograde amnesia, certain forms of learning remain conspicuously intact, and this apparent dissociation between spared and impaired learning capacities has proved of particular interest in the development of current concepts of the

neurobiology of memory, in implying the existence of at least two (and perhaps multiple) memory systems.

The amnesic syndrome may occur for a variety of reasons. Herpes simplex encephalitis, for example, is a rare but severe form of acute necrotising encephalitis which shows a predilection for medial temporal lobe structures. Postmortem and radiological studies reveal extensive lesions in hippocampus, amygdala and uncus, while diencephalic structures are left intact (Parkin 1987). Such patients therefore share similar pathology to those unfortunate enough to have undergone bilateral temporal lobe surgery, described above. Scoville & Milner's (1957) post-temporal lobectomy series suggested, following analysis of operative procedures, that all amnesic subjects had both hippocampus and amygdala removed. However, there is evidence that amygdalectomy alone does not cause amnesia (Parkin 1987), while the amnesic case R.B., described by Zola-Morgan et al (1986), was shown to have damage restricted to a bilateral lesion of the CA1 cell field of the hippocampus (demonstrated by an extensive postmortem neuropathological survey – the lesion in this case was caused by an ischaemic episode). Unfortunately, the study of brain damage leading to human amnesia in an effort to elucidate the biology of memory will always be hampered by the vagaries of 'uncontrolled' illness, varieties of clinical presentation and deficits additional to postulated 'core' or 'critical' damage. Animal models of the amnesic syndrome have permitted some of these difficulties to be overcome.

Efforts to produce a non-human analogue of amnesia have been dominated by two important considerations: the kinds of test required to demonstrate impaired learning and memory in animals; and the nature of brain damage required to produce such deficits. While early attempts to localise memory function in animals were unsuccessful, later studies consistently demonstrated, initially in primates and later in other mammals, that specific cortical damage could cause deficiencies in the acquisition and performance of discrimination tasks. Such tasks involved the discrimination of simultaneously presented cues, one of which was consistently associated with reward. Lesions were initially made in the inferotemporal cortex (non-primary, visual association areas), and the deficit produced was specific to visual discrimination learning. Subsequent studies demonstrated analogous isolated deficits in tactile and auditory modalities, placing lesions in the relevant cortical association areas. Control tasks used in these studies demonstrated that the deficits were associative in nature, and not due to impaired sensory or motor function. While the studies generally supported the principle that specific brain areas might subserve aspects of learning and memory, the findings did not mirror the pattern of global, multisensory deficit seen in human amnesia. Efforts to produce a global amnesia in primates and lower mammals, by destroying the limbic areas to which the cortical association areas project (and which are damaged in some amnesic humans), were initially disappointing, as the kinds of discriminative tasks used were largely, although not entirely, unaffected.

Significant progress was made, however, following the development of new types of memory task. These new tasks, initially developed by Gaffan (1974), differed from the earlier tasks in employing trial-unique visual stimuli, necessitating single-trial acquisition of information. A version of this new class of task, 'delayed non-match to sample' (DNMS), was found to be sensitive to limbic lesions (Mishkin 1978). The task consists of two phases. In the first ('sample') phase, the monkey is presented with a distinctive object, under which it finds a reward. The object is then removed and, after a variable interval, the second phase ('choice') begins. The animal is now confronted with two objects, one of them the object seen earlier, the other an unfamiliar object. The food is now concealed under the new object and the monkey must choose to displace it rather than the familiar object to obtain reward. Each trial makes use of a new pair of objects, such that the information needed to perform successfully changes from trial to trial, with none of the cues repeatedly associated with reward.

Normal monkeys performed the task with greater than 90% accuracy over an interval of 1–2 minutes between the sample and non-match phases of the trial, while animals with combined amygdalohippocampal lesions performed almost at chance. Importantly, however, the impairment does not occur in lesioned animals when the delay between sample and non-match phases is short (less than 20 seconds), indicating not only that sensory and motor systems are intact but also that the 'rule' of choosing the unfamiliar object is successfully learned and remembered. The effects of limbic damage on this task (Mishkin 1978) are not restricted to the visual modality. Similar impairments have been observed in tactile versions of the task (Murray & Mishkin 1984), suggesting that the learning deficit is global. In sharp contrast, and in confirmation of the earlier work discussed above, repeated-trial visual discrimination learning (where cues are repeatedly presented and consistently associated with reward) is largely unimpaired in lesioned monkeys, even at long delays between individual trials.

In interpreting these findings, Mishkin and his colleagues (1984) have proposed the operation of two learning systems, only one of which is impaired by limbic lesions. The impaired system is considered to subserve both recognition memory (as measured by the DNMS task) and associative recall (for example, one-trial object–reward association). The spared system is viewed as 'involving the gradual development of a connection between an unconditioned stimulus object and an approach response, as an automatic consequence of reinforcement by food' (Mishkin et al 1984). Mishkin designated this particular capacity as 'habit formation', which he described as a 'non-cognitive' form of learning operating independently of limbic structures and therefore unaffected by limbic lesions. Contemporary formulations draw an analogy between explicit memory in humans and the function impaired by limbic lesions in the DNMS task in monkeys.

The nature of the critical limbic lesion has, however, been disputed. In Mishkin's (1978) original report, combined bilateral damage to both the amygdala and hippocampus was required to produce a severe delay-dependent deficit in the DNMS task, the degree of impairment being significantly greater than that produced by damage to either structure alone. This result was taken to indicate that circuits through both the hippocampus and amygdala contribute to those aspects of recognition memory which are assessed by the DNMS task. However, in the creation of the combined hippocampus and amygdala lesion, periallocortex ventrally adjacent to both structures was removed. Interpretation of the experiment was therefore confounded by damage to additional tissue.

In an effort to determine the relative contributions of these various structures to the memory impairment, Murray & Mishkin (1986) compared the effects of damage to the cortical tissue subjacent to both hippocampus and amygdala combined with either bilateral hippocampal lesions or bilateral amygdala lesions. They found impairment after both lesion combinations, with greater impairment seen in the condition involving the amygdala. The finding was taken to support the notion that damage to both amygdala and hippocampus was necessary, given that removal of the cortical tissue in the condition involving the amygdala would have effectively deafferented the hippocampus.

Zola-Morgan and his colleagues have conducted a series of studies examining the performance of monkeys with a variety of more selective lesions on the DNMS task (reviewed by Zola-Morgan et al 1991). They developed a useful notation to indicate the nature of the various lesions: 'H' refers to the hippocampus, 'A' to the amygdala, and the optional suffix '+' to adjacent cortical damage, such that Mishkin's original combined lesion would be designated 'H+A+'. The lesion 'H+' includes, for example, the hippocampal formation and much of the parahippocampal gyrus but excludes the most anterior portions of the entorhinal cortex. This lesion caused a significant delay-dependent impairment on the DMNS task, but less severe than that seen with the 'H+A+' lesion, consistent with Murray & Mishkin's (1986) result. The 'A' lesion constitutes a lesion of the amygdaloid complex, sparing the surrounding cortex (periamygdaloid, entorhinal and perirhinal cortices), while the 'A+' lesion includes all of these structures. Monkeys with the selective 'A' lesion performed normally on the DNMS task, while monkeys with the 'H+A' lesion were significantly impaired, but no more so than monkeys with the 'H+' lesion alone. Further studies examining the effects of lesions restricted to perirhinal ('PR') cortex and perihippocampal ('PH') gyrus alone resulted in performance deficits apparently as severe as those seen in the 'H+A+' lesion, but could not be directly compared as the monkeys required a modification of the DMNS procedure in which the sample stimulus was presented twice in succession prior to the choice phase of the trial. The same subjects performed normally in pattern discrimination. Taking these findings together, Zola-Morgan and his colleagues suggest that the deficit seen following the 'H+A' lesion results from damage to the hippocampal formation and related cortex, rather than to the hippocampus and amygdala as proposed by Mishkin's group. Furthermore, because the 'PRPH' lesion may cause a greater deficit than the 'H+' lesion, Zola-Morgan has concluded that the impairment cannot simply represent a hippocampal disconnection phenomenon, and suggests that these cortical areas are implicated in aspects of normal memory function in their own right (Zola-Morgan et al 1991).

It should be noted that diencephalic limbic structures are also implicated in memory function. The most common form of human amnesia is seen in the Wernicke–Korsakoff syndrome, most frequently a sequel to chronic alcoholism, though the syndrome may result from any situation in which thiamine deficiency occurs, such as chronic malnutrition or malabsorption. Neuropathological surveys of such subjects consistently reveal damage to diencephalic structures, particularly the dorsomedial nucleus of the thalamus and the mamillary bodies, rather than temporal lobe structures such as the hippocampal formation and amygdala. There is disagreement as to which of these structures is critical to the disorder of memory function. Victor and colleagues (1971) suggest that the most consistent factor is disorganisation of the dorsomedial nucleus of the thalamus. On the other hand, Kahn & Crosby (1972, in a review by Parkin 1987) describe two patients rendered amnesic following tumour resection largely restricted to the region of the mamillary bodies, while Squire & Moore (1979) detail the amnesic effects of a stab wound destroying (as far as can be determined on the basis of radiological evidence) the left dorsomedial nucleus of the thalamus in

the patient N.A. (More recent functional imaging studies suggest, however, that N.A. may have had additional temporal lobe dysfunction).

Although superficially similar, the neuropsychological consequences of medial temporal and diencephalic damage have been suggested to differ in detail (Parkin 1987). This is likely to be due, in part, to the variable sequelae of additional damage incurred dependent upon precise aetiology. In herpes simplex encephalitis, for example, damage can be so extensive that the Klüver–Bucy syndrome supervenes – deficits never seen after diencephalic damage. Similarly, patients suffering from the Wernicke–Korsakoff syndrome following prolonged alcohol abuse are frequently found to have widespread cortical atrophy (presumably as a consequence of the toxic effects of prolonged alcohol consumption, and not specific to the Wernicke–Korsakoff syndrome) and occasionally evidence of repeated head injury, these factors conspiring to extend neuropsychological deficits beyond the 'core' amnesic syndrome and exaggerating perceived neuropsychological differences between diencephalic and medial temporal syndromes. In particular, deficits on frontal tasks are frequently reported in Korsakoff patients. Despite these potential confounds, there is some evidence that differences exist. Parkin (1987) reviews a series of studies bearing on this issue and draws particular attention to the fact that patients with diencephalic amnesia often have a less well circumscribed retrograde amnesia, and that temporal lobe amnesics may forget new information more rapidly than diencephalic amnesics. Squire (1986) reviews studies showing cognitive deficits in Korsakoff patients rarely found in bitemporal amnesics (such as impaired 'metamemory skills', failure to release from proactive interference, disproportionately large impairments of judgement of temporal order, and 'source' amnesia) which do not correlate with the degree of anterograde amnesia, and are therefore perhaps unrelated to the 'core' amnesic syndrome. These differences may reflect different aspects of cognitive function processed by separate limbic circuit components.

Studies of the internal physiology of the hippocampus in both whole animals and isolated slices have provided clues as to how the hippocampus may form memories. An electrophysiological phenomenon known as long-term potentiation (LTP) – the ability of neurones to change their strength of connection with one another – is readily demonstrated in the hippocampus. The changes in connection strength occur rapidly and are long lasting – important properties for a candidate memory mechanism. The process is mediated by a subclass of excitatory amino acid receptor, the NMDA receptor complex, which (though distributed throughout the brain) is found in greatest density in the hippocampus. Pharmacological blockade of the receptor, or genetic manipulation using knockout techniques (Morris & Morris 1997), results in memory impairment in rats and mice.

Morphological studies of the hippocampus implicate the structure in schizophrenic disorder. Quantitative in vivo structural imaging techniques, such as MRI, demonstrate significant reductions in medial temporal lobe grey matter, most pronounced in amygdala and anterior hippocampus (reviewed by Roberts 1991). Neurohistological studies conducted post mortem suggest that pyramidal cell number (Falkai & Bogerts 1986) and orientation (Kovelman & Schiebel 1984) may be abnormal in the hippocampus of some schizophrenic subjects. Though such studies require replication, they imply a neurodevelopmental pathology in schizophrenia, and may account for some of the neuropsychological abnormalities observed.

The hypothalamus

The hypothalamus has been considered a way station between the cognitive and the visceral, communicating on the one hand with higher structures such as the thalamus and limbic cortex, and on the other with the ascending fibre systems from the brainstem and spinal cord. It represents a major centre for control of the autonomic nervous system, and responds not only to neural information but also to chemical information in the circulating blood. The hypothalamus is a bilateral structure, bounding the third ventricle on each side, below the thalamus. It extends posteriorly to the mamillary bodies and anteriorly to the optic chiasm. Below, attached by the stalk of the infundibulum, is the pituitary gland. The hypothalamus consists of a number of important nuclei with diverse functions related to the maintenance of homeostasis, such as the regulation of food and water intake, and plays an important role in sleep, and sexual and defensive function. The hypothalamic–pituitary–adrenal axis, controlling corticosteroid activity, plays an important role in affective disorder. Neuroendocrine function is described in more detail in Chapter 14.

The passage of the fornix to the mamillary bodies divides the hypothalamus into medial and lateral sections. The lateral region consists mainly of lateral hypothalamic nucleus and fibre tracts, including the medial forebrain bundle carrying, amongst others, monoaminergic pathways from brainstem nuclei to neocortex. The medial component contains several well-defined nuclei, including the supraoptic and paraventricular nuclei in the anterior portion, which produce the neurohormones vasopressin and oxytocin.

The hypothalamus has long been believed to play an important role in basic emotional expression. Primitive rage responses appear to be coordinated by the hypothalamus: stimulation of the lateral hypothalamus in cats results in reactions analogous to anger, while lesions of region render animals placid and poorly responsive to threatening stimuli. Decortication has similar effects to stimulation, resulting in non-specific, non-directed, but coordinated defensive responses, described as sham rage by Walter Cannon in his studies conducted in the 1920s. If decortication is combined with hypothalamic damage, sham rage does not occur. These early findings led to the idea that higher structures, and input from higher limbic structures in particular, provided the analytical, directive components of emotional reactions and inspired the speculations of Papez, McLean and later theorists. Extensive projections from the amygdala to the hypothalamus (via the stria terminalis and the ventral amygdalofugal pathway), and from the hippocampus via the fornix, convey descending neocortical influence; while connections from the hypothalamus to prefrontal cortex and from mamillary bodies via the anterior thalamic nucleus to the cingulate gyrus complete McLean's modified view of the Papez circuit.

More selective, chemical stimulation and lesion techniques are refining understanding of the role of the hypothalamus as an emotional output station. Using microinjection of excitatory amino acids to destroy cells bodies, but to spare fibres of passage, it is becoming clearer that older, less specific electrical stimulation or more extensive mechanical destruction has produced some misleading findings. Effects ascribed to damage to, or stimulation of, the hypothalamus itself may be due instead to the interruption or stimulation of fibres passing through the structure. Contemporary findings emphasise the involvement of projections from the amygdaloid complex (see below) through the hypothalamic area to other brain regions (such as the central grey region) in defensive behaviours, though autonomic responses to threatening situations do indeed appear to be mediated by the hypothalamus itself (reviewed by LeDoux 1996).

The amygdaloid complex

The amygdaloid complex is an almond-shaped (L. *amygdala*, almond) collection of subcortical nuclei which lie in the anterior pole of each temporal lobe, above the tip of the inferior horn of the lateral ventricle. The anatomy of the AC is indeed complicated: the various nuclei and areas are a heterogeneous group, each distinguished by specific cytoarchitectural, histochemical and internal and external connectivity features. Classification of the various elements has become increasingly sophisticated: contemporary surveys (for example, Amaral et al 1992) recognise at least 12 major subdivisions comprising nuclear and cortical structures. There are three main groups: the deep nuclei (including lateral and basal nuclei); superficial nuclei and areas, including cortical elements (such as the periamygdaloid cortex); and the central nucleus. The lateral nucleus is an important input station in the amygdala, while the central nucleus has output functions.

The amygdaloid complex has widespread interconnection with subcortical and cortical areas. Subcortical projections range across autonomic and visceral centres in the diencephalon and brainstem, while there are numerous reciprocal neocortical–amygdaloid connections via the external capsule.

Two major extrinsic fibre systems project from the central nucleus of the amygdala to the hypothalamus and the dorsomedial nucleus of the thalamus (the stria terminalis and ventral amygdalofugal pathway respectively). The deep nuclei have important projections to the nucleus accumbens and striatum proper; and both superficial and deep nuclei have interconnections with the hippocampal formation, directly with the hippocampal subfields (CA1 and CA3) and also via the entorhinal cortex and subiculum. Neocortical areas have an extensive reciprocal connection with the amygdaloid complex: the superficial nuclei receive higher order uni- and polymodal sensory information from widespread cortical areas, in addition to input from prefrontal and cingulate paralimbic cortex. The amygdaloid complex in turn projects back even more widely to cortical areas, including, for example, those subserving the very early stages of visual processing in the occipital lobe. The cells in the amygdaloid complex receiving information from the cortex are not the same cells that project back: the amygdala therefore appears to take part in a processing loop, receiving highly processed sensory information, performing further computation, and then modulating the earlier stages of cortical sensory input.

This brief anatomical overview clearly indicates that the amygdaloid complex must play an important role in cognitive and emotional function. It has been known since the late 19th century that bilateral damage to the anterior portion of the temporal lobes, including the amygdala, results in gross behavioural (emotional, cognitive and perceptual) abnormalities. This syndrome was formally described by Klüver and Bucy in monkeys in 1937. It now bears their names, and consists of visual agnosia (inability to recognise objects by sight: psychic blindness); strong oral tendencies (the inappropriate oral investigation of objects); loss of fear and aggressiveness; and hypersexual and misdirected sexual behaviour). Aspects of the syndrome have been described following a variety of neurological disorders affecting the temporal lobes in humans (e.g. meningitis, temporal lobe surgery).

Subsequent, more refined neurobiological investigations in non-human primates indicated that damage to the amygdala was critical to the development of the syndrome (for example, Weiskrantz, 1956), though temporal cortical lesions are also necessary. A remarkable experiment conducted by Downer (1961) clarified the role of the amygdala in processing emotional features in visual input. He restricted input from each eye to its ipsilateral hemisphere (by division of the optic chiasm and forebrain commissures) in monkeys with unilateral amygdala damage. In this way, one eye projected exclusively to its ipsilateral hemisphere with an intact contribution from the amygdala to visual processing; while the other eye projected exclusively to the other hemisphere without amygdala input. Threatening stimuli presented to the intact system elicited normal fearful and defensive reactions, while the same stimuli presented to the other eye, though detected, did not elicit an emotional response. The idea that the amygdala contributes to the processing of the emotional significance of sensory input thus developed, and begins to explain aspects of the Klüver–Bucy syndrome – such as lack of fearfulness.

Recent studies indicate that the amygdala makes important and specific contributions to fear responses and anxiety. Joseph LeDoux and his colleagues (reviewed, LeDoux 1996) have examined the role of the amygdala in fear conditioning in rats, in which formerly neutral stimuli come to evoke fear responses (such as 'freezing' in rats) after repeated pairing with aversive events. Using a combination of anatomical, lesion and physiological techniques, they have tracked the processing of auditory stimuli in the development of fear conditioning from the earliest stages of auditory input in the brainstem, via the amygdala, through to the initiation of fearful motor responses. There are at least two pathways to the amygdala. There is a relatively direct route from the auditory thalamic relay (medial geniculate nucleus) to the lateral nucleus of the amygdala which bypasses primary auditory cortex, and a longer route via auditory cortex to the lateral nucleus. Simple auditory stimuli paired with aversive experience can thus be rapidly processed and associated, while more complex stimulus discrimination may require the contribution of the cortical route. LeDoux (1996) has suggested that the direct pathway provides a fast rough representation of threatening stimuli, which may prepare the amygdala to receive and evaluate more detailed information from the cortex. The central nucleus of the amygdala then orchestrates motor responses to the conditioned stimulus, activating autonomic systems via the lateral hypothalamus, and fear responses via the central grey matter.

Using a rather different experimental paradigm, Michael Davis and his colleagues (Davis et al 1987) have studied the role of the amygdala in the development of the increased startle response in rats which occurs in the presence of cues previously associated with aversive events. They suggest that the amygdala represents a critical integrative brain site where neural activity produced by conditioned and unconditioned stimuli converge, and is essential for the expression of the startle response via connections with the brainstem nuclei which mediate startle. Interestingly, there is evidence that NMDA receptor-mediated synaptic plasticity (encountered above in the hippocampus) is essential for the acquisition of the startle response, though not for its expression once acquired (Miserendino et al 1990).

These findings in rats relating to aversive experiences may shed light on the neural basis of human anxiety disorders. There is also a body of evidence implicating amygdala function in reactions to rewarding stimuli, which may in turn relate to the neural substrates of affective disorder. Such studies (for example, Everitt & Robbins 1992) emphasise projections from the basolateral amygdala to the ventral striatum – and the nucleus accumbens in particular – in the expression of voluntary responses to reward. The nucleus accumbens has been considered a 'limbic–motor' interface, modulated by dopaminergic input from the ventral tegmental area (see below). Electrical stimulation of such brain areas is innately rewarding, and they may play an important role in the appreciation and expression of hedonic tone in concert with the amygdala. Amygdalostriatal interactions may thus represent an alternative limbic output pathway, operating in parallel with amygdala–hypothalamic pathways, but more concerned with voluntary aspects of emotional response (Everitt 1997) rather than the reflexive fear responses discussed above.

The amygdaloid complex has also been specifically implicated in explicit memory function. Though the relative contributions of amygdala and hippocampus have been much debated, as we have seen, they may in fact make independent contributions to different aspects of memory. For example, amygdala, but not hippocampal lesions have been shown to impair a cross-modal DNMS task (Murray & Mishkin 1985). In the sample phase of this task, cues are presented in the tactile modality (by presenting the cues in the dark), but in the choice phase the same cues are presented in the visual modality. The monkey must therefore use information gained via touch in the recognition of a visually presented object in order to perform successfully. This impairment of cross-modal association may

explain elements of the visual and oral abnormalities observed in the Klüver–Bucy syndrome. Conversely, the hippocampus plays an important role in tasks requiring the use of spatial information, but the amygdala does not. Monkeys trained preoperatively to associate objects with locations performed at near chance levels following hippocampectomy, while their amygdalectomised counterparts performed as well as they had on the task prior to surgery (Parkinson et al 1988).

The amygdala is also thought to play a crucial role in social behaviour in primates (Kling & Brothers 1992, Brothers 1996). Single-unit recordings from the amygdala of monkeys indicate that specific neural responses are tuned to individual social stimuli, such as faces and their expressions, aversive and arousing events and so on. Direct stimulation of the amygdala in monkeys results in patterned social displays, and in humans may elicit subjective feelings of fear or pleasure. It seems likely that the amygdala subserves aspects of the reception of, and response to social signals. Recent PET studies in humans indicate that neural responses in the amygdala may be modulated by photographs showing varied intensities of emotional facial expressions, such as happiness and fearfulness (Morris et al 1996). Given the implication that the amygdala is involved in the 'neural representations of the dispositions and intentions of others' (Kling & Brothers 1992), it is hardly surprising that dysfunction of the amygdala has been implicated in schizophrenic disorder, particularly paranoid states.

Summary

Put crudely, the various components of the limbic system can be thought of as working together to generate important elements of the emotional and cognitive basis of everyday normal mental life: memories, fears, hopes and feelings. The hippocampal formation appears to produce explicit records of events, the amygdala provides emotional tone and responses, the hypothalamus directs neuroendocrine and autonomic output, while the frontal lobes monitor, control and plan activities on a moment by moment basis. Clearly, an evolving understanding of the detailed functions of limbic structures promises a rich and sophisticated scientific psychopathology (see Andreasen (1997) for a recent synthesis).

CHEMICAL NEUROANATOMY

In understanding brain–behaviour relationships, we are only beginning to grasp the complexities of the pattern of neurochemical brain function. The notion that there may be a simple relationship between single neurotransmitter systems and psychiatric disorders, by analogy with the relatively successful analysis of Parkinson's disease, is likely to be overoptimistic. This is exemplified by the increasing uncertainties surrounding the dopamine hypothesis of schizophrenia. In developing comprehensive theories or descriptions of the biological basis of normal brain function and dysfunction, a number of conceptual dimensions or levels must be considered and eventually synthesised. These range from the analysis of molecular aspects of receptor function, through patterns of synaptic connectivity and computational aspects of information processing, to functional macroanatomy and ultimately neuropsychology. A crucial piece of this jigsaw lies in the anatomy of neurotransmitter systems. The range and specific functional properties of neurotransmitters and modulators are considered in Chapter 3. Here, we provide a brief survey of the anatomy of classical neurotransmitter systems of special relevance to psychiatric disorder: dopaminergic (DA), noradrenergic (NA), serotonergic (5-HT, 5-hydroxytryptamine) and cholinergic (ACh, acetylcholine) systems. It is important to be aware that, despite their prominence in the psychiatric literature, these 'classical' systems account for only a fraction of the synaptic activity in the brain: most of the work is done by the amino acids glutamate and GABA, to say nothing of the efforts of a bewildering array of other transmitters and neuromodulators.

In anatomical overview, each 'classical' system consists of defined nuclei or groups of cell bodies – mostly in the brainstem – with associated projection targets throughout the central nervous system. For monoamine-containing systems, the cell body group designations in the brainstem follow the convention established by Dahlström & Fuxe, 1964 (for example, A1–A15 for catecholamine containing neurones; B1–B9 for serotonergic neurones).

Anatomy of the dopamine neurones

Groups of dopamine-containing neurones have been described and classified anatomically in a number of ways: in terms of distinct cell body groups (designated A8–A17); in terms of their efferent projection length characteristics (ultrashort, intermediate and long – Cooper et al 1996) and in terms of the course of their projections through the brain (e.g. mesolimbic, nigrostriatal).

Cellular groups A16 and A17 represent 'ultrashort' projection systems found in the olfactory bulb and retina respectively. These dopamine-containing cells act as intrinsic neurones (hence the designation 'ultrashort') in both olfactory bulb and retina. They thus form part

of the networks of neurones involved in initial sensory processing. In the retina, for example, the cells represent a subclass of amacrine cell, a cell type we encountered when considering visual processing above. It is conceivable that dopamine deficiencies in the retina and olfactory bulb account for some of the visual and olfactory abnormalities encountered in Parkinson's disease.

The cell bodies of the 'intermediate length' projection systems (A11–A15) lie in the diencephalon. The majority of axons from this group remain within the diencephalic region (hence 'intermediate length': an exception is the efferent fibres from A11 to the spinal cord). Principal cell groups include the ventromedial and arcuate hypothalamic nuclei (sometimes termed the tuberohypophyseal cells) projecting to the intermediate lobe of the pituitary and the median eminence; and the incertohypothalamic neurones which bridge dorsal posterior and anterior hypothalamus. Prolactin release from the anterior pituitary is inhibited by dopamine release from hypothalamic dopaminergic neurones: blockade of postsynaptic dopamine receptors here by antipsychotics raises serum prolactin levels, which may result in such adverse effects as breast enlargement, galactorrhoea and amenorrhoea.

Dopamine cell bodies located in the mesencephalon constitute the 'long length' projection system. Three cell groups are recognised: A8 (the retrorubral nucleus); A9 (the pars compacta of the substantia nigra); and A10 (the ventral tegmental area). The projections from these cells make up three important 'long' dopaminergic tracts: the nigrostriatal pathway; the mesolimbic pathway; and the mesocortical pathway. The relationship between cell body group and tract is not straightforward, with cell groups contributing heterogeneously to the main projections. There is however a degree of topographic organisation, such that adjacent cell bodies tend to project to adjacent target sites.

The nigrostriatal tract, mainly carrying fibres from the A8 and A9 groups, projects to the caudate and putamen of the neostriatum and plays a major role in motor control. Parkinson's disease results from a loss of dopaminergic cells from substantia nigra, with a consequent reduction in striatal dopamine – though dopaminergic projection loss in the condition is not exclusive to the nigrostriatal tract. Neuroleptic induced pseudoparkinsonism and other adverse motor effects of antipsychotic drugs are mediated by effects on this system.

The mesolimbic and mesocortical projections arise from all three mesencephalic cell groups, with a principal contribution from A10 neurones. Limbic projection targets include the nucleus accumbens, the central nucleus of the amygdala and the hippocampus. Cortical targets include the medial prefrontal and anterior cingulate cortices, and the piriform and entorhinal cortices. Frontal activation abnormalities observed in schizophrenia may partly be mediated by dysfunction in the mesocortical dopamine system, while projections from the ventral tegmental area to the nucleus accumbens – increasingly implicated in rewarded behaviour – may play an important role in affective disorder.

The mesencephalic dopaminergic systems are functionally heterogeneous, with electrophysiological, biochemical and metabolic factors distinguishing the mesocortical, mesolimbic and nigrostriatal projections. Indeed, functional differences are described even between mesoprefrontal and mesocingulate systems. Differing dopaminergic system responses to classical and atypical neuroleptics may explain the variations in side-effect profile and efficacy observed amongst these drugs (Cooper et al 1996). It is likely that continuing study of such heterogeneity will prove a potent stimulus to the development of safer and perhaps more effective antipsychotic agents.

Anatomy of the noradrenergic neurones

The cell bodies of the noradrenergic neurones lie in the lower brainstem, designated A1 to A7. They form two main cell groups: a rostral group at the level of the pons known as the locus coeruleus (A6 – LC) forming a prominent dark patch in the floor of the fourth ventricle; and a diffusely scattered medullary/medullopontine group found more caudally throughout the ventral lateral tegmentum. The LC itself contains 50% of the central noradrenergic neurones.

Though major input to the central noradrenergic system is highly restricted, both groups of neurones have very widespread efferent ascending projections to higher centres, in addition to descending projections to the spinal cord.

The ascending LC neurones (sometimes called the dorsal noradrenergic bundle) project widely to midbrain structures, the thalamus, limbic system and branch diffusely throughout the entire cortex. A further projection innervates cerebellar cortex. The descending projections course down through the mesencephalon, sending collaterals to motor nuclei in the brainstem, and then into the spinal cord (the coerulospinal pathway), innervating the ventral horn and basal part of the dorsal horn. Ascending projections from the diffuse tegmental cells (the ventral noradrenergic bundle) innervate brainstem, hypothalamic and some limbic cortical targets. Descending projections terminate in the grey matter of the spinal cord. In overview, though there is a degree of overlap, LC neurones contribute the main noradrenergic input to cortex, while the tegmental group provide principal noradrenergic innervation to the brainstem and spinal cord.

LC neurones appear to play a role in the detection of suddenly changing or aversive sensory input. In such circumstances, the neurones increase activity in a rapid and coordinated way (Role & Kelly 1991), and abnormalities in central noradrenergic systems may play an important role in anxiety disorders (Brawman-Mintzer & Lydiard, 1997). LC neurones respond in a similar way to novel sensory input. This in turn appears to increase cell excitability in subfields of the hippocampus via limbic noradrenergic projections, and may thus influence memory processing (Kitchigina et al 1997).

Anatomy of the serotonergic neurones

The cell bodies of serotonergic neurones are also found in the brainstem (cell groups B1 to B9). They constitute the most extensive monoaminergic system, with larger cell numbers than either noradrenergic or dopaminergic systems. The most caudal cell groups (B1–B4) have descending projections to the spinal cord, where they modulate spinal sensory and motor neurones. There are small, separate projections of serotonergic cell groups to the cerebellum and the LC. The raphe nuclei of the midbrain and pons (B7 and B8) play an important role in psychiatric neurobiology. The two main nuclei, the dorsal raphe nucleus (DRN) and median raphe nucleus (MRN) have ascending projections to striatum, limbic system and cortex. The DRN is found at a similar level in the brainstem to the dopamine-containing neurones of the ventral tegmental area, and has similar projection targets: the basal ganglia, nucleus accumbens, amygdala, and frontal cortex; while the MRN is located near the LC, with projection targets in thalamus, anterior temporal neocortex and hippocampus.

Deakin (1996) has suggested that the MRN and DRN serotonergic systems mediate different coping responses to acute and chronic aversive events, consistent with the long held view that serotonergic systems play an important part in the genesis of depressive disorder. It is proposed that DRN neurones modulate forebrain circuits concerned with evaluative and motor aspects of avoidance behaviour, while MRN neurones modulate sensory and memory processing of aversive events. Dysfunction of these putative normal serotonergic activities is hypothesised to result in depressive disorder, which is in turn corrected by serotonin reuptake inhibition by chemical antidepressants.

Appreciating the anatomical distinction between groups of cell bodies in the brainstem and their distant widespread projection fields is essential in understanding contemporary formulations of the action of serotonin specific reuptake inhibitors (SSRIs). These drugs act at reuptake sites both at cell bodies and terminals, but with different effects over time. It has been suggested that 5-HT_{1A} autoreceptors at the cell body shut down cell firing in the short term, acting against expected increases in synaptic 5-HT in the projection field. Once the cell body autoreceptors desensitise in the face of chronic reuptake blockade, and cell firing increases again, then the effect of reuptake inhibition at the terminals now results in an increase in synaptic 5-HT availability (Goodwin 1996). This may explain the delay in response to antidepressants seen in clinical practice, and informs recent attempts to accelerate antidepressant action using 5-HT_{1A} autoreceptor blockers.

There are morphologically distinct serotonergic axon types: fine axons with small varicosities project from the DRN; while beaded axons, with large spherical varicosities originate in the MRN. While the functional significance of the different types remains speculative (see Deakin 1996), they have a differential sensitivity to the neurotoxic effects of MDMA (ecstasy), such that the fine axons may be permanently damaged (for example, Green et al 1995).

Anatomy of the cholinergic neurones

Central cholinergic neurones fall into two principal groups: those that do not project from the regions in which they are located (i.e. local circuit cells like the ultrashort projection dopaminergic neurones described above); and projection neurones which link different brain regions.

Local circuit cells are represented by the cholinergic interneurones of the caudate and putamen, and those found in the nucleus accumbens and olfactory tubercle.

Projection neurones fall into two main groups of nuclei: a more caudal pontine group (the pontomesencephalotegmental cholinergic complex); and the more rostral basal forebrain cholinergic complex. The pontine group have both ascending projections (to the thalamus, basal ganglia and ventral diencephalic structures) and descending projections to the reticular formation, cerebellar nuclei, vestibular nuclei and cranial nerve nuclei. It is believed that these neurones have a role in arousal processes, amongst other activities.

The basal forebrain cholinergic complex consists of a group of nuclei, including the medial septal nucleus, the diagonal band nucleus, the substantia innominata, the magnocellular preoptic field and the nucleus basalis. Cells from these nuclei have a very widespread projection throughout limbic and neocortical targets.

Cholinergic neurotransmission has long been implicated in memory function in general, and in the pathology of Alzheimer's disease in particular, including the suggestion that there is a specific degeneration of the nucleus basalis. Reductions in concentrations of acetylcholine and choline acetyltransferase (an important enzyme involved in the synthesis of acetylcholine) have been observed at postmortem examination in brains from patients with Alzheimer's disease. However, neurotransmitter deficits in Alzheimer's disease are not restricted to the cholinergic system (Ch. 11) and the notion that the cholinergic system has a specific role in learning and memory has been increasingly challenged. The use of more recently available neurotoxins which selectively destroy cholinergic neurones in studies of animal memory indicate that the nucleus basalis projections are probably more concerned with visual attentional processes (reviewed by Wenk 1997). None the less, there is some evidence that hippocampal cholinergic projections from the medial septal nucleus may be more specifically involved in short-term working memory, while basalis–amygdala projections may influence affective learning. Projections from the diagonal band nuclei to the cingulate cortex may also contribute to learning processes (Everitt & Robbins, 1997).

REFERENCES

Alexander G E, Crutcher M D, DeLong M R 1990 Basal ganglia-thalamocortical circuits: parallel substrates for motor, oculomotor, 'prefrontal' and 'limbic' functions. Progress in Brain Research 85: 119–146

Amaral D G, Price J L, Pitkänen A, Carmichael S T 1992 Anatomical organisation of the primate amygdaloid complex. In: Aggleton J P (ed) The amygdala. Wiley, New York.

Andreasen N C 1997 Linking mind and brain in the study of mental illness: a project for a scientific psychopathology. Science 275: 1586–1593

Baddeley A 1986 Working memory. Oxford University Press, London

Barinaga M 1997 Visual system provides clues to how brain perceives. Science 275: 1583–1585

Baxter L R, Saxena S, Brodie A L et al 1996 Brain mediation of obsessive–compulsive disorder symptoms: evidence from functional brain imaging studies in the human and non-human primate. Seminars in Clinical Neuropsychiatry 1: 32–47

Brawman-Mintzer O, Lydiard R B 1997 Biological basis of generalized anxiety disorder. Journal of Clinical Psychiatry 58 (suppl 3):16–25

Brothers L 1996 Brain mechanisms of social cognition. Journal of Psychopharmacology 10: 2–8

Brown S, Schaefer E A 1888 An investigation into the functions of the occipital and temporal lobe of the monkey's brain. Philosophical Transactions of the Royal Society of London. Series B: Biological Sciences 179: 303–327

Chesselet M-F, Delfs J M 1996 Basal ganglia and movement disorders. Trends in Neurosciences 19: 417–422

Cooper J R, Bloom F E, Roth R H 1996 The biochemical basis of neuropharmacology, 7th edn. Oxford University Press, New York

Corbetta M, Miezin F M, Dobmeyer S, Shulman G L, Petersen S E 1990 Attentional modulation of neural processing of shape, color, and velocity in humans. Science 248: 1556–1559

Corsellis J A N, Janota I 1985 Neuropathology in relation to psychiatry. In: Shepherd M (ed) Handbook of psychiatry. Vol 5: The scientific foundations of psychiatry. Cambridge University Press, Cambridge

Crick F H C 1994 The astonishing hypothesis. Simon & Schuster, London

Dahlström A, Fuxe K 1964 Evidence for the existence of monoamine-containing neurones in the central nervous system. I. Demonstration of monoamines in the cell bodies of the brain stem neurones. Acta Physiologica Scandinavica Suppl 232: 1–55

Damasio A R 1994 Descartes' error: emotion reason and the human brain. Putnam, New York

Davis M, Hitchcock J M, Rosen J B 1987 Anxiety and the amygdala: pharmacological and anatomical analysis of fear potentiated startle. In: Bower G H (ed) The psychology of learning and motivation. Academic Press, San Diego

Deakin J F W 1996 5HT, antidepressant drugs and the psychosocial origins of depression. Journal of Psychopharmacology 10: 31–38

Downer J D C 1961 Changes in visual gnostic function and emotional behaviour following unilateral temporal lobe damage in the 'split-brain' monkey. Nature 191: 50–51

Drevets W C, Price J L, Simpson J R et al 1997 Subgenual prefrontal cortex abnormalities in mood disorder. Nature 386: 824–827

Ebert D, Ebmeier K P 1996 The role of the cingulate gyrus in depression: from functional anatomy to neurochemistry. Biological Psychiatry 39: 1044–1050

Ebmeier K P 1995 Brain imaging and schizophrenia. In: Den Boer J A, Westenberg H G M, van Praag H M (eds) Advances in the neurobiology of schizophrenia. Wiley, Chichester, pp 131–155

Everitt B J 1997 The emotional brain. Trends in Cognitive Sciences 1: 40–41

Everitt B J, Robbins T W 1992 Amygdala–ventral striatal interactions and reward related processes. In: Aggleton J P (ed) The amygdala. Wiley, New York

Everitt B J, Robbins T W 1997 Central cholinergic systems and cognition. Annual Review of Psychology 48: 649–684

Falkai P, Bogerts B 1986 Cell loss in the hippocampus of schizophrenics. European Archives of Psychiatry and Neurological Sciences 236: 154–161

Feger J 1997 Updating the functional model of the basal ganglia. Trends in Neurosciences 20: 152–153

Friston K J 1994 Statistical parametric mapping. In: Thatcher R W, Hallett M, Zeffiro T, John E R, Huerta M (eds), Functional neuroimaging: technical foundations. Academic Press, San Diego, pp 79–93

Gaffan D 1974 Recognition impaired and association intact in the memory of monkeys after transection of the fornix. Journal of Comparative and Physiological Psychology 86: 1100–1109

Goldman-Racic P S 1995 Architecture of the prefrontal cortex and the central executive. Annals of the New York Academy of Sciences 769: 71–84

Goodwin G M 1996 How do antidepressants affect serotonin receptors? The role of serotonin receptors in the therapeutic and side effect profile of the SSRIs. Journal of Clinical Psychiatry 57(suppl 4): 9–13

Grasso M G, Pantano P, Intiso D F et al 1994 Mesial temporal cortex hypoperfusion is associated with depression in subcortical stroke. Stroke 25: 980–985

Green A R, Cross A J, Goodwin G M 1995 Review of the pharmacology and clinical pharmacology of 3,4-methylenedioxymethamphetamine (MDMA or 'ecstasy'). Psychopharmacology 119: 247–260

Hubel D H, Wiesel T N 1979 Brain mechanisms of vision. Scientific American 241: 150–162

Hubel D H, Wiesel T N, Stryker M H 1978 Anatomical demonstration of occular dominance columns in macaque monkey. Journal of Comparative Neurology 177: 361–379

Jacobsen J F 1935 Functions of the frontal association area in primates. Archives of Neurology and Psychiatry 33: 558–569

Kitchigina V, Vankov A, Harley C, Sara S J 1997 Novelty-elicited, noradrenaline-dependent enhancement of excitability in the dentate gyrus. European Journal of Neuroscience 9: 41–47

Kling A S, Brothers L A 1992 The amygdala and social behaviour. In: Aggleton J P (ed) The amygdala. Wiley, New York

Klüver H, Bucy P C 1937 'Psychic blindness' and other symptoms following bilateral temporal lobectomy in rhesus monkeys. American Journal of Physiology 119: 352–353

Kovelman J A, Schiebel A B 1984 A neurohistological correlate of schizophrenia. Biological Psychiatry 191: 1601–1621

LeDoux J 1996 The emotional brain. Simon & Schuster, London

Lund J S 1988 Anatomical organisation of macaque monkey striate visual cortex. Annual Review of Neuroscience 11: 253–288

Macko K A, Jarvis C D, Kennedy C et al 1982 Mapping the primate visual system with [2-^{14}C]deoxyglucose. Science 218: 394–397

McLean P D 1949 Psychosomatic disease and the 'visceral brain'. Recent developments bearing on the Papez theory of emotion. Psychosomatic Medicine 11: 338–353

Martin J H 1996 Neuroanatomy – text and atlas. Prentice-Hall, London.

Miserendino M J D, Sananes C B, Melia K R, Davis M 1990 Blocking of acquisition but not expression of conditioned fear potentiated startle by NMDA antagonists in the amygdala. Nature 345: 716–718

Mishkin M 1978 Memory in monkeys severely impaired by combined but not by separate removal of amygdala and hippocampus. Nature 273: 297–298

Mishkin M, Malamut B, Bechevalier J 1984 Memories and habits: two neural systems. In: Lynch G, Weinberger N M (eds) Neurobiology of learning and memory. Guildford Press, New York

Morris R G M, Morris R J 1997 Memory floxed. Nature 358: 680–681

Morris S, Frith C D, Perrett D I et al 1996 A differential neural response in the human amygdala to fearful and happy facial expressions. Nature 383: 812–815

Murray E A, Mishkin M 1984 Severe tactual as well as visual memory deficits following combined removal of the amygdala and hippocampus in monkeys. Journal of Neuroscience 4: 2565–2580

Murray E A, Mishkin M 1985 Amygdalectomy impairs cross-modal associations in monkeys. Science 228: 604–606

Murray E A, Mishkin M 1986 Visual recognition in monkeys following rhinal cortical ablations combined with either amygdalectomy or hippocampectomy. Journal of Neuroscience 6: 1991–2003

Neary D 1995 Neuropsychological aspects of frontotemporal degeneration. Annals of the New York Academy of Sciences 769: 15–22

Pandya D N, Selzer B 1982 Association areas of cerebral cortex. Trends in Neurosciences 5: 386–390

Papez J W 1937 A proposed mechanism of emotion. Archives of Neurology and Psychiatry 38: 725–743

Parkin A J 1987 Memory and amnesia: an introduction. Blackwell, Oxford

Parkinson J K, Murray E A, Mishkin M 1988 A selective mnemonic role for the hippocampus in monkeys: memory for location of objects. Journal of Neuroscience 8: 4159–4167

Pascual-Leone A, Grafman J, Hallett M 1994 Modulation of cortical motor output maps during development of implicit and explicit knowledge. Science 263: 1287–1289

Penfield W, Rasmussen T 1954 The cerebral cortex of man: a clinical study of localization of function. Macmillan, New York

Petrides M 1995 Functional organisation of the human frontal cortex for mnemonic processing: evidence from neuroimaging studies. Annals of the New York Academy of Sciences 769: 85–96

Phillips C G, Zeki S, Barlow H B 1984 Localisation of function in the cerebral cortex: past, present and future. Brain 107: 327–361

Rao S C, Rainer G, Miller E K 1997 Integration of what and where in the primate prefrontal cortex. Science 276: 821–824

Roberts G W 1991 Temporal lobe pathology and schizophrenia. In: Kerwin R (ed) Neurobiology and psychiatry. Cambridge University Press, Cambridge, vol 1

Role L W, Kelly J P 1991 The brain stem: cranial nerve nuclei and the monoaminergic systems. In: Kandel E R, Schwartz J H, Jessel T M (eds) Principles of neural science, 3rd edn. Elsevier, New York, pp 693–699

Scoville W B, Milner B 1957 Loss of recent memory after bilateral hippocampal lesions. Journal of Neurology, Neurosurgery and Psychiatry 20: 11–21

Shallice T 1982 Specific impairments in planning. Philosophical Transactions of the Royal Society of London. Series B: Biological Sciences 198: 199–209

Squire L R 1986 Mechanisms of memory. Science 232: 1612–1619

Squire L R, Moore R Y 1979 Dorsal thalamic lesion in a noted case of chronic memory dysfunction. Annals of Neurology 6: 503–506

Stuss D T, Shallice T, Alexander M P, Picton T W 1995 A multidisciplinary approach to anterior attentional function. Annals of the New York Academy of Sciences 769: 191–212

Tanaka K 1993 Neuronal mechanisms of object recognition. Science 262: 685–688

Tatemichi T K, Desmond D W, Prohovnik I 1995 Strategic infarcts in vascular dementia – a clinical and brain imaging experience. Arzneimittel-Forschung/Drug Research 45-1: 371–385

Tessier-Lavigne M 1991 Phototransduction and information processing in the retina. In: Kandel E, Schwartz J H, Jessel T M (eds) Principles of neural science, 3rd edn. Elsevier, New York

Victor M, Adams R D, Collins G H 1971 In: Plum F, McDowell F H (eds) The Wernicke–Korsakoff Syndrome. Blackwell, Oxford

Weiskrantz L 1956 Behavioural changes associated with ablation of the amygdaloid complex in monkeys. Journal of Comparative and Physiological Psychology 49: 381–391

Wenk G L 1997 The nucleus basalis magnocellularis cholinergic system: one hundred years of progress. Neurobiology of Learning and Memory 67: 85–95

Wickelgreen I 1997 Getting a grasp on working memory. Science 275: 1580–1582

Wiesel F A, Wik G, Sjögren I, Blomqvist G, Greitz T, Stone-Elander S 1987 Regional brain glucose metabolism in drug free schizophrenic patients and clinical correlates. Acta Psychiatrica Scandinavica 76: 628–641

Wilson M A, Tonegawa S 1997 Synaptic plasticity, place cells and spatial memory: study with second generation knockouts. Trends in Neurosciences 20: 102–106

Zola-Morgan S, Squire L R, Amaral D G 1986 Human amnesia and the medial temporal region: enduring memory impairment following a bilateral lesion limited to field CA1 of the hippocampus. Journal of Neuroscience 6: 2950–2967

Zola-Morgan S, Squire L R, Alvarez-Royo P, Clower R P 1991 Independence of memory functions and emotional behavior: separate contributions of the hippocampal formation and the amygdala. Hippocampus 1: 207–220

3

Neuropharmacology

Gordon Arbuthnott

INTRODUCTION

Neuropharmacological studies contribute extensively to the evaluation of drug treatments in psychiatry and may provide useful insights into the neurobiology of mental illnesses. The fact that mental illnesses cannot be fully understood from a pharmacological perspective is in part attributed to their complexity but is to some extent related to the present stage of development of neurobiology as a science. Molecular mechanisms, especially those involving drug–receptor interaction and the control of genetic expression in the brain, form the focus of much current research in neuropharmacology. It is to be expected that as these studies progress the source of symptoms in psychiatric disorders will be understood and rational treatment will become possible, in the same way as understanding the cause of peripheral diseases such as diabetes made the symptoms accessible to rational therapy.

BRAIN METABOLISM

The first attempts to apply chemical methods to the study of brain function were made several hundred years ago and information concerning the inorganic constituents of the brain was obtained as early as 1719. With the development of suitable chemical fractionation techniques in the 19th century, detailed investigations of the organic constituents of neural tissue became feasible. Julius Schlossberger in his *General and Comparative Animal Chemistry* devoted 135 of its 616 pages to the chemistry of neural tissues. This work stimulated a number of more extensive studies of the nervous system by the methods of organic chemistry, culminating in the most comprehensive of 19th century studies of brain composition: Thudichum's *Treatise on the Chemical Constitution of the Brain*, published in 1884 (see McIlwain 1990). As early as 1833 attempts were being made to relate mental disorders to alterations in the chemical composition of the brain.

The emphasis on studies of brain constituents in the early phase of the development of neurochemistry was due in part to the widely held, but erroneous, view that brain metabolism was a very slow process. Subsequently, with the advent of isotopic tracer techniques, it became apparent that the brain had one of the highest metabolic rates of any tissue and that most cerebral constituents are in a dynamic state, undergoing rapid changes in association with changes in cerebral functioning. Knowledge of the chemical composition of the brain does not, therefore, in itself, afford much understanding of cerebral function. Although the composition of the brain is altered significantly in a number of conditions (such as some of the inborn errors of lipid and amino acid metabolism), most present-day research on the neurochemistry of mental disorders concentrates on dynamic processes such as synthesis, turnover, release, uptake and transport of neurotransmitters. Formidable practical obstacles still exist, including the structural and functional complexity of the brain, its cellular heterogeneity and the enormous range of timescales over which reactions can occur.

There are, for example, two major cell types in the brain, neurones and glia, and the difference in their functional roles is reflected in their very different chemical composition and metabolic properties. However, even small samples of brain tissue will contain several types of neurone and glia, usually in close juxtaposition, and it is extremely difficult to separate the contributions of each cell type to the metabolism of the tissue as a whole. A further complication is that the intracellular concentrations of many chemicals within brain cells are not uniform. Each cell is composed of many types of organelle, each having a different chemical composition and different metabolic properties. The existence of different metabolic 'pools' within cells is known as compartmentation and is particularly pronounced in the brain. Many brain constituents, e.g. amino acids such as glutamate, are found in several intracellular pools which can differ in size and turnover rate.

For these reasons classical biochemical methods for

studying metabolism (for example, the use of tissue slices and homogenates in vitro) can, when applied to the brain, yield data that are extremely difficult to interpret. Although some of the problems can be overcome by use of such techniques as histochemistry (to assist in precise localisation of substances), it has been necessary to develop fractionation and analytical techniques to enable the study of the metabolism of different cell types in isolation and the study of metabolism at the subcellular level. The successful development of such methods, particularly micromethods of single-cell analysis and fractionation methods that permit the study of isolated nerve endings ('synaptosomes'), has contributed greatly to progress in neurochemistry.

Although the tasks performed by the cells of the brain are less conspicuously energy consuming than those of many other cells, since they do not involve mechanical work, osmotic work or significant external secretory activity, there are, nevertheless, many functions of brain cells that are energy intensive: the maintenance of membrane potentials, active transport and the synthesis and axoplasmic transport of cellular materials. It is not surprising, therefore, that, with its organisational complexity and wide range of endergonic activities, the brain has a high metabolic rate. Although it comprises a mere 2% of body weight it accounts for approximately 10% of the energy expenditure and 20% of the oxygen consumption of the body at rest. In children this percentage is even higher; the brain of a 5-year-old accounts for approximately 50% of the resting total body oxygen consumption. The oxygen consumption of a typical neurone is between 10 and 100 times greater than that of a glial cell.

Energy metabolism is not responsible for absolutely all the oxygen consumption of the brain, as the brain contains a variety of oxidases and hydroxylases that have a role in the synthesis and metabolism of a number of neurotransmitters. However, important though these are, they account for a negligible proportion of the total oxygen consumption of the brain.

As a consequence of its high energy requirement the brain is extremely sensitive to disturbances in the supply of its energy sources and many clinical conditions associated with disturbances of brain function can often be traced back to a deficiency in the production or utilisation of energy. Furthermore, in view of the poor regenerative abilities of nerve cells, an energy deficiency of any duration can have long-term implications for both functional and structural integrity.

PRIMARY ENERGY SOURCES

The brain, like the rest of the body, obtains its chemical energy by the oxidation of foodstuffs. The energy derived from this oxidation is stored in a utilisable form as high-energy phosphate in molecules of adenosine triphosphate (ATP). The primary energy source of the central nervous system (CNS) is glucose, and in this the brain differs from other tissues which are able to utilise lipids and, to a lesser extent, protein. There is little storage of either lipid or glycogen. The glycogen content of brain is only 2–4 μmol/g and therefore the metabolism of the brain cannot be sustained by its carbohydrate reserves. Consequently, it is dependent on a constant blood-borne supply of glucose. Under normal conditions, the brain utilises approximately 16–20 μmol of glucose per gram of brain per hour and cessation of the blood supply of glucose and oxygen results in loss of consciousness within less than 10 seconds (the time taken to consume the oxygen within the brain and its blood) and irreversible brain damage within minutes.

In nutritional studies, a commonly used index for estimating the proportion of fat and carbohydrate being utilised is the respiratory quotient (RQ; calculated by dividing the volume of carbon dioxide produced by the volume of oxygen consumed). The RQ for fat oxidation is 0.71 and the RQ for carbohydrate oxidation is 1.00. The RQ calculated for the adult brain is 0.99. Under normal conditions, the amount of oxygen consumed in the brain is equivalent to that of the glucose removed from the blood (McIlwain & Bachelard 1985).

The normal arterial blood glucose concentration is approximately 80 mg/100 ml. When hypoglycaemia occurs, brain glucose consumption is reduced more than its oxygen utilisation and the total carbon dioxide produced by the brain can be increased to twice the basal level. Isotope experiments have shown that this increased carbon dioxide production is due to the oxidation of non-carbohydrate substrates, probably amino acids and lipids. As a result, hypoglycaemia may be associated with marked neurological manifestations, including convulsions. In insulin-induced hypoglycaemia the blood glucose concentration may fall to as low as 8 mg/100 ml and coma can result because, under these conditions, the reduced production of ATP is inadequate for normal brain function.

The pre-eminence of glucose as the substrate supporting the energy-requiring activities of the mammalian brain was first established over 50 years ago and remains unchallenged by more modern research. For reviews, see Bradford (1986) and Sokoloff (1989).

Nervous tissue contains all the enzymes and metabolic intermediates of anaerobic and aerobic carbohydrate metabolism and is also able to utilise lipid and protein in vitro. The dependence of the brain on glucose as its primary energy source in vivo is due to the fact that the availability of other substrates is severely limited by the set of diverse homeostatic mechanisms known as the blood–brain barrier. Whereas glucose has an unimpeded entry from the blood into the brain and rapidly reaches tissue levels adequate for maintaining normal metabolism, the entry of fructose, lactate, pyruvate, succinate and glutamate is restricted and tissue levels comparable to those achieved by glucose are not reached.

Glucose metabolism

The manner in which the potential chemical energy of glucose is captured and utilised for the synthesis of ATP in the brain is broadly similar to that in other tissues. It is achieved in three main stages. Firstly, glucose is converted to pyruvic acid by the glycolysis (Embden–Meyerhof) pathway in the cell cytoplasm. Although this glycolytic pathway is the main pathway of glucose utilisation, the pentose phosphate pathway is also functional and accounts for approximately 1% of the metabolic flux of glucose in human brain. Its primary role is to generate reduced coenzymes for use in biosynthetic pathways but the pentose phosphates it produces are also important for local nucleotide synthesis, as, in the adult, there is a restricted entry of nucleotides from the blood to the brain. In the second stage of glucose breakdown, pyruvic acid is oxidised in the mitochondria to carbon dioxide via acetyl coenzyme A (acetyl-CoA) and the Krebs or tricarboxylic acid cycle. In the third stage, the electrons produced by the Krebs cycle enter the electron transport chain (flavoprotein–cytochrome system) where they are used in the reduction of oxygen. This process is coupled with the generation of ATP and is known as oxidative phosphorylation. A summary of glucose metabolism in brain is shown schematically in Figure 3.1.

ATP production

During glycolysis, direct transfer of high-energy phosphate from 1,3-diphosphoglyceric acid and phosphoenolpyruvate to adenosine diphosphate (ADP) results in the formation of two ATP molecules. Under anaerobic conditions, therefore, there is a net synthesis of two ATP molecules as glucose breaks into two triose molecules, and two ATP molecules are used in the formation of glucose 6-phosphate and fructose 1,6-diphosphate. Under aerobic conditions, however, the reduced coenzyme nicotinamide-adenine dinucleotide (NAD) produced in the oxidation of glyceraldehyde phosphate is reoxidised through the flavoprotein cytochrome system, with the formation of three ATP molecules. Further oxidation of each pyruvate molecule to carbon dioxide and water via the tri-

carboxylic acid cycle yields a further 15 molecules of ATP, i.e. a further 30 molecules per molecule of glucose. This ATP is produced by the reoxidation of reduced NAD, NAD phosphate (NADP) and flavinadenine dinucleotide (FAD) by the electron transport chain, but ATP is also produced by reaction of ADP and guanosine triphosphate (GTP) formed in the conversion of succinyl-CoA to succinate. Thus during the complete oxidative breakdown of glucose to carbon dioxide and water there is a net production of 38 molecules of ATP. This represents a theoretical efficiency of 42% in capturing the energy latent in the glucose. However, in practice, approximately 15% of brain glucose is converted from pyruvate to lactate and does not enter the Krebs cycle and therefore the net gain of ATP is nearer 33 molecules per molecule of glucose utilised (Clarke et al 1989).

Regulation: metabolism in relation to functional state

Anaerobic metabolism of glucose, yielding as it does a mere two molecules of ATP, cannot supply the energy requirements of normal cerebral function and, as a result, the brain is very dependent on the efficient working of the Krebs cycle. This dependence is reflected in the neurological dysfunctions which can ensue as a consequence of interference with its normal operation. Deficiency of thiamine, a cofactor in the conversion of pyruvate to acetyl-CoA, has profound effects on the CNS, as does a deficiency of niacin (required for NAD synthesis). However, carbohydrate metabolism in brain is relatively insensitive to a number of factors that have pronounced effects on other organs. Thyroid hormones have been shown to have no effect on the cerebral respiration rate in the adult human, although the development of the adult pattern of cerebral glucose metabolism is retarded after neonatal thyroidectomy. There is even doubt whether insulin affects glucose transport and utilisation in nervous tissue directly, although there have been reports that insulin does facilitate the entry of glucose in nervous tissues.

Cerebral carbohydrate metabolism exhibits considerable flexibility to supply energy according to functional need. For example, during anaesthesia glucose utilisation is of the order of $0.15 \, \text{mmol} \, \text{kg}^{-1} \text{min}^{-1}$ but during convulsions utilisation can increase to more than $10 \, \text{mmol} \, \text{kg}^{-1}/\text{min}^{-1}$. Such flexibility in the cerebral metabolic rate is possible because cerebral glucose metabolism is regulated at a number of different levels: by changes in cerebral circulation; by changes in glucose transport from the blood; and by changes in the rate of individual enzyme reactions brought about by environmental influences on the activity of key regula-

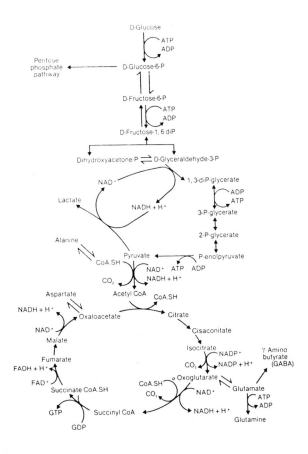

Fig. 3.1 Principal metabolic pathways of the brain.

high rate of incorporation of glucose carbon into free amino acids. In this respect the brain differs markedly from other organs such as the liver, kidney, lung, muscle and spleen. The explanation of this phenomenon is that the metabolism of certain glucose metabolites is closely related to that of the 'glutamate group' of amino acids. Members of this group (glutamate, aspartate and GABA) have a special role in the CNS and account for 75% of the free amino acids in the brain. They are found primarily in the grey matter and are associated with neuronal mitochondria. Glutamate, by its energy-dependent conversion to glutamine, plays an important role in the detoxification of ammonia in the brain, and both glutamate and GABA function physiologically as transmitters.

Aspartate and glutamate are glycogenic since they are readily and reversibly converted into oxaloacetate and α-oxoglutarate by transamination reactions. These reactions allow the extensive synthesis of non-essential amino acids from Krebs cycle intermediates and aid in regulating the concentration of metabolites entering this cycle. Another possible regulator of the Krebs cycle in the CNS is the metabolic sequence known as the 'GABA shunt' shown in Figure 3.2. This is a bypass around the cycle from α-oxoglutarate to succinate and accounts for approximately 10% of the total glucose turnover. Although this pathway is found at extremely low levels in some other tissues such as kidney, heart and liver, it is, by far, most active in the brain. This is due to the relatively high levels in the CNS of the enzyme responsible for catalysing the decarboxylation of glutamate to GABA. This enzyme, glutamate decarboxylase, in common with the transaminase enzyme, requires vitamin B_6 phosphate (pyridoxal phosphate) as a cofactor. The importance of these interrelationships between the glutamate group of amino acids and glucose metabolism

tory enzymes such as the glycolytic enzymes hexokinase and phosphofructokinase. Energy output and oxygen consumption in the brain are associated with high levels of enzyme activity in the Krebs cycle. The actual flux through the cycle depends on a number of factors: the rate of glycolysis and acetyl-CoA production which can 'push' the cycle; the activity of the pyruvate dehydrogenase complex which controls the rate of pyruvate entering the cycle; and the local ADP level, which is the prime activator of oxidative phosphorylation to which the cycle is linked. Another factor contributing to the flexibility in metabolic rate is the fact that the substrate levels found under normal physiological conditions are generally well below those required for maximum enzyme activities. For example, under normal conditions only half of the brain pyruvate dehydrogenase is active.

The γ-aminobutyrate (GABA) shunt

The metabolism of the adult brain is characterised by a

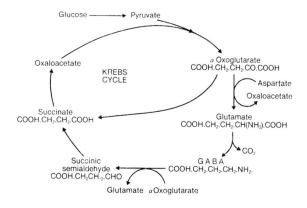

Fig. 3.2 The GABA shunt, a minor but important metabolic route in brain cells.

is illustrated by the deleterious effects of vitamin B_6 deficiency. Glutamate decarboxylase and transaminase inhibition caused by such a deficiency results in seizures. These seizures may be alleviated by the administration of GABA, suggesting that they are primarily due to the dysfunction of glutamate decarboxylase.

Earlier in this chapter it was noted that metabolic compartmentation is an important feature of brain metabolism. There is good evidence (Baxter 1976) that this is true of the Krebs cycle and the GABA shunt. It is believed that there are at least two pools – one associated primarily with nerve endings and another associated primarily with glial cells.

METABOLIC IMAGING

The powerful dependence of brain metabolism on glucose and on oxygen supply has advantages for those who want to study the activity of areas of brain. There are methods for the direct study of both blood flow and glucose utilisation in animal brain. The animals are treated with 2-deoxyglucose, which enters the brain on the glucose uptake pathways but is not metabolised, so that, if it is radioactively tagged, the amount of radioactivity in a brain area reflects the metabolic activity in the area. Similarly iodo-^{14}C-antipyrine follows the blood into brain and can be detected autoradiographically (Sokoloff 1989). It is extremely unusual for these two markers to be discordant and both usually mark areas of brain active during the drug application. Recent human brain imaging studies have used these principles in order to detect the areas of human brain active dur-

ing various sensory, motor or cognitive tasks. Results from these methods are presented in greater detail in Chapter 16.

PHARMACOKINETICS

The effective concentration reached by any applied substance in the relevant tissues depends upon its absorption, distribution, biotransformation and excretion, and those in turn depend upon its movement across cell membranes. This is determined by a substance's physical characteristics and the presence or absence of specific mechanisms to facilitate its passage across membranes. Passive movement of water-soluble substances of low molecular weight (less than 200 Da) is by filtration through aqueous channels, but these are too narrow (less than 4 Å) for most drugs which must pass through the cell membrane to enter a cell. Many drugs are organic electrolytes and are weak acids or bases. The extent to which a drug is ionised is determined by the pH of its solution and the dissociation constant (K_d) of the drug. The un-ionised portion is usually 10 000 times more lipid soluble than the ionised portion and consequently much more soluble in the lipid bilayer of the cell membrane. The pharmacokinetics of drug entry into the CNS are complex and summarised in Figure 3.3. The fraction labelled 'free' in this diagram is available to pass into the brain and its rate of movement is proportional to its concentration gradient from plasma to the extracellular fluid of the nervous system. The effective concentration in brain is also controlled by active mechanisms of both accumu-

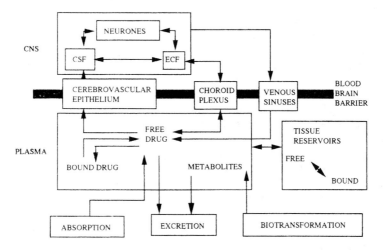

Fig. 3.3 Pharmacokinetics of drug entry into the central nervous system. (CSF, cerebrospinal fluid; ECF, extracellular fluid.)

lation into, and elimination from, the cerebrospinal fluid (CSF).

Absorption and distribution

The passage of drugs into the brain is governed by the general principles of drug absorption and also by the specific 'active' properties of the blood–brain barrier. One important general principle is that drugs given in aqueous solution are absorbed more quickly than those dissolved in oils or given as solids. Most drugs are given by mouth and the wide pH range encountered in the gastrointestinal tract influences absorption. Oral ingestion is the most convenient and economical method of administration and, because drugs are absorbed relatively slowly from the gut, is also relatively safe because adverse effects also develop slowly. Intravenous administration rapidly produces the desired plasma concentration of a drug, but, because the effects are immediate, so are adverse reactions. Table 3.1 summarises the properties of common routes of drug administration. After a drug is absorbed into the bloodstream, it is distributed between extracellular and intracellular fluids. At first, distribution is determined by the relative blood flow to the various regions of the body, so that highly perfused organs can reach peak concentrations within the first few minutes. Except in the brain, capillary endothelial membranes are highly permeable, allowing molecules as large as albumin (67 000 Da) to pass through intercellular aqueous channels.

The most immediate reservoir for drugs is formed by binding to plasma proteins, particularly albumin. Binding is relatively non-selective, so drugs compete for these binding sites. Drugs can also accumulate in other reservoirs such as muscle, fat or bone, and as the plasma concentration of a drug falls, it may be released from body compartments, which would allow its action to be sustained. Many drugs are highly lipid soluble and so they can be stored in body fat. In obese persons, this is an important drug reservoir.

The blood–brain barrier

The brain and CSF are separated from the blood by the blood–brain barrier, which regulates the movement of substances into and out of the nervous system. It is represented structurally by the capillary endothelium of the brain, and functionally by a complex set of active transport mechanisms. The cells of cerebral vessel walls are so tightly bound together that diffusion between cells is negligible and the cells function as a single continuous sheet, behaving like a lipid membrane. Lipid-soluble substances pass readily through this membrane, whereas non-lipid-soluble substances and proteins enter the brain much more slowly.

In some specialised areas of brain the capillary endothelium is permeable – in the subfornical organ, the area postrema in the medulla, and in the region of the median eminence – and these areas are often said to be outside the blood–brain barrier. These high permeability areas may allow transfer of compounds such as peptides which cannot cross into brain elsewhere.

The permeability of the blood–brain barrier to drugs (when there is no specific mechanism of entry) is determined by the general principles set out above. A ready guide to a drug's entry into the nervous system is provided by the 'pH partition hypothesis'. This states that the permeability of a cell membrane to a drug is propor-

Table 3.1	Properties of common routes of drug administration		
Route	Absorption	Advantages	Problems
Oral	Variable	Convenience Safety	Drugs of low solubility or high hepatic clearance have low oral availability
Subcutaneous	Quick in aqueous solution	Useful for some insoluble drugs and pellets	Pain, local necrosis Unsuitable for large volumes
Intramuscular	Quick in aqueous solution	Useful for low to medium volumes and some preparations of irritating drugs	Slow from depot Contraindicated during anticoagulant therapy
Intravenous	Often immediate	Useful in emergency and suitable for large volumes	Can have immediate adverse reactions Unsuitable for oily or insoluble preparations

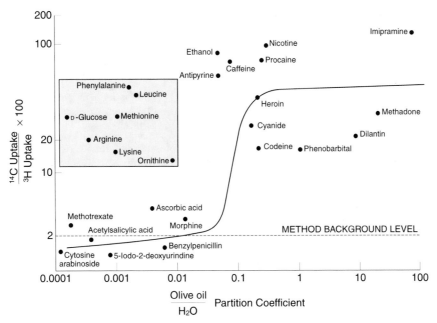

Fig. 3.4 Percentage clearance of radiolabelled substances plotted against their lipid/water coefficients during a single brain passage following carotid arterial injection. Drugs with a partition coefficient greater than about 0.03 show nearly complete clearance. The substances inside the box have very low lipid affinity but penetrate the blood–brain barrier by virtue of specific carrier transport systems. (After Oldendorf (1974) and Bradbury (1979).)

tional to that drug's partition coefficient, which is the product of two fractional concentrations, one of the un-ionised drug in aqueous solution and the other the lipid solubility of the un-ionised drug. The latter is usually measured as the optimal lipid/water partition coefficient. The pH of CSF can be regulated independently of plasma pH because un-ionised carbon dioxide passes across the blood–brain barrier much more readily than bicarbonate ions. CSF pH is usually 0.1 of a unit lower than plasma pH and, at equilibrium, concentrations of weak electrolytes may differ on either side of the blood–brain barrier, so that weak bases tend to accumulate in the CSF whereas weak acids tend to be excluded. The pH gradients between plasma and CSF can, therefore, produce concentration gradients at equilibrium for dissociated compounds. Figure 3.4 illustrates these principles by showing the relationship between the uptake by the brain of radiolabelled substances and their lipid/water partition coefficients. When a drug has a partition coefficient greater than 0.03, it is almost completely cleared from the blood after carotid artery injection during a single brain passage. A group of substances is enclosed within a box in Figure 3.4 and these exceptions to the general rule show high clearance yet have very low partition coefficients.

Specific carrier transport systems related to lipid affinity are available for these substances. Amino acids, essential for brain function, are not usually synthesised in the brain and so need to be transported from the blood. For example, the rate of entry of tryptophan into the brain is directly proportional to the ratio of its plasma concentration to the sum of the concentrations of phenylalanine, leucine, valine and isoleucine. These other amino acids all compete with tryptophan for the same transport system. Amino acid transport mechanisms are stereospecific, preferring the laevo- to the dextro-isomer. Active transport can operate in both directions and against concentration gradients, either from the brain to the blood or from the blood to the brain. The carrier which removes drugs and metabolites from brain has many properties in common with the acid transporter in the kidney, and may be a closely related mechanism. Some nervous system metabolites do not have specific mechanisms to clear them from CSF, and so are removed when CSF passes back into the blood (the 'sink action' of CSF).

Biotransformation and excretion

Biotransformation of most drugs takes place in hepatic

microsomal enzyme systems, though other systems – including plasma, gut, lung or kidney – may be involved. Lipid-soluble drugs are more readily metabolised by hepatic microsomes because of their ease of entry into the cell. Considerable individual variation in biotransformation can be related to genetic factors, the effects of age, hepatic disease or induction of microsomal enzymes by other drugs or environmental agents. The processes of biotransformation can lead to activation or inactivation of a drug and may involve numerous drug metabolites. Unchanged drugs or their metabolites are removed from the body by excretory organs such as the kidney or lung. Substances with high lipid solubility are not readily excreted until they have been metabolised to more polar compounds. The kidneys remove most drugs or their metabolites by renal excretion involving glomerular filtration, active tubular secretion and passive tubular reabsorption. Like all cell membranes, tubular cells are less permeable to the ionised portion of a drug, and more permeable to lipid-soluble compounds. Excretion of drugs in other body fluids is relatively unimportant, with the exception of breast milk.

Clearance

In psychiatric practice, the usual aim is to maintain the concentration of a drug within its presumed therapeutic range. 'Steady-state' concentrations are attained when the rate of drug elimination (clearance) equals the rate of drug administration. When complete bioavailability of a drug can be assumed, the rate of drug administration is, therefore, determined by its clearance. For most drugs used in psychiatry, clearance is typically constant within the range of concentrations seen in clinical practice. This arises because clearance mechanisms are not usually saturated and drug clearance is observed to be a linear function of the drug's blood concentration. A constant fraction of most drugs is cleared per unit of time, and when this happens the drug is said to follow *first-order kinetics*. When clearance systems for a drug are saturated, the pharmacokinetics of the drug become *zero order* and a constant amount of that drug is cleared per unit of time. Clearance is calculated as the total volume of blood (or other body fluid) from which a drug must be completely removed, not as the total amount of drug removed. Total clearance represents the sum of clearance by each organ of elimination (kidneys, liver, lung, etc.).

In some circumstances, clearance of a drug by a specific organ becomes a matter of clinical concern, for example the renal elimination of lithium. Clinical investigation of renal function of a patient on long-term lithium therapy might, therefore, use an alternative definition of clearance. Clearance can be defined by the blood flow to the organ under investigation (Q), arterial concentration (C_A) and venous concentration (C_V). The difference between the products of blood flow and blood concentration gives the clearance by an organ (CL_{organ}):

$$\text{elimination} = QC_A - QC_V = Q(C_A - C_V)$$
$$CL_{organ} = Q(C_A - C_V)/C_A$$
$$= QE.$$

The expression $(C_A - C_V)/C_A$ defines the *extraction ratio* (E) for a drug by a specific organ.

Some drugs show dose-dependent clearance that varies with drug concentration in blood. Dosing schemes for these drugs can be difficult:

$$\text{total blood clearance} = V_M/(K_M + C_B)$$

where K_M is the blood concentration at which 50% of the maximum rate of elimination is reached (in units of mass/volume) and V_M is the maximum rate of elimination (in units of mass/time).

Drugs such as chlorpromazine and imipramine are mostly cleared by the liver. Hepatic clearance is largely determined by hepatic blood flow, i.e. the rate at which the drug can be transported to hepatic sites of biotransformation and/or excretion in bile. Although changes in drug binding to blood components and other tissues (Fig. 3.1) may influence hepatic or renal clearance, in present circumstances, when a drug's extraction ratio (E) is high, changes in protein binding due to disease or competitive processes should have little effect on drug clearance. However, when the extraction ratio is low, changes in protein binding and intrahepatic functions will substantially alter drug clearance, but changes in hepatic blood flow will have little effect. Because a drug bound to blood proteins is not filtered and thus not subject to active glomerular secretion and/or reabsorption, renal clearance is substantially influenced by protein binding and thus by those diseases that affect protein binding.

NEUROTRANSMISSION

Almost 40 years ago, intracellular recording techniques established beyond reasonable doubt the neurochemical nature of synaptic transmission in the CNS. Chemical neurotransmitters were shown to produce inhibition or excitation of neurones by briefly and rapidly increasing neuronal membrane permeability to specific ions. Table 3.2 shows the 'classical' criteria for the identification of neurotransmitters that were once widely accepted. Later, studies on single neurones identified noradrenaline, acetylcholine, serotonin, dopamine, γ-aminobutyric acid (GABA), glycine and

Table 3.2 Criteria for identification of neurotransmitters
1. The transmitter must be shown to be present in the presynaptic terminals of the synapse and in the neurones from which those presynaptic terminals arise
2. The transmitter must be synthesised in the presynaptic neurone
3. The transmitter must be stored in an inactive form in the presynaptic terminal
4. The transmitter must be released from the presynaptic nerve concomitantly with presynaptic nerve activity
5. The effects of the putative neurotransmitter when applied experimentally to the target cells must be identical to those of the presynaptic pathway
6. The amount released by nervous activity (4) should be comparable to that required to produce postsynaptic action (5)
7. A method for control of the postsynaptic concentration which is capable of terminating the action of the transmitter is required, e.g. a presynaptic uptake system or an enzymatic degradation at the synapse

glutamate as transmitters at synapses in the CNS. A major development in understanding the function of neurotransmitters in neural networks was provided by Yamamoto & McIlwain (1966) who demonstrated the feasibility of recording from transverse hippocampal

slices. This structure contains numerous neurotransmitters and their receptors and electrophysiological preparations preserve the precise laminar structure and much of the neuronal circuitry of the hippocampus. Although many accounts of neuropharmacology present information in terms of a single synapse (the functional unit of the nervous system) the data summarised in such accounts have often been obtained and characterised in model neuronal systems such as the hippocampal slice preparation (Bloom 1990). It is still an open question whether the properties of functional groups of neurones are completely specified by such 'single synapse' models but in practical terms they are the basis of most neuropharmacology.

Neurotransmitters may open or close ion channels in the neuronal membrane and can do this directly or by activating adjacent proteins (Fig. 3.5). Initially, it was inferred that neurotransmitters caused a brief hyperpolarisation or depolarisation of the postsynaptic membrane. Now, it is known that neurotransmitters may have a much longer time-course of action produced by their altering the properties of voltage-sensitive (or 'voltage-gated') ion channels that are involved in the regulation of neuronal excitability. This is especially important in the case of K^+ and Ca^{2+} ion channels.

The release of neurotransmitters represents the 'final common pathway' of all neuronal functions. Table 3.3 summarises the properties of substances active at synapses. Neurotransmitters stored in presynaptic vesicles fuse with the presynaptic membrane at the nerve terminal. Synaptic vesicles are coated on their cytoplasmic face by synapsins, a particularly abundant group of

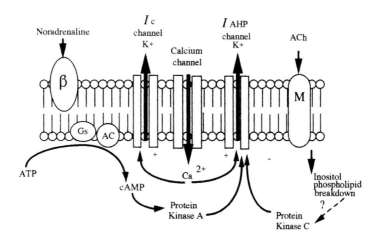

Fig. 3.5 Proposed mechanisms of action of noradrenaline and acetylcholine (ACh) in blocking the slow Ca^{2+}-activated K^+ conductance. Similar mechanisms are proposed for the actions of many G protein-coupled receptors which act on ion channels.

Table 3.3 Substances active in neuronal signalling

Substance	Properties	Example
Neurotransmitter	A substance found in neurone type A, secreted from it and acting on target neurone type B	Acetylcholine
Neurohormone	Peptide secretions of neurones directly into the blood that also act on other neurones as neurotransmitters	Corticotrophin-releasing factor (CRF)
Neuromodulator	A substance that influences neuronal activity and originates from non-synaptic sites	Steroid hormones
Neuromediator (second messenger)	Postsynaptic compounds that participate in generation of postsynaptic responses	Cyclic adenosine monophosphate (cAMP)
Neurotrophin	Substances released by postsynaptic structures which 'maintain' presynaptic neuronal structure	Nerve growth factor

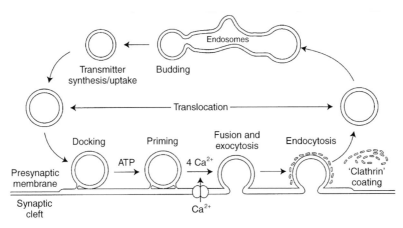

Fig. 3.6   Life history of synaptic vesicles. Synapsins are involved in every phase of vesicle function shown (After Südhof 1995.)

extrinsic membrane proteins (Südhof et al 1989). The four synapsins appear to connect synaptic vesicles to each other and to the neuronal cytoskeleton and probably regulate vesicular position in the nerve terminal. Synapsins share many common structural features and seem likely to comprise a single family of proteins with a common ancestor. Careful study of the molecular biology and physiology of synaptic transmission has provided a complex life history of synaptic vesicles (Fig. 3.6).

Calcium channels

Neurotransmitter release is Ca^{2+} dependent and study of entry of Ca^{2+} across surface membranes is of intense interest to neuropharmacologists. In part this interest stems from technological developments and the availability of specific agents with which to study Ca^{2+} channels. The interest is also based on the ubiquitous nature of neuronal Ca^{2+} and its clinical relevance. Ca^{2+} channels open in response to membrane depolarisation and generate electrical and chemical responses. Ca^{2+} entry into the neurone carries a depolarising charge that contributes to paroxysmal phenomena such as epileptiform or pacemaker activity. It also causes the intracellular Ca^{2+} concentration to rise, and this in turn alters Ca^{2+}-dependent mechanisms involved in neurotransmitter release from synaptic vesicles, enzyme activation, Ca^{2+}-sensitive ion channels and intracellular Ca^{2+} stores which are themselves sensitive to cytosolic Ca^{2+}. Thus, many diverse aspects of neuronal metabolism can be changed by Ca^{2+} entry.

Multiple types of Ca^{2+} channel exist in neurones and it is important to distinguish between them in order to understand neuronal function and its modification by drugs and neurotransmitters. Early electrophysiological studies demonstrated two classes of Ca^{2+} channel: 'low-voltage activated' (LVA) and 'high-voltage activated' (HVA) (Llinas & Yarom 1981). Subsequently, the HVA Ca^{2+} channel was found to comprise N and L subtypes (Nowycky et al 1985), yielding three subtypes designated T (or LVA), N and L. These acronyms should not be taken too literally but do have some mnemonic value: T for 'transient', L for 'long-lasting' and N for channels that are 'neither T nor L' (Tsien et al 1988). At present, none of the subtypes of Ca^{2+} channel is assigned an exclusive physiological role. However, T channels are important in pacemaker depolarization in heart cells and are the primary voltage-sensitive entry points for Ca^{2+} on contraction of certain smooth muscle cells. Ca^{2+} entry by L channels is associated with heart muscle contraction and substance P and noradrenaline release in the CNS. Only L channels are sensitive to blockade by the dihydropyridine Ca^{2+} channel-blocking drugs (nicardipine and nimodipine and diltiazem, nifedipine and verapamil). Recently, the list of Ca^{2+} channels has expanded by two (at least): the P channel was first described in Purkinje cells and seems to be more common on central neurones than in smooth muscle, and in central neurones a 'residual' or R channel has been proposed to include current carried by none of the channels so far described.

The complexity of the regulation of Ca^{2+} entry into neurones is not surprising in view of the central importance of intracellular Ca^{2+} in so many aspects of neuronal function. The fact that there are multiple types of voltage-sensitive Ca^{2+} channel and, as will be described later, multiple types of receptor-operated Ca^{2+} channel, indicates the adaptability available to the neurone in 'fine-tuning' intracellular Ca^{2+} concentrations (Miller 1987).

Pharmacological studies of the Ca^{2+} channel blockers have shown that each binds to a different recognition site on a single protein–receptor complex. Although these drugs do not influence neurotransmitter release, their diverse chemical structures resemble many other clinically useful compounds (Snyder 1989). The neuroleptic drugs comprise several chemical classes: phenothiazines, butyrophenones and diphenylbutylpiperidines. This last class is a Ca^{2+} channel antagonist equipotent with the Ca^{2+}-blocking drugs listed above. Ca^{2+} channel blockade probably also accounts for some neuroleptic side-effects.

Electrocardiogram (ECG) changes produced by thioridazine are similar to those produced by verapamil. Impaired vas deferens contraction and ejaculation observed in experiments using Ca^{2+}-blocking drugs probably explains a common side-effect of thioridazine that is rarely encountered with phenothiazines or butyrophenones. Cardiac and ejaculatory side-effects of thioridazine are probably caused by thioridazine-induced Ca^{2+} channel blockade.

Phosphatidylinositol (PI) metabolism

Protein kinase C (PKC) is a Ca^{2+}-dependent enzyme concentrated at synapses. It is activated by diacylglycerol (DAG), a cleavage product of a group of membrane lipids called phosphatidylinositols. PKC activation in turn potentiates neurotransmitter release. These events are important components of the regulation of neurotransmission and are affected by lithium. Initially, in response to extracellular signals, lipases including phospholipase C (PLC) degrade phosphatidylinositols into precursors of two intracellular 'second messengers'. These are inositol phosphates (IPs) and DAG. Inositol 1,4,5-triphosphate (IP_3) synthesis is the major product of phosphatidylinositol degradation. The pathway is shown in Figure 3.7 (Majerus et al 1988). The PLC enzyme that initiates this cascade of events in fact comprises a group of at least five structurally dissimilar enzymes (Rhee et al 1989). This highly conserved diversity of enzyme structure is poorly understood but probably allows distinct pathways (e.g. through IP_3 and arachidonic acid) to respond selectively to specific extracellular signals and to be negatively influenced by products of these pathways. PKC activation by phorbol esters mimics the action of DAG and is blocked by lithium (Fig. 3.7). Since PKC activation also potentiates serotonin and noradrenaline release, this effect of lithium at therapeutically relevant concentrations suggests a possible mode of action in the treatment of mania and prophylaxis of manic–depressive illness (Wang & Friedman 1989).

PHARMACODYNAMICS

Pharmacodynamics concerns the mechanism of action of drugs. Knowledge of drug pharmacodynamics in psychiatry is basic to their clinical use. Studies of drug action aim to identify chemical and physical interactions between drug and neurone. A proper understanding of the temporal order and scale of drug–neurone interactions provides the basis for understanding drug effects. It can be used to help design improved drugs and, potentially, may provide information of relevance

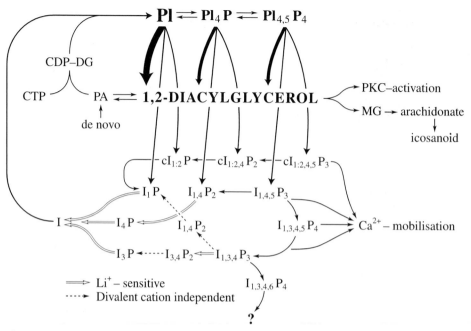

Fig. 3.7 Intracellular phosphatidylinositol (PI) metabolism. Lithium blocks the pathways indicated. (After Majerus et al 1988.)

to understanding neurobiological components of psychiatric disease.

Receptors

Receptors are conceptualised as large, functional molecules that change cellular function. The physical and chemical features of receptor molecules may vary substantially. Some are protein constituents of the cellular membrane, others are proteins that are important in the maintenance of subcellular architecture and some are intracellular enzymes or proteins concerned with cellular transport. Likewise, interactions between drugs and receptors are of multiple types and include covalent, ionic, hydrophobic and van der Waals binding. Covalent binding tends to be of long duration, while noncovalent high-affinity binding is usually reversible. The physical configuration of the receptor largely determines the structural requirements of a drug designed to interact with that receptor. Several clinically important drugs in psychiatry have been developed from deliberate chemical changes to the structure of the endogenous ligand (*physiological agonist*). Additionally, small changes of structure can alter the pharmacokinetic properties of drugs.

Most drugs produce their effects by interaction with receptive macromolecules (drug receptors) and so start a sequence of biochemical and physiological events.

Receptor mechanisms include recognition of the neurotransmitter (usually by a cell surface protein) and transduction of the message into alterations of cellular function that may involve changes in ionic permeability and the formation of *second messengers*.

Drugs that bind to receptors and initiate a response in neuroeffector tissue are *agonists*. Drugs that produce a maximal response are *full agonists* and those producing less than maximal response are *partial agonists*. Drugs that have no intrinsic pharmacological activity but produce effects by preventing an agonist initiating a response are *antagonists*. Some antagonists can produce a partial pharmacological response ('partial agonist activity') at receptor binding sites where they compete with endogenous ligands. Some drugs combine both agonist and antagonist properties as *mixed agonist–antagonists*, and understanding these properties may have therapeutic potential. For example, a mixed opiate agonist–antagonist might have the advantage of providing relief of pain with much less risk of addiction than a full agonist such as morphine. Pharmacological antagonism is distinct from physiological antagonism produced by substances initiating an opposing response in neuroeffector tissue. For example, noradrenaline can act as a physiological antagonist of acetylcholine but has negligible action at acetylcholine receptors.

Classical receptor theory assumes that the effect of a drug is proportional to the number of receptors with

Table 3.4	Criteria for identification of receptors

- 'Possible': Radioligand binding sites
  - Saturability and reversibility of radioligand binding
  - Homogeneous population of sites
  - Regional and species variation
  - Pharmacological properties
- 'Probable': Functional correlates
  - Identification of special messenger links
  - Delineation of physiological effects on membranes
  - Behavioural or other models of action
- 'Definite': Structural identification
  - Unique amino acid sequence
  - Cloned sequences mimic actions of natural receptor

After Peroutka (1988).

Table 3.5	Examples of 'superfamilies' of receptors
Superfamily	Neuroreceptor/ion channel
G protein-coupled receptors	Visual pigments Adrenergic Muscarinic, cholinergic Serotonergic
Ligand-gated ion channel receptors	Nicotinic cholinergic GABA$_A$ Glycine Glutamate
Tyrosine kinase-linked receptors	NGF Neurotrophins BDNF CNTF GDNF

NGF, nerve growth factor; BDNF, brain-derived neurotrophic factor; CNTF, ciliary neutrophic factor; GDNF, glial cell-derived neurotrophic factor.

which that drug interacts. The ease with which a drug attaches to a receptor is termed the *affinity* of the drug for that receptor. Receptors for neurotransmitters are components of the neural membrane. They are able to recognise specific neurotransmitters and produce physiological responses in neuroeffector tissues. Receptors can, therefore, be defined both in terms of their ability to recognise specific ligands and by the physiological responses they initiate (Table 3.4).

Receptor sensitivity

Drug–receptor interactions may be modified by changes in receptor sensitivity. The sensitivity of receptors is influenced by complex regulatory and homeostatic factors. When receptor sensitivity changes, the same concentration of a drug will produce a greater or lesser physiological response. Changes in sensitivity occur, for example, after prolonged stimulation of cells by agonists and the cell becomes refractory to further stimulation. This is also termed 'desensitisation' or 'downregulation'. Underlying mechanisms of desensitisation may involve receptor changes (e.g. phosphorylation) or the receptor may be concealed within the cell so that it is no longer exposed to the ligand. Long-term desensitisation may involve negative-feedback mechanisms that inhibit new receptor synthesis or cause a structurally modified receptor to be synthesised. Desensitisation involves at least two distinct 'closed' states of the nicotinic receptor. Both 'closed' states display a higher affinity for acetylcholine

than does the resting (or 'active') conformation. Structural studies show that a specific segment of the lumen-facing part of the ion channel is crucial in the process of desensitisation in response to prolonged agonist exposure (Revah et al 1991). This segment of the ionic channel is highly conserved in other receptor types (e.g. GABA$_A$ and glycine receptors) where it may play a similar role. Supersensitivity ('upregulation' or 'hypersensitivity') was first described after removal of the presynaptic element but often follows prolonged receptor blockade. This may involve synthesis of new receptors so that an increased number of receptors is exposed on the cell surface to their physiological ligands. In the case of supersensitivity following the destruction of the presynaptic terminal the loss of mechanisms that terminate transmitter action (e.g. uptake, enzymatic degradation) also contribute to the increase in response to agonist.

Receptor families

Historically, there has been considerable debate about criteria for the characterisation of receptor subtypes. Practically, the identification of new receptor types has quickly followed the development of specific, potent agonists and/or antagonists that selectively bind to the new receptor. Molecular, biochemical and physiological techniques indicate the existence of several 'superfamilies' (probably less than 10) of receptor macromolecules (Table 3.5). Molecular biological techniques have

Table 3.6	Neurotransmitter ligands acting through G protein-coupled receptors	
Neurotransmitter	Receptor subtypes	Examples of effectors
Catecholamines	$\alpha_1, \alpha_2, \beta_1, \beta_2, \beta_3$	Adenylate cyclase;
Cholinergic	M_1, M_2, M_3	PLC; phospholipase A_2;
Dopamine	D_1, D_2	phosphodiesterases;
Serotonin	$5\text{-HT}_{1A-F}, 5\text{-HT}_2$	Ca^{2+}, K^+ channels;
Histamine	H_1, H_2, H_3	guanylyl cyclase;
GABA	$GABA_B$	PKC
Glutamate	mGLUr(1–5)	
Angiotensin	$A_1\ A_{2A}\ A_{2B}$	

provided the best classification of subtypes within receptor superfamilies. Progress in this field has consistently led to revision of classification systems based on biochemical and physiological studies. Within each superfamily of receptor types there can be considerable structural diversity of their endogenous ligands. Receptors within each receptor family, however, have many structural similarities with other members of the same family and share common mechanisms of signal propagation.

G protein-coupled receptors A family of cellular proteins called 'G proteins' (guanine triphosphate (GTP)-binding) link cell surface receptors to a variety of enzymes and ion channels. By far the largest known class of receptor (summarised in Table 3.6) functions by stimulating a membrane-bound G protein. Members of this protein family are composed of three homologous subunits: α, β and γ. Figure 3.8 shows the likely organisation of receptors, G proteins and effectors (such as ion channels, adenylate cyclase and enzymes involved in phosphatidylinositol metabolism). Receptors coupled to G proteins have similar structures that include seven transmembrane helices (Fig. 3.8a). Sequence homology among the G protein-coupled receptors is found largely in the membrane-spanning regions. The cytoplasmic regions and loops between spans 5 and 6 show minimal sequence homology (Ross 1989). Neurotransmitter and hormonal ligands bind to G protein-coupled receptors in the pocket formed by the seven helices in Figure 3.8b. The G proteins are located on the intracellular surface of the plasma membrane and it is likely that part of the receptor which regulates G proteins is also on the intracellular face. Binding of the ligand to the extracellular part of the receptor distorts the binding site to an extent sufficient to alter the cytoplasmic part of the receptor and to transform it from its passive to active state. The cytoplasmic loop between spans 5 and 6 is probably the G protein regulation site, as G protein regulation is sensitive to mutations in this region. The ligand-binding

domain of the β-adrenoceptor lies within the core of the receptor molecule. Structure–activity analyses of adrenoceptor ligands and the amino acid sequences in the receptor core have been greatly helped by the synthesis of 'mutant' receptors. These studies point the way toward the development of new drugs. They are also important in understanding molecular mechanisms of receptor desensitisation (Strader et al 1989).

Figure 3.9 shows the process of signal transduction by G proteins. A ligand binds at its receptor and produces a change in receptor–G protein interaction. This change allows GTP (in the presence of Mg^{2+}) to replace guanosine diphosphate (GDP) on the α subunit of the G protein. Now activated, the α-GTP subunit dissociates from the $\beta\gamma$ subunit allowing one or both subunits to interact with an effector (e.g. adenylate cyclase). The α subunit possesses intrinsic GTPase activity and hydrolyses GTP to GDP, releasing inorganic phosphate (P_i), and the cycle is terminated by α-GDP recombining with a $\beta\gamma$ subunit. Throughout this cycle, the $\beta\gamma$ subunit remains a single functional unit and all phases of the cycle take place in the cytoplasmic compartment. $\beta\gamma$ subunits released in the cycle can interact with other effectors such as phospholipase A_2 (PLA_2) in some cell systems. The α subunit is thought to remain attached to the inner surface of the plasma membrane throughout this cycle (Neer & Clapham 1988).

There are very many G proteins and they can be subdivided by their susceptibilities to bacterial toxins. There are subtypes specific for:

- cholera toxin only
- pertussis toxin only
- both toxins
- neither toxin.

Cholera toxin-susceptible G proteins were initially thought to stimulate adenylate cyclase (G_s) and the pertussis toxin-susceptible G proteins to inhibit adenylate cyclase (G_i). These toxins modify different types of α subunit (α_i and α_s) which then act upon a wide range of

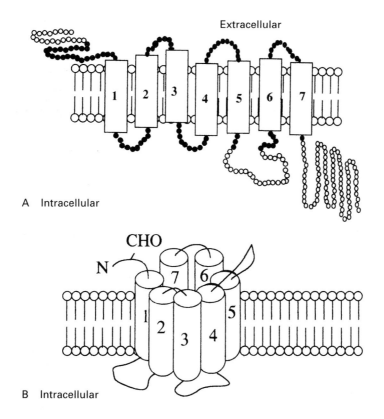

Fig. 3.8 A The peptide chains of the β-adrenergic receptor (G protein-coupled receptors in general) are assumed to span the extracellular membrane as shown. **B** A three-dimensional array of the seven membrane-spanning helices shown in A.

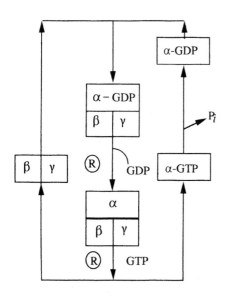

effectors. Structural analysis of the α and β subunits has revealed more subtypes than there are presently known functions. The α_i subtype alone is divisible into α_0, α_i-1, α_i-2 and α_i-3. These are highly conserved and their individual genes probably derive from a common ancestor. The β and γ subtypes are also heterogeneous and the overall picture is of a loose spatial organisation of receptors, G proteins and their effectors. Receptors can interact with a single G protein and the same G protein can interact with several receptors or effectors. Probably up to 15 distinct kinds of receptor can stimulate adenylate cyclase through G_s. Interactions between

Fig. 3.9 The G protein cycle of activation in transmembrane signalling. The αβγ complex is stable only with GDP bound to the α subunit. Binding GTP to the α subunit dissociates the complex, which can only reassociate after dephosphorylation of GTP to GDP. The free βγ complex acts on many cellular subsystems, including ion channels and intracellular signalling pathways. (After Sternweis & Pang 1990.)

G proteins and effectors, however, seem to be much more specific so that, for example, only G_s and not G_i or G_o can stimulate the most common of the adenylate cyclases found in neurones. This capacity of G proteins to interact with multiple effectors underlies the advantages of G proteins as signal transducers. Multiple receptors, G proteins and effectors make up a complex signalling network. These networks sort extracellular signals and integrate incoming information (Birnbaumer 1990). The effector enzyme, adenylate cyclase, can be stimulated or inhibited by numerous hormones or transmitters either directly or along the G protein pathway. Structural studies have revealed multiple forms of adenylate cyclase that, surprisingly in view of its intracellular functions, contain numerous transmembrane spans (Krupinski et al 1989). The structure has many features shared with G protein-regulated Ca^{2+} channels and transporter molecules. These structural similarities probably relate to hitherto unrecognised functions of adenylate cyclase. The cyclases differ in their sensitivity to calcium and to G proteins so that they too will eventually need to be specified in the description of the action of any receptor, G protein, adenyl cyclase cascade. Molecular cloning has isolated many proteins with good homology to these seven-transmembrane segment receptors but their ligands remain unknown. These 'orphan' receptors may represent a source of future drugs for psychiatry as their expression pattern and pharmacology are elucidated.

Ligand-gated ion channels Many of the best-known transmitter actions are mediated by this super-family of receptors. Acetylcholine acts at the neuromuscular junction on just such a receptor and the major receptors for glutamate and for GABA in brain are also of this type. The nicotinic acetylcholine receptor, because of the ease of its purification from the electroplax of fish, was the first to be isolated and its molecular structure is now described in some detail. The molecular biology of this receptor allowed the investigation of the other receptors of this class. They all have ion channels formed from several subunits (usually five) and the pentamer may be formed of many combinations of the individual subunits – thus perhaps conferring a variety of subtle properties on the receptors formed with different combinations.

The pentameric structure of the nicotinic receptor formed of two α, two β and one γ subunit is shown in Figure 3.10. It is thought that as acetylcholine binds to the α subunits the channel opens wider and allows the passage of cations, thus depolarising the membrane. The resulting excitatory postsynaptic potential (EPSP) may reach threshold for the voltage-sensitive Na^+ channel to open and an action potential be generated.

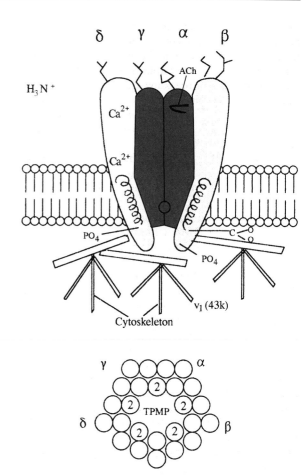

Fig. 3.10 Model of the ion channel of the nicotinic acetylcholine receptor. **A** Longitudinal section (ACh, acetylcholine). **B** Cross-section at the level of the site labelled by TPMP. (After Guy & Hucho 1987.)

Not all the receptor operated ion channels are excitatory, however, and although the structure of the receptor shares many features in common with the nicotinic channel the GABA receptor tetrameric channel opens to allow K^+ and Cl^- to pass through, with the consequence that the membrane resting potential is 'clamped' at Cl^- equilibrium potential and so it is harder to change the membrane potential and the generation of action potentials is inhibited. One note of caution is perhaps warranted at this stage: since each of the subunits of the receptor exists in many forms, it seems likely that there may be some combinations which never occur in vivo, otherwise the numbers of different GABA receptors would be astronomical!

Finally, some ligand-gated ion-channel receptors

may have a major effect intracellularly, in spite of the fact that the agonist opens an ion channel. This is particularly the case if the ion channel allows the entry of Ca^{2+}. This Ca^{2+} is just as able as the Ca^{2+} liberated by phosphatidylinositol breakdown to initiate cascades of intracellular signalling pathways, and indeed it seems likely that the potency of the N – methyl – D – aspartate (NMDA) glutamate receptor depends on just such a cascade.

Steroid and thyroid hormone receptors Receptors for steroid and thyroid hormones are members of a single family of receptor macromolecules. These are physiological regulatory proteins that each possess a region ('ligand-binding domain') that recognises steroid and thyroid hormones (ligands) and a structural part that couples the receptor to intracellular metabolic processes. Receptors for steroid and thyroid hormones, vitamin D and the retinoids are all part of this 'receptor family' (Evans 1988). The part of these receptors that binds to the hormone is crucial to the receptor's function. Removal of this part of the receptor produces an active receptor fragment almost as effective in the regulation of genetic transcription as the natural hormone-bound receptor. Binding of the natural hormone to its receptor removes the inhibitory effect of the remainder of the receptor structure. The second of the three parts of the receptor binds to regulatory sites on nuclear DNA. These DNA-binding regions are soluble proteins that in their inactivated state inhibit transcription of the related gene. They are highly receptor specific so that each type may mediate the effects of a specific endogenous ligand with the relevant ligand-responsive gene. The third component of the steroid/thyroid receptor is ill understood but probably serves to promote the regulatory activity of the receptor macromolecule.

Tyrosine kinase-linked receptors The receptors for nerve growth factor (NGF) have long been a puzzle but the recent description of the receptors for NGF and for a range of neuronal growth and survival factors called *neurotrophins* has revealed a set of receptors which are rapidly growing to become another superfamily. In this case the molecular structure is unlike any of the above receptors and usually include a tyrosine kinase region as well as a membrane attachment domain. The receptors are relatively specific to their neurotrophin agonist and get the imaginative names of *trk* (for tyrosine kinase) A, B and C. The next step in the intracellular signalling pathway is unclear but a range of compounds which act downstream of these receptors is beginning to be developed (inhibitors of tyrosine kinases for example), which may well lead to a deeper understanding of the molecular action of these receptors in the near future.

AMINO ACID NEUROTRANSMISSION

Inhibitory amino acid neurotransmission (IAA)

GABA and the amino acid glycine are the major inhibitory neurotransmitters. GABA receptors are more abundant at inhibitory synapses in the brain, whereas glycine receptors are more numerous in the brainstem and spinal cord.

Postsynaptic inhibition is mediated by the opening of ion channels in the postsynaptic membrane. These are selectively permeable to Cl^- and small monovalent cations. Electrophysiological studies show that glycine and GABA receptors have similar properties.

Glycine receptors

Recent pharmacological and molecular biological studies of receptors for GABA and glycine have established that several receptor macromolecules are involved. The postsynaptic glycine receptor (GlyR) is a large membrane-spanning glycoprotein complex which on binding with glycine forms an anion-selective transmembrane channel (Fig. 3.11). GlyR is a member of the ligand-gated ion channel superfamily of receptors (Betz 1987). Although these receptors are plentiful throughout the CNS and are of presumed biological importance, the neuropharmacology of glycine remains poorly understood. The amino acids taurine and β-alanine are effective agonists at GlyR but alanine, proline and serine are less effective. No non-amino acid agonists at GlyR have been detected but GABA has little effect at GlyR at physiological concentrations. GlyR antagonists include strychnine (a potent neurotoxic convulsant), which is believed to have its own specific binding site on GlyR close to the integral ion channel.

Like other ligand-gated ion channels GlyR is composed of a core made up of four subunits, two of which are the same (Fig. 3.11). The role of GlyR in neurodegenerative disease is largely unexplored. In Parkinson's disease and motor neurone disease, GlyR–strychnine binding sites are reduced.

GABA receptors

GABA is the main cortical inhibitory neurotransmitter. Its inhibitory actions are Cl^- dependent and are blocked by the plant alkaloid bicuculline. Some effects of GABA are, however, insensitive to bicuculline, indicating the existence of two different types of GABA receptor. The classical $GABA_A$ receptor is a 'ligand-gated ion channel' that has an integral transmembrane Cl^- channel that mediates GABAergic transmission by opening and

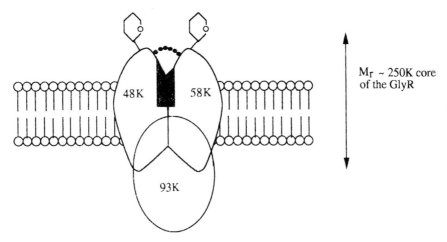

Fig. 3.11 The postsynaptic glycine receptor (GlyR). The core of the receptor is likely to be made up of four subunits, but only one copy of each subunit is shown here. (After Betz 1987.)

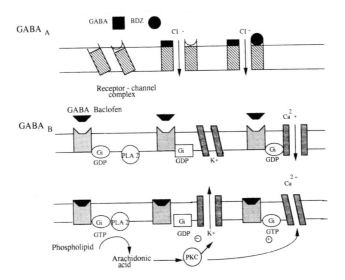

Fig. 3.12 GABA$_A$ and GABA$_B$ receptors. The GABA$_A$ receptor complex with its central Cl$^-$ ion channel is modulated by benzodiazepine binding (BDZ), which may increase Cl$^-$ currents (shown by a thicker arrow). GABA$_B$ receptors are coupled to two G proteins affecting K$^+$ and Ca^{2+} permeabilities in opposite directions.

allowing Cl$^-$ entry. Less is known about GABA$_B$ receptors. They are coupled to G proteins and linked to Ca^{2+} or K$^+$ channels (Fig. 3.12).

The GABA$_A$ receptor is the major inhibitory molecule in brain. It is present on most brain neurones, exists in several forms, and has at least four different sites at which ligands may bind (Fig. 3.12). These sites are for:

- the GABA agonist/antagonist
- picrotoxin (where agents that block GABAergic transmission may bind)
- benzodiazepine drugs
- CNS depressant drugs (these are multiple) where agents may bind and prolong GABAergic activation of the integral channel.

Each of these sites may be occupied simultaneously by their respective ligands, implying that each is a physically distinct part of the same receptor molecule. A group of molecular biologists led by Eric Barnard achieved the first purification and then sequenced the $GABA_A$ receptor protein. The purified protein contains subunits of the types α (about 53 000 Da) and β (about 57 000 Da). The receptor is composed of the combinations of four subunits, which may be either α or β (i.e. it is a heterotetrameric protein). Electrophysiological studies show that occupation of both of the two binding sites for GABA is necessary to open the integral Cl^- channel. These sites are on the two β subunits and binding sites for benzodiazepine drugs are on the two α subunits. Receptor complementary DNA (cDNA) cloning and functional expression of full-length α and β subunits provide conclusive evidence that the α and β subunits constitute the receptor and its chloride channel. The genes for α_1, α_2, α_3, and β_2 subunits of the $GABA_A$ receptor have been cloned and expressed in cell lines to produce reconstituted ion channels. These have been made up of combinations of single $GABA_A$ receptor subunits and have characteristics (ion permeability and ligand binding) of the native receptor (Blair et al 1988) that suggest these characteristics are determined by substructures of the subunits that are shared by all subunits. The gene encoding the α_3 subunit of the $GABA_A$ receptor is on the X chromosome in a region previously linked to susceptibility to manic–depressive illness. The $GABA_A$-α_3 gene is a possible candidate gene for this group of disorders (Bell et al 1989). The constituent amino acid segments of the receptor comprise parts that are sufficiently large to span the membrane and are also hydrophobic. Both α and β subunits contain four such parts and have a cytoplasmic loop. The β subunit loop is longer and probably serves to modulate receptor function. The entire receptor thus contains 16 transmembrane subunits (α_2, β_2) and these crowd around the integral ion channel of 506 Å diameter. Five α subunits could make up the necessary diameter but the likeliest solution is that one helix from each of four different subunits together form a single ion channel (Barnard et al 1987, Schofield et al 1987).

Benzodiazepine drugs are widely used as anxiolytics and anticonvulsants. They bind with high affinity to sites at the $GABA_A$ receptor and potentiate the actions of GABA. Pharmacological studies of benzodiazepine-binding sites show that the $GABA_A$ receptor may contain variants of α and β subunits. Expression of recombinant subunits produces functional receptors. When variants of the α subunit are coexpressed with standard β subunits the receptors produced are differentially distributed in the CNS (Lüddens et al 1990).

Inverse benzodiazepine receptor agonists of the β-carboline type decrease $GABA_A$ receptor-induced Cl^- flow through the central channel. Epileptogenic agents like picrotoxin and t-butyl bicyclophosphorothionate (TBPS) block the Cl^- channel by binding at a site close to the channel (Fig. 3.12). The convulsant actions of penicillin G and pentylenetetrazole involve blocking $GABA_A$ receptor function by an unknown mechanism. Barbiturates prolong $GABA_A$ receptor channel burst duration but do not affect conductance and directly activate Cl^- channels. The synthetic steroid alphaxalone has similar actions to barbiturates and points to the possibility that endogenous steroid metabolites may modulate $GABA_A$ receptor function. The regulation of $GABA_A$ receptor function by intracellular mechanisms is little understood. $GABA_A$ receptor sensitivity is substantially reduced after a rapid increase in intracellular Ca^{2+} concentration and this suggests that Ca^{2+} may alter $GABA_A$ receptor function in vivo (Inoue et al 1987). The cytoplasmic loops of the α and β subunits contain phosphorylation sites for cyclic adenosine monophosphate (cAMP)-dependent protein kinase, and their presence indicates interactions between the $GABA_A$ receptor and protein phosphorylation of a second messenger system.

$GABA_B$ receptors are pharmacologically differentiated from $GABA_A$ receptors. They are unaffected by bicuculline and are not stimulated by GABAergic drugs such as isoguvacine. GABA binds at both $GABA_A$ and $GABA_B$ receptors, but only $GABA_B$ receptors are selectively stimulated by (–)-baclofen (β-p-chlorophenyl GABA). There is, however, a paucity of specific antagonists at $GABA_B$ receptors with which to explore its pharmacology.

The $GABA_B$ receptor is not associated with an integral Cl^- channel. Instead, it is coupled to adjacent Ca^{2+} channels by G proteins and its structure shows it to be a member of the seven helices membrane-spanning superfamily of receptors. Binding between GABA or its agonist baclofen at the $GABA_B$ receptor selectively opens K^+ channels and closes Ca^{2+} channels (Deisz & Lux 1985). The $GABA_B$ receptor activates two membrane-bound G proteins. There are thus two likely routes along which the $GABA_B$ receptor can modify K^+ and Ca^{2+}: one involves G_i protein and the other involves G_o. G_i inhibits adenyl cyclase which opens K^+ channels, while the activation of G_o results in the closing of the Ca^{2+} channels.

$GABA_A$ and $GABA_B$ receptors share inhibitory functions in the CNS. They represent distinct receptor populations whose physiological functions are as yet poorly understood. The $GABA_B$ receptor may be more important in the regulation of Ca^{2+} entry and has been shown to have a role in the modulation of Ca^{2+}-dependent neurotransmitter release, and to be present presynaptically. $GABA_A$ receptors are more widely distributed than $GABA_B$ receptors and may have important roles in the control of receptor sensitivity (Bormann 1988); they appear to be mainly postsynaptic in location. Thus, like many other transmitters, GABA has receptors which are members of both of the major superfamilies, whose location in brain is different.

Excitatory amino acid neurotransmitters

Excitatory amino acid neurotransmitters (EAAs) are the focus of considerable current research. There is extensive evidence that EAAs provide the CNS with many useful functions that are essential in learning and memory, in the structural and functional organisational changes (plasticity) that occur in neural development and in the neurodegeneration of ageing. The most abundant EAAs are glutamate and aspartate and, together with cysteic acid and homocysteic acid, are the most frequently encountered excitatory neurotransmitters in the brain.

EAA effects are mediated through at least five different receptor systems. The first four are ligand-gated ion channels and the fifth is coupled to G proteins and stimulates the $IP–Ca^{2+}$ intracellular signalling pathway. The properties of these receptors are shown in Table 3.7

(Sladeczek et al 1988) and are pharmacologically defined as:

- N-methyl-D-aspartate (NMDA)
- quisqualate (Q)
- kainate (K)
- L-2 aminophosphorobutyric acid (AP4)
- the metabotropic glutamate receptor (mGluR).

Non-NMDA receptors (Q or K) are widely distributed. They are highly concentrated in the cerebellum, and elsewhere in the brain their density is markedly different from NMDA receptors (Henley & Barnard 1990).

NMDA receptors include a binding site for glycine and also for phencyclidine (PCP). Interactions between these receptor sites and the ion channels they regulate may prove as complex as the GABA-benzodiazepine ion channel. Although initially introduced as an anaesthetic, PCP is a potent psychotomimetic ('angel dust') and its drug-induced psychosis has been advanced as a useful model of schizophrenia. A similar psychosis can be induced by benzomorphan drugs, which are synthetic opiates (such as cyclazocine) that activate σ opiate receptors. PCP and σ opiate receptor activation antagonises the excitatory effects of NMDA activation but does not affect Q or K receptors (Sonders et al 1988).

Table 3.7	Ionotrophic excitatory amino acid receptor subtypes					
Receptor type	Agonists (most selective)	Competitive antagonists	Non-competitive antagonists	Allosteric agonist	Ions involved in ionotropic functions	Second messengers
NMDA	NMDA IBO	APV APH CPP	Ketamine MK-801, PCP SKF 10047 Mg^{2+}	Glycine	Ca^{2+} K^+ Na^+	Ca^{2+}(***) $1,4,5-IP_3$(**)/ cGMP? (**)
K	K Domoate	γDGG, GDEE, GAMS, FG9065	JSTX		Na^+, K^+	Ca^{2+} (*) $1,4,5-IP_3$ (*)
Q	Q AMPA	γDGG, GDEE, GAMS, FG9065	JSTX		Na^+, K^+	$1,4,5-IP_3$ (?) Ca^{2+} (?)
Qp IBO_P	Q IBO	No antagonist APB, phosphoserine				$1,4,5-IP_3$ (***) $1,4,5-IP_3$(***)

APH, D-2-amino-4-phosphorobutyrate; PCP, phencyclidine; AMPA, α-amino-3-hydroxy-5-methylisoxazole-4-propionic acid; cGMP, cyclic guanosine monophosphate. (*,**,***), level of efficiency in producing second messengers.
After Sladeczek et al (1988).

Glutamate and its analogues are potent neurotoxins (Olney 1989). Exogenous NMDA agonist compounds are established neurotoxins. The legume *Lathyrus satirus* contains β-*N*-oxalylamino-L-alanine (BOAA) which, if ingested chronically, causes neuronal degeneration by excessive excitatory neuronal stimulation. This model of excitatory neurotoxicity by exogenous compounds (as in lathyrism) or endogenous compounds (as proposed for Huntington's disease (Beal et al 1986)) has been extended to include other neurodegenerative disorders, including Alzheimer's disease, head trauma, brain ischaemia and epilepsy (Olney 1989). Antiexcitoxic agents are currently in development and some may soon enter clinical trials of their value in selected neuropsychiatric disorders (Honoré et al 1988).

Kainate receptors also mediate excitatory neurotransmission and are present on both neuronal and glial membranes, especially in the cerebellum. Their pharmacological and structural characteristics are those of the superfamily of ligand-gated ion channels (Gregor et al 1989). Because the NMDA receptor channel is normally blocked by the binding of a Mg^{2+} ion, it seems likely that it is normally silent and that the normal signalling function of glutamate must take place via these other receptor types. In cells with both K and NMDA receptors, the depolarisation due to K receptor activation may reach levels where the Mg^{2+} is released from the NMDA receptor and its activation, with the consequent influx of Ca^{2+} ions, leads to the intracellular cascade already described above and whose final action may well be to change the sensitivity of the cell to excitatory transmission for a very long-time (long-term potentiation or LTP).

CHOLINERGIC NEUROTRANSMISSION

Acetylcholine is a widely distributed neurotransmitter present in the brain in the neostriatal interneurones and septal–hippocampal pathway. Some effects of acetylcholine can be mimicked by muscarine and antagonised by atropine. These are termed 'muscarinic effects'. Other effects of acetylcholine are mimicked by nicotine, not antagonised by atropine but selectively blocked by tubocurarine. These are 'nicotinic effects'. The two types of cholinergic effect are mediated through two classes of cholinergic receptor: muscarinic and nicotinic. Cholinergic neuropharmacology is summarised in Table 3.8.

Nicotinic receptors are ligand-gated ion channels and, when activated by ligand binding, produce a rapid increase in cellular permeability to Na^+ and K^+. Muscarinic receptors are G protein-coupled and are not necessarily only linked to ion channels. The structures of nicotinic and muscarinic receptors show that they belong to two distinct superfamilies of receptor types. The channel of the nicotinic cholinergic receptor is composed of five homologous subunits (Guy & Hucho 1987). The neuromuscular nicotinic receptor contains four distinct subunits (α, β, δ, γ) arranged as a pentamer (the γ subunit is replaced by an ε subunit in adult muscle). Nicotinic receptors in the CNS are also pentamers but comprise only two subunits (α and β). Brain nicotinic receptors are open to complex variation as there are multiple forms of both α and β subunits and it appears that different parts of the brain contain different combinations of α and β subtypes. The structure of the nicotinic receptor is shown in Figure 3.10. The four genes encoding the $α_2$, $α_3$, $α_4$ and $β_2$ subunits of the nicotinic cholinergic receptor are differentially distributed in vertebrate brain. All four mRNAs are present in the cerebellum, whereas only $α_2$ and $β_2$ mRNAs are found in lateral spiriform nuclei (Morris et al 1990). This indicates that neurones are capable of differential expression in vivo of nicotinic receptor subunits and points to nicotinic receptor heterogeneity in the CNS. The mRNAs for these subunits also show different temporal patterns of expression during brain development (Moss et al 1989).

Muscarinic cholinergic receptors also exist as various subtypes. Pharmacological studies had supported the subdivision of muscarinic receptors into M_1, M_2 and M_3. Structural studies have determined three corresponding receptor subtypes termed m_1, m_2 and m_3. Two further molecules termed m_4 and m_5 have been detected, but little is known of their functions and distribution. Like all other G protein-coupled receptors, there are seven transmembrane domains; the characteristics of muscarinic receptors are shown in Table 3.9 (Bonner 1989).

Muscarinic receptors M_1 and M_3 activate a G protein that stimulates PLC activity. PLC stimulates hydrolysis of phosphatidylinositol phosphates to IP_3, which can release intracellular Ca^{2+}. DAG is also produced by PLC and this leads to PKC activation. Ligand binding to M_2 and M_4 receptors activates G_i proteins which inhibit adenylate cyclase, and open K^+ and close Ca^{2+} channels.

Drugs affecting acetylcholine synthesis

Acetylcholine is synthesised in a single step from acetyl coenzyme A (produced in neuronal mitochondria) and choline (from the liver), which is catalysed by choline acetyltransferase. Synthesis of acetylcholine can be increased by choline administration because the synthetic enzyme is not fully saturated.

Table 3.8 Cholinergic pharmacology

Presynaptic

Site of action	Effect	Drug	Use
Synthesis	Increases	Choline	Experimental
	Decreases	Hemicholinium	Experimental
Storage	Inhibits acetylcholine vesicle transport	Vesamicol	Experimental
Release	Increases	Black widow spider venom	Experimental
	Blocks	Botulinum toxin	Experimental

Postsynaptic

Receptor	Tissue	Agonist responses	Agonist	Antagonist	Molecular mechanisms
M_1	Cerebral cortex	?	Oxotremorine	Atropine	$\uparrow$PLC
	Sympathetic ganglia	Depolarisation		Pirenzepine	$\uparrow$Ca^{2+}
M_2	Heart	Slowed depolarisation		Atropine	$\uparrow$K$^+$ channels
	Sinoatrial node	Hyperpolarisation			$\downarrow$Adenylate cyclase
	Atrium	Shortened action potential			
	Atrioventricular node	Decreased contractile force			
	Ventricle	Decreased conduction velocity			
M_3	Smooth muscle				$\uparrow$PLC
	Secretory glands				$\uparrow$Ca^{2+}

Degradation

Cholinesterase inhibitors (e.g. physostigmine)

Table 3.9 Properties of cloned muscarinic receptors

Property	m_1	m_2	m_3	m_4	m_5
Molecular weight	51 387	51 681	66 085	53 014	60 120
Pirenzepine affinity	High	Low	$\longleftarrow$ intermediate $\longrightarrow$		
Phosphatidylinositol response	Stimulates	None	Stimulates	None	Stimulates
cAMP response	Stimulates	Inhibits	Stimulates	Inhibits	Stimulates
Arachidonic acid response	Stimulates	None	Stimulates	None	Stimulates
Ca^{2+}-dependent K_A^+ channel	Opens	No effect	Opens	No effect	?
mRNA distribution	Brain	Brain	Brain	Brain	?
	Glands	Heart	Smooth muscle		
		Smooth muscle			

After Bonner (1989).

Drugs affecting acetylcholine release

Newly synthesised acetylcholine is preferentially released on stimulation from storage in presynaptic cholinergic terminals. Black widow spider venom produces a rapid release of acetylcholine and also causes morphological changes in the presynaptic storage vesicles.

Drugs affecting nicotinic receptors

Nicotinic receptors are excitatory and function by opening ionic channels. They are specifically blocked by α-bungarotoxin. Nicotinic receptors are present in the brain, particularly in the thalamus and cerebellar cortex. Outside the brain, the cholinergic input from the spinal cord synapses on to nicotinic receptors at the neurotransmitter junction. Most nicotinic receptor antagonists have profound effects at the neuromuscular junction. The best known agent is (+)-tubocurarine, which does not easily cross the blood–brain barrier. Decamethonium and succinylcholine are also nicotinic receptor antagonists but, instead of competing with acetylcholine for the receptor site, they bind to the receptor for a long period, making it insensitive to acetylcholine. Like (+)-tubocurarine, decamethonium and succinylcholine have almost no central effects. Agonists at nicotinic receptors include nicotine, dimethyl-phenylpiperazinium (DMPP) and phenyl-trimethylammonium (PTMA).

Nicotine is present in tobacco (*Nicotiana tabacum*) and most smokers identify 'stress reduction' as a major determinant of their habit, saying that smoking helps them to relax. Small, repeated injections of nicotine, similar to those received while smoking, produce increased cortical release of acetylcholine and electro-cortical arousal. Adrenergic blockade has no effect on this action of nicotine but both muscarinic and nicotinic blockade prevent nicotine from activating the cortex. Lesion studies suggest that tobacco smoking increases electrocortical arousal by acting at sites of the cholinergic projections to the cortex. Low doses of nicotine produce stimulation in the periphery, while higher doses block nicotinic receptors and cause paralysis of neuromuscular junctions.

Drugs affecting muscarinic receptors

M_1 receptors are concentrated in the sympathetic ganglia, stomach and corpus striatum. They are selectively antagonised by pirenzipine and are closely associated with K^+ channels. M_2 receptors are concentrated in the hindbrain, cerebellum and heart. They are regulated by gallamine and GTP and inhibit adenylate cyclase. Muscarinic receptor antagonists, therefore, have both central and peripheral actions. Atropine and scopolamine are the best known and, in the periphery, they decrease secretion from the gut, nasopharynx and respiratory tract and increase the heart rate. Their central effects include confusion, lassitude and drowsiness, and

higher doses can cause delirium ('atropine psychosis'). Agonists at muscarinic receptors include muscarine, pilocarpine, arecoline, methacholine and carbachol.

The tricyclic antidepressants commonly cause anticholinergic side-effects. These include dry mouth, excessive sweating, blurring of vision and urinary retention, which may be especially troublesome in the elderly. It is important, therefore, to know the relative potencies at muscarinic receptors of antidepressant drugs to guide prescribing, for example, in patients with glaucoma or prostatism. Amitriptyline has about 5% of the anticholinergic potency of atropine, but, as it is used in much greater doses (100–150 mg daily) than the well-known anticholinergics (0.6 mg), its therapeutic administration can produce an extensive blockade of cholinergic receptors.

Parkinsonism

Until the introduction of L-dopa and decarboxylase inhibitors, anticholinergic drugs formed the mainstay of treatment for parkinsonism. These drugs remain useful for patients in the early stages of Parkinson's disease, for patients unable to tolerate L-dopa and in addition to L-dopa in selected patients. They can be especially useful in drug-induced parkinsonism.

The anticholinergic drugs used to treat drug-induced parkinsonism are tertiary amines (benztropine, trihexyphenidyl and procyclidine). Their extra-CNS antimuscarinic effects are much weaker than atropine. Diphenhydramine is an antihistamine drug that has slight anticholinergic properties and is especially well tolerated by old people.

Anticholinesterases

Anticholinesterase drugs cause acetylcholine to accumulate at cholinergic synapses. These drugs inhibit the enzyme acetylcholinesterase, and the prototype drug is physostigmine. Others were developed as insecticides and investigated for use in chemical warfare. These latter types cause irreversible inhibition of acetylcholinesterase. The mechanism of action of anticholinesterases (including physostigmine) is based on their binding with the enzyme and, in the case of physostigmine and neostigmine, hydrolysing slowly. The terms 'reversible' and 'irreversible' as applied to anticholinesterases are only relative and refer to the speed at which the enzyme recovers function. In psychiatry, the main use of physostigmine is experimental in Alzheimer's disease, where it may transiently produce a modest improvement in mental functions. Rarely, intravenous physostigmine may be used to reverse a brief psychosis induced by antimuscarinic drugs.

Physostigmine does not reverse the anticholinergic cardiotoxic effects of tricyclic antidepressants.

NORADRENERGIC NEUROTRANSMISSION

An understanding of the classification and properties of the different types of adrenoceptor is essential to understanding the diverse effects of catecholamines and the neuropharmacology of this system. Physiological studies by Ahlquist (1948) supported the distinction between two types of adrenoceptor, termed α and β. This initial distinction was supported by observations on adrenergic antagonists at α adrenoceptors (e.g. phenoxybenzamine) and β adrenoceptors (e.g. propranolol). Subsequently, β receptors were subdivided into β_1 and β_2, and later structural studies identified a third type, termed β_3. The relative number of each of these subtypes varies with tissue type. α Adrenoceptors are present in the iris where they stimulate contraction of the radial muscle, thus producing dilation. They are also present in the eyelid where their stimulation raises the lid. The heart contains β_1 receptors which mediate increases in both the rate and force of cardiac contractions. All β receptors are coupled through G proteins to the enzyme adenylate cyclase.

Table 3.10 summarises the sites of action, effects and uses of drugs that act on noradrenergic neurotransmission. Some drugs act specifically at noradrenergic synapses, while others affect several monoamines. Tricyclic antidepressants are believed to have mood-elevating actions because of their inhibition of uptake of monoamines, particularly noradrenaline and serotonin, from the synaptic cleft. These actions of antidepressants have led to the 'monoamine hypothesis of affective disorders', which, simply stated, postulates that in depressive illness there is reduced efficiency of neurotransmission at noradrenergic and/or serotonergic synapses and that this may involve abnormalities in the affinity of monoaminergic receptors for their endogenous ligands (Ch. 14).

Drugs inhibiting noradrenaline synthesis

Noradrenaline is synthesised from L-tyrosine by the following steps: L-tyrosine is hydroxylated to L-dopa (by tyrosine hydroxylase), L-dopa is decarboxylated to dopamine (by aromatic-L-amino-acid decarboxylase) and dopamine is then hydroxylated to noradrenaline (by dopamine β-hydroxylase). Tyrosine hydroxylase is inhibited by α-methyl-p-tyrosine, and this drug is used experimentally to prevent the synthesis of dopamine, noradrenaline and adrenaline. Carbidopa inhibits aromatic-L-amino-acid decarboxylase at sites outside the CNS and can be given at the same time as L-dopa, when it will prevent enhancement of dopamine synthesis outside the CNS. Dopamine β-hydroxylase is inhibited by disulfiram and by FLA63. Synthesis of noradrenaline can also be disrupted by the structurally similar precursor α-methyldopa. This is synthesised to α-methylnoradrenaline, which then acts as a 'false neurotransmitter', that is, it is released by the usual mechanisms involved in noradrenaline release but it is much less effective at noradrenaline receptors.

Drugs affecting the storage of noradrenaline

Most noradrenaline is stored in a presynaptic complex of noradrenaline, adenosine triphosphate (ATP), metallic ions of magnesium, calcium, copper and proteins called chromogranins. Dopamine β-hydroxylase is present in noradrenergic storage vesicles, probably in association with the vesicular limiting membrane. Noradrenaline is taken up into storage by an active transport mechanism that is magnesium dependent and requires ATP, although a little noradrenaline is available in the cytoplasm. The *Rauwolfia* alkaloids (e.g. reserpine) and tetrabenazine disrupt noradrenaline storage and inhibit noradrenaline uptake into storage vesicles; reserpine causes irreversible damage to granules, whereas tetrabenazine has reversible effects. These processes can be relatively slow so that noradrenaline released from storage may be degraded by intracellular monoamine oxidase before it can bind with postsynaptic receptors. Reserpine can initially produce postsynaptic adrenoceptor stimulation by releasing noradrenaline, and in the presence of monoamine oxidases it releases the relatively large storage pool on to the postsynaptic receptors.

Drugs affecting the release of noradrenaline

Noradrenaline is released from storage vesicles by a calcium-dependent process involving fusion of the vesicles with the presynaptic membrane and also involving prostaglandins (PGE_2 inhibiting and $PGE_{2\alpha}$ facilitating release). Release may be regulated by prostaglandins and other local hormones acting on noradrenergic nerve terminals. Presynaptic receptors (autoreceptors) are important in the regulation of impulse-induced noradrenaline release and such receptors may be sensitive not only to the local concentration of noradrenaline but also to acetylcholine, cAMP, prostaglandins and neuropeptides like thyrotrophin-releasing hormone.

Drugs that release noradrenaline quickly enough to bind with postsynaptic receptors are called 'indirectly acting sympathomimetic amines'. Examples are

Table 3.10   Noradrenergic pharmacology

Presynaptic

Site of action	Effect	Drug	Use
Synthesis	False transmitter Decreased	a-Methyldopa a-Methyl-*p*-tyrosine	Hypotensive Experimental
Storage	Decreased (irreversible) Decreased (reversible) Increased	Reserpine Tetrabenazine Monoamine oxidase inhibitors (MAOIs)	Hypotensive Chorea Antidepressant
Release	Increased Increased Decreased	Amphetamine Tyramine Debrisoquine	Euphoriant Experimental Hypotensive

Postsynaptic

Receptor	Tissue	Agonist responses	Agonist	Antagonist	Molecular mechanisms
α_1	Vascular smooth muscle	Contracts	Isoprotenerol Phenylephrine	Prazosin	↑PLC ↑IP$_3$ ↑K$^+$ channels ↑Intracellular Ca^{2+}
	Heart	Increased contractile force			
α_2	Neural↓	↓Noradrenaline release	Clonidine	Yohimbine	↓Adenylate cyclase ↑K$^+$ channels ↓Ca^{2+} channels
	Vascular smooth muscle	Contracts			
β_1	Heart	Increased contractile force			↑Adenylate cyclase ↑Ca^{2+} channels
β_2	Smooth muscle	Relaxation	Salbutamol		↑Adenylate cyclase

Degradation

Site of action	Effect	Drug	Use
Reuptake	Inhibits Inhibits Inhibits	Desipramine Amitriptyline Cocaine	Antidepressant Antidepressant Euphoriant

amphetamine, tyramine and ephedrine. Some drugs inhibit noradrenaline release from storage, for example antihypertensive agents such as debrisoquine, bethanidine and guanethidine. These drugs do not readily cross the blood–brain barrier (their lipid solubility is low) and therefore have few psychotoxic effects.

Drugs acting on adrenergic receptors

There are two main types of receptor for noradrenaline, α and β adrenoceptors. The existence of these two types was deduced from studies on smooth muscle where catecholamines produce both excitatory and inhibitory effects. Later studies of drug-binding to adrenoceptors supported the original division into α and β receptor types. Phenoxybenzamine produces selective blockade of α receptors and propranolol blocks β receptors. The development of more selective antagonist and agonists allowed these receptors to be further subdivided into β_1, β_2, α_1 and α_2 receptors. The relative number of the various subtypes of adrenoceptor varies with each tissue. Stimulation of α adrenoceptors in blood vessels causes vasoconstriction. Additionally, the pilomotor muscles and salivary glands are stimulated through their α adrenoceptors. The gastrointestinal tract has both α and β adrenoceptors and the smooth muscle in the tract relaxes in response to stimulation of either receptor type. Sphincter muscles, however, contract in response to excitation of α adrenoceptors.

The heart contains β_1 receptors which mediate increases in both rate and force of cardiac contraction. Stimulation of β_2 receptors in bronchial smooth muscle produces bronchodilatation. They are also present in the gastrointestinal tract, uterus and bladder, where their stimulation produces smooth muscle relaxation. β Receptors are also involved in the regulation of certain metabolic processes such as increasing lipolysis or gluconeogenesis and reducing insulin release. All β receptors are linked to the enzyme adenylate cyclase, so that stimulation of β receptors increases the synthesis of cAMP from ATP. Phosphodiesterases degrade cAMP to non-cyclic 5'-AMP. Drugs that inhibit phosphodiesterases (such as caffeine, aminophylline and theobromine) enhance the physiological responses to β adrenoceptor stimulation. α Adrenoceptor agonists include noradrenaline and adrenaline. Noradrenaline acts mostly through α adrenoceptors and adrenaline largely through β adrenoceptors. Phenylephrine and clonidine are directly acting α adrenoceptor agonists with few β adrenoceptor effects, and their actions are therefore similar to noradrenaline. Isoprenaline is a synthetic catecholamine acting only on β receptors, where it is more potent than either adrenaline or noradrenaline. Salbutamol is a selective β_2 adrenoceptor agonist and has been used as an antidepressant. The rationale leading to this application is derived from the 'amine hypothesis of depression', where a postulated reduction in the functional efficiency of neurotransmission at synapses involving monoamines concerned with the regulation of mood is accompanied by increased postsynaptic sensitivity to those monoamines. Administration of a selective monoaminergic receptor antagonist such as salbutamol might, therefore, allow re-establishment of more efficient neurotransmission. α Adrenoceptor antagonists are used mostly in experimental work, though phentolamine (a reversible α adrenoceptor antagonist) is useful in the emergency treatment of hypertension and the diagnosis of phaeochromocytomas. Some β adrenoceptor antagonists may have local anaesthetic-like activity on membrane fluidity as well as actions at adrenoceptors. These drugs are used mostly in the control of hypertension and the relief of angina. Their exact mode of action in the control of hypertension is unknown. Non-selective β adrenoceptor antagonists include propranolol and atenolol. Atenolol and metoprolol are selective β_1 adrenoceptor antagonists that in large doses affect all β receptors. These drugs act at both pre- and postsynaptic adrenoceptors. Presynaptic β_1 receptors facilitate noradrenaline release while presynaptic β_2 receptors are

inhibitory. These receptors may be involved in the pathogenesis of affective symptoms and effective antidepressants could exert some or all of their effects at these sites.

Antidepressants and adrenergic receptors

There is a close relationship between the potencies of tricyclic antidepressants to occupy postsynaptic α_1 adrenoceptors and their sedative–hypotensive effects. The tertiary amines (e.g. amitriptyline) are more potent at these sites than secondary amines (e.g. nortriptyline) and are only slightly less potent than the better known α adrenoceptor antagonist phentolamine. Chronic administration of antidepressants, but not short-term treatment, reduces noradrenaline-coupled adenylate cyclase activity and also reduces the number of β receptors in brain tissue. These effects do not seem to be limited to one type of antidepressant treatment but are found with tricyclic drugs, mianserin, iprindole, monoamine oxidase inhibitors and also in an animal model of electroconvulsive therapy (ECT). Some antidepressants may act, therefore, by initially increasing the synaptic concentration of noradrenaline, which in turn reduces the sensitivity and/or number of β adrenoceptors. The initial increase of noradrenaline may be caused by inhibition of noradrenaline uptake, blockade of presynaptic inhibitory autoreceptors, or actions at other sites.

Drugs affecting noradrenaline uptake

Antidepressants and euphoriants such as cocaine and amphetamine act rapidly on the presynaptic reuptake of noradrenaline. The structure of the noradrenaline transporter is known and has much in common with other members of the superfamily of neurotransmitter transporters. The structure is shown schematically in Figure 3.13. Distribution of the transporter matches the localisation of noradrenaline cell bodies in the CNS (Pacholczyk et al 1991). The transporter may be important in neurodegenerative diseases. Potent neurotoxins (such as 1-methyl-4-phenylpyridinium (MPP^+) and 6-hydroxydopamine (6-OH-DA)) can be actively taken up by the noradrenaline transporter and, if allowed to accumulate in neurones, cause selective neuronal death. The transporter is an important site of action of mood-affecting drugs and its further study (e.g. binding to novel, potentially antidepressant compounds) may facilitate new drug development. It may also prove relevant to understanding the genetic contribution to affective disorders.

Uptake of noradrenaline from the synaptic cleft is an energy-consuming process that is sodium dependent

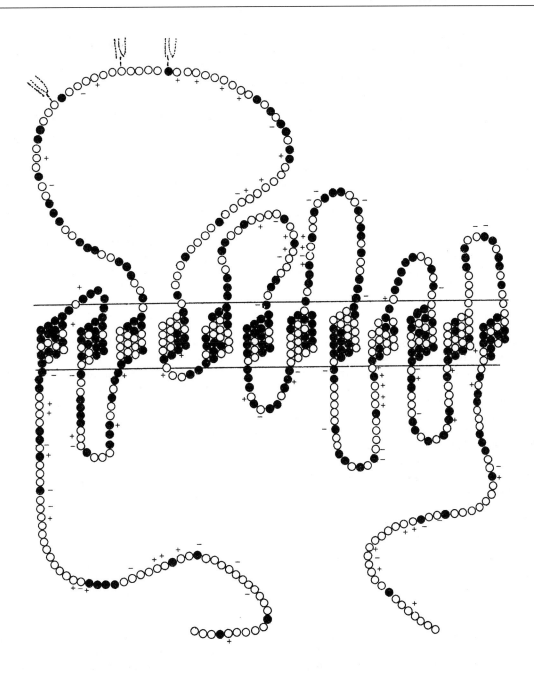

Fig. 3.13 The noradrenaline transporter showing proposed orientation with 12 sections spanning the plasma membrane. Solid circles represent residues conserved with the GABA transporter. Glycosylation sites and charged residues are also indicated. (After Pacholczyk et al 1991 and Snyder 1991.)

and involves ATP. Some drugs inhibit the uptake of monoamines from the synaptic cleft and this is thought to be the principal action of tricyclic antidepressants. These drugs affect both noradrenaline and serotonin uptake but have little effect on dopamine. The tertiary amines imipramine and amitriptyline mostly affect the uptake of serotonin. Secondary amines like desipramine and nortriptyline largely affect noradrenaline. Many tertiary amines are metabolised to secondary amines, so in reality the tertiary amines often affect both noradrenaline and serotonin uptake. A number of drugs have been developed to act selectively on serotonin or noradrenaline uptake but there are no clear differences in antidepressant activity between the two. Inhibition of uptake is evident from pharmacological studies within 24 hours of administration of the drug, but clinical effects are not typically seen for about 10–20 days. Because the tricyclic drugs and their related compounds were derived from the phenothiazines, they share several pharmacological properties with them. In particular, they have anticholinergic and antihistaminergic effects. The anticholinergic effects are evident within hours of first administering the drug and tolerance usually develops before the onset of the antidepressant effect. For these reasons, the anticholinergic effects of the tricyclics are probably not relevant to their antidepressant action. Further, the incidence of anticholinergic side-effects does not differ between patients who respond and those who do not respond to a tricyclic. The antihistaminergic effects of tricyclic drugs may prove relevant to their antidepressant actions. The commonly prescribed tricyclic drugs are amitriptyline, clomipramine, desipramine, dothiepin, doxepin, imipramine, iprindole, nortriptyline, protriptyline and trimipramine.

Drugs affecting degradation of noradrenaline

Noradrenaline that is not taken up by the presynaptic terminal from the synaptic cleft can be fused into the postsynaptic membrane, where it is degraded by the enzymes monoamine oxidase and catechol-O-methyltransferase (COMT). Monoamine oxidases are a group of enzymes that are present in a wide variety of tissues in which their substrate specificity and physical properties may differ. There are two types, known as A and B. Type A is more effective in the degradation of noradrenaline, serotonin and dopamine. Tyramine (a naturally occurring amino acid present in many foods) is a substrate for both forms and the use of a monoamine oxidase inhibitor is associated with the hazard of toxic reactions to excessive amounts of tyramine. The antidepressant actions of monoamine oxidase inhibitors such as tranylcypromine, pargyline, phenelzine and clorgyline (a selective type A inhibitor) are produced largely by their inhibition of monoamine oxidase. They also affect aromatic-L-amino-acid decarboxylase and various other oxidases and inhibit uptake of noradrenaline and serotonin, but the clinical relevance of these effects is not known. The metabolism of concomitantly administered drugs may also be affected by monoamine oxidase inhibitors so that the action of barbiturates may

be prolonged and the effect of amphetamine exaggerated.

Monoamine oxidase inhibitors also reduce the 'first-pass' presystemic degradation of tyramine after its intestinal absorption. Tyramine is selectively taken up into adrenergic neurones (by a high-affinity system), where it releases stored noradrenaline. Monoamine oxidase inhibitors thus potentiate the effects of tyramine and other indirectly acting sympathomimetic agents. New monoamine oxidase inhibitors have been developed that are selective for monoamine oxidase A and there are claims that these do not potentiate the tyramine response and are also effective antidepressants. Moclobemide is a novel reversible inhibitor of monoamine oxidase A. Since it spares the monoamine oxidase A present in the gut as a defence against ingested amines, it is potentially a useful antidepressant (Callingham & Ovens 1988).

DOPAMINERGIC NEUROTRANSMISSION

The modern era of pharmacotherapy in psychiatry began with the introduction of phenothiazine antipsychotics in 1952 and was quickly followed by the development of phenothiazine-derived tricyclic antidepressants. At first, the mode of action of these drugs was unknown, but during the past 30 years the effects of antipsychotic drugs on central dopaminergic transmission have been established as an important component of their antipsychotic actions. The neuropharmacology of dopaminergic neurotransmission is summarised in Table 3.11.

Dopamine synthesis

Dopamine is synthesised from the amino acid L-tyrosine by the following steps: L-tyrosine is hydroxylated to L-dopa (by tyrosine hydroxylase) and then decarboxylated (by aromatic-L-amino-acid decarboxylase) to form dopamine. Oral administration of L-dopa increases dopamine synthesis. In Parkinson's disease, dopaminergic neurones are damaged and have a much reduced capacity to synthesise dopamine. Adjacent glial cells retain dopamine synthetic capacity and, during L-dopa therapy, dopamine may leak out from these glial cells to stimulate surviving supersensitive dopamine receptors. Alternatively the serotonin nerve terminals in the basal ganglia contain a closely related decarboxylase which could also supply dopamine from applied L-dopa.

Dopamine storage

Dopamine is stored in presynaptic complexes of

Table 3.11 Dopaminergic pharmacology

Presynaptic

Site of action	Effect	Drug	Use
Synthesis	Inhibits	α-Methyltyrosine	Occasionally in phaeochromocytoma
	Increases	L-Dopa	Parkinson's disease
Storage	Inhibits	Tetrabenazine	Chorea
		α-Methyltyrosine	As above
		Reserpine	Occasionally in treatment of refractory psychoses
Release	Increases	Amphetamine	Experimental
	Inhibits	γ-Hydroxybutyrate	Experimental

Postsynaptic

Receptor	Tissue	Agonist	Antagonist	Molecular mechanisms
	Renal Mesenteric/ coronary vessels (vasodilatation) Pituitary–hypothalamic axis			↑cAMP
D$_1$	Cell bodies and presynaptic terminals of intrinsic striatal neurones	Pergolide SKF 38393	Lisuride SCH 23390	↑Adenylate cyclase
D$_2$	Neuronal cell bodies of striatum and presynaptic terminals of dopaminergic striatal neurones	Bromocriptine Pergolide Lisuride Apomorphine	Butyrophenones Sulpiride	↓Adenylate cyclase or no effect

Degradation

Site of action	Effect	Drug	Use
Uptake	Inhibits	Benztropine	Parkinson's disease
		Nomifensine	Experimental
		Cocaine	Experimental
		Amitriptyline	Antidepressant

dopamine, ATP, magnesium, calcium, copper and chromogranins. Drugs that disrupt the storage of noradrenaline, like *Rauwolfia* alkaloids and tetrabenazine, also disrupt dopamine storage complexes, and many of the behavioural sequelae of their administration may be related to the action of dopamine storage rather than on noradrenaline.

Dopamine release

Dopamine is released from central dopaminergic terminals by two discrete mechanisms that differ in their sensitivity to dopamine uptake inhibitors (Raiteri et al 1979). An energy-dependent transport mechanism for dopamine uptake is inhibited by nomifensine, benztropine and cocaine. A second carrier-independent mechanism for dopamine release is dependent upon extracellular Ca^{2+} concentrations and involves fusion of dopamine-containing vesicles with the presynaptic membrane upon the Ca^{2+} influx which follows action potentials. This type of release is facilitated by amphetamine at concentrations much lower than those required for amphetamine to stimulate postsynaptic catecholaminergic receptors. Amphetamines stimulate rapid release of dopamine, inhibit its uptake from the synaptic cleft and also inhibit its degradative enzyme monoamine oxidase.

The dopamine hypothesis of schizophrenia

The 'dopamine hypothesis of schizophrenia', simply stated, postulates that certain dopaminergic pathways are overactive in schizophrenia and so cause the symptoms of an acute schizophrenic episode. Clinical studies indicate that drugs like L-dopa or amphetamine which potentiate dopaminergic activity may induce or exacerbate schizophrenic symptoms.

When the neuroleptic drugs were first introduced, their mode of antipsychotic action was unknown. At first, studies in the peripheral nervous system suggested that the antiadrenergic effects of chlorpromazine probably explained its antipsychotic action, perhaps by reducing arousal. However, the fact that potent antiadrenergic agents had no antipsychotic benefit clearly did not support this hypothesis. Carlsson & Lindqvist (1963) first suggested that dopamine receptor blockade was the basis of neuroleptic effects. The low activity of butyrophenone antipsychotics at dopamine receptor sites linked to adenylate cyclase stimulation was seen as evidence against this idea. It was supported, however, by the recognition of two types of dopamine receptor. One (called D_1) was linked to adenylate cyclase stimulation and another, higher affinity one (called D_2) sometimes associated with adenylate cyclase inhibition and for which there was preferential binding of butyrophenones.

Neuropharmacological studies provide virtually all the evidence to support the 'dopamine hypothesis of schizophrenia'. Although some of the newer 'atypical' antipsychotic agents are weak dopamine receptor antagonists, all effective antipsychotics are believed to share the ability to impair dopaminergic neurotransmission. Postmortem studies of schizophrenic brains have demonstrated increased dopamine receptor (D_2) densities, but these densities are probably considerably influenced by antemortem drug treatments. Positron emission tomography studies on D_2 receptor binding in neuroleptic-naive schizophrenic patients have provided conflicting results. Wong et al (1986) reported a 2–3-fold increase in D_2 receptor densities of drug-free patients when compared with controls, but a later more extensive study by Farde et al (1990) did not support the earlier finding.

The CNS location of the site of antipsychotic action of neuroleptic drugs is unknown. Dopamine receptors are present in the basal ganglia, the mesolimbic system, the tuberoinfundibular region and, to a much lesser extent, in the cerebral cortex. Studies on the effects of dopaminergic transmission of psychotomimetic agents such as amphetamine, PCP and benzmorphan point to a possible common mechanism of psychotic action. Carlsson (1988) has proposed that 'information overload' and 'hyperarousal' are integral features of many psychotic illnesses. He postulates that these features arise because of impairment of the protective effects on cortical function of the mesolimbic system. In health, Carlsson argues that mesolimbic glutaminergic neurones oppose mesolimbic dopaminergic pathways and maintain this protective function. It is true that drug-induced psychoses are caused by blocking glutaminergic function (e.g. by PCP or benzmorphan) or by increasing dopaminergic activity (e.g. amphetamine). Recent anatomical investigations show that dopamine synapses are present on, or close to, the necks of spines on dendrites in the basal ganglia where glutamate synapses are present on the heads of the same spines. This close anatomical association may well be the substrate for the dopamine–glutamate interactions which many authors associate with psychotic symptoms.

Dopamine receptors

Pharmacological studies show that there are at least two types of dopamine receptor: D_1 and D_2. There is very good agreement between the affinity of a standard antipsychotic drug for D_2 receptors and the average daily dose of that drug used to treat schizophrenia. The structures of D_1 and D_2 receptors are now established and when expressed in cell lines are seen to possess the pharmacological properties predicted in earlier studies.

Blockade of D_2 receptors is the likely cause of unwanted extrapyramidal system (EPS) effects and, therefore, if blockade of the D_2 receptor is also the site of antipsychotic action, all effective neuroleptics should be equipotent in the induction of EPS symptoms and in antipsychotic efficacy. Some newer drugs used to treat schizophrenia (sometimes termed 'atypical') have a lower tendency to produce EPS effects than older neuroleptics such as haloperidol. (Atypical antipsychotic drugs include thioridazine, sulpiride and clozapine.) Pharmacological studies have not detected differences between postsynaptic D_2 receptors located in the striatum (where EPS effects arise) and in the mesolimbic system (where the antipsychotic action is presumed to be located).

Structural analysis of dopamine receptor types has revealed a family of at least five similar G protein-coupled molecules (Sunahara et al 1990). The mRNA for D_1 is most abundant in the caudate, nucleus accumbens and olfactory tubercle, with little in the substantia nigra (Dearry et al 1990). Structurally, D_1 receptors are most like the β adrenoceptor (Sunahara et al 1990, Zhou et al 1990) and are functionally coupled to adenylate cyclase (Monsma et al 1990). Subsequently, similarities between the known structures of G protein-coupled receptors helped to isolate and characterise the D_2 receptor (Bunzow et al 1988). Structural studies also identified two D_2 receptor isoforms; one predicted by pharmacological studies but the other appearing to be novel (Giros et al 1989) and probably an alternative product of a single D_2 gene (Monsma et al 1989). The D_2 receptor isoforms are termed $D_2(414)$ or D_{2short} and $D_2(443)$ or D_{2long}. Discovery of D_2 isoforms suggests a means by which different dopaminergic neuronal populations might adjust responses to stimuli (such as chronic exposure to neuroleptics) or be a source of genetically determined receptor variability of possible relevance to the aetiology of schizophrenia. However, no abnormalities of D_2 isoform structure in schizophrenia have been described, though linkage between the D_2 receptor gene (located in the q22–q23 region of human chromosome 11) has been reported in alcoholism (Blum et al 1990).

In in situ hybridisation it has been shown that the spiny output cells of the caudate/putamen are in two classes. In one, the mRNA for D_1 receptors predominate and they also make enkephalin and project to the globus pallidus and thence to the output nuclei of the basal ganglia (substantia nigra and the globus pallidus externa). The other class make D_2 receptors and substance P and dynorphin and project directly to the substantia nigra. The balance between these two output pathways is vital for the normal expression of movement, and loss of dopamine increases synthetic activity in the enkephalin-containing cells and reduces the activity of the others.

Further subtypes of dopamine receptor have been revealed by structural analysis. The D_3 receptor is located in the limbic system. It is present on both postsynaptic and presynaptic membranes and may mediate the therapeutic effects of neuroleptic drugs (Sokoloff et al 1990). The neuropharmacology, CNS localisation and, possibly, connections with intracellular signalling systems of the D_3 receptor subtype all differ from D_1 and D_2. For example, butyrophenones are 10–20 times more potent at D_2 than at D_3 receptors but sulpiride, thioridazine and clozapine are only 2–3 times more potent at D_2 than D_3. These observations probably account for differences between antipsychotic drugs in their ability to induce EPS effects. The D_3 receptor forms the basis of current attempts to design new antipsychotic drugs with fewer EPS effects and to develop new drugs for Parkinson's disease (Snyder 1990).The novel antipsychotic clozapine does not cause 'tardive dyskinesia'.

Recently, a further subtype of dopamine receptor termed D_4 has been described and found to bind clozapine preferentially (Van Tol et al 1991). It is structurally related to other members of the G protein-coupled receptor 'superfamily' and, as for D_3, understanding of its structure and functions may facilitate development of novel antipsychotic drugs. Sunahara et al (1991) have also described a further subtype of dopamine receptor (termed D_5 or D_{1b}) that is also primarily located in the limbic system and may be involved in D_2 regulation by D_1 activation which has been reported in vivo. On the other hand a recent report of its localisation in hippocampus suggests as yet unknown actions.

Administration of dopamine receptor-blocking drugs can produce supersensitivity of dopamine receptors. The mechanism(s) underlying supersensitivity following chronic administration of neuroleptics are largely unknown. In some patients (postmenopausal women seem most susceptible) continuous administration of neuroleptics can cause a syndrome of involuntary movements to emerge. This 'tardive dyskinesia' characteristically affects buccolinguomasticatory musculature but may also involve choreic movements of limbs and dystonic contractions of the trunk. The syndrome is of major clinical importance (Ch. 4) and usually starts during therapy, but may worsen on cessation. Occasionally, the symptoms are relieved by reintroduction of neuroleptics, but no generally satisfactory drug treatment is available for this condition.

Dopamine uptake

Amphetamine and other drugs which release dopamine also inhibit its uptake and so potentiate the action of dopamine. Nomifensine and cocaine are also well-established dopamine uptake inhibitors. Benztropine and to a lesser extent benzhexol and orphenadrine inhibit the uptake of dopamine and also block cholinergic receptors, actions that contribute to the effects of these anticholinergic drugs in the treatment of parkinsonism. In a very recent pair of letters to *Nature* (Volkow et al 1997a,b) the action of cocaine was localised to the dopamine system in the basal ganglia. The number of dopamine receptors (estimated from positron emission tomography of antagonist binding) was shown to be reduced in chronic cocaine users, and the extent of the 'high' obtained by cocaine doses closely correlated to the binding of cocaine to the dopamine uptake sites in the brains of the users. Such data reinforce the idea that dopamine receptors certainly have an action in the control of drug-taking behaviour, although the relationship to therapeutic actions of dopamine blockers is less clear.

Drugs affecting degradation of dopamine

Monamine oxidase inhibitors like tranylcypromine reduce the degradation of dopamine by monoamine oxidase. Tranylcypromine also reduces uptake of dopamine, but this is probably not relevant to its antidepressant action because drugs such as benztropine (a potent dopamine uptake inhibitor) are not effective antidepressants. In contrast the actions of the monoamine oxidase B inhibitor deprenyl seems to be less on the metabolism of amines and more on the reduction of oxidative stress and its concomitant neurotoxicity. A recent multicentre trial suggests strongly that pretreatment with deprenyl slows the progression of symptoms of Parkinson's disease.

Parkinsonism

There is a substantial reduction of dopaminergic innervation of the basal ganglia in Parkinson's disease. The loss of dopamine leads to parkinsonian signs and symptoms, and restoration of dopaminergic neuro-transmission is the aim of all effective treatments. The neural connections of the basal ganglia are shown in Figure 3.14. The pathways that connect the caudate nucleus–putamen to the substantia nigra are of most importance in parkinsonism. Dopamine-containing cell bodies in the pars compacta of the substantia nigra degenerate in Parkinson's disease. The afferents of these cell bodies in normal brain synapse on all types of output cell in the caudate–putamen. The effect of dopaminergic inputs to the caudate–putamen is the modification of its output to other structures. In particular, loss of dopamine results in the reduction of the synthesis of substance P in those cells which make D_1 receptors and project directly to the substantia nigra, and in an increase in the synthesis of enkephalin in the indirectly projecting, D_2 receptor-synthesising cells. Current surgical treatment in parkinsonian patients aims to redress the imbalance in the two pathways by surgically reducing the activity of the indirect pathway with a lesion in the globus pallidus interna. Reserpine and phenothiazines can produce parkinsonism; the first by depletion of dopamine storage granules and the sec-

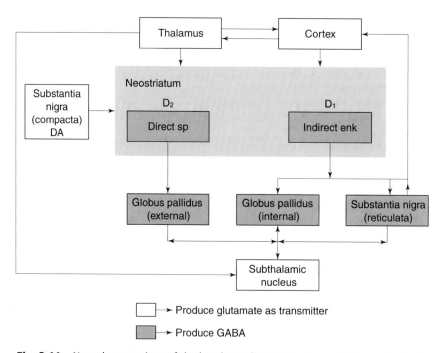

Fig. 3.14 Neural connections of the basal ganglia. Dopamine, cortical and thalamic inputs (glutamate) reach all of the cells in the neostriatum, although the spiny output cells form at least two output pathways from neostriatum. Dopamine D_1 receptors predominate on the direct pathway, while the indirectly projecting cells make D_2 receptors.

ond by blocking dopamine receptors. Both these treatments also produce the expected changes in synthesis in the two output pathways.

In health, dopaminergic and excitatory cholinergic activity in the caudate–putamen is balanced, and because cholinergic cells are spared in Parkinson's disease there is a relative excess of cholinergic activity. Blockade of cholinergic activity has therefore been used in the treatment of parkinsonism. Anticholinergic drugs (muscarinic antagonists) are commonly used in psychiatry to relieve drug-induced parkinsonism. Currently they are regarded as less effective than L-dopa in idiopathic Parkinson's disease but can often be usefully combined with L-dopa in patients who have not fully responded. Restoration of dopaminergic transmission by oral supplementation of L-dopa, a dopamine precursor, is also effective. Dopaminergic agonists that are useful in parkinsonism are mostly ergot derivatives: bromocriptine (often as an adjunct to L-dopa), lisuride, and pergolide mesylate. In experimental animals, deprenyl (a selective inhibitor of monoamine oxidase B) can prevent neurotoxin-induced parkinsonism by preventing the conversion of MPTP (1-methyl-4-phenyl-1,2,3,6-tetrahydropyridine) to its toxic metabolite MPP^+ by monoamine oxidase B. It has also been demonstrated to slow the progression of parkinsonian symptoms in patients.

SEROTONERGIC NEUROTRANSMISSION

Serotonin (5-hydroxytryptamine, 5-HT) is present in the enterochromaffin granules of the intestines and in blood platelets. Less than 2% of the total body serotonin is in the CNS. Early studies of serotonin indicated that disturbances of its physiology could produce abnormal behaviour, at times strongly suggestive of mental illness. Substances with marked structural similarities to serotonin possess considerable pharmacological potency. Examples are N,N-dimethyltryptamine (DMT) and bufotenine (both present in the cahobe bean). Mexican hallucinogenic mushrooms also contain serotonin-related substances such as psilocybin. All three have a long history of abuse.

Serotonin, like noradrenaline and dopamine, is localised within specific neuronal pathways in the brain and serotonin-containing cell bodies are found in discrete brain nuclei, especially the midbrain and brainstem raphe nuclei.

Serotonin synthesis

Serotonin is synthesised from L-tryptophan, being first hydroxylated to 5-HTP (by tryptophan hydroxylase), which is then decarboxylated to 5-HT (by aromatic-L-amino-acid decarboxylase). The capacity of the brain to synthesise serotonin is greatly in excess of requirements. Serotonin synthesis can be increased by oral tryptophan and takes place in neurones in both somata and nerve terminals.

Serotonin storage

Serotonin is transported to the terminals of axons where it forms a readily releasable pool of serotonin. It is stored in presynaptic complexes comparable to those storing catecholamines. The *Rauwolfia* alkaloids and tetrabenazine reduce serotonin stores by disrupting these granules. When serotonin storage is disturbed, large quantities of serotonin are released and outside the CNS this causes side-effects such as diarrhoea and abdominal cramps.

Serotonin release

Serotonin release is a Ca^{2+}-dependent process and there is some evidence, as with dopamine, that release takes place by two separate mechanisms. The amphetamines and some tricyclic antidepressants release serotonin from storage granules. Amphetamine analogues containing halogen atoms (e.g. fenfluramine) are more effective in stimulating serotonin release than those without.

Serotonin receptors

Receptors for serotonin are found in the CNS as part of a diffuse serotonergic network. There are multiple 5-HT receptors (currently at least a dozen) and the neuropharmacological study of 5-HT receptor function in the CNS is a rapidly expanding field.

Subtypes of serotonergic receptors

Physiological responses to serotonin are mediated through multiple serotonin receptor subtypes. Individual serotonin receptor subtypes activate different intracellular signalling systems. $5\text{-}HT_{1A}$ and $5\text{-}HT_{1B}$ receptors regulate adenylate cyclase or couple to G proteins that directly activate ion channels. $5\text{-}HT_{1C}$ and $5\text{-}HT_2$ receptors activate PLC and stimulate phosphoinositol metabolism. 5-HT receptor classification is shown in Table 3.12. Continuing problems in receptor classification arise because of a lack of compounds with sufficient specificity to demonstrate differences between putative receptor subtypes. The $5\text{-}HT_{1A}$ receptor is specifically activated by 8-hydroxy-2-(di-N-propylamino)tetralin (8-OH-DPAT). $5\text{-}HT_{1A}$ receptor densi-

Table 3.12 Serotonergic pharmacology

Presynaptic

Site of action	Effect	Drug	Use
Synthesis	Increases	Tryptophan	Antidepressant
	Blocks	p-Chlorophenylalanine	Experimental
	Blocks	5-Fluotryptophan	Experimental
Storage	Depletes	Reserpine	Experimental
	Depletes	Tetrabenazine	Chorea
Release	Increases	Amphetamine	Experimental
	Increases	Tricyclic antidepressants	Antidepressant
	Increases	Fenfluramine	Experimental

Postsynaptic

Receptor	Tissue (example)	Agonist responses	Agonist	Antagonist	Molecular mechanisms
5-HT_{1A}	Postsynaptic 5-HT neurones	Inhibits neuronal firing	LSD (partial) 8-OH-DPAT	Pindolol Metergoline Methysergide	↓Adenylate cyclase
5-HT_{1B}	Presynaptic 5-HT autoreceptor	Inhibits 5-HT release	RU 24969	Methysergide Metergoline	↓Adenylate cyclase
5-HT_{1C}	Choroid plexus and brain	Induction of specific behaviours (e.g. feeding)	TFMPP ICI 169369	Ritanserin	↑PI
5-HT_{2}	Postsynaptic 5-HT neurones	Induces slow wave sleep	LSD (partial)	Metergoline Ritanserin	↑PI
5-HT_{3}	Area postrema Limbic system	Emesis Modulation of dopamine and acetylcholine release	2-Methyl 5-HT	Ondansetron Granisetron Raclopride Zacopride	Via ionic channels

Degradation

Site of action	Effect	Drug	Use
Uptake	Inhibits	Zimelidine	Experimental
		Clomipramine	Antidepressant
		Fluoxetine	Antidepressant
		Fluvoxamine	Antidepressant
		Paroxetine	Antidepressant
		Citalopram	Antidepressant

Monoamine oxidase (A and B) inhibition

ty is highest in the CA1 region and dentate gyrus of the hippocampus and in the raphe nuclei. Clinically useful drugs that are selective partial agonists at the 5-HT_{1A} receptor are buspirone and ipsapirone, both effective antianxiety agents. 5-HT_{2} receptors probably mediate excitatory effects; 5-HT_{3} receptors may act similarly but their exact functions are unknown. The distinct ligand-binding properties of each subtype of serotonin receptor are based on important structural differences between them. Lübbert et al (1987) isolated a complementary DNA (cDNA) clone that coded for a substantial portion of the 5-HT_{1C} receptor and, subsequently, Julius et al (1988) cloned the entire 5-HT_{1C} receptor. This receptor shares much in common with other members of the G protein-coupled superfamily of receptors. There are seven membrane-spanning regions, the amino terminus is located on the extracellular side of the membrane and the carboxyl terminus is intracellular.

The 5-HT$_2$ receptor has also been characterised by Julius et al (1990). It is homologous with the 5-HT$_{1C}$ receptor and is also a member of the G protein-coupled superfamily. About 50% of the amino acid sequences are common to both 5-HT$_{1C}$ and 5-HT$_2$ receptors. These two receptors are further examples of the evolution of receptor subtypes within families that bind the same ligand (5-HT) and are coupled to the same signalling system (G proteins). However, the distinct structural differences between family members may provide the means for selective activation of intracellular pathways by different concentrations of the endogenous ligand or may be relevant to a comprehensive understanding of the genetic regulation of neurotransmitter function. Because the many CNS effects of serotonergic drugs are mediated through subtypes of 5-HT receptors, these structural studies are required in order to clarify individual differences in response to psychotomimetic drugs (e.g. LSD or other 5-HT agonists) and may in turn lead to a better understanding of some psychotic illnesses.

Chronic treatment with a wide range of antidepressant drugs (including the tricyclics, monoamine oxidase inhibitors and atypical antidepressants such as mianserin) is known to reduce the number of 5-HT$_1$ and 5-HT$_2$ receptors. Electroconvulsive shocks also decrease 5-HT$_{1A}$ receptors but increase 5-HT$_2$ receptor numbers. This difference may possibly explain why some depressive illnesses do not respond to a therapeutic course of oral antidepressant therapy but later respond to ECT.

Antidepressant drugs produce substantial decreases in 5-HT$_2$ receptor numbers after long-term treatment and these effects may be greater than their actions in catecholaminergic systems. For example, amitriptyline and imipramine reduce β adrenoceptor binding by about 20% but reduce 5-HT$_2$ binding even more, by about 40%. Monoamine oxidase inhibitors also reduce serotonin binding site numbers after chronic treatment, selective monoamine oxidase A inhibitors being most effective.

Abnormalities in serotonin receptor function have been put forward as part of the pathophysiology of depressive illness. Limited support for this hypothesis has been found in studies of [3H] serotonin binding to platelets and [3H] serotonin and [3H] spiroperidol binding to cortical tissue in suicide victims. The hypothesis has been extended to involve increased release of serotonin acting upon hypersensitive postsynaptic serotonin receptors and this has been suggested as a possible cause of depressive illness.

Cyproheptadine and methysergide are the most commonly used serotonergic antagonists. Structurally, cyproheptadine resembles the phenothiazines and also blocks histaminergic (H$_1$) and cholinergic (M$_1$) receptors. Methysergide is structurally similar to LSD, which can stimulate some serotonergic receptors and, especially in the periphery, be an antagonist at others. The physiological and biochemical actions of serotonergic receptors appear complex and study of their properties has been hindered by lack of specific antagonists or agonists. The recent development of such drugs is certain to add substantially to knowledge of the serotonergic system and will probably lead to better understanding of the mode of action of antidepressants as well.

Drugs affecting serotonin uptake

The reuptake systems for serotonin resemble those for the catecholamines and are influenced by many antidepressant drugs. These may differ markedly in their relative affinities for serotonergic and catecholaminergic reuptake mechanisms. The structure of the serotonergic transporter is known (Blakely et al 1991) and has much in common with other members of the superfamily of neurotransmitter transporters. The tricyclic antidepressant clomipramine was the first drug to inhibit serotonergic without also inhibiting noradrenergic reuptake, although its metabolite (desmethylclomipramine) is a strong inhibitor of noradrenergic reuptake. The first truly specific serotonergic uptake inhibitor was zimelidine which, though an effective antidepressant, was withdrawn because of its hepatotoxic effects.

The currently available inhibitors of serotonin uptake comprise a class of antidepressants known as 'selective serotonin reuptake inhibitors' (or SSRIs). Table 3.13 summarises potency and relative selectivity data. These show paroxetine to be the most potent inhibitor of serotonin reuptake and citalopram to be the most selective. In vivo, the pharmacological profile of each of these drugs is changed by the formation of active metabolites, which may possess pharmacokinetic properties that differ markedly from their parent compound. For example, fluoxetine is metabolised to norfluoxetine with a half-life of 7–15 days. Since norfluoxetine is equipotent with fluoxetine and is equally selective, it probably contributes importantly to the antidepressant effects of fluoxetine. However, the metabolites of sertraline, fluvoxamine and paroxetine are considerably less active than their parent compounds and probably do not affect their clinical actions.

These drugs also interact with monoaminergic receptors (Table 3.14) but have considerably fewer effects on

Table 3.13 Relative potencies of antidepressants after oral administration to rats for inhibition of noradrenaline and serotonin uptake

Drug	Inhibition of serotonin uptake	Inhibition of noradrenaline uptake
Paroxetine	0.4	—
Citalopram	2	>10
Fluoxetine	8	>100
Fluvoxamine	5	>30
Sertraline	—	—
Clomipramine	15	30
Imipramine	50	7
Amitriptyline	120	50
Desipramine	180	3

After Maitre et al (1982).

histaminergic, adrenergic and muscarinic cholinergic receptors than the tricyclic antidepressants.

Drugs affecting serotonin degradation

Most serotonin is oxidised by monoamine oxidase to 5-hydroxyindoleacetaldehyde and then to 5-hydroxyindoleacetic acid (5-HIAA) by aldehyde dehydrogenase. 5-Hydroxyindoleacetaldehyde is also reduced by alcohol dehydrogenase to 5-hydroxytryptophol. 5-HIAA is the major metabolite of 5-HT degradation. Monoamine oxidase inhibitors are the principal drugs to modify serotonin degradation.

PEPTIDERGIC NEUROTRANSMISSION

Advances in neurobiology have demonstrated that the neural and endocrine systems are closely linked. Previously, differences between the systems were apparent from a structural standpoint and seemed supported by the distinctive means of communication between the component parts of each system. Patterns of release following electrical activity in the nervous system were clearly not the same as the release of chemicals by endocrine tissue to act on distant target organs. The neural regulation of endocrine function is now seen to provide important insights into the working of the brain that are relevant to psychiatry. This view is based upon the following lines of evidence.

Firstly, there is extensive evidence showing that the neurotransmitter systems preferentially modified by effective psychotropic drugs (e.g. the dopaminergic and noradrenergic pathways) are also intimately involved in the limbic–hypothalamic integration and regulation of pituitary function. Putative abnormalities of these transmitter systems may extend from sites in the brain involved in the pathogenesis of mental illness to the hypothalamic–pituitary system and may therefore be detected in abnormal endocrine functioning.

Secondly, the hypothalamus regulates the anterior pituitary by synthesising and secreting releasing factors into the pituitary portal vessel system to act upon anterior pituitary cells. These releasing factors are synthesised and released at sites elsewhere in the nervous system without any obvious endocrine function and there is experimental evidence that they may function as neurotransmitters or neuromodulators, and thereby

Table 3.14 Inhibition of radioligand binding in rat brain membranes in vitro by different types of antidepressant

Antidepressant	Receptor subtype/radioligand							
	α_1/ prazosin	α_2/ clonidine	β/ DHA	D_2/ spiperone	5-HT$_1$/ 5-HT	5-HT$_1$/ ketanserin	Histamine H$_1$/mepyramine	Muscarinic/ QNB
Paroxetine	>10 000	>10 000	>5 000	>7 700	>10 000	>1 000	>1 000	89
Citalopram	4 500	>10 000	>5 000	>10 000	>10 000	>1 000	>1 000	2 900
Fluvoxamine	>10 000	>10 000	>5 000	>10 000	>10 000	>1 000	>1 000	>10 000
Fluoxetine	>10 000	>10 000	>5 000	>10 000	>10 000	>1 000	>1 000	1 300
Amitriptyline	170	540	>5 000	1 200	1 000	8.3	3.3	5.1
Imipramine	440	1 000	>5 000	2 400	8 900	120	35	37
Clomipramine	150	3 300	>5 000	430	5 200	63	47	34
Desipramine	1 300	8 600	>5 000	3 800	2 500	160	370	68

QNB, quinuclidinylbenzilate; DHA, dihydroalprenolol.
After Thomas et al (1987).

play important roles in the neural regulation of certain behaviours. The abnormalities characteristic of severe mental illnesses may, therefore, be caused by pathological changes in the non-endocrine functions of the releasing factors.

Thirdly, the hormones released by the pituitary regulate hormone production of target endocrine glands. These peripheral hormones can, in turn, act upon many aspects of neural function, for example by affecting neural development and classical neurotransmitters like noradrenaline. The actions on the brain of hormones such as testosterone, thyroxin and cortisol may be relevant to sex differences in the incidence of mental illnesses such as depression and the increased prevalence of psychological symptoms in endocrinopathies such as thyroid or adrenal cortical disease.

Fourthly, releasing factors and 'classical neurotransmitters' can coexist in the same nerve terminal (e.g. serotonin and thyrotrophin-releasing factor, TRF). In this circumstance, the releasing factor may modify (or 'modulate') the actions of the neurotransmitter and this may be of relevance, for example, to the serotonergic hypothesis of the mode of action of some antidepressant treatments.

Fifthly, stress responses to threatening or noxious stimuli include activation of the hypothalamic–pituitary system. These patterns of endocrine responses to stress are specific to the type of stressful stimulus. Since there is abundant evidence from clinical studies implicating stressful stimuli in the pathogenesis of mental illnesses, study of the neural regulation of endocrine responses to stress might elucidate important individual differences relevant to variations in vulnerability to mental illnesses.

Molecular biology of peptidergic transmission

Most regulatory substances released by the nervous system are peptides, i.e. they consist of amino acids joined by peptide bonds. Unlike classical neurotransmitters, these compounds are synthesised as parts of larger molecules that are cleaved by proteolysis and carboxylation into active fragments of amino acid chains at the point of release. Local tissue-specific differences in the activity of processing enzymes can yield important topographical variations in the proportions of peptide fragments derived from a single precursor. However, with the exception of pro-opiomelanocortin (POMC), the specific degradative, cleavage and post-translational processing enzymes involved are usually unknown. Fundamental questions relevant to proper understanding of the actions of drugs on the brain arise from this uncertainty. Neuropeptide fragments may be cleaved from widely available precursor molecules by enzymes

specific to that cleavage site and/or general-purpose enzymes that are locally regulated.

The chromosomal locations of neuropeptide genes are distributed widely throughout the human genome. Although some neuropeptides are close members of structurally related families, with the single exception of oxytocin and vasopressin, genes for these related family members are located on different chromosomes (Sherman et al 1989).

Neural regulation of neuropeptide synthesis and release

The hypothalamus controls the release of pituitary hormones in two ways, both of which involve neurones that synthesise and release neuropeptides. In the first, specialised neurones in the hypothalamus synthesise and secrete releasing factors. In the second, the magnocellular neurones of the hypothalamus synthesise precursor molecules (preprovasophysin and preproxyphysin) that are processed and transported to terminals in the posterior pituitary, from which vasopressin, oxytocin and their related neurophysins are stoichiometrically released. The neuroendocrine neurones of the hypothalamus are influenced by many types of neurotransmitter. Releasing factor-producing neurones are richly supplied with noradrenergic, dopaminergic and serotonergic connections.

Cotransmission of neuropeptides

Neuropeptides are present in the central nervous system in concentrations between 10^{-12} and 10^{-15} mol/mg of protein. These are much lower than the concentrations of the 'classical neurotransmitters', which vary from 10^{-9} to 10^{-10} mol/mg of protein. High concentrations of neuropeptides in the brain are found in the hypothalamic–pituitary system but some neuropeptides (e.g. cholecystokinin and vasoactive intestinal peptide) have their highest concentrations in the cortex. Other neuropeptides (e.g. oxytocin and vasopressin) are present in cell bodies only in the hypothalamus and their presence in other brain or spinal cord areas is accounted for by the long projections of these cells into those areas. Some widely distributed neuropeptides (e.g. TRF and substance P) are found in neurones in numerous areas.

Hökfelt et al (1987) have demonstrated the coexistence of neuropeptides and 'classical neurotransmitters' within the same neurone at many sites in the nervous system. The physiological importance of coexistence is not yet known but a number of models have been put forward, some of which may prove to be of relevance to hypotheses concerning changes in receptor sensitivity in mental illness. In one model, a nerve terminal containing serotonin, substance P and TRF responds to low-frequency electrical stimulation by releasing serotonin. The released serotonin attaches to the postsynaptic receptors, where it generates a small postsynaptic potential. Some serotonin also attaches to the presynaptic serotonergic receptors (autoreceptors) which inhibit further serotonin release. As electrical stimulation is increased, TRF and substance P are also released. TRF and serotonin then act synergistically on the postsynaptic serotonin receptor to generate an increased postsynaptic potential, while substance P blocks the serotonergic autoreceptor preventing inhibition of serotonin release. The three substances thus combine to produce prolonged postsynaptic activation without inducing compensatory responses at a presynaptic level. These interactions between a monoamine neurotransmitter and neuropeptides may be relevant to long-term changes in homeostatic mechanisms, neural learning and long-term potentiation of synaptic activity. They have also been related to the mode of action of antidepressant treatments (including ECT) and pathological alterations in receptor sensitivity that may occur in affective disorders and schizophrenia.

Peptide regulatory factors

CNS peptide regulatory factors are not the same as neuropeptides. They act through a different class of receptor and are important in the normal development of the nervous system, when they are usually called neurotrophins. These trophic substances are also important in neurodegenerative diseases, where they are necessary for the restoration of neural circuits and the coordination of glial responses to damage.

Nerve growth factor (NGF) is the best known trophic factor. It is a neurotrophic factor and influences the synthesis of neurotransmitters, cytoskeletal proteins and neuropeptides (Hanley 1989). The survival and functional maintenance of neurones depends upon the presence of specific neurotrophins. Cholinergic neurones damaged in Alzheimer's disease contain high concentrations of mRNA for NGF receptor and it is hypothesised that cholinergic loss in this condition may be reversed by NGF treatment (Perry 1990). Other neurotrophins include neurotrophins 2 and 3 (NT2,NT3), brain-derived neurotrophic factor (BDNF) (Maisonpierre et al 1990), glial cell-derived neurotrophic factor (GDNF, which may be important in Parkinson's disease), neuroleucin, glial nexin, insulin-like growth factors, platelet-derived growth factor (Williams 1989) and epidermal growth factor. Since the cellular mechanisms that regulate neurotrophin metabolism can be manipulated by noxious factors,

study of psychological stress in humans has been extended to include effects on functions influenced by trophic factors. Animal studies of electroconvulsive stimulation (ECS) of possible relevance to the mode of action of ECT have included direct measures of neurotrophin metabolism. Repeated ECS probably alters the expression of many neural genes along a time-course that is relevant to the actions of ECT (Leviel et al 1990). Interleukins 1 and 2 also have trophic actions and can be produced by the brain when stressed. Their functions may include integration of neural and immune responses to injury, studied in psychoneuroimmunology.

Peptidergic receptors

The receptors for most neuropeptides are less well studied but almost certainly will yield as many variations as are seen for the 'classical' transmitters. The products of the preprotachykinin genes (substance P, neurokinin A, neuropeptide K) seem to act on a group of at least three related receptors, all of which respond to substance P and which are labelled NK1, NK2 and NK3. The relationship between these receptors and the central actions of the tachykinins are still being elaborated. However, it seems certain that, as a group, neuropeptides appear to act on G protein-coupled receptors but the second messenger systems are largely unknown (Wollemann 1990). Opioid receptors appear linked to G_i and G_0 proteins (Wong et al 1989). Neuropeptides can function as:

- Neurotransmitters released by one neurone at a presynaptic terminal to act on the adjacent postsynaptic membrane.
- Neuromodulators that act by modifying the turnover, release or action of classical neurotransmitters.
- Neurohormones released by one neurone to act at a site distant to the point of release.

The most detailed understanding of a peptidergic receptor system currently available is provided by the pharmacology of opioid receptors. There is good evidence for the existence of three subtypes of opioid receptor.

Endorphins and enkephalins

The endorphins (literally 'endogenous morphine') are the endogenous ligands for the opioid receptors. Their study is a rapidly expanding field of research and has given rise to a confusing terminology. The term 'opiate' is used to describe drugs derived from the juice of the poppy *Papaver somniferum*. The word 'opioid' describes all substances with morphine-like actions. The word 'narcotic' is no longer used in pharmacology, although originally it described drugs that induced sleep and was later applied to morphine-like analgesics. The sites of action of opioid drugs in the nervous system appear to be the receptors for a number of endogenous ligands which include the pentapeptides, leucine-enkephalin (Leu-enkephalin) and methionine-enkephalin (Met-enkephalin). The amino acid sequence of Met-enkephalin is the same as the sequence contained in amino acid residues 61–65 in the pituitary hormone β-lipotrophin (β-LPH). Other opioid peptides are represented in fragments of the β-lipotrophin amino acid sequence. The carboxyl terminus of amino acid residues 61–91 is called β-endorphin. Sequences of amino acid residues 61–76 are called α-endorphin and amino acid residues 61–77 are called γ-endorphin. The enkephalins and endorphins derived from β-lipotrophin probably belong to separate physiological systems. β-Endorphin is present in the hypothalamic pituitary system, where it is derived from a larger precursor molecule, POMC, containing the amino acid sequences for both β-lipotrophin and adrenocorticotrophic hormone (ACTH). The enkephalins are not derived from POMC but are produced by cleavage of a separate precursor molecule.

The physiological role of endogenous ligands for opioid receptors is still unknown but they appear to be involved in the perception of pain and the neural control of certain aspects of endocrine function, the regulation of movement, mood and some aspects of behaviour. A large number of drugs are agonists at opioid receptor sites. Opioid agonist drugs appear to act largely at the μ receptor, with a few actions mediated at the κ receptor. Opioid agonists include morphine, heroin (diacetylmorphine), dihydromorphine, codeine, pethidine, methadone, pentazocine, levorphanol and meperidine. Many of these agonists are structurally related to morphine but some, like meperidine and methadone, are chemically quite dissimilar. Naloxone, naltrexone and nalorphine are antagonists at opioid receptor sites. Pentazocine has both opioid agonist actions and weak antagonist activity. All the compounds listed above have clinical applications and their specific use has been determined by their pharmacokinetics, pharmacodynamics and liability to produce dependence. All opioid drugs, when regularly administered, appear able to induce tolerance and dependence. Tolerance may be innate or acquired. Innate tolerance is subject to wide individual variation, determined presumably by genetic factors and the age and reproductive status of the individual. Acquired tolerance is observed as the need to increase the dose of the opioid drug if the same effects are to be obtained with repeated administration. The mechanisms underlying the development of tolerance are ill understood but may include the proliferation of new receptor sites or reduction in sensitivity of opioid receptors to their agonists. There is extensive cross-tolerance between opioid drugs. When they are administered regularly, tolerance frequently develops but this must not be taken to imply that withdrawal symptoms will always occur if the drug is removed. The manifestation of withdrawal symptoms (which may be either physical or psychological) demonstrates that an individual has become dependent (physically or psychologically) on the drug. Symptoms that can follow opioid withdrawal include insomnia, restlessness, anxiety, nausea and vomiting, abdominal cramps, myotonus, sweating, piloerection and rhinorrhoea. These symptoms may persist for several days and may be accompanied by a craving for the drug to be reintroduced. Tolerance may also develop to alcohol, barbiturates and hypnotic drugs. The withdrawal symptoms observed following prolonged administration of these substances are primarily rebound effects in the systems most affected by the drug. Depressant drugs tend to be followed by rebound hyperexcitability, and mood-elevating drugs like the amphetamines by lethargy and depressed mood. Epileptic seizures may be seen in withdrawal from drugs that raise the seizure threshold.

Theories of drug dependence and withdrawal usually attempt to explain withdrawal symptoms in terms of some form of rebound phenomenon. Pharmacological explanations have included modification of receptor sensitivity, change in numbers of receptors, the utilisation of otherwise redundant neural pathways and the induction of enzymes involved in the synthesis of neurotransmitters.

NEURONALLY-PRODUCED GASES

The most recent puzzle in neurochemistry is the discovery that some neurones possess the enzymic machinery to produce gases. The best-studied example is the enzyme called nitric oxide synthase (NOS). This is one of a family of NOS enzymes which occur in various sites in the body. The best known is perhaps the NOS of macrophages which may be involved in cell killing in the immune system. Why would neurones have evolved such a potentially lethal cargo? It seems that there are soluble GTPases in neurones that are appropriate receptors for NO formed when arginine is converted to citrulline by NOS. The NO is implicated in the control of NMDA receptor sensitivity, and by some is held responsible for the action of LTP-producing stimuli on presynaptic release. Endothelial cells also generate a NOS which is thought to provide a vasodilator tone in the CNS. The possibility for the control of these three enzymes independently exists but at present there are few NO receptor antagonists of any specificity and so the functional significance of these potentially toxic substances in neuropharmacology is still obscure. The fact that the cells in the caudate–putamen which produce NO are the last to die in Huntington's disease has led to the suggestion that they may cause, at least some of, the neurotoxic damage in that condition.

A suggestion that a heamoxygenase might be present in nerve cells which could then produce carbon monoxide is just one of the many challenges facing the continued battle to understand enough of the neurochemistry and neuropharmacology of the brain to be able to help alleviate the symptoms of mental disease.

REFERENCES

Ahlquist R P 1948 A study of the adrenotropic receptors. American Journal of Physiology 153: 586–600

Barnard E A, Darlison M G, Seeburg P 1987 Molecular biology of the GABA$_A$ receptor: the receptor/channel superfamily. Trends in Neurosciences 10(12): 502–509

Baxter C F 1976 Some recent advances in studies of GABA metabolism and compartmentation. In: Roberts E, Chase T N, Tower D B (eds) GABA in nervous system function. Excerpta Medica, Amsterdam

Beal M F, Kowall N W, Ellison D W, Mazurek M F, Swartz K J, Martin J B 1986 Replication of the neurochemical characteristics of Huntington's disease by quinolinic acid. Nature 321: 168–171

Bell M V, Bloomfield J, McKinley M et al 1989 Physical linkage of the GABA$_A$ receptor subunit gene to the DX5374 locus in human Xq28. American Journal of Human Genetics 45: 882–888

Betz H 1987 Biology and structure of mammalian glycine receptor. Trends in Neurosciences 10(3): 113–117

Birnbaumer L 1990 G proteins in signal transduction. Annual Review of Pharmacology and Toxicology 30: 675–705

Blair L A, Levitan E S, Marshall J, Dionne V E, Barnard E A 1988 Single subunits of the GABA$_A$ receptor form ion channels with properties of the native receptor. Science 242: 577–579

Blakely R D, Berson H E, Fremeau Jr R T et al 1991 Cloning and expression of a functional serotonin transporter from rat brain. Nature 354: 66–70

Bloom F E 1990 Neurohumoral transmission and the central nervous system. In: Goodman A G, Rall T W, Nies A S, Taylor P (eds) The pharmacological basis of therapeutics. Pergamon Press, New York, pp 244–268

Blum K, Noble E P, Sheridan P J et al 1990 Allelic association of human dopamine D$_2$ receptor gene in alcoholism. Journal of the American Medical Association 263: 2055–2060

Bonner T I 1989 The molecular basis of muscarinic receptor diversity. Trends in Neurosciences 12(4): 148–151

Bormann J 1988 Electrophysiology of GABA$_A$ and GABA$_B$ receptor subtypes. Trends in Neurosciences 11(3): 112–116

Bradbury M 1979 The concept of the blood–brain barrier. Wiley, London

Bradford H F 1986 Brain glucose and energy metabolism: the linkage to function. In: Chemical neurobiology. Freeman, New York, pp 118–154

Bunzow J R, Van Tol H H M, Grandy et al 1988 Cloning and expression of a rat D$_2$ dopamine receptor cDNA. Nature 336: 783–787

Callingham B A, Ovens R S 1988 Some in vitro effects of moclobemide and other MAO inhibitors on responses to sympathomimetic amines. In: Youdim M B H, Da Prada M, Amrein R (eds) The cheese effect and new reversible MAO-A inhibitors. Journal of Neurotransmission (suppl) 26: 17–29

Carlsson A 1988 The current status of the dopamine hypothesis of schizophrenia. Neuropsychopharmacology 1: 179–186

Carlsson A, Lindqvist M 1963 Effect of chlorpromazine or haloperidol on formation of 3-methoxytyramine and normetanephrine in mouse brain. Acta Pharmacologica et Toxicologica 20: 140–144

Clarke D D, Lathja A L, Maker H S 1989 Intermediary metabolism. In: Siegel G J, Alberto R W, Agranoff B W, Molinoff P B (eds) Basic neurochemistry: molecular, cellular, and medical aspects, 4th edn. Raven Press, New York, pp 541–564

Dearry A, Gingrich J A, Falardeau P, Fremeau R T, Bates M D, Caron M G 1990 Molecular cloning and expression of the gene for human D$_1$ dopamine receptor. Nature 347: 72–76

Deisz R A, Lux H D 1985 Gamma-aminobutyric acid-induced depression of calcium currents of chick sensory neurons. Neuroscience Letters 14;56(2): 205–210

Evans R M 1988 The steroid and thyroid hormone receptor superfamily. Science 240: 889–895

Farde L, Wiesel F-A, Stone-Elander S et al 1990 D$_2$ dopamine receptors in neuroleptic-naive schizophrenic patients. Archives of General Psychiatry 47: 213–219

Giros B, Sokoloff P, Martres M-P, Riou J-F, Emorine L J, Schwartz J-C 1989 Alternative splicing directs the expression of two D$_2$ dopamine receptor isoforms. Nature 342: 923–926

Gregor P, Mano I, Maoz I, McKeown M, Teichberg V I 1989 Molecular structure of the chick cerebellar kainate-binding subunit of a putative glutamate receptor. Nature 342: 689–692

Guy H R, Hucho F 1987 The ion channel of the nicotine acetylcholine receptor. Trends in Neurosciences 10(8): 318–321

Hanley M R 1989 Peptide regulatory factors in the nervous system. Lancet i: 1373–1376

Henley J M, Barnard E A 1990 Autoradiographic distribution of binding sites for the non-NMDA receptor antagonist CNQX in chick brain. Neuroscience Letters 116: 17–22

Hökfelt T, Millhorn D, Seroogy K et al 1987 Coexistence of peptides with classical neurotransmitters. Experientia 43: 768–780

Honoré T, Davies S N, Drejer J et al 1988 Quinoxalinediones: potent competitive non-NMDA glutamate receptor antagonists. Science 241: 701–703

Inoue M, Sadoshima J, Akaike N 1987 Different actions of intracellular free calcium on resting and GABA-gated chloride conductances. Brain Research 404: 301–303

Julius D, McDermott A B, Axel R, Jessell T M 1988 Molecular characterization of a functional cDNA encoding the serotonin 1c receptor. Science 241: 558–564

Julius D, Huang K N, Livelli T J, Axel R, Jessell T M 1990 The 5HT2 receptor defines a family of structually distinct but functionally conserved serotonin receptors. Proceedings of the National Academy of Sciences of the USA 87: 928–932

Krupinski J, Coussen F, Bakalyar H A et al 1989 Adenylyl cyclase amino acid sequence: possible channel- or transporter-like structure. Science 244: 1558–1564

Leviel V, Fayada C, Guibert F et al 1990 Short- and long-term alterations of gene expression in limbic structures by repeated electroconvulsive-induced seizures. Journal of Neurochemistry 54: 899–904

Llinas R, Yarom Y 1981 Properties and distribution of ionic conductances generating electroresponsiveness of mammalian inferior olivary neurones in vitro. Journal of Physiology (Cambridge) 315: 569–584

Lübbert H, Hoffmann B J, Snutch T P et al 1987 cDNA cloning of a serotonin 5-HT$_{1C}$ receptor by electrophysiological assays of mRNA-injected *Xenopus* oocytes. Proceedings of the Royal Academy of Sciences 84: 4332–4336

Lüddens H, Pritchett D B, Köhler M et al 1990 Cerebellar GABA$_A$ receptor selective for a behavioural alcohol antagonist. Nature 346: 648–651

McIlwain H 1990 Biochemistry and neurochemistry in the 1800s: their origins in comparative animal chemistry. Essays in Biochemistry 25: 197–224

McIlwain H, Bachelard H S 1985 Metabolism of the brain in situ. In: Biochemistry and the central nervous system, 5th edn. Churchill Livingstone, Edinburgh, pp 8–32

Maisonpierre P C, Belluscio L, Squinto S et al 1990 Neurotrophin-3: a neurotrophic factor related to NGF and BDNF. Science 247: 1446–1451

Maitre L, Baumann P A, Jaekel J 1982 5-HT uptake inhibitors: psychopharmacological and neurochemical criteria of selectivity. In: Ho B T (ed) Serotonin in biological psychiatry. Raven Press, New York, pp 229–246

Majerus P W, Connolly T M, Bansal V S, Inhorn R C, Ross T S, Lips D L 1988 Inositol phosphates: synthesis and degradation. Journal of Biological Chemistry 263: 3051–3054

Miller R J 1987 Multiple Ca channels and neuronal function. Science 235: 46–52

Monsma Jr F J, McVittie L D, Gerfen C R, Mahan L C, Sibley D R 1989 Multiple D$_2$ dopamine receptors produced by alternative RNA splicing. Nature 342: 926–929

Monsma Jr F J, Mahan L C, McVittie L D, Gerfen C R, Sibley D R 1990 Molecular cloning and expression of a D$_1$ dopamine receptor linked to adenylyl cyclase activation. Proceedings of the National Academy of Sciences of the USA 87: 6723–6727

Morris B J, Hicks A A, Wisden W, Darlison M B, Hunts S P, Barnard E A 1990 Distinct regional expression of nicotinic acetylcholine receptor genes in chick brain. Brain Research. Molecular Brain Research 7: 305–315

Moss S J, Darlison M G, Beeson D M, Barnard E A 1989 Development expression of the genes encoding the four subunits of the chicken muscle acetylcholine receptor. Journal of Biological Chemistry 264: 20199–20205

Neer E J, Clapham D E 1988 Roles of G protein subunits in transmembrane signalling. Nature 333: 129–134

Nowycky M C, Fox A P, Tsien R W 1985 Three types of neuronal calcium channel with different calcium agonist sensitivity. Nature 316: 440–443

Oldendorf W H 1974 Lipid solubility and drug penetration of the blood-brain barrier. Proceedings of the Society of Experimental Biological Medicine 147: 813

Olney J W 1989 Excitatory amino acids and neuropsychiatric disorders. Biological Psychiatry 26: 505–525

Pacholczyk T, Blakely R D, Amara S G 1991 Expression cloning of a cocaine- and antidepressant-sensitive human noradrenaline transporter. Nature 350: 350–354

Peroutka S J 1988 5-Hydroxytryptamine receptor subtypes: molecular, biochemical and physiological characterization. Trends in Neurosciences 11: 496–500

Perry E K 1990 Hypothesis linking plasticity, vulnerability and nerve growth factor to basal forebrain cholinergic neurons. International Journal of Geriatric Psychiatry 5: 223–231

Raiteri M, Cerrito F, Cervon A M, Levi G 1979 Dopamine can be released by two mechanisms differentially affected by the dopamine transport inhibitor nomifensine. Journal of Pharmacology and Experimental Therapeutics 208: 195–202

Revah F, Bertrand D, Galzi J-L et al 1991 Mutations in the channel domain alter desensitization of a neuronal nicotinic receptor. Nature 353: 846–849

Rhee S G, Suh P-G, Ryu S-H, Lee S Y 1989 Studies of inositol phospholipid-specific phospholipase C. Science 244: 546–550

Ross E M 1989 Signal sorting and amplification through G protein-coupled receptors. Neuron 3: 141–152

Schofield P R, Darlison M G, Fujita N et al 1987 Sequence and functional expression of the GABA$_A$ receptor shows a ligand-gated receptor super-family. Nature 328: 221–227

Sherman T G, Akil H, Watson S J 1989 The molecular biology of neuropeptides: neuropeptide genetics. In: Magistretti P J (ed) Discussions in neuroscience. Elsevier, Amsterdam, Vol VI, No 1

Sladeczek F, Récasens M, Bockaert J 1988 A new mechanism for glutamate receptor action: phosphoinositide hydrolysis. Trends in Neurosciences 11(12): 545–549

Snyder S H 1989 Drug and neurotransmitter receptors: new perspectives with clinical relevance. Journal of the American Medical Association 261: 3126–3129

Snyder S H 1990 The dopamine connection. Nature 347: 121–122

Snyder S H 1991 Vehicles of inactivation. Nature 354: 187

Sokoloff L 1989 Circulation and energy metabolism of the brain. In: Siegel G J, Alberto R W, Agranoff B W, Molinoff P B (eds) Basic neurochemistry: molecular, cellular, and medical aspects, 4th edn. Raven Press, New York, pp 565–590

Sokoloff P, Giros B, Martres M-P, Bouthenet M-L, Schwartz J-C 1990 Molecular cloning and characterization of a novel dopamine receptor (D$_3$) as a target for neuroleptics. Nature 347: 146–151

Sonders M S, Keana J F W, Weber E 1988 Phencyclidine and psychotomimetic sigma opiates: recent insights into their biochemical and physiological sites of action. Trends in Neurosciences 11: 37–40

Sternweis P C, Pang I-H 1990 The G protein-channel connection. Trends in Neurosciences 13(4): 122–126

Strader C D, Sigal I S, Dixon R F 1989 Structural basis of β-adrenergic receptor function. FASEB Journal 3: 1825–1832

Südhof T C, Czernik A J, Kao H-T et al 1989 Synapsins: mosaics of shared and individual domains in a family of synaptic vesicle phosphoproteins. Science 245: 1474–1480

Südhof T C 1995 The synaptic vesicle cycle: a cascade of protein – protein interactions. Nature 375: 645–646

Sunahara R K, Niznik H B, Weiner D M et al 1990 Human dopamine D$_1$ receptor encoded by an intronless gene on chromosome 5. Nature 347: 80–83

Sunahara R K, Guan H-C, O'Dowd B F et al 1991 Cloning

of the gene for a human dopamine D_5 receptor with higher affinity for dopamine than D_1. Nature 350: 614–619

Thomas D R, Nelson D R, Johnson A M 1987 Biochemical effects of the antidepressant paroxetinea specific 5-HT uptake inhibitor. Psychopharmacology 93: 193–200

Tsien R W, Lipscombe D, Madison D V, Bley K R, Fox A P 1988 Multiple types of neuronal calcium channels and their selective modulation. Trends in Neurosciences 11(10): 431–438

Van Tol H H M, Bunzow J R, Guan H-C et al 1991 Cloning of the gene for a human dopamine D_4 receptor with high affinity for the antipsychotic clozapine. Nature 350: 610–614

Volkow N D, Wang G -J, Fischman M W et al 1997a Relationship between subjective effects of cocaine and dopamine transporter occupancy. Nature 386: 827–830

Volkow N D, Wang G -J, Fowler J S et al 1997b Decreased striatal dopaminergic responsiveness in detoxified cocaine-dependent subjects. Nature 386: 830–833

Wang H-Y, Friedman E 1989 Lithium inhibition of protein kinase C activation-induced serotonin release. Psychopharmacology 99: 213–218

Williams L T 1989 Signal transduction by the platelet-derived growth factor receptor. Science 243: 1564–1570

Wollemann M 1990 Recent developments in the research of opioid receptor subtype molecular characterization. Journal of Neurochemistry 54: 1095–1101

Wong D F, Wagner H N, Tune L E et al 1986 Positron emission tomography reveals elevated D_2 dopamine receptors in drug-naive schizophrenics. Science 234: 1558–1563

Wong Y H, Bemoliou-Mason C D, Barnard E A 1989 Opioid receptors in magnesium-digitonin-solubilized rat brain membrane are tightly coupled to a pertussis toxin-sensitive guanine nucleotide-binding protein. Journal of Neurochemistry 52: 999–1009

Yamamoto C, McIlwain H 1966 Electrical activities in thin sections from the mammalian brain maintained in chemically-defined media in vitro. Journal of Neurochemistry 13(12): 1333–1343

Zhou Q-Y, Grandy D K, Thambi L et al 1990 Cloning and expression of human and rat D_1 dopamine receptors. Nature 347: 76–80

4

Clinical psychopharmacology

David G. Cunningham Owens

INTRODUCTION

The fact that human experience can be altered by drugs must rank, along with fire, as one of man's earliest discoveries. Accounts from the dawn of time bear witness to the use of plants and plant extracts for what might now be called recreational purposes. Furthermore, certain drugs came to occupy a central role in religious and cultural mysteries that remains evident to the present day. Even in medicine, the idea of medicaments having a 'tonic' or invigorating action, as much mental as physical, long antedated the arrival of psychiatry on the scene.

Despite this pervasive influence, psychiatry has had to work hard to gain acceptance for the range of pharmacological agents now available to it. Indeed the 'hard work' of modern psychiatric practice often seems to be equally split between advocacy for the use of medically recommended drugs and admonitions against the use of those not medically sanctioned!

The term 'psychopharmacology' is a relatively recent inhabitant of this ancient landscape, being attributed to the American pharmacologist, David Macht, in 1920. Although it has now achieved a pervasive professional acceptance, it is perhaps more a statement of an ideal and, as such, is to some extent a misnomer. Further more, for sections of the public it holds potentially sinister overtones. The way by which the drugs considered in this section achieve their effects is of course by actions on *brain* substrates, and the term 'neuropharmacology' is rather more neutral. None the less, the aim of drug treatments in psychiatric practice is to bring about efficacious changes in disorders affecting primarily the *mental state* and as such the idea of 'clinical *psycho*pharmacology' is not misplaced.

Drugs which produce mental state changes within a therapeutic context have been referred to by a series of generic names, though nowadays the most commonly used is *psychotropics* (i.e. acting on the mind). The term is not however specific. A number of compounds used

in medicine also affect mental state but are not given this generic classification, while contrariwise, some drugs utilised in psychiatric disorders have more peripheral than central actions. Also, an increasing number of illicit compounds are being manufactured specifically to produce alterations in mental state, though without medical sanction these are not conventionally referred to as 'psychotropic'.

Despite the value of medications in the treatment of psychiatric disorders, they are rarely if ever 'insulin' to a psychiatric 'diabetes'. They can bring about undoubtedly beneficial effects, but effects that are almost invariably partial. The complex interplay of biological and social factors that contribute to the development of psychiatric disorders is poorly understood and it remains the case that medication needs to be viewed as part of a treatment plan that incorporates a spectrum of approaches to management. None the less, psychopharmacology can be justly credited with a major – and increasing – positive contribution to the well-being of those afflicted with psychiatric disorders and to an understanding of the neurochemical basis of these.

All the major classes of drugs used in psychiatry comprise compounds whose clinical characteristics were identified empirically. It is often said that the discovery and introduction of these first-generation drugs was 'serendipitous' and, while this may be credible for some, a prior scientific lineage can be identified – however tenuously – in most.

The process began in 1949, when the Australian psychiatrist John Cade published the first account of the mood stabilising effects of lithium salts, though it would be many years before this could be brought to clinical realisation. The 'golden age' was however the decade of the 1950s. In December 1950, Paul Charpentier synthesised chlorpromazine, as the compound was initially called, and by 1952 its place was established as the foundation drug of the modern psychopharmacology era. In 1954 the *Rauwalfia* alkaloid reserpine, long a tool of Ayurvedic medicine, was introduced into Western psychiatry by Nathan Kline, who was also instrumental in the development of monoamine oxidase inhibitors, introduced in 1957 following observations of the mood-elevating actions of certain antituberculous agents. By the middle of the decade the first 'tranquilliser', meprobamate, became available and within 2 years rose to be the most widely prescribed drug in the USA. Also in 1955, the iminodibenzyl derivative of the renamed chlorpromazine was evaluated for antipsychotic efficacy, with somewhat disastrous results in that it seemed to promote manic-type symptoms in some patients. In 1957 however its efficacy in 'vital depression' was demonstrated by Kuhn and imipramine became the first tricyclic antidepressant, launched in 1958. In the same year, clozapine was synthesised and around that time the behavioural properties of the 1,4-benzodiazepines were identified by Randall, culminating in 1960 with the launch of chlordiazepoxide.

Golden ages are almost by definition time limited and so it was to be in psychopharmacology. For the next two decades what emerged was largely derivative. The next quarter century would be characterised by an increasing awareness of the therapeutic limitations of these empirically derived classes and the mounting dilemmas their adverse effects could present.

From the 1960s however, basic neuropharmacology started its exponential advance and in recent years psychotropic agents have for the first time started to emerge on the basis of specific hypotheses (though how accurate these 'hypotheses' are remains to be seen!). This first impacted on antidepressant psychopharmacology in the 1980s, though since the early 1990s has started to spread to the field of antipsychotics as well. This process is set to continue and, although it seems unlikely that this heralds a new 'golden age', these are certainly exciting times in psychopharmacology.

The following provides an overview of the major drug treatments used in current psychiatric practice, with clear priority given to pharmacology. This is done in the belief that an awareness of the pharmacology of the drugs we use daily should form the *starting point* for clinical practice, not an optional extra. It is no longer an adequate standard for therapeutic recommendations to be predicated solely on a reading of the *British National Formulary* or, worse, on the basis of mere habit or expediency. Should one share this belief, it is furthermore important to ensure that the major source of information is not the marketing literature for commercially available products.

There is however one caveat to bear in mind in the quest for pharmacological exactitude. The lifestyles of those who become 'users' of psychotropic medications differ in one crucial aspect from those of the volunteers from whom much of the pharmacokinetic data are acquired. Our patients are much more likely to smoke!

Smoking alters a number of the pharmacokinetic parameters pertinent to most psychotropic drugs, something the literature has only recently paid attention to. Furthermore, while diet is known to alter the kinetics of some drugs (e.g. valproate, see below), this aspect has been ignored in the literature on psychotropics. Thus the following data on pharmacokinetics might be seen for the most part as representing a set of baselines derived from a more 'ideal' population than the target one.

One of the consequences of the times being psychopharmacologically 'exciting' is that advances are occurring rapidly and some changes in the information presented here are almost inevitable before publication of the present volume.

ANTIPSYCHOTICS

Soon after the introduction of chlorpromazine in 1952 its use was noted to be associated with the development of parkinsonism, in the same way as reserpine. As this was largely a treatable and reversible phenomenon, it was for most psychiatrists not a matter of concern. Within a few years however, these neurological effects came to be seen as pointing to an *essential* element of the pharmacology and to offer a window on the drug's mode of action. To reflect these views, Jean Delay coined, in 1955, the term by which this new class of drugs has become universally known – 'neuroleptics', or compounds which forcibly 'grasp' or 'seize' neurones or the nervous system.

By the 1960s the idea that neurological effects were an essential herald of clinical efficacy had fallen into disrepute, though the term 'neuroleptics' has remained stubbornly entrenched. Nowhere else in pharmacology is a family of drugs classified on the basis of an adverse effect and the durability of the term is to be regretted.

The ideal would be to classify on the basis of a unique pharmacological characteristic that corresponds in some way to clinical usage. This is not yet possible. While all currently available compounds share in common dopamine blockade, not all drugs with this pharmacological profile are clinically effective in the management of major psychiatric disorders. In this situation, and again in line with convention, drugs effective clinically against psychotic disorders are best classified quite simply on the basis of this lead *clinical* function – that is descriptively, as 'antipsychotics'. These compounds exert unique effects that are *not* mediated via sedation, and any reference to them being 'tranquillisers' – major or otherwise – is erroneous. These unique effects are however evident at the *symptom*, not the syndromal, level so the class is diagnostically non-specific in its actions. It is therefore equally inaccurate to refer to them as 'antischizophrenics'.

An increasingly popular terminology is potentially a source of confusion. The idea of 'atypicality' has been applied to essentially all the new generation drugs. It remains unclear however on what parameters atypicality should be defined. The ideal would be if some clear pharmacological variable of difference could be linked to a pattern of clinical features that distinguished the atypical from the standard drugs, but this is not as yet possible. Essentially therefore atypicality is clinically defined and clozapine remains the benchmark. To be considered atypical, an antipsychotic should, like clozapine, have at least an exceptionally low or absent liability to promote extrapyramidal neurological disturbances throughout the therapeutic dose range, and not be associated with an elevation of serum prolactin or only produce a transient, ill-sustained increase (Lieberman 1993). Not all that is new in antipsychotic psychopharmacology is, by these criteria, atypical.

Structures

Despite being appropriately classified for the purposes of clinical pharmacology by a single term, antipsychotics in fact represent a chemically diverse group of compounds (Figure 4.1). The largest are the *phenothiazines*. The basic molecular structure was identified from methylene blue by August Bernthsen in 1883, and designated 'thiodiphenylamin'. Their modern name likewise reflects their essential composition – two benzene rings ('pheno'), linked by a central ring structure comprising a sulphur ('thio') and a nitrogen ('azo') atom, attached to which is a carbon side-chain terminating in a tertiary amine or a cyclic structural analogue of a tertiary amine.

Two types of substitution are important in the clinical pharmacology of phenothiazines. The first are substitutions of electronegative moieties, such as Cl or S-CH₃, at the so-called R1 site (position 2) which greatly enhances antipsychotic efficacy, probably independent of positive effects on potency (Baldessarini 1985). The second is the nature of the R2 substituted side-chains at position 10, which do affect potency but not efficacy and which form the basis of subclassification.

Dependent on the composition of these side-chains, phenothiazines can be subclassified as:

- *aliphatic* (or aminoalkyl), which have a straight chain of carbon atoms with methyl or alkyl substituents
- *piperidine*, in which the amino nitrogen is incorporated into a cyclic structure

- *piperazine*, in which the cyclic ring comprises two nitrogens and consequently is extended.

In all effective phenothiazines the side-chain comprises three carbon atoms.

As a rule, aliphatic compounds tend to be of low potency, with greater antiautonomic and sedative actions. They are therefore possessed overall of higher profiles of *general* adverse effects but have a lower liability to promote *extrapyramidal* adverse effects. Piperazine compounds on the other hand tend to be of high potency, with a relatively greater propensity to neurological adverse effects, but better general tolerability. Those with piperidine side-chains tend to adopt intermediate positions.

The *thioxanthenes* were synthesised in Denmark by Petersen and colleagues in 1958. Structurally they have been described as 'no more than a shift of emphasis' (Curry 1986) as they represent only a minor deviation from the phenothiazines in which the nitrogen of the latter's central ring is substituted by a carbon atom. The consequence of this structural change is that these compounds demonstrate stereoisomerism – that is, side-chain attachments can be mirror images of each other. This translates into considerable differences in pharmacology in that the affinity of different isomers for central dopamine (D₂) sites differs markedly. This group is represented by only a few compounds, including flupenthixol, the thioxanthene analogue of fluphenazine, and zuclopenthixol, the analogue of perphenazine.

The *butyrophenones*, which in structural terms may also be considered as *phenylbutylpiperidines*, represented an entirely new chemical group of compounds when the first of the group, haloperidol, was synthesised by Paul Janssen in 1958. They were subsequently shown to be amongst the most potent and selective D₂ antagonists. Thus these compounds possess a high propensity for induction of extrapyramidal side-effects but have overall very good *general* tolerability. Haloperidol, the major representative of the group, was to become the worldwide market leader antipsychotic, mainly due to its enthusiastic adoption in the USA. Droperidol is too short acting and sedative for routine use, but this latter property makes it a valuable tool in the management of emergency situations.

A modification to the side-chain structure of butyrophenones with the addition of an extra fluorinated benzene ring gives rise to the **diphenylbutylpiperidines** which have some of the longest half-lives of any antipsychotics. Since the withdrawal of fluspiriline in 1996 (for commercial reasons), only pimozide of this group has sustained a clinical presence, though some experimental compounds are also available, such as penfluridol.

Phenothiazine

Thioxanthene

Compound	R₁ substitution	R₂ substitution
Aliphatic		
Chlorpromazine	Cl	—CH₂—CH₂—CH₂—N(CH₃)₂
Piperidine		
Thioridazine	S—CH₃	—CH₂—CH₂— (N-methyl piperidine)
Piperazine		
Trifluoperazine	CF₃	—CH₂—CH₂—CH₂—N(piperazine)N—CH₃
Flupenthixol	CF₃	—CH—CH₂—CH₂—N(piperazine)N—CH₂—CH₂—OH*

Butyrophenone

Diphenylbutylpiperidine

Benzamide

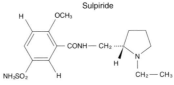

Dibenzazepine

Compound	R
Haloperidol	(4-chlorophenyl piperidine with OH*)
Pimozide	(benzimidazolone piperidine)

Sulpiride

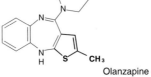

Dibenzo**diaz**epine

Clozapine

Dibenz**ox**azepine

Loxapine

Dibenzo**thia**zepine

Quetiapine

Thienobenzodiazepine

Olanzapine

* Depot esterification site

Fig. 4.1 Antipsychotic structures.

The exceptional half-lives of this group and the consequent possibility of infrequent (e.g. once weekly) oral dosing continues to make them an attractive clinical proposition.

Multiple substitutions of the basic benzene ring have been of pharmacological interest for many years. In the 1960s, modifications to the metoclopramide molecule (itself a modification of the antiarrhythmic, procainamide) produced sulpiride, the first of the antipsychotic *substituted benzamides*. The basic pharmacology of sulpiride appeared somewhat different from the other subgroups of antipsychotics, possibly indicating a dose-dependent action at presynaptic dopamine sites. Clinically it was also felt that, especially at low doses, its use may be associated with lower rates of extrapyramidal dysfunction. For these reasons sulpiride was the first antipsychotic to be talked of as 'atypical'. The substituted benzamides represent one of the largest group of psychotropic agents available worldwide, though only a few have effective antipsychotic properties and of these only sulpiride remains widely available. Remoxipride, an effective and successful drug immediately following its launch, was withdrawn in most countries in 1993 after the identification of a cluster of aplastic anaemia cases associated with its use. Amisulpride has been available in France for a number of years and may be due for a wider launch, and the highly potent raclopride, to date confined to experimental receptor binding work, has been shown to be effective clinically (British Isles Raclopride Study Group 1992).

Interest in the piperazine derivatives of the *dibenzazepine* tricyclic molecule goes back to the early days of psychopharmacology and is again in the ascendant. Those compounds with two nitrogen atoms in the central ring are termed *dibenzodiazepines*, the only currently available representative of which is also one of the most important compounds in the psychopharmacological canon, clozapine. Compounds in which one of the central ring nitrogens is substituted with an oxygen atom are *dibenzoxazepines*, of which loxapine is the sole marketed representative. Substitution of the same nitrogen with a sulphur atom gives rise to *dibenzothiazepines*. This group has traditionally been represented by compounds such as metiapine and clothiapine, which have never been available in the UK. However, one of the new generation antipsychotics, quetiapine (or Seroquel) is a novel representative of this group. A slightly more radical modification of the basic molecule involves substitution of one of the benzo rings with a thieno ring, creating a **thieno**benzodiazepine structure, of which the only current example is the recently launched olanzapine.

Other agents of more diverse chemical structure but with antipsychotic efficacy or potential include the *benzisoxazole* derivative risperidone, the first of the new generation drugs to achieve an international launch; the *benzisothiazoylpiperazine*, ziprasidone currently in late-stage development; and *indole* derivatives such as the long available oxypertine and the recently launched sertindole.

Pharmacokinetics

Oral formulations Surprisingly little is known about the mechanisms mediating *absorption* of antipsychotics but following *oral* ingestion most appear to be rapidly and completely absorbed from the proximal small bowel, with times to peak blood levels (T_{max}) in the range of 2–4 hours, though for reasons that are unclear wide discrepancies (0.5–6 hours) have been reported for haloperidol (Jorgensen 1986).

Orally administered antipsychotics are subject to *presystemic extraction* or *first-pass* effects with passage through the liver, the major clearing organ for these compounds. The extent of first-pass effects is dependent on a drug's *clearance* which, for almost all antipsychotics, is *flow*-limited and not capacity-limited (Greenblatt 1993). Thus the clearance depends only on the ability of the portal system to deliver drug to the liver and not on intermediate metabolism. The consequence of this is that the bulk of an orally administered antipsychotic dose does not reach the systemic circulation. Of that which does, only free drug is available for end-receptor activity. However, all antipsychotics are highly membrane bound and protein bound, especially to albumin, though also to other proteins such as α-glycoprotein. The bound fraction varies from around 90% to more than 98%. Free drug is rapidly and widely *distributed* due to a particular physicochemical property which is crucial to their effectiveness – lipophilicity. This not only means that unbound drug readily crosses the blood–brain barrier and is widely available to brain sites but also that uptake into peripheral organs is extensive. Antipsychotics therefore have a large *apparent volume of distribution*. Drug is reversibly and dynamically bound to peripheral sites, especially in lung and other organs with a rich blood supply, as well as adipose tissue, from where it is readily released back into the systemic circulation as excretion progresses, a factor underlying the persistence of efficacy and adverse actions and of active moieties in plasma long after cessation of treatment. As a result of these kinetic properties, standard antipsychotics have rather *low* bioavailability, which for chlorpromazine is in the region of 30%, though for haloperidol it appears to be higher at around 60% (Dahl and Strandjord 1977).

The elimination half-lives of antipsychotics, as with all drugs, bear a mathematical relationship to their hepatic clearance and volume of distribution. Despite their extensive clearance and wide distributions, the half-life of most antipsychotics is in the intermediate range at around 20 hours. Most are therefore suitable for once daily dosing regimens. However, wide distribution also means that following cessation of treatment drug can seep back into the systemic circulation over long periods. Thus the *terminal phase* half-life of some of these compounds is very long (in the case of chlorpromazine up to 60 days), resulting in the persistence of detectable drug moieties for many months – if not years – after exposure has ceased (Curry 1986).

Although antipsychotics cross the blood–brain barrier readily this does not mean they do so completely. Cerebrospinal fluid (CSF) levels have not been extensively studied but appear to represent only about 3–4% of plasma levels for chlorpromazine and haloperidol, which correspond approximately to free fractions in plasma, though they do seem to vary considerably in different individuals and with different preparations (Jorgensen 1986).

Metabolism is mainly in the liver for the simple reason that lipophilic compounds must be transformed into water-soluble ones in order to be excreted via the kidney. Antipsychotic metabolism is in general extensive, with little parent drug eliminated. The processes involved are for the most part unsophisticated ones, including oxidation, *N*-dealkylation and conjugation with glucuronic acid. Some metabolites are excreted in bile.

While some antipsychotics, such as flupenthixol and pimozide, do not appear to produce active metabolites, the majority do and some produce several which have clinically significant antipsychotic actions. This has profoundly complicated the field of therapeutic blood monitoring as the percentage of active metabolite varies considerably across individuals and these products have their own pharmacokinetic properties. Thus although therapeutic monitoring has been a recurrent theme of mainly the American literature over the past 20 years, it has not as yet led to anything that is clinically useful.

The exception to the above general principles is sulpiride, which appears to have somewhat different – and less favourable – pharmacokinetic parameters from other antipsychotics. Considerable amounts of sulpiride can be recovered unchanged from faeces, implying that part of its low bioavailability (around 27%) is a consequence of relatively poor absorption. Poor absorption and difficulty in crossing the blood–brain barrier are undoubtedly both a result of the fact that, unusually for an antipsychotic, sulpiride

is *water* soluble. The drug is subject to little first-pass effects and is substantially less protein bound than others of the class (approx. 40–50%). Estimated half-lives have been widely variable (Jorgensen 1986) but with an average of approximately 8 hours are in general shorter than those reported for other drugs and sulpiride is not suitable for once daily dosing. Benzamides as a group are subject to a number of metabolic steps which produce inactive products. They are none the less excreted to a considerable extent unchanged in the urine.

The specific therapeutic actions of antipsychotics are invariably delayed. It is usually stated that antipsychotic efficacy does not become evident till about the third week of treatment, though this may to some extent reflect methodological issues in the relevant studies. None the less it is clear that the desired effects inevitably emerge only after a week or two of regular exposure. This probably reflects partly receptor events that underlie the action of the drugs, though with antipsychotics, as with all drugs, it probably also reflects the time to steady state.

Steady state is achieved when the overall mean concentration of parent drug and active metabolites does not alter as long as the daily dose and factors influencing clearance do not undergo change. It is described by a constant relationship – namely that four half-lives are required to achieve within 10% of the steady-state condition (Greenblatt 1993). Clearly, drugs with very long half-lives, such as pimozide, will require much longer to achieve steady state than the likes of sulpiride, which has a much shorter half-life. This figure of four half-lives also applies to the time to achieve 90% elimination of a drug from plasma. Thus, in theory at least, drugs of short half-life may be associated with a more rapid onset of action but a swifter relapse rate on discontinuation. The trial evidence to support either of these assumptions is lacking, though at an anecdotal level the latter scenario might hold some truth.

Depot formulations   The kinetics of depot preparations are highly complex and markedly different from the above. Depots are manufactured by esterification of a terminal side-chain hydroxyl group to a long-chain fatty acid and the ester dissolved in an inert oil base. The most commonly utilised base is sesame oil, though the Lundbeck products (Depixol, Clopixol, Acuphase) use a synthetic triglyceride called Viscoleo. Following intramuscular injection, esters *slowly* diffuse from the oil base, though release may also be determined by partial metabolism of the oil, and are thereafter *rapidly* hydrolysed by plasma, and possibly muscle, esterases to release active drug.

Both the oily base and the fatty acid utilised in the esterification process are important in determining the kinetics of depot preparations. Viscoleo may be degraded more rapidly than sesame oil, which may be one reason why the decanoate of flupenthixol is detectable for a less protracted period after last injection than that of fluphenazine. The role of the fatty acid in determining the rate of drug release can be seen with zuclopenthixol which, when esterified with acetic acid (as Acuphase), gives plasma concentration curves closer to those of an aqueous solution than the characteristic depot curves found when the drug is esterified with decanoic acid (Clopixol).

These manufacturing principles radically alter the kinetics of depot preparations. This is because their pharmacokinetics are limited by the rate of drug absorption, not the rate of metabolism as is the case with other pharmaceuticals. Traditional pharmacokinetic models do not apply in such situations and that pertinent to depots has been christened a 'flip-flop' model, where the absorption rate constant is *less* than the elimination rate constant (Ereshefsky et al 1983, Jann et al 1985). Interpreting plasma curves in this situation is difficult as declines in blood levels reflect not only metabolism but also protracted absorption.

Most of the available long-acting depots (excluding zuclopenthixol acetate) share similar kinetic properties. Most achieve maximal plasma levels gradually over approximately 4–7 days, followed by a gentle decline in the subsequent few weeks. The exception is fluphenazine decanoate which uniquely achieves peak levels rapidly, within about 12–24 hours of administration, with an equally rapid decline to about one-third peak, followed by a more gradual reduction over the subsequent few weeks (Jann et al 1985). The reason for this rapid postinjection peak is not understood but may be related to the drug's vulnerability to muscle hydrolases. It probably underlies some difference in the pattern of early neurological adverse effects reported with depots (Owens 1998). Half-lives in the range of 5–7 days following single doses of depots appear to increase with multiple dosing to something in the range of 14–21 days (Jann et al 1985), though in a few individuals the half-life of flupenthixol decanoate has been found to be greatly extended (up to 112 days).

The pharmacokinetics of depots have clear clinical implications. The first is of course that drugs in this formulation do not undergo first-pass effects so the desired actions can be achieved with lower absolute doses. Of greater importance is the fact that depots take much longer than oral preparations to reach steady state and much longer to clear following discontinuation. Most achieve steady state after about 3 months, though again fluphenazine decanoate may be different, with a time of about 6 weeks reported (Jann et al 1985). This latter preparation can however be detected in plasma for up

to 12 weeks, and occasionally longer, after cessation of treatment, while the decanoate of flupenthixol has in general been found to be present for only about half this time.

The clinical implications are that depots are not as a rule suitable for acute phase management and that, after cessation, relapse may be substantially delayed by the actions of residual medication, a phenomenon perhaps more evident with Modecate than, for example, Depixol. Furthermore, dose regimens must be flexible and empirically derived in order to avoid detrimental cumulative effects in some patients.

Pharmacodynamics

Mode of action   As can be seen, from the chemical point of view antipsychotics represent a diverse class of compounds, diversity reflected in their clinical pharmacology. In general, those with more selective receptor-binding actions tend to be possessed of less extensive *general* adverse effects, both peripherally and centrally mediated. This may also extend to relatively stable general tolerability with increasing doses. In recent studies of the new generation drug, risperidone, in which data from two dose schedules of the comparator haloperidol and a placebo group were available, only 'nausea/vomiting' of 21 non-extrapyramidal adverse effects assessed in standardised fashion showed a dose-related increase in prevalence with a doubling of the dose of haloperidol from 10 mg to 20 mg per day (Owens 1996). A further general rule is that phenothiazines tend to be associated with higher levels of more varied adverse effects than other types of drugs (Edwards 1986), possibly a reflection of the known toxicity of the basic molecule that so hindered clinical development of the group for over half a century.

While peripheral actions of drugs are of practical importance in tolerability and safety, it is to the central pharmacology that we must look to understand efficacy. Again in line with their structural diversity, antipsychotics vary widely in their central pharmacology. Some examples are shown in Figure 4.2. In 1963, Carlsson and Lindquist suggested that antipsychotic drugs acted as postsynaptic dopamine antagonists, something that has now been clearly established. In 1979, Calne and Kebabian classified central dopamine receptors into two types – D_1 and D_2 – on the basis of the ability of the former to stimulate the synthesis of adenylate cyclase.

Whatever else these drugs may do in relation to other receptor systems, *all* currently known compounds of proven efficacy block central dopamine D_2 receptors at postsynaptic sites. While compounds acting at predominantly presynaptic (autoreceptor) sites and relatively selective D_1 antagonists may hold some potential, to date *no* strategies invoking other than postsynaptic D_2 antagonism have translated into effective antipsychotic treatments.

However, it has become clear that the situation is more complicated than any bald assertion regarding D_2 antagonism would imply. With the introduction of molecular biological techniques it has become clear that the D_1/D_2 classification represents at least two 'families' of receptor subtypes – the D_1 family comprising D_1 and D_5 isomorphs, and the D_2 family comprising the so-called long and short varieties of D_2, plus the D_3 and D_4 isomorphs. Antipsychotics differ considerably in their affinities for different isomorphs of the D_2 receptor, which has become a matter of some interest in recent years in the exploration of the detailed basis of the antipsychotic effect.

In addition, as Figure 4.2 shows, most antipsychotics are active at a range of other receptor types apart from dopaminergic ones. This was for many years felt to represent contamination contributing to adverse rather than therapeutic effects. The reason for this view springs from the inferences of the 'dopamine hypothesis of schizophrenia'. This is elaborated in three forms: that schizophrenia is a result of overactivity in central (mesolimbic) dopamine systems that is presynaptically mediated via increased turnover; or that is postsynaptically mediated via receptor supersensitivity; and that antipsychotic efficacy is mediated by (mesolimbic) dopamine D_2 antagonism. Despite the fact that only the last 'version' of this has any experimental support, the hypothesis has held a strong sway over perceptions concerning the pathogenesis of schizophrenia and the mechanism underlying its treatment.

The thrust therefore was to produce drugs that were increasingly selective D_2 antagonists and that acted preferentially on the mesolimbic as opposed to the nigrostriatal dopamine system. The benzamides represent to some extent the realisation of this. However this approach was turned on its head by the demonstration that clozapine, a highly *un*selective transmitter antagonist (Figure 4.2), was of superior efficacy to a standard drug (chlorpromazine) in at least treatment-resistant schizophrenia (Kane et al 1988). Drugs previously considered pharmacologically 'dirty' assumed the status of having a 'rich and challenging' pharmacology and, in the search for new treatments, the highly selective approach rapidly gave way to the highly unselective approach.

Of the many possible models that could be extracted from the complex pharmacology of clozapine, the one which has been thus far pursued to the market place focuses on serotonergic mechanisms and in particular

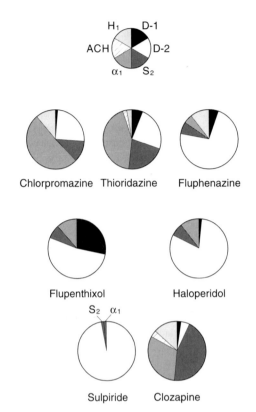

Fig. 4.2 Receptor-binding profiles of some commonly used antipsychotics.

the 5-HT$_{2A}$ receptor subtype. The new generation of antipsychotics all seek to combine D_2 antagonism with a powerful degree of 5-HT$_{2A}$ antagonism. However, it is also clear that if clozapine is now our model, the 'ideal' drug need not – indeed *should* not – be associated with the high levels of D_2 occupancy found with standard drugs. Using in vivo brain imaging, it has been shown that therapeutic doses of standard drugs are associated with 70–80% blockade of dopamine D_2 receptors. With clozapine, however, occupancy levels are only in the range of 50–60% (Farde et al 1992).

Thus our current model of antipsychotic efficacy is predicated on a combination of relatively weak D_2 antagonism with relatively potent 5-HT$_{2A}$ antagonism. All the new generation drugs either available or in late-stage development adopt this so-called serotonin–dopamine antagonist (SDA) approach. This interpretation of clozapine's benefits has resulted in a revivification of antipsychotic psychopharmacology by breaking us away from the confines of the classical dopamine hypothesis. It is however not the only model that can be proposed from clozapine's pharmacology and it is to be hoped that in future years other developments in the field will represent innovative explorations of these, rather than merely the repetitious production of further derivative compounds.

Adverse (or 'non-target') effects

General Antipsychotics can be associated with the production of a wide range of general adverse effects (Table 4.1). Despite this, these drugs are, as a class, remarkably safe. In other words, with regard to adverse effects of major medical significance, antipsychotics have in general a *wide* therapeutic index. However, with regard to adverse effects that may not be medically significant but are none the less unpleasant and intrusive for the patient, their therapeutic index is far less favourable. It is important for doctors to acknowledge that what to them may be minor, can be quite the opposite to the patient and may impact disproportionally on compliance.

Dry mouth, constipation, blurring of vision from impaired accommodation and, especially in males, *impaired urinary* and *sexual* function are not uncommon complaints from patients receiving antipsychotics, even those with little inherent anticholinergic activity. A background level of such symptomatology is to be found in patients on placebo and a proportion of these complaints undoubtedly reflect illness, rather than treatment, effects. Some are however likely to have more complex origins than 'single transmitter' pharmacology would lead us to believe and may be at least partially mediated by antiadrenergic as well as anticholinergic mechanisms. Problems of this sort are usually of little medical import but deserve to be taken seriously as they can be distressing or form the source of further medical problems. For example, a simple dry mouth can result in *stomatitis* which may be present in the majority of patients, especially those with dentures, and can lay the seeds of oral *candidiasis* and long-term *dental caries* and *gum disease* (Lucas 1993), while paralysis of accommodation can precipitate *closed-angle glaucoma* in those predisposed.

Clozapine may, in line with its potent anticholinergic actions, produce a dry mouth but more commonly its use is associated with *increased salivation*, The pharmacological basis for this is unknown but it is probably not an extrapyramidal phenomenon. It is therefore best referred to descriptively as hypersalivation rather than sialorrhoea, which is more intimately associated with the bradykinesia of parkinsonism. Hypersalivation increases in frequency with continued exposure and can affect up to three-quarters of those on clozapine (Lieberman et al 1994). It can be obviated by small starting doses and very slow increments but can remain a major obstacle to continued treatment.

Weight gain can be a major problem with all antipsy-

chotic drugs and is a further reason for non-compliance especially in women (Holden & Holden 1979, Silverstone et al 1988). The mechanism underlying this is usually ascribed to antiserotonergic actions but it is unlikely this provides the complete explanation as it was a phenomenon also reported in patients receiving remoxipride, a drug with little or no 5-HT actions (Owens 1996).

Antiautonomic actions result in an increase in resting *heart rate* which is usually of the order of 10 beats per minute or less and is not clinically significant. The more powerfully antiadrenergic drugs can also produce a significant fall in *blood pressure*, which is mainly *postural*. This is a potentially serious development that can precipitate myocardial ischaemia/infarction or cerebrovascular accident. For this reason such drugs, which are particularly represented by the low potency phenothiazines, should *never* be administered intravenously, and caution should *always* be exercised with intramuscular use.

Changes in the ECG include delayed ventricular repolarisation, as evidenced in prolongation of the QT interval, which is usually of no significance. In addition, ST depression, T wave flattening and on occasion the emergence of U waves can be found. Such changes seem to relate to the chemical structure of the drug and probably to potency. Hence they are more associated with phenothiazines, and with chlorpromazine and thioridazine more than trifluoperazine – approximately 50% versus 16% respectively (Lipscomb 1980). However, the development of ECG changes, and in particular the consequences of these, seem as much, if not more, related to the pharmacology of individual compounds and the doses used. High-dose thioridazine seems particularly associated with the development of tachyarrhythmias, including the particularly serious *torsade de pointes* (Smith & Gallagher 1980). Haloperidol has also been implicated in this potentially fatal dysrhythmia, though usually only when very high doses have been utilised in those with pre-existing heart disease, for example that associated with prolonged alcohol abuse (Metzger & Friedman 1993, Wilt et al 1993).

Such dysrhythmogenic potential may underlie the *sudden death syndrome* which has been reported in those receiving antipsychotics. This is a rare occurrence, usually involving apparently fit young males treated with higher dose regimens (Levinson & Simpson 1987). Whether it can be distinguished from the consequences of autonomic hyperarousal in general is unclear, though extreme muscular overactivity may indeed adversely alter the pharmacokinetics of certain agents (Jusic & Lader 1994), a factor emphasising the need for care when forcibly administering parenteral medications during psychiatric emergencies.

Table 4.1   Non-neurological adverse reactions to antipsychotic agents

Adverse reaction	Frequency	Comment	Adverse reaction	Frequency	Comment
General			*Dermatological*		
Sedation	++	Especially with low-potency drugs	Skin rashes	++	
			Erythematous	++	
'Torpor' ('ataraxy')	+++		Urticarial	Rare	
Dry mouth, blurred vision, constipation, urinary difficulties, impaired sexual function	+	Conventionally viewed as peripheral anticholinergic effects. Some probably include adrenergic actions	Contact	Rare	
			Photosensitivity	++	Can result in serious burning. Temperature less important than brightness
Priapism	Rare		Pigmentation	? Rare	Infrequently reported nowadays
Weight gain	+++				
Stomatitis/oral candidiasis	Very common	Rarely clinically significant	Alopecia	? Not uncommon	
			Haematological		
Cardiovascular system			Neutropenia	Rare	Except with clozapine: reversible neutropenia. Can progress to agranulocytosis if drug maintained
Increased heart rate	+++	Not clinically significant			
Hypotension	++	Can be fatal – caution with early exposure to low-potency drugs			
ECG changes	++	Quinidine-like effect			
Tachyarrhythmias	Rare				
Torsade de pointes	Very rare	Haloperidol but particularly thioridazine	Agranulocytosis	Very rare	
			Thrombocytopenia	Very rare	
			Haemolytic anaemia	Very rare	
Endocrine					
Hyperprolactinaemia	+++	Universal effect (standard drugs)	Aplastic anaemia	Very rare	? Except with remoxipride
Galactorrhoea	Rare	Rarely clinically significant	*Ophthalmic*		
Amenorrhoea	+	Rarely clinically significant	Lenticular deposits	Rare	Reversible with detection
Gynaecomastia	Rare	Rarely clinically significant	Pigmentary retinopathy	Rare	High dose, long term thioridazine; rarely with low doses
Hyper/hypoglycaemia	Rare	Rarely clinically significant			
Inappropriate antidiuretic hormone secretion	Rare	May present with oedema			
			Immunological		
Hepatic			IgM Isotype antiphospholipid antibodies	Very common overall (40–50%)	? All drugs but especially chlorpromazine. ? Clinical significance
Impaired liver function	++	Transient changes common. Jaundice especially with chlorpromazine (1–2%)	'Lupus anticoagulant' Antinuclear antibody Rheumatoid factor		
			Systemic lupus erythematosus	Very rare	

+, Infrequent; ++, frequent; +++, very frequent.
From Owens (1996).

Particular concern was raised following reports of 13 sudden, unexpected and apparently cardiac deaths in patients receiving pimozide, which in 1990 led the Committee on Safety of Medicines to issue strict guidelines for the use of this drug. There is in addition some epidemiological evidence that the risk of sudden death may be greater with thioridazine (Mehtonen et al 1991). A particular pharmacological action links these two drugs and may be of relevance – namely, that both have potent calcium channel antagonist properties (Gould et al, 1983, 1984). These cardiovascular system (CVS) actions make thioridazine a surprising drug to occupy the 'first choice' position it currently appears to enjoy in old age psychiatry.

During the phase III evaluations of the new generation antipsychotic sertindole, 27 deaths were reported, 16 due to adverse cardiac events (*Lancet*, 1996). This figure seems high (in a comparably sized sample, a single sudden death occurred in the phase III risperidone studies) and may be related to the drug's action in prolonging the QT interval, thereby rendering patients susceptible to torsade de pointes. As a result, ECG monitoring is currently a required accompaniment of sertindole prescription.

Isolated reports have suggested that long-term use of clozapine may be associated with development of a *cardiomyopathy*, though these may represent cases of incidental pathology. The question remains as yet unresolved but even if the association holds true, it represents a very rare occurrence.

Hyperprolactinaemia is an inevitable consequence of treatment with standard antipsychotics and results from blockade of tuberoinfundibular dopamine D_2 receptors. Rises in prolactin can be detected within a few hours of exposure, reaching a plateau within 4–7 days and remaining elevated for the duration of exposure (Meltzer & Fang 1976). Particularly high levels can be attained in patients on sulpiride. For the most part this is an asymptomatic phenomenon, though it may be associated with breast engorgement and *galactorrhoea* in both males and females. It may also contribute to *amenorrhoea*, though in the emotionally disturbed, disorder of the menstrual cycle has complex origins. It does not directly underlie the *gynaecomastia* encountered rarely in males on long-term treatment, as this is more related to disturbances in oestrogen:androgen ratios (Edwards, 1986).

Clearly many of these features can simulate pregnancy, a misattribution easily compounded by the tendency of phenothiazines to produce a false-positive pregnancy test.

Prolactin response is one feature that distinguishes new generation drugs from standard compounds. With one exception, the new generation drugs, in line with clozapine, produce either no increase or only a transient, non-significant increase throughout the dose range. The exception to some extent is risperidone which does produce a dose-related hyperprolactinaemia evident at the higher end of the therapeutic range (Ereshefsky & Lacombe 1993).

Phenothiazines unpredictably interfere with *glucose metabolism* and may promote both hypoglycaemia and, by inhibiting insulin secretion, hyperglycaemia, though only rarely does this complicate diabetic control. Likewise the *oedema* that can result from stimulation of antidiuretic hormone is usually mild and of little clinical significance. Other *endocrine changes* such as suppression of corticotrophin, growth hormone, thyroid stimulating hormone, follicle stimulating hormone and luteinising hormone are of uncertain and probably negligible clinical import (Edwards 1986).

Minor, transient *increases in hepatic enzymes* are not uncommon with antipsychotic treatment, especially chlorpromazine. These changes only result in clinical *jaundice* in 1–2% of exposures, which represents a striking decline from the drug's early days (Regal et al 1987). The reason for this fall is unclear, though it probably relates to better manufacturing processes, resulting in removal of contaminants present in the early samples. It is widely believed that the hepatic damage underlying these changes is allergic and indeed this is undoubtedly part of the aetiology. However, histological examination shows not only allergically mediated cholestatic change but scattered hepatic necrosis. Hence direct toxicity is also part of the mechanism. Phenothiazine-induced jaundice is usually benign and although symptoms may resolve with continued exposure this is not to be recommended and it is prudent in this situation to change to the dose equivalence of another compound. Cross-sensitivity among antipsychotics is rare so a switch to another phenothiazine is usually all that is required for resolution, though this may take 6–8 weeks. A few cases have been reported which progressed to a *primary biliary cirrhosis* type of picture, though this is very uncommon and the prognosis appears better than the idiopathic form of the condition (Regal et al 1987).

The risk of *skin rashes* with antipsychotics is high, especially with chlorpromazine. About 5–10% of patients on this compound develop a typical erythematous hypersensitivity-type rash within 10–14 days of first exposure, though sooner if previously exposed. This can be treated with antihistamines but again it is prudent to consider a change of drug. Contact dermatitis has been described in medical and nursing staff handling chlorpromazine, though this again appears to be an infrequent observation nowadays. *Photosensitivity* is on the other hand far from infrequent. Dermatological sources quote a prevalence figure in the range of 3% but this undoubtedly only applies to more severe cases. The pathology results from a mixture of phototoxicity and photoallergy with an action in the UVA range. It is not only the heat of the sun that is important, so patients can receive considerable burns in conditions that are subjectively relatively temperate.

Pigmentation is again a problem largely confined to phenothiazines and one rarely commented on nowadays. Earlier descriptions were of widespread deposition of a melanin-type pigment on mainly exposed areas. This imparted either a silvery or bluish-purple hue to patients, who were most often female, as a result of which the soubriquet 'purple people' was used. It may be that this was a phenomenon that resulted from chronic use of high-dose regimens, hence its decline. Deposition of pigment in the lens of the eye is still common and although this infrequently impairs vision the risk of *cataract* may be increased about 3–4-fold (Isaac et al 1991). Of much greater significance, though lesser prevalence, is retinal deposition of pigment. *Pigmentary retinopathy* has been most frequently associated with long-term use of high dose thioridazine (Weekly et al 1960, Marmor 1990) and, as it is an important though probably reversible development, guidelines now recommend that this drug should not be used in doses of more than 600 mg daily for longer than 4 weeks.

Hair loss is a not infrequent complaint of patients on psychotropics, especially women, and is a genuine observation, though it is more likely to be associated with tricyclics and mood stabilisers than antipsychotics (Warnock 1991). Usually it merely represents a speeding up of normal shedding and although the hair may thin it does not as a rule result in patches of complete loss, though full *alopecia areata* has been described (Kubota et al 1994).

Antipsychotics can potently suppress marrow function. Although any type of drug can be implicated, the problems are individually greatest with clozapine and collectively with phenothiazines. Clozapine-induced *neutropenia*, which is reversible on discontinuing the drug, has a cumulative incidence of 2.33% at 1 year, approximately 3% at 2 years, with a small (0.5–0.75%) but continuing risk thereafter (Owens 1996). *Agranulocytosis* with clozapine is also reversible following its early detection and discontinuation of the drug but can be fatal if allowed to persist. Data from long-term monitoring in the UK suggest an incidence of 0.73% at 1 year and 0.8% at 2 years (Atkin et al 1996). This certainly represents an idiosyncratic allergic response in affected individuals but as yet no clear predictors have been identified. It occurs early in exposure, with over 80% of cases developing in the first 3 months, with the peak in the third month. No cases have emerged after 2 years. Clozapine may also produce an eosinophilia which appears benign.

Although it is known that other antipsychotics, especially phenothiazines, can produce similar effects on the granulocyte cell line, accurate comparative data are surprisingly not available. In the only systematic evaluation, undertaken in the 1970s, patients receiving various phenothiazines were monitored over an 8 week exposure period. Transient leucopenia was noted in 10%, while agranulocytosis was estimated to occur in 1:1200 exposures (Pisciotta 1978). This is a higher risk than the 1:1400 exposures attributed to clozapine but the data from which these calculations are derived are not comparable. It is generally agreed that agranulocytosis is an established but *rare* complication of phenothiazine treatment, the risk being less than with clozapine.

Suppression of other marrow lines, such as erythrocytes and platelets, has been associated with antipsychotic exposure, but as with haemolytic anaemia, these comprise only sporadic reports and these adverse effects must be very uncommon. However, a cluster of eight cases of aplastic anaemia occurring in patients receiving remoxipride (though none was on this alone) was sufficient to lead to its withdrawal in most countries.

Clozapine (and remoxipride, at the time of writing still available in the UK) requires regular haematological monitoring as a mandatory part of its administration.

Antipsychotics can mediate change in a number of *immunological* parameters. The development of IgM isotype antiphospholipid antibodies can be detected in up to 50% of patients, again particularly those on chlorpromazine, though the significance of this is unknown, which is also the case for so-called 'lupus anticoagulant' (Canoso et al 1990, Zucker et al 1990). In the 1970s there was considerable interest in the high percentage of patients with major psychiatric disorders who were positive for antinuclear antibody. Interest waned when it became clear that rather than reflecting illness factors these changes could likewise be attributed to treatment. Very rarely, phenothiazines can cause a drug-induced *systemic lupus erythematosus*. These immunological abnormalities are poorly understood but speak of pervasive drug effects that would justify more detailed investigation than has been undertaken to date.

Finally, depot formulations may on occasion cause *reactions* at their injection site. These have been reported with fluphenazine decanoate and haloperidol decanoate and comprise a firm, tender and sometimes pruritic mass which can remain for up to 3 months (Hamann et al 1990). These may not relate simply to flawed injection technique but are more likely to be the result of impaired vascularisation with consequent delayed absorption. For this reason, injection sites should be rotated.

Neurological: non-specific Antipsychotics are not in classificatory terms 'sedatives' – that is, they do not bring about their desired effects in a barbiturate-like fashion. They can however produce *sedation* as a frequent adverse effect, especially the low potency phenothiazines and especially early in exposure. This is probably a consequence of a compound's antihistamine (H_1) activity. Although an adverse effect, this is a property that can be therapeutically advantageous in the control of behavioural disturbance, particularly in acute management.

Almost all antipsychotics alter the EEG. With remoxipride, changes are minimal, though they are particularly evident (in a dose-related fashion) with clozapine, where up to one-third of patients may demonstrate striking changes. The effect is toward a general slowing of waveforms with a decrease in α waves and an increase in θ and δ waves. Chronic exposure results in increasing synchronisation with increasing slow-wave activity and increasing amplitude. Spike and sharp waves can be superimposed and paroxysmal discharges similar to epileptiform activity may be seen. The reason why access to a detailed drug history is essential for the interpretation of an EEG will be clear.

As a consequence of these electrophysiological actions, antipsychotics lower the seizure threshold and there is overall approximately a 1% risk of the drugs precipitating *fits* (though this was not reported with remoxipride). The risk with low-dose clozapine (<300 mg per day) does not appear to be increased, though with doses above 300 mg a prevalence as high as 14% has been reported. This results in an average risk for clozapine of about 4% (Baldessarini & Frankenburg 1991).

It may be that antipsychotic-induced lowering of seizure threshold results in fits mainly in the context of some other predisposing factors, such as a past or family history of epilepsy, or pre-existing cerebral pathology. However, fits can be precipitated even in the absence of any such apparent predisposition and treatment variables such as polypharmacy, rapid increments and high-dose regimens may be relevant.

In terms of a rank order of risk, chlorpromazine appears to top the list, with thioridazine, pimozide, haloperidol and fluphenazine at the bottom, behind trifluoperazine which appears intermediate in liability (Cold et al 1990). Seizures in themselves are a potentially serious complication but, as they can usually be managed by a *gradual* switch to another preparation and the introduction of anticonvulsants, they do not represent a contraindication to antipsychotic use.

Antipsychotics can interfere with temperature control to produce two opposing clinical effects. Phenothiazines, and especially chlorpromazine, exert a *poikilothermic* action – that is they can lower core body temperature. This can result in clinical hypothermia, especially if the patient's alcohol intake is excessive, causing additional heat loss from peripheral vasodilatation.

Of greater interest in recent years has been the opposite action – namely, *hyper*thermia and the issue of *neuroleptic malignant syndrome*. This term has been applied to a syndrome of dramatic temperature rise sometimes amounting to hyperthermia, extrapyramidal symptomatology especially rigidity, confusion and autonomic lability. Creatine phosphokinase is usually strikingly elevated. The disorder has been reported most frequently in young males and most commonly early in treatment. This is a rare development but published prevalences, which range from 0.02 to 2.4%, help us little in deciding how rare. The largest study to date, of almost 10,000 Chinese patients, suggested a figure of 0.12%, which is more consonant with clinical practice than some of the more extravagant claims in the literature (Deng et al 1990). There is however a further problem with this concept, in that it has been shown that the diagnosis is often made in the presence of other medical conditions that could more readily explain the symptomatology (Levinson & Simpson 1986). Neuroleptic malignant syndrome has a reported mortality of around 20% (Shalev et al 1989) and can result in residual neurological deficits in survivors. It usually resolves, however, on discontinuation of the implicated antipsychotic and the instigation of palliative measures, such as rehydration, correction of electrolyte imbalance, and if necessary the use of benzodiazepines. Anticholinergics may be tried in those with profound rigidity but must be used with care as they may add to confusion and further impede heat loss by impairing sweat secretion. Non-selective drugs (see below) should be avoided. The dopamine agonist, bromocriptine, may be helpful in a dose of up to 60 mg per day but its use, and that of the peripheral muscle relaxant dantrolene (10 mg /kg) is empirical. Antipsychotics are not precluded in future by an episode of unequivocal neuroleptic malignant syndrome but it is wise to change to an alternative compound and, most importantly, to introduce it *ultra-slowly*.

Neurological: extrapyramidal Neuroleptic malignant syndrome is increasingly being classified as an 'extrapyramidal' adverse effect, though this heading usually refers to conditions that are purely disorders of movement.

Extrapyramidally mediated movement disorders represent *the* major set of adverse effects associated with the use of standard antipsychotics. Up to three-quarters of all patients exposed will experience some problem or problems of this sort – and even that may be an underestimate! Despite this, these syndromes remain poorly recognised and their full impact is rarely acknowledged. It is important to realise that, with the exception of the tardive syndromes, all these disorders comprise not only objective *signs* but subjective *symptoms*.

Drug-related movement disorders are best classified on the relationship their onset bears to the duration of drug exposure.

Acute dystonias are conventionally considered the earliest manifestation of drug-related neurological disorder, with some 90% coming on within 5 days of exposure or dose increment. They affect up to one-third of patients on high-potency standard drugs but fewer on low-potency compounds. No typical cases have yet been reported with clozapine. These disorders are heralded by increasing agitation and restlessness and awareness of discomfort and impaired function in the affected part, followed by the sudden onset of usually static postural distortions that in adults tend to be localised to the muscles of the head and neck, though in children may be generalised. The risk is inversely associated with age but relates positively to the potency, dosage and rate of increment of the particular agent. Acute dystonias respond readily to anticholinergics.

Parkinsonism associated with antipsychotic drug use comprises the same core triad of signs as are found in parkinsonism from all causes – namely, bradykinesia, rigidity and tremor, though in drug-related disorder the former predominates. Manifestations of motor slowing, loss of dexterity and postural instability emerge, with loss of pendular arm swing and postural tremor as early features. The typical flexed attitude of Parkinson's disease is uncommon except in the upper limbs, a more frequent posture in the trunk being mild hyperextension. Sialorrhoea, probably a result of impaired swallowing, may emerge, as may seborrhoea. The low-frequency, high-amplitude resting tremor so characteristic of idiopathic disease is an infrequent and late sign in drug-related disorder, while rigidity is usually mild and may require reinforcement to elicit.

It is important to remember that parkinsonism from whatever cause has a major *subjective* component which may precede the onset of overt objective signs. Subjectively, patients experience a weakness or ready fatiguability, usually in axial trunk muscles or proximal limbs, along with apathy and social disengagement. One must be alert to this component of symptomatology in order to maintain an adequately broad differential diagnosis in situations where other syndromes may present similarly.

The prevalence of drug-induced states is difficult to assess accurately but is usually quoted at between 15% and 40%, though with careful examination over time the true prevalence is likely to be higher. The impression with clozapine is much more favourable, with a prevalence at least half that of standard drugs. Onset can begin within a few days of exposure or dose increment, with the majority of cases evident within 2–3 months. Onset again depends on the potency of the chosen compound, the dose regimen and the rate of dose increments. No age group is exempt, though the risk is believed to increase with age. In this situation, antipsychotics may be releasing a tendency to Parkinson's disease.

The first step in management should be a reappraisal of the treatment plan, especially drug potency and rate of dose increases. Specific interventions for drug-related parkinsonism conventionally involve anticholinergics, and although subjectively patients may feel better, objective symptomatology often persists. Dopamine agonists have never found favour, though again this is largely due to the inferences of the dopamine hypothesis. The exception is amantadine, which was utilised to some extent in the 1960s and 1970s. Recent work has shown equal efficacy of amantadine compared with anticholinergics but less impairment in memory and learning. Amantadine is therefore worth considering, especially in the elderly and the very young.

Akathisia is a major source of non-compliance and comprises firstly, an unpleasant (i.e. dysphoric) inner restlessness and, secondly, an urge to move, either individual body parts or more commonly the whole body, in the form of non-goal-directed pacing, with the purpose, usually vain, of trying to ease the subjective distress. It has an incidence of up to 40% over 2 weeks in patients on standard drugs, though the incidence is substantially lower with clozapine. There is evidence that any advantages of drugs with potent 5-HT antagonist properties may be focused particularly on a lower liability to produce akathisia. Predisposing factors are again dependent on the variables of potency, dosage and rate of increment. Parenteral administration may also increase the risk. Reports from normal volunteer studies suggest this adverse effect may have a very early onset indeed – within a few hours of oral and 30 minutes of parenteral usage. Thus in acutely disturbed patients receiving emergency treatment by injection it is particularly easy for akathisia to be confused with mental state disorder.

Some patients may show restless, non-goal-directed behaviour without feeling particularly agitated subjectively. This situation tends to emerge with chronic symptomatology and is best classified as tardive akathisia. The alternative term, pseudoakathisia, is more appropriately reserved for patients who look akathisic but in fact are victims of tardive dyskinesia, usually of dystonic type.

Akathisia in acute form responds rather disappointingly to specific intervention. If, after a review of the treatment plan, specific medication is to be recommended, the usual first choice is again an anticholinergic. Results are however very variable and this approach is perhaps most efficacious in those who also demonstrate coincidental parkinsonism. An alternative strategy increasingly advocated involves a beta blocker, especially propranolol. Benzodiazepines are popular with some practitioners but their use rests on wisdom of the clinical rather than the scientific sort.

Tardive dyskinesia refers to a syndrome of involuntary movements developing in the course of long-term exposure to antipsychotic (and other predominantly antidopaminergic) drugs. Any type of hyperkinetic movement disorder – tics, chorea, dystonia, etc. – may comprise the syndrome, with the exception of tremor, which is specifically excluded. Eighty per cent of cases involve the muscles of the lower third of the face giving rise to involuntary activity in the tongue, which may sweep the inner buccal surface ('bon-bon' sign) or irregularly protrude from the mouth ('fly-catcher' sign). This can be combined with grinding/chewing lateral and/or anteroposterior jaw movements and puckering/pursing movements of the lips. The combination of these signs is referred to as the buccolinguomasticatory (BLM) triad. Despite the prominence of these features, symptomatology may involve any or all body areas, including internal muscle groups such as those of the oropharynx, larynx and diaphragm.

The prevalence of tardive dyskinesia depends on a series of variables, especially the age of the sample. Overall, it has been estimated at 20–25%. In special populations, it may be substantially higher. Incidence is in the region of 4–5% per year but, particularly in those first exposed in later life, may be as high as 30% in the first year. The risk appears greatest in the early years of exposure but disorder can emerge without warning at any time. Even after as long as 20 years incident-free exposure, a risk in the region of 10% persists. Once again, clozapine's profile appears unique in this regard, with only a handful of reported cases attributed to this drug.

Using retrospective study designs it has been difficult to establish clear predisposing factors beyond age, which is a robust association, though others suggested include alcohol abuse, metabolic disorders such as diabetes, and the mental state features of cognitive impairment, affective symptomatology and negative schizophrenia. Reported associations with female gender probably reflect the influence of interposing variables such as age. Prospectively, associations are emerging with antipsychotic dosage which are sufficiently strong to emphasise the need for cautious use of these drugs. In addition, intermittent exposure patterns (i.e. drug-free intervals of more than 1–3 months) are a further possible risk which should be considered with patients when recommending maintenance regimens. Associations with race (higher risk in Afro-Caribbeans and a lower risk in Asians, especially Chinese) are evident in some data sets, though it remains unclear whether these represent primarily genetic or treatment differences.

Tardive dyskinesia was for many years one of the major topics of research in the psychiatric literature, and was perceived as the most important extrapyramidal adverse effect of antipsychotic use. It is doubtful if such a perception can be sustained now, in view of an increasing awareness of the intrusive nature of other neurological adverse experiences and the realisation in recent years that the course and outcome of tardive disorders is less relentlessly progressive and pessimistic than was at one time thought. The majority of cases of tardive dyskinesia remain mild and unobtrusive and have a high likelihood of resolving or declining in prominence over time. However, the importance of the issue is that in a proportion of cases (probably less than 10%) symptoms can be extremely severe and may be irreversible, something that is more likely in patients over 40 years of age. Thus the degree of morbidity can be considerable, which may contribute to subjective distress and impair resocialisation. The clinical dilemma is that at point of onset the ultimate extent of the problem or the resultant incapacitation cannot be accurately predicted.

There remains a dearth of satisfactory treatments for tardive movement disorders and management remains heavily predicated on the principles of primary prevention. This involves strictly limiting the indications for antipsychotic drug use and utilising the lowest effective and the simplest dose regimens during all phases of management. In view of the fact that extrapyramidal motor disorders are intimately related to the degree of arousal the patient experiences, attempts should be made to treat incidental mental state disorder such as depression or anxiety. Benzodiazepines may be helpful both by virtue of their non-specific anxiolytic actions but possibly also by virtue of their γ-aminobutyric acid (GABA)-facilitatory actions, as the hyperdopaminergic state postulated to underlie the disorder may be inhibited by GABA-agonism. Further proposed but unproven interventions include the dopamine agonist bromocriptine and the presynaptic depleting agent tetrabenazine. Recently the free radical scavenger α-tocopherol (or vitamin E) has been reported as effective and, although the evidence is far from unanimous, this is a relatively safe intervention. The position of the new generation antipsychotics remains to be established but clozapine should always be considered, especially in those whose movement disorder is dominated by disorder of dystonic type as there is evidence that on this drug gradual resolution may take place, though over a protracted timescale of 2–2.5 years.

The above is only an outline of what are pervasive and important disorders, for detail of which the reader is referred to more specialist work (Owens 1998).

Therapeutics

Indications

In adult psychiatry it is possible to specify the indications for antipsychotics fairly clearly, though in other areas of psychiatric practice indications may be less defined. In adults the indications include:

- The treatment of acute schizophrenic episodes including schizophreniform disorders, acute exacerbations of chronic schizophrenia, and schizoaffective disorders.
- The acute management of delusional (paranoid) disorders.
- The maintenance of remission in patients with recurrent psychotic disorders of schizophrenic type. There is evidence however that the role of antipsychotics may be to delay rather than prevent subsequent episodes.
- The treatment of manic and hypomanic episodes with or without productive or positive symptomatology.
- The treatment of psychotic depression, characterised by the presence of productive or positive symptomatology.
- The maintenance of remission in patients with recurrent bipolar affective disorders in whom lithium or other mood stabilising medication is ineffective or only partially effective.
- The management of psychotic symptomatology occurring in the context of acute or chronic organic syndromes (though the tendency of antipsychotics to lower the seizure threshold reduces their value in withdrawal states).
- Clozapine is specifically indicated as a second or third line treatment in patients who are resistant to standard drugs given in adequate dose for an adequate time and in those who demonstrate extrapyramidal intolerance. Clozapine is the first antipsychotic to which enhanced efficacy has been attributed but it must be appreciated that although its benefits can in some patients be striking, in objective terms any advantages in efficacy are overall slight. Its neurological tolerability however makes this an exceptional antipsychotic compound.

There has been great debate in the literature over the past 15–20 years as to whether antipsychotics 'treat' the negative features of schizophrenia. This has largely concerned the standard compounds, though in recent years it has expanded to include the new generation drugs.

The problem is beset with conceptual problems as to what comprises 'negative' symptomatology. There is also the additional issue of whether, having agreed what constitutes it, such features can be distinguished clinically with any confidence from other similar but pathophysiologically distinct features, the most important of which are the anxiety and social withdrawal occasioned by positive features, the retardation of depression and the bradykinesia of parkinsonism. The authentic deficits of the illness have been referred to as *primary* negative features, while those states that appear similar but are the result of other illness mechanisms have been designated *secondary* negative states (Carpenter et al 1985). There is *no* evidence that antipsychotic drugs have any therapeutic actions on primary negative symptomatology – and this conclusion applies to the new generation compounds as much as to the standard ones (Moller 1993; Owens 1996).

Great care should be exercised in recommending the long-term use of antipsychotics solely as agents for non-specific behavioural control.

Strategies

There is no first-line antipsychotic for the treatment of acute psychotic states. The choice tends to be governed by the general professional culture and individual preference (usually the doctor's, not the patient's!). Thus high-potency compounds have traditionally been more favoured in North America, whereas in the UK a more eclectic approach has held sway.

Trial data do not confirm the intuitive belief that sedative low-potency drugs have advantages in the management of agitated, behaviourally disturbed patients, though this may be one of those examples in which the circumstances of a clinical trial do not allow all findings to be carried over to routine treatment environments. Even allowing for this, there are two big advantages of low potency drugs: they can impact immediately on non-specific symptomatology, such as agitation and insomnia, that patients themselves find unpleasant, and hence can produce some early signs of therapeutic advantage; and they have an inherently lower liability to produce extrapyramidal adverse effects. Their two major disadvantages are that their non-specific actions, such as sedation, may be intrusive to the patient, and they are as a rule possessed of a greater liability to produce a wider range of general adverse effects. However, while both doctors and patients are usually ever-alert to general adverse effects, there is strong evidence that neither parties are at all skilled in the recognition of extrapyramidal disorder, which means that the adverse experiences of patients on high-potency regimens may be persistently misattributed.

A further preliminary consideration is dose. There is clear evidence that in routine practice a climate of unnecessarily high dose schedules has become established for antipsychotics. This is especially the case for the high-potency compounds. It has been shown in America that in terms of dose equivalence, haloperidol regimens were approximately four times greater than for patients treated with chlorpromazine itself, while for fluphenazine the figure was six times (Baldessarini et al 1984). This may illustrate a further possible advantage of low-potency drugs, in that their general adverse effects may set a ceiling on over generous and unnecessary dose regimens. It probably also illustrates the error of prescribing according to fixed schedules as opposed to titrating schedules according to clinical need.

The new generation drugs are for the most part proving highly successful in commercial terms but the question of relative merits in relation to standard compounds remains at this stage unresolved, as a true understanding of the extent to which they may have shifted the cost:benefit ratio is not yet possible. It is however now incumbent on all clinicians to evaluate the cost:benefit ratio of every prescribing decision.

There are two principles governing the sympathetic use of antipsychotics:

- *Principle 1* is recognition that there is a *temporal dissociation* between the onset of adverse and therapeutic effects. Adverse effects may be evident after a single dose, and certainly within a few days, while the specific therapeutic action is *inevitably delayed* till at least the second week. The target actions *cannot* be accelerated by increasing doses rapidly, which will merely advance and escalate non-target actions, thereby seriously risking compliance.
- *Principle 2* is maintaining a *structure* to the management of major psychiatric disorders based on the formulation of plans which identify clear goals and recognise the evolution of these through different phases. With regard to the drug component of the treatment of schizophrenia, the primary aim of *acute phase* treatment is the control of acute or positive psychotic features and any behavioural disturbance that may be associated with them, using the *minimum tolerable* antipsychotic doses. In the *postacute phase*, the aim is *consolidation* and *rationalisation* of administration schedules, doses and redundant medications. In *maintenance*, the primary

role is *maximising* well-being on the *minimum* doses possible.

Both these principles are designed to ensure that throughout their illness the patient's exposure to antipsychotic drugs is confined to the *minimum effective* doses.

The evidence is that the majority of schizophrenic patients in the throes of an acute episode of illness will respond to doses in the range of 400–600 mg chlorpromazine per day or its equivalent (Kane 1987). The situation with their use in other clinical indications is less clear but the same principles apply. While the pharmacokinetics of most antipsychotics dictate that comparable efficacy probably accrues from single as from multiple dosing schedules (an exception being sulpiride which probably is unsuitable for single dosing), it is often useful to spread doses throughout the day to capitalise on any sedative effects that may ensue, at least during the acute phase.

Depots are widely used in the UK in maintenance treatment plans where they have been shown to enhance compliance (Davis et al 1994). There is however no evidence that they exert any preferential effects on outcome *independent* of compliance and their pharmacokinetics can make 'fine tuning' of regimens difficult. Furthermore, by virtue of their administration by another individual some patients feel that the element of choice in relation to their treatment is compromised. There is evidence that for maintenance purposes pimozide, a drug of exceptionally long half-life, may be effective in alternate day or four times a week regimens (McCreadie et al 1980).

The question of antipsychotic dose equivalence is more craft than science. Equivalence tables, such as Table 4.2, are not based on data from objective scientific tests but are largely derived from clinical studies which have adopted variable dose schedules. They therefore do not take account of varied actions at other than dopamine receptors, the higher doses of high-potency drugs used to achieve containment in acute situations and, for the most part, pharmacokinetic factors. They are crude, poorly reliable (especially for the high-potency compounds) and should be considered as representing no more than the median points in *ranges* at which comparable efficacy can be reasonably expected. Conversion tables between oral and depot formulations are even less reliable as most do not take into account pharmacokinetic factors which are particularly relevant to these formulations. These 'calculations' furthermore overlook the fact that depots are invariably used in maintenance management when overall dose requirements are less than during acute phase treatment.

Some treatment schedules are outlined in Figure 4.3.

Table 4.2 Antipsychotic dose equivalences	
Antipsychotic	Dose (mg)
Chlorpromazine	100/day
Orals	
Thioridazine	100/day
Pericyazine	24/day
Trifluoperazine	5/day
Fluphenazine	2/day
Perphenazine	8/day
Haloperidol	3/day
Pimozide	2/day
Flupenthixol	2/day
Sulpiride	200/day
Clozapine	50/day
Depots	
Fluphenazine decanoate	10–25/2 weeks
Flupenthixol decanoate	16–40/2 weeks
Zuclopenthixol decanoate	80–200/2 weeks
Haloperidol decanoate	40–100/4 weeks
Pipothiazine palmitate	20–50/4 weeks
From Atkins et al (1997).	

ANTIDEPRESSANTS

In the late 1940s and early 1950s physicians caring for patients with tuberculosis noted that when on treatment with certain antituberculous agents, most noticeably iproniazid, many patients seemed to experience an elevation of mood that was strikingly incongruent to their often parlous medical condition. These drugs were postulated, and subsequently shown, to non-selectively and irreversibly inhibit the action of monoamine oxidase, the major intracellular catabolic enzyme of biogenic amines, thereby resulting in an increase in the amount of transmitter available for recycling in neurotransmission. This laid the foundations for the first and most durable theory of the pathophysiology of affective disorders, though it is likely that the so-called 'biogenic amine hypothesis' is at best an oversimplification. None the less, with their launch in 1957 the monoamine oxidase inhibitors (MAOIs) became the first of the commercially available antidepressants.

Enthusiasm was however soon tempered by concern. Although these new drugs were less hepatotoxic than the parent iproniazid, it was evident that they could produce serious and occasionally fatal side-effects (see below). This, combined with the introduction of the tricyclics and the results of an influential trial sponsored by the Medical Research Council, showing no benefits over placebo, pushed these compounds into the thera-

peutic doldrums from which they have only emerged in the past decade or so.

As was noted, imipramine was initially investigated as a potential rival to chlorpromazine but it was its antidepressant properties that were identified by the Swiss psychiatrist, Roland Kuhn, and for a quarter of a century the position of the tricyclics was unrivalled. In the 1980s, however, a series of new generation antidepressants emerged, claiming as their justification a more selective pharmacology which translated into better tolerability and safety parameters than the tricyclics could offer. Furthermore, most of these new drugs could boast a theoretical foundation to support their efficacy, no matter that these foundations seem to tremble in proportion to the scrutiny imposed on the theory.

Unlike the antipsychotics, considerable differences exist within the class of antidepressants and are reflected in classification. Tricyclics continue to be classified on the basis of their *chemical structure*, while with the newer compounds (e.g. the SSRIs) classification reflects their putative *mode of action*. This extends to moclobemide, which is considered as an MAOI, although structurally it is in fact a substituted benzamide and in its mode of action is somewhat different from others of its group. Taking the tricyclics and MAOIs as the first-generation antidepressants introduced empirically, then those which have followed since the early 1980s might conveniently be considered together as simply 'new generation', as, although they may differ in their pharmacology, they share development on the back of at least some theoretical framework. It is accepted that the selective/reversible MAOIs sit uncomfortably within such a framework but for convenience they will be considered with the traditional MAOIs which they resemble more than the new generation drugs.

Tricyclics

Structures

As their group name implies, tricyclics comprise two benzene rings joined by a central ring which in the classical compounds is seven membered (Figure 4.4). Substitutions at position 5 can be either nitrogen, as with imipramine-type compounds, or carbon, as with amitriptyline. The former are therefore *dibenzazepine* analogues of phenothiazines, whereas the latter, technically a *dibenzocycloheptene*, is closely related to the thioxanthenes. On the basis of their side-chain attachments at position 5 they may be classified as either tertiary (e.g. imipramine, amitriptyline) or secondary (e.g. desipramine, nortriptyline) amines.

In general, most of the tricyclics vary only slightly in

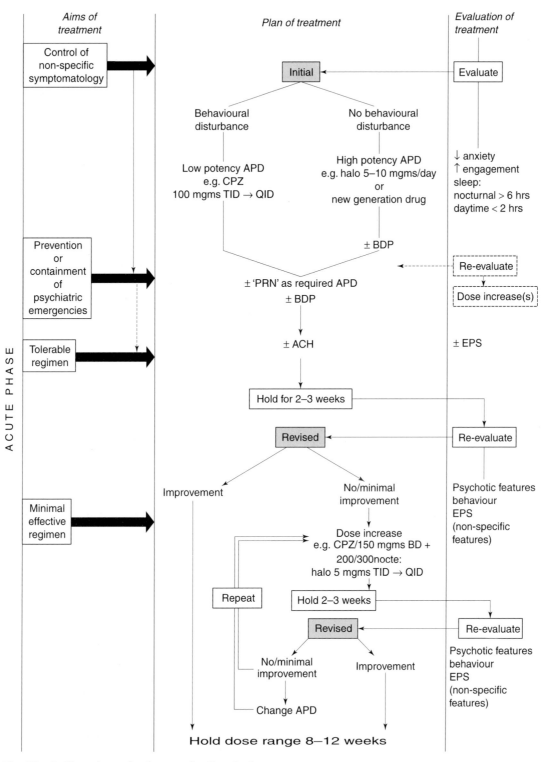

Fig. 4.3 Outline scheme for the use of antipsychotics.

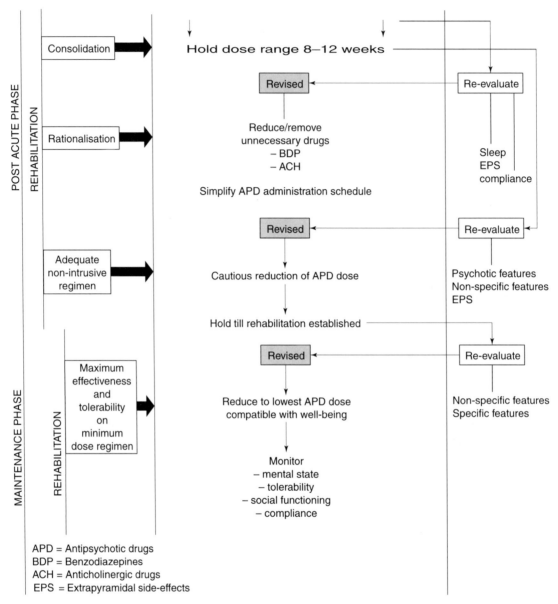

Fig. 4.3 *Cont'd*

APD = Antipsychotic drugs
BDP = Benzodiazepines
ACH = Anticholinergic drugs
EPS = Extrapyramidal side-effects

structure, based on modifications to their side-chains, despite some differences (essentially of emphasis) in their pharmacology. A few deviate somewhat more in their central ring structure. Amoxapine for example, is a metabolite of the dibenzoxazepine antipsychotic loxapine, and indeed might alternatively be referred to as norloxapine, while in maprotiline a six-membered central ring is stabilised by an ethylene bridge. This compound has been considered by some as a 'tetra-cyclic' but it is in fact merely a tricyclic variant.

Pharmacokinetics

Tricyclic antidepressants are all well absorbed from the gastrointestinal tract. The rate of absorption, and hence time to peak levels, is however more rapid for the ter-tiary amines (approximately 1–3 hours) than for the secondary amines (approximately 4–8 hours) (Preskorn 1993a,b). The speed of absorption (T_{max}) and the size of the post absorption peak (C_{max}) may be related to the likelihood of certain adverse effects developing, such as sedation, agitation and membrane stabilisation which

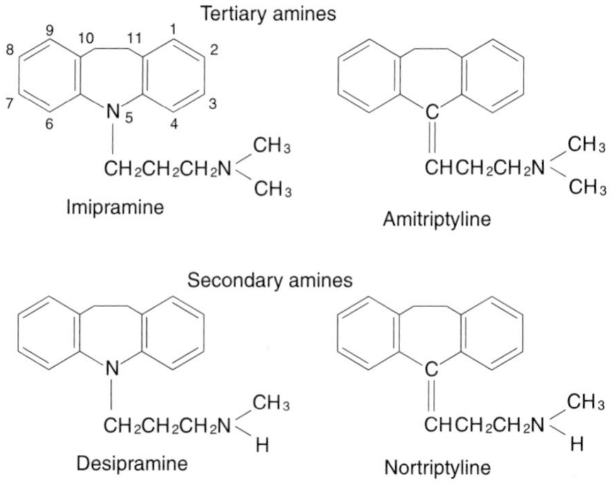

Fig. 4.4 Antidepressant structures: tricyclics.

underlies the cardiac actions. Although this has been used as an argument in favour of the preferential use of secondary amine preparations, this is probably only of clinical significance in selected individuals such as the elderly or those with a clear history of previous intolerance. Furthermore, divided dose regimens may be used to attenuate C_{max} without altering steady-state levels.

All tricyclics are subjected to heavy first-pass effects with only about 50–60% of an oral dose reaching the systemic circulation. The effect is particularly large with doxepin (average 70%). As with antipsychotics, at therapeutic levels clearance is flow dependent and decreased by hepatic diseases or states which impede hepatic through put. The major metabolic steps involve hydroxylation of the ring structures and demethylation of the terminal nitrogen (Baldessarini 1985). Hydroxylation appears to be the rate-limiting step and makes the largest contribution to breakdown, resulting in the formation of metabolites that in unconjugated form may be present in blood and brain in concentrations greater than the parent drug. Conjugated and unconjugated hydroxy metabolites account for up to 85% of an oral dose of imipramine and 55% for amitriptyline (Rudorfer and Potter 1987). The actions of hydroxylated tricyclic metabolites are however complex and difficult to study, especially for the tertiary amines. In vitro, and possibly in vivo also, they do appear to share reuptake inhibition actions similar in type and degree to their parent drugs and it seems increasingly clear that they make a contribution to efficacy and probably tolerability (Young 1991). There is a suggestion from animal studies that they may be more cardiotoxic than parent drugs, though it remains unclear if these data can be translated to humans.

Demethylation of the side-chain converts tertiary compounds to secondary amines and these to primary amines. Secondary amines are of course active compounds and a number are commercially marketed as such in their own right, whereas it appears that primary amines are not active. Tricyclic metabolism may however not be unidirectional as there is evidence that with administration of secondary amine compounds some 15% of patients may develop detectable levels of tertiary drug in plasma, e.g. desipramine to imipramine (Rudorfer and Potter 1987).

As will be noted, a number of drugs interfere with hepatic metabolism of tricyclics but of particular note is alcohol, which has a triphasic effect. Acute ingestion to intoxication in a non-dependent individual impairs metabolism by competition, resulting in a 2–3-fold increase in the amount of unaltered drug reaching the systemic circulation. This is one reason why combination overdoses can have such adverse medical consequences. A similar effect may be evident in chronically alcohol-dependent patients with coincidental hepatic cirrhosis and portocaval shunting. On the other hand, chronic alcohol ingestion without compromised hepatic blood flow increases the magnitude of first-pass metabolism via enzyme induction.

A second reason why tricyclic effects can be so toxic in overdose is that after hepatic transformation a large proportion of active metabolite is excreted via the bile to participate in an enterohepatic circulation. Bowel stasis accentuated by potent anticholinergic effects following overdose can protract this action and result in the maintenance of toxic blood levels for several days longer than the half-lives of the parent drugs would lead one to suspect.

Like antipsychotics, plasma protein binding for tricyclics is high (at around 90%), as is their lipophilicity. Elimination half-lives are on average in the region of 20–24 hours, with those for imipramine and desipramine somewhat less and for amitriptyline and nortriptyline rather longer. Protriptyline, with half-life values in the region of 75–80 hours, is exceptional in this regard and with daily dosing regimens accumulation is a possibility. Overall however, these half-lives are compatible with once daily dosing and steady state within 5–7 days. Amoxapine, with an average half-life in the region of 8 hours, may however be a doubtful candidate for single-dose regimens. Lofepramine also has a short half-life but since this compound appears to function as a 'prodrug', with rapid conversion to desipramine, the half-life figure is probably of less clinical importance.

The kidney is the major route for elimination of tricyclic antidepressants and the most important source of alteration in pharmacokinetic parameters by age, illness or other incidental factors (Rudorfer and Potter 1987).

Pharmacodynamics

Mode of action Tricyclic antidepressants with their wide range of actions are typical of so-called pharmacologically 'dirty' drugs. This, and an absence for many years of specific screening tests for antidepressant activity, made it difficult to advance the pharmacotherapy of affective disorders by isolating the essential component(s) of efficacy.

The amine hypothesis of affective disorders was handed down from on High on tablets of stone – or so it often seems, observing the presentations of its protagonists. In its generic format it states that depression is associated with a functional deficit of neurotransmitter amines at critical CNS synapses and mania with a functional excess. This was refined into two subhypotheses when in 1965 Schildkraut postulated that the disturbance lay with catecholamine (predominantly noradrenergic) mechanisms, while Coppen pointed the finger at serotonin. The theory/theories arose from observations made of the effects on mood of various compounds used in humans, initially the presynaptic depleting agents and the MAOIs, and while there is much that supports it, there is much that it does not as yet explain. It would be miraculous indeed if the complexities of mood and its disorders could be reduced to a simple disturbance in a single neurochemical system that we just happened upon, and it would seem prudent from a clinical perspective to view the amine hypothesis as a set of working proposals that provide for the testing of certain essentially therapeutic models.

Tricyclics modify transmission by, firstly, their receptor actions and, secondly, their effects on reuptake. As a group they have a strong affinity for histaminic (H_1), muscarinic cholinergic and α_1 adrenergic receptors (Table 4.3). They have only a weak affinity for dopamine D_2 receptors, with amoxapine, trimipramine and clomipramine the most potent tricyclics at these sites, though even these have only about one-tenth or less of the affinity of chlorpromazine (Richelson 1996).

Presynaptic reuptake is an important mechanism in neurotransmission in order to prevent receptor overstimulation. As early as the 1960s, Axelrod and colleagues identified, from amongst their many actions, reuptake inhibition of amine transmitters as a possible mode of tricyclic action. These compounds are however relatively non-selective in this, blocking to varying degrees the reuptake of both noradrenaline and serotonin, though with only as a rule minimal effects on dopamine. In vitro, the secondary amines (e.g. desipramine, nortriptyline, protriptyline) are more

Table 4.3 Binding affinities of various tricyclics for different receptor types (as *percentage* of reference compound)

Tricyclic	Receptor type			
	$H_1{}^a$	M^b	$\alpha_1{}^c$	D^d
Imipramine	128	2.6	16.4	0.9
Amitriptyline	1282	13.3	55.2	1.9
Desipramine	12.8	1.2	11.5	0.6
Nortriptyline	141	1.6	25.4	1.6
Clomipramine	45	6.4	38.8	10
Trimipramine	5211	4	62.7	10.6
Doxepin	5915	2.9	62.7	0.8
Protriptyline	56.3	9.5	11.5	0.8
Amoxapine	56.3	0.2	29.9	11.7

[a] Histaminergic receptors: reference diphenhydramine.
[b] Muscarinic cholinergic receptors: reference atropine.
[c] α_1 Adrenoceptors: reference phentolamine.
[d] Dopamine D_2 receptors: reference chlorpromazine.
Data from Richelson (1996).

potent and more selective inhibitors of noradrenaline reuptake than of serotonin, though there is doubt that any such selectivity operates in vivo (Frazer 1997). Clomipramine is exceptional in having reuptake characteristics in this regard that are comparable to the SSRIs.

While reuptake blockade of amine neurotransmitters is now accepted as the essential or necessary first step in tricyclic antidepressant action (Goodwin 1996), this rapid pharmacological action does not bear any relationship to the onset of clinical efficacy, and the nature of the secondary changes that seem likely to underlie the resolution of clinical symptomatology remains unclear.

Adverse effects A knowledge of the receptor antagonist properties of tricyclics can be helpful in understanding their adverse effect profiles. There are however few hard and fast predictions that are possible for individual compounds because of the limitations of extrapolating in vitro data to the clinical context, the interposing effects of pharmacokinetic variations and the fact that such data on parent compounds do not allow for the effects of active metabolites. The generalities can however be clinically useful.

Tricyclics as a group are potent antagonists of histaminergic H_1 receptors. Some, such as doxepin and trimipramine, bind with some 50–60 times greater affinity than reference antihistamines. Amitriptyline has approximately 10 times greater affinity than imipramine, which in its turn has approximately 2–3 times the affinity of protriptyline and clomipramine. Desipramine has, on the other hand, only very weak affinity for these receptors (Richelson 1996). Antihistaminic activity is thought to underlie the *sedative* side-effects of tricyclics, though it probably does not act alone in this regard. None the less, in clinical situations where anxiety and agitation are intrusive, capitalising on what is in effect an adverse effect can be a distinct aid to management.

It must be borne in mind that sedation associated with tricyclic use, as in all other therapeutic situations, diminishes *reaction time*. Lack of awareness of this by doctors, and consequent absence of appropriate advice concerning driving, is undoubtedly one reason why patients taking tricyclics are disproportionately represented amongst those involved in road traffic accidents. As a consequence of these sedative properties, tricyclics can also increase sleep time. They are not as a rule sleep-inducers but rather act to *maintain* sleep in those with early wakening. They may however be associated with prominent and distressing *dreams* (perhaps a result of anticholinergic effects). Antihistaminic activity may also contribute to what is for patients one of the most unwanted of adverse effects, namely *weight gain*. Increase in weight on these drugs can be considerable and a major reason for non-compliance. It is suggested that the likelihood is greatest with amitriptyline and least with the secondary amines (Fernstrom and Kupfer 1988). The mechanisms underlying it are undoubtedly complex and may involve factors such as carbohydrate craving.

Tricyclics also have clinically relevant affinity for muscarinic cholinergic receptors, with amitriptyline and protriptyline the most potent antagonists and nortriptyline and desipramine the least. Indeed these latter drugs have less affinity for cholinergic sites than paroxetine (Richelson 1996). Anticholinergic actions, mostly peripheral, make a major contribution to the adverse effects patients complain of most. Impaired salivary flow, results in an uncomfortable *dryness in the mouth* which, as with antipsychotics, may promote low-grade but potentially significant oral infection with dental caries. A similar reduction in *lacrimation* may also predispose to corneal infection and damage, especially in those who wear contact lenses. A relative paralysis of accommodation causes pupillary dilatation and *blurring of vision*, most marked with changes in focal length (e.g. in changing from distance sight to reading), and rarely, in predisposed individuals, may promote closed angle *glaucoma*. Inhibition of the cardiac sphincter may result in *oesophageal reflux* and heartburn. *Constipation* is of course a constant concern for the general public, though is rarely so for doctors. In the elderly, however, drug-induced bowel hypomotility may have major and sometimes catastrophic consequences, as for example

when *paralytic ileus* ensues. Impaired elimination and frank *urinary retention* is usually, though not exclusively, a problem in males, especially those with underlying prostatic hypertrophy. Sexual dysfunction can undoubtedly be associated with the use of drugs with anticholinergic actions. especially *poorly sustained erections*, but contrary to popular medical belief these effects are probably a relatively minor contributor. A lack of cholinergic balance on particularly noradernergic function may however underlie infrequent cases of *priapism*. Vagal blockade results in a mild *sinus tachycardia*, with an average increase of less than 10 beats per minute. This is rarely clinically significant but, especially when combined with a reflex tachycardia secondary to hypotension, may sufficiently increase oxygen demand in those with ischaemic heart disease to promote rate-related angina or so-called 'silent' ischaemia (Jefferson 1989). Central anticholinergic actions may produce *impairment of memory*, which is likewise usually not significant, though in the elderly this effect, exaggerated by pharmacokinetic changes, may promote learning and memory problems and frank *confusion* in those with a compromised brain substrate.

Separation of the tricyclics from the new generation drugs is less clear on the basis of anti-α_1 noradrenergic actions than with actions at other receptor types. Doxepin, trimipramine and amitriptyline all have strong affinity for α_1 receptors, with imipramine, clomipramine and nortriptyline intermediate and desipramine and protriptyline relatively weak. This compares with trazodone and nefazadone, which also have moderate affinity, and sertraline, which has little (Richelson 1996). As a result of these actions tricyclics can cause lightheadedness or a 'woozy' feeling on walking, especially when changing position consequent upon *postural* or orthostatic *hypotension*. This occurs in about 5–10% of even young healthy individuals on tricyclics and up to 20% of older populations, 4% of whom may sustain injuries (Frazer 1997). The best predictor of orthostatic drop during treatment is quite simply a postural drop prior to exposure (Glassman et al 1979). Although often viewed as an inconvenience by both patients and doctors, postural hypotension deserves to be taken for the potentially serious adverse effect that it is. It is a major cause of morbidity from falls, especially in the elderly, in whom hip fractures have been estimated to occur 2–3 times more often in those on tricyclics (Ray et al 1987), and on rare occasions can promote both cerebral and myocardial ischaemia of catastrophic degree. Noradrenergic antagonism at α_1 sites also mediates a reflex tachycardia and is probably the other major contributor to sexual dysfunction including impotence, impaired or premature ejaculation and anorgasmia.

Most tricyclics have little affinity for dopamine (D_2) receptors, the exceptions being amoxapine, trimipramine and clomipramine. In the case of amoxapine this can cause the gamut of extrapyramidal movement disorders and caution should be used in recommending long-term use of this drug or its use for any duration in the elderly. Clomipramine has been reported to produce the same clinical manifestations of hyperprolactinaemia as antipsychotics but in practice the prevalence of these is much lower and they only infrequently present a management problem. A higher risk of movement disorders has not been specifically attributed to either trimipramine of clomipramine.

Other important adverse effects of tricyclics do not relate directly to their properties of central receptor antagonism (Table 4.4). The increase in noradrenergic transmission integral to their action is probably behind the development of *anxiety* and *agitation* in some patients, especially within a few days of exposure. This has been referred to as the 'jitteriness' or 'early tricyclic' syndrome but to all intents and purposes appears phenomonologically similar to akathisia and might best be considered a variant of such. A similar mechanism is the likely explanation of the low amplitude, high frequency *tremor* that is not uncommon. Comparative studies suggest these symptoms are most frequent with desipramine and protriptyline (Cole and Bodkin 1990), which is in line with a pathophysiology based on the low affinity of these compounds for α_1 receptors in a climate of noradrenergic facilitation. In view of their reuptake inhibition properties it is perhaps surprising that reports of *hypertension* are few. This may reflect an absence of routine monitoring and it has been suggested that transient rises early in exposure are not uncommon, perhaps more with amoxapine and in those with pre-exiting hypertension (Jefferson 1989). Sweating, sometimes amounting to *hyperhidrosis*, can affect up to 10% of patients, and probably also reflects a basic group action. Even in mild degrees this can be subjectively distressing and is something worth asking about even if it is not volunteered spontaneously.

The most important and contentious of these actions not directly mediated via central receptor antagonism is the effects of tricyclics on *cardiac function*. For many years much of what was known about the cardiac effects of tricyclics was derived from studies of overdose, which no doubt contributed to the widespread belief that these drugs were uniquely toxic agents. It is only in the past 15 years or so that studies of the clinical pharmacology of these agents have been performed under therapeutic conditions, and a considerably more favourable impression has emerged. The direct actions on the heart show mainly in the two crucial areas of rhythm and conduction.

Tricyclics have properties of class I *antiarrhythmics*, promoting membrane stabilisation through inhibition of fast sodium channels. They share both type Ia effects, which are quinidine-like and result in decreased amplitude of Purkinje fibre action potentials and membrane responsiveness with slowed conduction, and type Ib lidocaine-like effects of decreased duration of action potentials and effective refractory period (Jefferson 1989). At therapeutic blood levels they are clinically effective in the treatment of supraventricular tachycardias and some dysrhythmias of ventricular origin. However, any drug with antiarrhythmic properties may be proarrhythmic in some patients, especially when blood levels are high or when two type I drugs are combined. Thus particular expertise is necessary in exposing patients already receiving a type I antiarrhythmic agent to a tricyclic.

Slight prolongation of the PR, QRS or QT intervals is not uncommonly seen on the ECGs of subjects receiving tricyclics, as on occasion is flattening of T waves. It is now known that tricyclics have little effect on atrioventricular (AV) nodal conduction but delay *intraventricular* conduction in the His–Purkinje system. In the most general terms the delay is related to blood levels and with these in the therapeutic range this action is for the most part of little clinical significance. The major potential issue consequent upon this action is precipitating or advancing the level of heart block. In an important prospective study of this issue however only 0.7% of patients (1 of 150) with normal pretreatment ECGs developed a 2:1 block and this was reversible on discontinuation of the drug (Roose et al 1987). In situ electrophysiology subsequently showed this patient to have a conduction deficit. Thus in patients with normal cardiac conduction the risk of tricyclics precipitating abnormality is extremely small. In those with confirmed pre-existing conduction disorder, no consequences of exposure to therapeutic levels of tricyclic were noted in this study in those with only first-degree block, but two of 22 (9%) of those taking imipramine who had pretreatment bundle branch block developed second-degree block during treatment, also reversible on discontinuation. In two others the QRS interval increased by more than 25%. Of 15 patients on nortriptyline, one developed sinus arrest requiring pacing and another, who had suffered a previous infarct, reinfarcted (Roose et al 1987). While the authours of this work acknowledged the increased risk of tricyclics exacerbating conduction disorders in those with pre-existing abnormality, they also pointed out that from a cardiological perspective tricyclics still represent relatively safe antiarrhythmic agents.

There remains debate about the effects of tricyclics on cardiac *contractility*, with animal studies suggesting

Table 4.4   Adverse effects of antidepressant drugs

Mediated by receptor antagonism					Not mediated by receptor antagonism
H$_1$	ACh	NA	D$_2$	Na fast channels	
Sedation[T,Mz] Lethargy[T] ↓Reaction[T] time ↑Weight[T] ↑Sleep[T] time	↑Dreams[T] Dry Mouth[T] Impaired accommodation[T] Oesophageal reflux[T] Constipation[T] Urinary difficulties[T] Sexual difficulties[T,(Mz)] Priapism[(T),Tz] Impaired memory[T]	Postural hypotension[T,Tz,(N),MP]	Hyperprolactinaemia[T] Movement disorders[T]	Delayed AV[T,(M)] conduction Delayed IV conduction[T] AV block[T] Cardiac dysrhythmias[T] Hypomania[M] Positive psychotic features[T,M]	Sedation[M,Mo,Mi,S,Tz,N] Agitation[M,Mo,S] Akathisia[(T),S] Insomnia[T,M,Mo,V,S] Dry mouth[M,Mi,Tz] Urinary difficulties[M] Sexual difficulties[M,S,Ve] Constipation[M] Seizures[T,Mp] Hyperhidrosis[T] Nausea[V,S,Ve] Vomiting[V,S,Ve] Diarrhoea[S,Mo] Headache[Mo,S] Migraine[V] Weight gain[M,Mz,Tz] Weight loss[V,S] Supine hypotension[Mp,M] Hypertension[T,Ve] Tremor[T,M,Mo,S] Movement disorders[S] Dizziness[Mo] Bradycardia[S] Rashes[(T),(S)] Hepatic dysfunction[(T),(M),(S)] Blood dyscrasias[(T),Mi]

M, MAOIs; Mi, mianserin; Mo, moclobemide; Mp, maprotiline; Mz, mirtazapine; N, nafazodone; S, SSRIs; T, tricyclics; Tz, trazodone; V, viloxazine; Ve, Venlafazine.

an augmenting (positive inotropic) effect on low doses but a depressant effect at higher doses. The position in humans, especially those with heart disease, however is still unclear. Studies in this field are clearly difficult to perform but the evidence, which is only suggestive, none the less does *not* support the view that tricyclics (nortriptyline, amitriptyline, imipramine and doxepin at least) adversely affect left ventricular performance (Glassman and Biggar 1981).

Thus the evidence to date is that at therapeutic levels tricyclics have *no* detrimental actions in the absence of pre-existing cardiac disease and in certain circumstances may actually have actions that are beneficial. With care, the evidence is that these drugs can also be used with a relative margin of safety in most patients with signs of cardiac failure.

These drugs do, like most antipsychotics, alter the EEG and lower the seizure threshold. Hence they can precipitate seizures but the risk is low, with prevalence rates estimated to be in the region of 0.1–0.5% of patients (Skowron and Stimmel 1992). The risk does however appear to be substantially higher with maprotiline and this drug should be avoided in those in whom any family or personal predisposition can be elicited. The likelihood of an individual developing fits appears related to dose and the rate of dose increment.

For a number of years controversy existed about whether or not antidepressants in general and tricyclics in paticular could precipitate *hypomania/mania* in non-bipolar depressed patients. The evidence is that this is unlikely and that those who do develop morbid elevation of mood while on treatment are predisposed to a bipolar disorder or are experiencing a withdrawal phenomenon (Kupfer et al 1988). A disorder of speech sometimes referred to as dysarthria, but better described as speech *blocking* or *hesitancy* has been described with a rarity that probably does not reflect its true frequency. This adverse effect, resembling stammer, is easily confused with agitation associated with the depression itself.

Other rarely reported adverse effects include skin rashes, blood dyscrasias, cholestatic jaundice and hepatic necrosis (though transient mild elevations in liver enzymes are not uncommon and are usually of no clinical significance), oedema from inappropriate secretion of antidiuretic hormone (ADH) and non-vibratory tinnitus.

Although sometimes marketed as a new generation drug, maprotiline is, as was noted, a modified tricyclic structure and in terms of its tolerability behaves, in general, similarly to amitriptyline. Two additional problems are however worthy of note. The first is an increased risk of skin rashes (approximately 3% in the first 2 weeks of treatment) and the second is a substan-

tially increased likelihood of precipitating seizures, even in the absence of predisposing factors (Blackwell and Simon 1988).

The prevalence of adverse reactions to antidepressant drugs is difficult to estimate from published studies which adopt differing methods and thresholds for recording. Their propensities would however seem to be less than clinical folklore indicates. The most systematic investigation reported a prevalence of 15.4% (Boston Collaborative Drug Surveillance Program 1972), which is comparable to the 18% or so found in comparative studies with newer antidepressants (see below).

Monoamine oxidase inhibitors

Structures

Although it is those monoamine oxidase inhibitors (MAOIs) with antidepressant activity that concern us here, it is important to appreciate that compounds acting by this mechanism have wide medicinal applications as antimicrobial, antineoplastic and antihypertensive agents.

Of the three traditional antidepressant MAOIs available in the UK, two are derivatives of hydrazine (NH_2NH_2): phenelzine, which represents a fairly simple manipulation of the molecule, and isocarboxazid, which represents a more complex analogue. The third, tranylcypromine, is a cyclopropylamine formed by substituting the isopropyl side-chain of amphetamine with a cyclopropyl side-chain (Fig. 4.5).

Advances in the pharmacology of drugs acting by inhibition of monoamine oxidase have resulted in a number of new compounds with a selectivity and/or reversibility of action not seen with the traditional drugs. Moclobemide, originally developed as a potential lipid-lowering agent, is chemically a substituted benzamide and is the only one of these new MAOIs currently available in the UK as an antidepressant. Selegiline (or −deprenyl), which is a metamphetamine derivative, is however pharmacologically within this group.

Pharmacokinetics

The pharmacokinetics of isocarboxazid have not been studied but phenelzine and tranylcypromine appear to have fairly comparable properties (Mallinger & Smith 1991). They are readily absorbed and reach peak concentrations in 1–2 hours. Elimination of both drugs is also very rapid, with half-lives in the range of 1.5–4 hours (especially short for tranylcypromine). This is due to rapid and almost complete hepatic metabolism.

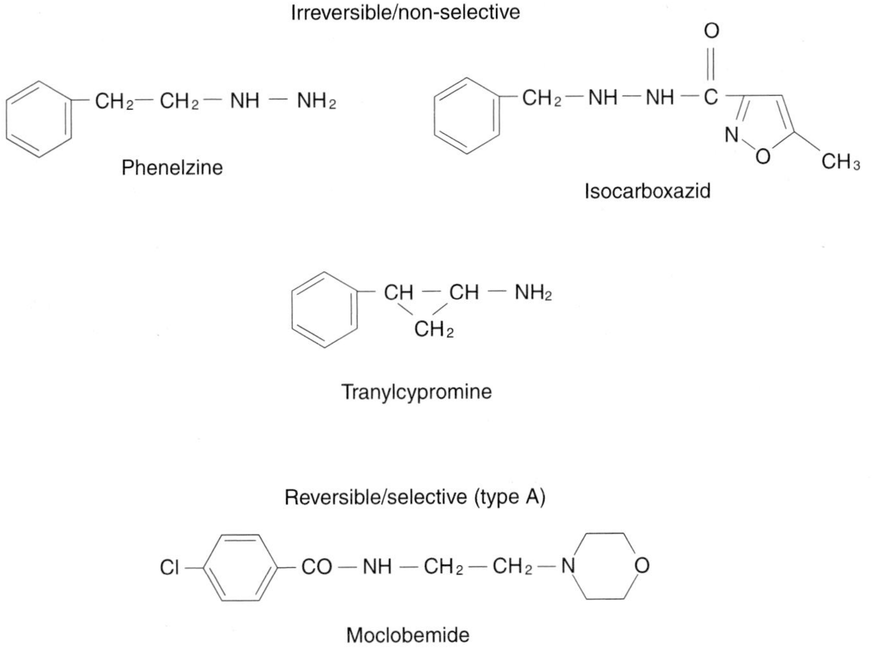

Irreversible/non-selective

Phenelzine

Isocarboxazid

Tranylcypromine

Reversible/selective (type A)

Moclobemide

Fig. 4.5 Antidepressant structures: monoamine oxidase inhibitors.

Even now the steps underlying metabolism of these drugs are poorly understood. Acetylation was at one time thought to be an important step in phenelzine metabolism, with acetylator status (slow or fast) a major determinant of efficacy and especially tolerability. However it is now unclear that acetylation is a predominant metabolic route for this drug. Plasma steady-state levels of phenelzine appear to rise over the first 6–8 weeks of exposure, which suggests that either the drug (or a metabolite) may inhibit its own metabolism.

To some extent the traditional irreversible and non-selective MAOIs are unique psychopharmacological agents, in that their clinical effects in fact bear little relationship to their pharmacokinetics. The reason for this is that these drugs mediate so-called *mechanism-based* reactions – that is, they are relatively inert compounds in themselves, but are converted by MAO into highly reactive intermediates which then inactivate the enzyme via a process of irreversible, covalent bonding (Amrein et al 1989). This results in what has been variously called a 'suicide' effect, in that the enzyme's affinity for the drug results in its irrevocable inactivation, and a 'hit-and-run' effect because the action of the drug can be detected long after the drug itself has been completely eliminated.

The newer MAOIs also have 'breakneck' kinetics. Moclobemide is readily absorbed and reaches peak plasma concentrations in approximately 1 hour.

Metabolism is rapid and complete and elimination half-life is in the range of only 1–3 hours. Some metabolites may be pharmacologically active but to clinically insignificant degree. Protein binding, at around 50%, is relatively low but bioavailability appears to increase with regular dosing (Amrein et al 1989). A mechanism-based reaction has been postulated for moclobemide but, even if true, the consequences are fundamentally different than with the traditional drugs, as enzyme binding is reversible.

Pharmacodynamics

Mode of action MAO is a flavin-containing enzyme situated mainly in the outer membranes of mitrochondria. It has a wide and dense distribution. It is the major intracellular enzyme catalysing the oxidative deamination of biogenic amines and in the CNS its function is intimately related to reuptake. By metabolising cytoplasmic amines and maintaining their concentration at a low level, its action facilitates inward-directed transporter activity from the synapse. However, the precise relationship between these intracellular events and concentrations of monoamines in the extracellular space is more complex than was originally thought and remains unclear.

In 1968, Johnston identified two subtypes of MAO, referred to as type A and type B. These subtypes differ in their preferential substrates and inhibitors. Thus the preferred substrates for type A include noradrenaline and serotonin, while phenethylamine, benzylamine and *N*-methylhistamine are preferential substrates for type B. Dopamine, tyramine and tryptamine have no preference for either subtype.

Some qualifications are necessary to the conventional wisdom about traditional MAOIs (Baldessarini 1985). The enzymatic hara-kiri that is the consequence of their mechanism-based action has allowed their effects to be viewed as irreversible, with inhibition only overcome by the manufacture of new enzyme. While this is in general true, a degree of reversibility is evident with tranlycypromine and recovery of enzyme function is somewhat more rapid (7–10 days) after discontinuation of this than it is after cessation of treatment with the hydrazine derivatives (2+ weeks). Secondly, although these drugs are considered non-selective, as is so often the case, this non-selectivity is relative. Thus phenelzine has an approximately 6:1 preference for type A, while tranylcypromine has a slight (2:1) predilection for type B. Only isocarboxazid has roughly equal affinity for both subtypes. It seems unlikely however that these differences translate into anything clinically meaningful. Finally, while mechanism-based reactions form the essential characteristic of the processes mediating efficacy, aspects of their adverse effect profile indicate that these drugs also partake in more conventional pharmacological interactions.

One of the problems in evaluating the place of traditional MAOIs in therapy has related to questions of dosing (see below). It has been suggested that in order to obtain therapeutic benefits blockade of MAO must be in the region of 80–85%, levels only achieved by doses of phenelzine in the range of 45–60 mg per day or above (Baldessarini 1985). This attempt at scientific exactitude is likely to be flawed however, as it refers to estimates of blockade performed on platelets, which contain only MAO-B. None the less it does emphasise the obvious point that even with drugs acting in the unique way that these ones do, adequacy of dosing is an essential prerequisite of therapeutic efficacy.

The identification of MAO subtypes led to the search for drugs with patterns of inhibition that were selective, particularly (in line with the biogenic amine hypothesis) to type A (Rudorfer 1992). The first of these, although selective, remained irreversible. For this reason, clorgyline, a selective inhibitor of MAO-A, has not found commercial sponsorship. The most prominent of the selective inhibitors of MAO-B, selegiline, is not useful in the treatment of depression because in the higher doses necessary for antidepressant activity its selectivity is lost. Because of its dopaminergic actions, it has however become an important tool in the management of Parkinson's disease.

A number of selective inhibitors of MAO-A that are also reversible have been developed in recent years, including brofaromine, cimoxatone and toloxatone. Of these so-called RIMAs (reversible inhibitors of MAO type A), only moclobemide has thus far received a wide launch. Despite producing a very similar plasma concentration time-course curve to tranylcypromine, the consequences of this with moclobemide are dramatically different, with maximum inhibition evident after the first dose (Mallinger and Smith 1991). Although moclobemide has a swift elimination half-life, it produces MAO-A blockade for 8–10 hours, though a decline in inhibition is already evident towards the end of even a t.i.d. dose schedule.

Traditional MAOIs and the RIMAs therefore produce very similar effects but over strikingly different timescales – some 2 weeks – with the former and almost immediate with the latter, yet there is no substantive evidence that the onset of clinical antidepressant action differs for the two types of drug. Once again the primary pharmacological action appears to represent only a necessary first step in the therapeutic process.

Adverse effects   Studies of the pharmacology of the traditional MAOIs have focused on their enzyme blocking action to the exclusion of other actions that may be more pertinent to some of their adverse effects (Table 4.4). Some adverse effects have been shown to relate to peak plasma concentrations, at least for tranylcypromine, the most studied of these drugs, and to be modifiable by alterations to methods of administration (Mallinger & Smith 1991). This is not compatible with the effects of exclusively mechanism-based activity.

The major adverse effect associated with the use of the traditional MAOIs is *hypotension*. Unlike the tricyclics, where the effects are largely if not exclusively postural, with the traditional MAOIs, lowering of *supine* blood pressure is also evident. Hence the overall clinical impact of any postural drop is more potentially disabling. The exact prevalence of reported postural hypotension varies considerably but may be in the region of 14% for tranylcypromine and slightly less for phenelzine (Rabkin et al 1985). The supine component of hypotension appears to develop relatively early (within the first week) but in a further difference with tricyclics, postural hypotension with traditional MAOIs may not be seen early in treatment but seems to build up, especially over the first 4 weeks or so of exposure. However, it may emerge at any point in the course of treatment and it is important that this is appreciated by both physician and patient. This may be one of the adverse effects that relates to pharmacokinetic parameters and therefore it may be useful to attempt to alter dose regimens as a first step in management.

The mechanism underlying the hypotensive actions

of traditional MAOIs is not clear, though it has been postulated to result from accumulation of biogenic amines because of their slowed metabolism, with a consequent increase in the activity of precursors. This is thought to result in the formation of amines with less direct sympathomimetic activity which in effect act as 'false transmitters' (Baldessarini 1985). This however remains a hypothesis.

Early in their use it was reported that these drugs possessed antianginal properties, probably mediated via a diminution in sympathetically regulated arteriolar tone. However, although acting to alleviate pain, they do not modify ischaemic changes on ECG, so are in fact merely converting symptomatic to asymptomatic ischaemia (Jefferson 1989). None the less, traditional MAOIs do not have any direct actions on cardiac rhythm, conduction or contractility and a reduction in basal heart rate usually accompanies treatment, so they may be useful in treating depressed patients with cardiac disease who are either on no, or compatible, medication.

It is surprising that drugs with little antimuscarinic actions should in practice be associated with the development of adverse effects conventionally viewed as anticholinergic in nature. These include *dry mouth, constipation* and *urinary difficulties*, including retention, and *sexual disturbance* such as impotence and orgasmic dysfunction. In fact such symptoms, established mainly with phenelzine but also found with tranylcypromine, can be very prominent, with even urinary retention occasionally affecting females. Rather than reflecting single receptor system (i.e. cholinergic) disorder, such adverse effects are probably manifestations of a peripheral cholinergic/noradrenergic imbalance with an excess of adrenergic sympathetic function.

Traditional MAOIs can produce *elevation of mood* in those not predisposed to bipolar disorders and hypomania/mania in those who are (Rudorfer 1992). They should also be avoided in schizophrenic patients as they may precipitate or exacerbate *productive* psychotic symptomatology. Tranylcypromine is the sole first-generation antidepressant to which *abuse* and *dependency* can be clearly attributed, a fact no doubt not unrelated to is close structural relationship to amphetamine, analogues of which are a product of its metabolism (Mallinger and Smith 1991).

As a result of their generally stimulant actions, traditional MAOIs may be associated with *insomnia* as well as agitation and general psychomotor 'arousal'. However, hydrazine compounds can be *sedative*, especially on first exposure. Prolonged phenelzine use has on occasion been reported to be associated with pyridoxine (vitamin B_6) deficiency, resulting in *peripheral neuropathy*. This appears to be reversible with B_6 supplements. Rare cases of diuretic resistant oedema,

probably associated with inappropriate ADH secretion, have been reported. The hepatotoxicity found with iproniazid does not appear to be an issue with the currently available drugs. However, tranylcypromine should be avoided in those with pre-existing liver disease, as there appears to be a risk of precipitating an encephalopathic-type picture (Blackwell and Simon 1988).

The adverse effect profile of moclobemide appears satisfactory and more favourable than tricyclics or the traditional drugs in the group. In particular, autonomic side-effects seem less prevalent, especially dry mouth. Restlessness, disturbed sleep, daytime fatigue and tremor can however occur, as can transient dizziness and headache (Baumhackl et al 1989). Confusion has been rarely reported; it appears reversible on discontinuation.

Hypertensive crises

Unquestionably the major source of concern with the traditional MAOIs is not strictly an adverse or toxic effect but rather a drug–drug (including food) interaction. This is the potential to precipitate a *hypertensive crisis*. These were described soon after the widespread introduction of the drugs and were crucial to the perception of risk that led to the side-stepping of the group from clinical practice for a quarter of a century. It was some years before the biochemistry of these potentially fatal reactions was understood (Blackwell 1963) and, although this offers some reassurances, an element of unpredictability remains. Because of their early association with ingestion of strong cheeses, the syndrome is still sometimes referred to as the 'cheese reaction', but this is an unjustified narrowing of the concept.

Hypertensive crises have two causes. The first, and traditionally the most common, results from the direct absorption of pressor amines formed as part of the bacterial decarboxylation of the amino acid constituents of certain protein-containing foods. Normally these amines, such as tyramine, phenylethylamine and histamine, are neutralised by MAO in the gut wall, but the loss of this protective effect by the action of enzyme inhibition allows free passage of the amines into the systemic circulation. The second cause is the ingestion of sympathomimetic drugs, including the likes of ephedrine and its derivatives and phenylpropanolamine, which are increasingly common in over-the-counter proprietary cold and cough remedies.

These compounds stimulate inappropriate release of noradrenaline from sympathetic nerve terminals and/or adrenaline from the adrenal medulla, resulting in symptoms similar to those of phaeochromocytoma. Patients develop pallor, and feel anxious, nauseated and sweaty, with pounding occipital headaches and palpitations from both forceful and irregular heart beat. These symptoms are associated with a dramatic paroxysmal rise in blood pressure. In severe cases death can ensue from either cerebrovascular accident or cardiac failure or arrest. The risk appears greatest with tranylcypromine.

When the mechanism of hypertensive crises was first delineated, an attempt was made to diminish the risk by defining the pressor amine content of foodstuffs with the aim of removing from the diet those foods with the highest contents. In the USA, this led to listings of over 700 items (Frazer 1997) and a recommended diet not much more palatable than bread and water! Problems of estimation contaminated much of this work and it is now clear that the dietary restrictions required of patients taking traditional MAOIs are in fact limited and rather prosaic, with only gastronomes of a faddy disposition finding them in any way burdensome (Baldessarini 1985). Clear proscriptions apply to pickled herring, yeast extracts like Marmite and fish and meat extracts, such as Bovril, and certain vegetable components such as broad bean pods and banana skins. It would also be prudent to go easy on the guacamole, and caviar should be kept for celebrating cessation of treatment. Most presentations of alcohol have low levels of pressor amines and the problems with coingestion relate more to potentiation. Chianti wines, prohibited in the past, appear to have been somewhat unjustly singled out. Red wines have in general higher amounts of pressor amines than white wines.

The position surrounding cheeses is less clear. Some, such as cottage or cream cheeses, are without risk, as also is sour cream and yoghurt. However the problem with other sorts of cheese relate not so much to the absolute amine values used in reference sources, which would indicate a limited source of concern, but to the fact that levels vary widely (up to 100-fold) and unpredictably in comparable samples. The fact is that the manufacturing process, especially of strong cheeses, lends itself to wide variations in amine content across batches and to a lack of uniform distribution within samples produced from the same batch. Hence caution should by exercised with all cheeses, especially matured ones. There is no particular proscription on 'blue' cheeses, as was once recommended, but the German Liederkranz, with its unusually high tyramine content, is verboten.

The risk of hypertensive crises with RIMAs is theoretically much reduced, though not completely eliminated. In practice however no specific dietary restrictions are necessary with moclobemide.

New generation antidepressants

Structures

There is no unifying chemical structure to drugs considered under this heading. Amongst the survivors of the first wave are mianserin, a distant tetracyclic cousin of cyproheptadine; trazodone, a triazolopyridine (or phenylpiperazine); and the mysterious viloxazine, a bicyclic oxazine structurally, though not pharmacologically, related to propranolol. Bupropion, available in the USA but not the UK, is an aminoketone whose efficacy appears predicated on reuptake inhibition – of dopamine!

The selective serotonin reuptake inhibitors (SSRIs) can be conveniently seen as comprising the second wave. They are, as a rule, novel and complex molecules (Figure 4.6) whose divergent structures help us little towards an understanding of their pharmacology.

A third wave is also now emerging: drugs which inhibit the reuptake of both serotonin and noradrenaline (venlafaxine), selectively inhibit noradrenaline reuptake (reboxetine), have complex receptor antagonist properties in addition to selective actions on serotonin reuptake (nefazodone, also a phenylpiperazine), or enhance serotonergic and noradrenergic transmission via antagonist actions at α_2-noradrenergic sites pre- and postsynaptically, such as mirtazapine, a close structural analogue of mianserin, also recently launched in the UK.

Pharmacokinetics

Mianserin is rapidly absorbed and is subject to very extensive first-pass effects. Its bioavailability is less than 30%. Time to peak is in the region of 3 hours and its half-life is between 10 and 20 hours, though is much extended in the elderly. It is completely metabolised and some products, such as desmethylmianserin, are weakly active.

Trazodone is rapidly absorbed (T_{max} = 1–2 hours) and is prone to first-pass effects. Between 60% and 80% reaches the systemic circulation. First-pass metabolism may be saturable and plasma levels may follow non-linear pharmacokinetics. The half-life is, for an antidepressant, relatively short, at 5–9 hours, and excretion is mainly renal. A major metabolite of trazodone, m-chlorophenylpiperazine (m-CPP), has anxiogenic properties counter to those of the parent which may produce clinical effects in patients who attain high blood levels (Preskorn 1993a,b).

Pharmacokinetic variables are the main things which distinguish the SSRIs. The major parameters for currently available compounds are shown in Table 4.5. All

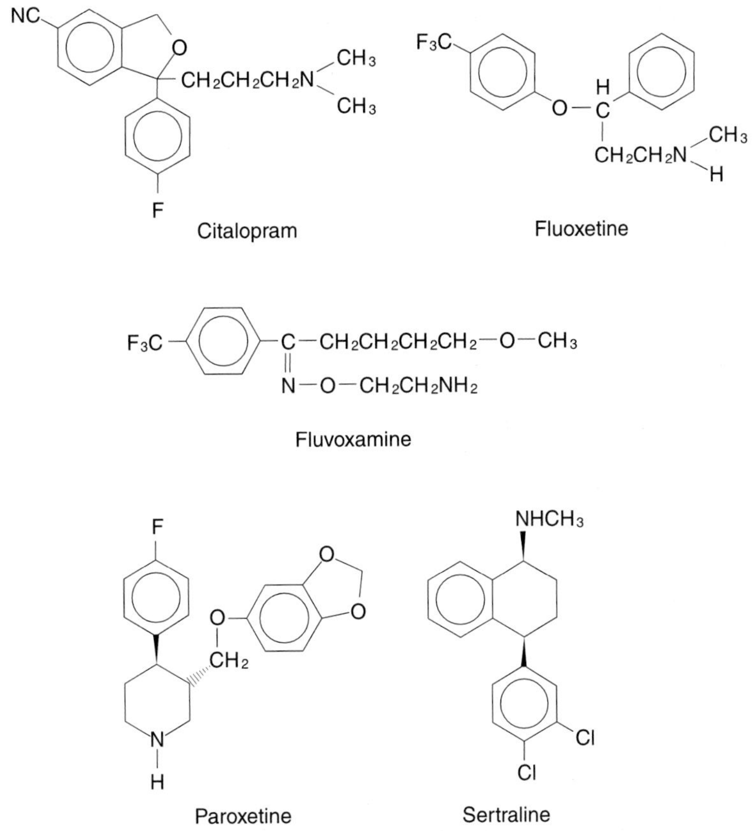

Citalopram

Fluoxetine

Fluvoxamine

Paroxetine

Sertraline

Fig. 4.6 Antidepressant structures: selective serotonin reuptake inhibitors.

Table 4.5 Some pharmacokinetic parameters of SSRI antidepressants

	T_{max}(h)	Protein binding(%)	Half-life (h)	Active metabolites
Citalopram	4–6	75 (or less)	36	+
Fluoxetine	6–8	94	24–72	+++
Fluvoxamine	2–8	77	15 (single dosing)	−
			17–22 (multiple dosing)	
Paroxetine	2–8	95	20	−
Sertraline	6–8	99	25	+

are well, if slowly, absorbed and with fluoxetine food may delay this further (Goodnick 1991). Likewise all are extensively metabolised. Both fluoxetine and paroxetine inhibit their own metabolism, so show *non-linear* pharmacokinetics, with increasing doses producing disproportionately large increases in blood levels (Preskorn, 1993a,b). In the case of fluvoxamine and paroxetine, metabolism does not appear to result in active metabolites. The others do produce pharmaco-

logically active breakdown products, though the contribution these make to efficacy is not uniform. Fluoxetine has as its major metabolite norfluoxetine, which is roughly equipotent in relation to serotonin reuptake inhibition to the parent drug. It also has an exceptionally long elimination half-life of 7–15 days. These variables may be extended in those with hepatic disease. In the case of fluoxetine, therefore, the metabolite has a major impact on the clinical action and on treatment decisions, especially following discontinuation. The mono- and di-methylated metabolites of citalopram are likewise serotonin re-uptake inhibitors, though are respectively four and 13 times less potent than the parent (Boyer & Feighner 1991). Desmethylcitalopram is however considerably more potent than its parent in inhibiting noradrenaline reuptake. The clinical impact of these in vitro findings is likely to be modified by the fact that both metabolites penetrate the brain poorly and, although opinions at present differ, it appears they make little contribution to the therapeutic package. Citalopram's half-life is extended in the elderly. The primary metabolite of sertraline, desmethylsertraline, is a weak serotonin reuptake inhibitor, being about 5–10 times less potent in this regard than the parent. Its elimination half-life however is, at over 60 hours, some two and a half times that of sertraline, and while in the elderly this variable is unchanged for sertraline, the half-life of the metabolite is prolonged.

It can be appreciated that for some members of this group steady state can take some time to achieve – for citalopram up to 2 weeks, for fluoxetine 2–3 weeks and for norfluoxetine anything from 4 to 8 weeks.

Venlafaxine is presented as a racemic mix of two active enantiomers. It is readily absorbed with T_{max} values in the range of 2–3 hours and first-pass effects are substantial. Protein binding is low compared to other antidepressants (<30%). Its half-life is also relatively short at approximately 5 hours, but that of its major metabolite, *o*-desmethylvenlafaxine – which is active – is about twice that of the parent. Excretion is almost exclusively renal.

Nefazodone is also rapidly and completely absorbed (T_{max} 1–3 hours) and is subject to substantial presystemic metabolism. It is uniquely highly protein bound (>99%) and is also unusual in its rapid elimination half-life which, at 2–4 hours, is more like those of the MAOIs. The pharmacokinetics of nefazodone are nonlinear and *m*-CPP is a metabolic product, though a minor one (Malik, 1996).

Reboxetine, recently launched in the UK, is structurally related to both fluoxetine and viloxazine. It is presented, like a number of the new antidepressants, as a racemic mixture of two enantiomers which appear to have similar kinetics. Riboxetine is rapidly absorbed (T_{max} approx. 2 hours) and its elimination half-life is in the region of 13 hours. It is highly protein bound, mainly to α_1-glycoprotein. Metabolism is extensive, with most excreted in the urine, though some may also be excreted in faeces in primates. The major interest of this drug may lie less with its mode of action than with its metabolism, for unlike most antidepressants it appears to have no (or little) inhibitory effects on the cytochrome P450 system (Dostert et al 1997). This,

together with its lack of action on serotonergic systems or against MAO, would indicate that its combined use with other drugs may be particularly uncomplicated, though this remains to be confirmed by clinical experience.

Mirtazapine is another recent recruit in the UK, and is referred to as a NaSSA – a noradrenergic and specific serotonergic antidepressant – which as an acronym has at least the benefit of familiarity! It is readily absorbed regardless of gastric contents, with a T_{max} value of around 2 hours, and the half-life, which varies from 20 to 40 hours, is sufficient for once daily dosing. It does not modify its own metabolism, which is mediated via several cytochrome P450 enzymes, and so in theory the drug is again less susceptible than many antidepressants to pharmacokinetic drug–drug interactions.

Pharmacodynamics

Mode of action Of these new generation drugs, the SSRIs have putatively similar modes of action and, although more diverse and intricate actions are claimed by the others considered here, the element of reuptake inhibition is common to most. The SSRIs selectively block the reuptake of serotonin relative to noradrenaline into the presynaptic bulb (Goodwin 1996, Frazer 1997). This selectivity is *relative* and all currently available drugs do to some extent also block noradrenaline reuptake, though for the majority this action is weak and probably not relevant to their efficacy. Citalopram is the most serotonergically selective of the current drugs and paroxetine the most potent (Richelson 1996). Viewed by the criterion of *relative* selectivity, clomipramine could be viewed as an SSRI. In addition, however, those drugs classified specifically as SSRIs are set apart by having little or no affinity for neurotransmitter receptors. Paroxetine has moderate affinity for muscarinic receptors with which sertraline, fluoxetine and citalopram also interact detectably, though very weakly. Sertraline also interacts with α_1 receptors and fluvoxamine with dopamine D_2 receptors. This however represents overall a fairly inert receptor-binding profile.

Venlafaxine appears to be a pure reuptake inhibitor with no affinity for the commonly studied amine receptor subtypes (Richelson 1996), while nefazodone, like its relative trazodone, is a fairly potent α_1 antagonist. The efficacy of nefazodone however is postulated to lie in the combination of serotonin reuptake inhibition with potent 5-HT_2 antagonism. Riboxetine is a selective reuptake inhibitor of noradrenaline but the newly launched mirtazapine does not appear to inhibit monoamine reuptake. It has a complex receptor binding profile involving antagonism at, especially, presynaptic α_2 adrenoceptors and 5-HT (2a, 2c and 3) sites and is postulated to work by enhancing noradrenergic transmission which is associated with a parallel increase in serotonergic function.

What essential components of action that can be extracted from the pharmacological mêlée that is antidepressant drugs in order to account for clinical efficacy is unknown, though there is no shortage of hypotheses. The fact is that antidepressant efficacy is associated with drugs which *selectively* block the presynaptic reuptake of noradrenaline *or* of serotonin, or are completely *non-selective* in inhibiting the reuptake of both. It may also by associated with the *facilitation* of serotonin reuptake, as with the atypical tricyclic, tianeptine. It may even be associated with inhibition of *dopamine* reuptake. It may occur in the context of direct receptor activity *or* no apparent receptor affinity. And of course one of our earliest lessons in antidepressant psychopharmacology was that it may occur in the *absence* of any direct effects on either reuptake or receptors. Indeed, it may in future be more rational to classify *all* antidepressants in terms of their putative functional characteristics (Table 4.6), though as far as our attempts to *refine* the biogenic amine hypothesis is concerned, the above does begin to look rather silly!

SSRIs, SNRIs, NaRIs or any other type of 'Is' are pharmacological tools for enhancing biogenic amine transmission in certain, probably specific, brain areas. This, it can be safely concluded, is the *necessary* first step. An advantage of these new drugs may lie in the precision with which they do this, as this may enhance tolerability and safety. This enhancement may be achieved solely by concentrating on serotonin or on noradrenaline separately, or may be achieved by utilising the relationships between serotonin and noradrenaline, which may extend efficacy to more severe disorders. However, *no* antidepressant drug, new or old, has a pattern of clinical response that parallels its primary pharmacological action. Therefore it must be concluded that *other* changes mediate the desired clinical effect – and these certainly involve receptors.

A number of receptor changes have been associated with chronic antidepressant exposure (Baldessarini 1985). These include desensitisation of cortical α_2-noradrenergic and presynaptic dopamine autoreceptors; upregulation at α_1 and downregulation at GABA$_B$ sites; desensitisation and downregulation of β-noradrenergic and 5-HT$_2$ receptors; and desensitisation and upregulation of limbic 5-HT$_{1A}$ receptors.

Moulding these into a coherent hypothesis of universal applicability to the mode of action of antidepressant drugs is beyond the capabilities of the present author to do and the needs of the present reader to know.

Adverse effects *Mianserin* is strongly sedative and despite having no anticholinergic actions can be associated with the development of dry mouth and a non-significant increase in pulse rate. It can also promote fits but the risk is, if anything, lower than with tricyclics.

The major advantage of mianserin is that, apart from the above, it appears to have very little effect on cardiac

Table 4.6   Classification of antidepressants by proposed modes of action

Enzyme inhibitors	
Monoamine oxidase	
Irreversible/non-selective	e.g. phenelzine, tranylcypromine
Reversible/selective (type A)	e.g. moclobemide
Reuptake inhibitors	
Serotonin selective	e.g. fluoxetine, paroxetine
Noradrenaline selective	e.g. riboxetine
Serotonin and noradrenaline non-selective	e.g. venlafaxine
Dopamine and noradrenaline	e.g. bupropion
Reuptake inhibitors with specific receptor actions	
Serotonin reuptake inhibition + 5-HT$_{2A}$ antagonism	e.g. nefazodone
Reuptake inhibitors (non-selective) with multiple receptor interactions	
	e.g. imipramine, amitriptyline
Reuptake inhibitors (selective) with multiple receptor interactions	
	e.g. desipramine, clomipramine
Receptor interactions (selective)	
5-HT$_{2A}$/5-HT$_{2C}$/5-HT$_3$/α_2-NA	e.g. mirtazapine

function. Prolonged PR interval and decreased T wave amplitude are inconsistent ECG findings with chronic treatment and there is even the suggestion of enhanced cardiac function (non-significant), as shown by an increase in the ejection fraction (Kopera 1980).

There is however also a potential problem. In 1979 the first case of blood dyscrasia associated with mianserin was described and in 1989 the Committee on Safety of Medicines issued a 'Current Problems' notice (No. 25) on a total of 239 cases received up to that time. Sixty-eight concerned patients with agranulocytosis and 84 granulopenia or leukopenia, 17 of whom had died. An excess of cases – and of deaths – occurred in the over-65s. Reports from Australia and New Zealand put the overall rate of agranulcytosis at between 1:2000 and 1:4000 exposures (Blackwell & Simon, 1988). These data remained controversial and, in a unique move, the manufacturer went to Court to prevent withdrawal of the drug in the UK. Mianserin requires close haematological monitoring for a least the first 3 months of use, particularly in the elderly, something which limits its value in the population in whom, because of its lack of cardiotoxicity, it might otherwise have been most useful.

Trazodone produces marked sedation and lethargy and indeed in some pharmacological test models has significant antianxiety effects. Once again it can be associated with dry mouth, blurred vision, etc. in the absence of cholinergic antagonist properties, probably relating to cholinergic–adrenergic imbalance promoted by its potent α_1-antagonist actions. This may also be the mechanism behind the uniquely high prevalence of *priapism* attributed to this drug (Warner et al 1987), though priapism is not something that correlates with antiadrenergic actions in general. This is a potentially extremely serious complication of trazodone, which may require surgical intervention, with impotence a not infrequent outcome. Male patients receiving this drug should be advised to stop treatment at the first signs of any increase in the frequency and duration of erections. Trazodone appears to have minimal effects on cardiac function at therapeutic doses.

Viloxazine has no 'anticholinergic' type side-effects and produces amphetamine-like stimulant changes on EEG compatible with its non-sedative profile and reported tendency to promote weight loss rather than weight gain. Gastrointestinal distress is more common than with other antidepressants and the drug has been implicated in precipitating migraine (Blackwell & Simon 1988). It has minimal seizure-inducing potential and no cardiac actions. Viloxazine has been popular with general practitioners in the UK, though it is a remnant of an era when clinical pharmacology was not seen as an essential part of drug development. Its durability is a triumph of marketing over substance.

Contrary to a developing lore, the *SSRIs* are not free from adverse effects (Table 4.4) but share a profile fairly characteristic of the group, though different from other antidepressants (Boyer & Feighner 1996). They all possess an increased liability to produce *gastrointestinal upset*, with *nausea*, the commonest adverse effect, recorded in 25–35% of patients. Nausea of sufficient severity to force discontinuation affects 5–8% of patients. Abdominal discomfort/pain, frank vomiting and diarrhoea also occur with greater frequency than with other antidepressants. These effects develop early in exposure, before the establishment of steady state, and tend to ease as this is reached. Hence they are likely to be mediated by local (gastrointestinal) rather than central actions. Dry mouth and constipation may be more frequent with paroxetine, reflecting its receptor-binding profile. A further common group effect is *headache*, which is usually occipital in situation and pounding in quality. This tends to increase in frequency with continued exposure (Frazer 1997).

While these drugs cannot be conveniently considered as stimulant or non-stimulant, fluoxetine appears to be particularly associated with *nervousness, anxiety* and *agitation*, which is likely to carry over into *insomnia* and reduced quality of sleep, even with the drug taken in the morning. The others, especially fluvoxamine and paroxetine, seem by contrast less likely to produce these effects and may indeed be associated with *sedation* and daytime fatigue.

It is not yet clear precisely where this restless state lies in relation to akathisia but, as with the tricyclics, it seems likely that it is phenomenologically very similar if not identical. What is clear however, is that SSRIs possess the potential to cause *acute dystonic reactions* and rarely *parkinsonism*, which are identical to those movement disorders caused by standard antipsychotic treatment (Owens 1998). The prevalence of these is not as yet known but is likely to be considerably lower than with antipsychotics. SSRIs have also been reported to exacerbate *tardive* movement disorders. These adverse effects have thrown new light on the mechanisms underlying drug-related extrapyramidal dysfunction and, although it is too early to say what the picture might be with long-term exposure, this is a question that will need to be addressed.

The other major set of adverse effects associated with the SSRIs relate to *sexual dysfunction* (Lane 1997). The frequency of side-effects of this sort is hard to specify and figures differ between studies but with widespread use it is becoming increasingly clear that problems such as abnormal ejaculation/orgasm, anorgasmia, impotence and decreased libido are common with this group, more so than with tricyclics. One review suggested that 34% of patients on fluoxetine reported sexual difficulties – 10% with reduced libido, 13% decreased responsiveness and 11% both (Jacobsen 1992). There may be genuine differences in prevalence with different compounds, though this cannot yet be concluded with certainty. Furthermore, the pattern may differ across drugs with some, such as sertraline, causing more sexual dysfunction in males than females (Frazer 1997).

SSRIs have a clearly different effect on *weight* than traditional antidepressants (Boyer & Feighner 1996). Fluoxetine and sertraline have an anorectic effect and are associated with a tendency to weight *loss*, especially in higher doses. Paroxetine appears unique in not possessing this property and indeed patients on long-term treatment may gain somewhat. The others tend to be more neutral in this regard, at least in standard doses. It appears that absolute declines in weight during treatment depend on initial body weight, with greater loss being found in more obese patients, though there is also a suggestion (unconfirmed) that the elderly may be more liable to this action.

This group also exerts virtually no effects on cardiac conduction and they are not dysrhythmogenic (Coupland et al 1997). However, they can produce *bradycardia* which may be clinically significant and symptomatic, especially in the elderly and those with certain forms of pre-existing heart disease.

A further uncommon adverse effect concerns the development of a *haemorrhagic diathesis* resulting in bruising and frank haematomata. This may be as a result of inhibition of platelet serotonin uptake and is more likely to be associated with laboratory abnormalities in platelet aggregation tests than in bleeding times. Intradermal bruising has been found in the offspring of laboratory animals exposed during pregnancy and is a strong reason for avoidance of this group of drugs during pregnancy until the position is clarified. Rarely, *skin rashes* and *hyponatraemia*, with or without inappropriate ADH secretion, have also been reported, as have *seizures*, but the liability of the group in this regard is minimal overall and less than tricyclics.

One way of evaluating the impact of adverse experiences is from data concerning discontinuation rates in comparative clinical trials. In two large meta-analyses of published studies (Montgomery et al 1994, Anderson & Tomenson 1995), fewer patients receiving SSRIs (14.9% and 14.4% respectively) than tricyclics (19% and 18.8% respectively) dropped out. In both these analyses the differences were *statistically* significant. However, as can be seen, they are far from dramatic and are unlikely to represent differences that are significant in *clinical* terms (Anderson & Tomenson,

1995). A further recent meta-analysis concluded that of every 100 patients treated with a tricyclic, 31 would be likely to drop out of treatment, while the comparable figure for those on an SSRI would be 28 (Hotopf et al 1997).

The other new generation drugs appear to share the relatively favourable adverse effect profile of the SSRIs, though at time of writing, data on riboxetine are sparse. Little in the way of drowsiness or sedation has been reported with *venlafaxine*, which is in line with its niggardly approach to receptor binding, and any early nausea appears for the most part to resolve rapidly. If anything it may cause a dose-related *increase* in blood pressure, though in less than 5% of patients and transient in about half (Frazer 1997). Effects on weight are inconsistent, with early tendency to lose being followed at 6–8 months by a slight increase, which may of course relate more to well-being than an adverse action. As with sertraline, sexual dysfunction may be more evident in males. *Nefazodone*, like its brother trazodone, is sedative despite being only weakly antihistaminic, and while both have potent anti-α_1-noradrenergic actions, the former seems to produce less postural hypotension than the latter. One of the marketing points with nefazodone is its apparently low liability to produce disorders of sexual function, and interestingly this drug does not appear to share trazodone's priapismic proclivities.

It is not yet possible to construct a reliable and detailed comparative adverse effect profile for the very recently launched drugs, something that must await a wider and longer experience. However, mirtazapine's receptor binding profile would allow the assumption that it may be associated with less in the way of nausea (5-HT_3 antagonism) but more in the way of daytime fatigue and impaired motor performance (H_1 antagonism) than the majority of the newer drugs.

Toxicity of antidepressants in overdose

For many years much of the little that was known about the clinical pharmacology of antidepressants was based on patients who had taken overdoses of tricyclic compounds. It is clear that, in overdose, the clinical pharmacology of tricyclics is different from that of their therapeutic use, transforming these drugs into potentially lethal agents. Even today, the toxicity of antidepressants remains largely the toxicity of the tricyclics.

The pharmacokinetic parameters of tricyclics change following overdose and this is the major factor underlying their toxicity in this situation (Jarvis 1991). Firstly, absorption is substantially delayed, probably as a result of anticholinergic effects. It is common at post mortem to find drug residues in the stomachs of patients dying from tricyclic overdose. Furthermore, as was mentioned, considerable enterohepatic recirculation takes place, contributing to the maintenance of high blood levels.

At excessively high levels tricyclics appear to shift from first-order to zero-order kinetics – that is, the amount metabolised is fixed rather than proportionate. This results from saturation of hepatic enzymes and in the case of tricyclics appears to relate to saturation of the rate-limiting hydroxylation pathways (Jarvis 1991). Thus high blood levels in a way sustain themselves by delayed absorption, enterohepatic circulation and saturated metabolism, thereby prolonging the half-life by as much as twofold.

Furthermore, metabolism is dependent on cardiac output and so any compromise in this will further impede metabolism. At high blood levels, tricyclics are profoundly cardiotoxic, mainly as result of their potent actions in delaying ventricular conduction time, resulting in QT prolongation, QRS elongation and ventricular premature beats, which may progress to ventricular tachyarrhythmias, which can in turn be associated with strikingly inefficient pump action. In addition, a clinically unimportant positive inotropic action at therapeutic levels inverts to a negative action at high levels, which may further contribute to output failure.

Furthermore, at high blood levels tricyclics can seriously impair gas exchange in the lungs. This is because of the central depressant effect common to the group, but also to increasingly recognised local alveolar damage (Roy et al 1989). The effect is acidaemia. Falls in pH are associated with a reduction in the amount of drug that is protein bound, and hence with an increase in the amount of pharmacodynamically-active free drug. Because such a large proportion of tricyclic is protein bound only very slight reductions in binding are necessary to greatly increase the percentage of free drug. For example, a reduction from binding levels of 95% to 93% could theoretically increase the free fraction by 50% (Jarvis 1991).

The major clinical manifestations of tricyclic toxicity are signs of CNS and cardiovascular depression. Patients may appear flushed and hot, with widely dilated pupils and peripheral tremulousness. Sedation and drowsiness, combined with motor signs of discoordination, progress to frank confusion as a prelude to coma. Breathing becomes rapid and shallow and tachycardia of sinus or supraventricular type is usually evident. Cardiac irregularities may also be apparent. Around 4–8% of patients may fit or go into status, though the risk of fitting may be as high as 36% with overdose of maprotiline (Knudsen & Heath 1984). Of note are reports of acute renal failure in approximately 10% of amoxapine overdoses (Jennings et al 1983) and permanent neurological damage in 2% of maprotiline over-

doses (Knudsen & Heath 1984), neither of which are features of uncomplicated overdoses of tricyclics in general.

For the reasons mentioned above it is always important to attempt gastric lavage in tricyclic overdose patients even if there has been a delay in discovering the individual. Otherwise treatment is essentially supportive. In view of the risks of antiarrhythmic drugs in the context of antiarrhythmic overdose and the fact that respiratory depression may require intubation, such supportive measures are for medical specialists. Even when the clinical situation appears stable, it is important for psychiatrists to be wary of the overzealous attempts of medical colleagues to return overdose patients to psychiatric units quickly. As a knowledge of the pharmacokinetics would suggest, half-lives – and risk periods – will extend for some days after a serious overdose.

The major advantage of the new generation antidepressants is undoubtedly their safety profile in overdose (Boyer & Feighner 1996). Although isolated reports of fatality have appeared, especially with the older drugs, these have usually been in association with polydrug ingestion in which the role of the antidepressant alone was unclear.

Antidepressant withdrawal/discontinuation syndromes

It has been known since 1959 that sudden cessation of treatment with tricyclics could be associated with the development of a withdrawal (or discontinuation) syndrome, though this was rarely commented on in the literature, and then only in the form of anecdotal reports. A similar phenomenon was also noted with MAOIs. The issue has however received greater prominence in recent years in connection with SSRIs (Lejoyeux & Ades 1997).

Sudden cessation of protracted and especially high-dose tricyclic regimens can be associated after a day or two with the development of symptomatology that can be considered in five categories (Dilsaver et al 1987):

- *somatic*, including nausea, vomiting, diarrhoea, sweating, malaise
- *sleep*, including poor quality, decreased duration and vivid anxiety-laden dreams
- *movement disorders*, especially akathisia and parkinsonian-type symptoms
- *'activation'* symptoms comprising mania/hypomania, anxiety, panic attacks and frank clouding
- *cardiac arrhythmias*.

Despite reported prevalence figures ranging from 16% to 100%, these are probably uncommon in a degree that merits clinical attention. It may be that prevalence is greater with tertiary amine compounds than with secondary ones, or alternatively that, as with antipsychotics, the risk may relate more to the potency of the drug's cholinergic antagonist properties, though neither of these possibilities has been established.

Withdrawal symptoms following MAOI treatment can be severe and include a 'rebound' depression or manic/hypomanic symptomatology with agitation, irritability, insomnia, myoclonic jerks and frank confusion/delirium. They seem particularly pronounced after sudden cessation of tranylcypromine (Halle & Dilsaver 1993).

The 'discontinuation syndrome' associated with stopping SSRIs is different from that associated with cessation of other antidepressants (Haddad 1997). It usually emerges within 24 hours of stopping and comprises anxiety and irritability, alteration in sleep and gastrointestinal symptoms, with in addition flu-like symptoms of coryza, myalgia and shaking chills. Particular features include 'dizziness' consisting of both true movement-sensitive vertigo and a 'spaced out' sensation akin to mild inebriation, ataxia and burning shock-like sensations, tingling or hypoaesthesias. It has also been suggested that aggressive and impulsive behaviour may represent a further novel SSRI discontinuation phenomenon but the few reports describing this are likely to represent coincidental phenomenology. These features can develop with all members of the group, though seem to be most likely to occur with compounds of shorter half-life. Thus they appear relatively uncommon following cessation of fluoxetine but may affect up to one-third of those coming off paroxetine (Haddad 1997). A similar situation has been described after sudden discontinuation of venlafaxine.

Withdrawal or discontinuation syndromes can sometimes be dramatic, especially when patients stop medication without medical advice. This is particularly the case with the traditional MAOIs. Although in the vast majority of instances they are brief and self-limiting events lasting only 2 or 3 days, they may be more protracted, especially with the older drugs. Most do not however require specific intervention. They do none the less emphasise the importance of gradual tapering of antidepressant regimens over days or preferably weeks, something which is made more problematic with the fixed dosing schedules of some of the newer drugs.

Therapeutics

Indications

There is currently much debate about the relative places of different groups of antidepressants in clinical practice. As a rule, these debates are not predicated on questions of efficacy as a superficial interpretation of the data would indicate that all antidepressants are equivalent in this regard (Frazer 1997). The debate rests largely on the balance of tolerablility and safety versus cost. There is however increasing evidence that in severe depressions, especially those conforming to the traditional picture of melancholia, SSRIs at least are not as efficacious as tricyclics (Perry 1996). The position of other new generation drugs remains to be seen. This apart, the indications for antidepressants in general can be summarised as:

- The treatment of acute episodes of major depression. Response is likely to be greater in depressions that are not secondary to other psychiatric disorders but these drugs, especially tricyclics, would also be indicated in secondary depressions, including postpsychotic (or schizophrenic) depressions.
- The prevention of relapse in recurrent, non-bipolar depressions.

Some compounds are in addition recommended in other or more specific situations:

- Obsessive–compulsive disorder: both the tricyclic clomipramine and the SSRIs, especially fluoxetine and paroxetine, have proven efficacy in this condition.
- Panic disorder: the work of Klein and colleagues established the efficacy of imipramine in the treatment of panic states where the lack of addictive potential makes it suitable for longer term use.
- Eating disorders, especially bulimia nervosa: in recent years fluoxetine in high dose (e.g. up to 80 mg per day) has been reported as effective.
- 'Atypical' depressions: researchers in New York have, over a number of years, refined this concept into what is now sometimes referred to as 'Columbia atypical depression', after the authors' institution (Quitkin et al 1993). Theoretically this is a somewhat uncomfortable concept for British audiences, combining as it does analytically based concepts such as 'hysteroid dysphoria' (covering narcissism, romantic preoccupation and disappointment in relationships) with biological symptomatology such as hyperphagia, hypersomnia, and profound fatigue associated with so-called 'leaden paralysis'. None the less the authors have presented data over the years to show that such patients respond preferentially to traditional MAOIs, especially phenelzine, compared with tricyclics.
- Attention deficit disorder with hyperactivity in

children: the strongest evidence relates to imipramine.

- Pain syndromes: tricyclics have clear efficacy in the management of chronic pain syndromes. One recent meta-analysis concluded that of every 100 patients with pain from such diverse causes as diabetic neuropathy, postherpetic neuralgia and atypical facial pain, 30 will experience a greater than 50% reduction of symptoms on a tricyclic, and that overall their efficacy is comparable with that of anticonvulsants (McQuay et al 1996).
- Enuresis in children (imipramine).
- Premature ejaculation (SSRIs).

Strategies

There has over the past few years been an effective – and *almost* convincing – campaign conducted against the use of tricyclics and in favour of new generation antidepressants, an argument which has been presented in stark terms that serve to oversimplify a complex balance of choices. There are several issues.

The statement is often quoted that all antidepressants are of equal efficacy, and that, by a modern reappraisal, includes the MAOIs (Frazer 1997). But as the above has illustrated, this does not mean that all are equally effective in all situations. Therapeutic choices must be finely balanced and include awareness of the increasing evidence that in some illnesses, especially the more severe ones conforming to the classical picture of melancholia, SSRIs may not be as effective as tricyclics (Perry 1996).

A second string to antitricyclic advocacy is tolerability. Meta-analyses of comparative studies have consistently shown better tolerability with SSRIs than tricyclics evaluated by patient withdrawals from trials. However, the differences are rarely marked and, although on statistical analysis they reach significance, it is unlikely that they are of significance *clinically* (Anderson & Tomenson 1995, Hotopf et al 1997).

Cost is an increasing consideration for doctors and a strong argument in favour of the new drugs is that, although costing more in themselves, they are in fact, for a number of reasons, more cost-effective in the long run. Considerable effort has gone into justifying this argument but it is clear that the outcome of such analyses depends crucially on the information fed into the analytical models. Thus far, such analyses have produced contrary conclusions (Hotopf et al, 1996).

The one argument on which there is no contest is safety in overdose. All the new generation antidepressants have a far more favourable toxicity profile than the tricyclics. Amongst the old drugs, amitriptyline, desipramine and dothiepin appear particularly associat-

ed with a fatal outcome after overdose (Cassidy & Henry 1987). The question then is the magnitude of the issue. Figures for the contribution made by the high-risk drugs to completed overdoses are variable. While some argue the contribution is substantial (Henry 1996), the data are open to different interpretations (Hotopf et al 1996).

Based on the figures of Montgomery and colleagues, derived from coroners' returns for England and Wales for the years 1975–1985, the two worst offenders, dothiepin and amitriptyline, were each associated with between 45 and 50 deaths per million prescriptions (Montgomery et al 1989). In absolute numbers, this translates into approximately 170 deaths per year between them.

What such data cannot tell us is to what extent these deaths in fact represent the outcome of *inadequate* treatment, still a problem with tricyclic prescribing, especially in primary care (Beaumont et al 1996), or poor supervision. It is furthermore not clear to what extent the suicide victims of tricyclic overdose might be saved by side-stepping these drugs and to what extent the well-described phenomenon of substitution would merely result in such individuals resorting to other means.

Not all tricyclics are however tarred with the same fatality risk in overdose as amitriptyline and dothiepin, with clomipramine, protriptyline and lofepramine apparently safer, though the data on which these conclusions rest are open to greater criticism. Perhaps the biggest problem with tricyclics is quite simply that a fatal overdose may comprise as little as 10–15 times the therapeutic dose, leaving the distressed patient little room for 'error'.

These points are not made in support of a Luddite approach to antidepressant prescribing choices but to apprise the clinician of the legitimate perception that such choices remain, in most situations, more finely balanced than is sometimes made clear.

There are several situations in which new generation antidepressants justify a first-line position:

- In patients in whom impulsive or planned misuse is an active or predictable issue.
- In primary care situations where depressive disorders may be more amenable and where, by virtue of time constraints, high levels of support and close monitoring are not feasible.
- In cases of medical complexity such as severe heart disease, recent CVA or coincidental complex drug regimens.
- In those in whom impaired motor performance may cause occupational restrictions.
- Previous intolerance to tricyclics.

- A pressing need to cultivate clearly tenuous cooperation by the avoidance of unacceptable adverse effects, e.g. a fear of weight gain, etc.

The elderly present special considerations because, although for pharmacokinetic and other reasons they are undoubtedly more susceptible to the riskier adverse effects of tricyclics, they may also be more prone to depressions which respond less favourably to newer drugs.

It might be argued that poor compliance with tricyclics has traditionally emanated as much from unsophisticated prescribing as from the problems inherent to the group and it remains the case that by the skilful application of some of the data presented above, tricyclics can be effectively and acceptably utilised if indicated.

The traditional MAOI's remain third-line drugs even in those with 'atypical' depressions and their use is best reserved for specialist settings. The role of the RIMA's remains uncertain, though the sole available representative, moclobemide, has as yet had some difficulty in establishing its niche.

The effective utilisation of antidepressants includes implementation of the following principles:

- *Principle 1*   Assess the appropriateness of pharmacological intervention in the knowledge that this may not be the most suitable first-line recommendation.
- *Principle 2*   Assess severity of the depression and the risk of self-harm independently. In general the risk of overdose of prescribed medication is likely to parallel the severity of the depression but attempts at self-harm may be impulsive and not necessarily related to severity of the mood disorder as assessed at interview, especially in those with comorbidity (e.g. personality disorders).
- *Principle 3*   Allow levels of anxiety/agitation and sleep disturbance to influence prescribing decisions. Notwithstanding medical probity, not all 'non-target' effects are 'adverse'.
- *Principle 4*   Specific antidepressant efficacy is inevitably delayed, and perhaps for longer than with antipsychotics. It is likely that about 10 days to 2 weeks will elapse before any specific benefits are evident, which may take 4–6 weeks to maximise. Patients must be advised of this as otherwise the tendency is for them to give up prematurely.
- *Principle 5*   The possible adverse effect profile of the chosen compound should also be discussed, as educating patients in this regard greatly enhances their willingness to tolerate the drugs and hence provides an enormous boost to compliance.
- *Principle 6*   Treatment must be adequate in terms

of doses. The most common cause of 'treatment-resistant' depression is inadequate dosage. This contributes to unnecessary morbidity and increases the risk of self-harm while exposing patients to the likelihood of needless side-effects. This is less of an issue with the SSRIs, which tend to a narrower therapeutic dose range, but is pertinent to other new generation drugs and especially to tricyclics, most of which have a therapeutic dose range between 150 and 225 mg per day.

- *Principle 7*   Suboptimal or non-existant response after 4–6 weeks on an adequate dose regimen should indicate a change of drug (and probably of group).
- *Principle 8*   Treatment should also be adequate in terms of duration. Successful management should be extended for at least 6 months, and for up to 1 year in some cases, in order to minimise the risk of relapse.

LITHIUM SALTS AND OTHER MOOD STABILISERS

Lithium

Lithium is an old, but not ancient, acquaintance of chemistry, being discovered in 1817 by the Swedes, Arfwedson and Berzelius, who identified the sulphate from the mineral, petalite. Elemental lithium was isolated by electrolysis in 1855. Lithium, a silvery-white alkali metal, is the lightest of all solids, occupying position 3 in the periodic table. As a highly reactive element it has found wide commercial application in everything from the processing of rubber to the manufacture of long-life batteries and from the strengthening of glass and ceramics to the construction of nuclear bombs. By contrast, only about 1% of annual supplies is devoted to medicinal use.

The medical applications of lithium salts began in 1841 when Lipowitz recommended their use in gout. Despite half a century of use, this was not in fact an effective treatment. From 1864 however, lithium was listed in the *British Pharmacopoeia* and the chloride, and especially bromide, salts were widely used as hypnotics throughout the latter part of the 19th and early 20th centuries. Lithium bromide was in addition one of the first compounds regularly employed as an antianxiety agent.

By the end of the 19th century the first reports of toxicity with the medical use of lithium began to appear but, despite this, unmonitored lithium chloride was enthusiastically endorsed in the 1940s as a salt substitute in the management of hypertension. In early 1949, considerable publicity in the USA surrounded a number of fatalities from toxicity which led to the Food and

Drug Administration (FDA) banning the use of lithium salts. This perception of hazard delayed the introduction of lithium in its current incarnation into the USA for over a decade.

In addition to their use in what might be called minor or non-specific psychiatric disorders, lithium salts were recommended early for the treatment of more severe forms of affective disorder. In the 1870s, for example, the American physician William Hammond recommended massive oral doses of lithium bromide for the acute treatment of mania and melancholia, while in the 1880s the Danish neurologist Carl Lange favoured alkaline salts for the treatment of what he called 'periodic depression'. This was part of a belief, prevalent at the time, that some forms of mood disorder were one manifestation of what was called 'the gouty diathesis', for which Lange recommended dietary restrictions, regular exercise – and prophylactic intake of alkaline salts!

The modern psychiatric use of lithium was begun by Dr John Cade of the Victoria Department of Mental Hygiene in Australia. He was interested in the possibility that mania might be the result of the build-up of some unidentified toxin, while depression might represent what he called 'a correspondingly deprivative condition'. Returning to purine metabolism, he noted that in guinea-pigs urea produced a state of hyperexcitability and wished to see if uric acid enhanced the toxicity of urea. He therefore administered lithium urate, the most soluble of urate salts, and found that, contrary to expectation, this protected the animals against the excitant properties of urea. On this flimsiest of bases, he administered lithium to excited patients in doses that he took from a 1927 text, Culbreth's *Manual of Materia Medica and Pharmacology*. In 1949, Cade published his results in a group of ten patients, most of whom had been chronically symptomatic with mania. The findings were dramatic, with mood stabilisation in a week or so. By contrast, six schizophrenic patients did not improve significantly. The doses Cade chose, courtesy of Culbreth, were very high (one of the original group eventually died of toxicity) and it has been suggested that what was observed as improvement in the psychiatric illness may in fact have been incipient toxicity. Be this as it may, this original publication stimulated some interest in Australia but, it must be said, in few other places. One of these was Denmark where Erik Stromgren suggested further exploration of the issue, thereby stimulating the work of the Aarhus group led by Mogens Schou, which was to be so influential in developing lithium as a safe and effective treatment.

Structure

The lithium atom is represented by a single electron circling a noble gas core (i.e. two electrons in a single balanced orbit around the nucleus). This outer electron is powerfully shielded from the attractive force of the nucleus so the energy required to displace it from the atom is very low, while the so-called second ionisation energy is much higher. Thus the chemistry of lithium is essentially that of the Li^+ ion. Furthermore, as the therapeutic benefits of different salts in psychiatric applications are identical, the same applies to the pharmacology.

The major bulk lithium chemicals are the sulphate and carbonate salts and lithium hydroxide, though of these only lithium carbonate is now used in psychiatric practice.

The lithium content of salts and of dosage formulations may vary: for accuracy, preparations should be compared on the basis of their lithium content in milliequivalent terms. In general, 37 mg of the carbonate salt is equal to 1 mEq. of lithium (Baldessarini 1985).

Pharmacokinetics

Unlike other psychotropic agents, lithium has a narrow therapeutic index and a knowledge of the pharmacokinetics of different formulations is important in maximising tolerability while minimising toxicity. There is however a difficulty with terminology in that different preparations are marketed as having discrete absorption characteristics that may not in practice be quite so discrete.

Lithium is readily and almost completely absorbed. Some 20% of an orally administered dose is absorbed from the stomach, a process not apparently dependent on gastric acidity. Absorption is however predominantly (>70%) from the small bowel and occurs by passive diffusion through the lateral intercellular spaces and the absorptive pores of the epithelial tight junctions (Diamond et al 1983). Absorption is hence fastest when concentrations in the bowel lumen are highest. The rise in plasma levels is rapid with standard preparations, peak levels being reached in 1–2 hours. Lithium is not protein bound and its volume of distribution is approximately that of total body water. Oral bioavailability is 90% or above.

Unlike sodium and potassium, lithium shows no strong preferential distribution across cell membranes but the rate of passage is not uniform across all body tissues and at equilibrium there are some differences in a variety of tissue–plasma concentration gradients (Cooper 1987). Thus in the liver the concentration of lithium tends to be lower than in extracellular fluid, while in muscle, bone and thyroid it is 2–4 times higher. The concentration in brain is roughly the same as that of extracellular fluid, which is approximately 50%

of the plasma concentration. It has been suggested that this might indicate that in pharmacokinetic terms lithium is best represented by a two-compartment model (Poust 1987).

Half-life values vary considerably even after single dosing, something to which age may contribute. The shortest half-lives are generally found in young adults (e.g. 18–20 hours). Overall the half-life is regarded as being in the region of 22–24 hours and does not vary with different salts. Steady state is therefore achieved within 4–7 days. However it seems clear that the half-life of lithium increases with long-term treatment by as much as 25–30% (Goodnick et al 1981). This has obvious clinical relevance in that accumulation may occur over time, with consequent increase in the risk of toxicity.

There are no metabolic steps in the body's handling of lithium, almost all of which is excreted via the kidneys, with less 5% accounted for by loss in faeces and from insensible sources. Lithium is secreted in most body fluids, including sweat, saliva, tears, ejaculate and breast milk and possibly also intestinal secretions. Being unbound, it is freely filtered by the renal glomerulus along with other cations such as sodium and potassium. Also, like sodium, some 70–80% of filtered lithium is reabsorbed in the proximal tubules by a mechanism which is competitive with sodium. However, while filtered sodium undergoes further reabsorption in the distal nephron (loop of Henle, distal tubule and collecting ducts), lithium does not. The speed at which lithium is excreted – i.e. the lithium clearance – is therefore linked to proximal tubular fluid output and as such is not constant. Clearance is increased with extracellular volume expansion, as for example during pregnancy, but more significantly it decreases with either water or sodium depletion. Thus in terms of increasing the risk of toxicity, not only must disorders that impair glomerular filtration, such as renal disease and increasing age, need to be kept in mind, so too do states of decreased sodium intake or increased extrarenal loss, salt-depleting medications such as diuretics and dehydration. The adverse effects of water deficiency may be militated against somewhat if dehydration is acquired via increased sweating, such as with inadequate fluid intake in hot climates or with fever, as increasing blood lithium levels will be associated with increased loss of lithium in sweat. However this 'homeostatic' mechanism must not be counted on to provide adequate protection and patients must be given prudent advice.

The advantages of single dosing have long been evident to pharmacologists as well as clinicians. Single daily dosing of *standard* lithium is not as a rule possible in healthy individuals as, in order to maintain adequate

levels over a 24 hour dosing interval, unnecessarily high average doses are required and peak levels would be well into the toxic range. Assuming a half-life of 24 hours a single dose regimen of a standard preparation can be expected to produce 12 hour blood levels approximately 25% higher than those with the same daily dose given in a t.i.d. schedule. Furthermore, giving a single dose of 900 mg standard lithium can result in peak levels almost four times those of trough levels, whereas on a t.i.d. regimen the same daily dose results in a less than twofold difference (Baldessarini 1985).

In order to minimise the size of the postabsorptive peak a number of formulations have been introduced over the years and have gone by a number of names, such as 'slow release', 'controlled release', 'sustained release', etc. Various ingenious methods have been used to try and achieve the aim of a delayed rise to a lower peak level, including decreasing the solubility, embedding the drug in a non-digestible porous carrier or gel, using ion exchange resins or controlled disintegration coatings, amongst others. These now (after some hairy starts) appear to have resulted in preparations that have at least some of the desired characteristics which, unlike the early attempts, are attained at little or no cost to bioavailability (Goodnick & Schorr-Cain 1991). In general, peak levels with these formulations are achieved after 3–6 hours, with Liskonum delayed somewhat more than others. Camcolit 400 and Priadel appear to have similar characteristics, while lithium citrate achieves the lowest peak levels but also appears to have the lowest 12 hour plasma levels (Shelley & Silverstone 1987). Although data are contradictory, there is a suggestion that the area under the curve (AUC) is less with the citrate syrup than carbonate in tablet form, which suggests lower bioavailability. None the less, liquid citrate may be an option to consider in those who find tablets difficult to swallow.

One complication in presenting the pharmacokinetic profile of lithium is that most studies have been done on normal volunteers, whereas there is evidence that the disorders for which the drug is being taken (i.e. affective disorders) may themselves alter pharmacokinetic data (Goodnick & Schorr-Cain 1991). This is something that has only been recognised in recent years and, while not altering the basic contention that an understanding of the drug's pharmacokinetics is an important aid to rational clinical practice, it does illustrate the need to utilise such information as a guide only.

Pharmacodynamics

Mode of action The mode of action of lithium is unknown. As a widely distributed and highly reactive cation, lithium influences chemical processes at a series of levels of central neurophysiology, yet clinically it seems to produce effects that are fairly focused. However, the lack of a tenable theory on the pathophysiology of affective disorders makes the task of unravelling the mode of action a 'needle in a haystack' job.

Lithium acts at three main neurochemical 'levels'. The *first* is at the level of membrane electrophysiology. Lithium shares many of the physical properties of other physiologically active cations such as sodium, potassium and calcium and can pass readily through ion channels associated with these. One of the earliest suggestions therefore was that it may stabilise electrolyte balances across neuronal membranes, something that may be disturbed in affective disorders. It may do this by stimulating Na/K-ATPase, the energy-dependent enzyme responsible for controlling the balance of sodium and potassium across cell membranes via the sodium pump mechanism. Lithium cannot however substitute for sodium in the pump arrangement and so excessive replacement of sodium by lithium, as might happen for example in toxicity, could result in a failure of membranes to maintain polarisation and to conduct an action potential (Baldessarini 1985). This could underlie the catastrophic CNS collapse seen with severe and escalating toxicity.

The *second* level that lithium acts at is on neurotransmitters. It has been shown, as an acute effect, to increase neuronal uptake of catecholamines and with chronic administration to potentiate serotonergic and noradrenergic function, effects on the latter being less in degree though more consistent (Manji et al 1991). Lithium treatment may also prevent or modify the receptor supersensitivity response to chronic catecholamine antagonists such as antipsychotics (Baldessarini 1985). However, this 'receptor-stabilising' hypothesis, once a promising theory, has been blighted by inconsistent data, especially at the clinical level. While it is likely that lithium's actions on catecholamine transmitter systems are regionally selective within the brain, there seems no doubt about this in relation to serotonin transmission. Short-term, lithium stimulates release of serotonin, especially in the hippocampus, and longer-term, may increase activity in presynaptic hippocampal neurones, resulting in receptor downregulation. While some of these changes may be taken as consistent with the biogenic amine hypothesis, they leave unexplained the compound's mode of action in these states.

The *third* and most complex level at which lithium may act is on so-called second messenger systems (Manji et al 1995). Neuronal membrane receptors mediate two sorts of events – those involving the propagation of electrical potentials on the membrane surface and those that result from the translation of receptor events into modifications in intracellular functioning. The agents mediating the first set of events – i.e. the neurotransmitters themselves – might therefore be considered as the 'first' messengers in neurophysiological processes, while those substances mediating the transduction of electrical information at the receptor into changes at the level of intracellular effectors might then be thought of as 'second' messengers. These intracellular messengers, which include adenylyl cyclases, inositol 1,4,5-triphosphate, arachidonate, protein kinase C isoenzymes, guanine nucleotide binding (or G) proteins and calcium, act on specific target proteins to initiate signalling cascades. It is clear that lithium affects a number of signal transduction pathways.

Inositol phospholipids are relatively minor components of cell membranes but none the less major participants in receptor-mediated signal transduction pathways. The activation of a number of receptor subtypes induces the hydrolysis of membrane phospholipids, a process involving the complex interaction of transmitters, including adrenaline and 5-HT, with G proteins which stimulate isoforms of the enzyme phospholipase C. These in their turn result in production of two intracellular second messengers, *sn*-1,2-diacylglycerol (DAG) and inositol 1,4,5-triphosphate. The brain is dependent on the recycling of inositol phosphates to maintain inositol levels and lithium, which inhibits the intracellular enzyme inositol monophosphatase, results in a depletion of free inositol. While these appear to be robust findings they seem unlikely in themselves to explain lithium's delayed and targeted actions.

A further receptor-coupled second messenger system which lithium acts on is the cAMP generation system. A further robust finding is that lithium inhibits the accumulation of noradrenaline-induced cAMP. Indeed this attenuation of amine-induced coupling to adenylyl cyclase may also occur in peripheral cells and may underlie some of the drug's adverse effects, such as nephrogenic diabetes insipidus and possibly thyroid impairment. These effects of lithium may be mediated acutely via competition with magnesium for a binding site on the adenylyl cylase molecule but with chronic exposure mediation seems to be via G proteins (Manji et al 1995). G proteins are a complex family of molecules that comprise an important signal transduction pathway. Long-term lithium exposure attenuates the actions of G proteins by inhibiting their coupling to receptor proteins. It has further been suggested that it is by this mechanism of G protein attenuation that lithium may prevent the development of receptor supersensitivity, though this is unproven at present.

The final intracellular system that has been of interest with regard to the mode of action of lithium concerns a widely distributed and highly active set of enzymes collectively known as protein kinase C. These operate postsynaptically but are also crucially important in presynaptic events. While acute administration of lithium activates this family of isoenzymes, chronic ingestion decreases the responses they mediate, including neurotransmitter release (Manji et al 1995).

Membrane events have been the traditional focus of neurophysiology but increasing understanding of intracellular events has opened an exciting new window on the complex systems that characterise intercellular communication. It is not yet clear precisely how the pervasive effects of lithium on the intracellular part of this communication highway relate to its therapeutic benefits – or for that matter to the pathophysiology of affective disorders – nor in what ways these may relate to other actions of the ion, as for example in modifying early gene expression. None the less, unravelling these complex events is likely to inform us more about the mechanisms underlying the modes of action of many psychotropics, including lithium, than approaches hitherto have done, as well as pointing the way to rational theories of pathophysiology at the molecular level.

Adverse effects Lithium is a highly toxic ion and has the lowest margin of safety of any of the classes of drugs used in clinical psychopharmacology. Although therapeutic monitoring has reduced the risk of toxicity dramatically, treatment can still be associated with a wide range of adverse effects (Table 4.7). Indeed with close monitoring it has been suggested that only a very few of those on standard lithium (around 10%) are likely to escape completely (Vacaflor 1975). The prevalence of most side-effects is however lower with 'slow' or 'sustained' release formulations, which are now the most commonly used.

To some extent many of the adverse effects of lithium and those of toxicity develop on a predictable continuum and are but matters of degree. Thus while it is usually possible to distinguish between the major adverse effects that occur therapeutically and those indicative of toxicity, an overlap exists and the distinction is, in the early stages of transition at least, largely a quantitative one. In fact, even with patients considered on the basis of a standard 12 hour blood level to be within the therapeutic range, adverse symptomatology can still be reported. This reflects both the rate of rise to, and the maximum height of, the postabsorptive peak. For purposes of emphasis the features of toxicity are highlighted separately below but it is important to appreciate that in practice they may not represent a discrete symptomatic break.

The most frequently reported adverse effects are gastrointestinal. The vast majority of patients – if not all – will experience a degree of *nausea*, especially evident after starting lithium and before the establishment of steady state. For the reasons noted, some may continue to experience this for an hour or two after each dose. However, it appears that this almost invariably abates with long-term treatment (>1 year)(Schou et al 1970). Alternatively, patients may complain of a bloated type of *epigastric discomfort*. Pain, on the other hand, is very uncommon. Nausea seems to relate to the biochemical changes effected by lithium in the cells of the gut wall and as such is unlikely to be helped by taking the tablets with or after food.

Occasionally nausea may be associated with frank *vomiting* in the absence of toxicity, though this also usually rapidly settles. It appears that even small amounts of the lithium ion are irritant to the lower bowel and *loose motions* are also a common experience. Watery *diarrhoea* can be found at therapeutic levels but in view of its potentially sinister implications, toxicity is usually a safer first assumption in this situation. Unlike most other adverse effects, lower intestinal symptomatology may be *more* frequently found with 'slow' or 'sustained' release products, as their mode of action, by significantly delaying absorption, delivers more ion to the lower bowel. It is important to take note of vomiting and diarrhoea that are sustained, if only for a few days, even in the presence of therapeutic blood levels, because of the consequences of fluid and sodium loss. Rarely patients may complain of *constipation*, especially with chronic exposure.

Disturbed salivary flow in the form of either an *increase in salivation* or *dryness* in the mouth are also described. The former is the more frequent complaint, something that with objective measurement is evident in over three-quarters of patients, and may be associated with salivary gland enlargement. The latter is however potentially the more troublesome. For a number of years concern was expressed about the high prevalence of dental caries in patients on lithium, which was thought to in some way reflect interference with enamel production. Lithium does not however appear to interfere with aspects of tooth development or maintenance (Curzon 1987) and it is now thought that a decline in dental status is the consequence of a chronically dry mouth. Infrequently patients may complain, sometimes bitterly, of a *metallic taste* in the mouth, no doubt the result of salivary secretion of the ion.

The diuretic properties of lithium were noted by Garrod in the middle of the last century and *polyuria* with compensatory *polydipsia* is commonly noted today, affecting up to 50% of patients in some surveys (Walker & Kincaid-Smith 1987). The problem relates to a failure of concentration and with laboratory evaluation it has been suggested that the majority of patients on lithium will show some increase in urine production on a normal fluid intake. Lithium appears to interfere with

Table 4.7 Adverse and toxic effects of lithium

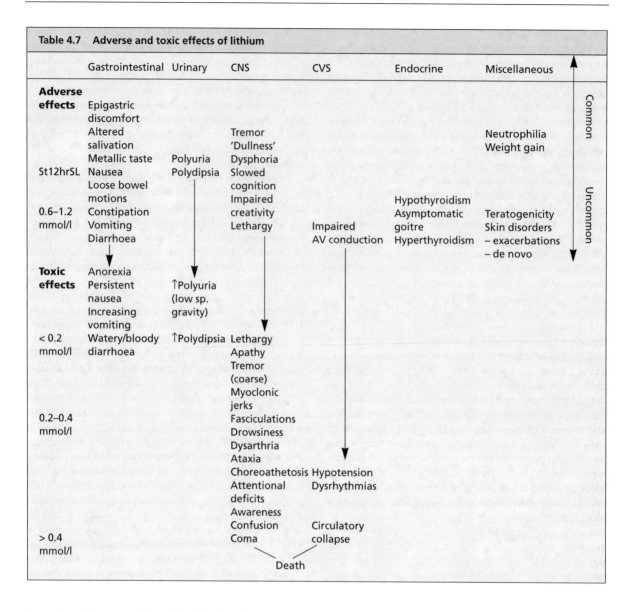

	Gastrointestinal	Urinary	CNS	CVS	Endocrine	Miscellaneous	
Adverse effects St12hrSL 0.6–1.2 mmol/l	Epigastric discomfort Altered salivation Metallic taste Nausea Loose bowel motions Constipation Vomiting Diarrhoea	Polyuria Polydipsia	Tremor 'Dullness' Dysphoria Slowed cognition Impaired creativity Lethargy	Impaired AV conduction	Hypothyroidism Asymptomatic goitre Hyperthyroidism	Neutrophilia Weight gain Teratogenicity Skin disorders – exacerbations – de novo	Common
Toxic effects < 0.2 mmol/l 0.2–0.4 mmol/l > 0.4 mmol/l	Anorexia Persistent nausea Increasing vomiting Watery/bloody diarrhoea	↑Polyuria (low sp. gravity) ↑Polydipsia	Lethargy Apathy Tremor (coarse) Myoclonic jerks Fasciculations Drowsiness Dysarthria Ataxia Choreoathetosis Attentional deficits Awareness Confusion Coma	Hypotension Dysrhythmias Circulatory collapse			Uncommon

Death

the action of vasopressin on the distal nephron, probably by inhibiting the adenylyl cyclase-mediated increase in the conversion of ATP to cyclic AMP. The effect can be a mild increase in urinary volume that is largely asymptomatic or shows mainly as nocturia, through to full and profoundly incapacitating vasopressin-resistant *diabetes insipidus*. The natural assumption would be that this might be helped by spreading the administration of particularly slow release preparations over the day to attain lower peaks. There is however a suggestion that in the long-term, the lower *troughs* associated with single daily administration may be more protective to the kidney and at a clinical level the most effective way of dealing with polyuria may be to utilise single dosing

regimens (Perry & Alexander 1987). An alternative strategy is the addition of the potassium-sparing diuretic, amiloride, which decreases urinary output without reducing lithium clearance. Thiazide diuretics may also achieve a reduction in urine volume but at much greater risk of producing rises in lithium blood levels which can be in the region of 20–25% and so require closer monitoring.

Impairment in urinary concentrating ability was for long thought to be reversible and of little consequence. This complacency was however shattered in 1977 with the publication of the first of a series of reports suggesting a strong correlation between the duration of exposure to lithium and impaired concentrating ability

(Hestbech et al 1977). Of particular concern was the demonstration that the functional deficit correlated with histological abnormalities in the form of a chronic focal *interstitial nephropathy*. Long-term administration of lithium has been confirmed to be associated with structural changes, though the changes originally causing concern may in part be non-specific as similar findings have also been reported in psychiatric patients not treated with lithium (Kincaid-Smith et al 1979). A common factor therefore may be long-term exposure to maintenance medications. However, it now seems clear that a potent predisposing factor to these 'non-specific' structural changes is *acute lithium toxicity*. In this situation, permanent renal damage that is associated with progressive impairment of concentrating ability may ensue. Lithium treatment does appear to be associated with a specific histological change in the form of distal tubular dilatation, following both acute and chronic exposure, though the long-term significance of this remains unclear.

Thus with prolonged and stable exposure to lithium the likelihood of impairment of glomerular filtration rate and the risk of permanent or progressive renal damage is *slight*, though this risk is increased by episodes of *acute toxicity* (Hetmar et al 1991).

A low-amplitude/high-frequency *tremor* of predominantly postural type is a common complaint which may also be exceedingly inconvenient and embarrassing to patients. This is one of the adverse experiences that most clearly relates to the rate and height of the postabsorptive peak and which may be helped by a change in preparation and/or schedule. It appears to be at least in part adrenergically mediated and may respond to a beta blocker. Although tremor may be pronounced at therapeutic levels, moderately severe degrees of disorder or greater should arouse suspicion of toxicity. A further sign is that the quality of the tremor may change to one with coarser characteristics, although a coarsening with increase in amplitude may be simply a feature of ageing.

Lithium can affect *cardiac conduction*, though this is only very rarely a matter of clinical concern (Martin et al 1987). The most common ECG finding is a notched, flattened and occasionally inverted T wave which is not significant. However, conduction deficits at both the level of the sinoatrial and atrioventricular nodes have been reported. The former may result in sick sinus syndrome or sinus node arrhythmias which may be asymptomatic or present with faintness or paroxysmal tachycardia, while the AV block associated with the latter is usually asymptomatic. Premature ventricular beats may occur from slowing of conduction in the Bundle of His. Those with pre-existing cardiac disease, especially conduction disorders, are at greater risk

and require closer monitoring but in general such changes are reversible on stopping the drug.

Long-term ingestion of lithium can, as with so many psychotropic drugs, be associated with substantial *weight gain*. Reported prevalence rates vary widely from 20 to 75% and the increases can in some cases be striking. This clearly can have major medical as well as cosmetic implications and is a further source of non-compliance, especially in females. The mechanism is unknown.

Lithium interferes with a number of hormone functions, the most prominent of which surround the thyroid gland. Within a few months on treatment slight falls in thyroxine (T_4) with compensatory rises in thyroid-stimulating hormone (TSH) are common. These do not usually take values outwith the reference range for normal and they usually stabilise within 12 months, though TSH may remain on the high side. Early in treatment, patients may develop signs of *hyperthyroidism*, though this is very uncommon. Of much greater frequency is the gradual development of *hypothyroidism*. Antithyroid antibodies are present in just under 10% of the general population but are more prevalent in females. Their presence rises sharply after the middle of the fifth decade. Of those who demonstrate both autoantibodies and an elevated TSH, approximately 5% per year will develop hypothyroidism, with females about three times more represented than males (Myers & West 1987). Thus it is likely that lithium is acting to promote disorder in predisposed individuals. The mechanism remains unclear but it is likely that there is no single pathway to lithium-induced hypothyroidism. One possibility is that in some patients with a predisposition to autoimmune thyroiditis it may alter directly the rate of antibody formation. It may therefore be possible to identify the group most at risk as comprising females over 45 with circulating antithyroid antibodies and a sustained elevation of TSH. The risk of hypothyroidism necessitates regular (e.g. annual) monitoring of thyroid function which should be extended to examination of the gland itself.

Lithium-induced *goitre* is rare and may not herald hypofuncton but it is better the physician discover it than the patient. Again the mechanism is unknown but appears to reflect an impairment of iodine uptake and/or incorporation into thyroid hormone. The development of asymptomatic goitre or biochemical, or even clinical, hypothyroidism are not contraindications to continued use of lithium as the thyroid disorder can be readily managed by supplements in the usual way.

Lithium can alter a number of other endocrine functions, though not in ways that are clinically relevant. In a small number of patients it can be associated with a rise in serum parathyroid hormone with associated hypercalcaemia but the number of such cases is so low that these may merely reflect patients with some predisposing disorder of parathyroid function. Despite possessing some insulin-like properties, lithium probably does not alter glucose metabolism to any clinically significant degree, even in those with diabetes mellitus.

A series of skin disorders can develop in the course of lithium treatment, though the reported total prevalence of around 1% (Lambert and Dalac 1987) would seem to represent a considerable underestimate. The most common is *acne vulgaris* which may present as a worsening of pre-existing disorder in the usual distribution or as a recrudescence of symptomatology long in abeyance. It may however also develop without prior abnormality, when the distribution may be eccentric involving thighs or upper arms. It tends not to come in cycles as does idiopathic acne and may cause profound embarrassment which can lead to patients discontinuing treatment. It may improve slightly with dose reduction but this in itself is unlikely to be sufficient. Treatment should be conservative in view of a possible interaction between lithium and tetracyclines.

Of more serious import is *psoriasis* which also may represent an exacerbation of prior disorder or, less commonly, the first manifestation of disorder. All types of psoriasis have been described and the condition may be associated with characteristic nail changes. This does not usually respond well to conventional treatment, and once again may be a reason for cessation of treatment. Other skin disorders include seborrhoeic dermatitis, follicular keratosis and pruritic maculopapular erythematous eruptions. As with other psychotropic drugs, lithium treatment may be associated with *hair loss*, and frank alopecia may be a more frequent – though still rare – event than with previously discussed compounds.

While some patients with a relevant dermatological history may show increasing signs over the first 12 months of exposure, not all those with such histories experience exacerbations, so development of these problems is unpredictable. The pathophysiological mechanisms are unknown.

Increases in white blood counts of up to 40%, reflecting mainly a *neutrophilia*, are common in the first week of lithium exposure. A similar stimulatory effect may apply to platelets. Lithium has been suggested as a treatment of various marrow deficiency disorders but this action becomes less evident with prolonged use. It may be most apparent with lower doses. From a psychiatric perspective this finding is an interesting curio, only worthy of note in order to prevent the enthusiastic going off down investigative blind alleys.

Controlled studies in normal volunteers have suggested that lithium in these groups produces a slight but detectable *impairment of cognition* and *subjective affective symptoms* of mental slowness, lethargy and dysphoria, sometimes with accompanying restlessness (Judd et al 1977a,b). Some of this may be related to the increasingly appreciated tendency of lithium to promote or exacerbate mild pre-existing extrapyramidal dysfunction and hence may represent the subjective manifestations of a subclinical parkinsonian-type disorder. In line with this is the descriptive language used by some patients to describe these types of features, such as feeling like 'a zombie'. Particular problems may be encountered by those whose occupation requires the display of creativity.

Lithium does accumulate in bone but earlier concerns about the possibility of prolonged treatment exacerbating osteoporosis seem unfounded. Caution should still be exercised with its long-term use in children and adolescents in whom bone is still developing. There are rare reports of lithium worsening the symptoms of *myasthenia gravis*.

Although not strictly a side-effect, there has been concern in recent years about the risk of *rebound mania* occurring with greater than expected frequency following abrupt discontinuation of lithium treatment (Faedda et al 1993). While this may relate to a possible 'withdrawal'-type phenomenon, it may equally speak of the drug doing what is expected of it in holding off manic episodes which would have developed earlier in its absence. Certainly lithium, in line with all other psychotropics, should be discontinued gradually and never stopped suddenly.

There has been much discussion over the years about the *teratogenicity* of lithium and, although the potential exists, the magnitude of the risk remains unclear. Lithium seems particularly prone to disrupt early morphogenesis and especially development of the cardiovascular system. It therefore exerts its most serious effects during the first trimester. It was originally suggested that 11% of pregnancies exposed to lithium may result in a congenital malformation, almost three-quarters of which involve the cardiovascular system. In particular a 2–3% risk appeared to attach itself to the particularly serious Ebstein's anomaly (Weinstein 1980).

These data on the teratogenicity of lithium come from cases reported to the international lithium baby register maintained for a number of years in the 1970s. The problems with this sort of methodology are legion and relate particularly to the preferential registration of abnormalities while pregnancies resulting in a normal infant are less likely to be reported.

There is no doubt that lithium is a potentially teratogenic compound, though the risks resulting from maternal ingestion are less than were at one time thought. Although the overall risk of congenital malformations does not appear to be greatly increased, the risk of first trimester fetal exposure resulting in major cardiac malformations is increased, but no accurate figure can be placed on this at present. None the less, patients need to be informed about this potential risk and strongly advised to avoid unplanned conception. Should the patient wish to become pregnant, lithium should be discontinued in the preconceptive period and for at least the first trimester. There is no specific information to guide the clinician thereafter but common sense would suggest the merits of, wherever possible, maintaining the immature central nervous system free from exposure to such a pervasively active compound.

Toxicity

The upper therapeutic limit for the standard 12 hour lithium level in most laboratories is 1.2 mmol/l. With modern methods of estimation the test is readily standardised and the margin of error slight. Hence this is now a fairly widely agreed figure. Accepting this as the upper limit does not of course mean that a value of 1.21 equals toxicity. There is no clear point of transition and in fact some patients may get substantially above this level before developing clinical features. None the less, patients showing an upward trend or a single reading above this level which represents an uncharacteristically high value and who develop a change in their pattern of tolerability should be suspected of moving to toxicity. Most patients will show an altered tolerance by the time their blood levels are in the range of 1.4–1.5 mmol/l. With levels over 2 mmol/l the patient will be obviously unwell with clear signs of toxicity.

Most cases of lithium toxicity occur in the context of long-term administration and hence represent a relatively *insidious* departure from a stable situation. While symptomatology can emerge swiftly, their antecedents can usually be traced back over 24–48 hours.

Gastrointestinal features comprising anorexia and persistent or obtrusive nausea culminating in vomiting are usually the first signs of impending trouble (Table 4.7). At the same time patients may experience a dry mouth and insatiable thirst associated with production of voluminous amounts of dilute (i.e. low specific gravity) urine which may contain glucose. Diarrhoea may then develop, which may be bloody. With this combination of disturbances, dehydration can rapidly ensue. Tremor accentuates with a coarse, jerky quality emerging, which may extend to all body parts. Patients feel increasingly weak. In addition, as levels rise, an appearance of restlessness is contributed to by muscle fasciculations and myoclonic-like jerks or typical choreoathetoid movements associated with generalised hypertonicity. With progression, a general breakdown in neuromuscular coordination may ensue, evidenced in dysarthria

and ataxia. Disruption of higher mental functions is a sign of serious toxicity, with victims becoming increasingly lethargic and drowsy with lack of interest and awareness, attention deficits and frank confusion/delirium. Incipient circulatory failure is signalled by hypotension and irregularities of cardiac rhythm. Fits are likely to emerge at this stage which leads on to stupor and eventual preterminal coma.

It is important to bear in mind that because of delayed brain penetration and egression of lithium, clinical signs of CNS toxicity may not occur in unison with escalating blood levels and may persist when levels are declining and even after they are back to the therapeutic range.

It is essential to educate patients on the often simple measures that can be effective in avoiding lithium toxicity, such as maintaining hydration and salt intake, and in being sensitive to any *change* in tolerability. In particular, the onset of gastrointestinal symptoms should always be emphasised as an important 'warning' where patients themselves can effectively intervene by simply stopping lithium for 1, or at most 2, days. Based on the half-life of lithium, blood levels can be expected to drop by about 50% in 24 hours, assuming maintenance of normal renal function, and discontinuation is an effective as well as necessary strategy in the management of toxicity of whatever degree.

Where clinical symptomatology is in keeping with established toxicity a so-called 'forced' diuresis is recommended (Thomsen & Schou 1975). This amounts to 1–2 litres of isotonic saline intravenously over a 6 hour period. The aim is volume repletion and a consequent increase in glomerular filtration and hence lithium clearance. In patients with hyponatraemia the use of saline is furthermore beneficial, by decreasing proximal reabsorption of lithium. Even with clinical improvement over the initial treatment cycle, intravenous fluids should be maintained to obviate the effects of delayed absorption, especially with slow release preparations. A recommended aim is infusion at a rate sufficient to produce a 20% decline in lithium levels every 6 hours (Gomolin 1987). It must be borne in mind that a large urinary output in response to fluid replacement may reflect renal damage in the form of impaired concentrating ability and so electrolyte balance must be closely monitored. Some authors have recommended that the best results from diuresis are achieved when the urine is alkalinised ('forced alkaline diuresis') but the increased hazard is not necessarily offset by an increased response and a number of authorities now no longer recommend this.

Where toxicity is mild to moderately severe and unaccompanied by significant renal failure, such steps may be sufficient. However, with serum levels over

4 mmol/l or renal incompetence due either to pre-existing chronic failure or acute tubular necrosis related to the immediate problem, then such methods are unlikely to be adequate or fast enough. In this situation dialysis is the recommended management. This can take the form of peritoneal dialysis but haemodialysis is the more efficient.

Lithium tends to be a drug patients treat with respect but, like all other drugs, it can be a medium for overdose resulting in *acute* toxicity. In this situation gastric lavage and induced emesis are widely utilised, especially when slow release preparations have been ingested. One point in advocacy of these formulations has been that because of their slow release characteristics such interventions are more likely to be worthwhile than with standard formulations. This is unlikely to be rational. As we have seen, little lithium is absorbed from the stomach and the mechanism of slow release is to delay absorption from the *small* bowel. The only advantage of gastric lavage beyond 2–3 hours of any overdose is to remove excess lithium *secreted* in gastric fluid. The amounts that can be removed by this means are relatively small and there is the very real risk of adding to any evolving electrolyte disturbance. Efforts at this stage are more profitably concentrated on measures to accelerate excretion, outlined above.

Other mood stabilising agents

Anticonvulsants

The recognition that certain anticonvulsant drugs exerted effects on mood symptoms was noted in the 1960s when patients receiving carbamazepine for epilepsy reported themselves to feel less anxious. The first report of their use in major affective disorders was by Takezaki and Hanoaka in 1971, though it was the report of Ballenger and Post nine years later that stimulated widespread interest. To date, most work has concerned the long available carbamazepine and sodium valproate but with the introduction of a new generation of anticonvulsants, such as lamotrigine and gabapentin, interest is widening. Anticonvulsants now occupy an important place in the treatment of major affective disorders, something that is set to increase.

Carbamazepine is a tricyclic compound closely related structurally to imipramine (Figure 4.7) It was synthesised in 1953 on the crest of the psychopharmacological excitement that followed the introduction of chlorpromazine. It was hoped that the new compound would emulate the actions of chlorpromazine but it did not. It was clear however that it possessed unique features of its own and in the 1960s it was introduced as a highly effective anticonvulsant.

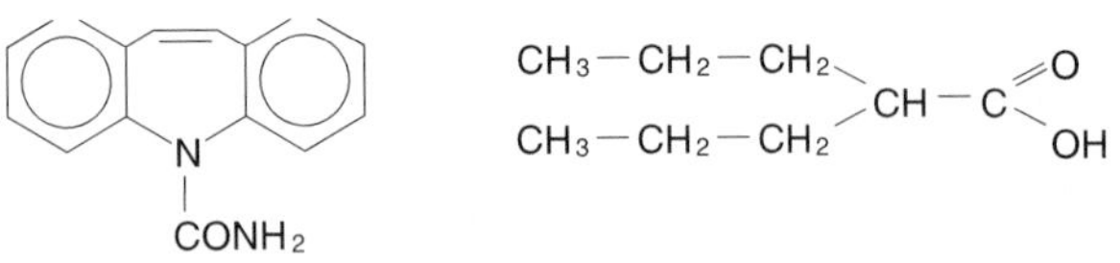

Fig. 4.7   Mood stabiliser structures.

Carbamazepine is rather slowly and erratically absorbed, with peak levels attained in 4–6 hours, though with Retard formulations T_{max} may be up to 24 hours. Bioavailability is in the range of 80–90%. There are substantial first-pass effects. Its apparent volume of distribution is in the moderate range. At around 75%, it is relatively less protein bound than most psychotropics. Its half-life is dependent not only on its complex metabolism but also on the fact that for the first 2–3 months of chronic treatment it induces its own metabolism to a substantial degree. Thus with single doses, half-life values are in the region of 25–45 hours, whereas with chronic administration these fall dramatically to 7–24 hours. After 1 month, the initial steady-state levels may have fallen by as much as 25% (Brodie 1987).

The major metabolic pathway in the liver is epoxidation by the enzyme arene oxidase to form carbamazepine-10, 11-epoxide, which has a shorter half-life than the parent but is a pharmacologically active and toxic intermediate. This is in its turn metabolised by epoxide hydroxylase to the inactive *trans*-carbamazepine-diol (or carbamazepine-10, 11 dihydrodihydroxide) which is excreted in the urine. Between 15 and 20% of a carbamazepine dose is metabolised by direct conjugation with glucuronic acid. Epoxide hydroxylase is inhibited by a number of drugs, notably valproate, coadministration of which can result in a dramatic increase in the ratio of carbamazepine to its epoxide metabolite (from 10:1 to 2:1). As a consequence, patients can experience signs of toxicity while still showing blood levels within the therapeutic range (Wilder 1992). Carbamazepine furthermore increases hormone clearance and can therefore negate the actions of the contraceptive pill, especially low oestrogen formulations.

Sodium valproate is the soluble sodium salt of valproic acid, a poorly soluble branched chain carboxylic acid (Figure 4.7). Absorption is rapid with unmodified formulations, peak levels being attained in 30–60 minutes. The drug is however a powerful gastric irritant and a number of slow release formulations such as enteric coated tablets are widely used which have T_{max} values in the region of 4–6 hours. Protein binding is up to 95% but is inversely dependent on the fat content of the diet. Binding of valproate is saturable within the therapeutic range, thus rapid increases in dose can be associated with disproportionately large increases in free drug levels which rapidly undergo metabolism with consequently lower than expected blood levels. Valproate displaces carbamazepine from protein-binding sites and its introduction can result in transient toxicity of the latter. Half-life varies with preparation but is in the range of 5–20 hours (Wilder 1992).

The metabolism of valproate is complex. One pathway is via the microsomal cytochrome P450 system which produces two potentially toxic metabolites, 4-en- and 2,4-en-valproate. The more significant pathway – at least when the drug is administered alone – is via mitochondrial β oxidation, the pathway extensively utilised in the degradation of fatty acids in general. This produces 3-hydroxy- and 3-oxo- derivatives and 2-en-valproate which has anticonvulsant properties and a long half-life. Therapeutic environments that stimulate P450 metabolism, such as coadministration of inducers like carbamazepine or phenobarbitone, can lead to excessive build up of toxic metabolites, which may be the mechanism underlying the infrequently reported but potentially fatal hepatic necrosis. Another rare but potentially serious scenario to be wary of is in those with inherited or acquired metabolic diseases who may be deficient in carnitine, an important constituent of fatty acid metabolism (Coulter 1991). Valproate decreases carnitine levels and in this situation may precipitate encephalopathy.

Both these drugs can produce significant adverse effects. Both can cause gastrointestinal upset and are sedative and can be associated with drowsiness. Carbamazepine can, like all tricyclic drugs, slow intracardiac conduction and produce arrhythmias. Hypocalcaemia can occur and inappropriate ADH secretion may be associated with hyponatraemia and oedema. Idiosyncratic reactions include marrow suppression, hepatotoxicity, (morbiliform) skin rashes, photosensitivity and rarely Stevens–Johnson syndrome and a lupus-type syndrome.

Valproate can cause tremors, skin rashes and hair loss and may also be associated with oedema. Of greater importance are rare cases of acute pancreatitis, hepatotoxicity and hyperammonaemia, possibly progressing to coma, which may be related to the kinetic factors noted above. This drug can also affect ovarian function, and recently concern has been expressed about its chronic use and the possible development of polycystic ovaries and hyperandrogenism (Isojarvi et al, 1993, 1996). Although apparently reversible, this is an important potential association in the context of the drug's increasing use as a mood stabiliser and, if confirmed, may severely restrict its future long-term use in women of childbearing age.

Both carbamazepine and valproate are potentially teratogenic, with the latter probably the more so (Wilder 1992). They should both be avoided in pregnancy if possible.

In recent years a new generation of largely 'add on' anticonvulsants has become available, with novel modes of action. Their use as mood stabilisers remains anecdotal but this is likely to be an area of increasing research interest in the next few years. *Lamotrigine* appears to inhibit the release of glutamate and possibly other excitatory amino acids from presynaptic terminals, while the evidence is that *gabapentin* attaches to high-affinity binding sites that, despite the drug's structural similarity to GABA, do not appear to be GABA recognition sites nor benzodiazepine receptors.

Calcium channel antagonists

In 1981, Dubovsky and colleagues reported antimanic properties in a patient treated with the *calcium channel antagonist*, verapamil. Since then a number of reports have appeared suggesting that this group of compounds may have clinical utility in bipolar affective disorders, though most of the evidence to date is anecdotal or based on small or open studies (Dubovsky 1993). Much of the early interest remained with verapamil whose value may be limited to patients with relatively mild disorder and/or patients who, for whatever reason, are unable to taken lithium. More recent evidence has suggested that drugs of the dihydropyridine type, such as nifedipine and nimodipine, may be particularly useful in rapid cycling bipolar disorders.

The calcium channel antagonists reduce calcium influx through potential-dependent calcium channels during cell stimulation. The actions of lithium on intracellular transduction pathways include desensitisation of the receptor-stimulated phosphatidylinositol cycle that mobilises calcium, and inhibition of calmodulin, the calcium activation protein. Furthermore, both carbamazepine and at least some antipsychotics also antagonise calcium cellular influx. There is therefore good reason to explore the therapeutic application of these compounds, though the justification for their use at present remains largely empirical.

Therapeutics

Indications

The indications for lithium are more tightly circumscribed than those for other psychotropic agents. They are:

• the treatment of manic/hypomanic episodes

- the prophylaxis of bipolar affective disorders
- the prophylaxis of recurrent unipolar depressions
- as an adjunctive agent in the treatment of major depressive disorders not responsive to antidepressants alone.

The place of anticonvulsants remains under review. Despite the benefits of the standard drugs, carbamazepine and valproate, anticonvulsants still tend to be reserved for second or third line, or combined use in treatment resistant situations, especially the prophylaxis of bipolar affective disorders. Their place in the adjunctive treatment of resistant depressions and the prophylaxis of recurrent unipolar depressions has not as yet been established.

Calcium channel antagonists have not been sufficiently investigated for their relative place to be established with clarity (despite their widespread use, and empirical efficacy, the same might incidentally also be said of antipsychotics!). They should therefore be reserved at present for treatment of refractory bipolar disorders, especially of rapid cycling or ultradian (ultra-ultra rapid) cycling type.

Strategies

The role of lithium in the treament of major affective disorders has been the subject of considerable revision in recent years. Long-term follow-up studies have suggested a less favourable impact on outcome than was at one time thought and although this is still the first-line approach, in especially the prophylaxis of recurrent bipolar illnesses, some have even challenged its use in this situation (Moncrieff 1997). None the less, having decided on its use, there are two major principles that must be adhered to:

- *Principle 1*   Because of its narrow therapeutic margin, it is important when starting lithium to establish a series of baseline parameters. These include routine haematological and biochemical screens, with particular attention to electrolytes, though baseline thyroid function is probably optional at this stage except in high-risk patients. Routine ECG is also most pertinent to older age groups or those with pre-existing heart disease. It is, furthermore, important to be aware of the patient's renal status, or, more accurately, whether any significant pretreatment renal incompetence is present. Strictly speaking this should be assessed by undertaking a *lithium* clearance but in practice a routine creatinine clearance is the usual method. It is questionable however whether in the presence of a normal serum creatinine a full creatinine clearance actually provides meaningful additional information.

Pregnancy should always be excluded in women of childbearing age.

- *Principle 2*   Treatment plans must be geared around the maintenance of blood levels within a defined range. This is done via the standardised 12 hour serum lithium (12H-stSLi) (Amdisen 1977). The assessment was originally validated with patients on multiple dosing regimens but is in fact equally applicable to once daily, nocte regimens. The major requirement, apart from the obvious one that the patient is reliably compliant, is that they must be in steady state. A plain blood sample is removed 12 hours after the last (nocte) dose and, if the patient is on multiple dosing regimens, *before* the first dose of the morning. Therapeutic levels are now fairly standardised internationally within the range 0.6–1.2 mmol/l, although in the context of maintenance, levels in the range of 0.45–0.5 mmol/l may be adequate (Jerram & McDonald 1978).

There are two subsidiary principles worth bearing in mind:

- *Principle 3*   Adverse effects may be obviated by flexibility, both in the use of preparations and dosing schedules, with the aim of trying to reduce the rate and height of the postabsorptive peak.
- *Principle 4*   Patients must be educated on an ongoing basis about the need to avoid dehydration and to maintain where possible relatively stable salt intakes.

There is no hard and last rule about how frequently serum lithium levels should be assessed but in patients who are stable and compliant three or four times per year is probably adequate. Thyroid function should be evaluated annually as routine, or 6 monthly in those at higher risk, such as middle aged/elderly females with circulating autoantibodies. The advantages of routine monitoring of renal function are unclear, though this remains a conventional recommendation. It would certainly be indicated in the wake of an episode of frank toxicity. Following the decision to discontinue, lithium doses should be tapered downwards gradually over several weeks.

There are no such clear principles that apply to the use of other mood stabilisers and although blood monitoring is often undertaken with carbamazepine, its only value is in pointing to high levels which will increase the likelihood of toxicity. The most sensitive pointers to this are however probably clinical. There is as yet no clearly established therapeutic range for affective disorders that is comparable to that for lithium. There would seem to be little value in routine monitoring of valproate levels.

BENZODIAZEPINES AND OTHER SEDATIVE/HYPNOTICS

Benzodiazepines

There is, even today, no single antianxiety compound but the search for medicaments which relieve anxiety and promote sleep is ancient and continuing. In the last century, alcohol and marijuana, opium and laudanum (tincture of opium) served this purpose. Later, specific compounds structurally and pharmacologically similar to alcohol, such as chloral hydrate and paraldehyde, were introduced and bromide salts found vogue well into the 20th century.

The first drugs to be termed 'sedatives' were the barbiturates which became available with the synthesis of diethylbarbituric acid in 1903. A large number of barbiturates were synthesised and widely used until the 1960s but this group of drugs is blighted by a high dependency-producing potential and very narrow therapeutic index, problems which also afflict their various analogues such as guanethidine and methaqualone, which temporarily found medical application in the 1960s and 1970s. Barbiturates are now obsolete except in a very few cases of epilepsy, though even here their use is minimal. They and their kin have however held on with remarkable tenacity as the 'downers' of illicitly supplied, recreational usage.

The first so-called 'tranquilliser' was meprobamate, a propanediol derivative synthesised in 1951. By the mid-1950s it was the most prescribed drug in America. However, although somewhat safer than barbiturates, it was still a drug with a relatively narrow therapeutic index and could also produce dependency. The world of instant composure was ready for something new.

No class of psychotropic agent illustrates better the triumphs and failures of psychopharmacology than the benzodiazepines. By the end of the first decade of their use they were the most prescribed group of drugs in the developed world; by the end of the second they were amongst the most vilified, an emblem of the public's perception that psychopharmacology was all about 'sorting' the ills of modern living with a pill. Neither of these two positions was – or is – justified. Benzodiazepines were undoubtedly excessively prescribed for problems that would have been better dealt with in other ways. But neither is psychopharmalogy society's policeman. This class of drugs is highly effective as part of the management of specific *medical* conditions and, with the same levels of *supervision* demanded of any drug treatments, they remain valuable therapeutic agents.

The 1,4-benzodiazepine structure was discovered by the chemist Leo Sternbach who, in the mid-1950s, was searching for behavioural properties among a group of compounds thought to be benzheptoxdiazines, which he had investigated previously for their potential as dyes. In fact the compounds being investigated turned out not to be benzheptoxdiazines but a new analogue of quinazoline, a compound known since the 1890s. These investigations were not getting anywhere and Sternbach was in fact in the throes of what he later referred to as a 'house cleaning' operation when in 1957 he submitted, without enthusiasm, one such compound for pharmacological screening (Sternbach 1983). This compound was later shown to have a different structure from the one that had been expected when it was created, and hence its production can indeed be seen as pure serendipity. However, the pharmacologist Lowell Randell noted that in animals this derivative possessed a similar psychopharmacological profile to meprobamate. Confirmation of this in humans led in 1960 to the launch of the first commercial product, chlordiazepoxide, which was to become the vanguard of a veritable pharmaceutical avalanche.

These were also the first drugs in which the influence of marketing strategies could be seen. Benzodiazepines have four main actions relating to antianxiety, hypnotic, anticonvulsant and muscle relaxant effects. There is however no evidence to support the view that different compounds have differential clinical profiles in these areas (Baldessarini 1985). Benzodiazepines differ in some pharmacological parameters – most notably potency – but not in terms of their differential effects. Yet even today professional wisdom has it that different drugs in the class should be prescribed for different clinical indications.

Structures

The basic components of the majority of compounds in this class comprise a benzene (or A) ring chlorinated at the R7 position, joined to a seven-membered diazepine ring (or B ring), the two nitrogens of which are sited at the R1 and R4 positions (hence 1,4-benzodiazepines) and to which is attached a phenyl (or C) ring at position 5 (Figure 4.8). The major variations in chemical substituents that characterise different drugs largely involve the B ring.

In recent years this basic structure has been modified somewhat. The simplest modification is the transposition of one of the nitrogens from the R4 to the R5 position. The major representative of the 1,5-benzodiazepines is clobazam. Clonazepam is a 7-nitrobenzodiazepine. Other modifications produce compounds that, although originally described as 'non-benzodiapines', are in fact more appropriately considered as benzodiazepine variants. These include the triazolobenzodiazepines, as exemplified by alprazolam

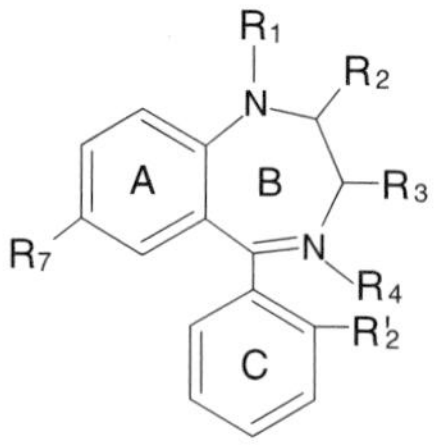

1,4-Benzodiazepines

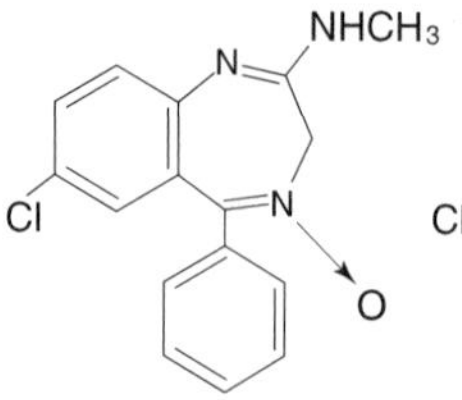

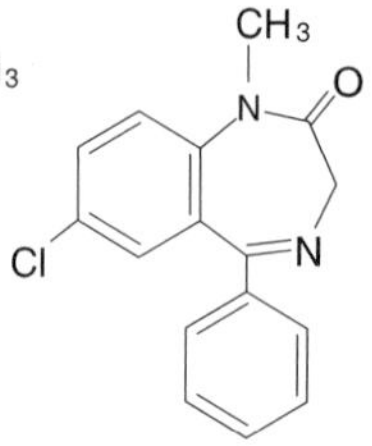

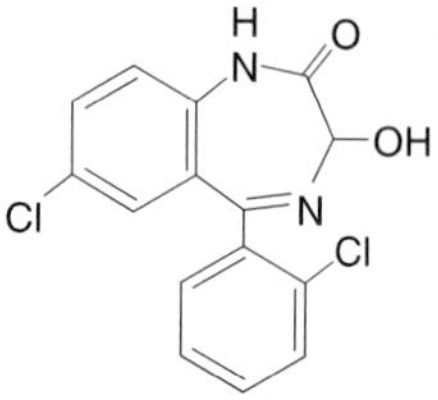

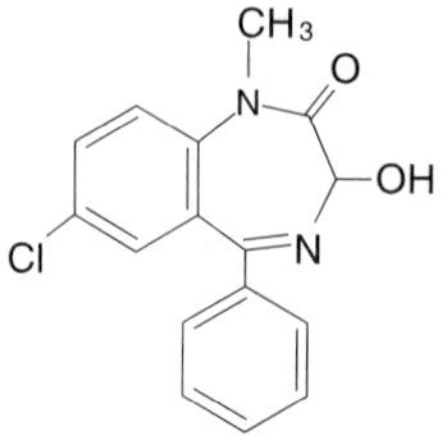

Chlordiazepoxide Diazepam Lorazepam Temazepam

7-Nitrobenzodiazepine

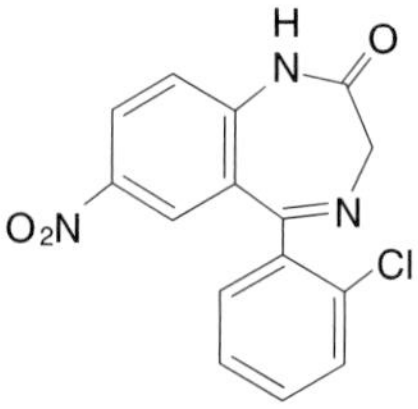

Clonazepam

1,5-Benzodiazepine

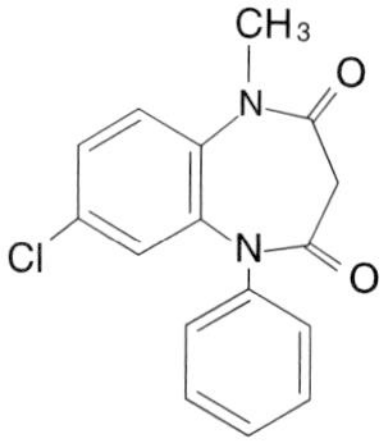

Clobazam

Triazolobenzodiazepine

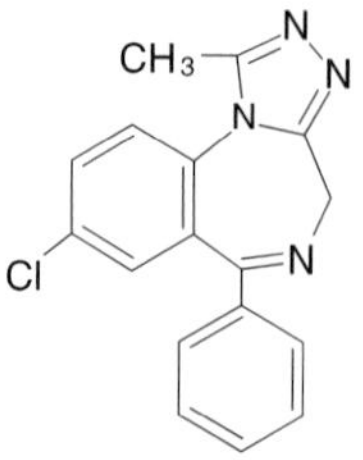

Alprazolam

Fig. 4.8 Structures of the benzodiazepines.

and triazolam (now withdrawn in the UK) and the thienodiazepines such as brotizolam, in which the benzene ring is replaced by a thiophene ring.

Pharmacokinetics

As was noted with the SSRIs, the benzodiazepines differ most from one another in their pharmacokinetic properties, which are in general not only varied but complex. Many of these variations relate to the differing physicochemical properties imparted by structural differences.

All benzodiazepines are weak organic bases which, when subjected to physiological buffering, become lipid soluble to varying degrees ranging from moderate to high. This variability in lipid solubility is one of the major factors contributing to pharmacokinetic – and most importantly, clinical – distinctions between compounds. Of the drugs encountered in psychiatric practice, flurazepam is approximately 10% more lipid soluble than diazepam, whereas temazepam and lorazepam are only about 50% as lipid soluble. Midazolam, used in anaesthetics, is the most lipid soluble of all (50% more so than diazepam) (Greenblatt & Shader 1987).

Absorption from the gastrointestinal tract is complete and followed by extensive first-pass metabolism for most compounds. For reasons that are not altogether clear, absorption is as a rule unpredictable from injection sites, especially in patients on continuous dosing regimens. The exception may be lorazepam, which appears to be rapidly absorbed from intramuscular sites (Richens 1983). The rate of absorption, which is the rate-limiting step in the onset of action, varies but is overall rapid. Diazepam and flurazepam are amongst the most rapidly absorbed, while temazepam, despite its licensed indication, is amongst the slowest (Greenblatt & Shader 1987). In general, absorption can be slowed but not decreased by food, which delays gastric emptying and time to reach the proximal bowel. For some compounds absorption may not only be delayed but also impaired by aluminium-based antacids. Peak levels are usually achieved in 30–90 minutes with the rapidly

absorbed compounds and 2–4 hours for the slower ones. Rectal administration, in the UK mainly confined to children with epilepsy (though 'popular' in France), is a highly efficient administration route, especially if liquid formulations are used. Peak levels in this situation can be achieved within 15 minutes (Richens 1983).

All the group are as a whole highly protein bound, mainly to albumin, with levels of up to 98% for diazepam and 94–97% for chlordiazepoxide. Lorazepam and nitrazepam are less protein bound at 85–90% and alprazolam is the least with a free fraction in the range of 30% (Moschitto & Greenblatt 1983).

Benzodiazepines are widely distributed, to an extent that is dependent on each drug's lipophilicity. Thus compounds such as diazepam which are highly lipophilic have large apparent volumes of distribution (V_d) and are widely and rapidly distributed, while drugs such as lorazepam have lower V_d values and are more slowly and less extensively distributed. The kinetics therefore technically conform to a two-compartment model with the plasma concentration curve reflecting distribution as well as metabolism. Distribution characteristics have considerable clinical importance, especially with single parenteral dosing. Half-lives also vary greatly across compounds and individuals and are susceptible to the range of variables that influence both the delivery of drug to hepatocytes and to the functional integrity of these, a point of particular note in predicting the susceptibility of neonates to these drugs. Flurazepam has a half-life that, at approximately 1–2 hours, is as short as any psychotropic agent, while that for clonazepam, at 50–70 hours, is as long as any. Figures for chlordiazepoxide in the range of 6–30 hours are shorter than those for diazepam, which are in the region of 20 hours in most healthy adults but may extend as high as 70 hours in some individuals.

Metabolism is hepatic, virtually total and for most compounds, complex, though often incestuously interrelated (Figure 4.9). For a few, such as lorazepam and temazepam, which share in common shorter half-lives, metabolism comprises simply conjugation with glucuronic acid which produces the water solubility neces-

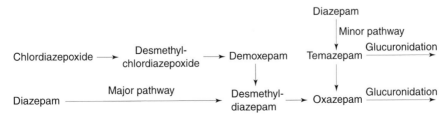

Fig. 4.9 Interconnected biotransformation pathways for some commonly prescribed benzodiazepines.

sary for renal excretion (Richens 1983). These drugs therefore produce no active metabolites. For compounds undergoing more extensive metabolism the fastest and hence first step involves dealkylation of alkyl substituents of the B ring, a process that strongly determines the half-life. Thus drugs in which the alkyl group is large or sited far from the ring itself undergo rapid dealklyation and have short half-lives (e.g. flurazepam), whereas those with small alkyl substituents positioned close to the ring, such as chlordiazepoxide, undergo slow dealkylation and have longer half-lives (Kaplan & Jack 1983). For those with methyl substituents at the N1 position demethylation takes place; this is a relatively slow process. Perhaps the most important aspect of metabolism is hydroxylation at the R3 site which, for a number of drugs, produces desmethyldiazepam, a fully active metabolite which undergoes slow oxidation before excretion and thus has a very long half-life (30–100 hours).

A knowledge of the pharmacokinetics of benzodiazepines illustrates the powerful impact that a drug's physicochemical properties and its intermediate metabolites have on clinical expectations and explains some apparent paradoxes. We have seen, for example, the ultrashort half-life of flurazepam, yet a knowledge of the fact its major metabolite, desalkylflurazepam, is active and has a half-life of 50–100 hours allows one to predict the sometimes potent hangover and even toxicity effects that can be seen with this drug, especially in the elderly. Indeed, cumulative effects are to be anticipated with those drugs, such as diazepam, which have desmethyldiazepam as a metabolite, and advice on driving and contact with machinery is particularly important when recommending these.

The conflicting impact of distribution and half-life is particularly evident with single intravenous use, a practice to which benzodiazepines lend themselves and that is widespread. Going by half-life values, it would be reasonable to expect that in the management of an acute situation intravenous diazepam would have a longer action than lorazepam, a drug with a much shorter half-life. This is not in fact the case, as diazepam is rapidly distributed, resulting in a swift decline in plasma levels to as low as one-fifth peak, and consequent loss of acute action. The less widely distributed lorazepam will maintain a longer action in this situation, despite its significantly shorter half-life (Greenblatt & Shader, 1987).

Pharmacodynamics

Mode of action In 1977, a frisson of excitement spread through the neuroscience community with the almost simultaneous discovery, by Braestrup and Squires in Denmark and Mohler and Okada in Switzerland, of specific benzodiazepine receptor sites in the mammalian brain that bound labelled diazepam with high affinity. Since then these sites have been characterised in some detail and are now known to represent part of a GABA receptor–chloride ionophore complex.

Receptors for the major inhibitory amino acid neurotransmitter, GABA, come in two forms. These were delineated by Hill and Bowery in 1981 by the fact that one group was sensitive to the drug bicuculline (GABA$_A$) while the other was bicuculline insensitive (GABA$_B$). These receptors have different distributions in the CNS and different patterns of agonist/antagonist interactions. Baclofen is the major agonist at GABA$_B$ sites which may be predominantly presynaptic in location and are coupled to their signal transduction mechanisms by G proteins. However benzodiazepines do not interact with GABA$_B$ receptors.

The GABA$_A$ complex comprises a ring-shaped collection of transmembrane proteins which include representatives of at least 16 subunit proteins arranged in five groups (Figure 4.10). These are given the Greek designations α, β, γ, σ and ρ. The α subunits are the sites at which benzodiazepines act as agonists, while the β subunits are the GABA sites. The α and β subunits interact insofar as each stimulates binding to the other, a relationship in which the γ subunits appear to be crucial. It appears that coassembly of an α, a β and a γ subunit is the minimum requirement for the production of a high affinity benzodiazepine-binding site, a motif sometimes referred to as the ω (i.e. benzodiazepine)-1 receptor.

These receptor components can be seen as the gatekeepers to the functional element of the complex which comprises a gated ion channel for chloride. Despite the close functional relationship between subunits, it is solely the GABA-related subunits which control the channel. Stimulation of these results in opening of the ion channel and an influx of calcium into the cell, inducing a state of hyperpolarisation and hence a decreased firing rate of critical neurones. Benzodiazepines facilitate GABA inhibitory effects in the CNS by increasing the number of channels opened rather than by prolonging the duration of opening of a few. The mechanism whereby GABA stimulation opens the chloride channels is thought to involve an element of physical distortion of the complex, which is a relatively new phenomenon referred to as *allosteric modulation*.

The elucidation of these intricate structural and functional relationships is one of the most impressive undertakings in modern psychopharmacology but it leaves unanswered two critical questions. How does

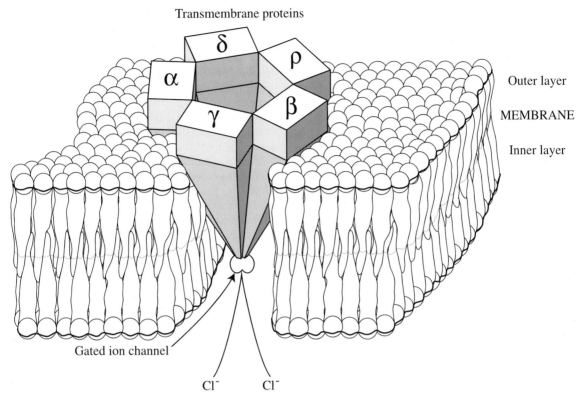

Transmembrane proteins

Outer layer

MEMBRANE

Inner layer

Gated ion channel

Cl⁻ Cl⁻

Fig. 4.10 GABA$_A$–benzodiazepine ionophore complex.

this at the end of the day relate to the pathophysiology and alleviation of anxiety? What are the elusive endogenous ligands (or ligand) – the so-called 'endozepines' – that in the absence of man's intrusions normally couple with the benzodiazepine recognition sites?

Adverse effects Benzodiazepines have perhaps the highest therapeutic index of all psychotropic drugs. And of course they are also extremely effective. In view of their actions it therefore becomes problematic as to whether patient complaints about 'side-effects' represent adverse effects as such or merely the drug carrying out its intended function.

These drugs have little of no autonomic actions, though they may promote mild hypotension with overzealous intravenous administration. Some patients complain of dry mouth and blurred vision, though whether these are drug effects is unclear. Patients may however complain of 'dizziness' or 'wooziness' which lacks the rotational and impelled qualities of vertigo and is probably related to mild blood pressure changes. Benzodiazepines do not alter the electrical or mechanical functioning of the heart. At therapeutic doses they do not interfere with respiration but when given rapidly by the intravenous route they can produce significant respiratory depression and even arrest, especially those which are distributed swiftly. This can be reversed by the benzodiazepine antagonist, flumazenil.

The most common patient complaint is also the prime example of the efficacy versus tolerability question – namely, a feeling of decreased mental acuity or frank daytime drowsiness and sedation. This can be evident early in exposure when it usually eases. It may however also emerge later in the course of chronic exposure as a result of the accumulation of drugs/metabolites of long half-life. Despite this however there seems to be a remarkable tolerance to such clinical consequences of accumulation (Baldessarini 1985).

Impaired psychomotor performance is an undoubted adverse effect which results from a primary deficit in information processing as well as a phenomenon secondary to sedation (Hindmarch 1980). As a group effect, benzodiazepines impair reaction times to a degree which can lead to significant functional deficits. Some performance deficits can be demonstrated soon after exposure and, although some do appear to ease with the passage of time, deviations from the norm can also become evident, again as a consequence of accumulation. Even those drugs with the shortest half-lives and marketed as hypnotics are still associated with significant residual daytime blood levels, so one cannot take solace in the fact of the drug's ingestion the night before. It is therefore imperative that doctors advise *all* patients taking a benzodiazepine of the impact this can have on daily tasks such as driving or operating machinery. Those requiring high degrees of motor responsiveness, such as airline pilots, must be specifically apprised of the implications of residual blood levels on daytime performance.

Benzodiazepines also impair short-term memory. Although the traditional view is that this comprises a retrograde amnesia, controlled studies have in fact shown that the problem is almost exclusively an anterograde one, with impairments of recall relating solely to events *after* administration of the drug (King 1992). It furthermore appears to be secondary to sedation. Patients on routine treatment schedules are usually unaware of this effect but after intravenous administration it can be striking. This is often used to therapeutic benefit in, for example, cardioversion and minor surgery, where patients given a benzodiazepine beforehand may not recall or have only a hazy recollection of basically unpleasant interventions afterwards.

In addition to the 'dizziness' noted above, patients occasionally develop unsteadiness which much more clearly relates to discoordination. In fact ataxia, dysarthria and a general breakdown of coordination are signs of the profound CNS depression that comprise intoxication and such features should be viewed in this light even if the regimen recommended has been 'therapeutic'.

Rare reports have appeared over the years of skin rashes, blood dyscrasias, headache, gastrointestinal upset, weight gain, impaired sexual function and dyskinetic movement disorder associated with use of benzodiazepines but in most instances these probably represented incidental disorder unrelated to the drug. Certainly such problems, if genuine, are extremely rare.

Two other side-effects are however important. Shortly after the introduction of chlordiazepoxide a 'syndrome' of paradoxical behavioural disinhibition or 'dyscontrol' was described (Ingram & Timbury 1960). The problem appears to be more frequent in women and, although reported most with chlordiazepoxide, is probably not unique to this preparation. The usual scenario is one of confinement, where the individual perceives themselves as trapped, and is then challenged. Confrontation in this situation can be met with a rage response associated with intemperate and assaultive behaviour. This is perhaps a better recognised phenomenon with other CNS depressants, especially alcohol, but it is important to bear in mind in psychiatric practice as professional interventions, and especially inpatient environments, might easily be perceived by patients as confining and restrictive. By using benzodiazepines in an attempt to achieve behavioural containment one might in fact unwittingly produce quite the opposite.

The final adverse effect to be considered is potentially the most serious and was the one that forced a radical reappraisal of the risk:benefit ratio of benzodiazepines in the most public way. This is physiological dependency.

As early as the 1970s it was clear that long-term use of benzodiazepines could be associated with tolerance effects. For example, patients frequently, if not usually, lost the sedation associated with early exposure, and this was known to happen rapidly over a few days. Also, the phenomenon of rapid eye movement (REM) rebound was known to be found in sleep EEGs of patients who had stopped long-term benzodiazepine hypnotics (Oswald & Priest 1965). More than this, withdrawal-type features, including fits, were well recognised after sudden cessation in some patients. However, full physiological dependency was thought to be a problem only in those who abused medication, and doubts continued as to whether these phenomena could occur at all with the regimens used clinically. A further problem was that complaints from patients suddenly stopping these drugs had a familiar resonance with those of the conditions for which the drugs were used in the first place.

The issue was thrown into stark relief when Petursson & Lader (1981) showed conclusively that a withdrawal syndrome – and hence physical dependence – could develop with benzodiazepine regimens that were considered to be in the therapeutic range.

The symptoms of benzodiazepine withdrawal are unusual in that their onset is, as a rule, delayed for longer than in most withdrawal states. They are also unusual in that they combine affective features with unique perceptual disturbances. Some 5–7 days after stopping, patients start to feel increasingly unsettled with an anxious dysphoria. Sleep diminishes in both quality and duration and daytime fatigue is prominent. Flu-like symptoms supervene, such as sweating, listlessness, anorexia, muscle aches and headache. Perceptual changes are evident in the form of heightened sensitivity to sounds, light and touch and may develop a 'temporal lobe'-type quality of distorted environmental relationships. Thus patients may experience doors as one sided or fireplaces that slope to one side. Surroundings can seem alien and frank depersonalisation may occur. In addition, bizarre paraesthesiae may be experienced, such as numbness, tingling or a feeling of movement or characteristically the sensation of walking on cotton wool. Fits are rare on withdrawal from therapeutic regimens.

There was a time when outpatient clinics were besieged by patients claiming persistence of such features many months after cessation of their medication, but this is clearly untenable. Features of benzodiazepine withdrawal last for 1–2 weeks at most. Belief in the endurance of symptoms was – and is – a reflection of their impact, the patient's expectation and a context of recurrent anxiety.

The risk of dependency with chronic benzodiazepine use is even now not something that can be confidently quantified, as it depends on individual factors such as personality type, the duration of exposure and pharmacokinetic parameters of the drug used. Overall the best estimate is that after 6 months of continuous exposure, a risk in the region of 45% can be anticipated (Tyrer et al 1981). However, features such as withdrawal anxiety/sleep disturbance may be found in some patients after only 6 weeks of treatment (Power et al 1985). The risk must therefore be adjudged as substantial, though it appears to be greatest, as would be predicted, with drugs which have relatively short half-lives, such as lorazepam.

If the problem has resulted from use of a short half-life compound, treatment should start by switching to diazepam, which, with its relatively long half-life, should make the ultimate task of tapered reduction easier (Higgit et al 1985). Beyond this however, management rests essentially on the good practice principle of slow or ultra-slow reduction, preferably over weeks. Although a number of drugs have been recommended as useful in easing withdrawal symptomatology, propranolol is probably the only one with any merits, and even these are slight.

Benzodiazepines are very safe. Even in overdose, fatality is usually only associated with combined ingestion with other drugs, especially alcohol.

Other sedative/hypnotic agents

In recent years other compounds have been identified that structurally do not belong to the benzodiazepine group yet appear to act within the GABA$_A$-benzodiazepine-chloride ionophore complex.

The imidazopyridines bind selectively to the ω-1 motif, unlike benzodiazepines which bind non-selectively to each of the three types of ω receptor units (ω-1–3). This preferential and targeted binding is advocated as a substantive point of difference between the drug types. However, imidazopyridines can be displaced from their binding sites by the selective benzodiazepine antagonist, flumazenil. At present this group is commercially represented by *zolpidem*, marketed as a hypnotic. There is some evidence that notwithstanding zolpidem's marketed indication, this group may have more specifically targeted antianxiety actions.

The cyclopyrrolones likewise bind with high affinity to different elements of the same receptor complex and are postulated to mediate their response across the sedative/hypnotic range by producing a different pattern of allosteric modulation of calcium channels than other compounds. The only commercially available member of this group so far is *zopiclone*, also marketed as a hypnotic. Preliminary clinical evidence is that this drug (and hence probably the group) needs to be treated with the same care as standard benzodiazepines.

Much has been made of the focused mode of action of these non-benzodiazepine drugs with the expectation that their use will not be associated with the same likelihood of physical dependency. It remains unclear however that with long-term or unsupervised use such optimism is justified.

An alternative approach to anxiety reduction is utilised by *buspirone*, an azapirone (or azaspirodecanedione). This does not act on the GABA$_A$-benzodiazepine-chloride ionophore at all, though its complex actions are incompletely understood. It is a partial 5-HT$_{1A}$ agonist and a relatively weak antagonist of dopamine, apparently at predominantly presynaptic sites. It is rapidly absorbed, undergoes extensive presystemic effects and has a very short half-life of only 2–4 hours. Buspirone's spectrum of action is restricted to anxiety management and it has no hypnotic, anticonvulsant or muscle-relaxant properties. In a further departure from benzodiazepine pharmacology, its action is not instantaneous but requires some 10 days to become apparent and up to 3 weeks to develop fully. It should not be used to substitute for benzodiazepines or alcohol in withdrawal regimens and in view of a proconvulsant action should be avoided in those at risk of fits. Its use may be associated with mild gastrointestinal upset and dizziness and, notwithstanding that its putative dopaminergic actions are on autoreceptors, it also elevates prolactin and can precipitate or exacerbate extrapyramidal disturbances. It must be avoided with traditional MAOI's. Because of its relative lack of interactions with other drugs, especially alcohol, and its apparent safety in overdose, buspirone may sometimes be useful in the management of chronic anxiety states but its effectiveness remains a matter of debate and it has as a rule found only limited clinical favour.

A disparate variety of other drugs are sometimes useful in the range of disorders covered by sedative/hypnotics. The 'old stand-bys' *chloral hydrate* and *triclofos* are still sometimes used in those rare situations in which hypnotics are indicated in children and can, in desperation, be tried in adults. Chloral, which added to alcohol comprised the original 'Mickey Finn', can be quite irritant to the stomach and triclofos is in general better tolerated. The highly sedative antihistamines such as *promethazine* can sometimes be useful sleep inducers but the thiamine analogue *chlormethiazole* is a potentially addictive and unpleasant compound whose use should be avoided.

Therapeutics

Indications

The indications for the use of sedative/hypnotics must be strictly circumscribed to:

- Short-term management of anxiety states, especially generalised anxiety disorder without depressive, hypochondriacal or other features.
- Short-term management of panic disorder, especially without agoraphobia, the presence of which may necessitate inadvisably prolonged exposure before efficacy accrues. Nowadays, however, imipramine is often considered a preferential strategy for the drug treatment of panic states.
- Short-term management of insomnia, especially when characterised by nocturnal anxiety and delayed initiation of sleep.

For these indications, 'short-term' is usually defined as 2–4 weeks.

- The emergency and prophylactic treatment of seizure disorders. The major value of benzodiazepines as a group is in the emergency treatment of status epilepticus, in which they are highly effective. They are also of great value in preventing seizure activity in states, such as withdrawal, where the seizure threshold is lowered. In the long-term prophylaxis of epilepsy their ability to obstruct generalisation of a fit and to maintain an elevation of the seizure threshold tends to undergo tolerance and they are of less value in this situation, although some, such as clonazepam which has an extremely long half-life, appear to be more effective in this regard.
- The containment of psychiatric emergencies. In such situations their ease of administration, rapidity of onset and safety make them ideal for the management of severe behavioural disturbance associated with usually psychotic disorders, where they are safer than parenterally administered antipsychotics.
- It has been proposed that in high doses (e.g. diazepam up to 100 mg per day) benzodiazepines have a primary antipsychotic action (Lingjaerde 1991). The evidence for this remains unconvincing but where these drugs may be helpful is as *adjunctive* treatments of acute psychotic states, particularly

schizophrenia. In this situation their value may be in lessening the subjective anxious/dysphoria of akathisic-type adverse effects which have themselves been implicated in exacerbating the positive features of the illness (Owens 1998).

- In the treatment of non-extrapyramidally mediated rigidity/spasticity.
- As preoperative or inducing agents in relation to minor surgery.

Strategies

The clinical use of sedative/hypnotics, and especially benzodiazepines, is difficult, largely because it is at one level so easy. Because they are so effective and have a very high therapeutic index, they appear to offer panaceas in relation to their target disorders which are in fact illusory. More than any other type of psychotropic agents, these drugs must be seen as part of a comprehensive package of management, with the drugs very much the junior partner.

The principles of their use in psychiatric contexts have already been alluded to:

- *Principle 1* Continuous treatment should be time-limited, as far as possible to 2–4 weeks.
- *Principle 2* An intermittent pattern of recommended use is preferable where possible, particularly in relation to insomnia.
- *Principle 3* The risks of dependency should be explained to the patient prior to implementing treatment – but should be done in relation to the facts. A single dose of temazepam on a long-haul flight is not the makings of a junky!
- *Principle 4* Intramuscular use as a rule offers little advantage over the oral route in emergency situations, while application of some of the pharmacokinetic data can contribute to maximising their effects with emergency, 'stat.' intravenous use.

While the new generation drugs may offer some advantages none of the compounds used for sedative/hypnotic purposes can at present be freed from the major risk of dependency.

MISCELLANEOUS DRUGS

Anticholinergics

Anticholinergics are among the most prescribed drugs in psychiatric practice yet are amongst the least studied. They are synthetic analogues of the belladonna alkaloids and have extensive applications in medicine in general, including cardiology, respiratory medicine and urology.

These drugs act as antagonists at muscarinic cholinergic receptors. They have little action at nicotinic sites. They have been used in the treatment of Parkinson's disease since the 1920s but have to a large extent been superseded by dopamine agonists. They are none the less effective in mild disorder and remain a cornerstone of the treatment of drug-related extrapyramidal disorders.

The pharmacokinetics of anticholinergics have been surprisingly little studied, and what is known has often been derived from patients with Parkinson's disease. The effects of coincidental administration of antipsychotics are largely unknown. In general, those commonly used in psychiatry are of three main types.

Tertiary amines related to diphenhydramine
Orphenadrine is of this group and combines antimuscarinic with antihistaminic properties. It has a variable therapeutic margin but can be fatal in overdose with amounts as low as 10 times the therapeutic dose (Dutz 1992). Little is known about its pharmacokinetics, although with a reported half-life in the range of 14–18 hours it is suitable for twice daily dosing. It is doubtful if the combination of actions found in this drug offer any advantages for its indicated psychiatric use, and reports of its relative toxicity would suggest that it is best avoided.

Compounds combining atropine-like and diphenhydramine-like actions The only widely used member of this group is benztropine which is also the least selective, combining both atropinic and antihistaminic actions. Because of its wide spectrum of actions it is particularly likely to interact with other drugs sharing a similar broad spectrum, of which the low potency antipsychotics are of course the most obvious examples. It is hard to see how such an unfocused compound could offer any clinical advantages. Furthermore, it may be worthy of note that heat stroke has been described in association with benztropine use (Adams et al 1977) and it should be avoided in those living in hot climates or who have a prior history, or current suspicion, of neuroleptic malignant syndrome.

Trihexyphenidyl-related compounds These include trihexyphenidyl itself (known in the UK as benzhexol) as well as biperiden and procyclidine. Several different types of muscarinic receptors have now been identified, of which the M_1 type is located in the CNS and is the desired target of anticholinergic drugs used to treat antipsychotic-related extrapyramidal disturbance. Of this group of compounds, biperiden is the most M_1 selective and benzhexol the least, with procyclidine only somewhat less selective than biperiden. The advantage of choosing a more selective drug is the lower likelihood of its use producing peripheral anticholinergic side-effects. A further disadvantage of benzhexol is that it may be more prone to cause excitement (Dutz 1992).

Biperiden is rapidly absorbed with a T_{max} of 1–2 hours. Its elimination half-life, in the region of 18 hours, might be compatible with once daily dosing. Procyclidine is also well absorbed but more slowly, with a T_{max} varying from 1 to 8 hours. It has a relatively short half-life (8–16 hours), suggesting that twice daily dosing is most appropriate, though the routine practice of three times daily administration would seem unnecessary.

In general, anticholinergics should not be used in fixed dose schedules but should be started in low doses (e.g. procyclidine 2.5 mg b.d.) and increased *flexibly* until resolution of target symptomatology (Owens 1998). Although they can sometimes produce sedation, the more usual response in low doses is excitement and they should not be given after tea-time. Even on such schedules they can significantly interfere with sleep (Johnstone et al 1983), though this action may undergo tolerance. They should furthermore be used *sparingly*: firstly, because even relatively selective drugs may produce their own pattern of side-effects, especially in combination with low potency antipsychotics; secondly, because they can produce an exacerbation of positive psychotic features; and thirdly, because they are euphorogenic and have a well-established potential to be abused.

L-tryptophan

L-tryptophan is an essential amino acid derived from dietary sources and is the precursor of serotonin. It has been known for 30 years to have antidepressant properties, though not of sufficient efficacy for it to be used as a first-line treatment. It has however an established adjunctive role, usually in combination with a tricyclic, in the management of treatment-resistant depression. It should be avoided in combination with an SSRI in view of the possibility of precipitating a serotonin syndrome.

In 1990, reports emerged of a serious multisystem allergic disorder, called *eosinophilia myalgia syndrome*, occurring in patients who had taken tryptophan from herbal sources, some of which proved fatal. No cases were reported with its medical use but as a precaution the purified preparation was also withdrawn. It was reintroduced in 1994, though its use remains strictly circumscribed to specialist settings. Patients and prescribers are required to be registered, clozapine-like, with the Optimax Information and Clinical Support Unit (OPTICS) via the manufacturer.

β-Noradrenergic antagonists

One of the oldest unresolved questions in psychology relates to the basis of anxiety symptoms – are they mediated by primarily central (Lange–James) or peripheral (Cannon–Bard) disturbances? Pharmacology has been of limited value in resolving the issue as the most appropriate clinical tools tend to act both centrally and peripherally.

Beta-blockers, and particularly propranolol, have been widely used in psychiatry for the treatment of the somatic manifestations of anxiety, though in general results are disappointing. Their major benefit may be in the management of anxiety symptomatology that is specifically environmentally triggered, such as performance anxiety in musicians or actors.

Propranolol was at one time advocated as an adjunctive treatment in severe or resistant schizophrenia but this could be a risky undertaking in the high-dose regimens often advocated. It was subsequently shown that any benefits might well have been the result of a pharmacokinetic interaction of propranolol in increasing antipsychotic blood levels, and this approach has faded.

There has however been interest in recent years in the use of propranolol in the treatment of akathisia. The greater the volume of trial literature on this topic the more sober the appraisal of efficacy, but in the low doses suggested (20–60 mg per day) propranolol is, in the absence of a history of asthma, safe, and if it is going to work, it is likely to do so within a few days. This might however be seen as the first-line approach primarily in patients who develop akathisia in the absence of coincidental parkinsonism.

Drugs used in the treatment of dementia

The magnitude of the health problems presented by dementia, not only now but for the future, demand effective pharmacological strategies which to date have proved elusive. Deficits in cholinergic transmission underlie the cholinergic hypothesis of dementia (Bartus et al 1982) which has formed the major starting point for the development of drug treatments. The approach most pursued has been towards compounds which inhibit the enzyme acetylcholinesterase, with the aim of extending the action of acetylcholine itself. The first widely studied acetylcholinesterase inhibitor was tacrine (or tetrahydroaminoacridine). Results have however been disappointing, especially so in view of the drug's hepatotoxicity (approx. 28%), and although licensed in the USA, tacrine remains an experimental drug in the UK.

Recently, donepezil has been licensed for use in early dementia. This is a reversible inhibitor of central acetylcholinesterase, with very little effect on peripheral butyrylcholinesterase, which is better tolerated than tacrine (Schneider 1996). It also appears to have more stable, linear pharmacokinetics. Results look far from

dramatic at this stage – but at least there appear to be some, though ill-sustained, beneficial effects on cognitive ability (Rogers et al 1996). Its place remains to be secured.

Although intuitively sound, acetylcholinesterase inhibitor strategies may be inherently limited, as experimental evidence suggests that the often profound decreases in the synthesis of M_1 receptor-linked phosphoinositides found in the neurones of demented patients not only reflect a reduction of M_1 receptor numbers but point to a loss of functional competency in those which remain (Shvaloff et al 1996).

Other strategies involving cholinergic agonism with drugs such as arecoline, pilocarpine and carbachol have been unsuccessful because of serious peripheral adverse effects, and the grandly named 'no-otropic' agents (drugs which enhance cognitive performance) such as piracetam appear of little value in the context of a degenerate substrate. The use of nerve growth factors and senile plaque inhibitors are interesting departures from conventional approaches but have yet to prove themselves.

Patients with rheumatoid arthritis appear to have lower rates of Alzheimer's disease (Schneider 1996) and there is considerable interest in the efficacy of anti-inflammatory agents in the management of dementias. There is evidence that non-steroidal anti-inflammatories such as indomethacin, and even aspirin, might delay the onset and progression of dementia, and such simple strategies, which might also include calcium channel antagonists which increase cerebral perfusion, may be the best available for some time to come (Schneider 1996, Shvaloff et al 1996).

Drugs used in the treatment of dependency states

In line with trends elsewhere in psychiatry there is increasing interest in the use of pharmacological methods to manage disorders of dependency. Disulfiram therapy is one of the more established techniques for attempting to maintain abstinence from alcohol. It is an inhibitor of hepatic aldehyde (including alcohol) dehydrogenases, resulting in the accumulation in the presence of alcohol of acetaldehyde, which produces a gamut of unpleasant symptoms such as flushing, nausea, vomiting, lightheadedness and, in severe cases, collapse. Disulfiram has other complex actions that may underlie some of its effects. It can be a powerful spur to motivation but requires a deal of motivation in the first place. Reactions can be potentially dangerous and patients must be advised of the need to avoid proprietary preparations containing alcohol and even the overgenerous use of alcohol-based toiletries.

A different approach which has some support from recent controlled trials is the reduction of intake by controlling cravings for alcohol. Strategies for attempting this have included the use of the synthetic opiate antagonist naltrexone, and the GABA agonist, acamprosate. Whether such strategies will define an established place in management remains to be seen.

DRUG INTERACTIONS

Polypharmacy is common across medical practice nowadays, including psychiatry, thus making drug interactions very likely. Most encountered in psychiatric practice do not fortunately have serious consequences but even these may delay or obstruct the target effect or increase the likelihood of non-target effects. Some, as we have seen, can be fatal.

Interactions may be of two kinds. In *pharmacodynamic* interactions a target action is magnified or diminished on the basis of the action of a second drug operating at the same target. These can produce responses that are strikingly different qualitatively from that of either drug alone. The *hypertensive crises* with MAOIs noted above is one example, where the second 'drug' can be food constituents. A further example is the serious interaction that can result from substituting fluoxetine with an MAOI or a tricyclic with serotonin reuptake inhibitory properties, such as clomipramine. The long half-life of fluoxetine and norfluoxetine results in an excess of serotonin in the synapse which may cause a so-called *serotonin* or *serotonergic* syndrome. This is characterised by agitation, excitement, diaphoresis, hyperthermia, extrapyramidal signs especially rigidity, hyperreflexia, tachycardia, hypotension, confusion and coma. It may prove fatal. For this reason, a washout of at least 5–6 weeks is now recommended after stopping fluoxetine and before commencing these types of preparation.

In *pharmacokinetic* interactions one drug produces an alteration that is usually quantitative in the target action of a second drug by altering its absorption, distribution and especially its metabolism or elimination.

In psychiatric practice, pharmacokinetic interactions are not uncommon, as Appendix 1 of the *British National Formulary* demonstrates. The efficacy of most psychotropics correlates poorly or not at all with blood levels and the relationships with tolerability are only slightly more secure, so these have traditionally been seen as rarely producing problems of significance to routine practice. However, a more detailed understanding of the bases of such interactions may throw light on important clinical issues such as differences in response rates and patterns of tolerability.

Occasionally it may prevent potentially toxic elevations in blood levels.

Recently, this area has expanded dramatically following advances in understanding of the cytochrome P450 system. These enzymes are of two types, *mitochondrial* which mediate steroid synthesis, and *microsomal* which mediate the metabolism of exogenous compounds. Although predominantly sited in the liver, it is increasingly clear that P450 enzymes have a wider distribution, including gut wall and brain.

The cytochrome P (CY-P) isoforms are characterised according to a genetic format, where the first number refers to the gene *family*, followed by the gene *subfamily letter* and finally the *gene number* itself, e.g. CYP-2 -D-6. In humans, most drugs are metabolised by four isoenzymes – CYP1A2, CYP2C comprising 2C9/10 and 2C19, CYP2D6 and CYP3A3/4 – though at present many isoenzymes remain to be characterised (Ketter et al 1995, Ereshefsky et al 1996). The latter two of these appear to be particularly important with regard to the metabolism of psychotropics with the CYP3A3/4 system the most abundant, especially in intestinal mucosa. The activities of these enzymes are determined genetically and striking interindividual differences in drug levels and tolerabilities of many psychotropic agents can to some extent be attributed to polymorphisms within these systems, especially the CYP2D6 genotype. About 7% of Caucasians can be characterised as 'poor' (as opposed to 'extensive') metabolisers of drugs undergoing oxidative metabolism via this enzyme, while the corresponding figure for Orientals is only 1% (Bertilsson 1995).

An outline knowledge of those drugs which are metabolised by P450 enzymes and some of the commoner inhibitors and inducers can be helpful in predicting patterns of interaction that may have clinical relevance (Table 4.8). One might for example predict that fluoxetine, a potent inhibitor of the CYP2D6 isoenzyme and less so of the CYP3A3/4 group, would produce elevations in the blood levels of other psychotropics such as tricyclics, certain antipsychotics (e.g. haloperidol) and benzodiazepines such as alprazolam, which is the case. It may in addition increase carbamazepine levels. It can also be recommended that for example nefazodone, a potent inhibitor of the 3A3/4 group, should not be coadministered with alprazolam in view of the high levels of the latter that are likely to ensue. Of particular importance is the avoidance of combination of tricyclics with potent inhibitors of CYP2D6, as tricyclics are dependent on this enzyme for their hydroxylation. It has been shown, for example, that the combination of a tricyclic (desipramine) with paroxetine or fluoxetine can result in a 3–4-fold increase in plasma desipramine levels, whereas co-

Table 4.8 Psychotropic drug interactions: substrates and inhibitors for different isoforms of the P450 system

Substrates	CYP1A2	CYP2D6	CYP2C9	CYP2C19	CYP3A3/4
Antidepressants	Tertiary amine tricyclics (*N*-demethylation)	Tertiary and Secondary tricyclics (hydroxylation) Fluoxetine Paroxetine Nefazodone Venlafaxine (*O*-demethylation) m-CPP		Tertiary amine tricyclics (*N*-demethylation) Citalopram Moclobemide	Tertiary amine tricyclics (*N*-demethylation) Sertraline Nefazodone *O*-desmethylvenlafaxine
Antipsychotics	Clozapine	Haloperidol Thioridazine Perphenazine Risperidone			Clozapine
Sedative hypnotics				Diazepam (*N*-demethylation) Hexobarbital Mephobarbital S-mephenytoin	Diazepam (*N*-demethylation and hydroxylation) Alprazolam Clonazepam
Miscellaneous	Caffeine Propranolol Paracetamol Theophylline	Beta blockers Codeine Type Ic antiarrhythmics	Warfarin Phenytoin Tolbutamide	Propranolol Omeprazole	Carbamazepine Calcium channel antagonists Terfenadine Androgens/oestrogens Ethosuximide Cisipride Lidocaine Quinidine Erythromycin Cyclosporin
Inhibitors Strong ↓ Weak	Fluvoxamine Fluoxetine Nefazodone Paroxetine Sertraline	Quinidine Paroxetine Fluoxetine Norfluoxetine Sertraline Desmethylsertraline Fluvoxamine Nefazodone Venlafaxine Moclobemide Thioridazine Haloperidol Perphenazine Erythromycin Ketoconazole	Fluoxetine Fluvoxamine	Ketoconazole Omeprazole Fluvoxamine Fluoxetine Venlafaxine	Ketoconazole Erythromycin Nefazodone Fluvoxamine Norfluoxetine Fluoxetine Sertraline Desmethylsertraline Paroxetine Venlafaxine Quinidine Diltiazem Verapamil Dexamethasone Naringenin
Inducers	Cigarettes (? nicotine) Omeprazole			Rifampicin	Carbamazepine Phenobarbital Phenytoin Rifampicin Dexamethasone

administration with sertraline, a weaker inhibitor, produces only modest increases in desipramine levels.

A further non-psychiatric example is naringenin in grapefruit juice inhibiting the CYP3A3/4 system on which cyclosporin and a number of calcium channel antagonists, amongst others, depend for metabolism, resulting in significant elevations in blood levels. Although unidentified as being of clinical importance as yet, several similar examples pertinent to psychiatry could be postulated.

Most drugs have several potential metabolic pathways and even now the necessary details of oxidative metabolism are still not known for the majority (~80%), so clinically it is not yet possible to apply information on the P450 system in a mathematical way. This is none the less an area that will become of increasing importance.

PREGNANCY AND LACTATION

Most psychotropics can produce fetal maldevelopment when administered to pregnant laboratory animals and the possible translation of such data to humans led at one time to considerable concern. This is reflected in the conservative recommendations usually offered by clinicians and by the *British National Formulary*.

Systematic clinical evaluation of the question has however been sparse (Altshuler et al 1996). Meta-analysis of published data suggests that first trimester exposure to low potency phenothiazines imparts a small but significant increase in the risk of organ dysgenesis. The *additional* risk has been quantified at approximately 4 per 1000 live births. No specific increase in risk can be attributed to high-potency antipsychotics or tricyclics, and although SSRIs also appear safe, their limited use precludes definitive conclusions at present. Data from the lithium baby register has already been noted, which placed the rate of Ebstein's anomaly at 400 times that of the general population. However, more recent appraisal puts the risk at 10–20 times, which translates into an overall risk of approximately 0.1%. First trimester exposure to carbamazepine is associated with a risk of spina bifida in the region of 0.5–1%, while the risk of this abnormality with valproate is around 2–5 times greater. Finally, although the data are somewhat contaminated, first trimester exposure to benzodiazepines may be associated with a twofold increase in the risk of oral cleft abnormalities.

While these data would support caution in the use of most psychotropics during early pregnancy, they probably reflect relative rather than absolute risks, as the conditions for which these drugs are prescribed are themselves often associated with an increased risk of fetal maldevelopment. Any drug with sedative properties should be avoided in the prenatal period as this may complicate delivery.

The lipophilic properties of the great majority of psychotropic agents results in them being secreted in breast milk. However, the large apparent volume of distribution of such drugs means that the fraction of a maternal dose that is available for secretion in breast milk is small. The levels attained are also dependent on the lipid content of the milk sample. Thus levels are as a rule higher in later expressed (or hind-) milk with its higher fat content than in initial (or fore-milk) samples.

Formal study of the passage of maternal psychotropic drugs to breast-fed infants has also been slight and differences in drug assay methodologies makes comparisons difficult. In view of immaturity of the liver, breast-feeding should be *contraindicated* with babies born *prematurely* or who have *neonatal illness*. Otherwise the evidence to date suggests that for mothers receiving most of the major classes of psychotropics the decision to breast-feed can, in terms of *safety*, be left to them (Yoshida & Kumar 1996).

There is a suggestion from a single case report that doxepin may cause toxicity (Matheson et al 1985) but other tricyclics, although transferred, appear to be associated wih very low or undetectable levels in infants. On the limited evidence to date, SSRIs also appear safe. Antipsychotics do attain measurable levels in breast-fed infants and isolated reports of acute dystonic episodes and 'restlessness' with standard drugs have appeared. However, in general these too seem relatively safe. Despite its teratogenicity, there is no evidence that carbamazepine need be contraindicated *post*natally (Yoshida & Kumar 1996). Care should be exercised with benzodiazepines as they may impair suckling from neonatal sedation and contribute to a 'floppy' baby.

The one possible proscription is on *lithium*, which is readily secreted and may attain plasma levels in the infant that are as high as one-third to one-half those of the mother. Because of immaturity of regulatory mechanisms, these may present a pharmacologically greater impact than comparable levels in adults and cases of toxicity in breast-fed infants have been described. The consensus for avoiding breast-feeding with lithium has been challenged (Linden & Rich 1983), but in the situation where a mood stabiliser is indicated an alternative to lithium during the period of breast-feeding would still seem the most prudent advice.

It is further reassuring that, as far as is known, there is no evidence that exposure of the neonate to psychotropics produces any detectable early developmental delays (Altshuler et al 1996), though the question has only been systematically evaluated in relation to tricyclics (Yoshida et al 1997).

Thus, overall, the evidence is that the decision to breast-feed can in most instances be left to individual mothers without undue influence being brought to bear from psychopharmacological sources. The issue then becomes a gut one – whether as a matter of principle the mother or the clinician has reservations about exposing the immature brain to centrally acting drugs of diverse and pervasive pharmacological actions. Placed in terms of such imponderables, it is likely most individuals would still opt for a pragmatic plan of avoidance.

REFERENCES

Adams B E, Manoguerra A S, Lilja G P et al 1977 Heat stroke associated with medications having anticholinergic effects. Minnesota Medicine 60: 103–106

Altshuler L L, Cohen L, Szuba M P et al 1996 Pharmacologic management of psychiatric illness during pregnancy: dilemmas and guidelines. American Journal of Psychiatry 153: 592–606

Amdisen A 1977 Serum level monitoring and clinical pharmacokinetics of lithium. Clinical Pharmacokinetics 2: 73–92

Amrein R, Allen S R, Guentert D et al 1989 The pharmacology of reversible monoamine oxidase inhibitors. British Journal of Psychiatry 155 (suppl 6): 66–71

Anderson I M, Tomenson B M 1995 Treatment discontinuation with selective serotonin reuptake inhibitors compared with tricyclic antidepressants: a meta-analysis. British Medical Journal 310: 1433–1438

Atkin K, Kendall F, Gould D et al 1996 Neutropenia and agranulocytosis in patients receiving clozapine in the UK and Ireland. British Journal of Psychiatry 169: 483–488

Atkins M, Burgess A, Bottomley C et al 1997 Chlorpromazine equivalents: a consensus of opinion for both clinical and research applications. Psychiatric Bulletin 21: 224–226

Baldessarini R J 1985 Chemotherapy in psychiatry. Harvard University Press, Cambridge

Baldessarini R J, Frankenburg F R 1991 Clozapine: a novel antipsychotic agent. New England Journal of Medicine 324: 746–754

Baldessarini R J, Katz B, Cotton P 1984 Dissimilar dosing with high-potency and low-potency neuroleptics. American Journal of Psychiatry 141: 748–752

Bartus R T, Dean R L, Beer B et al 1982 The cholinergic hypothesis of geriatric memory dysfunction. Science 217: 408–417

Baumhackl U, Biziere K, Fischbach F et al 1989 Efficacy and tolerability of moclobemide compared with imipramine in depressive disorder. British Journal of Psychiatry 155 (suppl 6):78–83

Beaumont G, Baldwin D, Lader M 1996 A criticism of the practice of prescribing subtherapeutic doses of antidepressants for the treatment of depression. Human Psychopharmacology 11: 283–291

Bertilsson L 1995 Geographical/interracial differences in polymorphic drug oxidation. Clinical Pharmacokinetics 29: 192–209

Blackwell B 1963 Hypertensive crisis due to monoamine oxidase inhibitors. Lancet ii: 849–851

Blackwell B, Simon J S 1988 Antidepressant drugs. In: Dukes M N G (ed) Meyler's side effects of drugs, 11th ed. Elsevier, Amsterdam, pp 27–69

Boston Collaborative Drug Surveillance Program 1972 Adverse reactions to the tricyclic-antidepressant drugs. Lancet i: 529–531

Boyer W F, Feighner J P 1991 Pharmacokinetics and drug interactions. In: Feighner J P, Boyer W F (eds) Selective serotonin reuptake inhibitors. Wiley, Chichester, pp 81–88

Boyer W F and Feighner J P 1996 Safety and tolerability of selective serotonin re-uptake inhibitors. In: Feighner J P, Boyer W F (eds) Selective serotonin re-uptake inhibitors, 2nd edn. Wiley, Chichester, pp 291–314

British Isles Raclopride Study Group 1992 A double blind comparison of raclopride and haloperidol in the acute phase of schizophrenia. Acta Psychiatrica Scandinavica 86: 391–398

Brodie M J 1987 Carbamazepine: pharmacokinetics and interactions. International Clinical Psychopharmacology, 2 (suppl 1): 73–81

Canoso R T, de Oliveira R M, Nixon R A 1990 Neuroleptic-associated autoantibodies: a prevalence study. Biological Psychiatry 27: 863–870

Carpenter W T, Heindrichs D W, Alphs L D 1985 Treatment of negative symptoms. Schizophrenia Bulletin 11: 440–452

Cassidy S, Henry J 1987 Fatal toxicity of antidepressant drugs in overdose. British Medical Journal 295: 1021–1024

Cold J A, Wells B G, Froemming J H 1990 Seizure activity associated with antipsychotic therapy. DICP, Annals of Pharmacotherapy 24: 601–606

Cole J O, Bodkin A 1990 Antidepressant drug side effects. Journal of Clinical Psychiatry 51 (suppl 1): 21–26

Cooper T B 1987 Pharmacokinetics of lithium. In: Meltzer H Y (ed) Psychopharmacology: the third generation of progress. Raven Press, New York, pp 1365–1375

Coulter D L 1991 Carnitine, valproate and toxicity. Journal of Child Neurology 6: 7–14

Coupland N, Wilson S, Nutt D 1997 Antidepressant drugs and the cardiovascular system: a comparison of tricyclics and selective serotonin reuptake inhibitors and their relevance for the treatment of psychiatric patients with cardiovascular problems. Journal of Psychopharmacology 11: 83–92

Curry S H 1986 Applied clinical pharmacology of schizophrenia. In: Bradley P B, Hirsch S R (eds) The psychopharmacology and treatment of schizophrenia. Oxford University Press, Oxford, pp 103–131

Curzon M E J 1987 Teeth. In: Johnson F N (ed) Depression and mania—modern lithium therapy. IRL Press, Oxford, pp 203–206

Dahl S G, Strandjord R E 1977 Pharmacokinetics of chlorpromazine after single and chronic dosage. Clinical Pharmacology and Therapeutics 21: 437–448

Davis J M, Metalon L, Watanabe M D, et al 1994 Depot antipsychotics: place in therapy. Drugs 741–773

Deng M Z, Chen G C, Phillips M R 1990 Neuroleptic malignant syndrome in 12 of 9792 Chinese inpatients exposed to neuroleptics: a prospective study. American Journal of Psychiatry 147: 1149–1155

Diamond J M, Ehrlich B E, Morawski S G et al 1983 Lithium absorption in tight and leaky segments of intestine, Journal of Membrane Biology 72: 159–183

Dilsaver S C, Greden J F, Snider R M 1987 Antidepressant withdrawal syndromes: phenomenology and physiopathology. International Clinical Psychopharmacology 2: 1–19

Dostert P, Benedetti M S, Poggesi I 1997 Review of the pharmacokinetics and metabolism of reboxetine, a selective noradrenaline reuptake inhibitor. European Neuropsychopharmacology 7 (suppl 1): s23–s35

Dubovsky S L 1993 Calcium antagonists in manic-depressive illness. Neuropsychobiology 27: 184–192

Dutz W 1992 Drugs affecting autonomic functions or the extrapyramidal system. In: Dukes M N G (ed) Meyler's side effects of drugs, 12th edn. Elsevier, Amsterdam, pp 307–334

Edwards J G 1986 The untoward effects of antipsychotic drugs: pathogenesis and management. In: Bradley P B, Hirsch S R (eds) The psychopharmacology and treatment of schizophrenia. Oxford University Press, Oxford, pp 403–441

Ereshefsky L, Lacombe S 1993 Pharmacological profile of risperidone. Canadian Journal of Psychiatry 38 (suppl 3): s80–s88

Ereshefsky L, Saklad S R, Jann M W, et al 1983 Pharmacokinetics of fluphenazine by high performance thin layer chromatography. Drug Intelligence and Clinical Pharmacy 17: 436–437

Ereshefsky L, Riesenman C, Lam Y W F 1996 Serotonin selective reuptake inhibitor drug interactions and the cytochrome P450 system. Journal of Clinical Psychiatry 57 (suppl 8): 17–25

Faedda G L, Tondo L Baldessarini R J et al 1993 Outcome after rapid vs gradual discontinuation of lithium treatment in bipolar disorders. Archives of General Psychiatry 50: 448–455

Farde L, Nordstrom A-L, Wiesel F-A et al 1992 Positron emission tomographic analysis of central D_1 and D_2 dopamine receptor occupancy in patients treated with classical neuroleptics and clozapine. Archives of General Psychiatry 49: 538–544

Fernstrom M H, Kupfer D J 1988 Antidepressant-induced weight gain: a comparison study of four medications. Psychiatry Research 26: 265–271

Frazer A 1997 Antidepressants. Journal of Clinical Psychiatry 58 (suppl 6): 9–25

Glassman A H, Biggar J T 1981 Cardiovascular effects of therapeutic doses of tricyclic antidepressants. Archives of General Psychiatry 38: 815–820

Glassman A H, Biggar J T, Giardina E V et al 1979 Clinical characteristics of imipramine-induced orthostatic hypotenision. Lancet i: 468–472

Gomolin I H 1987 Coping with excessive doses. In: Johnson F N (ed) Depression and mania—modern lithium therapy. IRL Press, Oxford, pp 154–157

Goodnick P J, Fieve R R, Meltzer H L 1981, Lithium elimination and duration of therapy. Clinical Pharmacology and Therapeutics 29: 47–50

Goodnick P J 1991 Pharmacokinetics of second generation antidepressants: fluoxetine. Psychopharmacology Bulletin, 27: 503–512

Goodnick P J, Schorr-Cain C B 1991 Lithium pharmacokinetics. Psychopharmacology Bulletin 27: 475–491

Goodwin G M 1996 How do antidepressants affect serotonin receptors? The role of serotonin receptors in the therapeutic and side effect profile of the SSRIs. Journal of Clinical Psychiatry 57 (suppl 4): 9–13

Gould G M, Murphy K M M, Reynolds I J et al 1983 Antischizophrenic drugs of the diphenylbutylpiperidine type act as calcium channels antagonists. Proceedings of the National Academy of Sciences of the USA 80: 5122–5125

Gould R J, Murphy K M M, Reynolds I J et al 1984 Calcium channel blockade: possible explanation for thioridazine's peripheral side effects. American Journal of Psychiatry 141: 352–357

Greenblatt D J 1993 Basic pharmacokinetic principles and their application to psychotropic drugs. Journal of Clinical Psychiatry 54 (suppl) 9: 8–13

Greenblatt D J, Shader R I 1987 Pharmacokinetics of antianxiety agents. In: Meltzer H Y (ed) Psychopharmacology: the third generation of progress. Raven Press, New York, pp 1377–1386

Haddad P 1997 Newer antidepressants and the discontinuation syndrome. Journal of Clinical Psychiatry 58 (suppl 7): 17–22

Halle M T, Dilsaver S C 1993 Tranylcypromine withdrawal phenomena. Journal of Psychiatry and Neuroscience 18: 49–50

Hamann G L, Egan T M, Wells B G et al 1990 Injection site reactions after intramuscular administration of haloperidol decanoate 100mg/mL. Journal of Clinical Psychiatry 51: 502–504

Henry J A 1996 Suicide risk and antidepressant treatment. Journal of Psychopharmacology 10 (suppl 1): 39–40

Hestbech J, Hansen H E, Amdisen A et al 1977 Chronic renal lesions following long-term treatment with lithium. Kidney International 12: 205–213

Hetmar O, Juul Povlsen U, Ladefoged J, et al 1991 Lithium: Long-term effects on the kidney. A prospective follow-up study ten years after kidney biopsy. British Journal of Psychiatry 158: 53–58

Higgitt A C, Lader M H, Fonaghy P 1985 Clinical management of benzodiazepine dependence. British Medical Journal 291: 688–690

Hindmarch I 1980 Psychomotor function and psychoactive drugs. British Journal of Clinical Pharmacology 10: 189–210

Holden J M C, Holden U P 1979 Weight changes with schizophrenic psychosis and psychotropic drug therapy. Psychosomatics 11: 551–651

Hotopf M, Lewis G, Norman C 1996 Are SSRIs a cost-effective alternative to tricyclics? British Journal of Psychiatry 168: 404–409

Hotopf M, Hardy R, Lewis G 1997 Discontinuation rates of SSRIs and tricyclic antidepressants: a meta-analysis and investigation of heterogeneity. British Journal of Psychiatry 170: 120–127

Ingram I M, Timbury G C 1960 Side effects of Librium. Lancet ii: 766

Isaac N E, Walker A M, Jick H et al 1991 Exposure to phenothiazine drugs and risk of cataract. Archives of Ophthalmalogy 109: 256–260

Isojarvi J I T, Laatikainen T J, Pakarinen A J et al 1993 Polycystic ovaries and hyperandrogenism in women taking valproate for epilepsy. New England Journal of Medicine 329: 1383–1388

Isojarvi J I T, Laatikainen T J, Knip M et al 1996 Obesity and endocrine disorders in women taking valproate for epilepsy. Annals of Neurology 39: 579–584

Jacobsen F M 1992 Fluoxetine-induced sexual dysfunction and an open trial of yohimbine. Journal of Clinical Psychiatry 53: 199–122

Jann M W, Ereshefsky L, Saklad S R 1985 Clinical pharmacokinetics of the depot antipsychotics. Clinical Pharmacokinetics 10: 315–333

Jarvis M R 1991 Clinical pharmacokinetics of tricyclic antidepressant overdose. Psychopharmacology Bulletin 27: 541–550

Jefferson J W 1989 Cardiovascular effects and toxicity of anxiolytics and antidepressants. Journal of Clinical Psychiatry 50: 368–378

Jennings A E, Levey A S, Harrington J T 1983 Amoxapine-associated acute renal failure. Archives of Internal Medicine 143: 1525–1527

Jerram T C, McDonald R 1978 Plasma lithium control with particular reference to minimum effective levels. In: Johnson F N, Johnson S (eds) Lithium in medical practice. MTP Press, Lancaster, pp 407–413

Johnstone E C, Crow T J, Ferrier I N et al 1983 Adverse effects of anticholinergic medication on positive symptoms. Psychological Medicine 13: 513–527

Jorgensen A 1986 Metabolism and pharmacokinetics of antipsychotic drugs. In: Bridges J W, Chasseaud L F (eds) Progress in drug metabolism. Taylor & Francis, London, pp 111–174

Judd L L, Hubbard B, Janowsky D S et al 1977a The effect of lithium carbonate on affect, mood, and personality of normal subjects. Archives of General Psychiatry 34: 346–351

Judd L L, Hubbard B, Janowsky D S et al 1977b the effect of lithium carbonate on the cognitive functions of normal subjects. Archives of General Psychiatry 34: 355–347

Jusic N, Lader M H 1994 Post-mortem antipsychotic drug concentrations and unexplained deaths. British Journal of Psychiatry 165: 787–791

Kane J M 1987 Treatment of schizophrenia. Schizophrenia Bulletin 13: 133–156

Kane J M, Honigfeld G, Singer J et al 1988 Clozapine for the treatment-resistant schizophrenic: a double-blind comparison with chlorpromazine. Archives of General Psychiatry 45: 789–796

Kaplan S A, Jack M L 1983 Metabolism of the benzodiazepines: pharmacokinetic and pharmacodynamic considerations In: Costa E (ed) The benzodiazepines: from molecular biology to clinical practice. Raven Press, New York, pp 173–199

Ketter T A, Flockhart D A, Post R M et al 1995 The emerging role of cytochrome P450 3A in psycho-pharmacology. Journal of Clinical Psychopharmacology 15: 387–398

Kincaid-Smith P, Burrows G D, Davies B M et al 1979 Renal biopsy findings in lithium and prelithium patients. Lancet ii: 7001–7002

King D J 1992 Benzodiazepines, amnesia and sedation: theoretical and clinical issues and controversies. Human Psychopharmacology 7: 79–87

Knudsen K, Heath A 1984 Effects of self-poisoning with maprotiline. British Medical Journal 288: 601–603

Kopera H 1980 Cardiac effects of mianserin: results of clinical pharmacological investigations. Current Medical Research and Opinion 6 (suppl 7): 36–43

Kubota T, Ishikura T, Jubiki I 1994 Alopecia areata associated with haloperidol. Japanese Journal of Psychiatry and Neurology 48: 579–581

Kupfer D J, Carpenter L L, Frank E 1988 Possible role of antidepressants in precipitating mania and hypomania in recurrent depression. American Journal of Psychiatry 145: 804–808

Lambert D, Dalac S 1987 Skin, hair and nails, in: Johnson F N (ed) Depression and mania–modern lithium therapy. IRL Press, Oxford, pp 232–234

Lancet 1996 Safety concerns over antipsychotic drug, sertindole (news item in Science and Medicine section) 348: 256

Lane R M 1997 A critical review of selective serotonin reuptake inhibitor-related sexual dysfunction: incidence, possible aetiology and implications for management. Journal of Psychopharmacology 11: 72–82

Lejoyeux M, Ades J 1997 Antidepressant discontinuation: a review of the literature. Journal of Clinical Psychiatry 58 (suppl 7): 11–16

Levinson D F, Simpson G M 1986 Neuroleptic-induced extrapyramidal symptoms with fever: heterogeneity of the 'neuroleptic malignant syndrome'. Archives of General Psychiatry 43:839–848

Levinson D F, Simpson G M 1987 Serious nonextrapyramidal adverse effects of neuroleptics: sudden death, agranulocutosis and hepatotoxicity. In: Meltzer H Y (ed) Psychopharmacology: the third generation of progress. Raven Press, New York, pp 1431–1436

Lieberman J A 1993 Understanding the mechanism of action of atypical antipsychotic drugs: a review of compounds in use and development. British Journal of Psychiatry 163 (suppl 22): 7–22

Lieberman J A, Safferman A Z, Pollack S et al 1994 Clinical effects of clozapine in chronic schizophrenia: response to treatment and predictors of outcome. American Journal of Psychiatry 151: 1744–1752

Linden S, Rich C L 1983 The use of lithium during pregnancy and lactation. Clinical Psychiatry 44: 358–361

Lingjaerde O 1991 Benzodiazepines in the treatment of schizophrenia: an updated survey. Acta Psychiatrica Scandinavica 84: 453–459

Lipscomb P A 1980 Cardiovascular side effects of phenothiazines and tricyclic antidepressants: a review with precautionary measures. Postgraduate Medicine 67: 189–196

Lucas V S 1993 Association of psychotropic drugs, prevalence of denture-related stomatitis and oral candidiasis. Community Dentistry and Oral Epidemiology 21: 313–316

McCreadie R G, Dingwall J M, Wiles D H et al 1980 Intermittent pimozide versus fluphenazine decanoate as maintenance therapy in chronic schizophrenia. British Journal of Psychiatry 137: 510–517

McQuay H J, Tramer M, Nye B A et al 1996 A systematic review of antidepressants in neuropathic pain. Pain 68: 217–227

Malik K 1996 Nefazodone: structure, mode of action and pharmacokinetics. Journal of Psychopharmacology 10 (suppl 1): 1–4

Mallinger A G, Smith E 1991 Pharmacokinetics of monoamine oxidase inhibitors. Psychopharmacology Bulletin 27: 493–502

Manji H, Hsiao J K, Risby E D et al 1991 The mechanism of action of lithium. I. Effects on serotonergic and noradrenergic systems in normal subjects. Archives of General Psychiatry 48: 505–512

Manji H, Potter W Z, Lenox R H 1995 Signal transduction pathways: molecular targets for lithium's actions. Archives of General Psychiatry 52: 531–543

Marmor M F 1990 Is thioridazine retinopathy progressive? Relationship of pigmentary changes to visual function. British Journal of Ophthalmology 74: 739–742

Martin C A, Dickson L R, Kuo C S 1987 Heart and blood vessels. In: Johnson F N (ed) Depression and mania–modern lithium therapy. IRL Press, Oxford, pp 213–218

Matheson I, Pande H, Alertsen A P 1985 Respiratory depression caused by N-desmethyldoxepin in breast milk. Lancet 16: 1124

Mehtonen O-P, Aranko K, Malkonen L et al 1991 A survey of sudden death associated with the use of antipsychotic or antidepressant drugs: 49 cases in Finland. Acta Psychiatrica Scandinavica 84: 58–64

Meltzer H Y, Fang V S 1976 The effects of neuroleptics on serum prolactin in schizophrenic patients. Archives of General Psychiatry 33: 279–284

Metzger E, Friedman R 1993 Prolongation of the corrected QT and torsades de pointes cardiac arrhythmia associated with intravenous haloperidol in the medically ill. Journal of Clinical Psychopharmacology 13: 128–132

Moller H J 1993 Neuroleptic treatment of negative symptoms in schizophrenic patients: efficacy, problems and methodological difficulties. European Neuropsychopharmacology 3: 1–11

Moncrieff J 1997 Lithium: evidence reconsidered. British Journal of Psychiatry 171: 113–119

Montgomery S A, Baldwin D, Green M 1989 Why do amitriptyline and dothiepin appear to be so dangerous in overdose? Acta Psychiatrica Scandinavica 80 (suppl 354): 47–53

Montgomery S A, Henry J, McDonald G et al 1994 Selective serotonin reuptake inhibitors: meta-analysis of discontinuation rates. International Clinical Psychopharmacology 9: 47–53

Moschitto L J, Greenblatt D J 1983 Concentration-independent plasma protein binding of benzodiazepines. Journal of Pharmacy and Pharmacology 35: 179–180

Myers D H, West T E T 1987 Hormone systems. In: Johnson F N Depression and mania—modern lithium therapy. IRL Press, Oxford, pp 220–226

Oswald I, Priest R G 1965 Five weeks to escape the sleeping pill habit. British Medical Journal ii: 1093–1095

Owens D G C 1996 Adverse effects of antipsychotic agents: do newer agents offer advantages? Drugs 51: 895–930

Owens D G C 1998 A guide to the extrapyramidal side effects of antipsychotic drugs. Cambridge University Press, Cambridge

Perry P J 1996 Pharmacotherapy for major depression with melancholic features: relative efficacy of tricyclics versus selective serotonin reuptake inhibitor antidepressants. Journal of Affective Disorders 39: 1–6

Perry P J, Alexander B 1987 Dosage and serum levels. In: Johnson F N (ed) Depression and mania-modern lithium therapy. IRL Press, Oxford, pp 67–73

Petursson H, Lader M H 1981 Withdrawal from long term benzodiazepine treatment. British Medical Journal 283: 643–645

Pisciotta V 1978 Drug-induced agranulocytosis. Drugs 15: 132–143

Poust R I 1987 Kinetics and tissue distribution. In: Johnson F N (ed) Depression and mania–modern lithium therapy. IRL Press, Oxford, pp 73–75

Power K G, Jerrom D W A, Simpsom R J et al 1985 Controlled study of withdrawal symptoms and rebound anxiety after six week course of diazepam for generalised anxiety. British Medical Journal 290: 1246–1248

Preskorn S H 1993a Introduction–Pharmacokinetics of psychotropic agents: why and how they are relevant to treatment. Journal of Clinical Psychiatry 54 (suppl 9): 3–7

Preskorn S H 1993b Pharmacokinetics of antidepressants: why and how they are relevant to treatment. Journal of Clinical Psychiatry 54 (suppl 9): 14–34

Quitkin F M, Stewart J W, McGrath P J et al 1993 Columbia atypical depression. British Journal of Psychiatry 163 (suppl 21): 30–34

Rabkin J G, Quitkin F M, McGrath P et al 1985 Adverse reactions to monoamine oxidase inhibitors: II. Treatment correlates and clinical management. Journal of Clinical Psychopharmacology 5: 2–9

Ray W A, Griffin M R, Schaffner W et al 1987 Psychotropic drug use and the risk of hip fracture. New England Journal of Medicine 316: 333–339

Regal R E, Billi J E, Glazer H M 1987 Phenothiazine-induced cholestatic jaundice. Clinical Pharmacy 6: 787–794

Richelson E 1996 Synaptic effects of antidepressants. Journal of Clinical Psychopharmacology 16 (suppl 2): 1s–9s

Richens A 1983 Clinical pharmacokinetics of benzodiazepines. In: Trimble M R (ed) Benzodiazepines divided. Wiley, Chichester, pp 187–205

Rogers S L, Friedhoff L T and the Donepezil Study Group 1996 The efficacy and safety of donepezil in patients with Alzheimer's disease: results of a US multi-centre, randomized, double-blind, placebo-controlled trial. Dementia 7: 293–303

Roose S P, Glassman A H, Giardina E G V et al 1987 Tricyclic antidepressants in depressed patients with cardiac conduction disease. Archives of General Psychiatry 44: 273–275

Roy T M, Ossorio M A, Cipolla L M et al 1989 Pulmonary complications after tricyclic antidepressant overdose. Chest 96: 852–856

Rudorfer M V 1992 Monoamine oxidase inhibitors: reversible and irreversible. Psychopharmacology Bulletin 28: 45–57

Rudorfer M V, Potter W Z 1987 Pharmacokinetics of antidepressants. In: Meltzer H Y (ed) Psychopharmacology – the third generation of progress. Raven Press, New York, pp 1353–1363

Schneider L S 1996 New therapeutic approaches to Alzheimer's Disease. Journal of Clinical Psychiatry 57 (suppl 14): 30–36

Schou M, Baastrup P C, Grof P et al 1970 Pharmacological and clinical problems of lithium prophylaxis. British Journal of Psychiatry 116: 615–619

Shalev A, Hermesh H, Munitz H 1989 Mortality from neuroleptic malignant syndrome. Journal of Clinical Psychiatry 50: 18–25

Shelley R, Silverstone T 1987 Lithium preparations. In: Johnson F N (ed) Depression and mania–modern lithium therapy. IRL Press, Oxford, pp 94–98

Shvaloff A, Neuman E, Guez D 1996 Lines of therapeutic research in Alzheimer's Disease. Psychopharmacology Bulletin 32: 343–352

Silverstone T, Smith G, Goodall E 1988 Prevalence of obesity in patients receiving depot antipsychotics. British Journal of Psychiatry 153: 214–217

Skowron D M, Stimmel G L 1992 Antidepressants and the risk of seizures. Pharmacotherapy 12: 18–22

Smith W M, Gallagher J J 1980 'Les torsades de pointes' – an unusual ventricular arrhythmia. Annals of Internal Medicine 93: 578–584

Sternbach L H 1983 The discovery of CNS active 1, 4-benzodiazepines. In: Costa E (ed) The benzodiazepines: from molecular biology to clinical practice. Raven Press, New York, pp 1–6

Thomsen K, Schou M 1975 The treatment of lithium poisoning. In: Johnson F N (ed) Lithium research and therapy. Academic Press, London, pp 227–236

Tyrer P, Rutherford D, Huggett T 1981 Benzodiazepine withdrawal symptoms and propranolol. Lancet i: 520–522

Vacaflor L 1975 Lithium side effects and toxicity: the clinical picture. In: Johnson F N (ed) Lithium research and therapy. Academic Press, London, pp 211–225

Walker R G, Kincaid-Smith P 1987 Kidneys and the fluid regulatory system. In: Johnson F N (ed) Depression and mania–modern lithium therapy. IRL Press, Oxford, pp 206–213

Warner M D, Peabody C A, Whiteford H A et al 1987 Trazodone and priapism. Journal of Clinical Psychiatry 48: 244–245

Warnock J K 1991 Psychotropic medication and drug-related alopecia. Psychosomatics 32: 149–152

Weekly R D, Potts A M, Reboton J et al 1960 Pigmentary retinopathy in patients receiving high doses of a new phenothiazine. Archives of Ophthalmology 64: 95–106

Weinstein M R 1980 Lithium treatment of women during pregnancy and in the post-delivery period. In: Johnson F N (ed) Handbook of lithium therapy. MTP Press, Lancaster, pp 421–429

Wilder B J 1992 Pharmacokinetics of valproate and carbamazepine. Journal of Clinical Psychopharmacology 12 (suppl 1): 64s–68s

Wilt J L, Minnema A M, Johnson R F et al 1993 Torsade de pointes associated with the use of intravenous haloperidol. Annals of Internal Medicine 119: 391–394

Yoshida K, Kumar R 1996 Breast feeding and psychotropic drugs. International Review of Psychiatry 8: 117–124

Yoshida K, Smith B, Craggs M et al 1997 Investigation of pharmacokinetics and of possible adverse effects in infants exposed to tricyclic antidepressants in breast-milk. Journal of Affective Disorders 43: 225–237

Young R C 1991 Hydroxylated metabolites of antidepressants. Psychopharmacology Bulletin 27: 521–531

Zucker S, Zarrabi H M, Schubach W H et al 1990 Chlorpromazine-induced immunopathy: progressive increase in serum IgM. Medicine 69: 92–100

5

Research design, measurement and statistics

John C. Duffy   Diana P. Morrison   David F. Peck

RESEARCH DESIGN

There are few publications which cover this area in psychiatry. Most of those available date from the 1960s and 1970s, although Freeman & Tyrer (1992) have recently edited an excellent introductory textbook. It is clear from reviewing the available literature that there has been enormous change over the last few decades in the design of research in psychiatry, with increasing sophistication and a greater acceptance of the need for properly designed studies which utilise appropriate statistical methods.

The point has been well made by Pond (1975), that 'no amount of theoretical sophistication makes up for barrenness of ideas and sloppy ways of working' and that much clinical research is rightly little more than an extension of high quality but routine clinical work. The best research projects are often relatively simple.

It is important to discuss possible research projects as early as possible with experienced colleagues in order to seek advice and assistance. Some otherwise good research ideas may not be feasible because of lack of subjects, time or facilities (McGuire 1993).

Putting together a study protocol

Before writing the protocol it often helps to clarify the purpose of the study if the idea is condensed by describing the aims, design, hypothesis and methods on one side of an A4 sheet. It then becomes substantially easier to write the study protocol (Table 5.1).

Literature survey

This describes the background to, and rationale for, the study and supports the basis of the hypotheses to be tested. It involves an objective review (p. 191) of the relevant literature for the following reasons:

- To establish whether the questions to be studied have been addressed by others and, if so, the extent

Table 5.1   Components of a study protocol
<ul><li>Background and rationale (including a review of the relevant literature and description of pilot studies)</li><li>Aims</li><li>Hypotheses to be tested</li><li>Design (blindness, randomisation, controls, parallel group or other comparisons)</li><li>Method (population selection, dosage and duration of treatments, diagnostic classification, assessment of outcome , statistical analysis to be used)</li><li>Patient information sheet and consent form</li></ul>

to which they have been answered by previous research.
- To determine whether, if the questions have already been answered, there is any useful purpose in replicating earlier work.
- To assess if the hypotheses are compatible and consistent with published research.
- To describe, and provide the results from, any pilot studies which have been carried out.

Pilot studies are normally conducted in advance of the main study, with a small group of subjects. They allow researchers to familiarise themselves with the study procedure, including the administration of any scales which are to be used. The pilot study can also be a useful method of assessing whether it will be possible to recruit the number of patients required to permit the study to be carried out in the time available. This can allow for adjustment of the selection criteria if these prove to be too restrictive. Pilot studies can be used to ensure that the design is feasible, which is particularly important if substantial funding is required to complete the study. They allow the design to be adjusted before embarking on the main study and this can often save considerable time and effort in the longer term. If no major alterations to the protocol are required as a consequence of the pilot study, the results can also be amalgamated with the results of the main study. The results of pilot studies which support the hypotheses being tested lend considerable credence to the project as a whole (Fava & Rosenbaum 1992).

Aims

These must be described clearly and simply. The objectives should be limited to the smallest number possible, preferably no more than three. Similarly, in a treatment study there should be a small number of end-points and one of these should be selected as definitive. The objectives and end-points should determine the study design and should be followed through in the study's statistical plan. The only exception to this is in complex situations where multiple indices are required to describe outcome accurately. However, multiple indices will make it much more difficult to analyse the results (pp 174 and 190–191).

Hypotheses

The hypotheses to be tested in the study should be stated concisely, conventionally in the form of 'null hypotheses' (p. 168–169).

Study design

Observational studies

Traditionally, many studies in psychiatry and psychology have been non-experimental in nature. There is no treatment, and no allocation of subjects to particular conditions. Instead, a group of subjects is studied, and a number of measurements (variables) made on each. Interest may lie in establishing summary values of the variables for normative purposes, or in the associations between the variables, perhaps with a view to predicting values of one particular variable from the rest, or examining the structure of interrelationships between the variables. In an observational study there really is no possibility of establishing causal relationships between the variables, far less the direction of causality. However, such studies may give useful clues to causality, which may be followed up by experimentation, or more intensive observational study.

The points made later in connection with specification of populations and measurements to be made apply just as strongly to observational as to experimental studies – it is, after all, important that the researcher and the readers of research are quite clear as to whom the research purports to apply.

The simplest observational study would focus on a clearly defined group of individuals, and equally clearly defined measurements would be made on these individuals. Thus an observational study of students might be undertaken, but the question arises as to how to select students for study. In general, the ideal situation is that a specified target population is defined. This is the population to which the results of the research are to apply. A sample of this population is then taken, by statistical means, and many readers will have heard the expression 'random sample'. A simple random sample is a sample of individuals from the target population such that each possible sample is equally likely; the selection is by processes analogous to 'drawing names out of a hat'.

Realistically, however, this is an impossible counsel of perfection in much applied research. If one wished to study depressed individuals, how could one construct a list of people suffering from depression in order to sample from it? Presumably many undetected cases will exist in the community. If one were to be more specific, and decided to restrict attention to hospital-treated depression, there is still the problem of obtaining a list of all the people who have ever been treated in hospital for this condition. In practice, what is often studied is a convenience sample of individuals suffering from depression in a single hospital, or perhaps a few hospitals. It should be borne in mind that as a result the possibility exists that these individuals are unrepresentative of the population of hospital-treated depressives, and no amount of statistical manipulation can justify generalisation to this larger population.

Needless to say, such studies may often have a comparative aspect – pursuing the particular example further, the researcher might wish to compare male and female depressed patients. Once again, the results of such comparison might be seriously incorrect. Suppose, for example, that women were more likely to be hospitalised for depression than men who are equally ill. A study in hospital would show that female patients appeared to be less depressed than male. However, this result need not be true of depressed people in general.

There are of course more complicated types of descriptive studies than those considered above. Two designs of particular interest in epidemiology are the cohort, or prospective study, and the case–control study.

Prospective study One way of assessing the influence of a suspected risk factor on illness is to follow two groups over time, a group exposed to the factor, and the other group not exposed. If more of those exposed to the factor develop the illness, then this is evidence of association between the factor and the illness, and may be a result of a causal relation.

The rates of illness among the exposed and unexposed may be estimated from cohort studies, and the ratio of these rates is called the 'relative risk' due to exposure.

Case–control study In a case–control study the researcher compares a group of individuals with the disease in question (cases) with a group without the disease (controls) in terms of their status on a variable or a number of variables which are thought to be possible risk factors for the disease in question. The numbers in the case and control groups are determined by the investigator, and therefore such studies do not permit direct estimation of the rates of illness among those exposed or not exposed to the possible risk factors. Nevertheless, it should be clear that if the proportion of cases with the variable in question is higher than the proportion of controls with the variable, then the variable may indeed be a risk factor for the disease. In fact, the odds ratio, page 179, can be estimated from a case–control study, and if the disease in question is relatively rare, the odds ratio will approximate the relative risk. However, as noted earlier, case–control studies cannot by themselves prove causality.

Apart from the putative risk factors under investigation, other variables such as age, sex and unknown risk factors may affect the probability of developing illness, and may also be associated with presence of the risk factor. Such variables are said to be _confounding_ and one way to take account of known confounding factors is by individually matching each case to a control who shares the potentially confounding characteristics of the case. The resulting study design, the matched case–control study is rather different from the previous types considered, and data analysis is different also.

Experimental studies

The aim of study design is to increase precision, to control as many extraneous aspects as possible and to reduce the influence of bias and random variation. These aspects are most clearly illustrated by consideration of experimental studies.

Blindness Studies may be _open_ where the treatment is known to both subject and observer, _single-blind_ where the treatment is known to the observer only and _double-blind_ where neither the subject nor the observer knows which treatment the subject is receiving. Double-blind studies reduce inadvertent investigator bias in rating the response to treatment or adverse events.

Randomisation When comparing groups of subjects having different treatments, differences in outcome may be due to differences between the groups other than the treatment which they have received.

In clinical research, subjects are heterogeneous, both in their presentation and in their response to treatment. This can be taken into account if the assignment of treatment to any individual is done using a chance mechanism. This means that each subject has the same opportunity of receiving any of the treatments under study and neither the subject nor the researcher knows which treatment he or she will receive in advance. This eliminates bias on the part of the physician in the allocation of treatment and of subject self-selection for the various treatments on offer. It also helps to balance unknown biases amongst the treatment groups and is the foundation for statistical analysis of the data. Randomisation is an essential technique whether the study is open or blind (Zelen 1992).

Controls Controls are those research subjects who do not receive the treatment under investigation in order to afford a comparison group for those who do. If in a randomised trial there is a difference in therapeutic response so that those receiving active treatment do better than those not receiving it, it is likely that the improvement results from receipt of the treatment, as this is the only important difference between the circumstances of the two groups. Control groups allow the researcher to take account of spontaneous recovery in the case of transient or cyclic conditions, placebo effects, seasonal variation, etc. When a new treatment is under investigation control subjects may receive the standard treatment, but in some cases, controls receive a 'dummy' treatment known to be inactive. Such a treatment is known as a placebo.

Controls may be concurrent, where the control group is selected at the same time as the experimental group and where there is a prospective comparison with active treatment. When this is not possible, individual patients can be used as their own control – for example in the case of chronic diseases where each of two treatments being compared is given to the same patient at separate times. The order in which the treatments are given is usually chosen at random. Historical controls compare current subjects with others who have previously been treated and for whom the results are already known. Using historical or retrospective controls of this type is less than ideal, as many aspects of their care and treatment may have been different (e.g. supportive care, patient management, the diagnosis, the severity of the illness and the patient evaluations). There may not be sufficient information to allow proper comparison with the prospective sample. Using historical controls is likely to lead to an overestimate of the efficacy of a new treatment but can be useful if only a limited number of subjects are available for a prospective study (Everitt 1989). The use of matched controls attempts to take account of variables such as age, sex, severity and others which may affect outcome by individually matching each treated subject to a control who shares these characteristics. As will be seen later, data analysis for matched designs differs from that for unmatched designs.

Group comparisons

Having randomised subjects to treatment, treatment differences should not be confounded by differences in background factors with prognostic importance for efficacy or for adverse events. There are various forms of group comparisons.

Parallel groups Each subject is assigned to either the experimental or the comparative treatment, which continues throughout the study. This has certain advantages in that there is one treatment period per subject and few assumptions are required for the statistical analysis. However, variation between subjects is an important consideration and a greater number of patients may be required to achieve prescribed levels of statistical power (see p. 186).

Crossover design In a crossover study the experimental treatment and comparative treatment(s) are given to the same subjects in sequence. As the order in which treatments are given may affect the results, each patient receives the treatments in random order. There may be a 'carry over' of treatment effect from one period to the next so that the results of the second treatment are affected by the first. Subjects must complete all treatment periods, otherwise analysis of the data becomes very complicated. Keeping treatment periods as short as possible can help to reduce drop-outs (Altman 1991b).

Factorial design In the simplest case we may consider two treatments, A and B, which are to be compared with each other, their combination, and a control. Subjects are divided into four groups who receive the control treatment, A only, B only and A and B together. This type of design can be extended to the case of several factors, and each factor may be applied at a number of levels (e.g. doses of a drug). Statistical tests of associations between response and each factor and interactions between factors can be performed.

Sequential design Parallel groups are studied but the trial only continues until a clear benefit of one treatment is seen or it becomes clear that no difference between treatments will be found. If there is a large difference between the effectiveness of the two treatments the trial duration is shortened. The data are analysed as each patient's results become available and this technique is therefore only suitable when the individual outcome is known quickly. Blinding the study can be difficult. In a group sequential design the data are analysed after each block of patients has been treated. This allows the trial to be stopped early if a clear difference is seen between treatments (Altman 1991b).

Methodological problems

Study population

The population selected for study will usually be defined by certain attributes, e.g. age, sex, etc. Restriction of the population will result in difficulty in recruitment and can also produce an atypical population from which it is impossible to generalise to the majority of patients.

It is important to review recruitment sources as there is a general tendency to be overoptimistic about the number of subjects which can be studied. Once inclusion and exclusion criteria have been established, the number of subjects who are available for inclusion in the study tends to fall dramatically. It is important when constructing inclusion and exclusion criteria to avoid selection biases, e.g. the inclusion of many treatment-refractory subjects will lead to lower response rates and thereby decrease the chances of obtaining a statistically significant difference between groups. Conversely, advertising will produce a higher number of treatment-naive subjects who are more likely to respond to treatment or placebo.

If particular characteristics of groups are thought to be likely to influence the response to treatment, it is possible to stratify the groups prospectively and analyse appropriately. This aspect of design, if used, should be clearly specified in advance of data collection.

Placebo response / responders

These individuals show a substantial non-specific improvement within a few days of starting treatment. Including a phase where placebo is given, single-blind, at the beginning of the study can help to identify placebo responders who may sometimes be excluded from the active phase of treatment. Alternatively, pattern analysis can be used. That is, with many types of psychotropic medication specific drug effects are most likely to occur after approximately 2 weeks of treatment and responses thereafter are stable. Placebo responses by contrast tend to occur early and fluctuate. Analysing the pattern of response can be used to identify the subjects who are most likely to be placebo responders. Similarly, incorporating a placebo crossover phase in the study or extending the period of follow-up can both establish the contribution made by placebo responders to the result.

Parallel group designs in which an active treatment is

compared with placebo can demonstrate that the active treatment has an effect. However, the size of the effect can only be determined by comparison with standard treatment. The optimum solution therefore, when a sufficient sample size is available, is to compare new treatments with both placebo and an available standard treatment (Fava & Rosenbaum 1992). (For ethical implications see p. 154).

Establishing the diagnosis

It is critical to use a reliable and valid method for establishing diagnosis to reduce unwanted sample heterogeneity. The optimal classification system will define diagnostic groups correctly and decide which group any individual patient belongs to. Random misclassification biases results towards the null hypothesis (of no difference between groups) by diluting the effects of treatment. It also reduces the effective sample size and therefore the power of the study. Differential misclassification can lead to false conclusions being drawn, either positive or negative. However, the most important issue is whether the effects of misclassification are balanced across the groups studied.

The best way to deal with misclassification is to avoid it, using the following strategies:

- Standardised study procedures, e.g. specify clear diagnostic criteria using formal instruments and train raters in the use of these instruments.
- With studies which continue over a long period of time, it may be necessary to review inter-rater reliability periodically.
- Use multiple sources of information, e.g. clinical interviews, hospital records and family history data, when establishing the diagnosis.
- Successfully blinding studies means that participants' responses and investigative evaluations are not distorted by preconceptions about the study hypotheses (Blacker 1992).

Dose selection and duration of treatment

In drug trials, fixed-dose studies are those in which dosage is kept constant throughout. This ensures consistency across study groups. A dosage titration phase with a stepwise increase in dosage can be incorporated at the beginning of treatment to minimise side-effects and to reduce the number of patients who drop out of the study because of these. Flexible-dose studies incorporate a series of dose levels which patients can move through, depending upon the need to increase efficacy or reduce side-effects. Flexible-dose studies improve compliance and help to reduce the number of drop-outs due to adverse events.

Compliance can be improved further if transient concomitant medication to reduce side-effects is incorporated into the protocol. A high rate of drop-outs (see pp 201, 206) will increase the number of patients required to ensure that a sufficient number complete the study to permit statistical analysis. With oral treatment, compliance measures are essential to ensure that medication is being taken as prescribed. Poor compliance with treatment will undermine or invalidate study results. Compliance measures may be simple, e.g. counting tablets at each visit to check that medication has been taken as prescribed and questioning patients about their adherence to the study protocol. Alternatively, blood and urine samples can be taken to check for the presence of medication or its metabolites. In most cases this can only determine whether medication has been taken, not whether the subject has taken it according to the dosage schedule prescribed.

The duration of the study is normally determined by the time taken to achieve an effect with the medications/treatments being assessed. As indicated above, extending the length of the trial can help to reduce placebo response.

Assessment of efficacy and safety

Analysis of the results can be simplified by keeping the number of outcome variables as small as possible. If a large number of variables are compared across groups it is likely that some differences may be found by chance alone (pp 190 and 191).

The methods of assessment must be precise, reliable and administered consistently throughout the study. The selection of instruments depends upon the population being studied, the condition that patients suffer from and the treatments under investigation. The instruments must reflect the primary goals of the study and should normally be in general use in psychiatric research to facilitate comparison with published results. The measures used must be able to detect treatment effects, be repeatable, quick and simple to use and as objective as possible. The choice of instrument is discussed in more detail in the section on measurement.

Patients who withdraw from the study prematurely (often referred to as drop-outs) must be investigated carefully. Actual reasons for premature withdrawal must be ascertained and compared across the treatment groups.

Intention to treat analysis involves comparing the groups originally randomised, whether or not all the patients complete the treatment to which they are randomised. Any other policy towards drop-outs will involve subjective decisions and will create an opportunity for bias (Altman 1991b).

Sample size

It is essential to estimate in advance how many subjects will be required to permit the study to have a high probability of showing a significant difference between groups if that difference exists. It is just as important to avoid recruiting too many subjects as too few, as this is a waste of human and financial resources. Measurement error also decreases with increasing numbers. It is important that the instruments selected to assess the outcome of the study are specific and sensitive enough to detect statistically significant effects given the likely effect size of the treatments under study (p. 186).

Statistical analysis

It is essential to discuss the proposed study with a statistician as early as possible. The protocol must include a detailed description of the planned statistical analysis, including power calculations based on effect size for the relevant outcome measures. This is discussed in more detail in the section on statistics.

Ethics

Improperly planned and improperly conducted research is unethical, as are unnecessary studies. The foreseeable benefits of the research must be weighed against predictable risks, with the interests of the subjects prevailing over science and society. The ethical obligation to prevent deterioration is always paramount (Everitt 1989).

All research projects involving human subjects must be approved by an independent local Ethics committee before the study starts. Ethics committees consider the scientific soundness of the project, the risk versus individual and general benefits, the ability of the researcher to carry out the study, the medical supervision of subjects during and after the study, the patient information leaflet and consent form for the study and the procedures for confidentiality.

Informed consent

This should be obtained before any study-related procedures are undertaken. The term 'informed consent' implies that the patient is able to understand the information given and to draw relevant conclusions regarding the risks and benefits of the study. Information should be given both orally and in writing. Obtaining consent should normally be delegated to an independent clinician who is not involved in the research being

undertaken. This person can also serve as a source of impartial advice and information regarding the study for the patient. Difficulties arise in the case of patients who are too ill or damaged to give informed consent; these are not easily circumvented, and, in particular, it should not be assumed that proxy consent will be ethically sufficient.

Patient information sheet

This describes the purpose of the study, explains the benefits and risks to the patient of taking part, and should discuss the use of comparative treatments and, if appropriate, of placebo. The language in the patient information sheet and in the written consent form must be plain and technical terms avoided to make it easier for the patient to understand what is involved. The sheet must describe any inconvenience to the subject, e.g. dietary restrictions during the study, the number of visits expected at the clinic and the number of blood tests to be taken, etc. It must be made explicit that the patient does not have to take part in the study and that if they do take part they are free to withdraw at any time without giving any explanation. It must also be made clear that if patients withdraw or do not wish to take part, their current or future treatment will not be prejudiced in any way. Patients should be aware that personal information collected will be regarded as strictly confidential and will not be made publicly available.

The ethics of placebo control groups

It has been suggested that it is only morally justifiable to put patients into placebo-controlled studies if the following conditions are met:

- There is genuine uncertainty as to whether the proposed treatment is more likely to help patients than placebo.
- There is no agreed alternative treatment of more value than placebo.
- It must be important to know whether the new treatment is better than placebo.
- There must be a reasonable possibility that the proposed treatment will be better than placebo.
- The illness must not be so serious that any delay in receiving active treatment would be harmful or dangerous (Evans & Evans 1996).

Methods of data collection

Data may be obtained directly from the subjects concerned, or from staff or relatives, or examining subject records.

Personal interview

This approach can generate high-quality data with a high response rate and allows more data to be collected than with any other method. It is possible to ask probe and follow-up questions to obtain information with greater depth. Personal interviews require experienced interviewers, or else training and practice must be provided for interviewers before the study starts. This is the most expensive method of data collection and also the most time consuming.

Telephone interview

This is quick, convenient and reasonably cheap but the number of questions which can be asked is restricted and it may be is difficult to obtain highly sensitive information in a telephone call. Telephone interviews may be computer-assisted, whereby the interviewer asks questions indicated on the computer screen, and records responses directly into a computer file.

Computer interview

With the recent development of small portable computers it is now feasible for subjects to complete questionnaires by direct interaction with a computer program. This method may increase truthfulness of responses compared to direct personal interview if stigmatising or socially undesirable characteristics are being investigated.

Mailed questionnaires

These allow information to be collected from a large number of respondents very quickly. The main disadvantages are that follow-up questions are generally not possible and the response rate tends to be low. Even when self-addressed stamped envelopes and follow-up letters are used the response rate is normally only 40–60%, and can be much lower. This makes it very difficult to generalise from respondents to non-respondents.

Record reviews

This involves extracting data which was not originally collected for research purposes. This can be done in a prospective way but is more usually done retrospectively. The main problems are incompleteness and inaccuracy of the data. This method is best avoided unless comparable data are unavailable from other sources.

The main principle is not to collect more information than is required. It can often be helpful to go through the list of data to be collected item by item, checking on the purpose of each and considering how the data collected will be analysed statistically. No single study can resolve all the unanswered questions in an area and it is better to address one issue comprehensively than several superficially.

If self-report measures are to be used (e.g. visual analogue scales, see p. 162) the wording must be clear and unambiguous and the vocabulary used must be comprehensible to the subject. A pilot study can be helpful in achieving this aim. It is important to use clear instructions, including what the subjects should do if they do not know the answer to a particular question or do not feel the question is applicable to them. Response rates can be improved by making participation as attractive as possible – for example, by explaining the importance of the study at the outset and giving the respondent a realistic estimate of the time it will take to complete the questionnaire. Again it can often be helpful to reassure subjects that responses will be anonymous and confidential.

Screening for psychiatric morbidity in community samples

Use of self-administered questionnaires allows large numbers of the population to be screened (Table 5.2).

General Health Questionnaire (GHQ) (Shepherd et al *1981)* This is used to screen for non-psychotic illness. The GHQ has 60 items and takes approximately 10–15 minutes to complete. The instrument has satisfactory sensitivity and specificity – these terms are defined on page 156. A high score indicates that psychiatric morbidity is likely but need not equate to a specific diagnosis. A shorter (32 item) version is also available.

Iowa Structured Interview (Tsuang et al *1980)* This was developed for epidemiological research in the general population. It assesses current psychiatric symptoms. There are 20 core screening questions for depression, mania, schizophrenia and neurosis. It can be used by trained non-medical personnel. It has good validity and inter-rater reliability for depression, mania and schizophrenia but less so for neurosis. It is particularly recommended for long-term follow-up and family studies of affective disorders and schizophrenia.

Achieving diagnostic homogeneity

The reliability of diagnosis relates to agreement (between scales or raters or tests on different occasions) and implies diagnostic consistency. The validity of diagnosis describes the extent to which it corresponds to a gold standard or, if a gold standard does not exist, how

Table 5.2	General morbidity scales		
Name	Authors	No. of items	Main features
General Health Questionnaire (GHQ)	Goldberg (1972)	60 12, 20 and 30 item versions also available	Self-administered screening tool Questions refer to past 4 weeks Detect non-psychotic psychiatric illness Cut-off point of 11 (60 item) and 5 (30 item) identifies a case
Iowa Structured Interview	Tsuang et al (1980)	235	Extensive personal and family history section Administered by trained non-medical interviewer Designed for epidemiological research in general population Twenty core questions for mania, schizophrenia, depression and neurosis

well these diagnoses correspond with external validators such as concurrent symptoms, course of illness, diagnostic stability, treatment response, familial pattern and biological markers. High reliability does not necessarily imply high validity.

The reliability of diagnosis can be estimated by assessing test–retest reliability, in which interviews of the same subject on two occasions are compared, and by inter-rater reliability in which the same interview is rated independently by two raters and the results compared. It is important to realise that the latter is simply a measure of agreement between the raters concerned – that is the raters may agree, but both may be in error.

Validity can be assessed in comparison to a gold standard which Spitzer (1983) has suggested is LEAD, i.e. Longitudinal Expert All Data Diagnosis. The sensitivity of the instrument is the probability of diagnosing disease when present; the specificity is the probability of not diagnosing disease when absent. Establishing the number and duration of symptoms required for diagnosis involves a trade-off between sensitivity and specificity. As the threshold for making the diagnosis is lowered, the sensitivity of the measure increases but the specificity is reduced. There are many other measures of validity, including:

- Criterion validity: how valid is the diagnosis when judged against one or more external validators ?
- Face validity: are the criteria used overtly related to the diagnosis?
- Construct validity: the conceptual soundness of the diagnosis and its consistency with available data.
- Predictive validity: can the diagnosis be used to accurately predict outcome or other patient-related events?

Diagnostic instruments usually have published estimates of reliability and validity, and the sensitivity and specificity of the instruments can be checked on a subsample of the population (Blacker 1992). It cannot be assumed that an instrument which is reliable in one particular situation will be so in all others.

Structured and semistructured interviews

Data on psychiatric disorders may be collected using specific diagnostic criteria. Their effectiveness has a major impact on the validity of research results. In the past, as different clinicians used different diagnostic criteria, it was difficult to compare patients diagnosed by different clinicians. Some of the most commonly used interviews are summarised in Table 5.3.

Present State Examination (PSE) (Wing et al 1974) The PSE is a structured interview which identifies both symptoms and behaviours and has precise rules for classification to ensure consistency of diagnosis. The PSE has been used to standardise the recording of mental state examinations from patients of different cultures, permitting comparison of research findings. It can also be used to measure change.

The PSE measures symptoms present during the previous month and there is also a syndrome checklist for symptoms present previously. At interview, symptoms are rated on the basis of affect, behaviour and speech.

There are 140 items which provide:

- a symptom score
- a syndrome score (on 20 psychotic and 16 neurotic syndromes)
- quantitative subscores derived from the syndrome score

Table 5.3 Diagnostic schedules

Name	Authors	Main features
Present State Examination and CATEGO Program (PSE)	Wing et al (1974)	Structured mental state interview which does not use historical information Provides descriptive symptom and syndrome profiles. Requires trained clinician CATEGO computer program classifies mental state data (can be compared to ICD groups)
Schedule for Affective Disorders and Schizophrenia (SADS)	Endicott & Spitzer (1978)	Interview designed to elicit information necessary for making RDC diagnosis Diagnosis is either present or absent Takes $1\frac{1}{2}$–2 hours to complete Three versions: SADS, SADS-L and SADS-C Requires trained psychiatrist, psychologist or social worker
National Institute of Mental Health Diagnostic Interview Schedule (NIMH DIS)	Robins et al (1979)	Designed to be used with Feighner's criteria – may be scored according to RDC Structured fixed phrasing interview, lasting 1–$1\frac{1}{2}$ hours. No diagnostic hierarchy imposed Diagnosis present, probable or absent Trained clinicians or non-clinicians
Structured Clinical Interview for DSM-IIIR (SCID)	Spitzer et al (1987)	Semistructured interview in two parts, i.e. present and past illness Diagnosis present or absent Requires trained clinician Takes 1/2–1 hour to complete
Composite International Diagnostic Interview (CIDI)	Robins et al (1988)	Combination of DIS and PSE. Incorporates Feighner, RDC, ICD-10 and DSM-IIIR criteria Trained clinicians or non-clinicians.

- qualitative total scores. A computer programme designates one of 12 CATEGO classes which are approximately equivalent to a diagnosis.

Raters must receive standardised training by established practitioners before the PSE is used. Reliability is good (Wing et al 1974).

Schedule for Affective Disorders and Schizophrenia (SADS) (Endicott & Spitzer 1978) A semistructured interview.

'Feighner Criteria' (Feighner et al 1972) These describe 15 psychiatric disorders in clear clinical terms which showed consistency over time.

Research Diagnostic Criteria (RDC) (Spitzer et al 1978) These were developed from the Feighner criteria which were expanded to include a further 10 diagnostic categories.

The SADS was designed to operationalise the RDC (Endicott & Spitzer 1978). Questions about each symptom are supplied, together with suggested probe questions. The interview is in two parts:

1. The current episode and function in the week before interview
2. Past psychiatric disturbance.

Interviewers decide on whether the symptom is present and, if so, its severity. It is intended for use by trained clinicians. Several versions are available for specific disorders and for making lifetime diagnoses.

Everyone using the SADS uses the same diagnostic criteria and has the same amount of information available on which to base the diagnosis (Robins et al 1979).

Diagnostic Interview Schedule (DIS) This was developed for a large epidemiological survey in the community where using clinicians as interviewers would have been too expensive. The DIS was devised for lay interviewers and operationalised the Feighner criteria (Helzer et al 1981). It is highly structured, i.e. all the questions are provided and are read out exactly as written. There is a set probing pattern and precise instructions about skipping questions. The DIS is respondent based and the respondent, not the interviewer, is responsible for the answer noted on the schedule.

Structured Clinical Interview for the DSM-IIIR (SCID) The SCID (Spitzer et al 1990) is less structured and considerable clinical knowledge is required to administer it. In research the SCID is usually used to ensure that the subjects in the study population have a disorder which meets DSM-IIIR criteria. It may also be used to exclude subjects with certain disorders and to obtain current and past psychiatric diagnoses.

The SCID begins with a brief overview of the present illness and an enquiry about past episodes of psychopathology. Open-ended questions encourage subjects to expand their answers. The interviewer is expected to make a clinical judgement rather than accept the respondent's views.

Composite International Diagnostic Interview (CIDI) (Robins et al 1988) This is a combination of the Diagnostic Interview Schedule (DIS) and the Present State Examination (PSE). It incorporates ICD-10, the Feighner, RDC and DSM-IIIR criteria (Reich 1992). It contains 276 symptom questions and also has probe questions. It is intended primarily for epidemiological studies but can also be used clinically. Test–retest and inter-rater reliability are good (Wittchen 1994).

MEASUREMENT

The most important consideration is the selection of an appropriate variable which will form the outcome of the study. Once selected, the measurement procedure used to assign numbers (scores) to that variable is normally evaluated with respect to its reliability and validity. The stability and precision with which an instrument can be used to assign scores is a function not only of the instrument itself but also of the situation and of the conditions in which it is used.

Developing a satisfactory measuring instrument can be a difficult and time-consuming part of the study, and it is normally more cost-effective to use an existing measure. Using a wide variety of instruments across different studies to measure the same variable can make generalising results and replicating the work of others extremely difficult.

Scales of measurement

Nominal or categorical data

Nominal measurement is the process of classifying different individuals or objects into categories based on a clearly defined characteristic. The categories are mutually exclusive (i.e. an individual can belong only to one category) and have no logical order. An everyday example would be colour of eyes, while in psychiatry type of disorder would be a nominal measure. Binary measures, which take only the values 0 or 1 (e.g. presence or absence of a symptom) constitute an important special case of categorical data.

Ordinal scales

This type of scale has the additional property that the categories are logically ordered and the numbers assigned to the categories indicate the amount of a characteristic possessed. For example, a psychiatrist may grade a patient on the Clinicians Global Impression scale as not at all ill, mildly ill, moderately ill, severely ill, or extremely ill, and use numbers to label the categories, with the lower numbers indicating lesser severity of illness. However, it cannot be said that the clinical difference between patients with scores of 0 and 1 is the same as for patients with scores of 4 and 5.

Interval scales

Differences between points in the scale reflect equal differences in the characteristic being measured. The zero point is simply another point in the scale and does not represent the starting point of the scale or the total absence of the characteristic, e.g. the Fahrenheit scale of temperature.

Ratio scales

This type of scale has a true zero point which represents an absence of the characteristic being measured, e.g. weight, where not only is the difference between 100 kg and 50 kg the same as that between 75 kg and 25 kg but an object weighing 100 kg can be said to be twice as heavy as one weighing 50 kg.

With nominal data the number of individuals falling into each category may be counted, and with ordinal data the individuals can be ranked in increasing or decreasing order. However, with interval and ratio scales the figures obtained can be further manipulated, permitting the calculation of means, etc. (Cliff 1982).

It is also important to point out the distinction between discrete and continuous measurements. A discrete measurement is one which naturally takes only whole number values, such as the number of admissions to hospital of a particular patient, the number of first-degree relatives of a patient and so on. This is not to be confused with qualitative data coded as whole number values (e.g. marital status might be coded single = 1, married =2, separated = 3, etc.). Continuous measurements may take any value in an interval – for example, height and weight are everyday examples of continuous data. Weekly income, even though it would actually be a whole number of monetary units, would have so many possible values that it is acceptable to consider it as continuous – and a similar argument is often employed to justify treating scores on rating scales as continuous measurements.

Error is inevitable in any form of measurement. As described earlier, it is important to be aware of this, to minimise it as much as possible and to be able to estimate with reasonable accuracy the extent of measurement error in any given study.

RATING SCALES

Psychiatric information is mainly descriptive and rating scales are used to convert this into numerical data which can be statistically analysed. Scales are often used to measure change during the course of the study. The sensitivity of the scale to small changes in symptoms is therefore important. It is also essential to take into account practical issues like how long the scale takes to administer, bearing in mind the frequency of administration required in the study, whether training is necessary before the scale can be used and finally whether a manual is available (Dennis et al 1992). Figure 5.1 provides an overview of the process involved in selecting an appropriate rating scale.

Rating scales used in schizophrenia

Positive symptoms

Brief Psychiatric Rating Scale (BPRS) (Overall and Graham 1962) This is based on information obtained and behaviour observed at interview. Each item is scored on a 7 point scale (not present, very mild, mild, moderate, moderate to severe, severe, extremely severe). Definitions are given for each item. Ratings are often expressed as the sum of all items. It is quickly completed and it is often used to determine treatment response in drug studies. Inter-rater reliability is high if raters are carefully trained.

Positive and Negative Symptoms Scale (PANSS) (Kay et al 1987) This measures both positive and negative symptoms and general psychopathology. The items are carefully defined in a manual. It takes much longer to complete than the BPRS. Both inter-rater and test–retest reliability can be high and it has been carefully validated against other instruments.

NOSIE (NOSIE 30) (Honigfeld et al 1966, McMordie & Swint, 1979) The Nurses' Observation Scale for Inpatient Evaluation (NOSIE) is designed to be completed by nursing staff and is often used to select patients for treatment programmes and assessment. Analysis produces three positive factors (personal neatness, social competence and social interaction) and three negative factors (manifest psychosis, retardation and irritability). These can be summed to give total scores.

Negative symptoms

Scale for the Assessment of Negative Symptoms (SANS) (Andreasen 1982) This has become the standard against which all other scales are compared. Each group of symptoms is given a global score from 0 to 5. A manual describes both the symptoms and anchor points for the scale. Raters should be clinically trained. Ratings take into account information obtained from staff and family members.

Some of the other most commonly used scales are summarised in Table 5.4.

Rating scales for mania

All the existing scales (Table 5.5) are for use in psychiatrically ill inpatient populations. The Mania Rating Scale (Young et al 1978) is an 11 item, clinician-administered scale which is based on the core symptoms of mania and includes abnormalities which cover the range from mild to severe illness. The scale is reliable, valid and sensitive and appears to function over the entire range of severity of manic illness. It is shorter and more sensitive than the other scales available. Four items (irritability, rate and amount of speech, speech content and disruptive aggressive behaviour) are weighted to compensate for poor cooperation.

The Manic State Rating Scale (Beigel et al 1971) was initially developed for use by nursing staff and is scored according to the frequency and intensity of symptoms.

Rating scales for depression

Hamilton Rating Scale for Depression (Hamilton 1960) This is probably the best known of the rating scales. (Table 5.6). It was not designed as a diagnostic instrument, although some studies use it as such by having a cut-off score to indicate presence of depression. It is

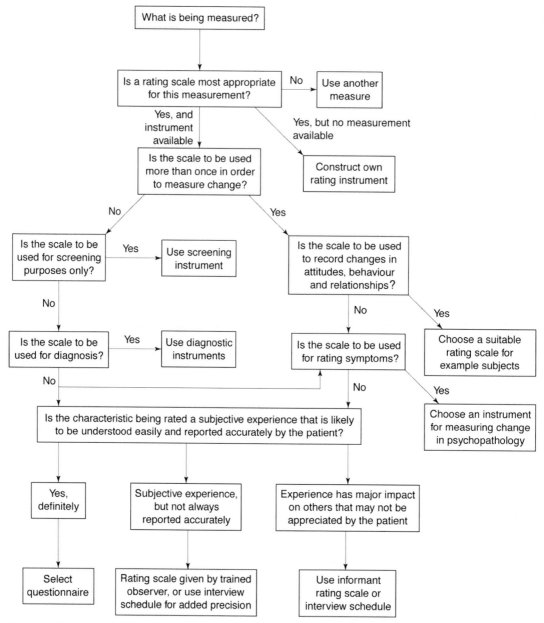

Fig. 5.1 Flow chart for selection of rating instruments in psychiatric research. (Reproduced with permission from Dennis et al 1992)

clinician administered and takes into account not only an interview with the patient but also information from all sources. The original version of the scale comprised 21 items but this was reduced to 17 because depersonalisation/derealisation, paranoia and obsessionality were found to be uncommon and the diurnal variation was felt to be more related to the form of the illness. Most items on the HRSD are graded 0 to 4 but some items, e.g.

insomnia, gastrointestinal symptoms, genital symptoms, insight, weight loss and general somatic symptoms are graded 0 to 2 because it is hard to make fine distinctions.

The main criticisms of the HRSD are that it has a heterogeneous and unstable factor analytic structure, that there is no general factor and that behavioural symptoms and somatic complaints are preferred over self-reported distress (Dennis et al 1992).

Table 5.4 Instruments for assessing negative symptoms in schizophrenia

Title	Authors	Main features
Rating Scale for Emotional Blunting	Abrams & Taylor (1978)	Clinical interview by psychiatrist. 16 items rated. Covers affect, behaviour and thought content
Negative Symptom Rating Scale	Iager et al (1985)	10 items 7 point scale Assesses thought processes, volition, cognition and affect 15 minute semistructured interview
Scale for Assessment of Negative Symptoms	Andreason (1982)	30 negative items Total score indicates level of severity 5 subscales of affective blunting, alogia, avolition, apathy, anhedonia, asociality, and attentional impairment

Table 5.5 Rating scales for mania

Title	Authors	Main features
Bech–Rafaelsen Life Scale for Mania (combined rating scale for mania and depression)	Bech et al (1979)	11 items Requires experienced clinical rater Scores based on clinical interview 5 point scale Total score may be used as index of severity, range 0–44
Rating Scale for Mania	Young et al (1978)	11 items (4 items receive double weighting) For use by trained rater Total score indicates level of severity
Manic State Rating Scale	Beigel et al (1971), modified by Blackburn et al (1977)	26 observable items Can be rated by nursing staff 6 of the items useful for measuring change Blackburn version modified for interview use with two additional scales

Table 5.6 Depression rating scales

Name	Authors	Mode of administration	No. of items	Main features
Hamilton Rating Scale for Depression (HRSD)	Hamilton (1960)	Clinical interview	21 (17)	Quantifies level of depression but not diagnostic tool
Beck Depression Inventory (BDI)	Beck et al (1961)	Self-rating administered by interview	21 (13)	Measures depth of depression and therefore used as a measure of treatment outcome
Montgomery–Asberg Depression Rating Scale (MADRS)	Montgomery & Asberg (1979)	Observer rating scale	17	Sensitive to change in depressive illness

Montgomery and Asberg Depression Rating Scale (MADRS) (Montgomery & Asberg 1979) The MADRS was derived from the Comprehensive Psychopathological Rating Scale (CPRS) (Asberg et al 1978). The CPRS is made up of 65 scaled items which cover a wide range of psychiatric symptoms. The 17 items which occurred most commonly in depressed patients were used as a basis for the MADRS. The 10 items most sensitive to change were then selected to form the final scale. The MADRS has good inter-rater reliability and is valid when compared with a global clinical assessment. The MADRS has fewer items to score than the Hamilton Rating Scale for Depression but has equally high reliability (Kearns et al 1982, Snaith & Taylor 1985). There is also less emphasis on somatic symptoms than in the HRSD and clear instructions on grading scores for individual items. The MADRS has high specificity for depression.

(Snaith et al 1986) have established score ranges for the MADRS which allow patients to be grouped into recovered, mild, moderate and severe categories.

Beck Depression Inventory (BDI) (Beck et al 1961) This self-completion inventory is clinically derived from observation of depressed patients. There are 21 items rated 0 to 3 according to severity. The BDI is prone to halo effects, i.e. the subject's general attitude can influence the response to many of the items and there is uncertainty as to what is actually measured (Dennis et al 1992).

Hospital Anxiety and Depression Scale (HADS) (Zigmond & Snaith 1983) This is a 14 item scale with each item scored 0 to 3 depending on the severity of the symptom. It is intended for the assessment of anxiety and depression in non-psychiatric medical outpatient populations. It has been shown to be a valid measure of severity and can assess change in mental state over time.

Rating scales for anxiety

Hamilton Rating Scale for Anxiety (HRSA) (Hamilton 1959) Assessment is made by an unstructured interview. There are 14 questions rated 0 to 4 on the basis of the subject's replies and behaviour at interview. The scale is somatically biased. It has been used extensively as a measure of change due to treatment.

Brief Scale for Anxiety (Tyrer et al 1984) This was derived from the CPRS and has 10 items, each rated on a 7 point scale.

Clinical Anxiety Scale (CAS) (Snaith et al 1982) The CAS was derived from the Hamilton Anxiety Scale. The CAS consists of six items largely confined to subjective anxiety and muscle tension. The HRSA and the CAS were both developed in clinical populations

suffering from anxiety neurosis. The authors of the CAS have suggested that, although it is intended for use in a clinical population, it may have wider applicability than the HAS and can also be used in patients with anxious personality disorder. The decreased emphasis on somatic anxiety compared with the HAS may make the CAS more valid in the assessment of anxiety in patients with medical rather than psychiatric disorders (Hamilton 1959, Snaith et al 1982). Score ranges which allow the severity of anxiety to be graded have been determined in the same way as for the MADRS described above (Snaith et al 1986).

Global rating scales

Visual analogue scales These are widely used as a quick and easy way of obtaining self-ratings of mood (Aitken and Zealley 1970). Subjects are asked to put a cross on a 10 cm line separating two extremes of mood at the point which best describes their own feelings. A score can be calculated by measuring the distance from the left-hand end of the line to this cross in millimetres.

INTRODUCTION TO STATISTICS

This section adopts the approach of helping the reader to understand statistical analyses as used in psychiatry, rather than how to conduct them. Therefore no worked examples, and few numbers, equations or symbols are given; the emphasis is conceptual rather than mathematical. Many excellent and readily available statistical packages exist that will carry out whatever analyses you may need, accurately, quickly and above all, simply, and it is assumed that the reader will have access to one of these packages.

Similarly, there are many excellent introductory texts. It would be redundant to repeat their contents here; several are recommended at the end. Accordingly this section will deal with introductory statistics relatively briefly, and will focus on explaining some commonly used methods in non-technical language. However, the reader will find it helpful to have some idea of the technical meanings of the terms 'probability' and 'independence'.

Probability is a relatively familiar everyday concept, but perhaps surprisingly its definition remains a matter of some controversy. There are those who hold that the probability of an event is a measure of the frequency with which that event will occur in a long sequence of trials, whereas others view probability as an expression of the degree of belief that a particular outcome will occur. If one considers tossing a coin, most people would intuitively be prepared to assume that the outcomes 'heads' and 'tails' are equally likely, and one could consider that as expressing a degree of belief. On the other hand, the frequentist view of the probability of obtaining a head when a coin is tossed, although not necessarily differing in numerical value, would be based on the idea that the coin could be tossed an infinite number of times and the outcome recorded. In any event, both would conclude that if the probabilities of heads and tails are equal then each would occur with probability 1/2. Since there are no other possible outcomes, and one of the two must happen, conventionally the sum of the probabilities of the outcomes is 1. This has the interesting consequence that if the probability of a particular outcome is P, the probability that that outcome does not occur is $(1-P)$ – often called the complementary probability.

The notion of independence is rather more difficult to explain, and in order to do so it is necessary to consider multiple outcomes. Thus, one could throw a six-sided die, and record the number shown topmost. Again, most people would be prepared to assume that each of the numbers 1 to 6 was equally likely, and hence assign a probability 1/6 to each. Now, if we think of the outcomes 'die shows an odd number' and 'die shows an even number' we would probably be prepared to consider these as equally likely, as each can happen in exactly three ways. But now, consider the probability that the die shows a 3, given that we are told it shows an odd number. Since the result is an odd number, it must be one of 1, 3 or 5. Thus the required probability is 1/3. But if we knew nothing at all about the number shown, we would calculate the probability of 3 as 1/6. Hence the events 'die shows a 3' and 'die shows an odd number' are not independent. Similarly, it is perhaps easy to understand that, if one tosses two coins simultaneously, obtaining a head or tail on one of the two is independent of the outcome of the other. But statistical independence is not the same as this physical independence. If, in a population of schoolchildren, 60% of boys have dark hair, 30% blonde hair and 10% red hair, and 60% of girls also have dark hair, 30% blonde and 10% red, then in that population the attributes hair colour and sex are statistically independent.

It is possible to construct various complex models of statistical dependence, but perhaps the simplest way to appreciate the importance of this idea is in considering the comparison of a group of treated individuals with a group of controls. If the outcome of interest is improvement, then the statement that 'outcome is independent of treatment status' is equivalent to 'treatment does not affect outcome'.

A major aim of this section is to demonstrate that the use of statistical analysis is not a mechanical, 'cook-book' application of techniques; rather, statistical analysis requires a great deal of planning, forethought and intellectual honesty.

Why statistics are important

Carrying out your own research

In most clinical research, enough data will be generated to require the use of statistics. It is important that the statistical analysis that you plan to conduct is taken into account at the stage of planning the research, and statistical considerations are likely to be crucial in determining the design. Any clinician undertaking research must have a good understanding of statistical methods, if only to communicate effectively with a professional statistician.

Evaluating published papers

Statistical errors are common in clinical research, sometimes to a degree that invalidates the conclusions drawn (p. 189). It is prudent for clinicians to adopt a sceptical approach when reading papers, so that the true value of the findings can be assessed; this is particularly important in treatment studies.

Ethical considerations

It is unethical to use erroneous statistics, especially in scientific publications. If the conclusions in a paper are not justified, clinicians may be encouraged to use harmful or ineffective treatments, or to avoid potentially useful treatments. In addition, a research publication containing misleading statistics would be wasteful of the subjects' time and of the resources consumed. Moreover, published papers are construed as authoritative, and the publication of apparently valid but erroneous conclusions may inhibit further investigations.

Professional and personal satisfaction

Analysing the data that you have collected to investigate a clinical hunch is professionally and personally stimulating, and is far from being the routine drudgery that it may seem initially.

The main purposes of statistics

There are three main purposes of statistical analysis; the distinction between them is not entirely clear-cut.

Data reduction

A prime reason for the need for statistics is that in clinical research there may be many measurements from hundreds of subjects. Simply viewing large sets of data will seldom permit the observer to spot trends or differences; statistics enables you to condense data to manageable proportions, thus facilitating interpretation.

Dealing with variable subject matter

In some areas of science, such as nuclear physics, the subject matter is highly predictable; one oxygen atom behaves much like another. But more variable behaviour is exhibited by people, and in particular people will differ in how they respond to interventions. When an effect of an intervention is observed it is important to know whether it is a real effect, or whether it arises simply from chance fluctuations because of your sample of subjects. Statistics is a tool to help you to make more clear-cut decisions, despite great variability.

Sampling and generalisation

In clinical research you are not able to include all subjects with, say, a particular diagnosis in research studies. A sample has to be taken. But we are seldom interested in the effects of an intervention on only the sample in our study. In order to be of real practical value, you need to assess how far the results are generalisable to all subjects to whom the intervention could be applied.

Typically statistics provides advice in a probabilistic way; for example, what proportion of discharged patients will need to be readmitted to hospital, and what are their characteristics? Seldom can you identify accurately all such cases, but you can obtain useful information about the proportion that might be expected to be readmitted, or about the probability of readmission for an individual.

The first purpose is approached by 'descriptive statistics'; the second and third purposes by 'inferential statistics'. Before moving on to these topics it is necessary to introduce some basic statistical concepts.

Basic concepts

Dependent and independent variables

A variable is, as its name implies, a measure or attribute that varies from instance to instance. In clinical research the dependent variable is the measure that is used to assess the changes that may have occurred in the study. For example, in a study on the treatment of obsessive–compulsive disorder, the dependent variable could be subjects' scores on the Maudsley Obsessional Questionnaire. An independent variable is a variable whose relationship with the dependent variable is being investigated; for example, the intensity of a treatment, the diagnosis, or the type of drug may be associated with the dependent variable of patient outcome. Research studies are concerned with examining the relationships between independent variables and dependent variables.

Although the terminology used to report statistical analyses may often make use of terms which tend to imply cause and effect – indeed even the terms 'dependent' and 'independent' applied to variables are readily interpreted in this way – causal relationships are difficult to establish unequivocally, and caution is always advisable in attempting to interpret statistical relationships as causal.

The normal distribution

A frequency distribution is a tabulation of a set of scores or values, showing for each value its frequency of occurrence. For binary data, that is observations taking values simply zero or one, the frequency distribution has only two classes, and is simply the number of zeroes and the number of ones in the data. For qualitative data with more than two classes the frequency distribution is the number of subjects in each class, and for discrete quantitative data, the frequency distribution is the number of subjects with each whole-number value.

The situation is slightly more complicated in the case of continuous data, as defined earlier, and frequency distributions are constructed on the basis of class intervals of values. For a particular interval, the number of values in the data lying in that interval is counted, and forms the corresponding frequency. Thus for data related to weight we might form 5 kg intervals, for example from 50 kg up to (but not including) 55 kg as one interval, from 55 kg up to but not including 60 kg for the next and so on. The corresponding frequencies would be the numbers of subjects with weights in the appropriate intervals.

A frequency distribution may be represented graphically. Frequency is usually plotted on the vertical axis, against intervals on the horizontal axis. The distributions can have a variety of shapes, but some biological and psychological variables, such as height, blood counts or IQ scores, tend to form what is called a normal distribution. However, by no means all variables are adequately described by the normal distribution, and it is always worth emphasising that the use of the word 'normal' in this context is to be understood in a specialised sense distinct from its everyday meaning of 'usual' or 'customary'. A normal distribution is symmetrical and 'bell-shaped' (Fig. 5.2). The centre or peak of a normal distribution is at the arithmetic mean

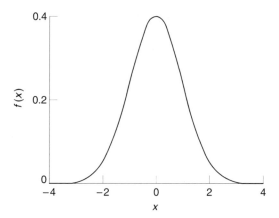

Fig. 5.2 The standard normal distribution

of the values, and as values get higher or lower they become increasingly less frequent and are located towards the 'tails' of the distribution. The distribution plotted in Figure 5.2 is the so-called 'standard normal' distribution, which has a mean of 0 and a SD of 1. The probability of a standard normal random variable exceeding any particular value is given by the area under the curve to the right of that value: the entire area under the curve is equal to 1.

Measurements that are determined by the addition of many small chance influences tend to form a normal distribution. This phenomenon is of great value to statisticians because much of statistics is concerned with deciding whether a research result is a chance finding or not, and models that reflect chance influences provide a basic framework for statistical analysis.

Distributions that are not symmetrical are termed 'skewed': when the peak of the distribution is to the right of the range of values, the skew is negative; when the peak is to the left it is positive. Bimodal distributions in which there are two peaks rather than one may also be found.

DESCRIPTIVE STATISTICS

In typical clinical research studies large amounts of data are gathered, and it is impossible to interpret the data without summarising them. Measures of central tendency, percentiles, and variation in the scores are the most useful ways of summarising the data.

Central tendency

Measures of central tendency are more commonly known as 'averages'. However, the term 'central tendency' is preferred because the term 'average' is often

but mistakenly taken to be the same as 'mean'. The mean is only one of several possible measures of central tendency.

The mean

This is calculated by adding all the scores in a set of data and dividing by the number of scores. It is familiar from elementary school maths as the average, or arithmetic mean, and is the most commonly reported summary statistic – under most circumstances in psychiatry it will provide the best indication of a 'typical' score in your data. There are several variants of the mean that are useful in specific circumstances. 'Trimmed' means may be useful if data contain one or more extreme scores that might distort the value of the conventional mean; a fixed proportion of extreme scores is omitted from the calculation. Thus the '5% trimmed mean' is the average of the data remaining after excluding 5% of the data values (the highest and lowest 2.5% of values).

The median

The median is the score at the point where 50% of scores are greater and 50% are smaller; that is, if all the data values are put in rank order, the median will appear precisely in the middle. Often the mean and the median of a data set are similar, but they will not be if the data are highly skewed. This notion of an ordered set of values is useful in defining other characteristics later.

The mode

The mode is the most common value in the set of values; it is not often used for continuous data, as it can be defined only by convention if all values are different from each other, and in those circumstances its value will typically depend on the class intervals used to construct the frequency distribution.

Percentiles and quantiles

A quantile is a value below which a certain proportion of observations occur in the ordered set of data values. Thus, the 10th percentile is a quantile, and is the value below which 10% of the observations lie. The first (or lower) quartile is the value below which 25% (a quarter) of the observations lie, while the median is also a quantile, being the value below which fall 50% of the observations. The upper quartile is the 75th percentile – 75% of the values in the data set are less than the upper quartile, and 25% greater than it. The interquartile range is the name given to the spread of the middle

50% of all the scores, which is thus the difference between the upper and lower quartiles. Percentiles and related summary statistics convey information about data easily and rapidly; several psychometric assessment devices present results in percentile form.

Variation

Standard deviation (SD)

This is one of the most important concepts in statistical analysis. To calculate the population SD, first calculate the mean, and subtract each score from it; these differences are squared and the result is divided by the number of scores. Finally, the square root of this is taken to compensate for having previously squared the differences. (The differences are squared in order to ensure that scores above and below the mean all contribute positively to the measure – it is easy to figure out that if the raw differences are added their sum is always zero!) If there is a wide spread of scores around the mean, the SD will be large. Thus the SD can be approximately defined as the mean deviation of all the scores from the overall mean. When calculating SD from a sample of observations rather than from all possible observations in a population, it is usual to divide by the number of observations minus 1. The SD should always be reported along with its respective mean; however, in a review of studies comparing selective serotonin reuptake inhibitors (SSRIs) and tricyclics, Song et al (1993) noted that only 20 out of 58 publications reported both.

The SD enables you to assess the position of a score relative to the mean. Because the SD is an index of the size of the mean difference between each score and the overall mean, it is possible to examine any individual score to see whether the difference between it and the mean difference is relatively high or low. For example, imagine a set of scores with a mean of 100 and an SD of 20; an individual score of 110 would be half an SD above the mean; and an individual score of 80 would be 1 SD below the mean. SD units are known as z scores. You can therefore describe the relative position of a score in terms of how far it differs from the mean, using SD as a measure.

The normal distribution has consistent properties in terms of mean and SD. Approximately 68% of scores fall between 1 SD above and 1 SD below the mean; 95% of scores fall between 1.96 SD above and 1.96 SD below; 99% of scores fall between 2.58 SD above and 2.58 SD below. These are general properties of all normal distributions, so it is possible to compare scores from distributions that have different means, different SDs, and different ranges of scores by what is called 'standardising' to a z score, as noted above. This is done by taking

an individual score, subtracting the mean of the normal distribution of these scores and dividing by the standard deviation. Thus if a patient has a z score of 2 on a depression scale (with a range of 0 to 30) and a z score of 0.75 on an anxiety scale (with a range of 0 to 100), one can conclude that the patient has a more extreme depression score than anxiety score (even if the anxiety raw score is higher). However, it should be borne in mind that transforming to z scores does not make clearly different quantities commensurable – in simple terms apples and oranges don't add together on the same scale. Although both are fruit, it doesn't make sense to ask how many apples make one orange, or how many apples and oranges will make a banana!

Variability, sampling distributions and 'standard error'

The problem of dealing with variability is the task of statistical analysis. It is commonplace to observe variability in many attributes of individuals, systems or other phenomena, and such variability may be, for example, between relatively permanent characteristics of individuals, or between the same individuals at different times. Models exist which form appropriate mathematical representations of variability – for example, we have earlier considered the normal distribution. In order to apply these models however, we have to take into account the methods by which individual values of the phenomenon modelled are observed. Central to the applicability of these models is the notion of randomisation – that is, individual values are selected from the model by a mechanism explicitly involving chance – this is not a haphazard mechanism, but one with prescribed and repeatable characteristics. In some applications it may be difficult to conceive of chance playing a part in the selection of subjects for study – for example, a research study might involve as subjects all available patients in a particular ward. Any generalisation to other patients, or application of a statistical model to the group of patients, is intrinsically open to question. The patients have been self-selected, in that they have sought treatment. However, let us suppose that a new treatment is to be compared with standard treatment using such a set of patients. The section on research design (see p. 151) suggests that patients be randomly allocated to either the standard or new treatment, and makes recommendations about blinding and so on. The basis of the statistical analysis of the data is the process of random allocation. If random allocation is used it is possible to apply a statistical model which enables conclusions to be drawn concerning the likely role of chance in influencing the results of the trial. Note that the extension of any conclusion to the population of all possible patients depends upon the assumption that the patients studied are the same as, or similar to, all the other patients that could have been studied. This would not need to be assumed if the patients in the trial had been drawn by a random mechanism from all possible patients.

The process of random selection is the basis of what is called the 'sampling distribution' of a summary statistical measurement. If a different sample had been drawn, different values would have resulted, and a different summary measurement would have been obtained. If we have a model of underlying variability, such as the normal distribution for continuous measurements, we can apply statistical reasoning which enables us to estimate what the distribution in repeated sampling of the summary statistic would be. This distribution is known as the sampling distribution, and its properties permit us to apply statistical reasoning to data which have been generated or collected by an appropriate randomised method. For example, if the population distribution of a particular measurement can be described by a normal distribution, then the mean of a random sample of n observations from this distribution has a particular sampling distribution. If the SD of the parent distribution is known, the sampling distribution of the sample mean is also normal, with the same mean as the population, but with standard deviation given by the standard deviation of the population divided by the square root of the sample size.

More usually however we know neither the mean nor the SD of the population distribution – on the contrary, the research being carried out aims to find out about these quantities. Again, staying with the example of a normal distribution of population values but with unknown SD, the 'standard error' of the sample mean is defined as the estimated SD of the sample values divided by the square root of sample size. With 64 subjects and a sample SD of 20, the standard error of the mean would be 20 divided by 8, or 2.5. Standard errors will be large if the sample is small and vice versa; in the previous example, if there were 25 subjects, the standard error would be 4, while if there were 400 subjects it would be 1.

The standard error of the mean is sometimes reported as an index of variability in data from research studies; this is not good practice because it reflects both sample size and the actual level of variability. The SD is the index of choice for reporting degree of variability in the data – the standard error of the mean reflects variability in the sampling distribution of the mean.

Different statistical models may lead to different sampling distributions and summary statistics. For example, in the case of a binary variable such as sex, a summary statistic of interest may be the proportion of males. In such a case the sampling distribution of the observed proportion of males will not be normal (although for large enough samples it may be assumed so). Nevertheless, statistical modelling permits us to calculate the standard error of this proportion.

Of what use is a standard error (SE)? It is not appropriate to go into the background rationale, but because of the consistent properties of normal distributions, for large samples the SE enables one to assess the range of likely difference between the sample mean and the 'true' population mean. That is, about 68% of sample means will be found within 1 SE above and 1 SE below the true mean.

As mentioned above, standard errors can be calculated for a variety of summary statistics. Their interpretation is always the same: an SE enables you to judge the reliability or accuracy of your sample data; or the range within which you might reasonably expect the statistic to fall if the study was repeated.

Confidence intervals (CIs)

CIs are a kind of reversal of the argument above concerning estimation of the range within which one might expect the actual value of a mean (or other statistic) to lie. We have seen that 95% of normally distributed values will be between 1.96 SD above and below the mean. Thus, if the normal distribution provides an appropriate sampling distribution for a sample mean, it follows that there is a 95% chance that this mean will lie in the range between 1.96 SE above and 1.96 SE below the true mean. Thus 95% of intervals centred on the sample mean, with a range of 1.96 SE either side will contain the population mean; such an interval calculated from a sample is known as a 95% CI.

For example, if an obtained mean is 40 (with an SD of 12), and there are 36 subjects, the SE mean will be 2 (12 divided by 6). The 95% CI will be between 43.92 and 36.08 (40 plus or minus 1.96 × 2); that is, there is a 95% chance that these limits contain the 'true' mean.

CIs can be calculated for most statistics, including the difference between means, medians, measures of association, and so on.

Conventionally, 95% CIs are reported. It is possible to calculate CIs for any percentage level; the higher the percentage, the wider the CI. In the above example the 99% CI would be between 45.16 and 34.84 (40 plus or minus 2.58 × 2).

Although in small samples the normal distribution will probably not provide the relevant sampling distribution, other statistical distributions will, and importantly, the ideas of the last two sections will still apply.

Points to check with descriptive statistics

- Present the SD rather than the SE mean as the index of variability for quantitative data.
- Do not report means of categorical variables (e.g. mean social class) – instead report frequencies or percentages in each category.
- Report the confidence intervals for population means of important variables.

INFERENTIAL STATISTICS

The essence of inferential statistics

Conventionally, inferential statistics encompass estimation – including interval estimation, or the construction of confidence intervals, and hypothesis testing. Thus inferential statistics are concerned with helping researchers to draw inferences from or to interpret their data, for example to estimate the mean number of re-admissions per patient (estimation), to decide whether an apparent difference or association is a real one, or whether it has arisen simply from chance factors (hypothesis testing). How does statistical analysis accomplish this? Although statistics can be used to address a variety of seemingly different questions, the underlying logic is similar. The essence of statistical analysis is:

1. To measure all the variability in the data; that is, to measure how far all the scores differ from each other.
2. To see how much of the variability can be explained (or accounted for) by the independent variables.
3. To estimate how far the explained variability is over and above the variability that might be explained in terms of chance factors (or in statistical terms, a significant effect).

Step (3) is the crucial one and relates again to the idea of a sampling distribution. For convenience, let us take as a concrete illustration a drug trial comparing the effects of two drugs on patients' scores on the Beck Depression Inventory (BDI). Suppose we randomly assign patients to one or other group to receive the particular drugs, and that in reality there is no difference between the drugs; perhaps both are inert placebos. We compare the outcomes on the BDI, and find that there are slight differences in the means between the groups. If we repeated our experiment again several times, using the same experimental conditions but with different randomisation, the results would be similar; but they would be unlikely to be precisely the same because of the variation induced by randomisation. Some would be higher, some lower (a similar argument relating to

natural variation between individuals could be used if our subjects were themselves randomly selected from a larger population of potential subjects).

If this is continued indefinitely, we would end up with a group of differences between means that gave a very good indication of the possible range of results that could be expected from a large number of similar studies. If there is no good reason to expect systematic differences, as in this example, the sizes of the findings of all the studies will show the distribution that would be anticipated if all the results were due only to chance factors. Some of these sizes of differences would be commonly found, whereas others would be rare; if plotted, they would form approximately a normal distribution.

Clearly it is not feasible to repeat studies indefinitely in this way, but fortunately this is not necessary. It is possible to derive an estimate of a chance-based distribution of differences from the results of a single study, in a way similar to calculating the SE mean. On the basis of a single sample (your study), you can estimate the distribution of many results that you would expect if there were no real effects at all, and compare your results with that distribution. If the magnitude of the difference between means that you obtained is so great that differences of that magnitude or larger are unlikely to have arisen purely by chance (in other words, in this hypothetical normal distribution of differences, differences as large as or larger than that obtained would be rare), your result is said to be *statistically significant*; chance would remain a possible explanation of the results, but it is unlikely. The evaluation of the relevant probability – the P value, or significance probability – is performed by consulting statistical tables of the appropriate distribution, or may be provided automatically by the computer package used to analyse the data.

The term 'statistical significance' is the one that is conventionally used to indicate the likelihood of a result as, or more, extreme than that obtained being drawn from a chance distribution. In many ways this is an unfortunate use of the term, because it seems to imply that the result is important or substantial. As will be discussed later, such implications may be unfounded.

This logic applies not just to differences between means of samples, but also to the differences in means between more than two samples, or to associations between variables, for example. The logic of estimating the reliability of a finding based on estimates from a single sample applies generally across all statistical analyses.

Null hypothesis

Hypothesis testing proceeds by testing the assumption that there is no real effect in the study; in other words that the data have come from a chance-based distribution. This 'null hypothesis' is then assessed in the light of the data collected, and the assessment shows how far the results are compatible with that assumption.

Levels of significance

Researchers acknowledge the possibility that erroneous conclusions may be drawn, but accept this only within well-defined limits. One type of erroneous conclusion is that you may decide that the null hypothesis is false when in reality it is not; this is known as the 'type 1' error, or a false positive. The risk of type 1 errors is normally set at a maximum of 5%. That is, you are willing to accept a 1 in 20 chance that you will conclude that an effect or statistical association is true or real when in fact it is due to sampling variation. The 5% level is arbitrary and based only on convention; some authorities consider it too generous, and recommend wide adoption of the 1% level.

When significance levels are reported they are normally of this form: $P = 0.05$ for 5% level; or $P = 0.01$ for 1% level. Researchers should whenever possible report the exact significance probability, that is, the probability of obtaining results as or more extreme than those actually obtained when the null hypothesis is true (e.g. $P = 0.0326$), rather than round it upwards to 0.05, 0.01 or whatever, as is common practice in clinical research publications. It is worth noting that there is a correspondence between the results of hypothesis tests and confidence intervals. Thus, if the 95% confidence interval for a mean difference contained the value zero, the null hypothesis that the population mean difference was zero would not be rejected at the 5% level. If, on the other hand, the 95% confidence interval for the true mean difference did *not* contain the value zero, then the null hypothesis of no difference *would* be rejected at the 5% level. You may notice that 95% and 5% add to 100%. It does indeed follow that if a 99% confidence interval did not contain the value zero, then the hypothesis that the true mean difference was zero would be rejected at the 1% level. Thus, expressing the result of a study in terms of a confidence interval permits the reader to infer the results of an appropriate hypothesis test, but more importantly conveys important information concerning the precision of estimation of the study.

One- and two-tailed tests

The 5% level of significance is usually divided into two parts: 2.5% in the upper tail and 2.5% in the lower tail. In, say, a drug trial comparing drugs A and B, the upper tail values lead to the conclusion (at the 5% level of significance) that A is better than B, and the lower tail that B is better than A. You may make a prediction that A will be the better drug, and maintain that you are not interested in whether B is better than A. The probability contained by the lower tail is in a sense 'wasted'. Accordingly, the probabilities in the two tails can be added together and put in the upper tail, making it a 'one-tailed' test; this would make it more likely that a significant result would be obtained. The upper tail would still contain only 5% of the total area under the distribution curve.

Theoretically this is a justifiable decision, but not all authorities agree. It is hard to envisage a situation in psychiatry when it would not be of interest if a significant finding emerged that was contrary to your prediction. If you did adopt a one-tailed procedure and obtained results in the opposite direction, the only honest course would be to ignore the result, or to repeat the experiment using a two-tailed procedure. If you do not do this, by bunching up the probabilities in one tail, you are effectively using a 10% significance level. The temptation would be great to change retrospectively the direction of your hypothesis, requiring an unusual degree of honesty to resist. It would also be tempting to revert to a one-tailed test if your two-tailed test produced a P value between 0.05 and 0.10.

In short, psychiatric research should seldom, if ever, use one-tailed tests, despite their popularity. If you are even vaguely interested in a result not consistent with your directional hypothesis, a two-tailed test should be used.

CHOOSING AN APPROPRIATE STATISTICAL TEST

There are many different applications of statistics but there are three main areas in which they are used to guide the interpretation of the results of clinical research studies. First, are the differences between groups significant? For example, is there a difference in outcome between two groups of depressed patients, one treated by drugs and the other by psychotherapy? Second, are these two measures related or associated? For example, what is the association between liver function tests and weekly alcohol consumption? Third, can one predict the value of one variable (or outcome) from knowledge of the values of other variables? For example, how far can one predict the need for readmission of discharged psychiatric patients, given knowledge of sociodemographic factors and clinical state?

No matter what questions are asked one should, as far as possible, keep to the principles of using as few tests as possible, and choosing the most simple tests possible. The availability of a wide range of tests in packages seems to have led to the unthinking and indiscriminate use of tests for no better reason than that they are available. The use of many complex analyses in a study opens the door to a multitude of problems, and probably goes some way to accounting for the notorious difficulties in replicating research findings in psychiatry.

The appropriate statistical tests to answer these kinds of questions are outlined in Table 5.7. First, however, it is necessary to introduce the concept of parametric and non-parametric statistics.

Parametric and non-parametric tests

Traditionally the term 'parametric statistics' has been used to refer to fairly elementary methods based on the normal distribution, which can only be used if the following assumptions are fulfilled:

- The populations from which your samples are taken should have a normal distribution.
- The SDs of the scores in the samples should be similar.
- The scale of measurement is at least interval (that is, the differences between scores are equal; thus the distance between 4 and 8 is the same as the distance between 13 and 17.
- The scores within each sample must be quite independent of each other.

Generally speaking one can violate the first three assumptions without the results being too misleading. Some of the major problems that can occur if the fourth assumption is violated are outlined on page 188. But if your sample is small (say, less than 30 per group), assumption violation is more serious; the use of standard parametric statistics would be invalid and consideration should be given either to using more advanced parametric statistics (beyond the scope of this chapter) or to using one of a group of methods that are known as 'non-parametric' or distribution-free. Non-parametric methods are not based on the same assumptions. They are often based on ordered values or data that are arranged in ascending (or descending) order – ranked data – and generally examine differences between groups in terms of medians rather than means. In a study with a small number of subjects where there is also severe assumption violation, they should normally be used. Obviously, non-parametric methods should also be used when the data are originally in ranked format (for example, a rank of prognostic features). Another useful application of non-parametric methods is in situations where your measurement device becomes less sensitive at extreme values (for example, an alcohol breath analyser with a limited ceiling); a non-parametric method does not require precise scores, only their relative ranks. However, non-parametric tests are less sensitive than parametric tests, and you are less likely to obtain statistical significance in your results.

In Table 5.7, the first column contains parametric methods, and columns 2 and 3 contain non-parametric methods. Although many of these are expressed as statistical 'tests' it is worth remembering that in every case the results of a study could also be legitimately expressible as estimates, and associated confidence intervals. This table is not an exhaustive list of all statistical methods or tests available. Many of the methods in the table have several variations for use under special circumstances, particularly when looking at the effects of many variables at the same time (multivariate analyses); key ones will be introduced later.

What are the most commonly used tests in clinical research?

Table 5.8 has been drawn up from published reviews of statistical analyses in research studies from various clinical disciplines in recent years. Unfortunately, reviews of statistical methods used in clinical research are not directly comparable, mainly because the reviews tend to categorise the tests in different ways. For example, some statistical reviewers have included simple and multiple regression together, whereas others have included simple regression with correlation, and multiple regression with 'multivariate' techniques. However the table does suggest that about 90% of methods used are relatively straightforward; thus an introductory knowledge of statistics will permit clinicians to be familiar with most of the methods used in clinical research publications. The table also suggests that the extent and range of methods used in psychiatry are at least as great as in other clinical disciplines.

The next section looks at these commonly used methods in more detail, and brief examples of their use, mainly from the psychiatric literature, are given.

Reporting relevant output

After the appropriate statistical method has been computed, the statistical package will automatically report the values of the statistic itself (e.g. 't'), of P, of the 'degrees of freedom' and appropriate 95% CIs. (The degrees of freedom (d.f.) relates to the number of subjects, depending on the test used.) Ideally, estimates of the quantities of prime interest, such as group means, proportion or medians, should also be provided, and when reporting the results of an analysis all this basic information should be presented. (Incidentally, in many of the examples from psychiatric studies given in this section, not all relevant output was reported in the original publication).

Table 5.7 How to choose an appropriate statistical method

Goal or question asked	Type of data		
	Continuous measures	Ranked measures	Categorical measures
Describing the data Summarise the data in this group	Mean, SD	Median, quartiles, percentiles	Proportions
Looking for differences Compare data from this group with hypothetical data	1-sample *t* test	1-sample Wilcoxon test	χ^2-squared
Is there a difference between these two independent groups?	Independent *t* test	Mann–Whitney test	χ^2-squared Fisher's exact test
Is there a difference between these two paired groups?	Paired (dependent) *t* test	Wilcoxon signed rank test	McNemar's test
Is there a difference between these three or more independent groups?	1-way analysis of variance (ANOVA)	Kruskal–Wallis test	χ^2-squared test
Is there a difference between these two or more independent groups, when they are categorised in several ways?	Multiway ANOVA	Friedman test (2-way distribution free ANOVA)	Log-linear analysis
Is there a difference between these three or more matched groups?	Repeated measures ANOVA	Friedman test	Cochrane Q test
Associations between variables Is there an association between two variables?	Pearson product moment correlation	Spearman rank correlation	Contingency coefficient Phi coefficient Kappa
Predicting Can I predict one value from another?	Univariate regression		Logistic regression Log-linear analysis
Can I predict one value from several others?	Multiple regression		Multiple logistic regression Log-linear analysis

Differences between groups

t test

There are two common uses of the *t* distribution. The two-sample *t* test is used to examine differences in the means between two populations on the basis of independent samples from each, when the data are continuous and approximately normally distributed with equal unknown SDs. Data from the same group measured on two separate occasions or from two different groups, where each individual member of one group is matched on key characteristics with an individual member of the other group (for example, in order to maximise similarities between the groups), should be analysed by considering differences in scores between occasions, or

Table 5.8 Statistical techniques used in clinical research (per cent of papers in which technique used)				
Technique	Psychiatry (McGuigan, 1995)	Rheumatology (Ruiz et al, 1991)	Ophthalmology (Juzych et al, 1992)	Radiology (Goldin et al, 1996)
None	33	38	34	47
Descriptive	17	16	65	
t test	19	—	17	20
ANOVA	12	4	7	3
χ^2-square	29	—	17	14
Pearson correlation	15	—	6	9
Non-parametric correlation	—	—	3	—
Other non-parametric (all non-parametric combined)	12	10	8	2
Regression (combined with correlation)	2	7	11	9
Advanced statistics	15	2	—	24

between members of each pair. In such cases the one-sample t test is applicable. You can also use a one-sample t test to compare a sample mean with a known population mean; for example, you could compare the mean age of patients with dementia with the mean age of all elderly patients in a general hospital.

If your sample size is large, you can safely use the t test even if some of the underlying assumptions are violated. Moreover, there is a variant of the two-sample t test (Welch's approximate t test) that can be used if the assumption of equality of variance is not upheld.

Points to check with t tests

- Ensure that the appropriate type has been used: paired or independent.
- Report the means, SDs and confidence interval of the difference between means.
- Check that there is no gross violation of underlying assumptions.

Example: Touyz et al (1993) examined the effects of an anaerobic exercise programme on weight gain in patients with anorexia nervosa in order to see if the exercise would adversely affect patients' ability to gain weight. Twenty patients received a behavioural programme only; 17 received the exercise programme in addition. They reported no significant difference in weight gain between the groups at 6 weeks (t = 0.51, d.f. = 35, P = 0.61; mean difference = 0.48 kg, 95% CI −2.31 to 1.35).

Mann–Whitney U test

This is the non-parametric equivalent of the indepen-

dent t test; it examines differences between medians rather than means. It should be used mainly in the case of severe violation of the assumptions underlying the t test. Group medians, the value of U and the P value should be reported.

Example: Castells et al (1996) had previously shown that some children with Down's syndrome suffer from growth hormone (GH) deficiency, and postulated that this may arise from hypothalamic dysfunction. They measured serum GH levels in response to levodopa and clonidine in 14 children with Down's syndrome and in 25 normal children. The distributions of serum GH were markedly skewed, and accordingly the Mann–Whitney U test was used. There was no significant difference between the groups (U = 134, P = 0.24).

The Chi-squared (χ^2) test

This test is used for data that are not continuous; rather, the data are in the form of frequency counts presented in a matrix or contingency table. The table can be 2 × 2, or 3 × 4, or any number of rows and columns, and in fact can be of more than two dimensions, although the two-way table is the simplest case. Very large tables make the results difficult to interpret. Essentially, χ^2 tests estimate how far the pattern of the obtained data in the cells differs from what one might expect if the probabilities related to row and column categories are independent. Thus, if row categories relate to treatments, and column categories to outcomes, as in Table 5.9, the null hypothesis is that outcome is independent of treatment – in other words,

Table 5.9 A 2 x 2 contingency table		
Treatment	Improved	Not improved
Drug	a	b
Placebo	c	c

there are no differences between the treatments in terms of outcome. An alternative formulation of the same null hypothesis is that the probability of patients improving is the same in both treatment categories.

Despite its apparent simplicity, χ^2 is often misused. Potential hazards can be overcome if the following rules are observed. First, the data in the cells must be in the form of a frequency count, and not percentages or other derivations from the raw data. Second, each subject must appear in one cell only. Third, the expected values should not be less than 5 in more than 25% of the cells, and no expected value should be 0. Adherence to rules one and two can be tested by adding the values in the cells to get sums of rows and of columns; the total of the sums of rows and the total of the sums of columns should be the same, and should equal the number of subjects in the study. Most packages will warn you if the expected values are too small; if so, a useful alternative, but for 2 × 2 tables only, is Fisher's exact test. For tables that have more than four cells, the best solution to the problem of low expected frequencies is to merge rows or columns together; for example, convert a 5 point scale of social class into a 3 point scale. Clearly you are likely to have low expected frequencies if the number of subjects is low, for example if it is below 30 in a 2 × 2 matrix.

If one of the variables has an underlying order (for example, if you have categorised height into short, medium and tall), a χ^2 for linear trend will examine if the effects of the order are significant.

Most packages automatically incorporate Yates' correction for continuity in 2 × 2 χ^2 tests; the reason for this correction need not concern us here but it is an important correction if the number of subjects is low. Without it, the obtained value of χ^2 is likely to be too high.

Several measures of association, for example the phi (φ) coefficient, can be calculated from χ^2.

Points to check with χ^2

- Ensure that the χ^2 has been calculated using raw data rather than transformed data (e.g. percentages).
- Check that the expected values are not too small.
- Check that subjects do not appear in more than one cell.

Example: Brown et al (1995) compared the influence of provoking events in the development of depression in two groups of women; one group (n = 58) were from a general population sample, the other from a sample of NHS treated women (n = 84). The provoking events were humiliation/trapped, loss/alone, and danger. No significant differences were found (χ^2 = 2.60, d.f. = 2, P = 0.273).

Fisher's exact test

Some authorities recommend that Fisher's exact test should routinely be used instead of χ^2 for a 2 × 2 table. It is not affected by low expected values, and as the name implies it reports the exact significance probability of your result if row and column categories are independent.

Example: Knauth et al (1997) investigated the effects of patent foramen ovale on the rate of multiple brain lesions amongst 87 sports divers, using magnetic resonance imaging (MRI) and ultrasonography. They reported that excess multiple lesions occurred in divers with large patent foramen ovale (Fisher's exact, P = 0.004).

Wilcoxon matched-pairs signed ranks test

This non-parametric test is the equivalent of the paired *t* test; as such it can be used for matched pairs or measures taken from the same subjects on two occasions. Being non-parametric, it is less powerful than the paired *t* test.

McNemar's test

This is a variant of the χ^2 test used to assess change in subjects before and after an intervention or when individual pair matching is used, when the data are qualitative. Once again the data are presented in the form of a contingency table, but the analysis differs considerably from the usual χ^2 test. Table 5.10 shows how the results of a before and after study would be tabulated for analysis where the measurement being investigated is either present or absent.

It is important to notice how this table differs from Table 5.9. The number of individuals with the attribute before treatment is (a + b), and the number with the attribute after treatment is (a + c). However, if the treatment has had an effect on the probability of an individual possessing the attribute, this will be evident from changes in status. Thus b individuals changed from having the attribute initially to not having it after treatment, and c changed from not having the attribute

Table 5.10   Contingency table for before and after studies or matched pair designs

		After	
		Present	Absent
	Present	a	b
Before			
	Absent	c	d

to having it. If the treatment is ineffective, one would expect the probabilities of such changes, given that change has occurred, to be equal in each direction, and this is the hypothesis tested by the McNemar test. When the test is used for paired categorical data, for example in a comparison of the effect of a treatment on a skin condition, in which an affected area of each subject is treated with a proprietary ointment, and another area with a placebo, the heading 'before' would be replaced by 'treatment', 'after' by 'placebo', and 'present' and 'absent' by 'improved' and 'not improved'. The entries in the table would add to the number of subjects in the trial, and the comparison of interest would again be b with c – that is, the number in which the treated area improved and the untreated one did not with the number in which the treated area did not improve and the untreated one did. Individuals in which both areas improved, or both areas stayed the same, do not enter the analysis, as they provide no information for the comparison of the treatments.

One-way ANOVA

This is similar to the t test, and can be used to determine if there are significant differences between means across three or more groups. ANOVA is based on a similar logic and procedure, but focuses more explicitly on the overall degree of variability or variance in a set of scores. Briefly, ANOVA examines how much of the variance in all the data can be explained by the variance between the groups; that is, looking at the differences between all the scores, is the degree of variance due to differences between the groups significantly greater than you might expect, given the amount of variance within groups? This is expressed in terms of a ratio: variance due to differences between the groups divided by the remaining variance from the whole set of scores. Equal numbers in each group are not required.

Because ANOVA results are expressed as a ratio (the F ratio), d.f. are needed for the numerator (the number of groups minus 1) and for the denominator (the total

number of subjects minus the number of groups) of the ratio.

Multiple comparisons

ANOVA is more complicated to interpret than a t test. With a t test only two groups are being compared; if you obtain a significant difference it is self-evident where the difference lies. ANOVA tells you only that somewhere in your data one or more of the means is significantly different from one or more of the other means. To find out where the differences may lie you will need to carry out a 'post hoc' test. Several are available in most packages, the most common being Tukey, the Dunnett, and the Scheffe. The Tukey is the usual method of choice; it is easy to interpret, ensures that an appropriate significance level is maintained despite looking at numerous comparisons, and is powerful at detecting differences. The Dunnett is preferred if you are only interested in comparing each of several interventions against a control group, and not interested in comparing the interventions with each other. The Scheffe is highly flexible and can seek out differences not only between all the groups but also between combinations of the groups (for example, group 1 + group 2 versus group 3 + group 4); it is a 'blunderbuss' method of approaching your data and is more difficult to interpret than the Tukey or the Dunnett.

You should report 'sum of squares' and 'mean square' as well as the usual data from the output.

Points to check with ANOVA

- Report group means, and the results of post hoc tests.
- Present d.f. for numerator and denominator of the F ratio
- Ensure that you have used repeated measures ANOVA if you have matched groups (see p. 171)

Example: Hayes and Halford (1996) proposed that schizophrenia and unemployment are often associated with poverty and lack of social role, and that there may be similarities in how people with schizophrenia and how people who are unemployed spend their time. They examined three groups with 16 subjects in each: males with schizophrenia, unemployed males and employed males. Various measures were taken of how time was spent, of pleasurable activities, and of self-perceived social difficulties (Social Situations Questionnaire, SSQ). Several differences were found; a key finding was that on the SSQ the males with schizophrenia reported significantly more social difficulties (mean = 47.31) than the unemployed males (mean = 24.5) and the employed males (mean = 19.19), who did not differ from each other (F = 13.97, d.f. = 2,45, P = <0.0001).

Kruskal–Wallis one-way analysis of variance by ranks

This test examines differences in three or more independent groups when the data are ranked. There should be at least five subjects per group; each group need not contain the same number of subjects. It is a non-parametric test and is therefore less powerful than a parametric ANOVA.

Example: Blair et al (1995) compared Expressed Emotion in the families of patients with anorexia nervosa (n = 26), cystic fibrosis (n = 29) and 'well' families (n = 31). The respective medians were 2, 2 and 0. The differences were significant (H = 25.97, d.f. = 2, P = <0.0001).

Multiway ANOVA tests

ANOVA tests can also be used in more complex ways. In particular you can examine the effects of more than one independent variable simultaneously; for example, in a drug trial you could explore the influence of dose, of time of administration, and of gender of subject. Moreover you can examine these influences not just by themselves but in all possible combinations; that is, you can look at the interactions between all the independent variables under investigation. Analysis of variance is the method of choice for analysing factorial designs, as described earlier. It should be noted however that unequal group sizes in multiway ANOVA pose special difficulties of interpretation.

The concept of interaction is very important in much clinical research because the influence of some variables can be attenuated or even reversed when looked at in combination with other variables. For example, it may be found that in a laboratory reaction time test, people with hypomania may perform better than non-patient controls, as may normal subjects when under laboratory-induced stress. But if you put people with hypomania under stress, their performance may deteriorate; the combination of the two variables reversed the effects of each taken alone. There are practical limits to the number of independent variables and their interactions that can be examined at the same time; interpretation of the results becomes very difficult if more than three are included.

Repeated measures ANOVA

This procedure examines differences between means when the data are from the same subjects (or matched subjects) assessed on three or more occasions. Like the paired *t* test, this is a powerful test because subjects act as their own controls and the error variance is reduced as there is no 'between-subjects' component. Repeated measures ANOVA also calculates *F* ratios. The Tukey post hoc test can be used to identify where significant differences may lie.

Example: Sanders et al (1996) conducted a preliminary analysis to determine if decreases were noted in a pain diary kept by 43 children during a 12 month follow-up after cognitive–behavioural treatment for recurrent abdominal pain. Pain diaries were kept over four time periods; a significant decrease was observed with a repeated measures ANOVA (F = 21.38, d.f. = 3, 117, P = <0.0005).

Other complex ANOVAs

There are many variants of ANOVA available for use in special circumstances. ANCOVA (analysis of covariance) can be used if you wish to control for or partial out the influence of a troublesome independent variable. For example, if you are comparing two treatment groups and you find that they differed substantially from each other on a critical variable (e.g. severity) before treatment started, you can hold the influence of that variable constant while examining the effects of other independent variables. The variable thus controlled is called the 'covariate'. It would be preferable to control for the influence of all relevant variables by the design of the experiment, for example by incorporating levels of the covariate as a factor in the design, but in clinical research such ideal conditions do not always exist and you may have to resort to using ANCOVA. Another common use of ANCOVA is to reduce the overall variance in your results by taking out variance due to one or more covariates, reducing the value of the denominator in the *F* ratio and thereby making your test more powerful.

MANOVA is used when ANOVA is conducted on many dependent variables in the same study. Similarly one can have a MANCOVA, or Multiple Analysis of Covariance. As a final complication, you can have multiway repeated measures ANOVA, MANOVA or MANCOVA, but such complex analyses should be avoided if possible.

Friedman two-way analysis of variance by ranks

As the name implies, this test is primarily for two-way analysis of variance on ranked scores; however, it can also be used for non-parametric repeated measures analysis of variance. The appropriate post hoc test is the Wilcoxon, but as before allowance must be made for multiple testing.

Log-linear analysis

Log-linear analysis is typically used for the analysis of multidimensional contingency tables, involving several categorical independent variables, with a view to examining the associations between them. With more than three or four variables many subjects are required, but each variable may have any number of categories. The analysis may focus on one of the variables as a 'dependent' variable if this makes clinical sense.

CORRELATION AND REGRESSION

How far is a score on a personality measure associated with prognosis after treatment for anxiety? Is parental depression linked to behaviour problems at school in the children? These are the types of questions that can be addressed using the statistical method of correlation. It is one of the most commonly used methods but also one of the most commonly misused. There are many different forms of correlation, but most express the degree of relationship between two variables as a value (or coefficient) between –1 and 1. Correlations can be positive, where an increase in one score is associated with an increase in another score; or they can be negative, where an increase in one score is associated with a decrease in another score. A correlation of 0 would indicate that there is no association; an example might be the association between cortisol levels and the number of positive symptoms in a group of psychotic patients. A correlation of +1 would indicate perfect agreement.

A correlation of absolute value 0.9 or above could be described as a very strong association; between 0.7 and 0.9 as indicating a strong association; between 0.4 and 0.7 as a moderate association; between 0.2 and 0.4 as a weak association; and below 0.2 as a very weak association.

Most forms of correlation assume that the association between the two variables is linear; that is, when the two variables change together the degree of change will be proportionately the same. In contrast, a small change in one variable may be associated with a large change in the other; or an association may be in different directions at different values of one of the variables (for example the association between age and arm strength would be positive in young people, non-existent in middle years, and negative in older people). In such cases, the association is not linear and the usual forms of correlation can not be used. It is possible to obtain a zero association if a linear test is applied to two variables that are in reality highly correlated but in a non-linear way.

Correlations can be diagramatically represented in a scatterplot. This is simply a graph of the pairs of values, on axes whose scales have been chosen so that the range of each of the two variables occupies approximately the same distance on each axis. The closer that the scores cluster around a line representing the trend, the higher the correlation; coefficients near to 0 will tend to be scattered approximately as a circle. Scatterplots give an instant picture of the nature of the association between two variables, and will often give a clear visual indication of linearity. A scatterplot should always be presented when a correlation is a key part of your results. There are also statistical methods that can be used to assess linearity. Special forms of correlation exist to deal with non-linearity; however, a common solution is to perform a transformation of the data (p. 185).

A scatterplot is also useful to determine if an apparent correlation has been spuriously generated by the existence of one or more 'outliers' (that is, an individual point that is considerably different from the rest). Outliers can have an undue influence on the magnitude of a correlation, sometimes to the degree that the correlation disappears if the outlier is omitted from the analysis. It is good practice to calculate the correlation with and without the outliers; it is often difficult to explain their existence, but clerical error may be responsible.

A useful way of interpreting a correlation is to convert it to a measure of the 'proportion of variance accounted for'. That is, how much of the variation in one variable is 'due to' or 'explained by' its association with another variable. This is achieved by squaring the coefficient. For example, Workman et al (1993) reported a mean correlation of +0.73 between perineal EMG levels and intravaginal pressure; thus about 53% (0.73^2) of the variation in intravaginal pressure is explained by its association with perineal EMG levels. Note that this does not necessarily mean 'caused by'. It is simply a measure of how much variance the two variables have in common.

If there are three variables that correlate with each other, clinicians may wish to remove the influence of one of these on the association between the other two. This is achieved by using partial correlations. For example, reaction time may be correlated with depression, but it may also be correlated with intelligence. Partial correlation will permit you to determine the association between reaction time and depression, having partialled out the confounding influence of intelligence.

A correlation between variable A and variable B does not mean that A causes B; or that B causes A. The association may arise because a third variable affects both A and B. There may be a causal relationship between A and B, but the correlation alone cannot tell you this; you will need data from another source or a systematic theory before inferences about causality can be drawn. Similarly, if A is correlated with B, and B is correlated with C, it does not necessarily follow that A is correlated with C.

Pearson product moment correlation (r)

This is the most commonly used parametric correlation, and it forms the basis of many more advanced statistical techniques. The assumptions underlying its use are similar to those underlying the use of the t test, but the key assumption which must not be violated is that the scores within each group are independent.

You should aim to have at least 30 subjects per group to calculate an r, because the confidence intervals are surprisingly wide for small samples. For example, even with 30 subjects and with an observed r of $+0.50$, the 95% CI is $+0.17$ to $+0.73$.

If one of the variables in a correlation is artificially restricted to a narrow range of scores, this will serve to attenuate the magnitude of the coefficient, underestimating the degree of association; for example, there may be a high correlation between adult age and scores on a memory test, but this may not emerge if the age range of your sample is only between 30 and 40 years. Correlations will also be attenuated if a continuous variable is recoded to a non-continuous variable; for example, if Hamilton depression scores are recoded as mild, moderate and severe. If two variables are correlated at $+0.60$, this will reduce to $+0.45$ if one variable is recoded into three categories.

The Pearson r is not sensitive to changes in absolute magnitude. If r is used to assess agreement between clinicians on a rating scale, you could not infer from a high correlation that the scores were comparable in terms of overall mean; only that the clinicians would rank order the scores in a similar way.

Example: Alaghband-Zadeh et al (1997) collected a variety of clinical and other variables, and MRI data, from 29 young people who had received a diagnosis of schizophrenia before the age of 12. They reported a correlation of −0.65 (d.f. = 27, p = <0.0001) between total score on the Scale for the Assessment of Negative Symptoms and total cerebral volume. They described this correlation between a rating scale score and a biological measure as 'striking', but cautioned that any conclusion should be tentative because of the small sample.

Spearman rank correlation (ρ)

This is the non-parametric equivalent of r, and is based on ranks. Mathematically it is derived from r; indeed if you calculate an r with ranked data, you will obtain exactly the same coefficient as if you had calculated a ρ.

Example: Krakow et al (1996) reported the results of an 18 month follow-up of 58 nightmare sufferers treated by cognitive–behavioural methods. A variety of pre- and post-treatment measures were used and related to nightmare reduction and to improved sleep. For example, improved sleep correlated strongly with decreases in total distress measured by the Symptom Questionnaire (ρ = −0.81, P = <0.0001). A Bonferroni correction was used (p. 191).

Other measures of correlation

The point-biserial correlation (rpb) is used when one variable is dichotomous and the other is continuous. It can be used to convert a t value to a correlation. This is useful because the t value itself imparts little information, but a correlation coefficient has a relatively standard meaning. Most packages do not routinely carry out this conversion but it is very straightforward. You square the t value, and divide the result by t squared plus d.f.; finally you take the square root. So with $t = 3.6$ and d.f. $= 32$, rpb $= 0.51$. If the dichotomous variable is in reality a continuous variable (if for example you have converted a continuous outcome measure to improved versus not improved), you should use the biserial correlation.

Similarly you can convert a χ^2 to a φ coefficient (for 2×2 tables), or a contingency coefficient (for larger than 2×2 tables).

Kendall's coefficient of concordance, a non-parametric test, is used when more than two people are ranking the same objects; it can only have a positive value. Kendall's tau (τ) is close to ρ, but has the additional advantage that it can be extended to carry out a non-parametric partial correlation.

Kappa (κ) is a useful measure of agreement; for example it can assess how far two or more clinicians agree with each other in allocating patients to the same diagnostic categories.

Simple linear regression

Regression is used to predict the score on a dependent variable from knowledge of scores on independent variables. If you are predicting from one independent variable, the appropriate technique is simple linear regression. If you are predicting from two or more variables, multiple regression is used. These techniques can be used only when the relationship between the dependent and independent variables is reasonably linear. If the relationship is non-linear, the data may have to be transformed. A further restriction in their use is that the dependent variable must be continuous; if it is not, you must use log-linear analysis or logistic regression (for binary variables) (p. 179).

The output of results from regression analysis is a formula enabling prediction of one score from another. This will always be in the format of: dependent variable = a constant + (the independent variable) × (a weight). The weight applied to the independent variable is known as the 'B' weight. The values of the constant and the weight are calculated to minimise the squared differences between the actual scores and the predicted scores. The analysis will also calculate a regression line; this is the 'best-fit' line that summarises the association between the variables. The slope of the regression line is the regression coefficient, and this is normally reported along with its standard error.

The results of a regression analysis do not permit inferences to be drawn of a causal relationship between variables, nor do they give any indication of directions of causality. Interestingly, a different regression formula will result if you regress variable A on variable B, than if B is regressed on A.

The computer output will indicate how much of the variance in the scores is explained by the regression. The statistical significance of this is expressed by the usual P value, based on the F ratio. There is a close mathematical relationship between regression and ANOVA.

Regression can be used when the dependent and independent variables are measured on scales that differ greatly in their ranges; for example, you might wish to predict duration of hospitalisation (a range of say 1 to 180 days) from scores on the HRDS (range of 0 to 30). It is possible to transform the variables to a common scale, by converting the raw scores into Z scores. The resulting weight is then known as a β (beta) weight. Incidentally the β weight in a simpler linear regression has precisely the same value as the correlation between the two variables.

Residuals

For each value in the data a residual may be calculated as the difference between the observed value of the dependent variable and the predicted value. Residuals provide a guide to 'goodness of fit', and can also be used to reduce the confounding association of one variable with another, in a way analogous to a partial correlation. The regression line summarises the association

between two variables; in other words it 'explains' or 'contains' the variance that they share. If that shared variance is subtracted from the remaining variance (that is, if the residuals are calculated), we have removed that part of one variable that is due to the other. For example, in a study of the prevalence of asthma in children, Austin et al (1994) used the residuals to obtain a measure of lung capacity uncontaminated by its relationship with body size. Similarly Price et al (1987) regressed body mass index (BMI) on age in order to remove the influence of age on BMI, in a study on the genetics of obesity.

Residuals can also be used to investigate whether the association between the variables is linear. The residuals are plotted against the independent variable. If the association is linear the values of the residuals should show no consistent pattern; but if the values appear to increase or decrease systematically, this demonstrates that the association is not linear.

The output will also indicate the presence of 'outliers' in the data; that is, unusual scores that do not conform to the pattern summarised by the regression formula. You should investigate the reasons for the outliers; they may be due to clerical error. If there are many outliers, this may suggest the presence of a subgroup in the data.

Multiple regression

Here two or more independent variables are put into the regression analysis, but the method is essentially the same. A formula is produced involving a constant, followed by each independent variable with its appropriate weight. The independent variables can be continuous or categorical, but for categorical variables with more than two categories 'dummy' variables must be introduced. A categorical variable with κ categories will require the construction of $(\kappa - 1)$ dummy variables. β weights are particularly valuable in multiple regression because, being on the same scale, they give an indication of the predictive power of the independent variables relative to each other.

Initially you should decide which variables from your data set should be examined, in advance of the analysis. You should pick those that are of particular interest on theoretical or clinical grounds, and not simply include all the independent variables in the study. The order of entering the variables can produce different solutions, although the underlying mathematical processes are equally valid. The order should reflect your hypotheses about associations between the dependent and independent variables. In many cases however, automatic variable selection methods are used. There are two main ways in which the multiple regression analysis selects which variables are predictive: forward selection and backward selection. In forward selection you start with the most predictive independent variable, and bring in others until you no longer account for significantly more variance. In backward, you start with all the variables and remove them one at a time until you reduce the variance accounted for. These methods may be combined so that at any step variables are examined both for deletion and entry into the predicting equation. Backward selection is probably the most appropriate of these simple methods, but it should be noted that whatever method is used a set of dummy variables representing a categorical variable should either all be in or all be out of the equation.

The output will normally present β and its SE, an *F* ratio and *P* value for each variable selected, and the cumulative proportion of variance accounted for as each variable is entered into the equation.

Variables are not necessarily selected according to the strength of the correlation between the independent and dependent variables, but according to how much additional predictive power they bring to the equation. If two independent variables are themselves highly correlated, only the more powerful of the two may be selected. If there is a high degree of association between the independent variables, a special form of regression, 'ridge' regression, can be used.

A large sample size is normally required for the valid use of multiple regression; there are no 'hard-and-fast' rules, but you should attempt to have at least 10 times as many subjects as independent variables. Note that this refers to each variable examined, not simply the number that is selected in the equation. As with simple regression, the output will indicate how much of the variance is accounted for by the equation; if you have few subjects and many independent variables the amount of variance accounted for will be massive but spurious. Outputs are unlikely to warn you of this, so be sceptical of particularly high values of variance accounted for (e.g. over 50%).

Example: This non-clinical example illustrates multiple regression in a readily understandable way. The record times of 113 Scottish hill races in a particular year is the dependent variable. The independent variables are the distance run and the height gained in each race. Multiple regression produced the following formula:

record time = − 8.65 + (distance × 5.39) + (height × 0.012).

This formula permitted the organisers to estimate the winning time of a new race run over 16 miles

and 6200 feet. Using this formula, the prediction was 2 h 32 min; the actual time was 2 h 34 min. The amount of variance accounted for was very high (over 95%). The results suggested that the influence of other variables (e.g. roughness of terrain) was not worth investigating because there was so little variance left to explain.

Logistic regression

Logistic regression is used to analyse data in which the independent variable has only two categories – known as a binary variable. In a particularly simple case we could consider a binary response and a binary independent variable, in which case the results could be expressed as a 2 × 2 contingency table as in Table 5.9. The appropriate method of analysis would then be a χ^2 test. However, the table may also be analysed by logistic-linear regression. The responses would be *a* out of *a* + *b* patients improved on active treatment, *c* out of *c* + *d* patients improved on placebo. The independent variable is treatment, and the regression model used attempts to predict the proportion of patients improving as a function of treatment. The regression coefficient corresponding to treatment is a little complicated in its interpretation – it is the estimated 'log odds ratio' of improvement between the two groups. It is perhaps helpful to explain this in some detail.

If we were to think of estimating the probability that a treated patient were to improve, the data would suggest a value of *a*/(*a* + *b*) for this. Similarly, for an untreated patient, the equivalent figure would be *c*/(*c* + *d*). Now, if instead of probabilities we think of odds, as defined by the relevant probability divided by its complement (i.e. 1− the probability), the odds that a treated patient improves would be estimated as *a*/*b*, and an untreated patient as *c*/*d*. The ratio of these odds is *ad*/*bc*, and the logarithm of this quantity, ln(*ad*/*bc*) is the log of the ratio of the estimated odds.

Although this may seem somewhat obscure, the great advantage of logistic-linear regression is that it provides a model for the probability of response which may be used for several independent variables of mixed categorical and continuous type. It is even possible to use the method to analyse data case by case, with the response for a single case being coded as 0 (absent) or 1 (present).

Example: Dawson and Archer (1993) examined the predictors of DSM-111R past year alcohol dependence in a large sample of drinkers. The response variable was binary – dependent/non-dependent. Using logistic-linear regression they found that the independent variables age, sex, ethnicity, marital status, family history, income, education, age of first drink, total body water, average alcohol consumption and frequency of heavy drinking were all predictive (some in a negative direction) of dependence.

SURVIVAL ANALYSIS

Survival analysis, as its name implies, was originally related to the drawing of inferences from numerical data on length of life. However, the methods of survival analysis may be applied to the amount of time elapsing before any particular event, such as relapse, in the history of an individual. Indeed more recent formulations of the survival approach have been applied to multiple, repeatable events, and this is often known as event history analysis (Allison 1984). Although the earliest developments in this area related to reliability theory in engineering applications, and were concerned with failure histories of industrial components, more recent methods have been developed in response to the need for efficient analysis of information from cancer trials, assessment of heart transplantation techniques, and so on. Parallel developments in the social sciences have seen applications of these methods to changes in marital status, occupational mobility and criminality among other topics (Diamond & McDonald 1991). A useful guide to more theoretical aspects of the subject is provided by Cox & Oakes (1984).

The quantity which is the subject of a survival analysis is the survival time of the individuals under study. The terminal event in psychiatric applications will not usually be death of the subject, but some other kind of event. Nevertheless, it is convenient to refer to the time interval between entry of an individual to the study and the individual's experience of the terminal event as survival time. Such time is not the same as the ages of the individuals, nor is it simply times/dates on the external calendar. Each one is the difference between two times/dates, and will usually be rounded to convenient units.

Censoring

It is not usually practicable to follow up all subjects selected for study until the occurrence of the terminal event. Individuals may be lost to follow-up through withdrawal of cooperation, because of geographical moves, or for other reasons. Standard practice is to study the respondents for a fixed period of time, and not all individuals will have experienced the event of interest at the end of this period. Thus, considering the outcome for a study member to be time from an appro-priate initial point (such as date on which an illness was diagnosed) to time of the event, for some cases the information available is only that the event had not occurred at time t_i, and we say that the observation is censored (or right-censored, as it sometimes happens that we may know the time of the event, but not the appropriate start time for an individual, in which case the observation is left-censored). This type of censoring is often called progressive censoring. A common type of censoring in industrial applications and also to some extent in laboratory experimentation on animals is single censoring. In this case all individuals start at the same calendar time, and the study finishes at a single suitable future time. Censoring occurs only because the event of interest has not taken place by the end of the study, and thus all censored values are equal to the duration of investigation.

A particular problem arises in the application of survival methods in investigations where direct follow-up is not undertaken. For example, in analysing a set of hospital admission records the event of interest might be the readmission of a patient after discharge. The survival time would simply be the time between discharge and readmission, and individuals not readmitted would be considered as censored, the corresponding time being the time from their discharge to the end of the study. However, there is a potential problem if the population is highly mobile, or is likely to be subject to high mortality rates. If migration from the area is associated with readmission elsewhere, or migration or mortality experience is associated with the factors under investigation, the possibility of serious bias exists. One way of attempting to deal with this is to consider shorter timescales following discharge, and restrict attention, for example to readmissions within 3 months of discharge, 6 months of discharge and so on. The use of several different periods of interest may give some indication of the likely scale of the problem of unrecorded loss to follow-up, at least in terms of its impact on the model estimates.

It could be suggested that an adequate description of survival experience would be given simply by estimation of the proportion surviving after a single particular period rather than by requiring all the individual survival times to be recorded. The difficulty with this relates to the appropriate choice of period, for if the period is long enough, all individuals will either have experienced the terminal event, or been censored. Further, with this approach it is not clear how to adjust for differential patterns of censoring in group comparisons.

Key statistical issues in survival analysis

• *Illustration and description* Survival methods should

provide an informative representation of the survival pattern of the population under study, in terms, for example, of the distribution of times to the event of interest from entry to the study.

- *Evaluation of precision* If we wished to estimate the average time to relapse from initial treatment we require to know how precise our estimate is. Within what range might we expect it to vary from the population true value?
- *Significance testing* For example, do male patients tend to relapse more quickly than female patients with a particular illness? If the survival times for male patients are shorter than those for females then we have to decide whether this represents merely the operation of chance, or is a reflection of a true systematic difference.

The aim of survival analysis is to model the survival experience of individuals and estimate associated quantities of interest. Models may include explanatory variables of several types, such as group membership, a discrete variable which might indicate different treatment regimens, age, a continuous variate which can be adjusted for in group comparisons, and other variables which may be of primary interest in themselves, or may be potential confounders of the relationships in question, and therefore need to be taken into account.

A brief description of some applications of survival methods in psychiatric research will help to give some idea of the potential utility of this approach, and also provide a framework to facilitate description of the methods in terms of appropriate events.

Fuller and Williford (1980) used survival methods in a 12 month follow-up study of 128 alcoholics to compare the treatment outcome of three groups: placebo control, a therapeutic dose of disulfiram, and a subtherapeutic dose of the same substance. The events considered of interest were:

1. relapse from abstinence
2. relapse to heavy drinking.

Analysis of group totals remaining abstinent at the end of the 12 month period failed to show significant differences between the groups, whereas the application of survival methods did produce statistical significance. Relapse was found to be significantly more frequent in the placebo group, while the two disulfiram groups were quite similar in outcome.

Keller et al (1980a) applied survival methods to recovery from major depressive disorder in 101 patients, and similarly (Keller et al 1980b) to relapse in major depressive disorder in 75 patients. In the former case 'survival' equates to remaining depressed, the terminal event of interest being recovery, while in the second

study these terms relate respectively to remaining well and becoming depressed.

Dean and Surtees (1989) followed up 125 breast cancer patients for periods of 6–8 years, in an assessment of the effect of psychiatric factors on survival. In this case, the terminal event is death, and the usual terminology of survival analysis is exactly appropriate.

Parametric and non-parametric approaches

Just as in other statistical methods, in survival analysis we may distinguish between parametric or distributional methods and distribution-free methods. The first type involve the assumption of a particular probability distribution governing times to death, and estimation of its parameters, whereas distribution-free approaches do not require the assumption of a particular distributional form. In this section we concentrate on the latter approach, and although we will concentrate on continuous time methods, it should be borne in mind that time will often be grouped into intervals.

We may describe the probability distribution of time to death from an appropriate initial point in a number of ways. The cumulative distribution function of time to death, T, that is the probability of dying before t, is defined as:

$$F(t) = P[\, T \leq t\,]: \quad t \geq 0 \qquad (1)$$

However, it is more usual to consider the survival function, the probability that an individual survives until at least time t, which is just the complement of $F(t)$:

$$S(t) = 1 - F(t): \quad t \geq 0 \qquad (2)$$

A function related to these and very widely used is the hazard function, also called the instantaneous death rate, failure rate or force of mortality. It may be denoted by $\lambda(t)$, and the probability of death in the infinitesimal interval $(t, t+dt)$, given survival to time t is given by:

$$\lambda(t)\, dt: \quad t \geq 0 \qquad (3)$$

Several explicit functional forms are commonly applied in the analysis (see p. 182) of survival data. For example, a constant hazard rate leads to the exponential distribution of times to death.

One interesting aspect of this particular distribution relates to the use of person-years at risk in meta-analyses (see p. 191) of studies. If the hazard rate is constant, as for the exponential distribution, then simply counting the number of deaths and dividing by the sum of the times at risk over all the individuals concerned will give a good estimate of the hazard. However, this procedure is not recommended in general for biomedical or social studies, precisely because hazard rates are unlikely to be constant. An example of the kind of bias which the procedure could induce is afforded by an analysis of suicide following discharge from treatment for alcoholism (Murphy & Wetzel 1990). In this case the hazard is markedly decreasing, so combining studies of different lengths of follow-up will lead to a greater or lower estimate of hazard depending on whether the studies are mostly short-term or long-term.

Clearly computational convenience alone would be an inadequate guide to choice of survival distribution. In some cases, particularly in engineering or other physical applications, a mathematical model of failure may be available which leads to the appropriate distribution, but in many applications in social and biomedical sciences empirical means must be used to assess the appropriateness of particular survival distributions. In general the problem of choosing the appropriate distribution in survival analysis is no different from the same question in standard statistical applications, but the presence of censoring makes for slight complications.

Estimating the survival function

Plotting the estimated survival function is a useful aid (among others) to decision in the case of censored data. In many cases suitable choice of axes will render the appropriate plots linear in appearance, the choice depending on the particular distribution, and therefore providing a useful diagnostic guide.

The object of many survival analyses is the comparison of two or more groups of patients, adjusted if necessary for the effect of confounding or possibly confounding explanatory variables. If, for example, it is desired to compare survival on a new treatment with a standard, it will sometimes be the case that the groups of individuals differ on background characteristics such as age, severity of illness, and so on. This will almost certainly be so when random allocation to groups has not been used, or for some reason has been inadequate. In these circumstances it is important to realise that attempting to control for these characteristics will not necessarily obviate the problems of inference, as the characteristics may be associated both with allocation and outcome or, in some cases be influenced by the treatment. Particular care must be taken when the explanatory variables are time dependent, when changes in these may be related to treatment and outcome.

In the simplest case we consider comparing two groups, and introduce an explanatory independent variable x taking values 0 and 1. One suitable model incorporating a difference in survival between the groups is the proportional hazards model in which the effect of a treatment is assumed to multiply the hazard by a constant. The proportional hazards model solves many of the problems of statistical inference on censored data with general hazard function in a particularly simple way.

As mentioned earlier, particular distributional assumptions regarding the form of the survival distribution may not be appropriate, for example when little previous investigation of a phenomenon has been performed and there is no model of failure leading to a particular distribution. It is unfortunate that in many survival applications no simple survival distribution may be applicable to the data, and in such circumstances it is advisable to use methods which do not depend on particular distributional properties of the data (i.e. non-parametric or distribution-free).

A set of survival data may be simply described by construction of a lifetable, and graphically represented by a survival curve. Data may be grouped into intervals by time of deaths, or considered as a set of individual observations.

For ungrouped data the Kaplan–Meier (Kaplan & Meier 1958) approach to estimation of the survival function proceeds as follows. Times of death, t_i, are ordered from smallest to largest, and for any particular ordered value t_i we may write the number of patients still at risk as n_i, which includes the patient dying at t_i. If one of the censored times is also equal to t_i the Kaplan–Meier method includes the censored patient in the n_i. The probability of surviving at least time t (between values t_i and t_{i+1} say) is estimated by:

$$\hat{S}(t) = \prod_{j=1}^{i} \frac{n_{j-1}}{n_j} \qquad (4)$$

This estimate is also often called the product-limit estimate, because the survival probabilities are calculated as the product of successive conditional probabilities. In fact this offers a particularly simple intuitive way of understanding the basis of the estimate. If $\hat{S}(t_{(j)})$ is the estimated survival function at time $t_{(j)}$, and the next death occurs at time $t_{(j+1)}$, the estimated survival function $\hat{S}(t_{(j+1)})$ is given by $\hat{S}(t_{(j)})$ times the probability of surviving during $(t_{(j)}, t_{(j+1)})$. This probability is the complement of the estimated probability of death in the period $(t_{(j)}, t_{(j+1)})$, which is estimated intuitively as the number dying (which is in fact 1, the death at $t_{(j+1)}$) in the interval divided by the number at risk of death in the interval.

Thus equation 4 above can be interpreted as the survival function at time 0, which is of course 1, times the complement of each of the death probabilities associated with the first i deaths. Note that if there is no censoring then for any particular value of t, the estimate reduces to the simple proportion of survivors at time t.

The importance of this method of estimating the survival function is that it does not require a distributional assumption about the form of $\hat{S}(t)$, and its robustness is one reason why it is still in common use many years after its development. To convey it in a more immediately apprehended form, it is usual to plot $\hat{S}(t)$ against t, although it should be noted that the estimates become less reliable as the numbers left alive diminish.

The Kaplan–Meier estimate is not without shortcomings. In particular, since it is not based on a particular distributional form it has a high variance, and so in a case where one might safely assume a particular distribution to be appropriate to the data, analysis should proceed on a parametric basis. In general, however, practical biomedical research requires a distribution-free approach, and the Kaplan–Meier method is most satisfactory.

In some circumstances individual times of death and censoring are not available, and it is necessary to work with data grouped into quite long time-periods, so that many events occur in a single period. The principle of analysis is very similar to that for the Kaplan–Meier estimator, but there is one important difference in the treatment of censored data. Instead of simply using as denominator the number of individuals present at the start of the interval, we calculate the person-years of exposure represented in the interval. Among other things this permits reasonably consistent analysis of a table in which the intervals are of different lengths. In calculating the person-years of exposure we count individuals censored during a time period as present for half the period, whereas in the Kaplan–Meier approach we considered individuals censored at the same time as a death as being in the population at risk at the time concerned. We consider individuals dying during a time interval as being at risk for the whole of the interval, by analogy with the procedure which we would follow in the absence of censoring. The actuarial survival curve is simply the graph of the resulting estimate of the survival function against t, but whereas the Kaplan–Meier estimate is graphed as a step-function, the actuarial graph is usually drawn as a succession of oblique slopes. This is equivalent to assuming that the death rate between the points corresponding to times j and $j+1$ is linear.

Statistical comparisons in survival analysis

If a numerical rather than a graphical summary of the data is required there are various possibilities. We might present 1 year, 5 year or 10 year survival rates, together with appropriately calculated confidence intervals. The choice of time-period will depend on the survival pattern itself, there being little point for example in quoting survival rates of 0 or 1 in most instances. The choice will also depend on available comparative data. If we wish to compare our results with other studies quoting 5 year survival, then clearly we will also quote 5 year rates.

It is often helpful to report a 'typical' survival time, and a suitable measure based on a distribution-free approach is the median survival time. The Kaplan–Meier approach readily provides an estimate of median survival time as the time point at which the horizontal line representing a constant probability of 0.5 crosses the Kaplan–Meier plot. If the value 0.5 is taken by a range of time points we use the midpoint of the range as our estimate.

A number of distribution-free tests have been adapted for the analysis of survival data. When there is no censoring the appropriate distribution-free test may be applied without modification to the times of death. For example, two groups may be compared by means of the Wilcoxon rank sum test, or equivalently the Mann–Whitney U test, while an appropriate test for several groups would be the Kruskal–Wallis analysis of variance by ranks. Censoring however necessitates adaptation of the tests.

The Wilcoxon test may be adapted following Gehan (1965) by considering the Mann–Whitney form of the test statistic. In this formulation all possible pairs of observations containing one member from each sample are considered, and a scoring system is adopted so that each pair in which, for example, the value for the sample 2 member is greater than that for the sample 1 member adds 1 to the total, those with the opposite relation subtracting 1, and tied pairs contributing 0. Where censoring is present pairs of censored observations do not contribute to the total and nor do cases in which the smaller member of the pair is censored. All other pairs are counted in the usual fashion. The distribution of the statistic may be constructed and used for statistical inference either directly or by means of a normal approximation. The approach generalises to κ groups, but the algebra involved is relatively complicated.

Perhaps the most widely used distribution-free test for this problem is the log-rank test (Peto & Peto 1972). The test is applicable to the comparison of any number of groups, but is most simply described for the two group case. The basis of the approach is to compare the observed numbers of deaths in each group with the numbers expected, assuming that at any time in the study any individual in one group has the same chance of dying as any individual in another group. Only intervals in which one or more deaths occur are used in the calculation, which essentially involves dividing the observed number of deaths in a particular interval into expected numbers of deaths in each group in accordance with the number of individuals at risk in the groups. If there are no differences between the survival functions for the groups we should find the total number of deaths observed in each group to be close to the expected number.

The test is most efficient in the case of constant death rate ratio, equivalent to the proportional hazards assumption. Departures from this assumption may be manifested in various ways: examples are Kaplan–Meier curves which cross, or which converge or diverge only after a certain non-negligible time. A possible explanation for such phenomena is an effect of a concomitant factor. In a comparison of two different treatments the ages of patients may be partially confounding the results, even if randomisation was used in assignment to groups.

Adjustment for concomitant factors in the log-rank test is in theory a simple matter, although typically involving calculations too laborious to be performed by hand. The data are stratified by each level of the concomitant variable and separate log-rank analyses performed to find observed and expected deaths in each stratum. These are then summed over strata, and the usual statistic calculated. If the variable to be adjusted for is continuous then it will be necessary to group it into appropriate strata. Simultaneous adjustment for several factors is possible by constructing the appropriate strata based on cross-classification by the factors, but usually this leads to small strata. It is advisable to avoid stratifying so finely as to have less than five patients per stratum.

When investigating a factor with several levels it may be natural to seek a progressive effect rather than a simple disparity between groups. Such an effect might be expected when comparing different levels of a treatment with a control substance, if survival is monotonically related to the treatment level. Hypotheses of this type (familiar from other statistical applications) are often called trend hypotheses. The log-rank test may be extended to cover this type of situation rather simply. However, in practice it is easier to use an explicit regression model for adjustment and testing of trends.

Cox regression

The proportional hazards model has been exploited to great effect by Cox (1972) in his development of a general methodology for the analysis of survival data. The approach permits estimation and testing in the case of many independent variables, including mixtures of categorical and continuous variates.

The distinctive feature of the method known as Cox regression is that the baseline hazard function, that is the hazard function corresponding to the reference level of the explanatory variables, is allowed to be of completely general form. The method is therefore distribution-free, although it does make the assumption that the explanatory variables act in accordance with a proportional hazards model. The approach obviates the need to estimate this baseline hazard, and the method of partial likelihood (Cox 1975) is used to estimate the parameters describing the relation between the explanatory variables and survival.

Partial likelihood fitting of models such as the above (of necessity involving use of computer program packages) leads to estimates of the parameters and corresponding standard errors for the independent variables.

In the simplest case there will be one of the explanatory variables which is of primary interest, a treatment variable for example, and the others may be considered as potential confounders of the effect of the treatment. Inference may be based on the estimate and standard error corresponding to this variable in the model including all possible terms.

A common method of model-fitting in exploratory analyses is backward elimination, as mentioned in the section on multiple regression. The first model fitted contains all the terms which might possibly be of interest, and is then compared with all the models obtained by omitting each one of the terms. If each term omitted turns out to be statistically significant then the full model cannot be reduced further. Otherwise the model omitting the term which was least statistically significant takes the place of the full model and the process is gone through once more.

It is important to point out that if a model contains interaction terms, these should be considered for deletion first. It does not make sense to delete a term from the model while including interactions involving the term.

OTHER ASPECTS

Principal components analysis (PCA)

PCA is used to explore the correlations between a large number of variables in a matrix, with a view to seeing how they relate to each other. The method produces a set of coefficients to be applied to each variable in the set to form 'components'. For example, if many bodily measurements are all correlated, it is likely that height, weight, neck circumference and foot length would correlate with each other and form a component that could be called 'body size'; similarly, heart rate, electrodermal measures, muscle tension and blood pressure would be likely to intercorrelate to form a component of 'autonomic arousal'. The components identified can be retained as new variables, and any of the original variables or items that do not feature in the newly formed components are sometimes discarded. The associations between the original variable and the components to which it relates are known as its 'loadings'.

A large number of subjects is required for PCA: at least 200 is normally recommended; more if there are many variables.

Components are hypothetical entities that emerge from the data entered into the PCA. There is no guarantee that with different subjects the same components will emerge. PCA should not be regarded as a technique that will reveal natural or true entities; rather it should be seen as a method for simplifying a complex series of associations between variables, or as an attempt to find the minimum number of components that can account for the intercorrelations.

PCA can produce several solutions; they will be equally valid mathematically, but some solutions will be more meaningful clinically. It is up to the researchers to choose which solution will best serve their purposes.

The PCA procedure will extract the same number of components as there are variables. The relative importance of the components in terms of variance explained is revealed by their corresponding 'eigenvalues'. If you specify that eigenvalues should be greater than 1, this will impose limitations on the number of components extracted. If the resulting components are unsatisfactory because they are too complex or are clinically uninterpretable, they can be 'rotated' until more satisfactory solutions are obtained. There are several methods of rotation, the most common in psychiatry being 'varimax'.

Components extracted are 'orthogonal'; that is, each is quite independent of all the others and there are no significant correlations between them. Alternatively, you can decide to extract 'oblique' components, where some degree of intercorrelation is accepted.

The key parts of the output from a PCA are the number of components extracted, the variable loadings, and how much of the original variance the factors can explain (the eigenvalues).

There are numerous problems associated with the use of PCA. It is a frequently misunderstood technique, and few clinicians are likely to develop a detailed knowledge of its complexities. Many of the problems are summed up by the acronym GIGO – 'garbage in, garbage out'. PCA results will depend on the variables entered, and the variables will need to be carefully selected by the clinician. Different solutions may be found when the same variables are analysed but with a different population. Finally, there are many optional procedures within PCA, which introduces an element of arbitrariness (and of capitalisation on chance) into the analysis.

Example: PCA is often a stage in the development of questionnaires and rating scales, enabling the original instrument to be shortened and refined. For example, Bleiker et al (1993) developed a questionnaire to measure emotionality for use in psycho-oncology. Eighteen items (e.g. 'When I feel afraid or worried, I smother my feelings') were completed by over 4000 women taking part in a screening programme for breast cancer. After rotation they extracted three components that explained 55% of the variance; all the items were loaded on at least one of the components.

PCA has also been used to examine how far symptoms within a diagnosis cluster together to indicate the existence or nature of diagnostic subgroups. For example Paykel (1971) used PCA to reduce the number of variables prior to performing a cluster analysis, in a study on the classification of depression.

Data transformations

As we have seen, parametric tests assume that the population sampled has an approximately normal distribution. Extreme skewness is a key way in which non-normality can render it invalid to use parametric tests. A solution is to alter the distribution of the scores, and make them more symmetrical, by subjecting them to mathematical transformations. This is a method widely used in natural sciences and engineering; for example, the Richter scale of earthquake severity is a logarithmic scale. Logarithmic transformations (to base 10 or 'natural' log) have a strong effect on the data, and so should only be used in case of severe skewness. A milder effect is produced by taking the square root of the scores; and a very strong effect is produced by taking the reciprocal (dividing scores into 1). The arcsine transformation is appropriate for proportions. It is possible to apply more than one transformation simultaneously (e.g. reciprocal log), but this is rarely needed in psychiatry. Transformations are particularly useful in correlations, when you may wish to 'pull in' extreme scores to reduce their influence on the coefficient.

Confidence intervals and inferential statistics

Over the last decade there has been a growing awareness of the drawbacks of conventional statistical analysis, especially in its overreliance on P values which, as we have seen, often leads to misinterpretation

(Borenstein 1994). Several alternative (or supplementary) methods have been proposed, including more systematic use of confidence intervals. A CI provides more comprehensive information than say a *t* test, in that you gain a better idea of the magnitude and reliability of a result and thereby the adequacy of the sample size, and the CI is based on the same unit of measurement as the original data.

CIs also provide information that can aid in the rejection or otherwise of the null hypothesis. Remember that a 95% CI of the difference between means provides an indication of the probable range of differences between means that might be expected, with 95% certainty. If the confidence limits encompass a zero difference, this is equivalent to saying that there is a reasonable chance (greater than 5%) that the difference between means may be zero and that the null hypothesis cannot therefore be rejected. Note that the appropriate way to use CIs to conduct comparisons, such as the difference between means, is to see if the 95% CI of the difference includes zero, rather than to examine the CIs of the two groups for the degree of overlap.

This is not to say that CIs can completely replace the use of *P* values. Researchers and clinicians are familiar and comfortable with *P* values, and advocating their demise may be too revolutionary, and may also be counterproductive. There is little evidence that more extensive use of CIs will necessarily improve the quality of clinical research publications; CIs themselves can also be misinterpreted (Walter 1995). The two approaches are not incompatible; indeed, mathematically they are closely related. Perhaps the easiest solution is to present both CIs and *P* values.

Interrelationships between statistical tests

Parametric tests derive from the same basic roots as do non-parametric tests; for example, all parametric tests are founded on the building blocks of the mean and the SD. It is therefore often possible to convert one test to another (for example, one-way ANOVA with two groups is equivalent to the two-sample *t* test – that is, it produces exactly the same significance level). It is of particular interest that a *t* test can be converted to a point-biserial correlation; a χ^2 can be converted to a ϕ coefficient or to a contingency coefficient; and an ANOVA can be converted to an Eta or an intra-class correlation. Thus tests of differences can be easily converted to tests of association.

There is a strong case for reporting such conversions in research reports. By themselves, a *t* or an *F* or a χ^2 are not informative. Interpretation of significant values of a statistical test depends on other factors, such as the group means, as well as the obtained value. However,

the interpretation of a measure of association is relatively consistent. Broadly speaking, a correlation of say +0.64 can be interpreted in the same way under all circumstances; and a correlation will also provide more information in terms of magnitude of experimental effect.

Power, sample sizes and effect sizes

The type 1 error, or the problem of false positives, has already been outlined. The converse is the type 2 error or false negative. This refers to the probability of concluding that there is no difference (or association) when in fact there is, but the study was not powerful enough to show it. Conventionally it is accepted that 5% (or less) is a reasonable risk to take of a type 1 error, but with a type 2 error the conventional level of accepted risk is usually permitted to be much higher, 20% being a commonly used value. Researchers are more willing to risk saying that there is no effect when there is, than to say that there is an effect when there is not. The term 'power' refers to the sensitivity of a test to detect an effect. If you accept a type 2 error rate of 20%, power is 0.80; an error rate of 10% means a power of 0.90, and so on.

Power bears a complex relationship to four considerations: sample size, size of effect, reliability of your measures, and adopted significance level. Adequate power is a function of large samples, large effect sizes, high reliability and the 0.05 significance level. Power can be increased by manipulating any of these; increasing sample size and adopting more reliable measures are obvious and uncontentious strategies. Effect sizes are more complex and refer to the minimal size of effect that would be of clinical value; a change in a mean HRDS score from 20 to 18 may be statistically significant, but the psychiatrist may consider the difference to be trivial and of little clinical or theoretical interest, and patients may not be aware of feeling different. You may decide therefore that you are only interested in a difference of 5 or greater, and that difference would be used in calculating how many subjects you will need in the study. It is relatively easy to achieve significance if the differences are large, even with few subjects; but the smaller the effect that you seek, the larger the required sample size. Similarly, the lower the significance level (for example, adopting $P = 0.01$ or less, rather than 0.05) the more subjects you will need for a given effect size. Two-tailed tests require larger samples than one-tailed tests.

Effect sizes for differences between continuous variables are often reported in terms of number of SD units that differentiate the groups. For example, if a measure has an SD of 15, and two groups differ by a mean of 5, the effect size is 0.33. A large effect size is considered to be 1.00; a medium effect size around 0. 50, and a small effect size is 0.20 or less. In order to maintain a power of 0.80 with a significance level of 0.05, you will need the following number of subjects in each group for a *t* test: large effect, 20 subjects; medium effect, 50 subjects; small effect, 300 subjects. If you are seeking at least a medium effect and you have only 20 subjects, there is less than 50% chance that you will detect the effect; and finally if you are seeking small effects and you only have 50 subjects, there is only a 16% chance of detecting the effect. There are equivalent methods of calculating effect sizes for categorical variables.

The required sample sizes are often much higher than clinicians might initially expect; if the decision has to be made not to proceed with the study because of difficulties in selecting enough subjects or because of inadequate resources, so be it.

The concept of effect size is useful in several other ways. For example, Lipsey (1990) presents a table (Table 3.6, p. 58) that illustrates how effect sizes can be converted into other ways of interpreting your results. In particular he shows how an apparently small effect size may be clinically useful, by converting the effect size into relative proportion of success in achieving change to a specific criterion. For example, in a trial of two drugs, a small effect size of 0.3 is equivalent to differential success rates of 42% versus 57% between the drugs; a difference of this magnitude would probably be of interest to clinicians. The equivalent figures for a large effect size (1) would be 26% and 74%.

Deciding on an appropriate effect size is a judgement that is specific to each study; there are no rigid rules. A further complication is that psychiatrists, other health care professionals, patients and carers may have quite different ideas about the degree of change in a patient's condition that is worth pursuing.

If several analyses are to be conducted, the sample size calculation should be based on the key comparisons with the main outcome variable; because this sample size may not be large enough for all additional analyses, power calculations should be reported for subgroup comparisons.

There are several ways in which required sample sizes can be estimated. Some text books contain tables (e.g. Stevens 1990), or formulae (e.g. Bourke et al 1985), and several statistical packages (e.g. Instat) contain relevant procedures.

Interaction, synergism and antagonism

There has been a great deal of interest over the past 20 years or so in the concepts of synergism and antagonism between causal agents in epidemiological

Table 5.11 Depression in women in Camberwell

| Severe event | Lack of intimacy | | | |
| | Yes | | No | |
	Yes	No	Yes	No
Case	24	2	9	2
Non-case	52	60	79	191
Total	76	62	88	193
Rates	0.32	0.03	0.10	0.01

From Everitt & Smith (1979).

research, and this has led to attempts to characterise certain modes of joint action as synergistic or antagonistic (Darroch 1997). For example Brown & Harris (1978) analysed data concerning the incidence of depression in women in Camberwell, London and claimed to have detected an interaction between the risk factors 'experience of a severe life event' and 'lack of intimacy' (in the sense of a confiding relationship with a partner). Some of their data on this subject are represented in Table 5.11.

Since this was a community study, the rates may be directly estimated by the proportions in each column. It can be seen that the observed relative risks due to experience of a severe event are approximately equal in each of the intimacy categories. That is, the ratio of the observed rate among those exposed to a severe event to that among those not so exposed is roughly the same in the two intimacy categories. Symmetrically, the relative risks due to lack of intimacy are similar in each of the event categories. Thus, in terms of relative risk, lack of intimacy is not a modifier of the 'effect' of a severe event. However, if we consider rate differences rather than ratios the rate difference due to experience of a severe event in those who lack intimacy is 0.29, compared with only 0.09 among those who have an intimate relationship. On an additive interpretation of effect, lack of intimacy *is* an effect modifier.

Brown & Harris (1978) noticed that among those not experiencing a severe event the χ^2 statistic for the relevant 2 × 2 table was not significant. From this they concluded that lack of intimacy was not itself a risk factor, and led to increased risk only in conjunction with a severe event. They accordingly identified lack of intimacy as a 'vulnerability factor', whereas experience of a severe event was considered a 'provoking agent'.

Statistical interaction depends on the scale of measurement. In the present example a multiplicative measurement of effect as in a logistic-linear model fits the data adequately without the need for an interaction term, whereas an additive model would require such a term. The scale of measurement of effect and model for combination of effects cannot be entirely at choice, since an additive model of risk difference may lead to difficulties associated with all risks involved in the model being required to lie between 0 and 1 as they are probabilities. Similarly, a multiplicative model for relative risk could lead to absolute risks of greater than 1, whereas a multiplicative odds ratio model such as the logistic-linear model will not lead to this inconsistency.

The application of statistical methods to data of this type cannot therefore be expected to yield definitive conclusions regarding synergism, antagonism or their absence. Rothman (1986) proposes a model for interaction which takes as axiomatic the measurement of effect in terms of rate difference. Walter & Holford (1978) present models of causation and joint action which give rise to additive, multiplicative and other models of joint action, showing in effect that there is no inherently 'natural' way in which causal agents act together.

Causal models giving rise to various forms of joint action can be elaborated, and to some extent tested. However, it is not always possible to test these with any degree of power on the basis of a single epidemiological study. In the example considered it seems that the main qualification of lack of intimacy as a vulnerability factor is that it does not increase the risk of depression except in conjunction with the provoking agent. One might therefore attempt to assemble a large sample of individuals free of the provoking agent, in order to perform a sensitive test of the potential effect of the vulnerability factor (a negative result being essential to the hypothesis). This approach will not work if there is misclassification of individuals as not exposed to a provoking agent when they are so exposed. It will also be ineffective if there exist other provoking agents which are unknown and which are potentiated by lack of intimacy. In both these cases there will be a higher rate of depression among those lacking intimacy because of the presence in the study of individuals exposed to an undetected provoking agent.

COMMON STATISTICAL DEFICIENCIES IN CLINICAL RESEARCH

Background

Reviews of the adequacy of statistical analyses published in clinical journals have highlighted many deficiencies, some of which have been sufficiently serious to invalidate the conclusions drawn (Altman 1991a). This is despite the efforts of journal editors to improve the quality of reported statistics (e.g. Gardner et al 1986). Some of the problems seem to arise from the thoughtless reproduction of the computer output of the results.

Deficiencies have been noted in the research literature in physical rehabilitation, psychotherapy (Dar et al 1994), ophthalmology, surgery, respiratory diseases, health services research (Balas et al 1995), inter alia, including psychiatry. On the whole the frequency and range of deficiencies are similar irrespective of the clinical discipline. Some of the more obvious deficiencies have been mentioned at the end of the description of the various tests. This section will highlight some of the more subtle ones.

Time series data and correlations

Paradoxically, obtaining a series of data over time from individuals (time series data) is one of the most simple experimental designs, but it requires some of the most complex methods of analysis. The paradox arises from the problem of 'serial dependency'. A useful way to think about dependency is to consider whether knowledge of one data point tells you anything about the value of any of the other data points. For example, if you are gathering heart rate data from a patient in the early stages of a session of exposure treatment for a phobia, you would expect the rate to increase rapidly. So if you were told the rate at one time and asked to guess the rate a few seconds later, you would be likely to be correct if you guessed that the rate is faster; thus knowledge of one value allows you to predict subsequent values. The data are not therefore independent. This is an important problem in statistical analysis; parametric and non-parametric tests are equally affected.

This problem has already been referred to in connection with t tests (p. 172). However, similar errors can occur if you try to perform correlations with time series data. For example, there is a very high correlation between foot size and reading ability in children; and there is a similarly high correlation between increases in unemployment and deterioration in health. It would not be logical to assume causality from these associations. The source of these possible interpretative errors is clear; in both examples the apparent correlation may simply reflect events that occur together over time – maturation, and changes in poverty levels, respectively. There may be a 'real' correlation (as there probably is in relation to employment and health), but other methods will need to be employed to confirm this. In much clinical research however the source of the logical error is less obvious.

One solution is to conduct a highly complicated method of analysis (ARIMA or Box–Jenkins analysis);

this method requires very long series of data and is complex to compute and interpret. A simpler method, especially when the set of data is small, is to use 'differencing'. With each variable you subtract one score from the next score, throughout the whole series. Thus the series 46, 57, 68, 87, 96, 102, 114 would become 11, 11, 19, 9, 6 and 12. This effectively eliminates the trend (at least for most time series found in psychiatry). For each series these differences are saved as a new variable, and the differenced variables can then be correlated. In effect, after differencing you are correlating the changes in each variable with each other; the more that the changes occur in the same direction and to the same degree, the higher the correlation.

Example: Carney et al (1989) reported high correlations (+0.70) between climatic variables (hours of sunshine and length of day) and hospital admissions for mania. However, these variables change together over time, and the association may therefore be spurious. Peck (1990) reanalysed their data having differenced the series. Some of the original conclusions were shown to be invalid (for example, the correlation between length of day and admissions dropped from +0.70 to +0.33 and was no longer significant), but the broad conclusion that there was an association between sunshine hours and admissions for mania was robust.

Correlation between initial score and clinical change

In psychiatry it is useful to be able to predict degree of clinical change, as measured by differences between pre- and post-treatment ratings. An obvious candidate for a predictor is the patient's initial severity. Thus it appears logical to correlate initial scores with change scores. For example, Kincey et al (1996) examined the effects of surgery for obesity, and reported that preoperative weight was correlated with postsurgery weight loss at 6 months ($r = +0.66$). However, if you do this you are likely to obtain high correlations even if the data are purely random. Describing the process in notation form makes the reason obvious: you are correlating x_1 with $x_1 - y$, where y is a random component.

It is preferable to address the question of predicting post-treatment outcome by using predictor and outcome variables of entirely different types, for example predicting days in work after discharge from a pretreatment score on a questionnaire.

Ecological fallacy

The ecological fallacy has several forms, but the under-

lying fallacy is to assume that phenomena that are associated at a macro level (e.g. from national or aggregated statistics) will be similarly associated at a micro or individual level.

Example: Potkin et al (1986) tested the hypothesis that the prevalence of seasonal affective disorder (SAD) would increase with latitude. They estimated the prevalence using postal questionnaires in 48 American states. The correlation between latitude of the state and prevalence was reported to be +0.85, a very high correlation. However, a more appropriate method of analysis is the point-biserial correlation (rpb) between the individual's suffering from SAD or not (dichotomous variable), and latitude of the individual's home (continuous variable). A later study (Rosen et al 1990) reported an rpb between latitude and SAD caseness to be substantially lower at about +0.20; when age corrected, this reduced to +0.18 or less.

Regression to the mean

For any measurement which is potentially variable in time, individuals with particularly high values of the measurement on one occasion are likely to have lower values on retest, and vice versa. Thus, if a group of high-scoring individuals are selected for follow-up, it is natural to find that their scores on retest are lower than their original values. An example of this phenomenon is afforded by a study of alcohol consumption on two occasions (Kendell et al 1981). The alcohol consumption of a group of individuals in the week before a survey at one point of time was recorded. Those who reported some consumption were reinterviewed some years later. The average alcohol consumption on the second occasion was less than on the first. Some of those reinterviewed had not had any alcoholic drink in the week before the second interview. However, some of those who had reported no consumption in the week before the first interview might well have reported consumption in the week before reinterview if they had been approached. The design defect of leaving out those reporting no consumption on the first occasion is considered sufficiently serious to call into question the results of the investigation (Altman 1991b).

Misinterpretation of *P* values

A major problem with *P* values arises from the binary (yes/no) nature of the approach. The 0.05 level of significance is arbitrary and reflects convention rather than logic. It is illogical to bemoan a result with a *P* value of 0.058, but celebrate a P value of 0.048; the actual difference being minute. Moreover the CI of a non-significant result might encompass some reasonably probable values that could be of major clinical interest. For example, suppose that a new treatment has been compared with an existing treatment, and the outcome variable is the percentage of patients whose scores drop below a cut-off point for caseness. The difference between the percentages (8%) is not significant, but the 95% CI of the difference is −4% to + 20%. Thus there is a reasonable chance that one treatment will improve 20% more patients than the other treatment; a substantial difference in effectiveness cannot be ruled out, and it would be clinically irresponsible to conclude that the two treatments were equivalent.

There is a further and related problem. If a result is not significant, it is tempting to conclude that there is no difference between groups, when in reality there is a difference but the study was not powerful enough to detect it. You cannot prove a negative, including a null hypothesis. As Dar et al (1994) note: 'We can only estimate the probability of obtaining the data given the truth of the null hypothesis, not the probability of the truth of the null hypothesis given the data' (p. 76). Non-significant P values tell you that chance may explain the results, not that chance does explain the results. This is important because in some studies, having shown that there are no significant differences between groups before an intervention, the authors have wrongly claimed that the groups were therefore equal at baseline; Dar et al (1994) report that over half of published studies in psychotherapy research in the 1980s contained this inappropriate interpretation of non-significant P values.

There is also some confusion between significance and importance. The P value tells you nothing about the importance, magnitude, replicability or validity of findings. With a large sample, very small effects may achieve statistical significance, although their clinical or theoretical significance is trivial or non-existent. For example with d.f. = 1025, a correlation as low as +0.07 is significant at the 0.025 level.

Multiple testing

The logic behind the null hypothesis and P values must be taken literally. With a significance level of 5%, there is only a 1 in 20 probability that, given the truth of the null hypothesis, your result may be explained by chance. If you conduct more than one test, the probability is no longer 1 in 20; the more tests that you perform, the more the actual significance level changes (if your hypotheses are independent of each other). A rule of thumb is that the actual significance level when several tests are performed can be estimated by multiplying the nominal level by the number of comparisons (or tests of association) conducted. If you adopt the 5% level, and conduct five comparisons, the actual significance level is approximately 0.25.

There are several ways in which this problem of multiple testing may occur. First, you may have multiple outcome measures, and perform univariate tests on each outcome whereas you should perform a multivariate test on all measures simultaneously. Second, you may have multiple end-points in the study. Third, you may compare several groups. Fourth, you may conduct several interim analyses. When more than one comparison is conducted, the problem of multiple testing arises.

A dramatic example of the dangers of multiple testing in clinical research was reported by Lee et al (1990, cited in Motulsky (1995)). A sample of patients with cardiovascular disease was allocated to one of two groups. Each group was further subdivided according to how many of the three coronary arteries were affected, and according to whether there were any abnormal ventricular contractions; each full group therefore contained six subgroups. The main groups were then given either treatment A or treatment B. No significant differences in survival were obtained between A and B in the full groups, nor in five of the subgroups. However, when the most seriously ill patients in each full group were compared (those with both three-artery disease and abnormal contractions), significant differences in survival were obtained in favour of treatment A ($P = 0.025$). The startling aspect of this study is that treatments A and B were identical, and allocation to A or B was random and therefore any differences were due to chance. If this were a 'real' study and an identical procedure had been followed the authors would probably have concluded that treatment A was superior, and would no doubt have found a (retrospective) convincing but tortuous explanation as to why A was better for the most ill patients. (We should not be surprised at this result, because with six comparisons there is a 26% chance that a 'significant' result at $P = 0.05$ will be found.)

Subgroup analyses should be prespecified and backed up by a strong convincing rationale; it is possible to conceive of multitudes of subgroups in most studies, and at least one of them is likely to produce 'significant' effects. Generally, only two or three major hypotheses, and certainly no more than five, should be tested statistically in a single study. This should include all planned tests, including those that you decide not to conduct after having examined the data; comparisons can be covert as well as overt. The main hypotheses to be tested should be explicitly stated before you start to collect the data.

A commonly advocated approach to the problem of multiple testing is the Bonferroni adjustment. This entails dividing the adopted significance level by the number of comparisons to be conducted. If the nominal significance level is 0.05, and you conduct four comparisons, the adjusted level would be 0.0125. This correction controls adequately for type 1 errors, but some authorities consider it too severe if it is applied to all comparisons. A reasonable approach would be to have a single prespecified hypothesis which would not require an adjustment to the significance level; but an adjustment should be applied to all subsequent analyses.

It is important to remember that, with many clinical trials being conducted, there is a serious risk that some of the 'significant' results are in fact 'false positives', or type 1 errors; hence the importance of publishing negative results as well as positive results, and of replication studies.

In short, given enough chances, chance will eventually produce a chance result that cannot be attributed to chance.

META-ANALYSIS

With the current emphasis on evidence-based medicine and clinical effectiveness 'systematic review' has grown into a fairly major industry. Whether or not the reader is likely to conduct such a review, some understanding of the process will be of help when reading and evaluating the relevant literature.

One should start by considering formulation of the topic to be reviewed – this should be as clearly defined as possible. Thus, a review of the use of SSRIs compared to tricyclic antidepressants in uncomplicated depression is a more clearly defined topic than 'drug therapies for depression'.

Finding the evidence

An interesting result of the recent emphasis on evidence-based medicine has been the realisation that the required evidence base is often missing or incomplete, with a consequent focus on the importance of rigorous searching for evidence. Typically, on-line bibliographies such as Medline and ISI Science Citation Index are searched by computer, selected journals are hand-searched, references in the literature found by these methods are followed up, and indexes to 'grey' literature such as conference proceedings, technical reports and so on investigated. Specific problems may arise in that some non-English-language literature may not be indexed, and even if references can be obtained from other sources it may be difficult to acquire copies of the relevant sufficiently detailed papers.

Publication bias

There is then the problem of 'publication bias'. Published research in an area is not representative of all research in that area, and, in particular, results which are 'statistically significant' are more likely to be reported, and to appear in the peer-reviewed literature. Thus, an analysis which relies only on published sources is likely to be biased in favour of 'statistical significance' or large effect sizes. This is one reason why it is important to attempt to trace all unpublished findings relevant to the issue under review, and to develop methods to assess the likelihood of the results of any analysis being affected by such bias, and if possible to correct for it.

Light & Pillemer (1984) described a simple and intuitive method of evaluating publication bias. For each study under consideration the estimated effect size is plotted against the study sample size. If there is no publication bias the resulting graph should be symmetrical and tapering inwards as the sample size increases. The points could be enclosed by a shape like a funnel, hence the name 'funnel plot'. Departures from this shape are an indication of potential publication bias. There are numerous variants of this idea – an obvious one being to plot effect size against its standard error. In this case the plot should taper towards the origin. Whichever method is used, publication bias will be reflected by points being markedly asymmetrical in the direction of overall effect.

Quality

Having obtained the source material for review there are a number of other issues to be considered. Quality may vary between studies. While the double-blind randomised controlled trial is the gold standard of experimental design, restricting attention only to such studies would be impractical, in that often there may only be a small number of them, and also unsatisfactory from the scientific point of view, as the results of a potentially very large number of (albeit weaker) studies would be ignored. Other design aspects may affect study quality, such as the definitions used for inclusion and exclusion of subjects, methods of control of extraneous variables and so on.

Studies will also differ in their level of reporting. Some may reproduce the original data, others give summary statistics, yet others 'effect' estimates and standard errors, while the least useful report only significant test results or even simply P values. All of these, apart from the raw data, may also be complicated by reporting figures adjusted for various possible confounders, differing from study to study. Another major complication is that studies may measure outcome in different ways. Although methods exist for combining the results of studies expressed in terms of different outcomes by means of Z scores, there must be a major question over whether this process makes sense. As mentioned earlier, incommensurables by their nature cannot be added together. Hence, while reporting in different units of the same measurement poses no problem, reporting different measurements does – e.g. if one study reports percentage patients improving, and another the test results of the subjects.

Analysis

When it comes to combining the results of the studies for review, the first thing to stress is that simple 'head counting' is inadequate. That is, simply noting, for example, that the majority of studies of a particular intervention showed statistically significant results and concluding that this indicates the effectiveness of the intervention, may be quite wrong. If the studies showing significant effectiveness are all small, while all the large studies fail to demonstrate statistical significance, then an obvious explanation of the data is afforded by publication bias. If there are differences in the conclusions of studies, then in combining their results we should obviously afford more weight to larger studies.

For the remainder of this section we shall consider the situation where M studies (the number of studies to be combined) provide estimates of effects, and these are to be combined in a meta-analysis. There are two basic models in common use for this purpose – the 'fixed effects' and 'random effects' models. Taking the fixed effects model first, a weighted average of the estimates from each study is obtained, using as weights the squared reciprocals of the appropriate standard errors. This gives the combined estimate of effect, and the standard error of the combined estimate can also be estimated. However, it is also possible to investigate variation between the estimates from the different studies, to see whether the studies provide a homogeneous set of estimates, or whether there is heterogeneity between studies. Without going into the details of the statistical test for heterogeneity, which is in any case not very powerful, it is worth remarking that from the point of view of classical statistical theory, heterogeneity implies that the results of the studies differ from one another, and therefore should not be combined.

In the random effects model however, heterogeneity between studies is in a sense 'expected' and built into the model. The result is that the combined estimate itself is different from the fixed effects estimate, and its standard error larger – often considerably so. There are many argu-

Table 5.12 Parameter estimates from two hypothetical studies		
	Odds-ratio estimate (OR)	Standard error of log (OR)
Study 1	1.1	0.05
Study 2	0.8	0.05

ments concerning which of the models, fixed or random effects, should be used. It might naively be assumed that the random effects model is the 'cure' for heterogeneity, in that instead of deciding the studies cannot be combined we simply incorporate the between-study variation into our estimation procedure. However, there are a number of arguments against ignoring heterogeneity. Two which are intuitively simple to understand relate to the principle of marginality, and the question of the population to which the combined estimate is supposed to apply.

The concept of marginality implies that it is pointless to speak of a main effect of a factor which interacts with another. To put this in the context of meta-analysis we could take the extreme example of two studies, as in Table 5.12 – in which the effects are expressed as odds ratios.

A standard meta-analysis – either fixed or random effects model – will produce an estimate of the pooled odds ratio of 0.93, despite the fact that the directions of effect are different in each study – that is, in study 2 the effect under investigation is in the opposite direction to the effect in study 1. But suppose study 1 was of men, and study 2 of women. Or suppose study 1 is of people aged 65 and over, and study 2 of people between 20 and 30 years of age. In these circumstances, what meaning does the pooled odds ratio have?

This leads naturally to the consideration of the population to which the results of the analysis purport to apply. Suppose a large number of studies have been conducted on men, and only one on women. If there is heterogeneity between the sexes, but we use a random effects model, then to what kind of population would the pooled estimate apply?

For the above reasons, amongst others, it is important to investigate heterogeneity between studies rather than just assume a random effects model. Thompson (1993) shows how suitable statistical modelling of heterogeneity between studies in terms of study characteristics can lead to improved understanding of the phenomenon under investigation, and in some circumstances permit interpretation of apparently heterogenous data. He suggests that the random effects analysis should be considered as a type of sensitivity analysis –

that is that rather than simply assuming random effects models and attempting to provide definitive conclusions, the results of various models should be compared, to assess the degree to which any conclusions drawn could be considered 'robust'.

STATISTICAL PACKAGES

Many statistical packages are available for clinical research. They differ markedly in the range of procedures that they contain, in price, and even in the algorithms used for calculation. Some procedures in some packages have been known to provide incorrect results, so it is important for the sake of repeatability that the package used for analysis is clearly stated in research reports and to specify the version used. The packages are continually updated, so some of the details below may be out-of-date. Some of the most popular used in psychiatry (which are all available for desk computers) are the following.

Statistical Package for the Social Sciences (SPSS)

SPSS is probably the most widely used package in academic clinical research in the UK. It is reasonably easy to use, and has a good 'help' facility. There is a basic version which includes virtually all the procedures that psychiatrists would wish to use; in addition there are 'advanced' and 'professional' options, as well as special versions for time series data and other uses. It also contains procedures for a wide range of graphs, and a host of facilities for editing, transforming data, recoding, selecting, and so on. Huge quantities of data can be accommodated. However, some aspects of SPSS are rather specific to social science, and a little idiosyncratic in terms of mainstream statistics.

Minitab

Minitab was originally developed as a teaching package, but the statistical procedures were so well thought out that it soon became popular for research applications. It is very simple to use, and contains most of the statistical procedures that clinicians may need, plus a good range of graphs. The output is simple to understand and there is an admirable written manual. The major drawback is that the procedure for selecting subsets of data is somewhat ponderous. There is sufficient capacity for data for most clinical research, except the largest surveys.

Instat

This small package is outstandingly useful. It is limited in capacity (maximum of 26 columns and 500 rows), and in the range of procedures (no complex ANOVAs or logistic regression); and you cannot select subsets of data. But it is extremely easy to use, has an excellent help facility, and the output is a model of brevity, containing the information needed for adequate reporting of the results and no more. It performs functions not contained in many of the more sophisticated packages, including sample-size calculations, and has the facility to perform tests on summary statistics without having access to the original data, extremely useful for checking the accuracy of statistics in publications or theses. Instat is also inexpensive.

SAS

This is a widely-used package in academia and industry. Apart from statistical programs, SAS contains an immense range of computer applications, and is an extremely powerful integrated system. However, it is less suited to the more naive user than Minitab or Instat.

BMDP

BMDP is a competitor to SPSS and SAS, developed specifically for biomedical applications, and as a result can be more immediately relevant to medical researchers.

There are numerous other packages, many specific to more advanced statistical methods, or to particular areas of application. In particular, as sample-size determination has become more important a number of packages have been developed to assist in this area.

REFERENCES

Abrams R, Taylor M A 1978 A rating scale for emotional behaviour. American Journal of Psychiatry 135: 226–229

Aitken R B, Zealley A K 1970 Measurement of moods. British Journal of Hospital Medicine 4: 215–224

Alaghband-Zadeh J, Hamburger S D, Giedd J N, Frazier J A, Rapoport J L 1997 Childhood onset schizophrenia: biological markers in relation to clinical characteristics. American Journal of Psychiatry 154: 64–68

Allison P D 1984 Event history analysis. Sage, Beverley Hills

Altman D G 1991a Statistics in medical journals: developments in the 1980s. Statistics in Medicine 10: 1897–1913

Altman D G 1991b Practical statistics for medical research. Chapman & Hall, London

Andreasen N C 1982 Negative symptoms in schizophrenia: definition and reliability. Archives of General Psychiatry 39: 784

Asberg M, Montgomery S, Perris C 1978 The comprehensive

psychopathological rating scale. Acta Psychiatrica Scandinavica 271 (suppl 5)

Austin J B, Russell G, Adam M G, Mackintosh D, Kelsey S, Peck D F 1994. Prevalence of asthma and wheeze in the Highlands of Scotland. Archives of Disease in Childhood 71: 21–216

Balas E A, Austin S M, Ewigman B G, Brown G D, Mitchell J A 1995 Methods of randomised controlled trials in health services research. Medical Care 33: 687–699

Bech P, Bolwig T G, Kramp P 1979 The Bech mania scale and the Hamilton depression scale. Acta Psychiatrica Scandinavica 59: 420–430

Beck A T, Ward C H, Mendelson M 1961 An inventory for measuring depression. Archives of General Psychiatry 4: 561–571

Beigel A, Murphy D L, Bunney W E 1971 The manic state rating scale. Archives of General Psychiatry 25: 256–262

Blackburn J M, Loudon J B, Ashworth C M 1977 A new scale for measuring mania. Psychological Medicine 7: 453–458

Blacker D 1992 Reliability validity and the effects of misclassification in psychiatric research. In: Fava M, Rosenbaum J F (eds) Research design and methods in psychiatry. Elsevier, Amsterdam.

Blair C, Freeman C, Cull A 1995 The families of anorexia nervosa and cystic fibrosis patients. Psychological Medicine 25: 985–993

Bleiker E M A, Van der Ploeg H M, Hendriks J H C L, Leer J-W H, Kleijn W C 1993 Rationality, emotional expression and control: psychometric characteristics of a questionnaire for research in psycho-oncology. Journal of Psychosomatic Research 37: 861–872

Borenstein M 1994 A note on the use of confidence intervals in psychiatric research. Psychopharmacology Bulletin 30: 235–238

Bourke G J, Daly L E, McGilvray J 1985 Interpretation and uses of medical statistics, 3rd edn. Blackwell, Oxford

Brown G W, Harris T 1978 Social origins of depression: a reply. Psychological Medicine 8: 577–588

Brown G W, Harris T O, Hepworth C 1995 Loss, humiliation and entrapment among women developing depression: a patient and non-patient comparison. Psychological Medicine 25: 7–21

Carney P A, Fitzgerald C T, Monaghan C 1989. Seasonal variations in mania. In: Thompson C, Silverstone T (eds) Seasonal affective disorders CNS (Clinical Neuroscience) Publishers, London 19–27

Castells I, Beaulieu I, Torrado G, Wisniewski K E, Zarny S, Gelato M C 1996 Hypothalamic versus pituitary dysfunction in Down's syndrome as a cause of growth retardation. Journal of Intellectual Disability Research 40: 509–517

Cliff N 1982 What is and isn't measurement. In: Keen G (ed) Statistical and methodological issues in psychology and social science issues. Erlbaum, Hillsdale, NJ

Cox D R 1972 Regression models and life-tables. Journal of the Royal Statistical Society B 34: 187–203

Cox D R 1975 Partial likelihood. Biometrika 40: 354–360

Cox D R, Oakes D 1984 Analysis of survival data. Chapman & Hall, London

Dar R, Serlin C, Omer H 1994 Misuse of statistical tests in three decades of psychotherapy research. Journal of Consulting and Clinical Psychology 62: 75–82

Darroch J 1997 Biologic synergism and parallelism. American Journal of Epidemiology 145: 661–668

Dawson D A, Archer L D 1993 Relative frequency of heavy drinking and the risk of alcohol dependence. Addiction 88: 1509–1518

Dean C, Surtees P G 1989 Do psychological factors predict survival in breast cancer? Journal of Psychosomatic Research 33: 561–569

Dennis M, Ferguson B, Tyrer P 1992 Rating instruments. In: Research methods in Psychiatry, 2nd edn. Gaskell, London

Diamond I D, McDonald J W 1991 Analysis of current status data. In: Trussell J, Hankinson R, Tilton J (eds) Demographic applications of event history analysis. Oxford University Press, Oxford

Dilks S L E, Shattock L 1996 Does community residence mean more community contact for people with severe, long-term psychiatric disabilities? British Journal of Clinical Psychology 35: 183–192

Endicott J, Spitzer R L 1978 A diagnostic interview: the schedule for affective disorders and schizophrenia. Archives of General Psychiatry 35: 837–844

Evans D, Evans M 1996 A decent proposal. Ethical review of clinical research. Wiley, Chichester

Everitt B S 1989 Statistical methods for medical investigations. Oxford University Press, New York

Everitt B S, Smith A M R 1979 Interactions in contingency tables: a brief discussion of alternative definitions. Psychological Medicine 9: 581–583

Fava M, Rosenbaum J F (eds) 1992 How to write a study protocol: a primer for the clinician. In: Research Designs and Methods in Psychiatry. Elsevier, Amsterdam

Feighner J P, Robins E, Guze S B, Woodruff R A, Winokur G, Munoz R 1972 Diagnostic criteria for use in psychiatric research. Archives of General Psychiatry 26: 57–63

Freeman C, Tyrer P 1992 Research methods in psychiatry: a beginner's guide, 2nd edn. Gaskell, London

Fuller R K, Williford W O 1980 Life table analysis of abstinence in a study evaluating the efficacy of disulfiram. Alcoholism: Clinical and Experimental Research 4: 298–301

Gardner M J, Machin D, Campbell M J 1986 Use of checklists in assessing the statistical content of medical studies. British Medical Journal 292: 810–812

Gehan E A 1965 A generalized Wilcoxon test for comparing arbitrarily single-censored samples. Biometrika 52: 202–223

Goldberg D 1972 The detection of psychiatric illness by questionnaire. Maudsley monographs. Oxford University Press, London

Goldin J, Zhu W, Sayre J W 1996 A review of the statistical analysis used in papers published in Clinical Radiology and British Journal of Radiology. Clinical Radiology 51: 47–50

Hamilton M 1959 The assessment of anxiety state by ratings. British Journal of Medical Psychology 32: 50–55

Hamilton M 1960 A rating scale for depression. Journal of Neurology, Neurosurgery and Psychiatry 23: 56–62

Hayes R L, Halford W K 1996 Time use of unemployed and employed single male schizophrenia subjects. Schizophrenia Bulletin 22: 659–669

Helzer J E, Robins L N, Croughan J L, Welner A 1981 Reliability and procedural validity of the Renard diagnostic interviews as used by physicians and lay interviewers. Archives of General Psychiatry 38: 393–398

Honigfeld G, Gillis R D, Klett C J 1966 NOSIE-30: a treatment sensitive ward behaviour scale. Psychological Reports 19: 180–182

Iager A C, Kirch D G, Wyatt R J 1985 A negative symptom rating scale. Psychiatry Research 16: 27–36

Juzych M S, Shin D H, Seyedsadr M, Siegner S W, Juzych L

A 1992 Statistical techniques in ophthalmic journals. Archives of Ophthalmology 110: 1225–1229

Kaplan E L, Meier P 1958 Nonparametric estimation from incomplete observations. Journal of the American Statistical Association 53: 457–481

Kay S R, Fiszbein A, Opler L A 1987 The positive and negative symptom scale for schizophrenia (PANSS). Schizophrenia Bulletin 13: 261

Kearns N P, Cruickshank C A, McGuigan K J, Riley S A, Shaw S P, Snaith R P 1982 A comparison of depression rating scales. British Journal of Psychiatry 141: 45–49

Keller M B, Shapiro R W, Lavori P W, Wolfe N (1980a) Recovery in major depressive disorder: analysis with the life table and regression models. Archives of General Psychiatry 39: 905–910

Keller M B, Shapiro R W, Lavori P W, Wolfe N (1980b) Relapse in major depressive disorder: analysis with the life table. Archives of General Psychiatry 39: 911–915

Kendell R E, de Roumanie M, Ritson E B 1983. Influence of an increase in excise duty on alcohol consumption and its adverse effects. British Medical Journal 287: 809–811

Kincey J, Neve H, Soulsby C, Taylor T V 1996 Psychological state and weight loss after gastroplasty for major obesity – some outcomes and inter-relationships. Psychology Health and Medicine 1: 113–118

Knauth M, Reis S, Pohimann S et al 1997 Cohort study of multiple brain lesion in sport divers: role of patent foramen ovale. British Medical Journal 314: 701–705

Krakow B, Kellner R, Pathak D, Lambert L 1996 Long term reduction of nightmares with imagery rehearsal treatment. Behavioural and Cognitive Psychotherapy 24: 135–148

Light R J, Pillemer D B 1984 Summing up: the science of reviewing research. Harvard University Press, Cambridge

Lipsey M W 1990 Design sensitivity: statistical power for experimental research. Sage, Newbury Park

Lucock M P, Morley S 1996 The health anxiety questionnaire. British Journal of Health Psychology 1: 137–150

McGuigan S M 1995 The use of statistics in the British Journal of Psychiatry. British Journal of Psychiatry 167: 683–688

McGuire R J 1993 Statistics and research design. In: Kendell R E, Zealley A K (eds) Companion to psychiatric studies, 5th edn. Churchill Livingstone, London

McMordie W, Swint E 1979 Predictive utility, sex of rater differences and interrates reliabilities of the NOSIE-30. Journal of Clinical Psychology 35: 773–775

Marder S 1995 Psychiatric rating scales. In: Kaplan H I, Sadock B J (eds) Comprehensive textbook of psychiatry, 6th edn. Williams & Wilkins, Baltimore

Montgomery S A, Asberg M 1979 A new depression scale designed to be sensitive to change. British Journal of Psychiatry 134: 382–389

Motulsky H 1995 Intuitive biostatistics. Oxford University Press, New York

Murphy G, Wetzel R D 1990 The lifetime risk of suicide in alcoholism. Archives of General Psychiatry 47: 383–392

Overall J E, Gorham D R 1962 The brief psychiatric rating scale. Psychological Reports 10: 799–812

Paykel E 1971 Classification of depressed patients: a cluster-analysis derived grouping. British Journal of Psychiatry 118: 275–288

Peck D F 1990 Climatic variables and admission for mania: a re-analysis. Journal of Affective Disorders 20: 249–250

Peto R, Peto J 1972 Asymptotically efficient rank invariant procedures. Journal of the Royal Statistical Society A 135: 185–207

Pond D A 1975 Choice of a subject for clinical research. In: Sainsbury P, Kreitman N (eds) Methods of psychiatric research. Oxford University Press, London

Potkin S G, Zetin M, Stamenkovic V, Kripke D, Bunney W E 1986 Seasonal affective disorder: prevalence varies with latitude and climate. Clinical Neuro-Pharmacology 9 (suppl): 181–183

Price R A, Cadoret R J, Srunkard A J, Troughton E 1987. Genetic contributions to human fatness adoptive study. American Journal of Psychiatry 144: 1003–1003

Reich W 1992 Structured and semi-structured interviews. In: Hsu L K, George Hersen M (eds) Research in psychiatry issues strategies and methods. Plenum Press, New York

Robins L N, Helzer J, Croughan J 1979 The National Institute of Mental Health diagnostic interview. National Institute of Mental Health, Rockville

Robins L N, Wing J, Wittchen H U 1988 The composite international diagnostic interview: an epidemiological instrument for use with different diagnostic symptoms and in different cultures. Archives of General Psychiatry 45: 1069

Rosen L N, Targum S D, Terman M, Bryant M J 1990 Prevalence of seasonal affective disorder at four latitudes. Psychiatry Research 31: 131–144

Rothman K J 1986 Modern epidemiology. Little Brown & Co., Boston and Toronto

Ruiz M T, Alvarez-Dardet C, Vela P, Pascual E 1991 Study designs and statistical comparisons in rheumatological journals: an international comparison. British Journal of Rheumatology 30: 352–355

Sanders M, Cleghorn G, Shepherd R W, Patrick M 1996 Predictors of clinical improvement in children with recurrent abdominal pain. Behavioural and Cognitive Psychotherapy 24: 27–38

Shepherd M, Cooper B, Brown A C 1981 Psychiatric illness in general practice. Oxford University Press, New York

Snaith R P, Taylor C M 1985 Rating scales for depression and anxiety: a current perspective. British Journal of Clinical Pharmacology 19: 175–205

Snaith R P, Baugh S J, Clayden A D, Husain A, Siple M A 1982 The clinical anxiety scale: an instrument derived from the Hamilton anxiety scale. British Journal of Psychiatry 141: 518–523

Snaith R P, Harrop F M, Newsby D A, Teale C 1986 Grade scores of the Montgomery Asberg depression and the clinical anxiety scales. British Journal of Psychiatry 148: 599–601

Song F, Freemantle M, Sheldon T A et al 1993 Selective serotonin re-uptake inhibitors: meta-analysis of efficacy and acceptability. British Medical Journal 306: 683–687

Spitzer R L, Endicott J, Robins E 1978 Research diagnostic criteria. Archives of General Psychiatry 35: 773–782

Spitzer R L 1983 Psychiatric diagnosis: are clinicians still necessary? Comprehensive Psychiatry 24: 399–411

Spitzer R L, Williams J B W, Gibbon M, First M 1987 Users guide for the structured clinical interview for DSM-111-R. Department of Psychiatry, Columbia University Biometrics Research, New York State Psychiatric Institute

Stevens J P 1990 Intermediate statistics: a modern approach. Erlbaum, Hillsdale, NJ

Thompson S G 1993 Controversies in meta-analysis: the case of the trials of serum cholesterol reduction. Statistical Methods in Medical Research 2: 173–192

Touyz S W, Lennerts W, Arthur B, Beaumont P J V 1993 Anaerobic exercise as an adjunct to refeeding patients with anorexia nervosa: does it compromise weight gain? European Eating Disorders Review 1: 177–182

Tsuang M T, Woolston R F, Simpson J C 1980 The Iowa structured psychiatric interview. Acta Psychiatrica Scandinavica 62 (suppl 282)

Tyrer P, Owen R T, Cicchetti D V 1984 The brief scale for anxiety: a subdivision of the comprehensive psychopathological rating scale. Journal of Neurology, Neurosurgery and Psychiatry 47: 970–975

Walter S D 1995 Methods of reporting statistical results from medical research studies. American Journal of Epidemiology 141: 896–906

Walter S D, Holford T R 1978 Additive, multiplicative and other models for disease risks. American Journal of Epidemiology 108: 341–346

Wing J K, Cooper J E, Sartorius N 1974 Measurement and classification of psychiatric symptoms: an instruction manual for the PSE and CATEGO programme. Cambridge University Press, London

Wittchen H U 1994 Reliability and validity studies of the WHO – composite international diagnostic interview (CIDI): a critical review. Journal of Psychiatric Research 28(1): 57–84

Workman D E, Cassisi J E, Dougherty M C 1993 Validation of surface EMG as a measure of intra-vaginal and intra-abdominal activity: implications for biofeedback-assisted Kegel exercises. Psychophysiology 30: 120–125

Young R C, Biggs J T, Ziegler V E et al 1978 A rating scale for mania; reliability validity and sensitivity. British Journal of Psychiatry 133: 429–435

Zelen M 1992 An introduction to concepts in clinical trials. In: Fava M, Rosenbaum J F (eds) Research designs and methods in psychiatry. Elsevier, Amsterdam

Zigmond A, Snaith R 1983 The hospital anxiety and depression scale. Acta Psychiatrica Scandinavica 67: 361–370

6

Epidemiology in psychiatric research

Glyn Lewis

INTRODUCTION

What is epidemiology?

Epidemiology began as the study of epidemics and infectious disease. John Snow is often credited with being the father of epidemiology because of his pioneering work on outbreaks of cholera in London in the 1850s (Snow 1936). Over the years, and especially since the Second World War, there has been an increasing recognition that similar principles of epidemiological research can also be applied to almost any medical condition. The term 'chronic disease epidemiology' has been coined to refer to the interest of epidemiology in non-infectious diseases. These developments accelerated after the 1940s and 1950s, much influenced by Bradford Hill. If John Snow is the father of epidemiology, Bradford Hill has a good claim to be the father of modern epidemiology. Hill was a statistician who worked in the London School of Hygiene and Tropical Medicine and made three important contributions (Doll 1992).

In a series of articles in the *Lancet* published in the 1930s, Bradford Hill persuasively illustrated the importance of statistics in the design and analysis of most types of medical research. It is extraordinary to imagine an era when medical journals were not full of statistics. Bradford Hill had a key influence in ensuring that random error is always considered as a possible explanation for research findings in medicine. Bradford Hill made important contributions in the understanding, design and analysis of case–control and cohort studies and is now regarded, along with Richard Doll, as amongst those who first established the association between smoking and lung cancer. Finally, Bradford Hill is credited with being the first scientist to carry out a randomised controlled trial in medicine studying the effectiveness of streptomycin in treating tuberculosis (Hill 1952).

Bradford Hill's contributions illustrate the way in which epidemiology has developed and broadened its remit from the early concern with the epidemics of infectious disease to its current role in studying all areas of medicine. It can now be defined as the quantitative, population-based study of the aetiology, prevention and treatment of disease. Increasingly epidemiology is being seen as the 'basic science' for investigating disease within human populations.

Epidemiological approaches have therefore also been applied to psychiatric disorders. The principles underlying the design, analysis and interpretation of epidemiological research, including randomised controlled trials, are the same whatever medical condition is being studied. There is nothing 'special' about psychiatric epidemiology and, as always, it is important to learn from our colleagues in other areas of medicine.

Causes and mechanisms

It is helpful first to distinguish between causes and mechanisms, a distinction more easily made in areas of medicine where there is greater knowledge. For example, research into the cellular mechanisms of carcinogens in tobacco smoke is not enough, on its own, to argue that tobacco smoke leads to lung cancer in humans. To establish cause requires the study of human populations. Epidemiological research is therefore needed to establish risk in the population, while more laboratory-based studies give clues as to likely mechanisms. John Snow found that drinking contaminated water was associated with cholera long before the *Vibrio* and mechanism was identified. Nowadays epidemiological researchers work in parallel with colleagues interested in mechanisms. For example, epidemiological work on parity and breast cancer (Miller & Bulbrook 1986) led to hormonal hypotheses concerning aetiology. Basic science on hormonal control of breast tissue then lead to a refinement of hypotheses that were tested using further epidemiological studies. Likewise, the current interest in human papilloma virus and cervical cancer arose because of epidemiological evidence (Munoz &

Bosch 1992). The interplay between epidemiological and laboratory-based biomedical research is an important source of scientific advance in most fields of medical research.

The range of potential 'environmental' causes of common mental disorders is particularly wide. It is likely that social, biological and psychological factors are of importance in the aetiology of almost all psychiatric disorders (Goldberg & Huxley 1992, McGuffin et al 1994). The division between 'social' and 'biological' psychiatry has been counterproductive because it is a classification based upon the nature of potential aetiological factors or mechanisms. It seems more productive to distinguish between biomedical and psychological approaches towards understanding mechanisms and epidemiological and genetic research concerned with the cause of disease within human populations. It makes more sense for those who are interested in the psychological mechanisms of psychiatric disease also to be interested in functional neuroimaging studies (David 1993). Likewise, a scientist investigating the possibility that pesticides cause depression should also be concerned about the psychosocial environment and its contribution. Both biological and psychosocial aetiological hypotheses need to be investigated using epidemiological methods. Epidemiologists interested in studying psychiatric disorder therefore need to be concerned with the whole range of likely causes of psychiatric disorder when planning studies and in generating hypotheses about likely mechanisms.

Uses of epidemiology

Aetiology of disease

One of the uses of epidemiology that has attracted most interest is the study of the aetiology of disease. There are two main reasons why the aetiology of disease is important. First, the causes of disease should be able to inform preventive policies. Prevention is better than cure and removing causal or risk factors should reduce the incidence of disease.

Aetiology is also important for a second reason, that it helps to improve understanding about the mechanisms of disease and these in the long term could lead to better psychopathological models and inform future treatments. Studying aetiology for these aims can also be described as basic science or 'blue skies' research and has to be carried out in tandem with laboratory-based research on psychopathology.

The main way in which aetiology is studied using epidemiological methods is by studying the association between possible environmental factors and onset of disease. Trying to infer cause from association is clearly a difficult task and this will be discussed at more length below.

Public health

Epidemiology has at times been described as the science of public health, though epidemiology is a far broader discipline. However, it is an essential component of public health. Finding the aetiology of disease should inform preventive approaches and epidemiological methods are also available to assess the population impact of causative factors in order to estimate the likely effects of preventive interventions. The evaluation of preventive procedures and screening also requires an epidemiological approach. The recent emphasis upon needs assessment within the UK has also highlighted the epidemiological contribution to determining needs for treatment and planning services.

Clinical effectiveness and evidence-based medicine

There is an overlap between the methods used in health service research and those used in epidemiology. Questions concerning clinical effectiveness, whether evaluated using randomised controlled trials or observational studies, tend to be investigated using epidemiological methods. Evidence-based medicine (Evidence-Based Medicine Working Group 1992) grew out of the interest of applying the epidemiological and statistical approaches developed in research to everyday clinical decisions. In the early days the term 'clinical epidemiology' described this general approach. The use of systematic reviews of the literature to generate evidence and extrapolating these to clinical situations tend to rely upon epidemiological principles and use some of the statistical analyses familiar to epidemiologists.

BASIC EPIDEMIOLOGICAL PRINCIPLES

Measures of disease frequency

Measuring disease

Referring to psychiatric disorder as 'disease' may seem old fashioned. However, this has been done to share a common terminology with that used in the rest of epidemiology and in the epidemiology textbooks. For the same reason, factors which are possibly associated with disease are referred to as 'exposures'. Disease and exposure are shorthand terms to describe the outcome (disease) with which you are interested and the possible variables (exposure) which might be related to that outcome. For example, the main outcome of a cohort study of schizophrenics may be relapse (the disease) and the association with various clinically derived variables (the exposure) would be investigated.

Standardisation of diagnosis Deciding whether someone has a psychiatric disorder is not a trivial matter and is one which has attracted a great deal of attention within psychiatry (Ch. 1). There have been innumerable demonstrations that diagnosis of medical conditions, including psychiatric disorders, show poor reliability when clinicians use unstructured assessments without diagnostic guidelines (Cooper et al 1972). Medical research workers have long recognised the need for standardisation in defining both symptoms of disease and diagnostic categories. Standardisation is a way of turning clinical judgements into explicit rules. The purpose of standardisation is to reduce between-observer variation and to allow comparability between and within studies when many interviewers are carrying out assessments. For a research worker the highest priority is reducing systematic error or bias as it can bias estimates in any direction (see below). In studying aetiology, the investigator is interested in comparing rates, so it is important to ensure that there is no bias in that comparison.

In most population-based studies disease is best described as a continuum (Rose & Barker 1978). This is also true in psychiatry, particularly when considering neurotic disorder, where there is continuum of distress between the normal ups and downs of emotional life and the severe depressions seen in psychiatric practice. There is no natural break between the normal and abnormal and case definitions are in that sense an arbitrary point above which the symptoms are severe enough to arouse medical concern.

Floating numerators Counting people with a disease can be of value, for example, in assessing the needs for treatment in a particular geographical area. However, numbers of cases alone are of limited value unless the numbers are related to the 'population at risk'. For example, discovering that there are more violent incidents towards nurses than doctors in a psychiatric hospital does not allow one to conclude that a nurse is more at risk of being attacked than a doctor. There are more nurses than doctors and calculating the proportions who are attacked encourages a more accurate interpretation of the data. This fallacy has become known as the floating numerator, as the number of violent incidents is not related to the population of nurses and doctors, the denominator.

Prevalence

There are two main measures of disease frequency: prevalence and incidence rate. The prevalence of a disease is determined using a cross-sectional survey. Prevalence is a proportion and can therefore be expressed as a percentage. For example, in the recent OPCS National Surveys of Psychiatric Morbidity it was found that about 15% of the population had a psychiatric disorder in the week before interview (Jenkins et al 1997). Prevalence has to be related to a time period, hence the terms weekly, monthly or even lifetime prevalence.

It is important to realise that subjects with longer illnesses are more likely to be selected in a cross-sectional survey. For example, if you were interested in the prognosis of people with schizophrenia, a sample that was already in contact with the service would underrepresent good prognosis schizophrenics who perhaps had only one admission.

Incidence rate

Incidence rates are a measure of new cases of disease. Incidence rates are not expressed as a proportion as the denominator is person-time. For example, the incidence rate of suicide in the UK is about 8 per 100 000 person-years. *Cumulative incidence* is the proportion of subjects who have developed a disease within a specified time period; for example, '20% of schizophrenics are readmitted to hospital within 12 months of discharge' is the cumulative incidence. As a rule it is preferable to use incidence rates rather than cumulative incidence. Cumulative incidence does not enable an accurate allowance for loss to follow-up or for new cases of disease no longer 'at risk'. If the disease is uncommon and loss to follow-up is small, then cumulative incidence will not introduce any major inaccuracy. Cumulative incidence depends upon the time period of follow-up and inevitably rises as the period of follow-up lengthens. In the long run we are all dead. The statistics required for the manipulation of incidence rates are usually based upon the Poisson distribution.

Measures of association

The epidemiological approach is based upon comparing prevalence or incidence rates of disease. This is true of all the epidemiological study designs discussed below. For example, in randomised controlled trials we are usually interested in comparing the rates of recovery of two or more groups. In case–control studies the odds of disease in the exposed and unexposed groups are compared. There are two main epidemiological measures of association between disease and exposure: relative risk and attributable risk.

Relative risk

Relative risk is a somewhat ambiguous term, though it is widely used. There are three ratio measures of association: risk ratios, odds ratios (Ch. 5) and incidence rate ratios, or rate ratios for short. Risk is used in this sense as a proportion. These three measures all share many properties as they compare either the prevalence, odds or incidence rates of one group against another. This family of measures is usually referred to as relative risk – as a shorthand term.

The relative risk gives an estimate of the 'aetiological force' of an exposure. For example, those who smoke cigarettes have a 10 times increased risk of developing lung cancer and double the risk of developing ischaemic heart disease. Those who experience an adverse life event have about five times the risk of developing depression within the next 3 months. The relative risk for winter birth and schizophrenia is about 1.1 and the recent associations between polymorphisms of the serotonin and dopamine genes and schizophrenia have a relative risk of about 1.2. These ratio measures therefore give a useful intuitive estimate of the size of association between disease and exposure. They allow easy comparability between studies, and experience in cardiovascular disease epidemiology suggests that the relative risk for an exposure tends to remain approximately the same whatever the base rates of disease. For example, smoking doubles the rate of heart disease in Scotland and in Japan, though the absolute rates of disease are markedly different in the two countries.

Odds ratios Odds ratios are frequently used as a measure of association in epidemiological studies. There are three main reasons for this. First, the mathematics of manipulating odds ratios is much easier than for risk ratios and it is therefore possible to conduct simple stratified analyses by hand. A second, related reason is that logistic regression, the multivariate method which is most commonly used when studying binary outcomes, also provides estimates of odds ratios between disease and exposure. By using logistic regression it is therefore possible to estimate odds ratios before and after adjustment for potential confounding variables. This approach aids the interpretation of findings. Third, in case–control studies odds ratios are the only measure of association that provide an unbiased estimate of the odds ratio in the population on which the case–control study was based. The simple algebra which demonstrates this is given in Schlesselman (1982, p. 38).

Odds ratios will approximate towards risk ratios and rate ratios as the incidence of the disease falls. This is because, for unlikely events, odds have approximately the same value as probability. This so-called 'rare disease assumption' means that for many studies the odds ratio can be interpreted as a rate ratio.

Standardised mortality ratios In the UK standardised mortality ratios (SMRs) are commonly used in describing routinely collected mortality data and the SMR gives the rate ratio in comparison with the England and Wales rates. SMRs are usually given after being multiplied by 100. For example, the suicide SMR for Central Manchester was about 285 in 1985, indicating that the rates there were 2.8 times the England and Wales average, after adjustment for the sex and age distribution of the area. SMRs are discussed further below.

Attributable risk

The attributable risk is an alternative measure of association that provides an estimate of the absolute difference in risk or rates between the exposed and non-exposed. The attributable risk therefore provides an assessment of the individual change in risk associated with the exposure. It is of use to patients and clinicians in assessing the benefits and risks for individuals.

Example: Suicide in psychiatric patients The suicide rate is about three times higher in men than women, a rate ratio of 3. In the general population, the suicide rate is about 4 per 100 000 person-years for women and 12 per 100 000 person-years for men. The attributable risk for men is $12 - 4 = 8$ per 100 000 person years and indicates an absolute increase in risk which is still infinitesimally small and of little value in making clinical decisions. In other words a man has a 0.008% increased chance of dying in the succeeding 12 months. However, in psychiatric patients the suicide rate is much higher than in the general population, probably with a rate ratio of about 30 (Goldacre et al 1993). It has been suggested that risk factors for psychiatric patients may differ from those in the general population (Dennehy et al 1996) but, assuming this is not the case, the attributable risk would be $360 - 120 = 240$ per 100 000 person years. As can be seen, the relative risk remains constant but the attributable risk increases as the absolute rates increase. However, this is still not much use in prediction as it corresponds to an increase in the chance of suicide of 0.24% in the subsequent year.

Acceptability of SSRIs The same principle applies to the interpretation of clinical trial results. For example, recent meta-analyses have indicated that serotonin reuptake inhibitors (SSRIs) have lower drop-out rates than tricyclic antidepressants in treatment trials of depressed subjects. On average there is about a 10% reduction in drop-out rates when SSRIs are compared with the older tricyclics (Hotopf et al 1997). Knowing this relative risk does not help a clinician or patient decide how advantageous this apparent increase in acceptability might be. In randomised controlled trials about 30% of subjects tend to drop out in the first 8 weeks. The attributable risk would then be about 3%. In other words, you are 3% less likely to drop out of treatment on SSRIs than tricyclics. However, if the same risk ratio were to apply to a group of patients with very poor compliance, say a group with an 80% drop-out, then the attributable risk rises to about 8%. More recently another way of expressing the attributable risk has been suggested. This is the number needed to treat to avoid one adverse outcome (Sackett & Cook 1995). The number needed to treat (NNT) is the reciprocal of the difference in risk between the compared groups. In the examples given above the NNT to prevent one person dropping out of treatment in the first 8 weeks are respectively 33 and 12.5. This is a more intuitive way of indicating attributable risks and it aids clinicians and patients in treatment decisions.

Population attributable fraction

Both the relative risk and attributable risk are assessing the strength of the association between disease and exposure in individuals. These measures, however, do not give an indication of the importance of an aetiological agent in the population as a whole. This is sometimes called the *impact* of an exposure in contrast to its *effect*. It can be estimated using a statistic with a variety of names, including 'population attributable fraction', 'population attributable risk per cent' and 'aetiologic fraction' (Last 1988, p. 141).

The principle behind the population attributable fraction (PAF) is to estimate the proportion of cases that can be attributed to the exposure. It answers the question: 'If the exposure were to be eliminated, what proportion of the disease would be prevented?' The impact expressed as a PAF is therefore dependent on the frequency of exposure and the size of the relative risk. A disease with large impact could result from a common exposure with a relatively small relative risk, or a less common exposure with a high relative risk (Fig. 6.1). If the relationship between the exposure has a causal relationship with the disease, and there is no residual confounding or bias in the relative risk estimate, the PAF gives the percentage reduction in the number of cases in that population which would be expected if the exposure were eliminated. PAFs can therefore be used to guide the development and assess the benefits of possible preventive strategies.

Example: Suicide and unemployment The unemployed have an increased risk of suicide and the rate ratio is about 3 (Moser et al 1984). At present, about 6% of the population is unemployed and, using a simple formula (Last 1988, p. 10), this corresponds to a

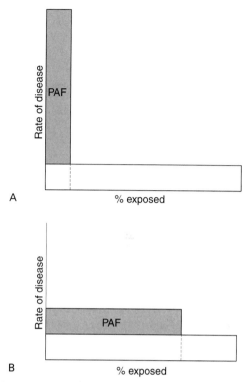

Fig. 6.1 Population attributable fraction (PAF) for a rare exposure with a large relative` risk (A) and a common exposure with a smaller relative risk (B). The magnitude of the PAF is illustrated as the shaded area.

PAF of 10.9%. This figure is an estimate of the potential importance of a risk factor in the population as a whole. If unemployment had a causal relationship with suicide, and the estimate of the rate ratio was unconfounded by any other variables, then eliminating unemployment should reduce the population suicide rates by about 10%.

STUDY DESIGNS

The main study designs used in epidemiological research are listed in Table 6.1.

Table 6.1   The main epidemiological study designs
Case–control
Cohort or longitudinal
Cross-sectional survey
Ecological studies
Randomised controlled trials
Systematic reviews

Cohort or longitudinal studies

The main distinction between the cohort and case–control study design is that in a cohort study the population is selected before the onset of disease. Cohorts can be defined in a variety of ways but often they use a classification based upon the exposure. In contrast, case–control studies are designed around subjects who are cases of disease and a comparative group of 'controls'. When deciding on the design of a study it is important to be clear about what is the disease or outcome and what is the exposure. For example, a study might examine the costs of treatment in those with postoperative wound infections and compare these with non-infected subjects. This is a cohort design and the 'exposure' is the wound infection and the 'disease' is the cost!

Cohort studies have a number of advantages over case–control studies as there is rarely any issue about whether the exposure predated the onset of disease and the exposure is measured without any bias in relation to the disease. However, cohort studies are usually more expensive and take longer than case–control studies. This is especially true for rare and uncommon diseases as large numbers of subjects need to be assessed, the vast majority of whom will not get the disease. For exposures that act a long time before disease onset, cohort studies can take so long to carry out that the results are no longer of interest or the exposure has become irrelevant. For example, a study of the toxic effects of dyes in the Fleet Street printing industry was published after this technology had become obsolete and replaced by computer-based systems.

Example: Cannabis and schizophrenia Schizophrenia is a relatively uncommon condition with an incidence rate of about 15 per 100 000 person-years. Therefore cohort studies are difficult to plan and carry out. However, many of the factors which might have some aetiological importance in schizophrenia are difficult to measure and are likely to be biased by the presence of the disease. There have been many reports that schizophrenics who smoked cannabis were at increased risk of relapse and it is possible that smoking cannabis might increase the risk of developing schizophrenia. Andreasson et al (1987) were able to perform a retrospective cohort study using data on 50 000 Swedish conscripts who were surveyed in 1969 when aged about 18. By means of record linkage to the National Psychiatric Case Register in Sweden they were able to identify about 200 subjects who developed schizophrenia and were admitted to hospital in the following 13 years. Their main results are shown in Table 6.2. There is a strong dose–response relationship with cannabis use reported at the age of 18. What are the possible explanations for this association?

Table 6.2   Cannabis and schizophrenia

No. of occasions on which cannabis was consumed	No. of subjects	No. of cases of schizophrenia	Odds ratios
0	41280	197	1
1–10	2836	18	1.3
11–50	702	10	3.0
>50	752	21	6.0

Cannabis smoking was recorded before the onset of schizophrenia but it is possible that a prodromal phase could have led to an increase in cannabis use. The other possibility might be that other aspects of the personality of the conscripts could be associated with both the onset of schizophrenia and with cannabis use; in other words, that the relationship was confounded by personality. The authors adjusted statistically for a number of other behaviours self-reported at 18, such as whether the individuals were in trouble with the police. They still found association with cannabis, though the association was reduced after this adjustment.

It is also worth noting that the analysis of this cohort study used odds ratios rather than rate ratios. Schizophrenia was so uncommon in this study that the rare disease assumption can be invoked and the odds ratios can therefore be interpreted as rate ratios.

Case–control studies

In a case–control study, individuals with a particular condition or disease (the *cases*) are selected for comparison with a series of individuals in whom the condition or disease is absent (the *controls*). Cases and controls are compared with respect to existing or past attributes or exposures thought to be relevant to the development of the condition or disease under study (Schlesselman 1982).

Case–control studies have a deceptively simple design. Subjects with the disease are compared in terms of the frequency of exposure with a comparison group. The function of the comparison group is thus to provide an estimate of the frequency of exposure in the population from which the cases were drawn. The word 'control' is thus a misnomer but one which has been adopted for many years. It is frequently overlooked that case–control studies are population based. Controls should be eligible for selection as cases if they were to become diseased. This is the most common design used

Table 6.3	An example of selection into treatment		
	No. with 3 or more children	No. with 2 or fewer children	Odds ratios (95% CI)
Patient cases	9 (8)	105	1.01 (0.47–2.19)
Community cases	9 (24)	28	3.77 (1.63–8.72)
Community controls	30 (8)	352	1.00[a]

[a]Baseline.
Values in parentheses are percentages.
From Brown and Harris (1978).

in medical and psychiatric research but the subtleties and difficulties are usually ignored.

Case–control designs are relatively quick and simple to carry out and can be used to study a variety of exposures for a single disease. However, they are susceptible to two important sources of bias, selection bias and recall bias.

Selection bias

Selection bias can occur in a case–control study when the controls give a biased estimate of the frequency of exposure in the population from which the cases were drawn. An example is given in Table 6.3, from the work of Brown & Harris (1978). Their study, identified cases, of depression using a cross-sectional survey, the 'community cases', and by contact with psychiatric services the 'patient cases'. Comparing the patient cases against the controls selected from the cross-sectional survey suggested there was no association between depression and having three or more children at home, with an odds ratio of 1.01. In contrast, when the community cases were compared with the community controls there was an association with having a young family (odds ratio 3.77). It is well known that the majority of cases of depression never get referred to a psychiatrist (Goldberg & Huxley 1992), therefore if one wanted to pick controls for cases seen in psychiatric services, a community sample would not be appropriate. There are many people in the community sample that would not get to psychiatric services even if they became depressed. In this sense there is a selection bias operating, and presumably having young children reduces the likelihood of receiving treatment from psychiatrists when someone is depressed. It should be noted in this example that the valid comparison uses results from a cross-sectional survey, a design that is relatively insensitive to selection bias.

Recall bias

Recall bias occurs when the measurement of exposure is biased by the presence of disease. In case–control designs the investigator often has to establish the frequency of exposure after the disease has occurred. This can involve the retrospective assessment of exposure, though it is possible on occasions to obtain exposure measurements that were made before the onset of disease even in a case–control design. One of the most common reasons for recall bias is the 'effort after meaning' that can occur in a sick individual or relative who seeks to have some explanation for an illness.

Matching in case–control studies

When the controls are matched to the cases on some variables, the control group becomes a biased sample compared to the population from which the cases were drawn. For example, if you have more women than men in your cases, by matching for sex you will also have an overrepresentation of men in the controls compared with the presumed population of the case–control study. This bias can be overcome if the analysis takes account of the matching (Hennekens & Buring 1987 p. 295) and in doing this the investigator has adjusted for any confounding effect of the matched variables. The use of the term 'control' often gives the impression that by close matching in case–control studies one can ensure a valid comparison. Matching is one of the strategies for adjusting for confounding and has the disadvantage that it makes the analysis of case–control studies more cumbersome.

The advantages and disadvantages of cohort and case–control studies are listed in Table 6.4.

Example: Fetal origins of schizophrenia O'Callaghan et al (1992) carried out a case–control study to examine the hypothesis that abnormalities in pregnancy and childbirth are associated with schizophrenia. They selected 616 schizophrenics attending a psychiatric hospital in Dublin and then traced the obstetric notes of 65 of their original sample. They used the next birth in the Dublin obstetric hospital as the control. They found an association between any obstet-

Table 6.4	Advantages and disadvantages of case–control and cohort studies	
Case–control	Cohort
Strengths Suitable for rare diseases Better for studying causes that are in the distant past Can examine many risk factors for a single disease Relatively quick and inexpensive	Suitable for rare exposures Recall bias and reverse causality are unlikely to explain an association Can examine many outcomes for a single exposure Can calculate incidence rates
Weaknesses Susceptible to selection bias Can be susceptible to recall bias and reverse causality Unsuitable for rare exposures and cannot directly calculate incidence rates	Usually unsuitable for rare diseases Can be expensive and can lead to a long delay before the results are available Losses to follow-up can affect validity

ric complication and schizophrenia, with an odds ratio of about 2.4 (95% CI 1.1 to 6.0). Using records made at the time of birth rules out the possibility of bias in the measurement of obstetric complications as long as the assessments were done blind. However, no account was taken in the design of the possibility of migration away from Dublin. Controls may have moved away and therefore, if they had developed schizophrenia, would not have been eligible as cases. It is difficult to know what influence selection bias might have on the results, but it is possible for example that 'sicker' individuals are less likely to migrate but stay in Dublin. A design in which the investigators had only included cases who still lived in Dublin would have reduced the chance of a selection bias. The authors also used prevalent cases of schizophrenia currently in contact with services. This tends to overrepresent chronic cases and so it is possible that obstetric complications are associated with a poor prognosis rather than causing schizophrenia.

Cross-sectional surveys

Cross-sectional surveys sample individuals from a population and then compare those with and without disease according to the frequency of exposure. Cross-sectional surveys are often used for descriptive purposes in estimating the prevalence of psychiatric disorder and the needs for treatment. They share some of the characteristics of case–control studies, in the sense that exposure is being determined after the onset of the disease. Recall bias is therefore a potential problem. However, selection bias is unlikely because a population is being randomly sampled.

Example: A national survey of psychiatric morbidity In 1994 the UK Department of Health commis-

sioned a household survey of Great Britain in order to investigate the prevalence of psychiatric disorder (Meltzer et al 1995, Jenkins et al 1997). One important question concerning neurotic disorder is its relationship with low income or wealth. One method of assessing wealth is by using indirect measures such as house ownership and whether a household has access to a car. In this survey there was a strong negative association between having access to a car in the household and the prevalence of psychiatric morbidity (odds ratio 1.5, 95% CI 1.3 to 1.7) and this association was independent of any association between occupational social class and psychiatric morbidity. Collecting information on car access should be fairly reliable and this is unlikely to be biased. However, there is a possibility of reverse causality, that those with neurotic disorders might earn less money and have less wealth. It is also not clear whether the association is with duration of episodes or onset, as a cross-sectional survey will have more chronic cases than a study that identifies incident cases.

Ecological studies

Ecological studies examine the association between disease and the characteristics of an aggregation of people rather than the characteristics of individuals. The main difficulty with this design has been called the *ecological fallacy*. The association between exposure and disease at an aggregate level may not be reflected in an association at the individual level. Put another way, ecological designs are more susceptible to confounding than other designs. For example, inner city areas in the UK with a higher proportion of residents from the Afro-Caribbean ethnic group also have higher rates of suicide. This apparent association is not seen in individual level data, in fact Afro-Caribbean individuals have a lower risk of suicide. The ecological association seems to result because inner cities have more people from ethnic groups and more people who live alone, and it is the latter who are at increased risk of suicide.

There have been reports of an association between schizophrenia and those born just after the 1958 influenza epidemic (Mednick et al 1988). This is also aggregate data as there is no information on individuals who did or did not have influenza. Carrying out studies of sufficient power with data on individuals would reduce the chance that these results are due to confounding.

There are also some potential advantages of studying population aggregations. Some variables can only be thought of in ecological terms. For example, Wilkinson (1992) and others have found an association between all-cause mortality and income inequality in Western market economies. Sainsbury (1955) found an association between his measure of alienation (the disorganisation of a community) and suicide rates in the London boroughs. Both these examples are studying variables that can only be considered in aggregate. It is also possible on occasions to examine whether such aggregate variables are better at explaining variation than the variables measured on individuals (Sloggett and Joshi 1994).

The other potential advantage of using aggregate data is that it might reflect long-term differences in lifestyle. For example, European countries with higher olive oil consumption have lower rates of heart disease, while there is little supporting evidence for an association between olive oil consumption and heart disease within the UK. This might be because olive oil has been consumed for many years in the southern European countries while it has only been used widely in the UK in more recent times. If diet were to reduce the chances of heart disease it would have to act over many years.

Example: Suicide and psychiatric services The UK Government's public health strategy *Health of the Nation* (Secretary of State for Health 1992) included a target for reducing suicide by 15% by the year 2000. The main proposals for achieving this target were to improve the effectiveness of health and social services and so there was a tendency for psychiatric services to be assessed in terms of the suicide rate in their area. Lewis et al (1994) examined the association between suicide rates in English health authorities and the resources available to psychiatric services in that area. There was a strong *positive* association before adjustment between the number of consultant psychiatrists in a district and the suicide rate (Table 6.5). For each consultant psychiatrist employed, the standardised mortality ratio for suicide rose by just over 6. This positive association was mostly accounted for by the fact that deprived areas have both higher suicide rates and more consultant psychiatrists. Inner city districts are also more likely to be teaching districts. The authors concluded that the sociodemographic characteristics of an area were more important in determining suicide rates than the resources provided for psychiatric services.

Table 6.5   Regression coefficients (95% CI) between the SMR for suicide and undetermined deaths across 191 English district health authorities and selected variables related to psychiatric service provision and sociodemographic factors

	Unadjusted		After Adjustment	
	Coefficient (95% CI)	P value	Coefficient (95% CI)	P value
Mental illness consultants (per 100,000 pop)	6.39 (3.99 to 8.79)	0.0001	1.70 (–0.07 to 3.46)[a]	0.06
Community psychiatric nurses (per 100,000 pop)	0.99 (0.26 to 1.73)	0.009	0.03 (–0.47 to 0.53)[a]	0.90
Available psychiatric beds (per 1000 pop)	0.28 (–1.41 to 1.98)	0.75	0.26 (–0.82 to 1.34)[a]	0.64
Mental illness nurses (per bed)	2.68 (–4.18 to 9.54)	0.45	–0.74 (–5.12 to 3.63)[a]	0.74
Teaching district	37.62 (28.35 to 46.88)	0.0001	8.13 (0.05 to 16.21)[b]	0.05
Underprivileged area score	0.90 (0.72 to 1.07)	0.0001	–0.05 (–0.27 to 0.18)[c]	0.69
Proportion of single person households	6.77 (6.00 to 7.53)	0.0001	6.42 (5.08 to 7.75)[d]	0.0001

[a]Adjusted for proportion of single households, regional health authority, underprivileged area score and teaching district
[b]Adjusted for underprivileged area score, proportion of single households and regional health authority.
[c]Adjusted for teaching district, proportion of single households and regional health authority.
[d]Adjusted for underprivileged area score, teaching district and regional health authority.

Randomised controlled trials

Case–control, cohort studies, ecological and cross-sectional studies are all observational studies in the sense that the investigator does not have any control over the allocation of the variables under study. In a randomised controlled trial (RCT), the investigator randomly allocates two or more interventions to the subjects in the trial. The main advantage of RCTs is therefore that they provide comparable groups in which confounding variables are equally likely to occur. An RCT can therefore be thought of as a matched cohort study in which the confounders that are unknown are also randomly allocated. There is still a possibility that an imbalance between the groups could arise by chance, though this becomes less likely as the sample size increases. RCTs are still susceptible to measurement bias and for this reason it is best for them to be double-blind, i.e. the randomised treatments are blind to both the subject and to the physician and/or research assistant who is making the assessments of outcome. It is also regarded as good practice to analyse the data blind to the treatment allocation – sometimes called 'triple-blind'.

Randomisation by group

There are many circumstances in which it is difficult or impossible to randomise individuals to an intervention. For example, if one were investigating the impact of an educational intervention on general practitioners' management of psychiatric disorder, randomising individual patients would not work very effectively. A stronger design would be to randomise general practice partnerships, or rather randomise the groups of individuals within practices. There will then not be contamination between the intervention and control conditions. The disadvantage of this design is that group randomisation reduces the statistical power and so these studies tend to be very large and expensive.

Analysis

One of the main difficulties in interpreting the results of an RCT concerns the difficulty in analysing data that are missing. As subjects drop out of an RCT, so the treatment groups depart from the balanced groups created at randomisation. If the drop-outs are substantial in number then there is a possibility that confounding is reintroduced. The main way in which this problem is circumvented is by use of an *intention-to-treat* strategy in the analysis. This involves using previous data in those subjects with missing data or assuming a poor outcome for drop-outs. This ensures that *all* the randomised individuals are used in the analysis.

The random allocation must also be checked for variables that would be expected to influence outcome. If there is an apparent difference between the randomised groups it is best to analyse the data after adjusting for the potentially confounding effects of those variables that appear to differ between the groups.

Example: Psychotherapy and pharmacotherapy for depression The NIMH Treatment of Depression Collaborative Research Program carried out an RCT (Elkin et al 1989) to compare the following interventions in depression: imipramine, placebo, cognitive behavioural psychotherapy (Beck et al 1979) and interpersonal therapy (Klerman et al 1984). The main findings were that all the active treatments seemed to be equally efficacious. The authors carried out an intention-to-treat analysis but also analysed data on those that had completed the 16 week course. Most of the argument about this trial concerned the statistical analysis and there was a considerable amount of correspondence about their strategy of only accepting probability (P) values of less than 0.017 as indicating statistical significance. However, this ignores the fact that in RCTs we are interested in the size of effect rather than the statistical significance of the results. The authors did not give confidence intervals for their findings, but the sample size in each group indicates that the confidence intervals would be broad and the trial was estimating treatment effects with little accuracy. This would be particularly so when comparing the three active treatments. This was a difficult and expensive trial to carry out but in order to inform clinical practice would need to be much larger. In cardiovascular disease, so-called 'megatrials' have been carried out in which tens of thousands of subjects are randomised. These trials can provide very accurate estimates of the effectiveness of treatments (Yusuf et al 1984).

Systematic reviews

Findings from a single study can rarely justify a change in clinical practice or in an aetiological theory. Though most scientific effort is expended on conducting individual research investigations, it is the conclusions from reviews upon which most clinical medicine, public health interventions and epidemiological associations are based. There has therefore been an increasing interest in using the methodological principles of primary research in conducting systematic reviews of the literature. Once these reviews are accomplished, the results can sometimes be subject to a meta-analysis that provides a quantitative summary estimate of the treatment effect in all the studies reviewed. The Cochrane Collaboration is an international network whose aims are to provide systematic reviews of all the RCTs carried out in medicine (Chalmers et al 1992).

The main advantage of systematic reviews is that they increase statistical power. They should also improve the generalisability of findings, as all the available evidence is included in the review. However, publication and citation bias can lead to erroneous conclusions (Davey Smith & Egger 1995) and it is important that a comprehensive search strategy is used to identify the literature. Plotting the sample size of the trial against the effect size (a funnel plot) can give an estimate of publication bias in the review, as one might expect smaller negative trials to be unpublished or published in less prestigious journals. Another important aspect of a systematic review is the information upon the methodological quality of the research. There are always concerns about giving the same weight to good and bad studies. Schulz and colleagues (1995) found that RCTs of poor methodological quality find larger treatment effects.

Example: acceptability of SSRI and tricyclic antidepressants There have been a number of systematic reviews of drop-outs from RCTs that compare SSRI and tricyclic antidepressants. The number of drop-outs have been taken as an assessment of acceptability, though this is undoubtedly a poor measure of treatment acceptability under service conditions. The most recent review compared SSRIs with three classes of alternative antidepressants: reference tricyclics (imipramine and amitriptyline), newer tricyclics and non-tricyclic antidepressants. A statistically significant difference in drop-out rates was only found when comparing SSRIs and the reference tricyclics (risk ratio 0.88, 95% CI 0.82 to 0.94). For the newer tricyclics the risk ratio was 0.92 (95% CI 0.81 to 1.03) and this was not statistically significant, however there was less statistical power and a type 2 error is a possibility. For the heterocyclic group the risk ratio was 1.02 (95% CI 0.83 to 1.25) (Hotopf et al 1997).

Genetic designs and epidemiology

Those designs that rely upon genetic linkage do not share much in common with the epidemiological designs described above. The design of genetic studies is discussed in Chapter 7. Studies that rely upon genetic association or linkage disequilibrium to establish associations between genetic polymorphisms and disease tend to be called 'association studies' by geneticists. These association studies are either case–control, cross-sectional survey or cohort studies and share the same methodological advantages and disadvantages. The term 'genetic epidemiology' is often used to refer to those who are concerned with the design and analysis of genetic studies, irrespective of whether those studies

are population based, in the sense used in epidemiology (Khoury et al 1993). An interesting development in methodology is the intrafamilial case–control study that uses the parents of the case to estimate the frequency of genetic polymorphisms in the population from which the cases are drawn (Schaid & Sommer 1994).

CAUSAL INFERENCE

Making the link between an association and cause is a difficult and crucial decision. It is inevitable, given the use of observational designs, that there is always a possibility that unknown confounders or unquantifiable biases may have distorted the association that has been observed. Furthermore, in deciding upon cause it is also important to look not at single studies but at a whole literature, including the basic science literature, on possible mechanisms. This section describes the main non-causal explanations for an association and also discusses evidence that might support causation.

Random error or chance

An association can arise by chance. The standard tests of statistical significance give an estimate of the probability (the P value) that the data (or more extreme data) could have arisen by chance assuming the null hypothesis (that there is no difference). A result which is significant at the 5% level will, on average, be found once in every 20 studies, even if there was no difference between the groups. This is known as a type 1 error. It is a particular problem when there is *multiple testing* when many statistical tests are conducted within a single study. Tests for statistical significance are of value when a study is testing a prior hypothesis with a single specified outcome. In studies which have no hypothesis and 'dredge' or 'trawl' the data the significance tests are very difficult to interpret.

Less commonly recognised is the opposite error. A research project may find no association, but a real association may have been missed because the study is too small and the random error correspondingly large. This is a type 2 error. A difference that is not statistically significant cannot be interpreted as showing 'no difference'. The routine use of confidence intervals would help to interpret such findings. Confidence intervals provide more information than the P value (Gardner & Altman 1986) as they indicate the statistical precision of an estimate as well as the probability of its having occurred by chance. Thus confidence intervals indicate not only whether an association is statistically significant but also whether a non-significant result is compatible with a clinically or scientifically important association.

Statistical power

The statistical power of a study gives the probability that a type 2 error will *not* occur. The power of a study depends on four factors:

- The strength of the expected association or difference in relation to the measurement error.
- The prevalence of exposure.
- The significance level, usually taken as 5%.
- The sample size.

For example, a case–control study, looking for an odds ratio of 2 at the 5% significance level where the prevalence of exposure is 15%, has a power of 80% when there are 200 cases and 200 controls (from tables in Schlesselman 1982). Unless the researcher is expecting a very strong association between the disease and exposure, a case–control study needs to be quite large to have sufficient statistical power. Many studies that use expensive measures such as brain scanning and some neuroendocrine and interview-based social measures tend to be very small. Small studies imply that the investigators only have sufficient power to look for massive differences. Smaller but perhaps important differences will remain undetected in underpowered studies.

Reverse causality

An association can result if the disease causes the exposure. This is more likely in studies that ascertain the exposure after the onset of disease, in case–control and cross-sectional surveys. For example, divorce and separation may lead to depression, or depression could lead to marital problems and so to divorce. Low social class is more common in those with schizophrenia and this is widely held to result from the illness rather than be a cause (Goldberg & Morrison 1963). Therefore, the timing of exposure and onset of disease is important. In life-events research much attention is paid to 'independent' life events as opposed to those which may be influenced by the illness under study (Brown & Harris 1978). Reverse causality is less of a problem in cohort studies, as they start by identifying exposed subjects who do not, at that stage, have the disease.

Confounding

Confounders are associated with *both* the exposure and disease and can lead to a spurious association or can eliminate a real association. A confounder is an independent risk factor or protective factor for the disease and one which varies systematically with the exposure of interest; it is not, however, on the causal pathway between exposure and disease. If confounding variables are considered in the design of a study, there are various means of adjusting for the likely effects that are described below.

A simple illustration is provided by the observation that more women have Alzheimer's disease than men. This arises from two associations: first, Alzheimer's disease, which becomes commoner with age; second, women are more likely to live longer than men. Thus age is said to confound the relationship between gender and Alzheimer's disease. Age is a common confounder and needs to be taken into account in most studies. Table 6.6 illustrates this with some hypothetical figures. The rates of Alzheimer's disease within each age band is the same in both sexes.

In randomised clinical trials subjects are randomised to the groups irrespective of their characteristics but people are not randomly allocated to possible causes of disease. Observational studies (cross-sectional, case-control and cohort) remain the only way to investigate environmental causes of illness in humans but confounding is an inevitable consequence. In attempting to interpret an association from an observational study it is often helpful to ask: 'What are the determinants of exposure in this group, why were some exposed, others not?' In other words: 'How does this study situation differ from a randomised trial?'

Methods for adjusting for confounders: design

Randomisation This is the most powerful method but not an ethical option in studies that are investigating risk factors for disease, though for protective factors it should be considered.

Restriction Subjects are only included if they have the same value of the confounding variable. For example, Jenkins (1985) was studying gender differences in the prevalence of neurosis and restricted the sample to a narrow socioeconomic band – the subjects were all civil servants of a particular grade. Any differences in the prevalence between the sexes would not therefore reflect the lower status jobs experienced by women.

Matching Matching has different implications in case–control and cohort studies. The difficulties of matching in case–control studies have been discussed above, though it is commonly used in case–control studies. Controls are chosen in order to have similar values as the cases on the matching variables. For example, controls might be chosen to have the same age and sex as the cases. It is more advantageous to match in cohort studies, though there is no necessity. In cohort studies, matching might be chosen when an exposed cohort is being compared with an unexposed cohort. In those cases, matching the exposed and unexposed subjects on selected variables might be advantageous.

Individual matching and frequency matching are usually contrasted. In the former, each individual case is matched with an individual control subject. In frequency matching, the groups are matched. For example, one might wish to ensure that the controls also have the same proportion of subjects in the age groups observed in the cases.

It is important to emphasise that matching is a method of adjusting for confounders. Decisions about matching are primarily concerned with the practicalities of carrying out a study. Unmatched studies are perfectly valid as there are usually alternative methods of adjusting for confounders. We have already discussed the need to perform an analysis in matched case–control studies that takes account of the matching.

Advantages and disadvantages of matching

The main advantage of matching is that it should increase statistical power in adjusting for confounding variables. Matching on variables that are not confounders will tend to reduce power. The second advantage is that by matching one might be able to adjust for confounders that are difficult or impossible to measure, for example by matching on neighbourhood or friendship.

The disadvantages are usually the increased administrative effort that is required, especially to individually match. Subjects may have to be screened and excluded and the investigator has to balance any advantages of matching against the extra time required to recruit subjects. In many cases it may be more efficient to recruit more cases rather than attempt to increase statistical power by matching.

An investigator cannot investigate the association between disease and exposure on the matched variables, though interactions with matched variables can be studied. In case–control studies, the analysis of matched studies is more complex and it reduces the

opportunity to perform simple stratified analyses that are often helpful in interpreting the results. There is also the phenomenon of *overmatching*. This is a somewhat ambiguous term that has been used to describe almost any of the disadvantages of matching (Last 1988). In this context it will be used when subjects are being inadvertently matched on the exposure variable. For example, matching on neighbourhood might also lead to the matched pairs having a similar social class. This will reduce the statistical power of a study investigating associations with social class, though it will not bias the association.

Example: Matching using the snowball method Lopes et al (Lopes et al 1996) used an unusual design in studying the association between psychiatric disorder and substance abuse. As substance abuse is an illegal activity, and dependence is relatively uncommon, it is difficult to select a sample of cases except from treatment facilities. Choosing an appropriate control group then becomes difficult. Lopes and colleagues chose to use the snowballing technique, developed by qualitative researchers concerned with accessing hidden populations. In this method identified subjects nominate others who have the desired characteristics. Lopes asked subjects to nominate others who either had or had not a substance abuse problem. In this way the cases and controls were matched on friendship and other aspects of lifestyle. One could be reasonably confident that if the controls had developed a substance problem, they would have been eligible to be selected as cases in the study.

Methods for adjusting for confounders: analysis

Stratified analysis The principle behind stratified analysis can be illustrated by reference to Table 6.6. In this example, age is confounding the relationship between Alzheimer's disease and gender. Stratifying by

Table 6.6 Hypothetical example of confounding: gender and prevalence of dementia				
	65–74 years	75–84 years	> 85 years	> 65 years
Men				
Percentage	2	8	16	5.3
No. of cases	2	4	3	9
Sample size	100	50	20	170
Women				
Percentage	2	8	16	7.7
No of cases	2	7	11	20
Sample size	100	90	70	260

the confounder, age in this example, removes the confounding effects and within each stratum the true relationship between gender and Alzheimer's disease emerges. By taking a weighted mean across the strata, one can provide an estimate of the association between gender and Alzheimer's disease that is adjusted for age. There are various methods for carrying out stratified analyses described in detail elsewhere (see Further Reading).

Standardisation of mortality or admission rates is a method of stratified analysis. There are indirect or direct methods of standardisation. Indirect standardisation tends to be used mostly in the UK, particularly in Government statistics, and this uses standard rates, usually the England and Wales rate, and applies these to the population of interest. Standardised mortality ratios (SMRs) then provide estimates of rate ratios adjusted for the age and sex distribution of the population. SMRs tend to be expressed after being multiplied by a 100. Therefore a rate ratio of 1.5 corresponds to an SMR of 150.

Multivariate analysis Multivariate statistical techniques can be used to adjust for a number of confounding variables simultaneously. There are a variety of multivariate methods that are used in studying different outcomes. The two main approaches are logistic regression and least squares regression. Logistic regression is used when studying binary outcomes, for example whether someone has a disease or is well. Least squares regression is used to model continuous outcomes, for example scores on a depression test. Least squares regression assumes that the dependent variables are normally distributed, and this is often not the case with many outcomes of interest in psychiatry. In order to study an association and the likely confounding effects, it is usually advisable to carry out simpler analyses before embarking on multivariate analysis.

Residual confounding

It is often impossible to measure confounding variables very accurately. In such circumstances it is likely that they will remain confounding, even after the analysis or design has apparently adjusted for the confounding effects. This is known as residual confounding. If an association is reduced when adjusting for a confounder but there still remains an association, residual confounding should be considered.

Adjusting for variables on the causal pathway

Statistical adjustment for a variable that is further along the causal chain between exposure and disease will reduce or eliminate the association between the expo-

sure and disease. When interpreting such results it is important to consider the likely causal mechanisms and carry out analyses that will help to decipher these relationships.

Confounding in genetic association studies

One of the main confounding variables in studies of genetic association is ethnic origin. The frequency of genetic polymorphisms varies between ethnic groups and such groups can also show marked variation in the incidence of disease, perhaps because of culture or lifestyle or other genetic risk factors. This is sometimes termed 'population stratification' by genetic investigators. One way of preventing confounding in this way is by restricting a study to an ethnically homogenous population. For example, by only having white British people in a study or by using Finnish subjects, a region where there has been very little inward immigration. An alternative and more powerful strategy is to carry out an intrafamilial case–control study (Schaid & Sommer 1994). In this design the parents of the case provide the estimate of the frequency of the genetic polymorphism in the population at risk. It is important to realise that this design still relies upon linkage disequilibrium and estimates the association between genetic polymorphisms and disease.

Bias

Bias is 'any process at any stage of inference which tends to produce results or conclusions that differ systematically from the truth' (Sackett 1979). There are two main sources of bias: selection bias and information or measurement bias. Sackett (1979) has given a more comprehensive classification of bias. Selection bias is mainly a problem for case–control studies and has been discussed above. Measurement bias will therefore be discussed here.

Random misclassification

There is an important distinction between random and systematic misclassification in measurement. Random error is usually used in epidemiology to refer to the role of chance. Random misclassification is used to indicate inaccurate measurement. The term 'random' is used to indicate that the misclassification is occurring irrespective of whether the subject has the disease or exposure. For example, using a brief questionnaire measure of neurotic disorder, such as the General Health Questionnaire (GHQ) (Goldberg & Williams 1988), will be less accurate than using a more detailed assessment. However, there is no particular reason to expect that 30-year-olds will be more likely to be cases on the GHQ than 40-year-olds, so a study looking at an association with age would only be subject to random misclassification.

Random misclassification tends to reduce the size of the observed association. In contrast, systematic misclassification or bias can bias an estimate in either direction, increasing or decreasing observed associations. When interpreting results, it is an important principle that associations cannot be spuriously increased because of random misclassification. Though one should strive to increase accuracy whenever possible, it is more important to ensure that measurements are unbiased as this will aid the interpretation of positive findings.

Subject-based measurement bias

One of the most important types of subject-based measurement bias is recall bias. This is a particular difficulty in interpreting the results of case–control studies and cross-sectional surveys when the measurement of exposure occurs after the disease has developed. There are a number of areas in psychiatry where one would expect the disease to affect the measurement of exposures. Depression would be expected to increase memory for aversive life events (Lloyd & Lishman 1976) and early aversive experiences (Wolkind & Coleman 1983). One would expect depressed subjects to give poorer ratings for social network (Sarason et al 1986), personality (Katz & McGuffin 1987) and marital discord.

There are several strategies for minimising recall bias and these should be considered in the design of case–control studies and cross-sectional surveys. Using a structured questionnaire and standardising the criteria for exposure is an essential prerequisite for reducing measurement bias, including recall bias. Relying upon recognition rather than recall, by supplying the subject with a comprehensive series of prompts, should also minimise this bias. This method is now routinely adopted in life-events research. It is less likely to occur if the illness is of recent onset, a further reason for favouring the study of incident rather than prevalent cases.

The validity of self-reported exposure data can be tested, for example by interviewing a close relatives or consulting medical records. Case–control studies can also be performed that use data obtained before onset of disease. This method is sometimes used for studying fetal origins of schizophrenia, as in the example discussed above (O'Callaghan et al 1992).

In cohort studies one is often more concerned about bias affecting the identification of disease. This can occur in psychiatry as the diagnosis tends to rest upon self-reported symptoms from patients. For example, in a study of exposure to organophosphate pesticides and psychiatric morbidity, one would be concerned that existing lay beliefs about these compounds would influence the reporting of symptoms.

Observer bias

Observer bias occurs when the measurement of disease or exposure is biased because of the observer. In RCTs it is recommended that observers make ratings blind to the treatment allocation to ensure outcomes are measured without bias. However, even in these circumstances it is often possible for observers to discover the randomised allocation if the treatments have distinctive side-effects, for example when comparing SSRI and tricyclic antidepressants. Maintaining blindness of the observer is also ideal for observational studies. Highly structured assessments and recording unambiguous information will also reduce bias.

Observer bias is eliminated by self-administered questionnaires and computerised assessments (Lewis 1994). On the other hand there is concern that subjects may not fully understand self-administered questionnaires, and that those who read poorly or are illiterate may be unable to respond. Self-reported diagnostic information in psychotic individuals is unlikely to be valid. Other sources of bias, for instance when the subject's responses are influenced by disease status, will remain when using self-administered measures.

It is often advisable to use non-medically trained interviewers as they are more likely to follow questionnaires exactly and not to use their own judgement in deciding on exposure and disease. It may also be possible to keep interviewers unaware of the purpose of the study, though it is often difficult to maintain motivation if this is done.

Measuring bias

One of the problems with bias is that it is usually difficult to measure. Unlike confounding, it is therefore difficult to adjust for bias. Efforts must be made in the design to reduce bias but often it is up to the judgement of the investigator and the readers to decide if bias has had an important effect on the result.

If it is possible to measure a bias then it can be treated as a confounder. Unquantifiable biases are a major problem because it becomes difficult to interpret the results of a study. A bias may have a trivial effect or alternatively lead to a major distortion. The only solution to this difficulty is to attempt to measure bias. Thus, in a randomised controlled trial patients may experience a distinctive and unusual side-effect when on the active agent. At the end of the trial both they and the investigators can be asked to say whether they think they were on the active drug or the placebo; the results can be taken into account in the analysis. However, 'Efforts to compensate for it [bias] in the analysis must be viewed with suspicion' (Rose & Barker 1978).

Criteria for causality

The concept of causality in medicine has evolved over the last century. Nineteenth century ideas were primarily concerned with infectious disease and implied that causes were both necessary and sufficient; in other words, for something to be a cause it had always to lead to disease (sufficient) and also was present in all cases of the disease (necessary). There has been an increasing realisation that such simple models do not fit most infectious diseases and in chronic disease epidemiology the emphasis has always been on a multifactorial model of disease in which causes are neither necessary nor sufficient. For example, some people who smoke never get lung cancer, and lung cancer exists in non-smokers. Smoking increases the risk of lung cancer and there are other factors, both environmental and genetic, that also affect susceptibility.

Bradford Hill (Hill 1965) discussed some criteria for deciding upon cause (Table 6.7). An essential prerequisite is that the cause should come before the disease, but Hill also suggested that the strength of association as measured by relative risk increased the likelihood of a causal relationship. An increase in risk as the degree of exposure increases, a dose–response relationship, also strengthens the case. Finally, it is important to examine the consistency of a finding with existing knowledge. Different study designs adopting different methodologies that all come to the same conclusion are an important element. A plausible mechanism is also needed

before one would accept an exposure as a causal agent. Of most importance is a degree of scepticism about causes. There are no hard and fast rules about inferring cause, though there are some examples, of which smoking and lung cancer is the most celebrated, in which epidemiological associations have provided the main evidence for causality.

EVIDENCE-BASED MEDICINE

Randomised versus non-randomised evidence

Evidence-based medicine has grown out of the application of statistical and epidemiological concepts to clinical medicine. Doctors have been using evidence upon which to base their clinical practice for many years, but if there is anything 'new' about evidence-based medicine it is in the suggestion that the production and synthesis of evidence should be done in a more explicit and quantitative way.

One consequence of this movement has been the increasing emphasis placed upon randomised controlled trials as providing the best evidence for clinical effectiveness. Clinical anecdote and experience is now largely discounted as a basis for clinical decision making, unless there is no evidence from other sources. Using observational designs, whether case–control or cohort, to investigate clinical effectiveness is of course fraught with the difficulties of identifying and adjusting for confounders. Sadly, the problem of confounding is rarely acknowledged in non-randomised studies of clinical effectiveness but there are circumstances under which non-randomised evidence is of potential value, as listed in Table 6.8 (Black 1996).

It is also of importance to recognise the limitations of RCTs in guiding clinical practice. Though randomisation should eliminate confounding, the internal validity

---

Table 6.7   Causal inference
Explanations for an association
Chance or random error
Reverse causality
Confounding
Selection bias or information bias
Evidence for causality
Time sequence
Strength of association
Consistency with existing knowledge
Dose–response relationship

Table 6.8   When is non-randomised evidence of value?
In the absence of randomised evidence
When randomised controlled trials are regarded as unethical because of a strong consensus
When the intervention is given on a geographic basis and randomisation is impracticable
When observational data is readily available and can provide some preliminary evidence
When there is good understanding of the confounding variables that affect prognosis

of an RCT can also be affected by chance, the possibility of measurement bias and losses to follow-up. Of more concern to health service researchers is the external validity, the difficulty in generalising the results from an RCT to real-life clinical situations. This has led to the development of the pragmatic randomised controlled trial. Anyone familiar with the arguments over the findings of randomised controlled trials (e.g. NIMH correspondence) will regard the idea that RCTs are gold standards as somewhat naïve. There are still serious difficulties in interpretation even after well-conducted studies.

RCTs often have a number of limitations in informing clinical practice. Many clinical trials have quite restrictive inclusion criteria. For example, trials of antidepressants almost always exclude those who are at suicidal risk, even though they are the group about whom most clinicians would like good evidence on clinical effectiveness.

Pragmatic randomised controlled trials

Schwartz & Lellouch (1967) are usually credited with contrasting explanatory and pragmatic attitudes in clinical trials. Explanatory trials are primarily aimed at providing evidence of efficacy or answering theoretical questions about treatments. For that reason it might be reasonable to analyse only data on those subjects who received the course of treatment, rather than adopting an intention-to-treat analysis. Pragmatic trials on the other hand are concerned with providing evidence for the effectiveness of treatments under real service conditions. Table 6.9 lists some of the questions one can ask when criticising pragmatic trials. One of the important principles is to ensure that the trial is addressing a dilemma faced by clinicians or health managers. It is also important to realise that the costs of treatments have to take account of use of other health and social services, and personal costs (Drummond et al 1987).

Research, guidelines and audit

There are always difficulties in generalising the results from single trials and there is always the possibility that the results of small trials, particularly the well-known ones, are a result of random error. Systematic reviews of research studies should be the backbone of providing advice to clinicians about treatment. These can therefore be used to provide guidelines for best practice. Audit is therefore about determining the extent to which guidelines are adhered to. There has been much talk also about measuring outcomes in routine clinical practice in the context of auditing services. This practice would produce unrandomised evidence, usually with a poor understanding of potential confounders. In

Table 6.9	Methodological aspects of pragmatic randomised controlled trials

Aims
Does the trial address a clinically important dilemma?
Are the subjects in the trial those patients in which the treatment would normally be considered in clinical practice?
Is the intervention a realistic reflection of likely good practice in the Health Service? Is it a 'Rolls Royce' service provided in a centre of excellence that would be difficult to sustain elsewhere?

Design
What was the method of randomisation and how did the investigators ensure that it was adhered to?
Who was blind to the randomised allocation – patient, physician, the research assistant measuring outcomes, the investigator who analysed the data? How was blindness ensured and how was it assessed? Did the experimenters include an assessment of 'quality of life'?
Is there an economic assessment that measures health and social service costs not directly concerned with the treatment?

Analysis
Was there an imbalance between the randomised groups in any important prognostic variables?
How is missing data analysed? Is an intention to treat strategy used or are other statistical methods used?
Have the investigators performed multiple statistical tests on a variety of outcomes? Was the main outcome specified before the trial was started? Is the power calculation from the research proposal described?
If a negative result, how large are the confidence intervals? Have the investigators ruled out the possibility of an important treatment effect?

the present author's view this is unlikely to be of much use to clinicians in deciding upon what treatments to use. If the research evidence is thought to be inadequate it is best to advocate carrying out pragmatic clinical trials that are relevant to practice in that locality.

PSYCHIATRY AND PUBLIC HEALTH

Preventive strategies and public health

Geoffrey Rose (Rose 1992) made the distinction between high-risk and population-based strategies for preventing disease. The high-risk approach identifies

Table 6.10 Number, mean rate and odds ratios for disability days in the days preceding the second wave of the ECA survey in North Carolina

	N	Mean rate (SD)	Odds ratios[a] (95% CI)	Excess disability days
Major depression	49	11.0 (29.0)	4.8 (1.6 to 13.9)	474
Dysthymia	62	3.0 (7.5)	1.9 (0.3 to 11.9)	51
Minor depression (with mood disturbance)	176	6.1 (21.4)	1.6 (1.0 to 2.4)	712
Minor depression (without mood disturbance)	696	4.0 (16.3)	1.3 (0.9 to 1.7)	1356
No symptoms	1997	2.0 (10.7)	1.0[b]	Baseline

[a]Adjustments include race, sex, age, 12 medical conditions, socioeconomic status.
[b]Baseline.
From Broadhead et al (1990).

individuals at high risk and any intervention is directed purely at them. An example might be the usual medical approach towards hypertension in which general practitioners screen and treat the hypertensive person. The population-based approach aims to reduce the frequency of risk factors in the whole population; for example, by encouraging everyone to exercise more and eat less salt in order to reduce blood pressure and the incidence of cardiovascular diseases. Unfortunately our knowledge of the aetiology of psychiatric disorder is such that we are not yet in a position to adopt preventive strategies.

High-risk strategies fit better with the medical model and restrict any intervention to those who would benefit most. However, Rose has repeatedly shown that there are many circumstances where high-risk strategies have rather modest effects in reducing the rates of disease because they exclude the large numbers of people at moderate risk. This point can be illustrated using data in Table 6.10 from the Epidemiologic Catchment Area Program study in the USA (Broadhead et al 1990). In this study the authors examined the association between disability days (e.g. days off work) and major depression, dysthymia and two categories representing those with neurotic symptoms that fell below the threshold for DSM-III (APA 1980) diagnoses. Those with major depression had higher rates of disability days. However, in aggregate there was more disability as a result of those with the less severe disorders. If one wanted to prevent the disability associated with psychiatric disorder, treating those with major depression and dysthymia would only reduce the disability associated with these neurotic disorders by a maximum of a limited degree.

Screening and case finding

Screening programmes have been set up for a variety of

conditions. For psychiatrists, the best examples are probably the neonatal screening for phenylketonuria and hypothyroidism, conditions that when treated can prevent the development of mental handicap. There has been a discussion about the principles that govern decisions about adopting screening programmes (Wilson & Junger 1968). There has been more interest in psychiatry in the possibility of case-finding subjects with neurosis, particularly in primary care where it is difficult to diagnose cases of depression and anxiety when patients do not complain of these symptoms.

As a general rule briefer tests need to be used in large populations and then confirmed with a more detailed diagnostic test in those screened positive. It is therefore important to know the accuracy with which screening tests can predict disease. This is usually measured by calculating the sensitivity, specificity and positive predictive value that are defined in Table 6.11. There tends to be a trade-off between sensitivity and specificity and, as the threshold for being positive on the test increases, so the false positives reduce

Table 6.11 Agreement between a screening test and a gold standard

		Gold standard	
		Yes	No
Screening test	Yes	a	b
	No	c	d

Sensitivity = a/(a + c); the true-positive proportion.
Specificity = b/(b + d); the false-positive proportion.
Positive predictive value = a/(a + b).

(increased specificity) in frequency and the false negatives increase in frequency (reduced sensitivity). Sensitivity and specificity tend to be called validity indices as they give a measure of the validity of a test in measuring a gold standard. Of course there is no such thing as a gold standard in psychiatry, and that is also true of most areas of medicine. Unreliability of the gold standard measure effectively places an upper limit on the sensitivity and specificity of a test.

Positive predictive value and prevalence

The positive predictive value (PPV) gives the probability that someone scoring positively on a test is really a case. This is the one the most important characteristics in considering screening and case-finding programmes. The PPV depends critically upon the prevalence of a case. As the prevalence falls then the positive predictive value also falls because of the increase in the number of false positives when there are few positives in the population. In Table 6.11, as the number in the second column increase then the cell frequency represented by b will increase and the PPV will fall. This was an expected problem in the OPCS National Survey of Psychiatric Morbidity that conducted a household survey in order to estimate the prevalence of psychosis. A psychosis screening questionnaire was developed (Bebbington & Nayani 1995) which had high specificity and sensitivity in a validity study. When used in the household survey the PPV dropped to about 10% because the prevalence of psychosis was low, around 0.5%.

Primary care psychiatry

Epidemiologists are population-based researchers and primary care is population-based medicine. The UK system of strong primary care with a defined list of patients encourages doctors to promote health and prevent disease. British general practitioners also see the whole spectrum of morbidity. Thus for epidemiologists that are interested in the health service there is often an interest in primary care and its care for neurotic disorders (Goldberg & Huxley 1992). Psychotic disorders usually lead to more disability for the individual than neurotic disorders but neurotic disorders are so common that in aggregate they also lead to a considerable burden on the community. This is reflected in general practitioners' concern for the effective treatment of this group of patients. In the long term, knowledge of the aetiology of these conditions may allow us to prevent morbidity using preventive strategies. Until that time we need to ensure that effective treatments are provided for those who would benefit.

FURTHER READING

This chapter can only touch on some of the main concerns of epidemiologists in designing and analysing studies. For a more detailed, though still introductory, text you could consult Beaglehole et al (1993), and Hennekens & Buring (1987) is recommended for reference. Pocock (1983) has written a text on clinical trials and the Department of Health have published a good summary of the main principles in designing pragmatic clinical trials and using other designs in evaluating the cost-effectiveness of interventions (Advisory Group on Health Technology Assessment 1992). Last's (1988) *Dictionary of Epidemiology* is a useful reference and explains most epidemiological terms. The BMJ Publishing Group has produced publications on critical appraisal (Crombie 1996) and on systematic reviews (Chalmers & Altman 1995).

REFERENCES

Advisory Group on Health Technology Assessment 1992 Assessing the effects of health technologies. Department of Health, London

Andreasson S, Allebeck A, Engstrom A, Rydberg U 1987 Cannabis and schizophrenia: a longitudinal study of Swedish conscripts. Lancet ii: 1483–1486

APA 1980 Diagnostic and statistical manual of mental disorders, 3rd edn. American Psychiatric Association, Washington, DC

Beaglehole R, Bonita R, Kjellstrom T 1993 Basic epidemiology. World Health Organization, Geneva

Bebbington P E, Nayani T 1995 The psychosis screening questionnaire. International Journal of Methods in Psychiatric Research 5: 11–20

Beck A T, Rush A J, Shaw B F, Emery G 1979 Cognitive therapy of depression. Wiley, New York

Black N 1996 Why we need observational studies to evaluate the effectiveness of health care. British Medical Journal 312: 1215–1218

Broadhead W E, Blazer D, George L, Tse C 1990 Depression, disability days and days lost from work. Journal of the American Medical Association 264: 2524–2528

Brown G W, Harris T 1978 Social origins of depression. Tavistock, London

Chalmers I, Altman D G (eds) 1995 Systemic reviews. BMJ Publishing, London

Chalmers I, Dickersin K, Chalmers T C 1992 Getting to grips with Archie Cochrane's agenda. British Medical Journal 305: 786–788

Cooper J E, Kendell R E, Gurland B J, Sharpe L, Copeland J R M, Simon R 1972 Psychiatric diagnosis in New York and London: a comparative study of mental hospital admissions. Oxford University Press, London

Crombie I K 1996 The pocket guide to critical appraisal: a handbook for health care professionals. BMJ Publishing, London

Davey Smith G, Egger M 1995 Misleading meta-analysis. British Medical Journal 310: 752–754

David A S 1993 Cognitive neuropsychiatry? Psychological Medicine 23: 1–5

Dennehy J A, Appleby L, Thomas C S, Faragher E B 1996 Case–control study of suicide by discharged psychiatric patients. British Medical Journal 312: 1580

Doll R 1992 Sir Austin Bradford Hill and the progress of medical science. British Medical Journal 305: 1521–1526

Drummond M F, Stoddard G L, Torrance G W 1987 Methods for the economic evaluation of health care. Oxford University Press, Oxford

Elkin I, Shea T, Watkins J T et al 1989 National Institute of Mental Health treatment of depression collaborative research program: general effectiveness of treatments. Archives of General Psychiatry 46: 971–983

Evidence-Based Medicine Working Group 1992 Evidence-based medicine. A new approach to teaching the practice of medicine. Journal of the American Medical Association 268: 2420–2425

Gardner M J, Altman D G 1986 Confidence intervals rather than p values: estimation rather than hypothesis testing. British Medical Journal 292: 746–750

Goldacre M, Seagroatt V, Hawton K 1993 Suicide after discharge from psychiatric in-patient care. Lancet 342: 283–286

Goldberg D, Huxley P 1992 Common mental disorders: a biopsychosocial approach. Routledge, London

Goldberg D P, Williams P 1988 The user's guide to the general health questionnaire. NFER-NELSON, Windsor

Goldberg E M, Morrison S L 1963 Schizophrenia and social class. British Journal of Psychiatry 109: 785–802

Hennekens C H, Buring J E 1987 Epidemiology in medicine. Little Brown, Boston

Hill A B 1952 The clinical trial. New England Medical Journal 247: 113–119

Hill A B 1965 The environment and disease: association or causation? Journal of the Royal Society of Medicine 58: 295–300

Hotopf M, Hardy R, Lewis G 1997 Discontinuation rates of SSRIs and tricyclic antidepressants: a meta-analysis and investigation of heterogeneity. British Journal of Psychiatry 170: 120–127

Jenkins R 1985 Sex differences in minor psychiatric disorder. Psychological medicine monographs 7. Cambridge University Press, Cambridge

Jenkins R, Lewis G, Bebbington P et al 1997 The national psychiatric morbidity surveys of Great Britain: initial findings from the household survey. Psychological Medicine 27: 775–789

Katz R, McGuffin P 1987 Neuroticism in familial depression. Psychological Medicine 17: 155–161

Khoury M J, Beaty T H, Cohen B H 1993 Fundamentals of genetic epidemiology. Oxford University Press, New York

Klerman G L, Weissman M M, Rounsaville B J, Chevron E S 1984 Interpersonal psychotherapy of depression. Basic Books, New York

Last J (ed) 1988 A dictionary of epidemiology, 2nd edn. Oxford University Press, New York

Lewis G 1994 Assessing psychiatric disorder with a human interviewer or a computer. Journal of Epidemiology and Community Health 48: 207–210

Lewis G, Appleby L A, Jarman B 1994 Suicide and psychiatric services. Lancet 344: 822

Lloyd G, Lishman A 1976 The effect of depression on speed of recall of pleasant and unpleasant experiences. Psychological Medicine 5: 173–180

Lopes C S, Lewis G, Mann A 1996 Psychiatric and alcohol disorders as risk factors for drug abuse: a case–control study in Rio de Janeiro, Brazil. Social Psychiatry and Psychiatric Epidemiology 31: 355–363

McGuffin P, Owen M J, O'Donovan M C, Thapar A, Gottesman I I 1994 Seminars in psychiatric genetics. Gaskell, London

Mednick S A, Machon R A, Huttenen M O, Bonet D 1988 Adult schizophrenia following prenatal exposure to an influenza epidemic. Archives of General Psychiatry 45: 189–92

Meltzer H, Gill B, Petticrew M, Hinds K 1995 OPCS Surveys of psychiatric morbidity. Report 1. The prevalence of psychiatric morbidity among adults aged 16–64 living in private households in Great Britain. HMSO, London

Miller A B, Bulbrook R D 1986 UICC multidisciplinary project on breast cancer: the epidemiology, aetiology and prevention of breast cancer. International Journal of Cancer 37: 173–177

Moser K A, Fox A J, Jones D R 1984 Unemployment and mortality in the OPCS longitudinal study. Lancet ii: 1324–1328

Munoz N, Bosch F X 1992 HPV and cervical neoplasia: review of case–control and cohort studies. In: Munoz N et al (eds) The epidemiology of cervical cancer and human papillomavirus. IARC, Lyon

O'Callaghan E, Gibson T, Colohan H A et al 1992 Risk of schizophrenia in adults born after obstetric complications and their association with early onset of illness: a controlled study. British Medical Journal 305: 1256–1259

Pocock S J 1983 Clinical trials: a practical approach. Wiley, Chichester

Rose G 1992 The strategy of preventive medicine. Oxford University Press, Oxford

Rose G A, Barker D J P 1978 What is a case? Dichotomy or continuum? British Medical Journal 2: 873–874

Sackett D L 1979 Bias in analytic research. Journal of Chronic Disease 32: 51–63

Sackett D L, Cook R J 1995 The number needed to treat: a clinically useful measure of treatment effect. British Medical Journal 310: 452–454

Sainsbury P 1955 Suicide in London. Chapman & Hall, London

Sarason I G, Sarason B R, Shearin E N 1986 Social support as an individual difference variable: its stability, origins and relational aspects. Journal of Personality and Social Psychology 50: 845–855

Schaid D J, Sommer S S 1994 Comparison of statistics for candidate-gene association studies using cases and parents. BMJ 313: 829–830

Schlesselman J J 1982 Case–control studies. Oxford University Press, New York

Schulz K F, Chalmers I, Hayes R J, Altman D G 1995 Empirical evidence of bias: dimensions of methodological quality associated with estimates of treatment effects in controlled trials. Journal of the American Medical Association 273: 408–412

Schwartz D, Lellouch J 1967 Explanatory and pragmatic attitudes in therapeutic trials. Journal of Chronic Disease 20: 637–648

Secretary of State for Health 1992 The Health of the Nation: a strategy for health in England. HMSO, London

Sloggett A, Joshi H 1994 Higher mortality in deprived areas. Community or personal disadvantage? British Medical Journal 309: 1471–1474

Snow J 1936 On the mode of communication of cholera, 2nd edn. Commonwealth Fund, New York

Wilkinson R G 1992 Income distribution and life expectancy. British Medical Journal 304: 165–168

Wilson J M G, Junger G 1968 Principles and practice of screening for disease. World Health Organization, Geneva

Wolkind S, Coleman E Z 1983 Adult psychiatric disorder and childhood experiences: the validity of retrospective data. British Journal of Psychiatry 143: 188–191

Yusuf S, Collins R, Peto R 1984 Why do we need some large, simple randomised trials. Statistics in Medicine 3: 409–420

7
Genetics

Douglas Blackwood   Walter Muir

INTRODUCTION

The discovery of the genetic basis of many diseases, including several involving the nervous system, has been one of the triumphs of recent science and the methods of genetic and physical mapping are being increasingly applied to common complex psychiatric disorders and, indeed, to the entire range of behavioural phenotypes. The genetics of specific psychiatric disorders will be found in the appropriate chapters of this volume. This chapter is an overview of the relevant genetic concepts and the methodologies used to identify genes for inherited disorders.

CHROMOSOMES AND CELL DIVISION

Chromosomes occur in the cell nucleus, and are a complex assemblage of deoxyribose nucleic acid (DNA) and proteins. DNA is coiled around pairs of histone protein subunits, with a cluster of four such pairs being termed a nucleosome. These units in themselves are coiled into the densely packed architecture of the chromosome which reaches its most compact form during the metaphase period of cell division, when the chromosomes are visible under the microscope. Each chromosome is divided into a long (q) and a short (p) arm by the centromere, which attaches to the spindle apparatus and plays a major role in chromosome assortment during cell division. The chromosome ends – the telomeres – are functionally specialised, stabilising the chromosome and preventing loss of DNA during its replication. In the acrocentric group of chromosomes the short arms are very small and contain little coding DNA. Individual chromosomes can be distinguished by DNA and protein stains (Verma & Babu 1995). One of the earliest methods, and still the most common, uses Giemsa (G-banding) to produce a series of dark bands interrupted by non-staining zones unique to each chromosome pair, allowing the fine structure of chromo-

somes to be studied. Banding methods led to the discovery of disorders associated with chromosomal deletions, insertions and movements of chromosomal material from one chromosome to another (translocations) or within the same chromosome (inversions).

Most human cells have 44 autosomes and two sex chromosomes (46; the diploid count) and sperm and ova have 23 chromosomes (the haploid count). Autosomes are numbered from 1 to 22 on the basis of overall length. The karyotype is a term expressing the total number of chromosomes, the sex chromosome complement, and the particulars of any abnormalities of an individual. Thus a normal human female would be 46,XX, whereas a man with Down's syndrome (trisomy 21) could be 47,XY,+21.

Somatic cells divide by mitosis, in which each chromosome is duplicated during prophase of the cell cycle to form double chromosomes joined at the centromere (sister chromatids) before the total complement is shared equally between the two daughter cells. Gamete formation by meiosis follows a different route. During prophase an initial duplication of chromosomes forms sister chromatids, which then pair together to exchange chromosomal material by the process of recombination, in which bridges of chromatin (chiasma) loop out to enact reciprocal exchanges from one chromatid to the other. Recombination is the first of three essential processes (recombination, random assortment of chromosomes at fertilisation, and DNA mutations) that establish the molecular individuality of the organism, maintaining the evolutionary diversity and strength of the gene pool. Recombination rate, the physical basis of linkage analysis, can be used as an estimate of the distances between two points on a chromosome because the greater the physical distance between two markers the more likely they are to be separated during meiosis. Meiosis proceeds to a second meiotic cell division, without duplication of chromosomal material, producing four gametes with a haploid count of chromosomes. In the formation of ova only one of the four gametes survives as an ovum, the others form polar bodies.

GENES AND DNA

The DNA in chromosomes

The well-known double helix is composed of a linear array of DNA forming two strands (a duplex) of linked nucleotides composed of a base – adenine (A), cytosine (C), thymine (T) or guanine (G) – linked to a sugar (deoxyribose) joined to the next nucleotide by a phosphate bond. Strands form complementary pairs (A to T and C to G) and the length of a DNA sequence is usually measured as numbers of base pairs. The average human genome is estimated to be around 3000 million base pairs (3000 Mbp) and to have up to 100 000 genes. Thus, ignoring differential lengths, each chromosome has on average 130 Mbp and will contain around 4000 genes, 30% of which may be related to the development and function of the central nervous system.

Genes are not evenly shared between chromosomes, nor homogeneously distributed within them (Bickmore & Craig 1997). Surprisingly most DNA, in some estimates over 90%, does not have a known coding function but includes stretches of repeat sequence nucleotides (tandem repeats). The centromeres are bracketed by long stretches of large repeats of several hundred nucleotides (satellite DNA) which form into dense heterochromatic non-coding regions (the C-bands). Smaller repeats are very frequent in the other areas of the chromosome, those of several tens of nucleotides are sometimes termed minisatellites, and those of a few nucleotides microsatellites. The total number of repeats of these monomers (and the overall size of the block) is often highly variable in the population, but stably inherited; they are used as polymorphic markers in linkage and association studies.

The function of genes

A gene (sometimes called a cistron) is a complex unit ranging from around 100 bp, as in the gene coding for a type of human transfer RNA molecule, to over 2 mbp for the dystrophin gene whose mutations lead to the Duchenne and Becker muscular dystrophies (Lewin 1997). Within any gene are stretches of DNA, called exons (dystrophin has 79 exons), which code for the amino acid units of a given polypeptide, separated from each other by non-coding intron sequences. Within an exon a sequence of three nucleotides (a codon) on one strand of DNA will define one specific amino acid for the polypeptide chain – the genetic code – and there is considerable redundancy with only 20 amino acids but 64 different codons. Some codons do not code an amino acid but instead act as signals for the cessation of polypeptide building (stop codons). The processes of transcription and translation by which the genetic code of DNA dictates the formation of specific proteins are mediated by messenger RNA (mRNA) and transfer RNA (tRNA). First mRNA is transcribed from a DNA template by the action of RNA polymerase enzymes in the nucleus, and subsequently the introns are excised and the exons spliced into a single linear sequence. The mRNA is further processed by the addition of sequences at each end (cap and polyadenylate tail) before passing from the nucleus to the cytoplasm, where it binds to a ribosome for protein synthesis. The mRNA moves through the ribosome like a tape through the head of a recording machine as tRNA assembles amino acids in the appropriate sequence until the completed polypeptide is released. In addition to coding sequences a gene also has regulatory elements, including a promoter sequence just upstream of the first exon, needed to initiate transcription, and enhancers that influence promoter effectiveness. The promoter and enhancer complexes are important in the control of transcription. The presence of an enhancer element up to several thousand base pairs away from the β-globin gene promoter has been found to produce a 200-fold increase in transcription activity. Homeodomain proteins are one important class of regulatory factors. The genes that code for these proteins are termed homeoboxes (or Hox boxes) and are important in controlling development. A series of human diseases occur with mutations in hox genes, including malformations of the eye (aniridia, anophthalmia, etc.) and brain (schizencephaly, X-linked mixed deafness, and a form of hypopituitarism). One type of homeobox, PAX6, is involved in a variety of human developmental eye and brain disorders (Freund et al 1996).

Mutations in genes

Gene mutation denotes a change in the coding information of a gene through changes in the sequence of nucleotides. The types of mutation are various, from single base pair changes, through to insertion or deletion of many bases. There are many detailed reviews of this important area (for example, Malcolm 1994, Cooper et al 1995). Mutation is an essential component of life and a source of molecular individuality, providing one mechanism for adapting to environmental changes. For instance, an immense number of haemoglobin variants have evolved under the selective environmental pressure of malaria infection. Over 120 mutations are known in the β-globin gene and others in α-globin which protect against malarial infection but also confer β- or α-thalassaemia, possibly the most common genetic disorder in the world (Weatherall 1996).

Mutations in coding regions of genes can take several forms. A single base pair substitution may occur in a codon. The base pair substitution may be due to a truly random stochastic error in the DNA replication mechanism – a simile would be a typographical error of one letter, in a word, when copying a long paragraph of text. The sense of that word may be completely different to the original. The cell has various error correction (proof-reading) mechanisms which pick up some mistakes, but these occasionally fail and allow the error to stand. The single substitution can have one of three outcomes: it create a new codon, causing the insertion of an incorrect amino acid into a protein (missense mutation – the most common); it can create a stop codon terminating the polypeptide chain prematurely (nonsense mutation); or it can create another codon coding for the same amino acid and thus have no overall effect (a silent mutation). All three forms of mutation (and many others) have been described in the gene for the cystic fibrosis transporter protein.

Coding region mutations can also arise from deletions. In the extreme, an entire gene or series of genes can be incorporated in deletions of many thousand base pairs. Small deletions have been shown to be important in several conditions comprising the contiguous gene syndromes (Ledbetter & Ballabio 1995). These often have highly variable phenotypes, and arise from chromosomal rearrangements involving several genes on a chromosomal segment, leading to gene dosage anomalies – partial monosomies and trisomies. These rearrangements are often subtle and below the level of classical chromosome banding methods. The most common of the rearrangements seem to be microdeletions as in the Miller–Dieker (17p13.3), DiGeorge/velocardiofacial (22q11.2), Smith–Magenis (17p11.3), Rubenstein–Taybi syndromes (16p13.3), or microdeletions with imprinting effects, described below for the Prader–Willi/Angelman syndromes (15q11–13). All these syndromes have learning disability as a component in conjunction with a set of other clinical features. Beckwith–Weidmann (11p15.5), by contrast, involves a duplication and paternal imprinting. The origin of the submicroscopic abnormalities can either be de novo or based on a cryptic parental translocation or inversion (e.g. in the Miller–Dieker syndome, and the Kallman syndrome on the X chromosome), leading to multiple cases in the same sibship. Unstable triplet repeats are duplication mutations that cause several neuropsychiatric conditions. Repeats within the coding regions cause Huntington's disease and the spinocerebellar ataxias. Triplet repeats outwith the coding frame cause a second group of disorders, including myotonic dystrophy and the recessive condition Friedreich's ataxia (Klockgether & Dichgans 1997). The first such condition described was the fragile X syndrome, and this is discussed in detail in Chapter 22.

Mutations in non-coding regions can also have phenotypic effects. Elimination or creation of splice sites can alter mRNA formation. Mutations have also been described in DNA coding for the capping and tailing of mRNA. A final site for mutation effects in genes is in the promoter and enhancer regulatory sequences, especially in the binding motifs. Such mutations can either upregulate or downregulate gene transcription.

PATTERNS OF INHERITANCE

Chromosomes containing genes, and the mutations they may harbour, are passed down from generation to generation. Complementary genes on both members of a pair of autosomes in a cell are usually (but not always) active. Thus a mutation silencing the transcription of a gene on one chromosome usually leads to a reduction (haploinsufficiency), not absence, of a gene product. The level of this product may be enough to allow the cell to function normally, and in such cases there would be no phenotypic consequences of the mutation, until the other gene was also made dysfunctional by a separate mutation. At the other extreme the silencing or downregulation of one gene of the pair is not compensated by the other, and a disease process results. These two conditions have implications for the phenotypic expression of a mutated gene in a family: the first will show classical recessive inheritance and the second dominant inheritance. It was the study of such patterns of inheritance in plants that led Mendel to propose that quantal genetic factors were being inherited, and disorders due to the inheritance of a single mutated gene (monogenic disorders) are often said to be mendelian. Recessive conditions rely on the second gene also being mutated (the person is said to be homozygous for the mutated gene; if the two mutations in the genes are different they are said to be compound heterozygotes). The chances of this occurring in a rare condition will be increased if the parents are related. Thus there is often an increased rate of consanguinity in families expressing a rare recessive disorder, and in certain ethnic groups where this is relatively common, recessive disorders may be vastly overrepresented. However, this does not apply to more common recessive disorders such as cystic fibrosis (1:2500 live births). Here the rate of carriage of mutant genes is high in the general population, and either new mutations are frequent, or carriage of the mutation confers a reproductive advantage of some form. If both parents have one copy of the mutant gene (are heterozygous for this gene), then, on average, one in four of their children will be affected. There may be no evidence of any other cases in previous generations, and the disease may apparently only appear in the children ('horizontal' inheritance). A theoretical example of a family showing recessive inheritance can be found in Figure 7.1. Overall, recessive conditions are rather rare, occurring in 2–3 per 1000 live births. Dominant disorders are more common (up to 7 per 1000 live births). Truly dominant disorders will be equally apparent in people carrying one (heterozygote) or two (homozygote) mutant genes. There are few, if any, completely dominant disorders, the closest probably being Huntington's disease (1:2500 live births). Dominant conditions, on average, affect subjects in all generations ('vertical inheritance') with around half of a sibship being affected (Fig. 7.1). Unless a new mutation has arisen, one of the parents of an affected child will express the condition. Most such disorders are not fully dominant however, and the expression of the disease state in heterozygotes and homozygotes can be very variable. The penetrance of the condition is the proportion of people with a mutated gene on one chromosome (i.e. heterozygotes) showing any feature of the disease. The third type of mendelian disorder is due to a mutated gene on the sex chromosomes. Males can only pass on their Y chromosome to their sons, so that there will be no male-to-male vertical inheritance in X-linked conditions but affected males are more common in X-linked pedigrees (Fig. 7.1). The mothers of an affected male will be carriers of the gene mutation, and either be unaffected (X-linked recessive) or affected (X-linked dominant). The fragile X syndrome has a modified inheritance pattern, and the most common mendelian X-linked disorders are probably the Duchenne muscular dystrophies (1:3000 live births).

Sometimes one gene may interact with another gene on the same or a different chromosome to influence the expression of a phenotype – a situation termed epistasis. An example of a gene–gene interaction affecting expression of a disease is the human leucocyte antigen (HLA) system on chromosome 6. Around 90% of people who have ankylosing spondylitis have the HLA-B27 allele, whereas only a small percentage of carriers of this allele in the general population will have the disease (Tomlinson & Bodmer 1995). In polygenic (literally many genes) or oligogenic (a few genes) conditions the clinical phenotype is the result of contributions from many different genes. A dozen different genes on nine different chromosomes contribute to the development of insulin-dependent diabetes mellitus (IDDM) of which one locus (IDDM1) contributes around 30% of cases and interacts with the HLA system. A second locus (IDDM2) is due to variation at a repeat sequence at the insulin gene – a case of a pathogenic polymorphism in a non-coding region (Cordell & Todd 1995). The power of genetic investigation in psychiatry is clearly shown by the recent findings in dementia. At one time it was seriously questioned whether genes could be found contributing to any but the rarest causes of this condition. It is now known that a proportion of presenile familial dementia of the Alzheimer's type can be caused independently by mutations in three different genes (presenilin I and II genes on chromosomes 14 and 1, and Alzheimer's precursor protein gene on chromosome 21). A locus for late-onset dementia has been found on chromosome 19 and further complexity is added by the apolipoprotein E gene (ApoE), specific alleles of which have an epistatic effect of increasing risk or of protecting against the development of dementia.

In addition to one disease arising from mutations in many different genes, there may be a host of different pathogenic mutations within one single gene. Almost 600 different mutations (mainly missense) have been found in the cystic fibrosis transmembrane conductance regulator gene (CFTR) associated with cystic fibrosis, and again there may be an important modifier locus altering the severity of the disease (Estivill 1996).

There has been an explosion of knowledge about other disorders also thought to be complex such as non-syndromic hearing impairment, which is hugely genetically heterogeneous and clinically variable with over 30 different chromosomal loci so far identified (Van Camp et al 1997), and inherited cancers including the common breast–ovarian and breast cancer syndromes. For almost all dominant forms of cancer the relevant genes have now been cloned (Brown & Solomon 1997). There is no overriding reason to believe that psychiatric disorders should be less amenable to investigation.

NON-MENDELIAN INHERITANCE

Anticipation

There are now many inherited disorders that do not conform to the simple rules formulated by Mendel. The classical case, fragile X syndrome, is described in detail in Chapter 22.

It has been long known that anticipation, the phenomenon in which a disease has an earlier age of onset and increased severity in succeeding generations, has been described in bipolar disorder (McInnis 1996). Triplet repeat expansion, the basis of anticipation in the fragile X syndrome, has not yet been convincingly found in major psychosis. Other unstable repeat sequences may be important. For instance, an expansion of a minisatellite on chromosome 21 in the promoter region of the crystallin B gene seems to be responsible for progressive myoclonus epilepsy type 1 (see Buard & Jeffreys 1997 for review).

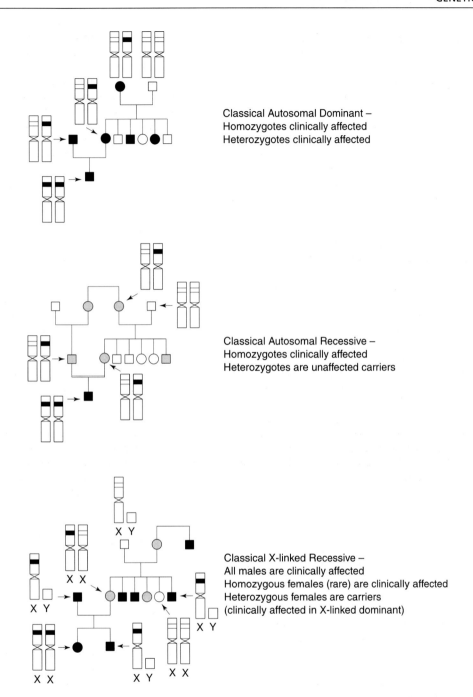

Classical Autosomal Dominant –
Homozygotes clinically affected
Heterozygotes clinically affected

Classical Autosomal Recessive –
Homozygotes clinically affected
Heterozygotes are unaffected carriers

Classical X-linked Recessive –
All males are clinically affected
Homozygous females (rare) are clinically affected
Heterozygous females are carriers
(clinically affected in X-linked dominant)

Fig. 7.1 Classical patterns of inheritance in mendelian disorders. The diagrams show hypothetical family trees and chromosome pairs for selected individuals. In the pedigrees circles represent females and squares males. Filled symbols are clinically affected individuals; a single dot in the centre of the symbol represents a clinically unaffected carrier. The double line in the autosomal recessive pedigree represents a first- cousin (consanguineous) marriage. In the chromosome diagrams a black band signifies that there is a mutated gene present, a white band that the chromosome carries a normal gene.

Parent of origin effects (imprinting)

Parent of origin effects, where different phenotypes are associated with paternal and maternal inheritance of a disorder, have been described in a variety of disorders. The mechanism of this effect is thought to lie in the differential contribution of genes from each parent through so-called imprinting of genes in the germline. Such inherited changes, affecting phenotype but not involving change in the genotype, are termed epigenetic. By some mechanism the germline DNA must initiate events at or after fertilisation that result in the selective activation or inactivation of genes originating from one parent rather than the other. It also follows that in the child's germline these imprints must be reset to allow new imprints to be acquired (Ferguson-Smith 1996). Again this has been described in the fragile X syndrome. Perhaps the most vivid illustration, however, is the locus on the long arm of chromosome 15, which is involved in two conditions associated with learning disability – Prader–Willi and Angelman syndromes. The Prader–Willi syndrome (PWS) occurs in 1:10 000–20 000 live births, and mild to moderate learning disability is associated with short stature, hypogonadism and a behavioural disorder that involves overeating, leading to severe obesity if unchecked. Angelman syndrome is rarer (around 1:30 000) and phenotypically very different, with severe learning disability, ataxia, epilepsy, inappropriate paroxysms of laughter, absence of speech and a characteristic facial appearance. PWS is caused by absence of activity of genes at 15q11–13 inherited from the father. Loss of paternally inherited gene function can occur by several means, and thus PWS is aetiologically heterogeneous. Most cases (75%) are due to a deletion of genes on the paternally derived chromosome 15. Most of the other cases are due to a phenomenon termed uniparental disomy (UPD), illustrating yet another form of non-mendelian genetic disorder. UPD results from the inheritance of a pair of chromosomes, both derived from the same parent. This is thought to occur in several ways. Non-disjunction of a haploid gamete at meiosis can lead to a duplication of chromosome 15. Fusion with sperm will result in a trisomic state in which two chromosomes 15 will be derived from the same parent. Further chromosome loss from the set may result in these two chromosomes 15 from the same parent being left in the cell. The diploid gamete may also fuse with a gamete that has completely lost chromosome 15, again causing both chromosomes to be derived from one parent. Finally there may be fusion of a gamete that lacks a chromosome 15 with a normal gamete. The resulting duplication of the single gamete gives a 'twin' of the gamete (a condition called isodisomy, as opposed to both chromosomes originating from the pair possessed by one parent). This novel genetic mechanism also occurs in other conditions, and, for instance, has been described for chromosome 7 in a case of cystic fibrosis. The implication of UPD and deletions for PWS is that the maternally derived homologues do not compensate for loss of the paternally derived genes. In essence the normal state of the relevant genes on chromosome 15 is that only the paternally derived gene is active – a functional monosomy – as opposed to the usual case for autosomal genes where both copies are expressed. The prime candidate for the gene involved is small nuclear ribonucleoprotein polypeptide N. Very rarely in PWS imprinting or deletions are not seen, and in such cases a point mutation in the relevant gene may be important. Angelman syndrome is the complement of PWS and results from silencing of a gene on the chromosome of maternal origin. Again most cases (70%) are due to a deletion at 15q11–13, but this time on the maternally derived chromosome. UPD (both chromosomes paternally derived) may account for a small number of cases (2%). The remaining cases may be due to direct mutations.

Cytoplasmic inheritance

The mitochondria contain DNA that resides outside the nucleus and thus does not segregate in meiosis. In man the mitochondrial DNA (mtDNA) is small (around 16.5kb), has been entirely sequenced and contains genes particularly involved with oxidative phosphorylation. Since sperm have no mitochondria, inheritance is purely maternal. However, most cells have several copies of this genome, and mutations have been associated with a variety of human neurodegenerative diseases, including a form of deafness. The mutation may only occur in some of the copies and the expression of the conditions can be very variable.

Quantitative trait loci

The methods of quantitative genetics may also help to elucidate the inheritance patterns of major mental illnesses and other common disorders including addictions, anorexia, reading disability and a vast range of behavioural and personality traits. In contrast to a 'one-gene, one disorder' hypothesis, these complex phenotypes may be considered as quantitative traits that are the result of an interplay of several (perhaps many) genes which individually are neither necessary nor sufficient to produce the phenotype. These multiple gene effects are of varying magnitude and act like risk factors, additively and interchangeably contributing to the vulnerability to the disorder. Genes contributing to the variance in quantitative traits are termed quantitative trait loci (QTL). The term QTL is almost synonymous with polygenic (many genes) or oligogenic (a few genes) but quantitative trait analysis considers genotypes to be distributed quantitatively as dimensions in a population and not as as dichotomous diagnoses (Plomin et al 1994).

The methods of QTL analysis have been particularly successful in leading to the detection of loci implicated in reading disorder (Grigorenko et al 1997).

FAMILY STUDIES

First-degree relatives (parents, siblings and offspring) share an average of 50% of their genes, and second-degree relatives (aunts, uncles, grandparents and grandchildren) share approximately 25%. To confirm genetic transmission of complex disorders, including most psychiatric conditions, epidemiological studies measure familial aggregation by comparing rates of illness in relatives of cases with relatives of controls. The rates of schizophrenia (Gottesman & Shields 1982, Kendler et al 1993), affective disorders (Tsuang & Faraone 1990), anxiety disorders (Mendlewicz et al 1993), personality disorders and a range of behaviours (Yeung et al 1993) are higher among relatives of affected probands than among relatives of controls, but segregation analysis, the statistical method by which the observed proportion of affected relatives is compared with the proportion expected according to a particular genetic hypothesis, fails to show classical mendelian modes of inheritance. In the case of major psychiatric illness it is possible that a variety of genetic and environmental factors can interact to produce phenotypes that are clinically indistinguishable; they are said to be genetically heterogeneous. Families showing apparent dominant, recessive and X-linked inheritance patterns have been described for these illnesses, and there is justification in supposing that all may truly coexist, acting through different mutations on different chromosomes.

Family studies are easy to carry out but their interpretation is limited because, in general, the closer the relationship, the greater the shared culture and environment. A family history of an illness is not enough to define a condition as being genetically based; for example, infection by tuberculosis may run in families entirely as a result of poor diet and housing and other purely environmental causes.

ADOPTION STUDIES

Adoption studies are one of the most powerful ways to

disentangle genetic from environmental influences on a disease. The three main designs of adoption studies are:

- *Parent as proband* Heston (1966) in the Oregon Schizophrenia Study was able to trace in adulthood 47 individuals who had been adopted shortly after birth when their mothers had been receiving institutional care for schizophrenia. Rates of illness were compared with 50 adopted offspring of mothers without psychiatric illness. The striking finding of this study was a significant increase in schizophrenia in the adoptees whose mothers were schizophrenic (5/47) compared with 0/50 in the control group.
- *Adoptee as proband* In this approach adopted children who become ill are ascertained and rates of illness are compared in their biological and their adoptive families. This design was followed in the Danish adoption study of schizophrenia whch showed a significantly higher rate of schizophrenia (20%) among 118 biological relatives than among 224 adoptive relatives (6%) (Kety et al 1976, Kety 1983).
- *Cross fostering design* This compares the rate of illness in two groups of adoptees, one group has ill parents, and after adoption has been raised by well parents; the second group has well biological parents but has been brought up in a family where a parent has become ill.

The choice of methodology will depend on the available methods of ascertainment. Children adopted shortly after birth will still have experienced the prenatal and perinatal environment provided by their biological mother and after adoption may suffer greater stress by virtue of being an adoptee. A criticism of adoption studies was that they could not exclude the possibility of strong shared environmental influences in utero. Kety et al (1976) addressed this by studying the rate of illness in a group of paternal half-siblings of schizophrenic adoptees and demonstrating an increased incidence of schizophrenia in paternal half-siblings that could not be attributed to prenatal and perinatal effects.

TWIN STUDIES

Monozygotic (MZ) or identical twins result from a single fertilized ovum and therefore share all genes, whereas dizygotic (DZ) or fraternal twins are the result of the implantation of two separate fertilized ova and generally share about 50% of genes and are no more alike than other siblings. Since, in general, twins share very similar cultural family and educational environment, a comparison of MZ and DZ twins allows an estimate of genetic as well as environmental contributions to their phenotype. Concordance rate measures the similarity of phenotype between twins. If both members of a pair of twins develop a disease they are said to be concordant for that condition. The simplest way to measure this is pair-wise concordance, defined as the number of pairs of twins where both are affected divided by the total number of pairs studied. More commonly the proband-wise concordance is quoted and this is the number of affected co-twins of an affected proband divided by the total number of co-twins in the study (Emery 1986). Clearly the mode of ascertainment of the sample of twins used in the study is all important and, unless an entire population has been systematically screened, proband-wise concordance will be different from pair-wise concordance because in that case some twins will be counted twice if they have been independently ascertained. In a classic study of schizophrenia, Gottesman & Shields (1972) found in their sample that there were 11 concordant and 11 discordant pairs of MZ twins and 3 concordant and 30 discordant DZ pairs of twins. This gives a pair-wise concordance rate of 11/22 (50%) for MZ and 3/30 (10%) for DZ twins. In the same sample, proband concordance was calculated to be 58% for MZ twins and 12% for DZ twins. The difference between the two methods arose because in 4/11 pairs of concordant MZ twins both of the twins were ascertained independently, so in effect were counted twice. Similarly 1/3 pairs of concordant DZ twins were ascertained independently. This illustrates the importance in these studies of the method of ascertainment of samples.

Environmental influences certainly include factors such as fetal nutrition, exposure to maternal metabolism, infections and birth trauma but also included are non transmitted genetic effects. Examples of these are somatic mutations, repeat sequence expansion, imprinting and variation in methylation which could effect the expression of inherited genetic factors. Gottesman & Bertelsen (1989) showed that the offspring of discordant MZ twin pairs had the same high rate of schizophrenia whether their parent was the schizophrenic or the unaffected co-twin. This observation could be explained by the operation of 'genetic' factors unique to each individual that influence the expression of the inherited disease-related genes, and thus alter the penetrance of the disease.

Family and twin studies have established evidence for a substantial genetic contribution to schizophrenia, bipolar disorder, Alzheimer's dementia, autism and reading disorder, and a weaker but important genetic contribution to panic disorder, alcoholism, anorexia and Tourette disorder. Twin studies have been particularly informative in measuring the size of the genetic contribution to nearly all aspects of behaviour and personality cognitive abilities, sexual orientation and even happiness. In these cases the intra (within) pair and the inter (between) pair, variances and the intraclass correlation are calculated (Emery 1986). For a variable under strong genetic influence, the correlation will be higher between MZ than DZ twins. In a recent study in which 1380 pairs of twins completed a personality questionnaire, correlations for a 'well-being' scale were 0.44 for MZ and 0.08 for DZ twins, leading to the remarkable conclusion that a person's baseline level of cheerfulness and contentment is largely a matter of heredity, with a heritability of 40–50% (Lykken & Tellegen 1996).

A systematic study of twins reared apart and assessed in adulthood, the Minnesota twin study, has provided an unusual opportunity for studying the effects of nature and nurture on personality, occupational and leisure interests, and social attitudes (Bouchard et al 1990). In this special situation the within-pair correlation of a trait is a direct estimate of the variance due to genetic factors.

MAPPING AND FINDING GENES

When quantitative genetic approaches suggest an important genetic contribution to a disease the strategy adopted to identify genes may follow one of two approaches. Functional cloning is possible if the cause of the disease is known with some certainty and a candidate gene can be examined directly. For most psychiatric conditions where we have no clear understanding of the underlying disorder the strategy of positional cloning is adopted. The position of the disease-related gene is first localised to a particular chromosomal site, using linkage analysis and association studies, and only then can the gene be characterised. This approach has been successful for identifying genes responsible for many single-gene disorders, including cystic fibrosis, Huntington's disease, muscular dystrophy and some familial cases of Alzheimer's disease. QTLs for reading disability have also been localised by similar methods.

Manipulating DNA

Many analyses require DNA to be handled in small lengths. DNA can be randomly fragmented by irradiation or ultrasound but the discovery in 1970 of bacterial enzymes – restriction endonucleases – that cut DNA only at definite, irregularly occurring base-pair motifs meant that lengths of DNA could be ordered into a highly specific map using the cut sites defined by such enzymes (restriction mapping). Within a year a restriction map locating the various enzyme cut sites had been made of the DNA from a virus (SV40). The fragments, after digestion with such enzymes, can be loaded into an agarose medium (a gel) and separated by electrophoresis. The separated fragments can be transferred from the gel to a membrane (usually nylon) in a blotting process, and subsequently fixed for further study. The whole process is termed Southern blotting after its originator in Edinburgh.

Amplifying DNA: the polymerase chain reaction

Undoubtedly the greatest technological advance in molecular biology in recent years has been the development of the polymerase chain reaction or PCR. Since its invention it has permeated all aspects of laboratory work, and has become a standard tool in DNA diagnostics. Duplex DNA can be caused to unwind (melting or denaturing) into single-stranded (simplex) DNA by heating to over 90°C. Cooling reverses the process (annealing). In the PCR small pieces of DNA are chemically synthesised that are complementary to unique DNA sequences that bracket the stretch to be amplified. Each such oligonucleotide primer of a pair is specific to an opposite strand of the duplex DNA template. Melting of the DNA allows these primers to bind to the separate strands and cooling reforms the duplex. Heat-stable DNA polymerases, isolated from bacteria that live in hot mud springs, allow the amplification of DNA between and including the primers when the DNA has been remelted by heating. The whole process is repeated in a cyclical fashion with an exponential amplification of the template DNA, and the reactions are automatically carried out in tubes in the wells of an efficiently controlled heating and cooling plate or thermal cycler. With the correct choice of primers the PCR allows the specific and highly sensitive amplification of DNA from tiny amounts of starting sample. The conservation in the use of valuable human material is immense; for example, over 250 separate amplifications of a DNA polymorphism can be done with the PCR on the same amount of DNA required for one analysis with a restriction enzyme digest. The PCR is also much faster than alternative amplification systems, and results can be obtained within hours rather than days. Its limitation, at present, is that it is usually restricted to templates of around 5 kbp or less.

LINKAGE ANALYSIS

Genetic mapping follows the descent down the generations of DNA markers in pedigrees and their segrega-

tion with illness. Either very large single pedigrees, or collections of smaller families where the effect of linkage is additive, are studied. Another method is to study pairs of affected siblings.

Linkage analysis exploits the characteristic of all chromosomes to recombine during meiosis. Recombination occurs when homologous chromosomes pair up during meiosis and exchange stretches of DNA. On average recombination takes place at about two stretches of DNA on each chromosome every meiosis or, put another way, if two points are separated by 1 mbp of DNA then recombination will occur between them roughly once in every 100 meioses; the statistical unit to describe this rate of recombination is termed the centimorgan (cM). Recombination ensures a mixing of genetic material so that two traits that are physically far apart on a chromosome or on separate chromosomes will assort independently of each other (Mendel's law of independent assortment). In general, the closer a polymorphic marker is to a disease locus on a chromosome, the more often the two will remain together from one generation to the next. If in a mating a marker and a disease become separated, we say that recombination has taken place. In a family or group of families the number of recombinants divided by the total number of offspring is called the recombination fraction; this is a useful quantity because over short distances the recombination fraction is proportional to the physical distance between the two loci, just as the chances of two cards becoming separated when a pack is cut is proportional to their distance apart in the pack. Genes on different chromosomes, or far apart on the same chromosome, cosegregate randomly and have a 50:50 chance of remaining together during meiosis and being transmitted to an offspring. The recombination fraction will therefore lie between 0 (which would indicate that a polymorphic marker was actually a physical part of the gene responsible for the disease, so the marker and the gene would never become separated) up to 0.5 (indicating completely independent assortment of marker and gene). The conventional statistical method of testing for linkage, is to calculate the LOD score from the recombination fraction (Morton 1982). The LOD score is the common logarithm of the odds that the recombination fraction has some given value, divided by the odds that the value is 0.5. For diseases where the mode of inheritance is known and the phenotype can be clearly defined, it is conventionally accepted that a LOD score of 3 (odds in favour of linkage of 1000:1) is considered proof of linkage, and conversely a LOD score of −2 (odds against linkage of 100:1) is accepted as exclusion. For conditions, including most psychiatric illnesses, where the mode of inheritance is uncertain and the phenotype far from clear, a stronger burden of proof is needed to avoid false-positive claims of linkage and LOD scores of 4 or greater would be preferred (Lander & Kruglyak 1995). Calculating a LOD score is simple for a small family where the mode of inheritance is clear, all cases of the disease are identified (fully penetrant) and all family members are available for study. This rarely happens in practice and certainly, as applied to psychiatric genetics, linkage analysis must make assumptions about mode of inheritance and deal with incomplete penetrance and must also cope with the probable situation that more than one gene may contribute to a disorder. Assumptions need also be made about defining the phenotype (e.g. in schizophrenia, whether to include only cases of definite schizophrenia or to include also schizotypal personality disorders and affective disorders in the same family). Allowances must be made for age-dependent penetrance, sex-linked diseases and other possibilities including imprinting (the differing phenotypes, depending on whether inheritance is from the mother or the father). In general, these complex situations that probably most closely match the reality of psychiatric genetics can be incorporated into the various linkage programmes available (Terwilliger & Ott 1994).

Genetic markers, to be useful for linkage analysis, must be polymorphic (have two or more alleles with a gene frequency of at least 1%). In the past, markers were limited to classical markers such as blood types and HLA, but now with very large numbers of genetic markers, closely spaced across the whole genome, linkage analysis has become a routine method of investigation. Repeat fragment length polymorphisms were the mainstay of early linkage studies in psychiatry, but have been largely replaced by various repeat length polymorphisms, including variable number tandem repeats (VNTRs) and short tandem repeats (STRs), usually based on the variable length of di-, tri- or tetra-nucleotide repeat stretches.

The fine mapping of a disease locus by linkage is limited in part by the available density of polymorphic markers, and sets of specific markers have now been created, spaced apart at an average of 10cM or less throughout the entire human genome. Over 5000 highly informative microsatellite markers varying in the number of repeats they contain have been produced through the Généthon initiative in France (Dib et al 1996). They can be directly amplified by PCR and visualisation after electrophoresis. Incorporation of fluorescent tags to the amplified product allows direct visualisation of the size of the segment during gel electrophoresis, and with automation the throughput of markers can be high. With such advances the time needed to place a disease gene on a chromosome and find its neighbouring markers has decreased consider-

ably. It has been noted that it took 17 years to map breast cancer to 17q21, but only two years to map prostatic cancer to 1q24–25 with around the same number of informative meioses (King 1997). Genetic mapping can constrain a disease mutation to within a few million base pairs, and paves the way for the identification of the gene itself by physical mapping of the region.

The availability of dense maps of markers and the development of adequate software for data analysis have made possible a large number of linkage studies in schizophrenia and manic–depressive illness, often involving whole genome scans using several hundred markers and large groups of multiply affected families (Baron 1997, Karayiorgou & Gogos 1997).

ASSOCIATION STUDIES

Linkage analysis is performed on families, whereas association studies involve populations of patients and healthy controls. In the search for genes these two approaches are entirely complementary. The idea of association is simpler and is well known through the long-established association between HLA subtypes and some common diseases, including diabetes, rheumatoid arthritis and ankylosing spondylitis. There are three interpretations of an increased frequency of a marker polymorphism in patients over controls:

- It could indicate linkage disequilibrium between the polymorphic marker and a gene responsible for the phenotype. An ideal setting for an association study would be a completely isolated island population where the disease had been introduced many generations previously by a single founder. Linkage disequilibrium between the disease gene and polymorphic markers close to the gene would be detectable in this population many generations on, because all affected individuals being descended from the same founder would have inherited the same mutated disease gene and flanking polymorphisms.
- Association could occur because the polymorphic marker itself is a functional variant that affects the phenotype (pleitropy). One example is the association of late-onset Alzheimer's disease with ApoE4. The frequency of ApoE4 is about 0.4 in individuals with Alzheimer's disease, compared with 0.15 in controls. This QTL increases the liability to develop dementia but is neither sufficient nor necessary to cause illness (Corder 1993).
- An apparent association could be due to population stratification and it is important to match populations carefully in this type of study.

Association strategies are useful in the study of quantitative traits and in large populations may detect genes of small effect that are not detectable by linkage.

PHYSICAL MAPPING

A combination of methods is used to pin down the exact locus of a mutated gene within the stretch of DNA identified by genetic mapping. Total genomic DNA can be fragmented and cloned into a variety of vectors, each harbouring one specific piece. A collection of such pieces is termed a library, and this, in theory, will include DNA fragments that derive from the region of interest. However, in making a library the order of the DNA fragments is completely lost. The goal of physical mapping is to assemble the correct DNA fragments from such a library into a continuous overlapping stretch (contigous DNA or contig map) which will contain the gene of interest. Yeast artificial chromosome (YAC) libraries with large insert sizes are ideally suited to such contig building. Linked marker probes from the genetic map can be hybridised to individual YACs in the library and the human DNA from these characterised. To define each piece of DNA uniquely, a variety of landmarks is used; for example, restriction enzymes, especially those that cut very rarely, can help provide a fingerprint of the YAC clone. A recent advance has been the generation of sequence tagged sites (STSs). These are stretches of unique DNA, up to 1 kbp long, for which oligonucleotide primers have been designed, and thus capable of PCR amplification. STSs are being independently assigned to specific chromosomal locations by a variety of methods, such as radiation hybrid mapping (Hudson et al 1995), and a dense map of over 30 000 STSs spaced at 100 kbp intervals is anticipated (Weatherall & Wilkie 1996). STSs can be used to characterise YACs and to identify them in libraries.

These approaches are illustrated by the analysis of a chromosomal abnormality associated with schizophrenia and other major mental disorder. A large family was described in which a balanced reciprocal translocation involving chromosomes 1 and 11 was significantly linked to the development of schizophrenia, schizoaffective disorder and major depressive disorder (St Clair et al 1990) and it was strongly suspected that the abnormality had affected a gene at one or other of the breakpoints, either by direct disruption, a microdeletion, or through a long range effect on gene regulation or chromatin structure (position effect mutations, see Bedell et al 1996). The linkage result was strong enough to justify positional cloning of the region. The boundaries of the translocation were established by fluorescent in situ hybridisation (FISH) with probes on to metaphase preparations, and a series of somatic hamster–human hybrid cell lines created, containing various portions of human chromosome 11 to act as mapping tools and marker sources (Fletcher et al 1993). The breakpoint defining the chromosome 1/11 boundary on the derivative chromosome 1 was found to be visible under phase contrast microscopy, and microdissection of unstained preparations generated large insert size libraries, all of which could be amplified directly by PCR (Muir et al 1995). The pooled clones were also used as a paint library to confirm the cut zone, and used directly to identify YACs as part of the construction of the physical map of both chromosomes 1 and 11 (Petit et al 1995). A YAC contig spanning the chromosome 11 breakpoint has been constructed (Evans et al 1995) – and more recently the equivalent contig for chromosome 1. Those clones that span the breakpoint should contain the mutated gene if this is directly disrupted.

Detecting genes

The process of physical mapping can be slow and labour intensive. If the major aim is to detect genes in a region, other complementary approaches can be taken. Exons code for mRNA and the level of this in a tissue correlates with gene activity. The turnover of mRNA is very variable, and most mRNA degrades rapidly after death. However, with fresh tissue collection and careful preparation, mRNA can be converted into its complementary form (complementary DNA or cDNA) and this can be cloned into an appropriate vector resulting in a cDNA or expression library. Cross-hybridisation of tissue cDNA libraries with other DNA pools can identify genes of interest in a region. For instance, a series of coding sequences were found on cross-linking fetal brain cDNA library with microclones obtained from the t(1;11) schizophrenia-associated translocation breakpoint (Brookes et al 1995). Other methods of DNA–DNA cross-hybridisation include the identification of the cross-species conservation of sequences which are likely to be important genes (zoo blotting). The establishment of the end-sequences of huge numbers of random cDNA clones has led to over 300 000 partial gene sequences being registered in a public computer database (db EST – see Boguski et al 1993). These stretches of genes are termed expressed sequence tags or ESTs and can be amplified by PCR from clones of interest. The mapping of ESTs on to chromosomes is a major part of the human genome project (see below). The partial EST sequence can be used to identify the complete cDNA in a cDNA library, or to screen YAC clones. The identification of all the genes in a given stretch of DNA would mean that after linkage is found the set of genes in the region could be directly examined for mutations, without having to walk through the intervening non-coding DNA. With the progress of the human genome project such a positional candidate gene approach is becoming a reality.

Detecting mutations

There are now a variety of methods of detecting gene mutations (Cotton 1997). Direct sequencing is the most obvious, but it is time intensive and expensive, especially if the gene is large and has many exons. Single-strand conformation polymorphism analysis (SSCP) relies on the different gel mobility of a mutated strand (even single base substitutions) from the wild type. Denaturing gradient gel electrophoresis (DGGE) relies on the differential melting of mutated duplexes versus the wild type by denaturant. If there is a gradient of denaturant concentration down the gel then the fragments will melt, and halt, at different levels on the gel. Other methods are based on mismatch between a mutated strand and a wild type strand in a duplex (heteroduplex), causing the formation of loops and cruciform arrangements which can be attacked by enzymes or chemicals (mismatch cleavage). A refinement of this using high performance liquid chromatography has been useful in detecting mutations in the breast cancer type 1 gene. The method chosen to scan DNA samples depends on the type of mutation and the error rate that can be supported. Ideally a 100% detection rate is desired, but is not currently available, even with direct sequencing.

THE HUMAN GENOME PROJECT AND THE HUMAN GENE MAP

The human genome project has the capacity to enormously facilitate and influence our understanding of the molecular basis of human disease, including psychiatric disorders. With the large scale mapping of DNA and genes it is likely that the time taken to identify disease mutations will shorten dramatically, in fact far faster than equivalent advances in the therapy of such conditions. This raises moral and ethical dilemmas around the control of and access to individuals' genetic information, and the use of genetic screening programmes in conditions that are not currently amenable to medical treatment. Because of the complexity of psychiatric disorders it is in this field that the most difficult problems will arise in the short term, but in the longer outlook it is with genetic advances that the hopes for a fuller understanding of the pathophysiology and treatment of these conditions lies.

REFERENCES

Baron M 1997 Genetic linkage and bipolar affective disorder: progress and pitfalls. Molecular Psychiatry. 2: 200–210

Bedell M A, Jenkins N A, Copeland N G 1996 Good genes in bad neighbourhoods. Nature Genetics 12: 299–232

Bickmore W, Craig J 1997 Molecular biology intelligence unit. Chromosome bands: patterns in the genome. Springer, Heidelberg

Boguski M S, Lowe T M J, Tolstoshev C M 1993 dbEST – database for 'expressed sequence tags'. Nature Genetics 4: 332–333

Bouchard T J, Lykken D T, McGue M, Segal N, Tellegen A 1990 Source of human psychological differences: the Minnesota study of twins reared apart. Science 250: 223–250

Brookes A J, Slorach E M, Evans K L et al 1995 Identifying genes within microdissected genomic DNA: isolation of brain expressed genes from a translocation region associated with inherited mental illness. Mammalian Genome 6: 257–262

Brown M A, Solomon E 1997 Studies on inherited cancers: outcomes and challenges of 25 years. Trends in Genetics 13: 202–206

Buard J, Jeffreys A J 1997 Big, bad minisatellites. Nature Genetics 15: 327–328

Cooper D N, Krawczak M, Antonarkis SE 1995 The nature and mechanisms of human gene mutation. In: Scriver C R, Beaudet A L, Sly W S, Valle D (eds) The metabolic and molecular bases of inherited disease. McGraw-Hill, New York, pp 259–291

Cordell H J, Todd J A 1995 Multifactorial inheritance in type 1 diabetes. Trends in Genetics 11: 499–504

Cotton T G H 1997 Slowly but surely towards better scanning for mutations. Trends in Genetics 13: 43–46

Dib C, Fauré S, Fizames C et al 1996 A comprehensive genetic map of the human genome based on 5264 microsatellites. Nature 380: 152–154

Emery A E H 1986 Methodology in medical genetics. An introduction to statistical methods, 2nd edn. Churchill Livingstone, Edinburgh

Estivill X 1996 Complexity in a monogenic disease. Nature Genetics 12: 348–350

Evans K L, Brown J, Shibasaki Y et al 1995 A three megabase contiguous clone map on the long arm of chromosome 11 across a balanced translocation associated with schizophrenia. Genomics 28: 420–428

Ferguson-Smith A C 1996 Imprinting moves to the centre. Nature Genetics 14: 119–121

Fletcher J M, Evans K, Baillie D et al 1993 Schizophrenia-associated chromosome 11q21 translocation: identification of flanking markers and development of chromosome 11q fragment hybrids as cloning and mapping resources. American Journal of Human Genetics 52: 478–490

Freund C, Horsford D J, McInnes R R 1996 Transcription factor genes and the developing eye: a genetic perspective. Human Molecular Genetics 5: 1471–1488

Gottesman I I, Bertelsen A 1989 Confirming unexpressed phenotypes in schizophrenia. Archives of General Psychiatry 46: 867–872

Gottesman I I, Shields J 1972 Schizophrenia and genetics: a twin study vantage point. Academic Press, New York

Gottesman I I, Shields J 1982 Schizophrenia, the epigenetic puzzle. Cambridge University Press, Cambridge

Grigorenko E L, Wood F B, Meyer M S et al 1997

Susceptibility loci for distinct components of developmental dyslexia on chromosomes 6 and 15. American Journal of Human Genetics 60: 27–39

Heston L L 1996 Psychiatric disorders in foster home reared children of schizophrenic mothers. British Journal of Psychiatry 112: 819–825

Hudson T J, Stein L D, Gerety S S et al 1995 An STS-based map of the human genome. Science 270: 1945–1954

Karayiorgou M, Gogos J A 1997 Dissecting the genetic complexity of schizophrenia. Molecular Psychiatry 2: 211–223

Kendler K S, McGuire M, Gruenberg A M, O'Hare A, Spellman M, Walsh D 1993 The Roscommon family study. 1 Methods, diagnosis of probands and risk of schizophrenia in relatives. Archives of General Psychiatry 50: 527–540

Kety S S 1983 Mental illness in the biological and adoptive relatives of schizophrenic adoptees: findings relevant to genetic and environment factors in etiology. American Journal of Psychiatry 140: 720–726

Kety S S, Rosenthal D, Wender P H, Schulsinger F, Jacobson B 1976 Mental illness in the biological and adoptive families of individuals who have become schizophrenic. Behaviour Genetics 6: 219–225

King M-C 1997 Leaving Kansas . . . finding genes in 1997. Nature Genetics 15: 8–10

Klockgether T, Dichgans J 1997 Trinucleotide repeats and hereditary ataxias. Nature Medicine 3: 149–150

Lander E, Kruglyak L 1995 Genetic dissection of complex traits: guidelines for interpreting and reporting linkage results. Nature Genetics 11: 241–247

Ledbetter D H, Ballabio A 1995 Molecular cytogenetics of contiguous gene syndromes: mechanisms and consequences of gene dosage imbalance. In: Scriver C R, Beaudet A L, Sly W S, Valle D (eds) The metabolic and molecular bases of inherited disease. McGraw-Hill, New York, pp 811–839

Lewin B 1997 Genes VI. Oxford University Press, Oxford

Lykken D, Tellegen A 1996 Happiness is a stochastic phenomenon. Psychological Science 7: 186–189

McInnis M G 1996 Anticipation: an old idea in new genes. American Journal of Human Genetics 59: 973–979

Malcolm S 1994 Mutations and human disease. In:

Humphries S E, Malcolm S (eds) Human gene mutation. From genotype to phenotype. βios, Oxford

Mendlewicz J, Papadimitriou G, Wilmotte J 1993 Family study of panic disorder: comparison with generalised anxiety disorder, major depression and normal subjects. Psychiatric Genetics 3: 73–78

Morton N E 1982 Outline of genetic epidemiology. Karger, Basel

Muir W J, Gosden C M, Brookes A J et al 1995 Direct microdissection and microcloning of a translocation breakpoint region t(1;11)(q42.2;q21) associated with schizophrenia. Cytogenetics and Cell Genetics 70: 35–40

Petit J, Bosseau P, Evans K et al 1995 Seeding of YACs over regions 1q41–42,3 and 11q14.3–q23 with microdissection clones. European Journal of Human Genetics 3: 351–356

Plomin R, Owen M J, McGuffin P 1994 The genetic basis of complex human behaviours. Science 264: 1733–1739

St Clair D, Blackwood D, Muir W et al 1990 Association within a family of a balanced autosomal translocation with major mental illness. Lancet 336: 13–16

Terwilliger J D, Ott J 1994 Handbook of human genetic linkage. Johns Hopkins University Press, Baltimore

Tomlinson I P M, Bodmer W F 1995 The HLA system and the analysis of multifactorial genetic disease. Trends in Genetics 11: 493–498

Tsuang M T, Faraone S V 1990 The genetics of mood disorders. Johns Hopkins University Press, Baltimore

Van Camp G, Willems P J, Smith R J H 1997 Nonsyndromic hearing impairment: unparalleled heterogeneity. American Journal of Human Genetics 60: 758–764

Verma R S, Babu A 1995 Human chromosomes. Principles and techniques, 2nd edn. McGraw-Hill, New York

Weatherall D J 1996 The genetics of common diseases: the implications of population variability. Ciba Foundation Symposium 127: 300–311

Weatherall D J, Wilkie A O M 1996 Genetics of disease. Current Opinion in Genetics and Development 6: 271–274

Yeung A S, Lyons M J, Waternaux C M et al 1993 A family study of self-reported personality traits and DSM3R personality disorders. Psychiatry Research 48: 243–255

8
Psychiatric interviewing

Linda Gask

INTRODUCTION: WHY IS THE INTERVIEW SO IMPORTANT?

...the occasion when, in the intimacy of the consulting room or sick room, a patient who is ill, or who believes himself to be ill, seeks the advice of a doctor whom he trusts. This is a consultation and all else in the practice of medicine derives from it (Spence 1949).

the psychiatric expert is presumed, from the cultural definition of an expert, and from the general rumours and beliefs about psychiatry, to be quite able to handle a psychiatric interview (Harry Stack Sullivan 1954).

The consultation or medical interview remains the indispensable unit of medical practice. Its success depends on how well doctors and patients communicate with each other (Simpson et al 1991). We know that this is frequently less effective than it could be. There is now a large body of research linking quality of communication to accuracy of diagnosis, memory for and understanding of the information and advice given, adherence to treatment and patient satisfaction. It has also been demonstrated that clinical outcome and competence in the skills of good communication are linked (Davis & Fallowfield 1991). Dissatisfaction with the quality of medical communication is often a factor in the decision to begin litigation (Richards 1990) and may be a reason why so many patients now seek alternative remedies. Changes in both society and the National Health Service in the last decade have resulted in real changes in what people expect from their doctors and how doctors view patients in the new 'consumer' or 'charter' culture. This is alien to many doctors who feel that their training has ill-prepared them for dealing with the 'new' patient. Good communication skills are essential if misunderstanding and dissatisfaction are to be avoided for both parties.

Psychiatry is no more or less successful than other medical specialities in this respect, yet, in our work,

perhaps more than any other, so much depends on what happens during our interview with the patient. It has been noted that 'one often observes a greater comfort and intellectual curiosity in the discussion of the psychopathology of the patient rather than exploration of the interview process' (McCready & Waring 1986). The psychiatrist who interrogates the patient about psychiatric symptoms or psychosocial problems without considering the interview process in greater depth is in fact little different from the surgeon or physician who interrogates the patient about physical symptoms. Both are adopting a style which will not endear them to the patient or ultimately assist in providing the best quality of care. So, whatever our ultimate therapeutic preference, we need to be able to communicate effectively. In order to be able to carry out the tasks expected of a clinical psychiatrist, we need to possess the clinical skill required to carry out a high-quality assessment. Furthermore, the medical interview does not end with diagnosis. Whatever the treatment, it has to be explained to the patient and his or her cooperation negotiated in the consultation. The skills involved in carrying out the basic therapeutic aspects of any clinical encounter (Novack 1987) are still seldom taught effectively.

This chapter will seek to demonstrate briefly how good interviewing skills provide a common basis for all medical specialities, including psychiatry, before exploring in more detail the specific skills needed to both assess and manage people suffering from mental health problems. We must approach all of this with the awareness that the illnesses which we, as psychiatrists, treat still carry an enormous amount of stigma for our patients within society and that many patients are vociferously dissatisfied (often with some justification) with what we offer (Rogers et al 1993). In the past, medical students received little or no training in interviewing patients, other than being given lists of questions to ask in order to clarify patients' initial complaints and to ensure that no other important symptoms had been missed. A barrage of routine questions can however seriously inhibit communication. In the course of the clinical years, students' interviewing skills may actually deteriorate rather than improve (Maguire & Rutter 1976). Recently, the General Medical Council (1993) has put considerable emphasis on the importance of this teaching, and, although until the last few years this played only a small part in the curricula of many medical schools, the picture is now changing rapidly. Communication skills training will ideally become a continuous process carried out alongside and within other teaching of all specialities, in hospital and in the community and not something simply carried out during psychiatry or general practice attachments. However, it will be some time before improvements permeate through into postgraduate medicine and the conditions in which people have to work may influence whether or not they feel able to put into practice what they have learned.

INTERVIEWING: SOME INFLUENTIAL MODELS

The importance of interviewing techniques in psychiatry has long been recognised. The biopsychosocial approach, described by Adolf Meyer, required the clinician to develop expertise in both structured approaches to the interview (to achieve a differential diagnosis) and a more 'free' or 'psychodynamic' style (in which psychological understanding of the patient might emerge) (Shea & Mezzich 1988). The latter approach was further developed by the various psychoanalytic schools, the interpersonal school of Harry Stack Sullivan (1954), the client-centred approach of Carl Rogers (1951) and the counselling model (Egan 1975). The advent of explicit diagnostic criteria has meanwhile led to a variety of structured interviews for use in research interviewing, such as the Present State Examination (PSE), first published by Wing et al in 1974, and now the Schedules for Assessment in Neuropsychiatry (SCAN) (WHO 1991).

A number of key models have been influential in the development of medical interview skills training over the last two decades. These are now having a major impact at the undergraduate level and on training in general medical and primary care settings, and they also have relevance to the basic tasks that a psychiatrist needs to master. The *Three Function Model* developed by Julian Bird and Steven Cohen-Cole (see summary in Epstein et al 1993) is probably the most comprehensive and makes the most immediate sense. The model highlights three core functions of the interaction between doctor and patient:

- gathering data to understand the patient

- development of rapport and responding to the patient's emotions
- patient education and behavioural management.

Another important and influential concept has been 'patient-centredness'. In *Meetings Between Experts*, David Tuckett and colleagues (1985) draw attention to the importance of understanding the patient's views of his problems. Increasingly, with the development of consumerism in medicine the views and needs of the patient or 'service user' have been brought to the fore. The *Patient-Centred Clinical Method* (Stewart et al 1995) focuses on how patients provide cues to their feelings, fears and expectations, which, if responded to appropriately, will lead to their expression. No person can be seen in isolation from his environment and the *Family Systems Approach* (McDaniel et al 1992) emphasises the importance of taking into account patients' family and social networks. Last but not least, the role of the doctor in this complex equation must not be ignored. Michael Balint (1964), a psychoanalyst who spent much of his career working with non-specialists to bring psychoanalytic insights into 'routine' medical practice through the development of *Balint Groups*, where doctors discuss the feelings generated by their patient, referred to the doctor as a 'drug' in his own right because he has the power to be therapeutic regardless of what he prescribes. Becoming aware of our own feelings and learning how to cope with them can help us to practise better and more effective medicine regardless of whether we choose to train more extensively in analytically oriented therapies.

In the next few sections, we will use insights gained from all of these traditions to delineate the skills that psychiatrists in training need to master.

PSYCHIATRIC INTERVIEWING: THE ASSESSMENT INTERVIEW

In psychiatry, the initial interview serves several quite different purposes (Rutter & Cox 1981):

- It is a means of asking questions to obtain factual information on historical events, happenings and activities.
- It serves as a stimulus to elicit emotions, feelings and attitudes.
- It begins to establish a relationship that will constitute the basis for further therapeutic contact.

In this section we will distinguish form from content. The form of the interview is determined by the range of skills employed by the clinician in response to what the patient has to say. The content of the interview is not only determined by the patient, but also by the specific topics addressed by the clinician. The quality of the information obtained under each topic heading will be greatly influenced by the skill of the interviewer. In other words, form has an impact on content. The skill of interviewing lies in getting the balance right between an 'open-ended' and 'checking out' style of interviewing which can encourage a patient to talk more, and may be essential in engaging a person who is finding it difficult to talk to express feelings (Hopkinson et al 1981), and a more probing and systematic style of interviewing, which seems to be important in getting good quality factual information (Cox et al 1981). A skilled interviewer is able to demonstrate flexibility and to switch between styles during the interview in order to carry out the three different tasks of the assessment interview, as listed above, as well as to respond to cues provided by the patient.

In any standard psychiatric assessment there are a number of key areas about which the clinician will seek to gain information. These 'content' topics are summarised in Table 8.1.

Beginning the interview

Before beginning to interview there are a number of important things to check that we usually group together as the tasks of 'greeting and seating' (Table 8.2). If a patient is clearly anxious about seeing a psychiatrist, address this early. You might ask something like 'How do you feel about talking to me?' or 'What do you think about coming up to the clinic today?' Addressing this will help you to find out more about the patient's beliefs and concerns about mental illness and its treatment (see below).

Getting the history of the presenting problem: the key tasks

At the beginning of the interview your first task will be to try and find out what the patient's presenting problems are. There may be more than one, and it may be necessary to draw up a *list of problems* and negotiate an order of priority for dealing with these. The problems may also be linked to each other. For each presenting problem establish as clearly as possible the items in Table 8.3.

Eliciting the patient's ideas about aetiology is important because it can help you understand what might be worrying the patient most. The stigma associated with psychiatric illness and fear of 'going mad' must not be underestimated and helping a patient to contain or deal

---

Table 8.1   Content of the psychiatric assessment (history)

History of the presenting problem(s) (see Table 8.3 for detail)

Past psychiatric history
  Nature, duration, treatment (what? where? adherence?)

Past medical history
  Nature, duration, treatment (what? where? adherence?)

Family history
  Information about immediate family members: age, sex, occupation, health, quality of relationships, cause of death, any family history of physical or psychiatric illness

Personal history
  Early development
  Childhood health, educational experience and social adjustment
  Education: achievements, relationships
  Work record: achievements, relationships, reasons for dismissal
  Psychosexual history: menstrual history, sexual development and attitudes, sexual relationships, age at marriage or establishment of partnership, age and occupation of spouse, quality of relationship
  Children: pregnancies including miscarriage and stillbirth. Age, sex, health of children, quality of relationships

Current social circumstances
  Living relationships, housing, economic circumstances, sources of support

Premorbid personality
  Temperament, ability to form relationships, attitudes, character, interests, source of social and spiritual support
  Drug and alcohol use.

---

with these anxieties is an important function of the interview. It is crucially important not to make assumptions about patient's health beliefs but to make a genuine attempt to find out what they are (Tuckett et al 1985).

A corollary to the need to discover patients' views is to encourage them to ask questions to which they want answers, but hesitate to ask. Many patients come away from an interview with doubts and questions. We can deliberately make it easy for our patients to ask such questions: answering them may remove anxieties and misconceptions of which we are unaware and also increase the educational function of the interview.

Table 8.2   Beginning the interview

- Arrange seating so that doctor and patient are conveniently close – not separated by a desk. Chairs placed at right angles allow the patient to make eye contact if he wishes.
- Introduce yourself and say what your role is
- Indicate the purpose of the interview
- Explain how much time it is likely to take
- If you are taking notes, stress confidentiality. If recording, say what will happen to the tape
- Check that patient is happy about all this
- Do not write immediately. Learn how to both make notes and ensure eye contact, particularly at the end of a question or statement

---

Table 8.3   History of the presenting problem(s)

- Nature of the problem
- Time of onset
- Development of the problems or symptoms over time
- Precipitating factors or possible links with life events
- Key events since the onset
- Alleviating or exacerbating factors
- What help has been given or offered?
- What is the *patient's view* of what is wrong, and what help has been offered so far? What help would the patient like?

Table 8.4   Information-gathering skills

Asking open-ended questions
Listening
Facilitation
Noticing and responding to verbal cues
    Clarification
    Asking for examples
Noticing and responding to non-verbal and vocal cues
Eliciting and dealing with emotion
    Reflection
    Use of empathic comments
    Understanding hypotheses
    Directly responding to emotion
Checking
Encouraging precision
Summarising
Controlling the flow of the interview
    Use of transition statements
    Summarising

Gathering information: key skills (Table 8.4)

Asking open-ended questions   These are questions which cannot be answered in one word. It is essential to begin the interview in an open-ended manner such as 'What are the problems that have brought you here?' A common error in interviewing is to ask too many questions which can only be answered by 'Yes' or 'No' too early in the interview, therefore not giving the patient space and opportunity to develop a description of how he is feeling. *Directive questions,* such as 'Tell me about how you have been sleeping', help to direct the patient to a particular topic without closing down the conversation. Closed questions have their place nearer the end of particular sections of the interview to fill in gaps in information. This pattern of open changing to closed questions is known as the *open to closed cone.* It may be self-evident to say that *listening* is a key skill. It is essential to allow the patient time to talk without interruption, both at the beginning of the interview and at crucial points where silence may be important. An effective interview, however, has periods of silence interspersed with times when the psychiatrist uses other skills in order to help the patient to focus on key topics or to dwell on specific experiences or feelings. These skills include the following.

Facilitation   This refers to encouraging the patient to continue talking by either verbal means, for example saying 'Go on', or by non-verbal means such as nodding. Facilitation is very important in interviews with patients who do not provide very much information without encouragement.

Noticing and responding to verbal cues   These are key words and phrases offered by the patient which indicate what he is worried about. One way of responding is to ask a question. Another, often more efficient, way is to *clarify* what the patient is saying by asking, for example: 'What do you mean when you say you have been having panic attacks?' Staying with the patient's own words is often much more efficient than embarking on a check list of questions about panic attacks immediately. Another alternative is to ask for a *specific example* of the problem: 'Take me through the last time you had one of these attacks ... tell me exactly what happened'. This too is often more efficient. You may also *delay* your comment until the patient has finished a particular story before saying something like 'A moment ago you said you had been depressed before you had this attack... can you tell me more about that?'

Noticing and responding to non-verbal and vocal cues   Non-verbal cues are, for example, changes in posture or eye contact when talking about particular problems; vocal cues are significant changes in tone of voice. Commenting on such cues can be very effective in helping to discover what is worrying the patient but such comments must be offered with sensitivity: 'You seemed quite tense when we talked about your father....'

Eliciting and dealing with emotion Reflection means 'stating or labelling the observed emotion'. Sometimes this is called *making an empathic comment.* Both of these mean letting the patient know that you have noticed, or are prepared to offer a suggestion about, what he seems to be experiencing. (Do not make the mistake of conveying the belief that you know exactly what someone is thinking. This can appear, at the very least, to be patronising.) Sometimes we make the mistake of assuming that patients know that we have taken on board what they are feeling but this may not be the case unless we are very explicit. Offering this as a suggestion based on your observation rather than a firm statement about what the patient is feeling, 'You seem quite upset when you are talking about this' rather than 'You are upset by this', allows the patient to either confirm or refute the suggestion and enter into a discussion about it, which will further aid clarification.

By empathy we mean:

- Learning to listen to your own inner feelings in response to what the patient is saying and to see things from the patient's point of view.
- Using expressions which demonstrate your understanding from the patient's point of view rather than talking authoritatively to the patient.
- Learning how to 'be with' rather than always 'doing to'.
- Communicating respect for the patient's opinions and decision-making abilities as well as bringing out his beliefs, attitudes, doubts and concerns.

Empathy differs from sympathy, which isn't always helpful because it really means how you would feel if you found yourself in that situation. Giving sympathy may result in the patient feeling patronised rather than understood. The combination of picking up a non-verbal cue, followed by an empathic comment, can be a very powerful way of giving a person 'permission' to talk about his feelings. For example 'You look quite sad...I can see that things must have been very tough for you recently.' You may use an *understanding hypothesis* to make an educated guess about what has been happening, given as a statement, to help in clarifying how events are linked. For example 'It seems as if the depression got worse after you broke up with your boyfriend.' As this is given in the form of a statement it again allows the patient to either agree with it or refute it. You may also *directly respond to emotion* by drawing attention to feelings you observe, for example, 'You look quite angry when you talk about that.'

Checking This allows you to review the information you have elicited and correct misunderstandings. Checking comments also indicate that you have been listening and so help to develop rapport, and they can also provide useful thinking space during which you can make a decision about where to go next.

Encouraging precision You may need to explain that you need to be as precise as possible about information. Be prepared to say something like 'I'm still not sure that I've got this quite right...can we try and sort this out before we go any further?'

Summarising Summarising statements can be used as the patient finishes talking about each problem to check out what the patient has reported and provide a link to the next part of the interview: 'Before we talk about the panic attacks can I just summarise what you've told me about the depression ... correct me as I go along', ending with 'Have I got that right?' Summarising can also be useful to help control the flow of the interview if a patient presents too much information at once (see below).

Controlling the flow of the interview There are three forms of control which you may need to consider.

Controlling the sequence of the interview It is disconcerting to be on the receiving end of a number of questions without understanding why there has just been a change of topic – for example, from depression to appetite. You might keep the patient informed, and therefore more willing to cooperate, by using a *transition statement* such as 'Now you've mentioned depression, there are a few other important things I just need to ask you about ... can I start off by asking about how your appetite is?'

The patient who finds it difficult to talk: increasing the flow There are a number of reasons why someone may find it difficult to talk. You can try employing facilitations (verbal and non-verbal), using silence, making supportive or empathic statements and putting your notes and pen to one side. If a person seems unwilling to talk because they look frightened, suspicious or upset, it may be necessary to comment directly on the feelings you observe: 'You seem very upset about this' or 'This is something that you find it difficult to talk about.' It may be necessary to restate issues dealt with under 'greeting and seating', particularly confidentiality.

The patient who talks a great deal: decreasing the flow You can try waiting for the patient to breathe in, and then ask a direct question. Alternatively try summarising – 'You've told me about the depression and the drinking and panic attacks and the difficulties at work; tell me more about how much you have been drinking', or prioritising – 'What shall we talk about first?', or bringing the patient back to the point – 'I wonder if we can just return to talking about how much you have been drinking. I think what you're saying about work is also important but we only have 20 minutes now and we can come back to that next.'

Using these skills in the mental state examination

During the mental state examination you will need to be able to observe systematically the patient's verbal and non-verbal behaviour, clarify the nature of the patient's experience and get the patient to describe exactly what he is preoccupied with or concerned about. This will mean employing precision when, for example, asking about the exact nature of hallucinations, and when assessing the degree of suicidal risk. Clarification in the patient's own words is also essential when trying to establish the quality and severity of mood disturbance and when examining the nature and intensity of depressive thoughts.

When a person begins to cry, it may be necessary to change the pace of the interview temporarily in order to ensure that it is able to continue effectively. Judicious use of empathic statements, verbal and non-verbal reassurance, can then be followed up with a gentle exploration of the thoughts and feelings that triggered off the tearfulness at that moment in the conversation. When a person is talking about frightening experiences, the flow of conversation may again be helped by the use of empathic statements such as 'That must have been very frightening . . . you must have wondered what on earth was going on.' When a person is very defensive is one of the occasions when leading questions are permissible. However, these must again be tempered with statements indicating your willingness to listen, to try and understand and an indication both verbally and non-verbally that you are not going to make premature judgements about the reality or otherwise of the patient's experience.

Finally, discussion of sensitive material, such as disclosure of suicidal ideas, homicidal thoughts or information about rape, assault or sexual abuse, require use of all the strategies above but most of all an indication of a willingness to listen, to make time and once again to avoid any suggestion of passing judgement.

Difficult assessment situations: the potentially violent patient

A person who is threatening to be violent, or has been so, is not necessarily mentally ill, but psychiatrists are often asked to make assessments in this situation. This is not the place to discuss what the content of such an assessment should be, but there are some general guidelines for interviewing (McGrath & Bowker 1987):

- Before seeing the patient, find out as much as you can from informants, other staff and notes, so that you are prepared.
- Always treat the patient rationally. State exactly who you are and indicate that you are there to try and understand what is going on and to try and help. Explain what is going on clearly at all times.
- Establish control early in the interview. It is always preferable to interview someone alone, sitting down, in a quiet setting but within easy calling distance of assistance. This of course is not always possible, but if it becomes apparent that the patient is not able to maintain control, you should strongly indicate that you are prepared to assist by summoning external controls if necessary.
- Avoid any form of challenging confrontation. Stay calm and indicate willingness to understand reasons for anger, fear or other strong emotions. This may involve gently commenting on feelings you observe and seeking clarification: 'You really are upset by all this.' Try not to indicate to the patient, either verbally or non-verbally, any feelings you may have about his personality, attitudes or behaviour.

When you have to talk to other staff it is better to do this well away from the patient to avoid risk of misinterpretation. Assessment can take time, and you should indicate your willingness to stay with the problem until it has been clarified and a course of action decided upon.

Difficult assessment situations: working with an interpreter

Communication with patients from another culture and/or who do not speak or understand your language is often difficult (Bal 1981, Putsch 1985). If they share no language with the doctor a fluent interpreter is essential for verbal communication, but the usual non-verbal expressions of interest and concern should be used. It is not ethical to use children as interpreters for their parents. Speak slowly, clearly and quietly, looking at the patient, not the interpreter. Explain your aims in both interview and discussion to the interpreter, who may have to amplify what you say. You should:

- Avoid using a family member as an interpreter (this is certainly not always possible, but preferable).
- Be patient.
- Address the patient directly.
- Use short questions and comments – avoid jargon and ambiguity.

- Use language and explanations your interpreter can handle.
- When lengthy explanations are necessary, break them up into sections.
- Provide instructions in the form of lists: have patients outline their understanding of the plans.
- Ask the interpreter to comment on the patient's word content and emotions.

It is important to remember that in a consultation there may be a number of ethnic gaps to bridge which do not stem entirely from communication difficulties. Death and bereavement are thought of and managed differently in certain ethnic groups and their wishes and fears should be carefully attended to (Black 1987).

SOME BASIC THERAPEUTIC SKILLS

A range of basic skills is required by any mental health clinician, whatever their orientation (Table 8.5). Some trainees will choose to develop higher level skills in one or other form of psychotherapy but is important not to focus on knowledge of the content of therapeutic interventions alone without addressing the skills that are needed to carry them out at even a basic level. Most interview skills training focuses only on the psychiatric assessment interview. Formal psychotherapy training can help to develop a trainee's pragmatic understanding

---

Table 8.5 Some basic therapeutic skills

- How to engage a person in a working treatment alliance of any nature
- How to provide information
- How to negotiate: this may involve getting a person to stop or start any form of treatment, stop having or start to have medical investigations, and either leave or be admitted to hospital
- How to help someone to talk freely about their thoughts, feelings, ideas, concerns and expectations
- How to manage someone who is in crisis
- How to help a person change, for example stop drinking or engage in some form of rehabilitation for any type of disorder
- How to deal with a range of potentially difficult situations where there is, for example, risk of violence, risk of self-harm, angry relatives, etc
- How to be able to talk to families and couples without necessarily learning how to do family therapy

---

of what happens in the human psyche and its relationships, but may fail to address the routine of the psychiatric outpatient clinic, where the reality may be less contact time than the patient is already having with their own general practitioner. To a new trainee, how one learns from this experience may seem a mystery: 'No-one except you and the patient really know what happens when you take him for an interview. You learn from your own mistakes behind the closed door' (Adams & Cook 1984). In the next few sections, a structure for developing these skills will be described.

ENGAGING A PERSON IN A TREATMENT ALLIANCE

If the assessment interview has been effective and has met all the criteria listed above, you should be fairly clear at the end whether or not you are going to successfully engage a patient in treatment. Some patients however are more difficult to engage. These include not only patients who clearly have no insight into their illness but also patients who:

- Because of the level of hopelessness they are experiencing are doubtful about whether or not their problems can be helped.
- Because of the degree of guilt they are experiencing do not feel that they deserve to be helped.
- Doubt that there is any emotional cause for their symptoms so doubt the validity of psychiatric treatment for their problems. This includes people presenting with somatic complaints who may be very difficult even to engage in assessment.
- Doubt the validity of psychiatric treatment in general, or the treatment they presume will be offered to them. This includes people who see their symptoms as not due to illness but due to life problems which psychiatry cannot solve.
- Have only attended because of pressure from family, general practitioner or the law.

It is crucially important to establish:

- The patient's perceptions of the problem. If you haven't obtained this information earlier in the interview, obtain it now. People almost always have some idea as to the cause of their symptoms, which can usually be elicited with a simple open-ended question such as 'What have you thought was wrong?' If you are able to address particular fears and anxieties immediately it can enable your interview to be not just more efficient but also more effective.
- The patient's views about its aetiology and the reasons for this.

- The patient's expectations of you. What does he expect from seeing you?

If you are fully aware of all the potential difficulties and misunderstandings it will make it easier to arrive at an agreement with the patient about treatment. It will also be possible for you to be clear and honest about what is and is not possible without inadvertently causing distress.

Difficult engagement situations: patients who present with somatic complaints

Patients presenting with somatic symptoms of emotional distress are frequently encountered in liaison settings such as general medical and surgical wards. Creed & Guthrie (1993) have reviewed this topic in detail and emphasise the importance of :

- Collaboration with the referrer. Find out what the patient has been told about the reason for seeing you. If possible talk to the referrer first to discuss what he is going to say.
- Review of the case notes. Find out about the patient's history in detail.
- Interviewing a relative. Who will be able to tell you about the patient's illness behaviour and the family's response to it.
- Employing a subtle and empathic approach to the interview. Patients who present with somatic complaints have difficulty talking about feelings and may be worried about being labelled as 'mad'. You need to be particularly sensitive to verbal and non-verbal cues. If you offer empathic or supportive comments this will help the patient to feel that you are taking his problems seriously, as will taking a full history of the complaints, both physical and psychosocial.

Various styles can then be adopted for the therapeutic content of the interview depending on therapeutic orientation, including the *reattribution approach*, which attempts to get the patient to accept a psychological view of their symptoms (Goldberg et al 1989), the *psychotherapeutic approach* which focuses on developing a close personal relationship with the patient (Guthrie 1991), and the behavioural or *directive approach* (Benjamin 1989).

PROVIDING INFORMATION

The main topics about which a psychiatrist may have to provide information include: diagnosis, aetiology, investigations, treatment, prognosis, how to prevent any recurrence and what social or psychological consequences of the illness there may be and how to cope with them.

The following framework contains the essential skills for discussing diagnosis:

- Establish the patient's (or carer's) perceptions of the problem, as described above. Establish also what they have been told already.
- Provide a basic diagnosis. It is terribly important that this information is given briefly and succinctly. Anxiety inhibits a person's ability to take in and retain detailed information.
- Respond to emotions. People will often respond emotionally to information. The stigma associated with psychiatric illness must not be underestimated. It is important to respond by making it clear that it is acceptable to talk about feelings and by acknowledging the emotions that are being expressed.
- Provide details of the diagnosis. Go on to provide more detailed information using language that the patient or carer will understand and short sentences that make the point very clearly. Indicate, if you can, whether this is a common problem.
- Check understanding and elicit questions. It is most important to stop frequently to check understanding and ask for questions. Equally, you should also check out that you have fully understood all concerns. Respond as truthfully as you can to questions about meaning, aetiology, likely treatment and prognosis. At the end you should ask 'Do you have any questions about what we have just discussed?' It may be useful to supplement what you have said with written or even audiotaped or video information and to offer to speak to others where appropriate, bearing in mind issues of confidentiality and permission.

NEGOTIATION AND MAINTENANCE OF A TREATMENT PLAN

The next step is to negotiate a clear plan. The skills of negotiation cannot be overestimated in importance and are useful at all stages of developing and maintaining the relationship with the patient. Various tasks must be carried out:

- Check baseline information. Find out what the patient already knows or believes about treatment.
- Describe treatment goals and plans with options (if any). For many disorders there are a range of treatment goals and possible interventions that can

be selected. Indicate if there is only one possible treatment strategy or whether such a range of possibilities exists. Again this information should be provided clearly and succinctly in words that the patient can understand.

- Check understanding. Make sure that the patient understands the range of possibilities by checking out as before.
- Elicit patient preferences and commitments. Ask the patient what he wants to do? Which option does he wish to choose?
- Develop plan. A treatment plan, once agreed, should preferably be written down. It is then important to spend time anticipating potential problems and discussing possible solutions before these arise. Written information may again be useful here.
- Maintenance and prevention of relapse. The plan needs to be followed up and reviewed regularly. What is the patient actually managing to do? What problems have been experienced? How can these be successfully overcome?

Negotiation

Buried in the stages described above is the word 'agreement'. Implicit in this is the understanding that, rather than the health professional deciding what is best and simply telling the patient, they will 'strike a deal'. This suggests there will be some concept of partnership or a shared role in decision making which develops out of sharing of ideas and values and a clear demonstration of respect for these ideas and values, even if the only agreement possible between doctor and patient on some issues is an agreement to differ. Try and get over to the patient that he has an equal role to play and will not have 'control' taken away from him. Of course there are situations within psychiatry when this inevitably becomes necessary, but in most cases, where treatment has been effectively negotiated this will ensure a clear commitment to treatment.

Not only will you need to negotiate treatment, but also expectations and priorities within treatment. Both patient and professional have their own agendas and these may diverge considerably so it is crucially important to explore with the patient what his hopes, concerns and expectations of treatment are.

Relationships between patients and professionals may reflect differing balances of power, control and responsibility. As commented earlier, there has been increasing recognition of the patient's right to decide what he wants from the relationship, but the *skill lies in determining the right balance within a particular relationship*. It is equally important to respect the wishes of the patient

who does not want to be involved and just wants you to decide and advise.

Mutual commitment to treatment

This is a better, if slightly clumsier term than 'compliance' because it reflects the partnership between patient and professional rather than compliance with the professional agenda (Trostle 1988). Nevertheless, few health care professionals check whether this mutual commitment exists, preferring, perhaps through lack of skill, embarrassment or simply arrogance, to assume that it does. Almost anyone, and perhaps especially doctors, can be a defaulter at some time or another. All of us may also, in some way, bear responsibility for failure to achieve commitment. It may not be that the patient has forgotten to take the medication, but that the doctor gave him inadequate or conflicting information.

Providing information about drug treatment

Good prescribing takes time. Patients want to know more than ever before about the drugs that they take. Longer interviews, taking time for explanation and reassurance could reduce the 'quick fix' of a prescription to end the meeting (Gilley 1994). Clear information should be offered and ideally, each patient should be told for each drug the information in Table 8.6. Remember that women may be pregnant or intending to become pregnant. If so, some drugs must be avoided. This is a lot of information to be given in a consultation or for patients to remember without writing it

---

Table 8.6   Information to be provided for each drug prescribed

Its name
What it is intended to do
Dose and frequency
How long to go on taking it. Importance of completing the course even if symptoms disappear
Any special precautions (e.g. before driving or using machinery)
Any interactions with other drugs, foods or alcohol
Possible side-effects and what to do if they occur
What to do if a dose is missed or an extra one taken
How to tell if the medicine is working and what to do if it is not

---

down. Pharmacists can play an important role here. Where possible, information should be supplemented with written notes which you may need to discuss further with the patient. This will be particularly important with patients who are illiterate, blind or cannot read English. They will have to be given the information verbally by you or by a friend who can tell them what the leaflets say.

Treatment must be explained clearly, without jargon, so that as far as possible informed consent can be given. Do not suppose that a signature implies comprehension (Byrne et al 1988). Always make sure that patients understand what is to be done. To be sure that there has been no misunderstanding you can ask patients to repeat back to you what you have told them about the treatment.

Providing information about investigations

If you are intending to arrange any investigations ensure that you explain their purpose, what will actually be done to the patient (including any discomfort it may cause), how soon the result will be known and how the patient will be told about this. Then ask how the patient feels about the tests. Any fears should be explored and truthful reassurance given. Ask if there are any further questions and answer them honestly without minimising common difficulties or using jargon. When you are short of time, it is best not to give a cursory opinion but to specify a later time when you can give full attention to the patient's problems and answer any question he wants to ask.

TALKING ABOUT FEELINGS, THOUGHTS, WORRIES AND EXPECTATIONS

Many of the skills which are necessary in order to help someone talk about difficult or painful feelings have already been described above. These include listening, asking open-ended questions, gentle clarification, commenting on non-verbal cues and expression of empathy. It may also be helpful to indicate that a protected amount of time is available for this. We all offer time to patients to allow expression of feeling but this form of interaction, which is commonly employed in many settings, is often undervalued (Holmes 1995) and the need for psychiatrists to be trained in 'talking skills' appropriate to their everyday role in multidisciplinary teams has been highlighted (Grant et al 1993).

Supportive psychotherapy is not simply about allowing someone to talk but also about offering interventions which assist in strengthening rather than breaking

down defences, to facilitate normal coping mechanisms. In our everyday conversations with patients in the clinic (and each other) these are:

- *Legitimation*: indicating not only that it is OK to talk about these feelings but that it is quite acceptable for the person to feel the way that he does.
- *Support*: indicating and emphasising the doctor's (or other person's) role in helping: 'I want to offer what help that I can.'
- *Respectful* statements which positively reinforce the person's ability to cope: 'I'm impressed by what you've managed to do despite all this.'
- *Offering hope* that a problem can be resolved: 'I think there are ways that we can work together to help you feel better.'
- *Provision of encouragement*: 'You have managed it before, you can do it again.'
- *Reassurance* (you cannot reassure if you do not first know what the person is actually worried about).
- *Facilitation*, for example of expression of feelings or even of self-forgiveness.

The topic of supportive psychotherapy is addressed in greater depth in Chapter 30.

HELPING A PERSON WHO IS IN CRISIS

A common situation faced by all psychiatrists, particularly when on call, in the casualty department or on an emergency domiciliary visit, is having to help someone who is in acute crisis. Assessment of suicidal risk is dealt with elsewhere (Chapter 26) but is clearly central here. Managing the patient in crisis employs a number of the skills described above and can be encompassed in the following broad strategies (Morriss et al 1997).

Allowing emotion to be released Show that it is all right if the patient wants to cry or shout. Crying can be a release which may give the distressed person some relief from suffering. However, do not tolerate aggression towards yourself, other people or furniture. Firmly discourage this and encourage the patient to tell you what is wrong. If necessary get the distressed, aroused person to take some deep breaths before proceeding further. Aggression can be a way of testing you out. Sometimes patients will tell you afterwards that they did not feel in control of themselves and remained so until they found someone who could be both assertive and supportive.

Taking control of the interview Do not let the patient leave the interview without ensuring that he is safe and calm and there is a practical plan for what he is going to do over the next few hours. Patients can get too distressed and overwhelmed by their problems and decide to leave while still distressed and suicidal. You can take control of the situation by distracting the patient. Ask more about other aspects of the patient's life that are positive or not so upsetting, or talk about unrelated issues. Such periods can often help to calm the patient down so that the interview may proceed or you can cope until more support arrives. Again you may need to calm the patient down by showing him how to take deep breaths if he starts to hyperventilate.

Addressing immediate problems   You should be aware of these from your initial assessment and you may need to try and address the most pressing problems as best you can. Try and clarify (either from the patient or others):

- What exactly has happened?
- What would be acceptable to the patient?
- What is the discrepancy between these two?
- Does the patient's view of the problem sound accurate and plausible?
- Is the patient's position realistic and achievable?
- Would the patient accept some form of compromise?
- Does the patient need more information to check out the practicalities of his viewpoint or goal?
- What practical problems prevent his goal or a suitable compromise from being achieved?
- Who else needs to be involved?

Look at past solutions the patient has employed in solving similar problems. Could these be used again (possibly with some modification)? You do not need to solve the patient's problems. In most cases all you need to do is persuade the patient that there is something realistic that he could do to help his situation – that is, it is not entirely hopeless.

Providing immediate support   Try and establish who can be available to support the patient through the next few hours or days. (It is when there is absolutely no solution here and suicide risk is judged as high that the question of admission will be addressed, but it is clearly not the only possible solution.)

Bolstering self-esteem   It can be important to compliment the person in crisis for being able to share painful feelings with you. This can help to bolster self-esteem and confidence.

Increasing hopefulness   When a person is expressing ideas of suicide it can be helpful to discuss the final and irrevocable nature of the act and also to challenge 'black and white thinking', where the situation is either seen as entirely hopeless or entirely satisfactory. Is there anything he can still look forward to? Explore how he sees the effects of suicide on those around them and how these ideas may conflict with his own beliefs and ideals.

Ensuring safety   Attempt to ensure safety over the next few days. This may or may not involve admission to hospital.

Use of families/friends/other professionals Assess what is necessary and possible in the given circumstances. Inform family or friends of the risks and what should be done if the situation gets out of hand. If necessary, offer access to other professionals or yourself, by telephone if possible.

The particular strategies and skills useful in dealing with a range of different types of crisis, from the suicidal patient to the bereaved and victims of crime, are described in detail in France (1996).

HELPING A PERSON TO CHANGE: EXPLORING AND INCREASING MOTIVATION

What do you do if the patient doesn't seem to be keeping to the agreement that you have made? What you must not do is assume that you know why without first attempting systematically to find out what is happening. There are a number of steps involved in assessing and trying to influence motivation.

Check adherence carefully   Help the patient to admit to any difficulties he may have been having without causing him to feel embarrassed about this: 'Most people have some problems taking tablets regularly . . . what problems have you had?'

Diagnose adherence problems   Clarify the reasons. Common problems are forgetfulness or side-effects but many people are very unhappy about taking psychotropic medication. With lifestyle changes, the most common problem is lack of motivation and this may need to be addressed specifically (see below). Alternatively the patient may have simply misunderstood the plan. Once the problems are clarified an approach to overcoming them can be negotiated.

Elicit statement of commitment   Before asking the patient to make a commitment to try again, it can be helpful to make a positive statement explicitly about the characteristics of the patient which make it more likely that you can achieve something: 'I know that it isn't easy to stick to this, but I also know that you are very worried about getting back to work...what do you want to aim for now?' An exploration of the pros and cons of tackling the problem from the patient's perspective (see below) may be very helpful here in providing useful 'hooks' on which to phrase your negotiation.

Negotiate solutions   Again, it is really important to start with the patient's ideas about what will work.

Clarify intentions and arrange follow-up   Once again, check out exactly what the patient intends to do and specify a time and place for a follow-up session.

There is too much literature on compliance and non-adherence to review here and much is not of practical help. However, there are various ways of helping patients stick more effectively to a treatment regimen that they have agreed to. We do know that if patients build up a relationship with a doctor over time, and see the same doctor, they find adherence easier (Ettlinger & Freeman 1981).

It also makes sense to try and look at the problem from the point of view of the patient in order to try and understand why it is so difficult for them to go on with the treatment. This may particularly be an issue in adolescence when a range of difficult feelings may be generated by the onset of an illness which threatens hopes and aspirations for the future. Powerful emotions such as anger and guilt may lead to defiance, rebellion, poor self-esteem and family disturbance. In contrast, older patients may be particularly at risk because of the sheer complexity of their problems and treatment regimens and lack of time spent by professionals in ensuring mutual understanding.

Motivational interviewing

Recent work in the field of helping people to cut down on drinking (Miller & Rollnick 1991) has highlighted the importance of good interviewing skills in actually helping to motivate people to change their behaviour. In other words, it is not enough to simply say that a patient is 'unmotivated'; recognise instead that health professionals can actually help people to change if they possess the right talking skills. This doesn't mean that the responsibility for that change no longer belongs to the patient, but that the professional recognises that he bears some responsibility for ensuring that the patient gets the best possible help in arriving at the decision. The skills and strategies involved in helping people to change are as follows.

Clarifying the patient's view of the problem Build rapport with the aid of the skills we have discussed earlier, in particular the use of good eye contact, listening, picking up verbal and non-verbal cues and making empathic comments. It is important to remain *neutral* with respect to the problem behaviour. Help the patient to draw up a problem list in order of priority, and if the topic of problem behaviour is not already on the agenda raise it sensitively and obtain clear information in a non-judgemental fashion. Discuss whether the patient considers the 'behaviour' to be a problem. If not, who does? At this point you may have to negotiate whether or not you are going to discuss things any further.

Exploring the necessity for change Help the patient to draw up a balance sheet of the *pros and cons* of the behaviour. To try and promote change you can empathise with the difficulty of changing ('It's hard giving up something that you enjoy'), reinforce (by repeating) statements which express a desire to change ('So you think you have to do something about it …') and resist saying why you think they ought to change.

It is helpful to *summarise* frequently and also to *highlight for discussion statements which are contradictory*. 'For examples: On the one hand you are telling me that alcohol is not a problem and you don't care what anyone says, but on the other, you've just said that your marriage means a lot to you and it will break you if your wife leaves you because of your drinking.'

Promoting resolution Indicate that your role is to provide information in order to enable the patient to make an informed decision. You can provide basic information about safety/risks of behaviour, results of any examination or tests, information about the potential medical, legal or social consequences and the likely outcome of potential choices. Then pause and ask for feedback. Give the patient responsibility for his own decision. If change is sought, negotiate plans in a *patient-centred* manner. If change is not sought, or the patient remains undecided negotiate if/when/how to review.

'DIFFICULT' SCENARIOS

We have already looked at some potentially difficult situations above, such as dealing with a person who is potentially violent or someone who is in crisis. Now let us consider another.

Talking to a person who is angry

When a patient or a relative becomes angry it is very important to try and avoid being defensive. This isn't always easy – especially if you have had no sleep or you feel that the anger is unjustified. You must:

- Stay calm.
- Acknowledge the anger but try and avoid this coming over as either patronising or just simply clichéd.
- Explore the depth of the feelings: 'How upset have you been about it?'
- Find out what the reasons are: 'What has happened?'
- If you can see that the reasons are quite reasonable or understandable in the circumstances, say so: 'I can quite understand why it has upset you so much.'
- Demonstrate you are prepared to take worries and concerns seriously: 'I'll look into what you have said… can we meet again?'

Usually this is enough to at least defuse the anger, but there may be occasions when you need to explore other possible causes of anger and consider whether some anger has been displaced on to you from another problem or worry. This is not uncommon after a person has died.

There are a range of potentially difficult situations that you will need to cope with and many of these are appropriately dealt with in other chapters. You will have to be able to talk to patients' relatives and discuss difficult issues with them without breaking confidentiality. You may have to give someone bad news, for example about the death of a relative. There will be a number of occasions when you have to talk about sensitive issues concerning taboo subjects such as sex, death and money. Most trainees get no opportunity to practice these skills. Audiotaping routine interviews can be helpful but often the most difficult situations occur outside the routine clinic appointments. The best way is to employ specific role play in order to set up and learn from a difficult scenario (see below).

TALKING WITH FAMILIES AND COUPLES

Partners and families often come with a patient to an appointment. You can employ a *family systems approach* without having to be skilled in family therapy. Perlmutter and Jones (1985) have described in detail how this can be usefully applied to assessment of the psychiatric emergency. However, some basic rules can be easily remembered (Table 8.7).

Table 8.7 Involving families
When you are interviewing an individual Ask how the family are involved in the problem Decide if / how to involve the family in the treatment process
When a family member comes in with the patient Develop a conversation with the family member first if you already know the patient Clarify the reasons for the family member coming Ask for the family member's observations and opinions of the problem Solicit their help in treatment if appropriate Do not take sides!
Adapted from Epstein (1993).

DEVELOPING SKILLS: THE RESEARCH

There are a range of ways that you can develop the skills described in this chapter. A considerable amount of research has been carried out in the last 20 years into the effectiveness of some of these approaches. Video or audiotape feedback is most effective in enabling psychiatrists (Harrison & Goldberg 1993), as well as other groups such as medical students (Maguire et al 1978) and general practitioners (Gask et al 1988, Whewell et al 1988), to develop their interviewing skills. It has also been effectively employed to teach psychotherapy skills to psychiatric trainees (Maguire et al 1984). The video feedback method involves watching video recordings of your own interviews so that you can see yourself as your patients see you. The tape can be stopped by any member of the group (including the facilitator) but group members should be encouraged not to simply criticise performance but offer instead what they would have said themselves at that particular point in the interview. In this way a repertoire of 'talking skills' is gradually acquired through rehearsal. It is particularly effective in helping you to appreciate the importance of noticing and using non-verbal communication. However, video feedback training does require skilled and sensitive facilitation (Gask et al 1992). Consultations videotaped for teaching purposes can be conducted with real or role-played patients. In the absence of suitable video recording facilities, audiotape recordings can be successfully used instead. These can be particularly useful for recording interviews in the outpatient clinic for supervision purposes. Either type of recording, if conducted with real patients, requires informed consent, and written consent should always be obtained for videotaped recordings. In the absence of video training, role-play can be a useful technique for improving skills, particularly some of the specific therapeutic skills, described above where the opportunities for learning these skills by watching interviews with real patients may be limited.

CONCLUSION

Psychiatric interviewing is not simply about learning how to take a psychiatric history and carry out a mental state examination. It is a set of skills which are required in a variety of face-to-face encounters with patients where the task at hand can range from initial assessment to complex intervention. Although there is no doubt that some people are born communicators, there is clear evidence that skills can be learned. Theoretical understanding does not necessarily lead to skill acquisition and it is easier to acquire such skills if they are clearly defined and delineated as demonstrated in this chapter. Training should build on the skills developed at an undergraduate level, and the new approaches to teaching communication skills which are now being developed in medical schools across the world should better prepare trainees for further developing therapeutic skills in postgraduate training.

The quality of information that you obtain, the satisfaction of patient and family with your care and ultimately the clinical outcome of the patient are all related to the expertise with which you communicate.

REFERENCES

Adams G, Cook M 1984 Beginning psychiatry. Bulletin of the Royal College of Psychiatrists 8: 53–54

Bal P 1981 Communication with non-English-speaking patients. British Medical Journal 283: 368–369

Balint M 1964 The doctor, his patient and the illness. Pitman, London

Benjamin S 1989 Psychological treatment of chronic pain: a selective review. Journal of Psychosomatic Research 33: 121–131

Black J 1987 How to do it: broaden your mind about death and bereavement in certain ethnic groups in Britain. British Medical Journal 295: 536–538

Byrne D J, Napier A, Cuschieri A 1988 How informed is informed consent? British Medical Journal 296: 839–840

Cox A, Hopkinson K, Rutter M 1981 Psychiatric interviewing techniques: III. Naturalistic study: eliciting factual information. British Journal of Psychiatry 138: 283–291

Creed F, Guthrie E 1993 Techniques for interviewing the somatising patient. British Journal of Psychiatry 162: 467–471

Davis H, Fallowfield L 1991 Counselling and communication in health care. Wiley, Chichester

Egan G 1975 The skilled helper: a model for systematic helping and interpersonal relating. Brooks/Cole, Monterey

Epstein R M, Campbell T L, Cohen-Cole S, McWhinney I R, Smilkstein G 1993 Perspectives on patient–doctor communication. Journal of Family Practice 37: 377–388

Ettlinger P R A, Freeman G K 1981 General practice compliance study: is it worth being a personal doctor? British Medical Journal 282: 1192–1193

France K 1996 Crisis intervention: A handbook of immediate person-to-person help, 3rd edn. Thomas, Springfield.

Gask L, Goldberg D, Lesser A, Millar T 1988 Improving the psychiatric skills of the general practice trainee; an evaluation of a group training course Medical Education 22: 132–138

Gask L, Usherwood T, Standart S 1992 Training teachers to teach communication skills: a problem-based approach. Postgraduate Education for General Practice 3: 92–99

General Medical Council 1993 Tomorrow's doctors: recommendations on undergraduate medical education. GMC, London

Gilley J 1994 Towards rational prescribing: better prescribing takes time. British Medical Journal 308: 731–732

Goldberg D, Gask L, O'Dowd T 1989 The treatment of somatization: teaching the techniques of reattribution. Journal of Psychosomatic Research 33: 689–695

Grant S, Holmes J, Watson J 1993 Psychotherapy training as part of professional training. Psychiatric Bulletin 17: 695–698

Guthrie E 1991 Brief psychotherapy with patients with refractory irritable bowel syndrome. British Journal of Psychotherapy 8: 175–188

Harrison J, Goldberg D 1993 Improving the interview skills of psychiatry trainees. European Journal of Psychiatry 7: 31–40

Holmes J 1995 Supportive psychotherapy. The search for positive meanings. British Journal of Psychiatry 167: 439–445

Hopkinson K, Cox A, Rutter M 1981 Psychiatric interviewing techniques: III. Naturalistic study: eliciting feelings. British Journal of Psychiatry 138: 406–415

McCready J R, Waring E M 1986 Interviewing skills in relation to psychiatric residency. Canadian Journal of Psychiatry 31: 317–332

McDaniel A, Campbell T, Seaburn D 1992 Family oriented primary care: a manual for medical providers. Springer, New York

McGrath G Bowker M 1987 Common psychiatric emergencies. Wright, Bristol

Maguire P, Rutter D R 1976 History taking by medical students: 1. Deficiencies in performance. 2. Evaluation of a training programme. Lancet ii: 556–560

Maguire P, Roe P, Goldberg D, Jones S, Hyde C, O'Dowd T 1978 The value of feedback in teaching interviewing skills to medical students. Psychological Medicine 8: 697–704

Maguire P, Goldberg D, Hobson R, Margison F, Moss S, O'Dowd T 1984 Evaluating the teaching of a method of psychotherapy. British Journal of Psychiatry 144: 515–580

Miller W R, Rollnick S 1991 Motivational interviewing: preparing people to change addictive behaviour. Guildford Press, New York

Morriss R, Gask L, Battersby L 1997 Helping people who are suicidal or at risk of harming themselves. Final report to North West Regional Research and Development Office NHSE

Novack D H 1987 Therapeutic aspects of the clinical encounter. Journal of General Internal Medicine 2: 346–355

Perlmutter R A, Jones J E 1985 Assessment of families in psychiatric emergencies. American Journal of Orthopsychiatry 55: 130–139

Putsch III R W 1985 Cross-cultural communication: the special case of interpreters in health care. Journal of the American Medical Association 254: 3344–3348

Richards T 1990 Chasms in communication: still occur too often (editorial). British Medical Journal 201: 1407

Rogers A, Pilgrim D, Lacey R 1993 Experiencing psychiatry: users' views of services. Macmillan: London

Rogers C R 1951 Client-centred therapy. Houghton Mifflin, Boston

Rutter D, Cox A 1981 Psychiatric interviewing techniques: I. methods and measures. British Journal of Psychiatry 138: 273–282

Shea S C, Mezzich J E 1988 Contemporary psychiatric interviewing – new directions for training. Psychiatry 51: 385–397

Simpson M, Buckman R, Stewart M et al 1991 Doctor–patient communication: the Toronto consensus statement. British Medical Journal 303: 1385–1387

Spence J 1949 The need for understanding the individual as part of the training and function of doctors and nurses. National Association for Mental Health. Reprinted 1962 in: The purpose and practice of medicine. Oxford University Press, London

Stewart M, Belle Brown J, Weston W W, McWhinney I, McWilliam C L, Freeman T R 1995 Patient-centered medicine: transforming the clinical method. Sage, Thousand Oaks

Sullivan H S 1954 The psychiatric interview. Norton, New York

Trostle J A 1988 Medical compliance as an ideology. Social Science and Medicine 27: 1299–1308

Tuckett D, Boulton M, Olson C, Williams A 1985 Meetings between experts: an approach to sharing ideas in medical consultations. Tavistock, London

Whewell P J, Gore V A, Leach C 1988 Training general practitioners to improve their recognition of emotional disturbance in the consultation. Journal of the Royal College of General Practitioners 38: 259–262

Wing J K, Cooper J E, Sartorius N 1974 Measurement and classification of psychiatric symptoms. Cambridge University Press, Cambridge

WHO (1991) SCAN Schedules for Assessment in Neuropsychiatry. World Health Organization Division of Mental Health, Geneva

9
Mental state examination

Allan I. F. Scott

INTRODUCTION

The term 'mental state examination' has a range of uses in the clinical practice of psychiatry. At one extreme it refers to no more than a simple description by one observer of a salient feature of a person's mental condition at one point in time; at the other extreme the term refers to a detailed systematic assessment by several different observers in different situations and over a period of days, such as might occur during admission to a psychiatric hospital. In this chapter the mental state examination will refer to the systematic evaluation and recording of features of mental disorder to enable the diagnosis of a clinical syndrome. The acquisition of the skills required for its successful completion distinguishes the psychiatrist from other medical doctors, and is necessary for the most important role of the psychiatrist in a multidisciplinary team.

Theoretical approaches

The mental state examination follows history-taking in a diagnostic process, which often leads to comparisons with the physical examination in general medicine. A simple comparison is not appropriate because the mental state examination is concerned with disorders of the mind. The study of the features of mental disorder is known as psychopathology, and there are distinct theoretical approaches to its study. *Descriptive psychopathology* emphasises precise description and categorization that involves both observation and a process known as *empathy*, where the observer learns to use personal experience and questioning to think himself into another person's experience. The development of descriptive psychopathology was strongly influenced by *phenomenology*, the study of subjective experience; the word has several different meanings in psychiatry (Sims 1995), but its most influential proponent was the German psychiatrist and philosopher Karl Jaspers who summarised phenomenology as the attempt to make subjective experience understandable without preconceived theo-

ry. The seventh edition of his classic textbook, *Allgemeine Psychopathologie (General Psychopathology)*, is available in an English translation (Jaspers 1963). In contrast, *explanatory* or *interpretative psychopathology* approaches the study of mental disorder from an explicit preconceived theory – for example, models of the aetiology of mental disorder that stress psychodynamics, cognition or learning. Few of the models are amenable to traditional scientific methods of testing a hypothesis. In contrast, *scientific psychopathology* uses traditional methods of scientific study to investigate the aetiology of mental disorders – for example, the experimental conditions that can induce hallucinations in otherwise healthy people.

Form and content

Descriptive psychopathology emphasises the difference between the form and content of subjective experience; for example, a definition of a delusion can be made without any reference to the nature of the belief itself. Much greater emphasis is placed on form in diagnosis. The diagnostic pre-eminence of form may be lost on the sufferer who, for example, is upset that other people talk unkindly of him and makes no distinction between an overvalued idea and delusion.

Approach in present chapter

The difference between a 'sign' and a 'symptom' of disease is clear in general medicine, but the terms are sometimes used interchangeably in psychiatric writing. Professor Kurt Schneider argued that the use of these terms is not justified in many mental disorders where the disease process is unknown; he suggested that these terms ought to imply no more than common or characteristic features of clinical syndromes (Schneider 1959). This chapter will refer only to associated, common or characteristic features of clinical syndromes. Descriptive psychopathology will predominate, and this will emphasise the form of subjective experience for diagnostic purposes. The skilled examiner discriminates the assessment of subjective experience from behaviour that may be verifiable by other observers, and routinely records a description of the positive finding; for example, 'He told me that he had stopped a woman unknown to him in the street to say that he had solved the mystery of cancer' is substantially more informative than simply writing 'delusion of grandiose ability'.

Each section will start with a definition of the major abnormalities, and end with practical suggestions for interview techniques. The Present State Examination (PSE) is a semistructured interview schedule developed for psychiatric research that has been influential in clinical practice because it included standard questions of particular relevance to the diagnosis of psychotic illnesses (Wing et al 1974); several of the practical suggestions are based on questions from the PSE. Discussion points have been included on topics of controversy or particular importance.

MENTAL STATE EXAMINATION (Table 9.1)

Appearance and behaviour

There have been attempts to develop general classifications of the disorders of posture, speech, movement and behaviour (for example, Hamilton 1974), but the classification of the complex behaviour that may accompany mental disorder is problematic. This section will concentrate on common disorders and those associated with clinical syndromes.

Agitation increases movement, which becomes repetitive and often ineffective because the task of the movement is never actually completed, or undone by repetition of the movement. It is not specific to any clinical syndrome, and can occur in severe anxiety, depression, psychotic illness, delirium or dementia. In the past it was accepted that most patients who displayed agitation also felt anxious, but that this was not invariably so; most contemporary writers now use the term simply to imply the motor restlessness that accompanies severe anxiety. *Psychomotor retardation* reduces movement by slowing the initiation and execution of both facial expression and movement; it is often accompanied by slowness in initiation and execution of thought and this is noticed by the sufferer. It is a common feature of severe depressive illness, although it can occur rarely in manic stupor. Psychomotor retardation can be so mild that it is only detected by the sufferer's friends or family, yet so severe that it is associated with stupor.

Certain disorders of posture and movement are of interest because they can be associated with acute or chronic schizophrenia; they are also seen in organic mental disorders. The disorders of posture include *waxy flexibility*, where the patient's limbs can be placed in a position in which they then remain because of increased muscle tone; this can lead also to 'psychological pillow', where the patient's head is maintained a few inches above the bed for a lengthy period. Disorders of facial expression include grimacing and *Schnauzkrampf* ('snout spasm'), that is, the rounded lips are thrust forward in a tubular manner. Many disorders of movement may occur. *Negativism* is when the patient does the opposite of what is asked, and resists efforts to make him do what was asked. *Mannerisms* are repetitive, voluntary, purposeful movements, which are distinguished from *stereotypes* that are repetitive, purposeless movements carried out in a uniform way. Both mannerisms and stereotypes can manifest through posture, facial expression, speech and movement, although the distinction between what is purposeful and purposeless may be difficult.

Perseveration is worthy of special mention. It too can occur in catatonic schizophrenia, but is much more commonly associated with acute and chronic organic mental disorders. It is usually thought of in connection with speech, but can affect any motor response; it occurs when a motor response is made appropriately at the first occurrence of a stimulus, but is repeated inappropriately to a second and different stimulus.

This section has not considered the motor disorders of overt neurological disease such as chorea or athetosis, nor the extrapyramidal disorders that may be associated with the intake of neuroleptic drugs.

Examination

This should begin with a description of the person in everyday language; comments such as 'appropriately dressed' are of little value. Self-neglect may be manifest by dishevelled hair, untidy clothing, or uncertain cleanliness. Body build should be noted. Facial appearance and expression are often informative about a person's

Table 9.1 Mental state examination
Appearance and behaviour
Speech
Mood
Abnormalities of thought
Thought content
Abnormalities of perception
Cognition
Interviewer's reaction to patient
Insight

mood, and may reveal the stigmata of physical disease. Posture and the quantity and speed of bodily movement may also reflect mood, as well as one of the specific disorders described above. Social behaviour can be assessed by the person's demeanour towards the interviewer. This may be typical of how the individual behaves towards other people and may be of relevance to the presenting problem; information from someone who knows the person will be required to confirm that the observed behaviour at interview is typical, and in its absence this assessment must be made with circumspection. Gross disorders of social interaction can occur in severe mental disorders; for example, threats of violence in dissocial personality disorder or attempted physical intimacy in hypomania. The possible presence of extrapyramidal disorders must be considered routinely in patients who have taken neuroleptic drugs, and it is important to record their presence or absence.

Speech

Disorders of thinking

The classification of these disorders is complex because there are different types of thinking (Hamilton 1974), and thought processes are inferred from speech. In this section of the examination it is conventional to focus on disorders in the form of thinking rather than its content. Such disorders can arise from overt brain disease and impairments of vocalization and articulation as well as mental illness; it is conventional to focus here on the disorders of form that can be broadly separated into disorders of the stream of speech and those concerning the structure of words and sentences, that is, etymology and linguistics. The disorders of the stream of thought can be divided into those concerning tempo and continuity. The major disorders of tempo are flight of ideas and psychomotor retardation; the latter was covered in the section above. *Flight of ideas* is accelerated or *pressurised* speech, where the associations between elements of speech are understood by the interviewer, but based on superficial association; this may be no more than alliteration, rhyming, punning or cliché. *Clang association* refers to the linkage of two or more words with a similar sound. Flight of ideas is characteristic of elation. The major disorders of continuity are thought blocking and perseveration of speech; the latter was also described above. In *thought blocking*, there is a sudden cessation in the train of speech, which the sufferer may be able to describe and associate with failure of apperception; in other words, he may complain that his mind suddenly becomes empty.

Disorders of the form of thought have been of interest since the development of the conception of the schizophrenias. Bleuler believed that the characteristic abnormality of these illnesses was an impairment of abstract thinking that led to a loosening of association among elements of speech; in its mildest form it might be no more than a lack of precision in the use of words, and in its most severe it might lead to incoherence. A personal mode of speech may develop; *metonyms* are imprecise approximations for a more exact word, and *neologisms* are new words that are constructed by the individual, or existing words that are given a personal meaning.

Thought disorder   This may refer to the totality of disorders of both form and content of thinking, which would for example include delusions, the totality of disorders of form only, which would include flight of ideas but exclude delusions, or an abbreviation for the disorders of form believed to be characteristic of the schizophrenias. Andreasen (1979) argued that the term be abandoned; she failed to confirm that loosening of association among elements of speech was unique to the schizophrenias because it also occurred in mania. Loosening of association was referred to as derailment in the fourth edition of the *Diagnostic and Statistical Manual of Mental Disorders* (DSM-IV) (APA 1994). She developed a rating scale for disorders of speech, and advocated that further research distinguish between so-called negative aspects of thought disorder such as poverty of speech and positive aspects such as derailment. Her writings also contain detailed examples of disorders of thinking.

Examination

This concerns how the individual speaks, rather than what he says. It considers whether the person talks only when spoken to or spontaneously, and with what rate or quantity of talk. Appropriateness and coherence ought to be considered as a matter of routine. Any disorder in the stream or form of thought should be recorded word for word. The identification of thought blocking requires care; the sufferer is aware of a sudden cessation in what were freely flowing thoughts such that there are 'none left' in his mind; this should have happened repeatedly. Thought blocking may be accompanied by a delusional explanation.

Mood

Disorders of mood

The terminology of these disorders is confusing because in everyday usage different terms are used interchangeably. Jaspers distinguished feelings, which were states of the self, from sensations, which were elements in the perception of the environment. Further classification depended on the intensity and duration of feeling. Individual, unique feelings were distinguished from *affects*, which were brief emotional processes of great intensity with conspicuous bodily changes. *Moods*, or more precisely mood states, were prolonged and coloured the whole of an individual's subjective experience and behaviour. These distinctions have not been consistently retained. Pathological mood states thought to be reactions to adverse life events are still classified separately in the tenth edition of the *International Classification of Diseases* (ICD-10) (WHO 1992) and DSM-IV, thus combining orthodox descriptive psychopathology with assumptions about aetiology. Fish defined *anxiety* as a fear for no adequate reason (Hamilton 1974). This raises the question about how one distinguishes a normal or appropriate mood from the pathological. Anxiety is an unpleasant state associated with feelings of threat and fearful anticipation (or worry) that is often associated with autonomic and somatic features of arousal – for example, awareness of tachycardia, sweating and muscular tension. A *panic attack* is a discrete period of intense anxiety associated with the onset of several of the somatic features of anxiety and usually accompanied by a fear of collapse, a heart attack or the like, to the extent that the sufferer feels compelled to take some form of action. Recurrent panic attacks are often, but not invariably, associated with phobic avoidance. A *phobia* is an intense fear that occurs in a specific situation or in response to a specific stimulus and leads to the avoidance of the situation or stimulus. The sufferer acknowledges that the fear is out of proportion to any actual threat. *Agoraphobia* can be particularly disabling because it also involves the anticipatory fear that panic will occur in a range of places or situations from which egress might be difficult or embarrassing. Pathological anxiety can arise without an obvious cause and vary little from situation to situation, in which case it is sometimes referred to as *free-floating*.

Depressed mood of sufficient severity to be considered a depressive illness is by convention required to last for at least 2 weeks and to be associated with social or functional impairment. Thinking may become restricted to a few gloomy topics, which may be self-reproachful or frankly guilt-ridden. The somatic features of depressive illness are well-known, but sufferers may in addition become unusually indecisive or dependent upon other people. Motor activity is reduced and in severe depressive illness this may lead to psychomotor retardation; agitation can also occur.

Elation can be conceptualised as the polar opposite of depressed mood, but it tends to be associated with more marked functional or social impairment; this is partly because it is usually not acknowledged as patho-logical by the individual. There is a clear onset of elevated mood that has persisted for at least several days; this may be complicated by irritability. The person is full of feelings of well-being and inflated self-worth, which is sometimes referred to as expansive mood. Talk and motor activity are increased, although actual task completion may be impaired by distractibility, that is, the attention is drawn to trivial or irrelevant stimuli. Somatic changes include a reduced need for sleep, impaired concentration and increased libido. *Euphoria* refers to exaggerated feelings of cheerfulness or well-being that can occur without any features of elation and in the absence of mental illness; it can also result from both acute and chronic organic mental disorder, in which cases the elevated mood is in no way infectious. *Ecstasy* is a private state of exalted mood in which themes of contemplation predominate. It can occur in the absence of mental illness, or be associated with delusional preoccupations or overt brain disease.

Reactivity of mood The first edition of this text provided a good historical review of this term (Ashcroft et al 1974), which has been used in two completely different ways. 'Reactive depression' was an abbreviation for a milder form of depressive illness that was brought about by external events of psychological significance for the sufferer and appropriately treated by psychotherapy. This was distinguished from 'endogenous' or 'manic–depressive' illness that was held to be a severe disorder that could arise without any obvious precipitant and was unlikely to improve with psychotherapy. Alternatively, the term was used to describe fluctuations in mood during a single day. This included the diurnal variation that was thought to be characteristic of severe depressive illness in which mood lifted and activity increased from morning to night, and other fluctuations brought about by external stimuli or pleasant diversion. The term was clearly ambiguous, and later ignored because attempts to distinguish so-called endogenous and non-endogenous depressive illness became discredited. Nevertheless, the consistency of depressed mood is an important clinical index of its severity. A respectable remnant of the conception is *anhedonia*, where there is a complete loss of interest of pleasure in former activities. The definition of anhedonia in DSM-IV is the only time that reactivity is mentioned by name; it is defined as 'a lack of reactivity to usually pleasurable stimuli'. Anhedonia is believed to be one of the clinical features of depressive illness most closely correlated with successful outcome after physical treatments.

Disorders of emotional expression are not unique to the schizophrenias (Hamilton 1974), but the more common abnormalities of mood in schizophrenia have acquired their own terminology. *Flattening of affect* refers to the lack of the normal fluctuation in mood that is common in chronic schizophrenia. This can be associated with an acquired insensitivity to social situations in which case it is sometimes referred to as *blunting of affect*. *Incongruous affect* is the expression of a mood that appears to the observer to be inappropriate to the person's thought content or surroundings. Diagnosis of these disorders should be made with care and preferably on more than one occasion. The expression of mood can be inhibited by anxiety or the sedative and other adverse effects of psychotropic drugs. A patient may apparently display incongruous affect by, for example, smiling about a negative life event, but this may result from social awkwardness; it is always necessary to ask the person why he smiled, and only consider incongruity of affect if he himself is puzzled why a sad thought should make him smile.

Examination

The expression of mood is a complex and personal matter that involves non-verbal communication as well as speech. Mood may be inferred from self-care, choice of clothing, posture, gesture, tone of voice as well as through more obvious expressions such as tearfulness or laughter. History-taking may already have provided clues about the person's mood and this may be confirmed by direct open questioning such as 'How are you in your mood or spirits?' It is always necessary to enquire about the possibility of suicidal ideas, which may begin with a question about 'things at their worst'. It may be necessary to proceed to ask about worries whether life is worth living, worries that the patient would be better off dead, suicidal ideas, the formulation in mind of a method for suicide, and actual acts of self-harm or attempts at suicide. It can be informative to enquire of patients with suicidal ideas what it is that helps them to resist these thoughts. Hopelessness may be approached through questions about the future. Elevated mood may be approached through questions about cheerfulness, energy or 'interesting or exciting' ideas or activities.

A few profoundly depressed people do not complain of low spirits, while some patients complain of deep depression and appear cheerful. The assessment of mood can usefully be divided into the subjective, that is, what the person says about his or her mood, and the objective, that is, what the examiner can infer about the person's mood from what is seen or heard. The depth and consistency of depression is an important clinical guide to severity. This can be assessed by reported fluctuations in mood in response to pleasurable or distracting activity and observed fluctuations during the interview.

Table 9.2   Abnormalities of thought
Obsessions and compulsions
Depersonalisation and derealisation
Thought content
Primary and secondary delusions
Symptoms of first rank

Abnormalities of thought (Table 9.2)

Obsessions and compulsions

Disorders in the form of thought were considered above, and disorders of the content of thought will be considered below. This section concerns what Fish regarded as disorders in the possession of thought, although Jaspers emphasised the loss of control over conscious thought.

An *obsession* is a thought that recurs despite the fact that the individual recognises it is a senseless product of his own mind and wishes to resist it. It is the sense of forced thinking and attempts to resist this that are important in the definition of obsessional thinking. Other writers have stressed that the content of thinking is usually repugnant or distressing to the sufferer – for example, recurrent thoughts of violence or unusual sexual acts. The thought can be an idea, an image, an impulse, or ruminative – for example, endless mental debates or fears about the effects of mundane actions. A *compulsion* is a repetitive action that is an attempt, albeit often unsuccessful, to reduce the distress associated with an obsessional thought. The repeated action may involve checking or counting, and when it has a symbolic quality, as in cleaning, it is often referred to as a *ritual*. Isolated or mild obsessional features can occur in otherwise healthy people or associated with an anankastic personality. The clinical syndrome of obsessive–compulsive disorder is an anxiety disorder. Obsessions can occur occasionally in depressive illness, schizophrenia or organic mental disorders.

A screening question for obsessional ideas is 'Do you get awful thoughts coming into your mind even when you try to keep them out?' A positive response should not be accepted on its own as the presence of an obsession, but a specific example should be assessed for the qualities of obsessional thinking. A screening question for compulsions is 'Do you repeat the same action time and time again?' or 'touch or count things over and over again?'

Depersonalisation and derealisation

These are disorders of the experience of the self and

they do not fit neatly under the other major headings of the mental state examination. *Depersonalisation* is a peculiar and unpleasant altered awareness of the self that sufferers find difficult to describe. The sufferer feels as if he or his surroundings have become strange or unreal. Some writers distinguish the feeling of unreality for self, depersonalisation, from unreality of the surroundings, *derealisation*; the two usually coexist. The sufferer is aware that this unpleasant and sometimes frightening experience is a product of his own mind; he is not deluded, in that it is *as if* everything was unreal. Depersonalisation can occur in people without any mental illness, particularly young people at times of fatigue.

People who have never experienced depersonalisation often misunderstand questions about it and may give misleading answers. Suitable screening questions include 'Have you felt unreal or that you were not a real person, or that you were outside yourself, or looking at yourself from outside?' A suitable screening question for derealisation is 'Have you ever had the feeling recently that things around you were unreal ... an imitation, or like a stage?' Most sufferers find these experiences puzzling and struggle to find an explanation, although one should be sought by the interviewer.

Thought content

Disorders of thought content

A standard undergraduate definition of a *delusion* is that it is a false unshakeable belief, which is out of keeping with the individual's social and cultural background. Postgraduate textbooks may stress that it is the result of morbid thought processes, and therefore held with remarkable conviction even in the face of counterarguments by other people. Fish noted that the falsehood of the belief is not the sole criterion; some people who express delusions of infidelity will be correct by coincidence. Wernicke distinguished true delusions from *overvalued ideas*, where a solitary abnormal belief preoccupies a person to the extent of dominating his experience and behaviour. These ideas are associated with marked affect, need not be false, and may even be understandable in the context of the individual's life experience. They can occur in the context of mental illness, but are more closely associated with abnormalities of personality. Fish suggested that overvalued ideas had more pervasive influence over behaviour than many forms of delusions because they could occur in people who had not suffered the 'disintegration of personality' associated with the morbid processes that led to true delusions; this presumably referred to the social withdrawal and impaired volition that occurs in the more severe schizophrenias. The distinction between a delusion and overvalued idea is not simple and the interested reader is referred to McKenna (1984).

Primary and secondary delusions Jaspers distinguished two types of delusion according to their presumed origin: *delusion-like ideas* or *secondary delusions* are always understandable from pre-existing experiences such as morbid mood states, abnormal experiences, derealisation or so on. For example, a manic person with elated mood and expansive thinking may come to believe that they have fantastic powers of healing or recuperation. In *delusions proper* or *primary delusions*, a new meaning arises that is largely non-understandable. The origins of delusions are poorly understood, although Sims (1995) has summarised a number of theories.

Primary delusions are believed to be characteristic of acute schizophrenia. *Autochthonous delusions* arise suddenly and yet are fully formed and held with conviction; they are sometimes referred to as *sudden delusional ideas*. Jaspers quoted a patient who reported that 'It suddenly occurred to me one night ....' and then went on to describe a complex system of persecution involving telepathy. The *delusional perception* is a primary delusion where the content of the belief makes reference to a normal perception, which is usually invested with unreasonable personal significance. Fish gave an example of a man who was offered a biscuit by his brother-in-law with a few encouraging words, and then suddenly realised that his brother-in-law was accusing him of being a homosexual and organising a gang to spy on him. Delusional perceptions and sudden delusional ideas can both occur as delusional memories, sometimes referred to as retrospective delusions. A *delusional atmosphere* may precede a primary delusion; the person believes the world around him has changed in some way that he finds hard to describe, but is believed to be of great personal significance; if this belief is accompanied by great fear or perplexity, it is usually known as *delusional mood*. Jaspers suggested that delusional atmosphere may be associated with the primary or original morbid experience that precedes the development of a delusion.

Content of delusions This is heavily dependent on the life experience, social background and culture of the individual. *Delusions of persecution* are the most common type of secondary delusion, and can occur in organic mental disorders, schizophrenia or severe mood disorders. The persecution can take many forms and is particularly influenced by social and cultural factors; the persecution may vary from simple slander to murderous intent, and may be attributed to a single person at one extreme, or an international organisation at the other extreme. The term 'paranoid delusion' is not synonymous with persecutory delusion because the term paranoid was previously used to mean mental illnesses in which a variety of delusions was prominent. *Delusions of reference* often coexist with persecutory delusions, but can also occur with grandiose delusions. Here the sufferer attaches great personal significance to a mundane object, person or event that is believed to have been deliberately arranged. For example, a deeply depressed patient known to the author said that he believed that the wording of a standard prompt on a computer screen actually made reference to his homosexual affair of some years ago. *Delusions of guilt* or *worthlessness* are typically associated with severe depressive illness; the sufferer attaches great significance to a past misdemeanour, or comes to the view that he is worthless or deserving great punishment. In contrast, *grandiose delusions* are beliefs of exaggerated self-importance and may concern both the person's identity and ability; for example, he may believe himself to be a famous celebrity or that he is endowed with supernatural powers. Such ideas occur today in mania and schizophrenia, but were seen associated with tertiary syphilis before the introduction of antibiotic drug treatment. *Nihilistic delusions* are denials of reality, or beliefs in nothing, and such themes can also occur in severe depression – for example, the sufferer may deny the existence of his body or his family. The term is sometimes broadened to cover bizarre hypochondriacal beliefs such as the complete blockage of the bowels. *Themes of infestation* concern beliefs that parasites or insects infest or burrow into the sufferer; delusions of infestation can be associated with tactile hallucinations or occur in bizarre form in schizophrenia, and a belief in infestation is one of the well-recognised types of overvalued ideas. *Hypochondriacal* ideas can occur as bizarre delusions in schizophrenia or overvalued ideas of bodily deformity or the presence of a specific disease in the absence of any confirmatory evidence. *Delusions of jealousy* are beliefs about infidelity in the person's partner, and are said to be more common among men. Beliefs of infidelity can also occur as overvalued ideas and are important because they can have a great impact on behaviour; the partner may be followed, questioned, searched or even subjected to violence. *Delusions of love* are said to occur more commonly in young women; she believes that a man she may never have met and who is typically of higher social status is actually in love with her. *Religious delusions* have aroused research interest because it has been suggested that they are becoming less prevalent as the importance of religion in modern society declines, although this is not a consistent finding.

Symptoms of the first rank

The English translation of the fifth edition of Professor Kurt Schneider's textbook *Klinische Psychopathologie (Clinical Psycho-*

pathology) was published in 1959 (Schneider 1959). He classified schizophrenia and cyclothymia separately from the psychoses associated with delirium and dementia. He believed that schizophrenia and cyclothymia, the so-called endogenous psychoses, could be distinguished on symptoms alone, and that some symptoms were of particular or 'first-rank' importance because they had a special value in diagnosing schizophrenia as distinct from cyclothymia or non-psychotic disorders. (Schneider himself had reservations about the use of the term 'symptom' as noted above, but the term 'first-rank symptom' is still widely used.) These symptoms of first-rank importance were the eight types of delusions described below and the three types of auditory hallucination described in the next section of the mental state examination. He stated explicitly that when any of these symptoms was undeniably present in the absence of overt brain disease, then the appropriate diagnosis was one of schizophrenia. Nevertheless, he accepted that a diagnosis of schizophrenia could be made in the absence of symptoms of first-rank importance, and he did not believe these symptoms of diagnostic importance explained the cause of schizophrenia. Schneider's opinions have been both influential and controversial. In fact he did not define the first-rank symptoms in detail, and researchers have had to develop operational definitions for use in semi-structured interviews. It has now been clearly established that first-rank symptoms can be diagnosed reliably in sufferers of schizophrenia from different countries and cultures across the world, but their prevalence varies. Contrary to Schneider's assertion, first-rank symptoms are not unique to schizophrenia; they can be features of affective disorders (usually mania) and occasionally other mental illnesses. They are of no help in attempts to predict the longer term outcome of the schizophrenias. The best assessment of their diagnostic value would be in a comparison of the diagnosis of schizophrenia made on the basis of the presence of first-rank symptoms with the diagnosis made completely independently; unfortunately no such diagnostic test exists (Geddes et al 1996).

Delusions of first rank The delusional perception was described above. In *delusions of control*, the sufferer believes that either his feelings, drives or acts are controlled by an outside agency; his will is replaced by some other force. These beliefs are sometimes known as passivity experiences or 'made' feelings, drives or acts. *Somatic passivity* is the belief that an external force penetrates the mind or body. It is not an hallucination of touch or sensation, although it can be a delusional explanation of an hallucination.

There are three types of delusions about the control of thought. In *thought withdrawal*, the sufferer describes his thoughts being taken away from him against his will; this may be associated with thought blocking. In *thought insertion*, the sufferer believes that some of his thoughts are not his own, but have been introduced by an outside agency. In *thought broadcasting*, the thoughts are widely known to other people; the PSE definition requires that the person hears his own thoughts spoken aloud in his head. Fish described these delusions about the control of thoughts as 'thought alienation' to distinguish them from obsessions, and they are often associated with bizarre explanatory delusions involving telepathy, aliens or the like.

Examination

This begins with a record of the individual's major concerns or preoccupations. It is always important to ask what the most distressing problem or worry is; it must not be assumed that this will have been mentioned spontaneously. The next task is to confirm the presence or absence of obsessional thinking and depersonalisation. The assessment of the presence or absence of delusions may well be much harder. Delusional ideas are unlikely to be spontaneous complaints, and some people are reluctant to share these ideas with other people. The interviewer may be alerted to their presence by information from other people or no more than hints from the person himself. A number of screening questions will be provided, but like those for obsessions and depersonalisation, these may be misunderstood; an answer of 'Yes' must not be taken to signify their presence without more detailed assessment of a specific example.

Delusions of control concern much more than the common notion that life is directed by some outside influence such as God or fate, and does not refer to command hallucinations. A screening question is 'Do you feel under the control of some force or power other than yourself ... as though you were without a will of your own?'. It is not uncommon for deluded patients to believe that others can infer what they are thinking by inspection of their expression or movements, but delusions about the control of thought are much more specific. 'Can you think quite clearly or is there any interference with your thoughts? Is anything like hypnotism or telepathy going on?' A suitable question for thought broadcasting is 'Do you ever seem to hear your own thoughts spoken aloud in your head, so that someone standing near might be able to hear them?'

The next consideration is to decide with what conviction the delusion is held, and to what extent it affects the patient's talk or behaviour. Questions about conviction require tact as it can be helpful to check out in a gentle manner whether or not someone accepts that his 'imagination might be playing tricks' on him, or whether there are any other occasional doubts. There is a gradient of influence over talk and behaviour from where the patient may discuss delusions only with close friends or family to openly discussing his thoughts with complete strangers. The degree of conviction does not always correlate closely with its influence on behaviour; all psychiatrists eventually meet patients with delusions of grandiose identity who nevertheless accommodate the daily routine of the hospital ward or hostel. Information from family and friends can be critical and is paramount in the assessment of specific kinds of delusions. If ever there is uncertainty about whether an apparently strange belief would be normal in a specific culture, it is essential to obtain information from a healthy relative or someone from the same cultural background. Violence to other people may be particularly associated with delusions of infidelity and impersonation. *Delusional misidentification* occurs when someone believes that a person close to him has been replaced by an impostor.

Other people usually argue with the deluded person, but rarely delusional beliefs may be shared. *Shared delusions* usually occur when someone has lived in relative isolation from the outside world for a long time with a more dominant deluded person; the delusional belief in the second person is called an *induced delusion*, and the situation *folie à deux*.

Abnormalities of perception (Table 9.3)

The disorders of perception are traditionally divided into sensory distortions, where real perceptual objects are perceived in a distorted way, and sensory deceptions, where new perceptions arise without adequate perceptual objects. The discussion will make reference to the conception of imagery.

Imagery

Healthy people usually have no difficulty in distinguishing their imagination from the perception of real objects. Unlike a true perception, imagery is recognised

Table 9.3 Abnormalities of perception
Imagery
Sensory distortions
Sensory deceptions
Illusions
Hallucinations
Pseudohallucinations

to originate in the internal world, dependent upon the observer, and with conscious effort. Unlike imagery, the observer realises that the existence of a true perceptual object can be confirmed, for example, by a perception through a different sense. Fish distinguished imaginative thinking, which does not go beyond the possible and rational, from fantasy thinking that does (Hamilton 1974).

Sensory distortions

The distortion may result in a change in the intensity, quality or spatial form of a perception. The intensity of perception may be heightened or diminished. For example, *hyperacusis*, heightening in the intensity of sound, is a recognised complaint associated with anxiety. This may be better understood as a decreased tolerance for ambient noise rather than heightened perception. *Visual hyperaesthesia*, where colours are perceived more intensely or with greater vividness, is a recognised feature of elation. Changes in quality usually affect vision – for example, distortions in colour perception are recognised adverse effects of several medicines. Changes in spatial form also affect vision, where objects are seen smaller or further away than they really are, *micropsia*, or its opposite, *macropsia*. *Dysmegalopsia* is distortion in shape and associated with diseases of the eye, cranial nerves or brain. The most common cause of sensory distortions in the general population is intoxication with drugs of abuse, and they are common features of complex partial seizures.

Sensory deceptions

Illusions An illusion is a combination of the perception of an external object and a mental image to produce a false perception. A *completion illusion* can occur at times of inattention when a stimulus that is only partly perceived is augmented by the individual to become meaningful in terms of his past experience. An illusion can also arise at a time of mood disturbance, the so-called *affect illusion*. Illusions are more likely to arise when aetiological factors combine – for example, when a fearful delirious patient 'sees' frightening illusions at night when the lights are dimmed.

Pareidolic illusions are not dependent on inattention or mood disturbance, and are regarded by some writers as closer to vivid visual imagination rather than proper illusions. Complex photographic images result from mundane visual stimuli; they are recognised as false perceptions, but may not disappear immediately with conscious effort. Vivid visual imagery occurs most commonly in children, but pareidolic illusions have also been reported in healthy adults, and in association with fever and intoxication with drugs of abuse.

Hallucinations Esquirol distinguished hallucinations, which were perceptions without an object, from illusions. Jaspers noted that this definition excluded certain types of hallucinations, for example, functional hallucinations, but included dreams; he suggested instead that an hallucination was a false perception, which was not a sensory distortion or misinterpretation, but which occurred at the same time as real perceptions.

Types of hallucinations Hallucinations can be categorised by their complexity, sensory modality and by special features. The term *elementary hallucination* is used for experiences such as flashes of light or whirring noises, whereas *complex hallucinations* would include visual experiences organised into figures or scenes and auditory experiences organised into music or voices. Hallucinations occur in all senses. *Auditory hallucinations* may be noises, music or voices. The description of voices varies; it may involve one voice, or many; the voice or voices may be indistinct or speak words, phrases, or sentences, which may or may not be located in space and may be ascribed to someone recognised or unknown. The voices may give instructions, the so-called *imperative* or *command hallucination*. Auditory hallucinations occur in organic mental disorders, schizophrenia and occasionally in severe mood disorders. Those that are in the form of voices are particularly associated with the schizophrenias.

Visual hallucinations are characteristic of organic mental disorders, but may occur rarely in the schizophrenias and severe mood disorders. These may be normal in size or affected by micropsia, for example, the fearful hallucinations of small animals seen in delirium tremens. Visual hallucinations of tiny people are sometimes referred to as *lilliputian*.

Olfactory and gustatory hallucinations, that is, hallucinations of smell and taste, can be difficult to distinguish from each other, and from sensory distortions or illusions. Healthy people often find the two senses difficult to distinguish, and the two types of perception often coexist. Some people complain of complex persecutory delusions that include ideas that they are being poisoned by gas or a substance in their food, and it is not always easy to clarify what exactly they smell or taste. Both types of hallucination are associated with complex partial seizures and can occur in schizophrenia or rarely in severe depressive illness.

The core definition of an hallucination is less easily applied to *hallucinations of touch* or *sensation*. All superficial hallucinations may be grouped together as *tactile hallucinations*, or superficial hallucinations of touch, *haptic hallucinations*, may be distinguished from other superficial sensations such as temperature and so on. They may be felt as movements on or just under the skin, and when this is ascribed to small animals or insects crawling over the body is known as *formication*. This is a common feature of cocaine psychosis, when it is known as 'the cocaine bug'. Formication in other settings is commonly associated with delusions of infestation. *Hallucinations of deep sensation* and *proprioception* can occur, for example, sensations of stretching, squeezing or pain. Complex hallucinations involving stimulation of the sexual organs may be perceived as forced orgasms or actual penetration. The extent of any delusional elaboration is of greater diagnostic significance than the nature of the hallucination itself – for example, bizarre explanations involving outside agencies are likely to be associated with the schizophrenias.

Hallucinations of first rank There are three of these. Two take the form of voices clearly heard as speaking to or about the subject. *Commentary hallucinations* consist of one or more voices that talk of the person's thoughts or actions. Two or more voices may be heard talking to each other, perhaps discussing the subject; when they refer to the person as 'he' or 'she', they are known as *third person hallucinations*. The hearing of one's own thoughts spoken aloud is called *thought echo*; this may anticipate, occur simultaneously, or repeat the thought.

Other special kinds of hallucinations A *functional hallucination* requires an external stimulus to initiate it, and it is perceived at the same time and in the same modality as the normal perception of the stimulus. The hallucination and true perceptions are discrete, and therefore distinguished from an illusion. *Synaesthesia* occurs when a sensory stimulus in one modality results in a sensory experience in a different modality; the usual example is of the squeak of chalk on a blackboard leading to a tingling of the spine. When the associated perception is not a true one, but an hallucination, this is called a *reflex hallucination*. *Extracampine hallucinations* are perceived beyond the limits of the sensory field – for example, the subject hears someone talking in a far away place. None of these special kinds of hallucination is of diagnostic significance. *Autoscopy* is the visual hallucination of seeing oneself, and is associated with advanced brain disease. An *hypnagogic hallucination* occurs on going to sleep, and an *hypnopompic hallucination* on waking. Both can occur in healthy people. The hallucination may be visual, auditory or tactile, but is usually brief and elementary.

Pseudohallucinations Taylor (1981) noted that pseudohallucinations had been distinguished from hallucinations in two completely different ways. First, the term had been used to refer to hallucinations of vividness and spontaneity, but that were not referred to external space, and secondly to vivid hallucinations that were recognised as such by the subject. He suggested more precise definition, although the distinction between the two types of pseudohallucination was not of any diagnostic significance. Pseudohallucinations that were experienced within the mind could be referred to as image pseudohallucinations, and those experienced as located in external space but recognised as unreal would be referred to as perceived pseudohallucinations. Jaspers had earlier recommended an alternative approach in which the core definitions of imagery and hallucination would be used as standards against which a perception would be compared. Although it is sometimes disputed, Jaspers himself acknowledged that different forms of abnormal experience can combine in severe mental illness, and that actual 'transitions' between pseudohallucinations and true hallucinations can occur (Jaspers 1963, p. 70). People who suffer florid hallucinations often struggle to make sense of their strange experiences and they may find it impossible to put them into words; consequently, the interviewer may not have the necessary information to make these diagnostic distinctions.

Examination

'Hearing voices' is to many lay people synonymous with madness. Screening questions for abnormal appearances often have to be asked with tact. 'I should like to ask you a routine question. Do you ever seem to hear noises or voices when there is no one about, and nothing else to explain it?' Specific questions for first-rank hallucinations include 'Do you hear several voices talking about you?' 'Do they refer to you as 'he' (she)?' 'Do they seem to comment on what you are thinking, or reading, or doing?' Auditory hallucinations in the form of voices can be located by asking 'Are these voices in your mind or can you hear them through your ears?' Specific examples must be recorded, and their form compared to the standard definitions of imagery and hallucination as described above. Other relevant information includes when they occur (particularly important for hallucinations on waking or falling asleep), associations with other external stimuli (relevant to functional hallucinations), the effect on the subject, and the subject's explanation for the experience. The effect of abnormal experiences may be obvious to the interviewer – for example, if the subject is terrified by frightening visual hallucinations, or shouts replies to auditory hallucinations. The subject's explanation may be of diagnostic significance if it is obviously delusional.

Cognition

Disorders of consciousness

Consciousness is the state of awareness of the environment. Sims (1995) described the three dimensions of consciousness: vigilance, lucidity and consciousness of self. Only the first two will be considered here. *Vigilance* refers to the physiological stages of wakefulness, from being fully awake to deep sleep. The level of vigilance is largely controlled in health by the ascending reticular activating system. While *lucidity* of consciousness is contingent on adequate vigilance, it is much more closely related to higher mental functions. A lucid individual responds appropriately in a coordinated manner to the surroundings by integrating past experience and learning to the current situation. *Attention* concerns the focus of the mind and can occur both with and without conscious effort. *Concentration* is the process where attention is sustained for a period of time. *Orientation* is the capacity of a person to gauge time, space and person, that is, their identity, in his current surroundings.

Impairments in attention and concentration, which can occur in otherwise healthy people at times of fatigue or anxiety, are non-specific features of mental illness. The combination of markedly impaired concentration and increased vigilance leads to *distractibility*, that is, when the person is diverted by almost all new stimuli irrespective of their relevance or importance. This can occur in elation, delirium or intoxication with psychostimulant drugs. Clear consciousness is always associated with the ability to apprehend or grasp the meaning of the environment or situation. Impaired consciousness, sometimes referred to in its milder forms as *clouding of consciousness*, is a pathological impairment of consciousness that in its most severe leads to coma, where there is no outward sign of mental activity and the person does not respond even to painful stimuli. Clouding of consciousness is a characteristic feature of acute organic mental disorders. Milder degrees of impairment are associated with reduced attention and concentration, slow muddled thinking, and impaired grasp of the environment. As the severity of impairment increases, this leads inevitably to disorientation, another characteristic feature of acute organic mental disorders. Orientation for time requires a conscious awareness of external events that mark the passage of time, and is more easily disturbed in clouding of consciousness. Orientation for place is usually better retained because of clues in the environment. Disorientation for person, that is, the inability to state one's own name or identity, only occurs in severe impairment. Disorientation also occurs in the absence of clouding of consciousness in mental handicap and chronic organic mental disorders. Confusion is a descriptive term with several different meanings, and its use has now been abandoned in the classification of organic mental disorders.

Examination

Impaired attention may have been apparent during history-taking if it was difficult to arouse the person's attention, questions had to be continually repeated, or the person had difficulty in shifting from topic to topic. Impaired concentration may have been obvious if the person was unable to sustain a train of thought or forgot the specifics of the question. In distractibility, the topic of talk may be deflected by a trivial noise from outside the interview room.

Concentration can be tested by asking the patient to recite the months of the year backwards, starting with December, or a more demanding test is to subtract 7 from 100 and subtract 7 from the answer and so on (serial 7s). If the latter task is too difficult, it can be substituted with serial 3s. People who show definite evidence of impaired attention and concentration will inevitably have difficulty with tests of short-term memory. This is assessed by the digit span test; the patient is asked to memorise and then repeat sequences of digits that have been spoken aloud slowly enough to allow memorisation. The task can begin with a sequence of three digits to ensure that the patient understands the task. Then the patient is asked to repeat five digits, and if this is achieved successfully the task is repeated with six digits and so on until seven digits have been attempted. Specific questions about orientation for time, place and person may not be required if the patient has made his orientation clear during history-taking. Many healthy people struggle to recall the date exactly, but have no difficulty with the day of the week, month and an estimate of the time of day. If someone is clearly orientated for time and place, it is simply embarrassing to ask them to confirm their identity.

Memory

A popular model of working memory is the assumption that normal memory can be held or stored in three different ways. *Immediate memory* concerns a limited amount of information from the sense organs that is retained for less than 1 second. Immediate memory is intimately involved with attention. *Short-term* or *primary memory* is limited to an average of seven items that can be stored for longer than 30 seconds only if they are consciously rehearsed. Items in the short-term memory will be forgotten unless they are selectively chosen for longer term storage in the *long-term* or *secondary memory*. In clinical practice it is common to divide long-term memories into those for recent events, that is, the previous 24–48 hours, and remote events. Severe impairments of memory may be associated with *confabulation*, when the person gives a reply that may sound plausible and which he believes to be true, but that is actually false.

Examination

Experienced examiners make selective use of memory tests. If there is no suggestion of memory loss from the presenting complaint or history-taking, and there is no evidence of inattention or impaired concentration, and the patient is clearly orientated, then the following screening tests are unlikely to detect any abnormality. Short-term or primary memory is tested by the digit span as described above. Recent memory can be assessed by giving the patient a fictitious name and address to memorise; the patient is asked to repeat it immediately and then asked to recall it 5 minutes later. The first repetition is to check that he has memorised the address correctly, and is also itself a test of short-term memory. Long-term memory is only assessed if indicated, and this can be done by asking about recent events such as day of hospital admission and so on. The assessment of remote long-term memory can be problematic and will be discussed again in the situation where there is a specific indication for detailed assessment of intellectual function.

Other aspects of intellectual function

Some textbooks suggest that general knowledge and intelligence be tested routinely. The appropriateness of routine testing is questionable, and also raises methodological problems. Tests of general knowledge are heavily dependent on educational opportunity and the interests of the individual himself. Experienced interviewers take account of the patient's general intelligence in assessing the presenting complaint, his coping strategies, their choice of wording in questions, and in the assessment of tests of intellectual function. While this is clearly an important aspect of the mental state examination, they rarely use tests of intelligence. General intelligence is usually estimated from educational attainment, occupation, social functioning and verbal skills.

Interviewer's reaction to patient

This section considers whether or not the patient communicates to the interviewer a particular mood, the ease or difficulty of control of the interview, and what the interviewer can learn of the patient's personality. It would be important for the interviewer to note, for example, when a depressed person brings about a mood of sadness in the interviewer, but any inferences about the person's characteristic behaviour is more problem-

atic. The two may meet only once and the person's behaviour may not be typical because of embarrassment or anxiety. Despite these reservations, it is the case that the interviewer may observe examples of behaviour or interpersonal style of relevance to the presenting complaint (see above). Repeated contact allows more careful consideration of these matters and whether or not a satisfactory working relationship is developing.

Insight

Professor Aubrey Lewis defined insight as 'a correct attitude to a morbid change in oneself' (Lewis 1934). This was an influential definition of insight, but the assessment of insight based on this definition would rely heavily on the judgement of the interviewer. There have subsequently been fundamental challenges to the basic conception of insight. The essential debate is whether or not insight can be defined as a distinct aspect of psychopathology, rather than the direct consequence of the presence of delusions and/or hallucinations. For example, a delusional belief is by definition usually false and held with conviction despite logical argument to the contrary. Other writers have argued also that insight may be more closely associated with the personal significance of the illness to the individual, rather than the illness itself; in this case factors such as life experience, education and personality would influence insight more than the illness itself. David et al (1995) listed reasons why the conception of insight merited research: it may influence treatment compliance and affect the likelihood of symptomatic and social recovery; markedly impaired insight is a common feature of schizophrenia, which in turn may be related to the cognitive impairments and brain imaging abnormalities described in severe forms of the illness.

Examination

Insight is not assessed adequately by a categorical approach, that is, as simply present or absent. It is better assessed along a continuum and the specific factors used as the scale will depend on the nature of the disorder and its treatment. A general psychiatrist may report with satisfaction that someone recovering from an acute episode of schizophrenia is gaining insight because he acknowledges he has been ill, accepts previous delusional beliefs were false, and welcomes the prospect of treatment. A psychoanalyst might refer to much more sophisticated psychological conceptions.

The first practical aspect in the assessment of insight is whether or not the patient accepts he is unwell, and whether or not this is acknowledged to be a mental illness. It is advisable to confirm that the most salient mental complaints are attributed by the individual to mental illness. For example, someone who has suffered a chronic delusional disorder characterised by complex delusions of persecution may readily accept the suggestion that he suffers from a nervous illness such as 'stress' or 'depression', but attribute this to the alleged persecution. A more sophisticated appraisal is the extent to which the individual understands the nature and possible causes of his illness; for example, can a severely depressed patient recognise that he has become more pessimistic as his mood has gradually sunk after a series of adverse life events and that this explains his preoccupations of hopelessness. Treatment compliance is not the most fashionable of themes, but the acceptance of treatment is a very important issue, and this is particularly true in the schizophrenias and manic–depressive illnesses.

SPECIAL SITUATIONS THAT NEED TO BE BORNE IN MIND (Table 9.4)

The unresponsive patient

The patient who will not or cannot talk to the interviewer poses a special problem. *Mutism* is the absence of speech in clear consciousness and can occur as elective mutism in children, where ordinary speech is produced only in specific situations, for example, at home but not at school. *Stupor* has a special meaning in psychiatry, which is different to that in neurology. It refers to a state where there is an inability to initiate speech or movement when awake and aware. Awareness may have to be inferred from no more than purposeful movements of the eyes, and sometimes can be confirmed only in retrospect by the sufferer's ability to remember events during the relevant period. Stupors can be classified into those of psychogenic and neurological aetiology, the former being associated with clear consciousness; unfortunately there are major practical difficulties in assessing consciousness, as already noted. They can be associated with severe emotional reactions, catatonic schizophrenia, depressive and, rarely, manic

Table 9.4	Special situations

The unresponsive patient
Suspected organic mental disorder
Problems of communication, e.g. deafness, language difficulties
The uncooperative or aggressive patient

illnesses, and organic mental disorders. *Locked-in syndrome* is a combination of tetraplegia and mutism with clear consciousness, which results from bilateral damage to the brainstem or bilateral damage to the cerebral peduncles; voluntary movement consists of no more than blinking or ocular movements. *Akinetic mutism* is a variety of stupor originally described in association with compression of the walls of the third ventricle by a craniopharyngioma. A normal sleep–wake cycle is preserved, but there is impaired consciousness; that is, a response occurs only after vigorous or continuous external stimulation.

Examination

Information from someone who knows the patient should always be sought, and this might usefully cover the time and speed of onset, progress of the disorder, past medical and psychiatric history, current mental and physical health and any recent or relevant life events that may have been associated with the onset. A physical examination will be essential. The neurological examination ought to pay special attention to possible signs of midbrain or upper brainstem disease, including pupillary function, eye movements and the quality of respiration. Stupor may be associated with hypotension and retention of urine and faeces. Medical investigations will be required to exclude metabolic causes of stupor (Walton 1993). The mental state examination itself may be limited to the assessment of the level of consciousness and a systematic review of appearance and behaviour. Information from relatives or nursing staff may provide valuable information about behaviour outwith the examination itself. Fish noted that excitement can occur in the same mental illness as stupor, and it is necessary to be wary because stupor can turn suddenly into excitement.

The level of consciousness can be inferred from what little motor or vocal response is made. Is the patient alert to daily routines such as meal times or other ward activities, and does he respond, albeit in a limited way, to contact with staff or relatives? Does he attend to activities of daily living, including personal hygiene and toileting? Are the eyes open or shut, and, if open, is the gaze fixed or does it follow moving objects? If shut, can the patient open them on request or actually resist their passive opening?

Posture and movement may be informative. Is the posture ordinary and comfortable, or awkward or bizarre; are any of the movement disorders associated with catatonic schizophrenia present? Is the facial expression bland or does it suggest an emotional state or is it disordered, as in grimacing or 'snout spasm'? The interviewer should allow sufficient time after any question to confirm that the patient is actually mute. Is it possible to obtain a brief reply to a simple or mundane question, but not one that is more complex or psychological? Does the patient vocalise without speaking? Will the patient make a verbal or non-verbal response to certain topics?

Is it possible to infer anything about the patient's inner world from his appearance and behaviour? Do certain topics of conversation bring about an emotional response, such as tears in the eyes? Does the patient appear frightened or responding, albeit in a limited way, to possible abnormal experiences?

Examination when an organic mental disorder is suspected

Detailed examination of cognition may be indicated from the presenting complaint itself, for example, increasing forgetfulness, when history-taking has revealed inconsistencies or gaps in the person's account, or when routine testing has detected intellectual impairment. A full physical examination will be essential. A thorough assessment of intellectual function may not be possible at one session because some patients will be unable to maintain their attention or will tire easily. The order of examination may have to be geared to individual patients, and this is particularly important if it is suspected that comprehension is impaired, when language function will be tested early. Information from someone who knows the patient well will be important in clarifying the nature and severity of any impairment. Examples of screening tests are available in the article by Folstein et al (1975), and a more detailed discussion is available from Walton (1993).

Level of consciousness

Acute and chronic organic mental disorders are distinguished by examination of consciousness, as described above. Unfortunately, a fluctuation in consciousness is also characteristic of acute organic mental disorders and it is important to question nursing staff or other informants about possible changes during the day and night. Impaired consciousness in incipient coma is more relevant to medical emergencies and is usually graded by the Glasgow Coma Scale (Teesdale & Jennett 1974).

Detailed assessment of memory

Verbal memory can be assessed by the name and address test, and the ability to repeat immediately a Stanford–Binet sentence after a single hearing. It is necessary to explain to the patient that you wish him to lis-

ten carefully, remember a sentence, and then repeat it word for word. Task difficulty can be adjusted to estimated intelligence. If the first repetition is accurate, a more difficult sentence can be tried; if the first repetition is not correct, an easier sentence can be attempted. One-half of subjects can recall the following sentences at the stated age: 'Yesterday we went for a ride in our car along the road that crosses the bridge' (11 years); 'The aeroplane made a careful landing in the space which had been prepared for it' (13 years); 'The red-headed woodpecker made a terrible fuss as they tried to drive the young away from the nest' (average adult); and 'At the end of the week, the newspaper published a complete account of the experiences of the great explorer' (above average adult).

Tests of non-verbal memory are also required and can be combined with tests of visuospatial ability – for example, asking the patient to recall a simple figure, such as a circle intersected with a diamond, after 5 minutes.

The assessment of long-term memory is more problematic because knowledge of historical events such as the dates of world wars is also affected by general knowledge, educational opportunity and general intelligence. Recall of autobiographical events is more sensitive to any impairment, but assessment of recall requires access to informants knowledgeable of the individual's personal history. Correct recall of historical events such as the dates of world wars excludes any gross impairment of long-term memory, and a failure to recall such events should be taken as an indication for further testing using autobiographical information.

Language function

Impairment of language function is classically divided into *sensory* or *receptive dysphasia*, where comprehension of speech is impaired, and *motor* or *expressive dysphasia*, where speech production is impaired with normal vocalising ability. (The terms aphasia and dysphasia are used interchangeably.) Comprehension of the spoken word can be tested by asking the patient to listen to a simple command and carry it out. Comprehension of the written word can be assessed by asking the patient to read aloud and carry out a simple command. Comprehension of the written and spoken word can be impaired independently. Gross expressive dysphasia will have been obvious in history-taking, but less severe impairment can be detected by tests of speaking and writing. In *nominal dysphasia* the sufferer is unable to produce names at will, but he may be able to talk relevantly of the object. Less severe impairment may be detected by difficulty in part-naming, where the person may be able to name a watch, but not its strap or buckle.

The precise description of the language impairment may be used to localise the site of brain disease, although this requires knowledge of cerebral dominance; impairment points to the involvement of the left cerebral hemisphere in right-handed people, but the location of pathology is more problematic in left-handed people (Walton 1993).

Visuospatial and constructional ability

The pathology of these impairments is not always known, but most suggest the localisation of cerebral disease to the parietal lobes (Walton 1993). *Agnosia* is the inability to comprehend the significance of sensation in the presence of full consciousness and the absence of any disease of the sensory organs. *Visual agnosia* can be detected by asking the patient to describe or name a particular object. The inability to recognise faces is known as *prosopagnosia*. In *finger agnosia* the sufferer is unable to point to individual fingers or distinguish his own fingers from those of the examiner. *Astereoagnosia* is the inability to identify a three-dimensional form, and is tested by asking the patient to identify objects placed in his hand while his eyes are closed. *Anosoagnosia* is the inability to recognise functional handicaps caused by disease, most commonly the denial of left-sided weakness and impairment of sensation after a cerebral vascular accident affecting the non-dominant parietal lobe. *Topographical orientation* is the ability to find one's way around the immediate surroundings. This can be tested by asking the patient to go to a particular location, and important information about topographical orientation may be obtained from relatives or nursing staff, for example, the ability to find the toilet. The ability to distinguish right from left may be impaired, and this can be assessed simultaneously with finger agnosia.

Apraxia is the inability to perform a voluntary motor act, the nature of which is comprehended, in the presence of normal consciousness and the absence of any musculoskeletal disability. *Constructional apraxia* is detected by asking the patient to draw simple geometric figures of increasing complexity, for example, a diamond intersecting a circle, a cube, or clock face. *Dressing apraxia* is detected by asking the person to put on his clothes. *Idiomotor apraxia* concerns the completion of complicated tasks upon instruction.

Patients with communication difficulties

The main problems that arise relate to deafness and language difficulties. Patients with late deafness who therefore have normal verbal/reading skills need present no major problem once the situation is appreciated. Patients with prelingual deafness are very difficult for most psychiatrists to assess, as adequate communication cannot usually be achieved. It is essential to obtain the assistance of someone who can communicate with the patient but where this is done adequate assessment of the mental state can be achieved. Indeed there is a standardised assessment available (Thacker 1994). Patients who present language/cultural difficulties are increasingly frequent in this era of world travel. Even for psychiatrists with a smattering of the relevant language it is helpful to obtain the assistance of an appropriate (adult) individual who can communicate adequately with the patient.

Patients who are uncooperative/aggressive

Such patients not infrequently present in emergency clinics. It is important to exclude organic mental disorders and the steps in examining disorders of consciousness have been described above. Having clarified this matter the important issues to be considered in such situations are whether or not the patient requires assessment and treatment and whether or not he will accept it. If the latter question is an issue, implementation of mental health legislation may have to be considered. Once these matters have been attended to, finer points of assessment can wait for a later date.

REFERENCES

Andreasen N C 1979 Thought, language, and communications disorders. Archives of General Psychiatry 36: 1315–1321

APA 1994 Diagnostic and statistical manual of mental disorders, 4th edn. American Psychiatric Association, Washington

Ashcroft G W, Blackburn I M, Cundall R L 1974 Affective disorders. In: Forrest A (ed) Companion to psychiatric studies. Churchill Livingstone, Edinburgh, vol II, ch IX, pp 187–195

David A, Van Os J, Jones P, Harvey I, Foerster A, Fahy T 1995 Insight in psychotic illness: cross-sectional and longitudinal associations. British Journal of Psychiatry 167: 621–628

Folstein M F, Folstein S E, McHugh P R 1975 Mini-mental state examination: a practical method for grading cognitive state of patients for the clinician. Journal of Psychiatric Research 12: 189–198

Geddes J R, Christofi G, Sackett D L 1996 Commentaries on 'first-rank symptoms or rank-and-file symptoms'. British Journal of Psychiatry 169: 544–545

Hamilton M (ed) 1974 Fish's clinical psychopathology, revised reprint. Wright, Bristol

Jaspers K 1963 General psychopathology, 7th edn. Translated by J Hoenig & M W Hamilton. Manchester University Press, Manchester

Lewis A 1934 The psychopathology of insight. British Journal of Medical Psychology 14: 332–348

McKenna P J 1984 Disorders of over-valued ideas. British Journal of Psychiatry 145: 579–585

Schneider K 1959 Clinical psychopathology. Translated by M W Hamilton. Grune & Stratton, London

Sims A 1995 Symptoms in the mind, 2nd edn. W B Saunders, London

Taylor F K 1981 On pseudohallucinations. Psychological Medicine 11: 265–271

Teesdale G, Jennett B 1974 Assessment of coma and impaired consciousness: a practical scale. Lancet ii: 81–84

Thacker A J 1994 Formal Communication Disorder – a sign language in deaf people with schizophrenia. British Journal of Psychiatry 165: 818–823

Walton J N (ed) 1993 Brain's diseases of the nervous system, 10th edn. Oxford University Press, Oxford

WHO 1992 The ICD-10 classification of mental and behavioural disorders: clinical descriptions and diagnostic guidelines. World Health Organization, Geneva

Wing J K, Cooper J E, Sartorius N 1974 The measurement and classification of psychiatric symptoms. Cambridge University Press, London

10
Diagnosis and classification

Eve C. Johnstone

INTRODUCTION

In psychiatry, as in the rest of medicine, the purpose of diagnostic classification is to bring order to the wide range of symptoms, signs and courses of illness that are encountered in clinical practice. It allows us to identify groups of patients who resemble one another in terms of their clinical features, response to treatment and outcome of their condition. In most branches of medicine the value of diagnosis is never questioned. Its importance is regarded as self-evident because treatment and prognosis depend upon it. In psychiatry the situation is rather different. With a few exceptions diagnoses continue to be based entirely on the clinical picture and, although it is possible to achieve a high degree of reliability in staff trained in particular styles of practice, overall the diagnoses are relatively unreliable. Furthermore, the therapeutic and prognostic implications of psychiatric diagnoses are relatively weak. In the light of this it is not surprising that the value of psychiatric diagnosis has been questioned. Indeed psychoanalysts such as Karl Menninger (1963) have suggested that the practice of psychiatric diagnosis be abandoned. Such ideas are not widely held in the way that they were at the time of the antipsychiatry movement of the 1960s (Szasz 1961, Turner 1995) but it is important to examine the arguments around the issue to appreciate why diagnosis matters and the ways in which the attaching of a diagnostic label may harm a patient as well as help him.

THE INEVITABILITY OF CLASSIFICATION

Every patient possesses characteristics of three kinds:

1. Those he shares with all other patients
2. Those he shares with some other patients, but not all
3. Those which are unique to him.

Insofar as the first of these three categories is dominant, classification or subdivision is pointless and unnecessary. All patients have fundamentally similar problems and even if there are a few superficial differences between them they all require the same treatment. Insofar as the third category is dominant, classification is impossible. Learning from experience and useful communication with others are also impossible. For if every patient is different from every other we can learn nothing useful from textbooks, from colleagues, or the accumulated wisdom of our predecessors. Indeed, we cannot even learn from our own personal experience if there are no significant similarities between our last patient and the next. Our attention has, therefore, to be focused on the second category. What is more, as soon as one begins to recognise features that are common to some patients but not all, and to distinguish those which are important from those, like eye colour, which are not, one is classifying them, whether one recognises it or not. And if we have more than one treatment available, as we have, and wish to use these different treatments with maximum efficacy, we must distinguish between one type of patient and another. Otherwise we are reduced to allocating different patients to different treatments by whim or the throw of dice. (Those who argued that diagnostic categories would be abandoned did indeed believe that all patients required the same treatment – the 'moral regime' of the asylum for Neumann and Prichard in the 19th century and psychotherapy for Rogers and Menninger in the 20th.)

A distinction between different kinds of mental disorder is therefore inevitable. The only open issues are whether this classification is going to be public or private, stable or unstable, reliable or unreliable, valid or invalid. Classifications of mental disorders may well be less useful than classifications of, say, cardiovascular disorders or gastrointestinal disorders, for they are still largely based on differences in symptomatology rather than on differences in aetiology, but the only viable option in this situation is to try to improve the classification we possess. It cannot simply be abandoned, and the idea that diagnosis can, or should, be replaced by a formulation is based on a fundamental misunderstanding of the nature of both. A formulation which takes account of the unique features of the patient and his environment, and the interaction between them, is often essential for any real understanding of his predicament, and for planning effective treatment, but it is unusable in any situation in which populations or groups of patients need to be considered. The essential feature of any population is that its members share at least one important characteristic in common. The essence of a diagnosis is that it embodies as many as possible of those characteristics which are common to several different patients (i.e. category 2 above), just as it is the essence of a formulation to embody those which are unique to the individual (category 3 above). Formulation and diagnosis are equally necessary, but for quite different purposes.

The shortcomings and disadvantages of diagnoses

If some form of categorisation or subdivision of mental disorders is inescapable, as it is, it is essential that we appreciate the limitations and potential ill-effects of allocating patients to diagnostic categories. In the first place, psychiatric diagnoses are often a very inadequate means of conveying what the clinician regards as the essence of his patient's predicament, and the better he knows the patient the stronger this feeling becomes. To say that a woman has a depressive illness does not explain why she became depressed or how she came to medical attention, nor does it establish whether she is on the brink of committing suicide or merely despondent and dejected. She may have been ill for anything from a few weeks to several years and may require electroconvulsive therapy (ECT) or antidepressant drugs or psychotherapy. Another important problem is that many patients do not conform to the tidy stereotyped descriptions found in textbooks. They possess some, but not all, of the characteristic features of two or three different diagnostic categories and so have to be allocated more or less arbitrarily to whichever syndrome they seem to resemble most closely. As a result, disagreements about diagnosis are commonplace and hybrid terms like schizoaffective and borderline state have to be coined and pressed into service.

Many psychiatric diagnoses also have pejorative connotations. Terms like hysteric, neurotic, schizophrenic and psychopath are sometimes used as thinly disguised expressions of contempt, and even when this is not so the aura surrounding such terms can very easily have harmful effects on the behaviour and attitudes of other people, and so on the patient's own attitude to himself. Attaching a name to a condition may also create a spu-

rious impression of understanding. To say that a patient is suffering from schizophrenia actually says little more than that he has some puzzling but familiar symptoms which have often been encountered before in other patients. Historically, of course, it has been very convenient for doctors to be able to conceal their ignorance from their patients by clothing it in Greek neologisms, but all too often they also deceive themselves. They 'reify' the diagnostic concept and treat the 'disease' instead of trying to relieve their patients' symptoms, anxieties and disabilities.

Diagnoses as concepts

It is important never to lose sight of the fact that all diseases and diagnostic categories are simply concepts. Schizophrenia and manic–depressive insanity were not discovered by either Kraepelin or Bleuler. It is closer to the truth to say that they were invented by them, and we continue to use the terms a century later only because the concepts they represent make it easier to comprehend the variegated phenomena of psychotic illness than it would otherwise be. The same is true, of course, of tuberculosis and migraine. To assert, as Szasz does, that 'there is no such thing as schizophrenia' is as trite an assertion as it would be to point out that there is no such thing as tuberculosis or poverty. None of these are objects; none has mass, velocity or position in space. All three are concepts which may in time lose their usefulness and pass out of use, as earlier concepts like phthisis and monomania have already done. But if this happens it will be because they have been replaced by other more useful concepts, not because of any sudden realisation that they do not exist. And, of course, to tell a bewildered patient who has been told he is suffering from schizophrenia that there is no such thing does not remove his disabilities, or prevent hallucinatory voices from tormenting him, any more than a man whose lungs have been destroyed by the tubercle bacillus would be prevented from dying by being told there was no such thing as tuberculosis.

Classification on the basis of symptoms

It is widely agreed that classifications of diseases should, wherever possible, be based on aetiology. This is so simply because physicians have learnt by experience that aetiological classifications are almost invariably more useful than others. Classifications of infections based on the identity of the infecting organism are, for example, more useful than those based on purely clinical phenomena – the patient's fever, tachycardia, malaise and limb pains, the appearance of his tongue and the fetor on his breath – because they provide more information about treatment, prognosis and the risk to others. Unfortunately, apart from a few conditions like delirium tremens, dementia due to human immunodeficiency virus (HIV) and Wernicke's encephalopathy, the aetiology of most psychiatric disorders is still unknown, or all that is known for certain is that both genetic and environmental factors are involved. For this reason, most contemporary classifications of psychiatric disorders are largely based on clinical symptoms, a term which is usually assumed to include abnormalities of subjective experience elicited by questioning and abnormalities of behaviour observed by the examiner or described to him by others, in addition to the symptoms of which the patient actually complains.

In all branches of medicine diseases usually start by being defined by their clinical symptoms, largely because these are the overt manifestations of illness. They are the reasons for the patient seeking medical attention in the first place, or being identified as ill by other people. But in most other medical disciplines, apart perhaps from neurology, this is no longer so. As their aetiology has slowly been elucidated they have come to be defined instead by the presence of some more fundamental characteristic – a distinctive morbid anatomy perhaps, or an infective agent or a biochemical defect. Phthisis, for example, which was originally defined by its symptoms and clinical course, became pulmonary tuberculosis, defined by a characteristic histology and the presence of the *Mycobacterium* tubercule, when it became clear that this organism was ultimately responsible for the symptoms; and myxoedema, originally defined by the patient's complaints and appearance, became hypothyroidism, defined by an abnormally low level of circulating thyroxine, when it was established that the syndrome was a consequence of thyroid deficiency. A few conditions, like migraine, dystonia deformans and spasmodic torticollis, are still defined by their symptoms, but during the last 100 years these have dwindled to a small minority. We assume that the same transition will eventually take place for psychiatric disorders also, as their aetiology is slowly unravelled, but so far this has only occurred for a few conditions. The majority are still defined by their clinical features. In Scadding's terminology their defining characteristic is still their syndrome (Scadding 1963).

This state of affairs has a number of important consequences. Decisions about the presence or absence of symptoms are relatively unreliable: and, because few psychiatric illnesses have pathognomonic symptoms, most conditions have to be defined by the presence of some or most of a group of symptoms rather than by the presence of one key symptom. In the jargon of nosology they are *polythetic* rather than *monothetic*. This invites ambiguity and lowers reliability still further unless operational definitions are adopted (see below). Another important consequence is that most psychiatric diagnoses can never be confirmed or refuted, for there is no external criterion to appeal to. If two clinicians disagree about whether a patient is suffering from Pick's disease or Alzheimer's disease their disagreement can eventually be resolved by postmortem examination of the brain, for the defining characteristic of both conditions is its histology. But if two clinicians disagree about whether a patient is suffering from a schizophrenic or an affective illness no comparable criterion is available, for both schizophrenic and affective disorders are defined by their clinical syndromes. There is therefore no way of resolving the disagreement except by appeal to authority. One can only conclude either that the two clinicians have elicited different symptoms, or that they have different concepts (or are using different definitions) of schizophrenia and affective illness.

For these and other reasons it has often been suggested that symptoms should be ignored and a new classification developed on an entirely different basis. Psychoanalysts have frequently advocated a classification based on psychodynamic defence mechanisms and stages of libidinal development. In the 1950s, clinical psychologists extolled the advantages of a classification based on scores on batteries of cognitive and projective tests. More recently, learning theorists have argued that we should classify patients on the basis of a comprehensive analysis of their total behavioural repertoire. In principle all of these approaches are perfectly legitimate. In practice, however, none of them has ever progressed beyond the stage of advocacy. Although a series of different professional groups has, each in turn, proposed new classifications based on the mechanisms, scores or behaviours they themselves were most interested in, none has ever made a serious attempt to develop, test and use the new classification they were advocating. It is likely that a classification based on psychodynamic defence mechanisms would be hamstrung by the low reliability common to all inferential judgements, that one based on cognitive and projective test results would yield even fewer useful prognostic distinctions than one based on symptoms, and that any classification aspiring to be based on an analysis of the patient's total behavioural repertoire would simply prove to be impracticable, but one can only suspect these things because such classifications have never been developed.

Two other alternatives are sometimes proposed: classification on the basis of treatment response and classification on the basis of the course or outcome of the illness. Unfortunately, neither is feasible. The fatal weakness of the treatment response proposal is that there are few if any specific treatments in psychiatry. Depressive, schizophrenic and manic illnesses may all respond to ECT; schizophrenic and manic illnesses both respond to antipsychotic drugs; depressions and anxiety states both respond to cognitive psychotherapy; and so on. Worse still, these therapies are not mutually exclusive. The patient who responds to ECT often responds equally well to an antipsychotic agent. In any case, the fact that two disorders respond to the same treatment does not imply that they share the same aetiology. Depression, panic attacks and nocturnal enuresis all respond to imipramine, and bruises, dysmenorrhoea, rheumatoid arthritis and rheumatic fever all respond to aspirin. Classification on the basis of outcome is equally impracticable, though for rather different reasons. One of the main functions of a diagnosis is to indicate the need for treatment, and the relative merits of different therapies. But if outcome was the defining characteristic one would, logically, have to wait until the outcome was known before making the diagnosis and therefore knowing which treatment to use. In any case most disorders, in psychiatry as in other branches of medicine, can have a wide range of outcomes. The fact that the patient recovered within a few weeks does not prove that he was suffering from chickenpox rather than smallpox, it merely makes it more likely. It is sometimes assumed that Kraepelin's classification, or at least his distinction between dementia praecox and manic–depressive insanity, was based on long-term outcome, but this is a misunderstanding. Kraepelin certainly emphasised the difference in the lifetime course of his two great rubrics, and perhaps subdivided the functional psychoses in the way that he did in order to maximise the difference in outcome between dementia praecox and manic–depressive insanity. But he used outcome as a validating criterion (i.e. as evidence that his two rubrics were fundamentally different disorders), not as a defining characteristic. Otherwise, when patients with dementia praecox recovered completely he would automatically have changed their diagnosis.

As things stand, therefore, we have no choice but to use a classification which is largely based on symptoms, despite its shortcomings and imperfections, because no practical alternative has yet been developed.

THE DIAGNOSTIC INTERVIEW

So far, we have discussed why psychiatric disorders have to be classified and why that classification is largely based on symptoms. We have also noted that all diagnoses are arbitrary concepts, liable to be altered or discarded as circumstances change; and that psychiatric diagnoses are particularly likely to be misunderstood and misused. We must now consider the important practical implications of these decisions; in particular, how to elicit the patient's symptoms as completely and as reliably as possible, and how to make the appropriate diagnosis when this has been done. As the general principles of psychiatric interviewing have been described in detail in Chapter 8, only matters bearing specifically on diagnostic interviews need be discussed here.

The conduct of the interview

Traditionally, psychiatrists, like other physicians, have usually detected symptoms by holding a free-ranging interview with the patient, and sometimes with his relatives also, and have assumed that the symptoms they elicited were present and that those they failed to elicit were absent. Unfortunately, these happy assumptions are unwarranted, as the many reliability studies carried out in the 1950s quickly revealed. A well-known study of the reliability of clinical ratings made under ordinary National Health Service working conditions illustrates the scale of the problem. A series of 90 patients referred to an English mental hospital were each reinterviewed by one of two research psychiatrists a few days after being seen as outpatients or on a domiciliary consultation by one of three consultants. All five of these interviewers recorded the presence or absence of 24 key symptoms in each patient. Despite having discussed their criteria for rating these items beforehand, the average 'positive percentage agreement' between the first and second interviewers was only 46% (Kreitman et al 1961). In other words, when one psychiatrist recorded a symptom as present there was less than a 50:50 chance of his colleague agreeing with him.

Many factors contribute to this low reliability. There are behavioural differences between one interviewer and another. They ask different questions, show interest and probe further in different places, establish different sorts of relationship with the patients, and so on. Their preconceptions are also important. If two interviewers are expecting to find different symptoms, both may succeed in fulfilling their expectations by means of subtle differences in the wording of their questions, and in the way in which they interpret ambiguous replies. Finally, important conceptual differences are often involved. Common terms like 'anxiety', 'delusion' and 'thought disorder' may be used in rather different ways by different psychiatrists without their being aware of the fact; and even when there is no disagreement over the meaning of a term, there is often disagreement over the extent to which graded characteristics, like worry or tension, have to be present to justify a positive rating.

Because of these problems, unstructured interviewing methods are no longer used for research purposes. Instead a variety of 'structured' or 'standardised' interviews are employed. These specify not only, as rating scales do, the way in which symptoms are recorded, but also the manner in which they are elicited. Definitions, implicit or explicit, are provided for each item, and, subject to varying degrees of flexibility, the questions the patient is asked, and their order, are predetermined and ratings are made serially as the interview progresses rather than collectively at the end. Examples of these diagnostic instruments, include the Present State Examination (Wing et al 1974) and the Diagnostic Interview Schedule (Robins et al 1981). With such instruments trained raters achieve considerably higher reliability than is possible under ordinary clinical conditions.

Structured interviews of this kind are generally unsuitable for ordinary clinical purposes, mainly because they are not sufficiently flexible. The need to cover a wide range of symptomatology makes them either too long or too sketchy, and they do not permit that rapid focusing on the patient's main difficulties that is the essence of a good assessment interview. Even so, much of the discipline involved in structured interviewing can be incorporated into any information-gathering interview. Most of the principles involved are simple enough, even self-evident, though this does not stop them being flouted, even by experienced clinicians who ought to know better. Knowing how to conduct a diagnostic interview – when to give the patient free rein and when to interrupt him, which areas to concentrate on, and how to phrase one's questions so as to focus the patient's replies without putting words into his mouth – is a skill which is best learned by experience, but which is not necessarily acquired with experience. Knowing how to interpret what the patients says and what information is necessary to establish the presence of particular symptoms is, or ought to be, a simpler matter. If the interviewer understands, and different interviewers agree, precisely what is meant by the technical terms like depersonalisation and delusion of control that are used to describe symptomatology, it will usually be clear to him what information he needs to establish the presence of the symptom in question. The problem is essentially one of definition. Adequate definitions are not provided in any systematic way in most textbooks, or even in psychiatric dictionaries or glossaries, and much of the low reliability of clinical ratings is attributable to this. A comprehensive list can be found in the manual of the Present State Examination (Wing et al 1974).

Information from relatives

It is a sound principle always to obtain collateral history from a relative or appropriate other, if possible, before making a formulation of the problem. Often 10 minutes will suffice to establish that the relative's perception of the situation is essentially the same as the patient's, but it is commonplace for his account to be different in important ways. He may describe a more alarming situation than the patient has admitted to, or make it clear that the symptoms the patient complains of are not a new development but have been present to a greater or lesser extent for years. It is particularly important to get an independent history from someone else if there is any suspicion of alcohol or drug abuse. The capacity of people with alcohol problems to minimise or gloss over the ways in which their drinking has disrupted their lives is difficult to exaggerate and the diagnosis will often be missed if the patient's account is accepted without corroboration.

THE RELATIONSHIP BETWEEN SYMPTOMS AND DIAGNOSIS

For reasons discussed previously, diagnoses are mainly based on symptoms – the patient's complaints and descriptions of abnormal subjective experiences and the behavioural abnormalities evident on examination or reported by others. Other factors, like the patient's age, sex and personality and the course of the illness in the past, are certainly taken into account, but the patient's symptoms, past and present, are the main determinants. Unfortunately, it is only comparatively recently that we have appreciated the need to specify the relationship between symptoms and diagnosis. Textbooks have always made it clear that the characteristic symptoms of schizophrenia were thought disorder, auditory hallucinations and delusions of control, that the characteristic symptoms of melancholia were severe depression, retardation and early morning wakening, that the characteristic features of obsessional illness were persistent and disabling compulsive acts or ruminations, and so on. They have not made it clear, however, which diagnosis should be given to someone with auditory hallucinations alone; or with obsessional ruminations in the presence of severe depression. As a result, psychiatrists frequently made different diagnoses when confronted with such situations and diagnostic reliability was low.

What was needed were *rules of application* or *operational definitions* specifying the appropriate diagnosis for every possible combination of symptoms. Instead of simply listing the typical features of diagnosis X as A, B, C and sometimes D, as they had generally done in the past, textbooks and glossaries needed to say something like this: before diagnosis X can be made A must be present, together with one or more of B, C and D, and E must be absent. As with symptoms themselves, the problem is primarily a matter of adequate definition. In the last 20 years, operational definitions of this kind have slowly come into everyday clinical use. In 1972 Eli Robins and his colleagues in St Louis published operational criteria for 15 major diagnostic categories (Feighner et al 1972) and since then many alternative operational definitions have been published for most of the main syndromes and their use has become the norm in clinical research. The most decisive change, however, was the American Psychiatric Association's decision to provide an operational definition for every diagnostic category in the third edition of its Diagnostic and Statistical Manual (DSM-III) (APA 1980). As a result, since 1980 American psychiatrists have been committed to using operational definitions for all their diagnostic terms, not just in research but in routine clinical practice as well.

DSM-III's successors DSM-IIIR (APA 1987) and DSM-IV (APA 1994) follow broadly similar schemes of sets of operational definitions. Until recently the system used by the International Classification of Diseases was an essentially descriptive one but in the latest edition ICD-10 (WHO 1992) the clinical descriptions are followed by specific operational criteria in a very similar style to that of DSM-IV. The terminology and definitions of the two systems are not of course the same but, as may be seen from Table 10.1, there is a good deal of common ground between them. Both classifications provide detailed subdivisions of the categories shown in Table 10.1 and the system by which ICD-10 divides what it still calls 'organic' including symptomatic mental disorders may be seen in Table 10.2. DSM-IV avoids the use of the term organic and, although ICD-10 does not, as described in Chapter 1 those responsible for this classification in their 'Notes on unresolved problems' (Cooper 1991) acknowledge that since the use of advanced imaging has revealed structural and functional findings outwith the normal range in conditions such as schizophrenia, affective disorder etc., we no longer know what to call organic. IDC-10 is a single

Table 10.1 Comparison of principal categories of ICD-10 and DSM-IV – Axis I	
ICD-10	DSM-IV – Axis I
F00–F09 Organic including symptomatic mental disorders	Delirium dementia and amnestic and other cognitive disorders
F10–F19 Mental and behavioural disorders due to psychoactive substance abuse	Substance-related disorders
F20–F29 Schizophrenia, schizotypal and delusional disorders	Schizophrenia and other psychotic disorders
F30–F39 Mood (affective) disorders	Mood disorders
F40–F48 Neurotic, stress-related and somatoform disorders	Anxiety disorders Somatoform disorders
F50–F59 Behavioural syndromes associated with physiological disturbances and physical factors	Eating disorders Sleep disorders Sexual and gender identity disorders
F60–F69 Disorder of adult personality and behaviour	Personality disorders
F70–F79 Mental retardation	Disorders usually first diagnosed in infancy childhood and adolescence includes
F80–89 Disorders of psychological development F90–F98 Behavioural and emotional disorders with onset usually occurring in childhood and adolescence	Mental retardation Pervasive developmental disorder Attention deficit and disruptive behaviour disorders and other disorders of infancy childhood or adolescence
F99 Unspecified mental disorder	Other conditions that may be a focus of clinical attention

Table 10.2 Classification of 'organic' disorders			
ICD-10 3 Character Classification of organic including symptomatic mental disorders		**ICD-10 4 Character** Classification of dementia in Alzheimer's disease F00	
F00	Dementia in Alzheimer's disease →	**F00.0**	Dementia in Alzheimer's disease with early onset
F01	Vascular dementia	**F00.1**	Dementia in Alzheimer's disease with late onset
F02	Dementia in other diseases	**F00.2**	Dementia in Alzheimer's disease atypical or mixed type
F03	Unspecified dementia	**F00.9**	Dementia in Alzheimer's disease
F04	Organic amnesiac syndrome not induced by alcohol		unspecified
F05	Delirium, not induced by alcohol or other psychoactive substances		
F06	Other mental disorders due to brain damage and dysfunction and to physical disease		
F07	Personality and behavioural disorders due to brain disease, damage and dysfunction		
F09	Unspecified organic or symptomatic mental disorder		

Table 10.3 Five Axes of DSM-IV multiaxial classification	
Axis I	Clinical disorders Other conditions that may be a focus of clinical attention (e.g. maladaptive behaviours affecting a medical condition)
Axis II	Personality disorders Mental retardation
Axis III	General medical conditions
Axis IV	Psychosocial and environmental problems
Axis V	Global assessment of functioning

axis classification but DSM-IV (like its predecessors) advocates the use of five axes to promote consideration of all relevant aspects of clinical situations. The five axes are shown in Table 10.3.

The introduction of these systems of operational definitions has provided a means of classifying clinical pictures in a way that can be clearly communicated to others and which, as we shall see below, greatly enhances the reliability of diagnostic classification.

Diagnostic hierarchies

Insofar as there is a formal structure to the relationship between symptoms and diagnoses it is a hierarchical one. At the top of their hierarchy come the organic psy-

choses. If there is evidence of organicity – perhaps clinical or EEG evidence of epilepsy or definite cognitive impairment – this overrides all other considerations, and whatever other symptoms the patient has, psychotic or neurotic, the diagnosis is organic. Schizophrenia has traditionally come next in the hierarchy. To many European psychiatrists certain symptoms are regarded as diagnostic of schizophrenia, regardless of which other symptoms are also present, provided only that there is no question of cerebral disease. The 'symptoms of the first rank' which Schneider (1959) regarded as pathognomonic of schizophrenia 'except in the presence of coarse brain disease' constitute an explicit statement of this convention, and other clinicians have attached a similar significance to symptoms like thought disorder and incongruity of affect. For Schneider and his successors, third place in the hierarchy is occupied by the affective disorders. Even if the characteristic features of mania or melancholia are unmistakably present, organic or schizophrenic symptoms take precedence. As a result, patients with both schizophrenic and affective symptoms are classified as schizophrenics, and were so classified in ICD-9. However, in ICD-10, schizophrenic and affective disorders are both at the same level. A diagnosis of schizophrenia cannot be made if the full depressive or manic syndrome is also present 'unless it is clear that schizophrenic symptoms antedated the affective disturbance'. Neurotic, stress-related and somatoform disorders come at the bottom of the hierarchy. As a result, patients with both neurotic and psychotic symptoms are regarded as having psychotic illnesses. Another consequence of the relative status of neurotic and psychotic symptoms in the hierarchy is that, for those who still employ the traditional distinction between psychotic and neurotic depression, the latter is characterised by the absence of the characteristic features of psychotic depression, rather than by the possession of typical symptoms of its own. In general, any given diagnosis *excludes* the presence of the symptoms of all higher members of the hierarchy and *embraces* the symptoms of all lower members.

It is no coincidence that the order in which diagnostic categories are arranged in the international and other classifications is the same as in this hierarchy, for both reflect the sequence of questions psychiatrists commonly ask themselves when making a diagnosis. Indeed, a very similar sequence is involved in the decision pathways of computer programs like Catego (Wing et al 1974). The psychologist Graham Foulds suggested that this structure was inherent in the nature of psychiatric illness but it is more likely that it is a man-made imposition. It is a firm principle in medicine that every effort should be made to account for the patient's symptoms in terms of a single diagnosis. In a situation in which most individual symptoms are liable to be encountered in the presence of a wide range of other symptoms this is not easy to achieve unless the defining characteristics of different illnesses are in a hierarchical relationship to one another, with the least common symptoms at the top and the most common at the bottom. There is also some empirical justification for this arrangement. For example, when schizophrenic and neurotic symptoms coexist, the patient's prognosis and response to treatment are determined more by the former than by the latter, so if only one diagnosis is allowable it is more appropriate to regard the patient as schizophrenic than as neurotic.

INTERNATIONAL DIFFERENCES IN DIAGNOSTIC CRITERIA

As described above, until comparatively recently the relationship between symptoms and diagnoses was vague and ill defined. Many technical terms – like thought disorder, dependency and immaturity – were also poorly defined. As a result, trainees were forced to learn how to make diagnoses by copying their teachers. In the absence of adequate rules the only way to learn which of their patients should be regarded as schizophrenics was to observe which patients their mentors gave this diagnosis to and do the same. As a result, diagnostic criteria were at the mercy of the personal views and idiosyncrasies of influential teachers, and also liable to be affected by therapeutic fashions and innova-

tions, and changing assumptions about aetiology. This led to the development of substantial differences in the way in which several key diagnostic terms were used in different centres. The less contact there was between two centres – and of course national boundaries and language differences were substantial impediments to such contact – the more likely it was that progressive differences in diagnostic usage would develop.

The best documented of these differences in usage were those that developed between Britain and the USA in the 1940s and 1950s. The comparative studies carried out by the US/UK Diagnostic Project in the 1960s established that, in comparable series of patients, psychiatrists in New York diagnosed schizophrenia twice as frequently as their counterparts in London. Patients regarded in London as suffering from depressive illnesses or mania, or even neurotic illnesses or personality disorders, were all diagnosed as schizophrenics in New York (Cooper et al 1972). The International Pilot Study of Schizophrenia confirmed that American psychiatrists had an unusually broad concept of schizophrenia, and also showed that the same was true, for quite different reasons, of Russian psychiatrists (WHO 1973). Of the nine centres involved, seven (London, Prague, Aarhus in Denmark, Ibadan in Nigeria, Agra in India, Cali in Colombia and Taipei in Formosa) shared a very similar concept of schizophrenia, but Washington and Moscow both had a much broader concept. In Europe the situation was complicated by the fact that Scandinavian psychiatrists, particularly the Norwegians and the Danes, made frequent use of a diagnosis of reactive or psychogenic psychosis which embraced many patients who would have been regarded as having schizophrenic or affective psychoses in Britain or Germany. And French psychiatrists used a number of categories like *délire chronique* and *bouffée délirante* which had no counterpart in other nomenclatures. These differences are now disappearing, and for the younger generation of psychiatrists are already a thing of the past. The very broad American concept of schizophrenia was psychoanalytic in origin and the decline of psychoanalytic influence in the 1970s, together with a renewed interest in descriptive psychopathology and classification, led to a rapid change. Indeed, the contemporary American concept of schizophrenia embodied in the operation criteria of DSM-IV is somewhat narrower than the current British concept. The widespread adoption of the operational definitions of DSM-III and DSM-IV by research workers in many different parts of the world has also played an important role in reducing international differences in usage.

It is important to realise that it is meaningless to ask who is right where any of these differences, past or present, are concerned. If two individual psychiatrists disagree about a diagnosis we are accustomed to assume that whichever of the two is more experienced, or whom we respect the more, is probably right. But if experienced psychiatrists in different centres disagree with one another when presented with identical information, all one can say is that they have different concepts of that condition. The same is true of two psychiatrists using different operational definitions of the same syndrome. One can check that they are both using their respective definitions appropriately, but beyond that one can only concede that the two definitions embrace different populations of patients. However, although it is meaningless to ask who is *right*, it is perfectly legitimate, and necessary, to ask which concept of definition is more *useful*. Essentially, the choice between alternative definitions is a matter of validity. If we knew more about the aetiology of psychiatric disorders we could easily decide which of the two alternative definitions of the syndrome correlated better with the underlying abnormality, just as we could easily decide which clinical definition of mitral stenosis was most reliably associated with narrowing of the mitral valve, or which clinical definition of Pick's disease was most reliably associated with the characteristic pathology of that condition. In the absence of this knowledge all we can do is ask which of the competing definitions most successfully meets some arbitrary criterion like homogeneity of outcome or treatment response. But as different criteria may be best satisfied by different definitions the problem is not resolved. For example, the definition of schizophrenia which most successfully identifies patients who subsequently develop a defect state and become chronic invalids is probably different from the definition which gives the highest monozygotic:dizygotic concordance ratio in twin populations. We must accept, therefore, that until we know more about the aetiology of the various syndromes we recognise and treat we cannot be sure how they should best be defined. As a result, we will probably have to accept the coexistence of a number of alternative operational definitions of syndromes like schizophrenia, and in some areas of alternative classifications, for some time to come.

CONTEMPORARY CLASSIFICATIONS

The international classification

International classifications of mental disorders have existed for over 100 years but had little influence until the late 1960s. In response to strenuous efforts by the World Health Organization (WHO), most countries were persuaded to sacrifice their own traditions and aspirations in the interests of international communication and to use the nomenclature and definitions of the eighth revision of the *International Classification of Diseases, Injuries and Causes of Death* (ICD-8) which came into use in 1969.

This eighth revision was replaced by a ninth (ICD-9) a decade later. If one compares the successive revisions of the ICD from the sixth in 1948 to the ninth in 1979, each was undoubtedly an improvement on its predecessor. The mental disorders section of ICD-6 was primarily a classification of psychoses and mental deficiency. Its successors provided much more adequate coverage of neurotic and stress-related disorders, of childhood disorders and of the range of conditions attributable to alcohol and drug dependence and abuse. Many new terms were introduced, a few obsolete ones like involutional melancholia were dropped and every category was provided with a brief definition (and sometimes a list of synonyms and another list of incompatible alternative diagnoses as a further aid to consistent usage). Despite these improvements the inherent problems associated with an international classification became more apparent with each revision. The definitions provided in ICD-8 and ICD-9 were not operational definitions. They were simply thumb-nail sketches of the clinical concept in question. They described its essential features well enough but did not provide rules of application. A more fundamental problem was that radical change of any kind was very difficult to effect, because every country had to be willing to accept whatever innovations were introduced, and any attempt to force the pace risked damaging the fragile international consensus on which the whole enterprise was based. Another major problem was that, because national representatives were always prepared to argue more forcefully for the inclusion of their own favourite terms than they were to oppose the efforts of others to do likewise, there was a constant tendency for the classification to expand by incorporating alternative and sometimes incompatible concepts. ICD-9 contained no less than 13 categories for patients with depressive symptoms, because in effect two or three different ways of classifying depressions were included alongside one another.

The tenth revision (ICD-10)

Preparation of ICD-10 started as long ago as 1983 but it did not finally come into use in the UK and most other countries until 1993. It has a new title – the *International Statistical Classification of Diseases and Related Health Problems* – and a new alphanumeric format (WHO 1992). The main purpose of the latter is to provide more categories (there are 26 letters in the alphabet but only 10 digits) and so leave space for future expansion without the whole classification having to be changed. The general format of the section entitled 'mental, behavioural and developmental disorders' (F00–F99) is very similar to that of the American Psychiatric Association's recent classifications because it incorporates many of the radical innovations introduced in DSM-III (see below). The traditional distinction between psychoses and neuroses has been laid aside, though the terms themselves are retained, and all mood (affective) disorders are brought together in a single grouping (F3). All disorders due to the use of psychoactive substances, including alcohol, have also been brought together under a common format (F1). Most categories are provided with both 'diagnostic guidelines' for everyday clinical use and separate 'diagnostic criteria for research'. It will probably remain in use for considerably longer than the 10 years for which ICD-6 to ICD-9 were each used. It is likely, therefore, to be the classification that today's young psychiatrists will use for most of their careers. Field trails of the 1986 draft text were held in 194 different centres in 55 different countries and the final text benefited greatly from the comments of users in these very varied settings, and the evidence they provided of the acceptability, coverage and inter-rater reliability of the provisional categories and definitions of that draft.

The American Psychiatric Association's classifications

The first edition of the American Psychiatric Association's *Diagnostic and Statistical Manual of Mental Disorders* (DSM-I) was published in 1952. Its format reflected the dominant Meyerian philosophy of the times and, although its influence was limited, it was the first official nomenclature to provide a glossary of descriptions of the diagnostic categories it listed. The second edition (DSM-II), published in 1968, was, like the corresponding English glossary (General Register Office 1968), a national glossary to the nomenclature of ICD-8, the American Psychiatric Association (APA) having been persuaded on this occasion to sacrifice its own diagnostic preferences in the interests of international conformity.

DSM-III

The third edition (DSM-III), published in 1980, was radically different from any previous classification (APA 1980). Its innovations were a response to the evidence that had accumulated over the previous 20 years that psychiatric diagnoses were generally unreliable, that there were systematic differences in the usage of key terms like 'schizophrenia' between the USA and other parts of the world, and that major changes were needed to the overall format of the international and other existing classifications. It was also evidence of a sea change in the orientation of American psychiatry; the end of the psychodynamic era and the dawn of a new biological or 'neo-kraepelinian' era. For the first time in any classification of disease almost every diagnostic category was given an operational definition to make it as clear as possible which patients were and were not covered by that rubric. Although this made the manual five times the size of its predecessors – and involved much discussion, argument and persuasion as well as extensive field trials in order to secure the necessary agreement – the result, as the field trials demonstrated, was that the reliability of most of its 200 categories was far higher than in any previous classification.

DSM-III was also a multiaxial classification with separate axes allowing the systematic recording of five different information sets: the clinical syndrome (Axis I); lifelong disorders or handicaps like personality disorders and specific developmental disorders (Axis II); associated physical conditions (Axis III); the severity of psychosocial stressors (Axis IV); and the highest level of social and occupational functioning in the past year (Axis V). The clinical syndromes coded on Axis I were also arranged in a novel sequence; in particular, the traditional distinction between neuroses and psychoses was abandoned to allow all affective disorders to be brought together. A further important change was that most, although not all, diagnostic terms were either explicitly divested of their aetiological implications or replaced by new terms devoid of such implications. As a result, many of the hallowed terms of psychiatry, like hysteria and manic-depressive illness, and even psychosis and neurosis, were discarded and replaced by stark, utilitarian terms like somatoform disorder, factitious disorder and paraphilia.

Classifications always tend to be controversial, if only because they involve fundamental concepts and important philosophical assumptions. Initially, DSM-III and its principal architect, Robert Spitzer, were bitterly criticised by many senior American psychiatrists for introducing what they regarded as a crude 'Chinese menu' approach to diagnosis.

Such objections were perhaps most elegantly expressed by Cancro (1983), who recommended that the following verse could usefully be printed on every copy of DSM-III:

> That false secondary Power
> By which we multiply distinctions, then
> Deem that our puny boundaries are things
> That we perceive and not that we have made.
> (Wordsworth, The Prelude, II)

Clinical researchers and the younger generation of American psychiatrists, on the other hand, welcomed the new classification with enthusiasm (Jampala et al 1986) and it was soon clear the DSM-III was going to have a major influence on American psychiatry, particularly on clinical and biological research. Indeed, within a few years of its publication it had become an all-time psychiatric best-seller and made huge profits for the APA. It had also been translated into 13 other languages and its definitions were being widely used throughout the world. DSM-III also led to important changes in American usage of several diagnostic terms (Loranger 1990). Fewer patients were labelled as schizophrenics and more were diagnosed as having unipolar or bipolar affective disorders. The creation of a separate axis for them also resulted in more extensive use of personality disorder diagnoses.

DSM-IIIR

DSM-III was replaced by an extensive revision, DSM-IIIR, in 1987 (APA 1987). No fundamental changes were involved but a substantial number of minor alterations were introduced. The classification of sleep disorders was expanded, mental retardation was moved from Axis I to Axis II, one or two categories were dropped and one or two new ones introduced. Schizoaffective disorders were given an operational definition for the first time; the definition of paranoid disorders was enlarged to include patients with grandiose, somatic and erotomanic delusions, as well as those with delusions, of persecution and jealousy; the inappropriate stipulation that schizophrenia must start before the age of 45 years was dropped; and 'agoraphobia with panic attacks' was replaced by 'panic disorder with secondary agoraphobia' in deference to the emerging view that panic attacks were the primary phenomenon. Most important of all, the definition of the majority of disorders listed in the glossary was altered, usually in fairly minor ways.

Individually, most of these changes were improvements. They involved either the correction of mistakes or misjudgements, or rational responses to new evidence or a change in the climate of opinion. Even so, it is doubtful whether it was wise to introduce a new classification after only 7 years, with all the disruption to newly established clinical concepts, to clinical research and to residency training programmes that new definitions inevitably involve.

DSM-IV

In 1987 the APA set up a new task force, to produce yet another revision of its Diagnostic and Statistical Manual, DSM-IV, 'concurrently and congruently' with ICD-10. It was assumed that DSM-IV and ICD-10 would both be introduced in 1993. Unfortunately, the APA did not appreciate that by 1987 the major elements of the format of the mental disorders section of ICD-10 had already been decided. As a result, the task force was forced to choose between accepting the, in some cases rather unsatisfactory, terminology and definitions of ICD-10 in order to harmonise the two classifications as much as possible; or alternatively to ignore ICD-10 and accept the recommendations of the 13 work groups it had set up to draft proposals for the format of each of the individual sections of DSM-IV (Kendell 1991). The latter course was chosen and because of this the differences between DSM-IV and ICD-10 are more extensive than they might have been if the DSM-IV task force had been set up 2 or 3 years earlier.

Future classifications of mental disorders

Until we know more about the aetiology of the major syndromes like schizophrenia, Alzheimer's disease and bipolar disorder it is unlikely that any future classification will be self-evidently superior to those now available. Literature reviews, follow-up studies, family studies, therapeutic trials and laborious analyses of sets of ratings derived from structured interviews with representative populations of patients can only take us so far. Apart from one or two under-researched areas like the personality disorders, we may already be approaching the limits of what can be achieved by traditional clinical and epidemiological means. We should not be in a hurry, therefore, to develop new versions of comprehensive, formal classifications like DSM-IV and ICD-10. It would be better to wait and see what novel concepts are introduced over the next decade by individual research groups, and what insights we gain from burgeoning developments in the neurosciences and human genetics. Other branches of medicine did not progress by a dogged pursuit of better and better classifications of their subject matter. They did so by acquiring new technologies, by developing radically new concepts and by elucidating fundamental mechanisms.

THE RELIABILITY AND VALIDITY OF PSYCHIATRIC DIAGNOSES

Reliability

The reliability of psychiatric diagnoses is usually measured in one of two ways. Either a diagnostic interview is watched by a passive observer who makes his own independent diagnosis at the end (*observer method*), or else a second diagnostician conducts an independent interview with the patient a few hours or days after the first (*reinterview method*). The former overestimates reliability because all variation in the conduct of the interview is eliminated; the latter may underestimate it because the subject's clinical state may change in the interval between the two interviews, and he may react differently to the second interview simply because it is a repetition of the first.

Many reliability studies were carried out in the 1950s and 1960s and most of them found reliability to be depressingly low. The studies of Beck in Philadelphia and Kreitman in Chichester are often quoted because they were well designed and the participants were all experienced psychiatrists. Both used the reinterview method. Beck obtained 54% agreement for specific diagnosis, compared with the 15–19% agreement that could have arisen by chance alone. Kreitman, using a restricted range of 11 diagnostic categories, obtained 63% agreement. There are three main ways of reducing disagreement: using structured or standardised interviews to minimise variation in the conduct of the interview, and providing definitions for all the items of psychopathology covered by that interview, which together will help to minimise disagreements about which symptoms the subject exhibits; and using operational definitions to ensure that any given combination of symptoms always leads to the same diagnosis.

It has been shown repeatedly that research workers using standardised interviews can obtain considerably higher diagnostic reliability than is possible with unstructured interviews, and that further improvement can be obtained by adopting operational definitions for all diagnostic categories. For example, the field trials of DSM-III carried out in various parts of the USA in the late 1970s gave values for the reliability of the major diagnostic categories varying from 0.65 to 0.83, compared with values ranging from 0.41 to 0.77 in comparable reliability studies carried out between 1956 and 1972. Organic and psychotic disorders generally have higher reliability than neuroses and personality disorders, and for this reason reliability studies based on inpatients tend to produce higher overall reliability than those based on outpatients. The comparatively low reliability of neuroses and personality disorders is probably due to the frequency of neurotic symptoms and maladaptive personality traits in the general population, and the fact that quantitative as well as merely qualitative judgements are therefore involved.

In summary, although the studies conducted in the 1950s and 1960s demonstrated that the reliability of psychiatric diagnoses was often very low, the introduction of structured interviews and operational definitions has transformed the situation. In skilled hands, psychiatric diagnoses are now as reliable as the clinical judgements made in other branches of medicine, and sometimes more so. But reliability still does not, and probably never can, match the reliability of laboratory tests where the human eye is only required to judge the position of a needle on a scale or the timing of a colour change. Clinical judgements, whether they concern depersonalisation or bronchial breathing, are inevitably imprecise and imperfect, and the best we can do is to understand what the problems are and do our best to minimise them.

Validity

Separate from the question of reliability of diagnosis is the matter of validity – that is, whether the diagnosis is a predictor of some independent variable such as outcome or response to treatment. Reliability sets a limit on validity but reliability may be high while validity remains low, and in this situation reliability is of little value.

Textbooks of psychology usually describe four different types of validity: concurrent, predictive, construct and content. Predictive validity is the most important of these where psychiatric diagnoses are concerned. In the last resort all diagnostic concepts stand or fall by the strength of the prognostic and therapeutic implications they embody. The ability to predict the outcome of an illness, and to alter this course of events if need be, have always been the main functions of medicine. Diagnoses like pulmonary tuberculosis and bronchial carcinoma are useful and valid, not because we understand what causes them – indeed, there is much about both that we do not understand – but because they enable us to predict fairly accurately what will happen to the patient, and which therapeutic measures will and will not improve that outcome.

Although numerous studies of reliability have been carried out in the last 30 years, few direct attempts have ever been made to assess validity, either predictive validity or validity of other kinds. Indeed, it is still an open issue whether there are genuine boundaries between the clinical syndromes recognised in contemporary classifications, or between these syndromes and normality (Kendell 1989). This is partly due to lack of agreement on how best to establish the validity of diagnostic concepts, and partly because much of the basic evidence for the validity of our diagnostic categories accumulated and became accepted before anyone began to ask questions about reliability and validity. Most psychiatrists, for example, accept that the distinction between schizophrenic and affective disorders is valid because they consider it to be well established that, generally speaking, the two respond differently to antipsychotics and lithium salts, and have different long-term outcomes, the former tending to run a progressive downhill course and the latter to relapse repeatedly but to recover fully each time. To demonstrate that this is really so it would be necessary to follow up a representative population of patients with schizophrenic and affective disorders for a decade or more and then show that the differences in outcome between the two were not simply, or mainly, due to other variables like age of onset, social class and treatment. Strictly speaking, this has never been done, though it has been shown many times that, although the overlap is considerable, there are substantial and consistent differences in outcome between schizophrenic and affective illnesses.

Family studies are a further source of evidence. The fact that the relatives of schizophrenics have a raised incidence of schizophrenia but not of affective disorders, and that the relatives of patients with unipolar or bipolar affective disorders have a raised incidence of affective disorders but not of schizophrenia even when the relatives' illnesses are diagnosed blindly (Tsuang et al 1980), is evidence for the validity of the two concepts, and of the distinction between them. There is also a good deal of evidence relevant to the issue of validity implicit in the results of the numerous therapeutic trials that have been conducted in the last 30 years. These clearly establish the existence of several effective treatments for psychiatric disorders: ECT, antipsychotics, tricyclic antidepressants, lithium salts, and some behavioural and cognitive techniques. They also establish that each of these therapies has a limited sphere of action. ECT is highly effective with severe depressions, rather less effective with schizophrenic or manic illnesses, and generally ineffective elsewhere. Antipsychotics are most effective with acute schizophrenic or depressive illnesses, and largely ineffective in neurotic states. Lithium and the antidepressants show the same general pattern: one or two diagnostic categories where their effect is greatest, others where it is weaker but still demonstrable, and others where it is negligible. The fact that each of these treatments has a limited range of action, and that diagnostic categories are helpful in predicting treatment response, is indirect evidence that the categories concerned are useful and valid. On the other hand, the fact that none of these therapies is specific to a single diagnostic category, and none is effective in more than perhaps two-thirds of the members of even that category in which its action is most powerful, clearly puts limits on their validity.

Cluster analysis also provides evidence for the concurrent validity of some diagnostic categories. This is a generic term for a variety of statistical techniques designed to sort heterogeneous populations into subpopulations of 'clusters' of similar individuals, similar, that is, in respect of the ratings on which the analysis is based. If clinical ratings derived from large populations of patients are subjected to such procedures the resulting clusters usually correspond quite well with diagnostic categories such as mania, paranoid schizophrenia and melancholia, suggesting that these concepts do correspond to genuine groupings in nature (see, for example, Everitt et al 1971).

In summary, the existing evidence for the validity of most psychiatric diagnoses is rather meagre, but by no means non-existent. It is also considerably better for major syndromes like schizophrenia, mania and depression than it is for other less well-defined syndromes, or for subcategories of the major syndromes such as catatonic or paranoid schizophrenia. Eventually, of course, we assume that validity will be established by elucidating the underlying pathology.

CATEGORIES OR DIMENSIONS

Traditionally, psychiatry has always used a categorical classification or typology. That is, it has divided its subject matter, psychiatric illness, into a number of separate and mutually exclusive categories like schizophrenia, mania and Alzheimer's disease. The reasons why it has done so are clear enough. Medicine is rooted in the biological sciences and physicians were deeply impressed by the advantages botany and zoology derived from the development of detailed classifications of their subject matter into species, genera and orders in the 18th and 19th centuries. More compelling still, the structure of our language is based on classification. Every common noun – like 'tree', 'star' or 'fairy' – denotes the existence of a category or class of objects. There is, however, an alternative way of expressing the relationship between the members of a heterogeneous population, namely to assign each to a position on one or more axes or dimensions.

There has been much debate about the relative merits of these two types of classification (Table 10.4). In general, theoreticians like Eysenck have favoured a dimensional approach, while most practising clinicians – though not Kretschmer or Jung – have preferred to use a typology. It is important to appreciate that, in principle, both options – dimensions and categories – are available; there is no statistical technique or other criterion capable of deciding which is 'right'. The choice between the two is essentially a matter of deciding which is more useful, and the answer may well vary with the purpose for which the classification is required.

Table 10.4   The relative merits of categories and dimensions

Advantages of categories
- They are familiar
- They are easy to understand, to remember, and to use
- Categorisation is a ready prelude to action, e.g. the diagnosis is X and X is treated with drug D
- They are more acceptable to a somewhat conservative profession

Advantages of dimensions
- They convey more information because finer distinctions are possible
- They are more flexible, because they can easily be converted into any desired number of categories, and back again
- They do not imply the presence of unproven qualitative differences between members of different subpopulations
- They do not impose boundaries where none may exist in reality, and do not distort the observer's perception of individuals lying near the boundary between adjacent categories

The main advantage of a dimensional classification is its flexibility. Consider, for example, the advantages of an IQ – a dimensional representation of intelligence – over a typology with two categories (clever and stupid). Two individuals with IQs of 120 and 160 would both, presumably, be allocated to the 'clever' category, but this would involve losing sight of what in many situations would be an important difference between them. Conversely, two individuals with IQs of 98 and 102 are in reality almost identical, yet one would be classified as stupid and the other as clever. Moreover, a distribution of IQs can always be converted to any number of categories as occasion demands, and the boundaries of these moved up or down the scale at will. But if the members of a population are all assigned to one of the three categories (clever, ordinary and stupid) to begin with, this cannot subsequently be increased to four categories or reduced to two, except by splitting or combining some of the existing groups; nor is there any possibility of converting them to a dimension.

Another important advantage of dimensions is that they do not distract attention from the atypical in favour of the typical, or distort the observer's perception of individuals lying near the boundary between two adjacent categories. One of the most serious drawbacks of categorical classifications is the way in which they cause individuals who seem to lie halfway between two disorders, or between a disorder and a healthy state, to

be overlooked or misrepresented. Patients exhibiting a combination of schizophrenic and affective symptoms illustrate this problem very clearly. Time and again in clinical research they have either been ignored, and the study confined to patients with typical schizophrenic or affective illnesses, or, if they were included, one or other component of their symptomatology was glossed over or ignored. In other words, using a typology leads us to expect, and so to perceive, our patients as fitting neatly into one or other of its categories, whether or not they do so in reality.

The great disadvantage of dimensions is that any system involving more than one dimension can only be handled geometrically or algebraically, and if there are more than three only the latter is possible. This is why the only dimensional systems used in everyday life are those like height, weight and intelligence which only involve a single axis.

The most important advantage of a typology, apart from its familiarity, is the ease of description and conceptualisation it provides. A description of a typical member of category provides a simple and easily remembered means of defining, and subsequently of recognising, the essence of that clinical concept, and of the essential differences between it and other categories. It is also difficult to ignore the fact that categorisation is the norm in most other areas of study and is inherent in the structure of all language. If we had good evidence that psychiatric illnesses were distributed in discrete clusters and that interforms between one disorder and the next were relatively uncommon, the arguments in favour of categorical classification would be very strong. Unfortunately, we still lack much evidence. Attempts to demonstrate by discriminant function analysis that interforms between psychotic and neurotic depressions, or between schizophrenic and affective psychoses, are less common than typical members of these categories have mostly been unsuccessful (for example, Kendell & Gourlay 1970a, 1970b). The frequency with which psychiatrists are driven to employ such terms as schizoaffective, anxiety depression, borderline syndrome and the like, and the difficulty they have agreeing where to draw the boundary between one category and the next, is further evidence that in reality patterns of symptoms merge into one another and are not separated by convenient 'points of rarity'. It is said that the art of classification lies in carving nature at the joints, but where psychiatric illness is concerned we cannot be sure that we have found the joints, or even that there are many to be found.

Despite the considerable theoretical attractions it is unlikely that psychiatry will adopt a dimensional classification for ordinary clinical purposes in the foreseeable future. Old traditions die hard, and there is little immediate prospect of the advocates of dimensional systems being able to agree how many dimensions are needed and what their identity should be. In the long run, though, it is difficult to believe that personality disorder, and perhaps also neurotic illness, will not be more conveniently and usefully portrayed by a set of dimensions than by the discrete types we attempt to delineate at present. There is already broad agreement that the protean variations of normal personality are better portrayed by dimensions, and the continuity between normal personality and the clinical categories of personality disorder and neurotic illness is increasingly difficult to ignore. Where psychotic illness is concerned, however, the balance of advantages and disadvantages is rather different and it may well be that here a typology will continue to be preferable, even though the names of the disorders we recognise, and their defining characteristics, may change considerably as we come to understand their aetiology.

Atypical presentations

The limitations placed upon psychiatric diagnoses by the fact that they are based upon the clinical picture and outcome of the various conditions have been emphasised in this chapter and it will be obvious that sometimes patients will be given diagnoses which in retrospect will appear to have been inappropriate. As diagnosis is a guide to prognosis and treatment, this can at times be very unfortunate and it is important to consider the sorts of atypical presentation that may give rise to such situations.

Atypical presentations may be classified as:

- 'Functional' disorders (principally affective and schizophrenic illnesses) which have a presentation suggestive either of a different functional disorder or of an 'organic' disorder.
- 'Organic' disorders which have a presentation suggestive of functional illness.

These issues have been dealt with in detail elsewhere (Coffey & Johnstone 1997) and only the main points are summarised here.

Atypical presentations of affective disorder most often concern depressive illness. In masked depression patients present their complaints in physical terms. The response of such patients to antidepressant therapy has been claimed as evidence that the disorders are depressive in nature (Paykel & Norton 1982). It is not however possible to sustain the view that the response to such drugs is specific to affective illness. None the less, in practical terms it is important not to miss depressive illness presenting in this way. A further area of difficulty is the matter of depressive illness presenting as dementia – so called 'pseudodementia'. Doubts have been expressed about this term (Folstein & Rabins 1991) but clinical experience supports the concept in that, of 19 patients diagnosed as having pseudodementia over a 10 year period, only one had an earlier diagnosis of pseudodementia revised to dementia (Sachdev et al 1990). Clinically important atypical presentations of elevated mood are probably less common but Tyrer et al (1993) have described patients where behavioural disturbance was initially ascribed to personality disorder requiring repeated admission but who later developed features of bipolar affective disorder. Following treatment with mood stabilisation further admissions were not required.

It is quite common for schizophrenic disorder to have been preceded by a manic or depressive episode (Lewis & Pietrowski 1954) and cynics may consider that this is due to reluctance to diagnose schizophrenia in a first episode. Schizophrenia can however present as behavioural disturbance which is not necessarily recognised as illness, and this may lead to inappropriate judicial action (Humphreys et al 1994) which is of course not in the patient's best interests (Department of Health and Home Office 1992). Reports of apparently typical 'functional' psychotic pictures of both a schizophrenic and affective nature being associated with organic brain disease have been found in the literature for some time (Davison & Bagley 1969, Krauthammer & Klerman 1978). Numerous physical conditions may underlie such situations (Davison 1983, Johnstone et al 1987, 1988) but all are uncommon. A recent problem is that of new variant Creutzfeldt–Jakob disease (Will et al 1996). This disorder has only very recently been defined and its frequency is yet to be established. At present it appears that the early manifestations of this ultimately fatal organic brain disease are anxiety and depression (Will et al 1996), and indeed it would appear that 'functional' psychiatric illness – principally affective disorder – has been the initial diagnosis in many of the young adults who are the main group affected by this dementing illness (Zeidler et al 1997). It may be hoped that this disorder will remain vary rare but, if it does not, the question of depressive features in a young adult being an atypical presentation of dementia may become one that will have to be considered in the practice of many psychiatrists.

REFERENCES

APA 1980 Diagnostic and statistical manual of mental disorders, 3rd edn. American Psychiatric Association, Washington, DC

APA 1987 Diagnostic and statistical manual of mental disorders, 3rd edn, revised. American Psychiatric Association, Washington, DC

APA 1994 Diagnostic and statistical manual of mental disorders, 4th edn DSM IV. American Psychiatric Association, Washington, DC

Cancro R 1983 Towards a unified view of schizophrenic disorders. In: Zales M (ed) Affective and schizophrenic disorders. Brunner Mazel, New York

Coffey I W, Johnstone E C 1997 Atypical illnesses. In: Bhugra D, Munroe A (eds) Troublesome disguises. Blackwell, Oxford

Cooper J E 1991 Notes on unresolved problems. In: Pocket guide to the IDC-10 classification of mental and behavioural disorders. Churchill Livingstone, London

Cooper J E, Kendell R E, Gurland B J, Sharpe L, Copeland J R M, Simon R 1972 Psychiatric diagnosis in New York and London. Maudsley monograph 20. Oxford University Press, London

Davison K 1983 Schizophrenia-like psychoses associated with organic cerebral disorders: a review. Psychiatric Developments I: 1–34

Davison K, Bagley C R 1969 Schizophrenia-like psychoses associated with organic disorders of the nervous system: a review of the literature, In: Herrington R N (ed) Current Problems in Neuropsychiatry. Headley, Ashford, Kent

Department of Health and Home Office 1992 Review of health and social services for mentally disordered offenders and others requiring similar services. Final summary report. HMSO, London

Everitt B S, Gourlay A J, Kendell R E 1971 An attempt at validation of traditional psychiatric syndromes by cluster analysis. British Journal of Psychiatry 119: 399–412

Feighner J P, Robins E, Guze S B, Woodruff R A, Winokur G, Munoz R 1972 Diagnostic criteria for use in psychiatric research. Archives of General Psychiatry 26: 57–63

Folstein M F, Rabins P V 1991 Replacing pseudodementia. Neuropsychiatry, Neuropsychology and Behavioral Neurology 4: 36–40

General Register Office 1968 A glossary of mental disorders. Studies on medical and population subjects no 22. HMSO, London

Humphreys M, Johnstone E C, MacMillan M 1994 Offending among first episode schizophrenics. Journal of Forensic Psychiatry 5: 51–61

Jampala V C, Sierles F S, Taylor M A 1986 Consumers' views of DSM-III: attitudes and practices of US psychiatrists and 1984 graduating psychiatric residents. American Journal of Psychiatry 143: 148–153

Johnstone E C, MacMillan J F, Crow T J 1987 The occurrence of organic disease of possible aetiological significance in a population of 268 cases of first episode schizophrenia. Psychological Medicine 17: 371–379

Johnstone E C, Cooling N J, Frith C D 1988 Phenomenology of organic and functional psychoses and the overlap between them. British Journal of Psychiatry 153: 770–776

Kendell R E 1989 Clinical validity. Psyhcological Medicine 19: 45–55

Kendell R E 1991 Relationship between the DSM-IV and the ICD-10. Journal of Abnormal Psychology 100: 297–301

Kendell R E, Gourlay J 1970a The clinical distinction between psychotic and neurotic depression. British Journal of Psychiatry 117: 257–260

Kendell R E, Gourlay J 1970b The clinical distinction between the affective psychoses and schizophrenia. British Journal of Psychiatry 117: 261–266

Krauthammer C, Klerman G L 1978 Secondary mania. Archives of General Psychiatry 35: 1333–1339

Kreitman N, Sainsbury P, Morrissey J, Towers J, Scrivener J 1961 The reliability of psychiatric assessment: an analysis. Journal of Mental Science 107: 887–908

Lewis N, Pietrowski Z 1954 Clinical diagnosis of manic–depressive psychosis In: Hoch P M, Zubin J (eds) Depression. Grune & Stratton, New York

Loranger A W 1990 The impact of DSM-III on diagnostic practice in a university hospital. Archives of General Psychiatry 47: 672–675

Menninger K 1963 The vital balance: the life process in mental health and illness. Viking Press, New York

Paykel E S, Norton K R W 1982 Diagnoses not to be missed: masked depression. British Journal of Hospital Medicine 28: 151–157

Robins L N, Helzer J E, Croughan J, Ratliff K S 1981 National Institute of Mental Health diagnostic interview schedule. Archives of General Psychiatry 38: 381–389

Sachdev P S, Smith J S, Angus Lepan H, Rodriguez P 1990 Pseudodementia twelve years on. Journal of Neurology, Neurosurgery and Psychiatry 53: 254–259

Scadding J G 1963 Meaning of diagnostic terms in broncho-pulmonary disease. British Medical Journal 2: 1425–1430

Schneider K 1959 Klinische Psychopathologie, 5th edn. Hamilton M W (trans). Grune & Stratton, New York

Szasz T 1961 The myth of mental illness. Hoeber-Harper, New York

Tsuang M T, Winokur G, Crowe R R 1980 Morbidity risks of schizophrenia and affective disorders among first degree relatives of patients with schizophrenia, mania, depression and surgical conditions. British Journal of Psychiatry 137: 497–504

Turner T 1995 Schizophrenia – social section In: Berrios G, Porter R (eds) A history of clinical psychiatry. Athlone Press, London

Tyrer S P, Brittlebank A D 1993 Misdiagnosis of bipolar affective disorder as personality disorder. Canadian Journal of Psychiatry 38: 587–589

WHO 1973 Report of the international pilot study of schizophrenia. World Health Organization, Geneva, vol 1

WHO 1992 International statistical classification of diseases and related health problems, 10th revision. World Health Organization, Geneva, vol 1, pp 311–387

Will R G, Ironside J W, Zeidler M et al 1996 A new variant of Creutzfeldt–Jakob disease in the UK. Lancet 347: 921–925

Wing J K, Cooper J E, Sartorius N 1974 Description and classification of psychiatric symptoms. Cambridge University Press, Cambridge

Zeidler M, Johnstone E C, Bamber R W K et al 1997 New variant Creutzfeldt–Jakob disease: psychiatric features. Lancet 350: 908–910

11

Organic disorders

Tom M. Brown

INTRODUCTION

This chapter groups together a number of topics which traditionally psychiatry has classified under the heading of 'organic psychiatry'. It includes the dementias, delirium, amnestic disorders and disorders arising from structural brain disease. It also includes epilepsy and psychiatric disorders arising from systemic pathology outside of the brain, for example endocrine disorders.

A major shift in paradigm is occurring in the way psychiatrists view the relationship between symptomatic mental disorders and brain function. This has been reflected in major changes in the classification of so-called organic disorders, particularly in the fourth edition of the *Diagnostic and Statistical Manual of Mental Disorder* (DSM-IV) (APA, 1994).

Historically psychiatrists have either viewed psychiatric disorder as a symptomatic manifestation of cerebral or systemic disease (organic) or considered it to be psychological in origin (functional). This approach has relied on the detection of structural lesions or the diagnosis of underlying disease processes as the basis of defining organic disorders. As has been discussed in Chapter 1, it is becoming increasingly evident that the idea of such clear-cut boundaries is a simplification of a complex function.

Most psychiatrists would concede that all behaviours have a cerebral substrate, though it should be cautioned that this does not equate with a biological reductionism, which ignores psychological, social, spiritual and cultural aspects of patients' experience. This shift in paradigm has been given momentum by the advent of the new technologies in medicine. For example, some patients with so-called functional psychoses (schizophrenia, bipolar affective disorder) are found to have central nervous system (CNS) abnormalities when studied by means of structural brain imaging (magnetic resonance imaging (MRI) and computerised tomography (CT)) or functional brain imaging techniques (positron emission (SPECT)) tomography (PET) and single photon emission computerised tomography (SPECT).

CLASSIFICATION

As can be seen in Table 11.1, ICD-10 (WHO 1992) has retained the term 'organic disorders'. It has been discarded by DSM-IV, which has taken a more radical approach in dealing with the difficult question of terminology in this area of psychiatry. The organic – functional divide has been jettisoned by DSM-IV in favour of a 'primary/secondary' classification. In abandoning the term 'organic', the DSM-IV manual states 'the term organic mental disorder is no longer used in DSM-IV because it incorrectly implies that non-organic mental disorders do not have a biological basis'. The relevant chapter in DSM-IV is now entitled 'Delirium, dementia and amnestic and other cognitive disorders'. DSM-IV is clearly attempting to move to a more aetiologically based classification. When a syndrome is known to be a manifestation of either cerebral or systemic medical disorder it is classified as being secondary to that disorder. By implication a patient has a primary (idiopathic) disorder only when all other underlying aetiologies have been ruled out by appropriate examination and investigation. In doing this DSM-IV has removed from this section of the manual some disorders which were formerly subsumed under the heading organic. These include mental disorders due to underlying general medical conditions, e.g. dementia caused by hypothyroidism, which are now classified in separate sections and not in the section entitled 'Delirium, dementia and other cognitive disorder'. ICD-10 by contrast subsumes disorders secondary to physical disease or brain damage under the section on organic disorders.

The classifications also differ in the way in which they deal with cognitive disorders caused by substance misuse. DSM-IV includes in the section on delirium, dementia and amnestic disorders a category for sub-

Table 11.1 Classification of organic mental disorders	
DSM-IV	ICD-10
Delirium, dementia, amnestic and other cognitive disorders	*Organic, including symptomatic mental disorders*
Dementia	Dementia in Alzheimer's disease with early onset
Dementia of the Alzheimer's type with early onset	Dementia in Alzheimer's disease with late onset
Dementia of the Alzheimer's type with late onset	
Vascular dementia	**Vascular dementia**
Dementia due to HIV disease	Multi-infarct dementia
Dementia due to head trauma	Subcortical vascular dementia
Dementia due to Parkinson's disease	
Dementia due to Huntington's disease	**Dementia in other disease, classified elsewhere**
Dementia due to Pick's disease	HIV disease
Dementia due to Creutzfeldt–Jakob disease	Parkinson's disease
	Huntington's disease
Amnestic disorders	Pick's disease
Amnestic disorder due to general medical condition	Creutzfeldt–Jakob disease
Substance-induced persisting amnestic disorder	**Organic amnestic syndrome, not induced by alcohol or other psychoactive substance**
Delirium	
Delirium due to a general medical condition	**Delirium, not induced by alcohol and other psychoactive drugs**
Substance-induced delirium	
Substance-withdrawal delirium	**Other mental disorders due to brain damage and dysfunction and to physical disease**
Delirium due to multiple aetiologies	Organic hallucinosis
	Organic delusional (schizophrenia-like) disorder
	Organic mood (affective disorders)
	Organic anxiety disorder
	Personality and behavioural disorders due to brain disease, damage and dysfunction
	Organic personality disorder
	Postencephalitic syndrome
	Postconcussional syndrome

stance-induced delirium, substance-induced dementia and substance-induced amnestic syndrome. ICD-10 records these in a separate section entitled 'Mental and behavioural disorders due to psychoactive substances abuse'.

NEUROPSYCHIATRIC ASSESSMENT

This section concentrates on aspects of neuropsychiatric assessment which require particular care and attention in patients with suspected cognitive impairment. Although many of the disorders which can underlie cognitive impairment are characterised by a wide variety of clinical manifestations, cognitive disorders are normally manifest by one, or more, of the following underlying clinical features :

- disturbance in consciousness (embracing arousal, attention and concentration)
- disturbance in mood
- perceptual abnormalities
- disturbance in intellectual functioning, e.g. memory, language and thinking
- personality change
- disturbance in motor function.

Neuropsychiatric evaluation should therefore pay particular attention to the following points.

A general description of the patient   This should include particular emphasis on dress, evidence of self-neglect, use (or lack of use) of sensory aids such as glasses or hearing aids, gait, motor abnormalities and responsiveness to the interviewer (including the ability to pay attention and cooperate).

Assessment of consciousness   This will be based on the level of arousal, orientation, behaviour, short-term memory, level of attention and distractibility.

Assessment of language and speech   This will include the ability to understand the spoken word, including commands, and will include some assessment of fluency and spontaneity of speech, coherence of speech and repetitiveness. Assessment of ability to name objects and body parts is also helpful. Speech must be assessed against knowledge of the patient's premorbid intellectual ability and social, cultural and educational background.

Assessment of thought There should be attention to both form of thought (as evidenced in speech) and content of thought, including the presence of hallucinations and delusions.

Assessment of mood in the context of cognitive impairment Particular attention should be paid to congruence between what the patient says about his mood and the demonstrated emotions. Lability of mood and exaggerated expression of mood are often seen in such patients.

Assessment of judgement and insight This should include an appraisal of the patient's awareness of his current circumstances and environment and an assessment of his appraisal of his physical and mental health and level of awareness of major social relationships and their current status.

Cognitive assessment This will include assessment of memory, which is often the first intellectual function to be impaired in organic brain disease. Normal practice is to divide memory into immediate, short-term and long-term memory. Unless cognitive deficits are severe, long-term memory is usually best preserved, with problems in short-term and immediate memory being more obvious. Patients may fill in memory gaps by confabulation. This term refers to the situation whereby when questioned about recent events a patient provides a reply which sounds plausible and which he appears to believe to be true but which is actually false. Sometimes these confabulations have a grandiose wish-fulfilling quality but they are more commonly genuine memories displaced in time. This is particularly characteristic of Korsakoff's psychosis. Where memory problems are thought to exist it is often wise to request fuller assessment from a clinical psychologist. Other cognitive functions which should be tested in patients suspected of cognitive impairment include ability to read, write and count, constructional abilities, right/left orientation, finger recognition and assessment of finer sensory function (astereognosis, agraphaesthesia, two-point discrimination).

Some instruments have been devised as aids to routine clinical assessment of cognitive impairment. Examples are Folstein's mini-mental state examination (Folstein et al 1975) and the cognitive capacity screening examination (Jacobs et al 1997). While these tests do help distinguish those with clear cognitive impairment from normal controls, they have not been shown to be more sensitive or specific than thorough clinical evaluation. Their main use is in providing a brief preliminary screening examination.

Assessing clinical features of focal cerebral lesions

It is important that the examining clinician has some understanding of the handicaps which result from focal damage to various parts of the brain. A brief account of this is given here. For further detail the reader is referred to Lishman (1987) and Kolb & Whishaw (1990).

Frontal lesions

Frontal lobe lesions can have widespread effects on mood, behaviour, temperament, motor function, speech and abstract thinking. Neurological signs associated with frontal lobe damage include the reappearance of primitive reflexes, including the grasp reflex and the sucking reflex. In frontal lobe lesions encroaching on the motor cortex or deep projections, contralateral spastic paresis and dysphasia can result. In bilateral lesions there may be incontinence of urine. Abstract reasoning is affected and patients often have diminished ability to plan tasks. Attention span is usually poor.

Personality change is characterised by a disinhibited, overfamiliar manner. Although the mood is often described as euphoric, emotional response is blunted. Patients may be egocentric with a lack of tact and concern for others. They exhibit lack of drive and initiative and poor judgement. In some there is marked apathy and inertia; others are aggressive and at times impulsive. There is evidence that this particular symptom cluster in an individual patient relates to damage in specific areas within the frontal lobes; for example, damage to orbital frontal regions seems more commonly to lead to disinhibition, distractibility, aggressiveness and impulsivity, whereas damage to the dorsolateral surface of frontal lobes leads to deficits in fluency of speech and to perseveration (Stuss & Benson 1983).

Temporal lobe lesions

Temporal lobe lesions (particularly those of the dominant hemisphere) lead to deficits in intellectual function, communication (speech, reading and writing) and occasionally to personality change. Deep temporal lobe lesions can produce neurological signs, including contralateral homonymous upper quadrantic visual field defects and mild contralateral hemiparesis. Temporal lobe lesions are associated with epilepsy and an increased risk of schizophrenia-like psychosis (Slater et al 1963). Bilateral lesions of the medial temporal lobe structures often lead to amnestic syndrome, with profound disturbance of memory. Posterior temporal lobe lesions are associated with dysphasia. There is a relationship between this dysphasia and handedness, though it seems clear that in both left- and right-handed subjects language is more commonly mediated by the left than the right hemisphere. Left-handed persons, however, are less severely dysphasic than right-handed persons after equivalent lesions. This suggests that in left-handed individuals language function is represented bilaterally.

Parietal lobe lesions

Parietal lobe lesions are less likely to cause psychiatric syndromes than frontal or temporal lesions. They are associated with a variety of neuropsychological disturbances, which can cause considerable functional impairment. The parietal lobe has a close functional relationship to both temporal and occipital lobes. Neurological signs associated with parietal lobe lesions include cortical sensory loss, agnosias and apraxia, and occasionally visual disturbance if the optic radiation is involved in the lesion. Cortical sensory loss is characterised by astereognosis, agraphaesthesia and loss of two-point discrimination.

Agnosia refers to a variety of disorders of body image, i.e. a person's awareness of his bodily self. Lesions of the non-dominant parietal lobe cause visuospatial problems, including neglect, whereas lesions of the dominant parietal lobe result in prosopagnosia (failure to recognise the faces of others, including close friends and relatives).

Gerstmann's syndrome is a specific form of body image disturbance characterised by right/left disorientation, agraphia, acalculia and finger agnosia. It seems more common in patients with left-sided lesions.

Apraxia includes the inability to imitate gestures and actions when asked to do so (assuming the patient can comprehend the request, and is not paralysed). It involves difficulties with carrying out complex actions requiring sequencing acts. Dressing apraxia refers to difficulties in putting on garments in the correct order and fastening buttons, belts and other parts of the clothing. It occasionally results from neglect of the left side of the body in non-dominant hemisphere lesions. Constructional apraxia refers to the inability to copy designs and to construct simple three-dimensional models, for example from bricks. It leads to difficulties in carrying out simple activities of daily living, for example setting a table.

Other features of parietal lobe lesions include the inability to find one's way around in familiar surroundings (topographical disorientation) and deficits in temporal awareness, leading to difficulties in estimating time.

Speech disorders

Speech disorders can result from lesions in frontal, temporal and parietal areas. Two main brain areas are involved in speech. The first is the posterior two-thirds of the inferior frontal gyrus (Broca's area) and the second the posterior third of the middle and central frontal gyri and the adjacent parietal lobe. Speech disorders are commonly divided into fluent and non-fluent dysphasias. In non-fluent dysphasia vocabulary is limited; the patient may use a few phrases, often incorrectly. This is also referred to as Broca's aphasia or expressive dysphasia. In fluent dysphasia fluency of speech is normal, as is sequencing of words, but the speech does not make sense. This is also referred to as receptive dysphasia, sensory dysphasia or jargon aphasia. In nominal dysphasia the patient has difficulty in naming common objects or people that he knows. He may be able to describe correctly the function of an object, but without being able to name it, e.g. 'this is something for keeping the time'. In non-fluent dysphasia (Broca's dysphasia, motor dysphasia, expressive dysphasia) there are significant difficulties in finding words and in motor control of the muscles of articulation. There may be some comprehension difficulties, but these are not prominent. The patient's speech may be unintelligible to the listener, even though the speaker knows what he wants to say and may be able to write it down. There are sometimes attendant behavioural manifestations because of the frustrations produced in the patient by his inability to communicate, despite reasonably intact comprehension. In fluent dysphasia (receptive or sensory aphasia) comprehension is usually severely impaired, though word fluency is not. As it was first described by Wernicke in 1881, it is sometimes also known as Wernicke's aphasia. Such patients are unable to repeat words or phrases when asked, their speech is littered with grammatical abnormalities and occasionally with neologisms, though it is fluent. Although the speech is usually fluent and containing many words, it is unintelligible and meaningless. Reading and writing are significantly impaired in this form of dysphasia. Such deficits usually occur with lesions in the posterior temperoparietal areas.

Occipital lobe lesions

These are usually characterised by complex visual disturbances, which can be misdiagnosed as 'hysterical'. Visual hallucinations can occur, leading to misdiagnosis of other mental disorder.

Diencephalic / brain stem lesions

Lesions of these midline structures most commonly produce amnestic syndrome and disturbances of sleep (usually hypersomnia) and appetite (usually hyperphagia). They may also cause progressive intellectual deterioration and emotional lability with outbursts of anger. Lesions of the posterior diencephalon or upper midbrain, e.g. tumours, infarcts, can lead to presentations with mutism and stupor. Other organic causes of mutism and stupor include uraemia, hypoglycaemia, fluid and electrolyte disturbance, endocrine disorder and intoxication with drugs and alcohol. The principal psychiatric disorders causing stupor are severe depression and schizophrenia. A good history and examination usually reveals the underlying cause, though EEG and CT may be required to distinguish between causes due to psychiatric disorder (depression and schizophrenia) from the many organic causes listed above.

Investigations of patients with suspected cognitive impairment

The range of investigations to be carried out in patients with suspected delirium, dementia and other cognitive disorders will be guided by the history and by careful physical examination. Judgement has to be exercised about the extent to which any given patient should be investigated. As well as being informed by clinical suspicion, investigation should also be led by an appreciation of the costs and benefits of each test. Plain radiographs of the skull, for example, rarely yield useful information, though they are not uncommonly requested. Table 11.2 lists baseline screening tests which should be carried out in virtually all cases. In many patients, history, examination and the results of these baseline tests will yield sufficient diagnostic information. The extent to which the further investigations listed in the table will be used is dictated by the clinical picture. In some cases, a variety of these investigations will be 'first line', for example CT, blood cultures and lumbar puncture. Testing for the human immunodeficiency virus (HIV) is not usually carried out routinely on ethical grounds, but may have to be performed in the presence of risk factors for this disease.

Electroencephalography

The advantages of electroencephalography are that it is non-invasive and very sensitive. It is, however, an investigation with very low specificity and its mains uses are in epilepsy, in the differential diagnosis of stupor and in the occasional case when there is difficulty in distinguishing delirium from dementia.

Table 11.2   Investigation of neuropsychiatric disorder

Baseline screening tests
Full blood count
Erythrocyte sedimentation rate
Urea and electrolytes
Blood glucose
Liver function tests
Calcium and phosphate
Thyroid function tests
Urinalysis
Urine culture
Urine analysis for drugs

Further investigations
Blood cultures
HIV testing
Serum heavy metals
Serum copper and caeruloplasmin
Serum B$_{12}$ and folate
VDRL and TPHA
Electroencephalogram
Lumbar puncture
   glucose
   protein
   cultures
   VDRL
Radiology
   CT
   MRI
   SPECT
Neuropsychological testing

Computerised tomography and magnetic resonance imaging

CT is now widely available in the UK, even in district general hospitals. MRI is largely confined to major teaching hospitals.

CT is particularly useful in excluding intracranial lesions in those with suspected dementia. These include:

- tumours, primary or secondary
- infarcts
- subdural/extradural haematoma
- normal pressure hydrocephalus.

It may also be used in:

- investigation of first episode psychosis of unknown aetiology
- investigation of stupor or catatonia
- behavioural and intellectual disturbance in patients with known or suspected HIV infections.

MRI provides much better definition than CT as it

readily visualises the posterior fossa, which is partially hidden by bone in CT scanning. It is useful in the investigation of movement disorders of unknown aetiology and in suspected posterior fossa lesions. Likewise, MRI better discriminates between grey and white matter lesions and is particularly helpful in detecting white matter lesions. This makes it a useful investigation in suspected multiple sclerosis and HIV infection.

Single photon emission computerised tomography and positron emission tomography

These techniques are physiologically based and image brain function. They involve the injection of radioactively labelled compounds, or radiopharmaceuticals, and measure cerebral blood flow, or the incorporation of the labelled compounds into metabolic pathways. They have been used in a variety of neurological and neuropsychiatric disorders. Geaney (1994) has suggested that SPECT is a useful investigation in the diagnosis of dementia. Its specificity, however, remains to be determined. PET is an expensive investigation available in very few centres and its uses are at present virtually confined to research.

Neuropsychological testing

Neuropsychological tests provide assessment of patients' cognitive abilities which are both standardised and quantitative. They are useful for baseline evaluations of patients with suspected cognitive impairment, and also for monitoring progress over a period of time. Tests depend on the patient's cooperation, and assessment can be made difficult by the patient's ability to understand and communicate, as well as by behavioural disturbance and anxiety. For this reason test results should not be evaluated in isolation, but in the light of clinical assessment and other investigations. Tests have been used in the assessment and monitoring of patients suspected of having early dementia, to monitor progress in patients with head injury and occasionally to help differentiate between symptoms which may be caused by brain injury or disease and so called 'functional' mental disorder.

Some tests are designed for specific purposes, for example, the Cambridge Mental Disorders of the Elderly Examination (CAMDEX) in dementia and the Wechsler Adult Intelligence Scale (WAIS) in the measurement of intelligence. Other tests are designed to assess specific brain functions, for example speech. For a more comprehensive account of the use of neuropsychological tests the reader is referred to the textbook by Kolb & Whishaw (1990).

DELIRIUM

The clinical syndrome of delirium has been recognised and described for the last 2000 years. The description of the core clinical features is found in the writings of Hippocrates (Chadwick & Mann 1950) and in other ancient works. The term itself has been used in different ways. Berrios (1995) states that it was only in the 19th century that the term was consistently used to describe a disorder of attention, cognition and consciousness. It had previously, for example, been used to describe a state of excited behaviour.

A large variety of terms has been used to describe the syndrome we now know as delirium. These include 'acute confusional state', 'acute organic reaction', 'acute brain syndrome' and 'acute brain failure'. With the advent of DSM-III, terminology became more consistent and operational diagnostic criteria for delirium were made explicit. DSM-IV subdivides delirium thus:

- delirium due to a general medical condition
- substance-induced delirium
- substance-withdrawal delirium
- delirium due to multiple aetiologies.

ICD-10 (WHO, 1992) takes a slightly different approach, separating out delirium induced by alcohol and other (non-prescribed) psychoactive substances which it codes separately as 'disorders due to psychoactive substance use'.

Clinical features

Delirium is a transient, organic mental syndrome characterised by disorder of cognition, attention, conscious level, psychomotor activity and sleep–wake cycle. It virtually always has an underlying physical cause, either due to systemic or cerebral disease. Regardless of underlying cause, the essential features of the clinical syndrome remain very similar. The onset is acute and occurs more commonly during the night than during the day (Lipowski 1989). Classically symptom severity fluctuates and is often worse during the night. These are patients who, not atypically, keep junior doctors out of bed at night and are considerably better by the time of the morning ward round. Impaired consciousness and disturbance in attention are invariably present. One difficulty here is that consciousness is a poorly defined concept (Taylor & Lewis 1993). It embraces wakefulness, alertness and awareness of one's environment. Lipowski has described three clinical variants of delirium: a hypoalert, hypoactive type, a hyperalert, hyperactive type and a mixed type. In the hypoalert/hypoactive variant the patient seems lethargic and drowsy, responds slowly to questions and other stimuli, and may be misdiagnosed as suffering from depression. The patient's general underarousal and underactivity often leads to the delirium being overlooked and Lipowski points out that it is important to bear in mind that not all delirious patients are hyperactive. In contrast a hyperalert, hyperactive patient is restless, agitated, often talking with pressure of speech and talking very loudly. This patient's agitation may result in physical overactivity, which can for example take the form of disconnecting himself (and others) from drips and monitors. This agitation is usually associated with other evidence of overactivity of the sympathetic nervous system. It is typical of patients withdrawing from alcohol or hypnotic drugs. In the mixed variety the patient shifts in an unpredictable way from underactivity to overactivity and vice versa. It is also important to point out that delirious patients may have lucid periods, during which their cognitive state seems normal. Disturbance of the sleep–wake cycle is invariable in delirium. Reversal of the normal cycle, with drowsiness occurring during the day and agitation during the night, is exceedingly common. The typical patient is awake, restless and overactive during the night and at these times may also have hallucinations and fleeting delusions. Such sleep as the patient does get is often accompanied by frightening nightmares, which can merge imperceptibly with the hallucinations the patient has on wakening.

Patients with delirium have reduced ability to focus and sustain attention. They find it difficult to shift from subject to subject. This is of crucial clinical importance, not only in the assessment but also in the management of such patients as things may have to be explained to them on more than one occasion. Failure to appreciate the patient's impaired attention, concentration and short-term memory span often underlies some of the difficulties which medical and nursing staff find in managing these patients.

The memory problem in delirium is one of immediate memory, though secondary short-term memory deficits result. Long-term memory is usually preserved, except in very severe cases. These memory difficulties are reflected in disorientation for time, place and person. Patients often have difficulty identifying the day of the week, the month or the year and even the time of day. Disorientation for place is common. Hospitalised patients may for example feel they are still at home or at a former place of work. Misidentification of persons is common. Levin (1956) has pointed out that this usually involves mistaking unfamiliar persons for those who are well known to the individual.

The patient's thinking is usually disorganised, incoherent and poorly directed. This results in difficulties with simple problem solving and the planning of the most straight forward of actions. Fleeting transitory delusions, often of a persecutory nature, are common. Hallucinations occur in all sensory modalities but are most often visual, or visual and auditory. Visual hallucinations are particularly vivid, and usually frightening, and can contribute to the behavioural disturbance often seen in patients with delirium. Illusions are also common and other perceptual distortions, including micropsia and macropsia, have been described.

The mood of patients with delirium can range from apathy and disinterest to anxiety, agitation and even terror. Depression, perplexity and suspiciousness are also not uncommonly observed. The mood of patients with delirium, and the consequent behavioural change, is markedly labile, shifting frequently and often rapidly from one state to another.

Differential diagnosis

The most important distinction to make is between delirium and dementia, though the two can, and commonly do, coexist. Other important differential diagnoses to be considered are of psychotic illness and occasionally dissociative disorders.

The patient's history provides the most important clues in differentiating delirium and dementia. In delirium the onset is invariably sudden and acute, whereas in dementia it is insidious. Delirium usually lasts for days to weeks, rather than for months. The course of delirium fluctuates much more wildly and it is invariably worse at night. Hallucinations and delusions, though found in dementia, are more common in delirium, particularly visual hallucinations. They are also fleeting in delirium, often varying with the state of arousal of the patient. Importantly the conscious level of patients with delirium is reduced, whereas in dementia consciousness is clear. Signs of underlying physical illness are also useful in distinguishing delirium from dementia. Particular difficulty can be found in distinguishing cortical Lewy body dementia from delirium, as its course is more fluctuating. The presence of parkinsonian symptoms in a patient apparently suffering from delirium points to possible underlying Lewy body dementia.

It is not uncommon to find patients with delirium misdiagnosed as suffering from psychotic illness. The patient's disturbance of sleep and affect, along with hallucinations and delusions, mislead many clinicians, particularly non-psychiatrists. These mental state abnormalities fluctuate more in delirium, and delusions in particular are less well systematised. Likewise in psychotic illness, conscious level, attention and memory are often unimpaired or only minimally impaired, whereas in the patient with delirium they are clearly abnormal.

Dissociative disorders are relatively uncommon, but the impairment of consciousness and amnesia which occur sometimes lead to difficulties distinguishing them from delirium. As is the case with delirium, these disorders are sudden in onset, which can again confuse the diagnostic picture. In dissociative states loss of personal identity occurs, whereas it does not in delirium. The memory loss tends to be circumscribed (for example to past personal memories). Dissociative disorder is often precipitated by stressful life events, which can help diagnostically. In cases of difficulty the EEG is a useful investigation. It is normal in dissociative disorder, whereas in delirium it usually shows diffuse background slow-wave activity.

Epidemiology

Most epidemiological studies of delirium have been carried out in hospital inpatients and reveal a high prevalence. Lipowski (1989) cites a figure of 10% for all medical and surgical inpatients. As Taylor & Lewis (1993) have pointed out this makes delirium the most common mental disorder in hospital inpatients. This figure rises in the elderly and Warshaw et al (1982) claim that as many as 50% of the hospitalised elderly meet the diagnostic criteria for delirium at some point during their stay.

Delirium is associated with considerable morbidity and mortality. Hodgkinson (1973) reports a doubling of the risk of death in patients with delirium. Folstein et al (1991) report an overall mortality of 25% in elderly hospitalised patients with delirium.

Aetiology

Delirium is a consequence of a wide range of organic factors, which can be either primary brain lesions or secondary to systemic illness and intoxication. Whatever the cause, there is widespread reduction in cerebral metabolism and widespread electrical and neurochemical disturbance (Lipowski 1989). The common causes are listed in Table 11.3. It is important to point out that in some cases more than one of these factors can occur concurrently, precipitating delirium. The most common single cause of delirium, particularly in the elderly, is intoxication due to prescribed drugs, particularly anticholinergic drugs or drugs with anticholinergic side-effects (for example tricyclic antidepressants or disopyramide). The elderly are particularly vulnerable to effects of prescribed anticholinergic medications because of the effects of ageing on the central cholinergic system, which are often exacerbated by degenerative cerebral disease (Blazer et al 1983). As Lipowski has pointed out, relative cholinergic deficiency is a major

---

Table 11.3   Causes of delirium

Drug intoxication
Anticholinergics
Psychotropic drugs
Anticonvulsants
Antiarrythmics, e.g. lignocaine, disopyramide
Steroids
Amantadine
Digoxin
Lithium
Alcohol
Illicit drugs

Drug withdrawal
Alcohol
Benzodiazepines

Infection
Chest
Urinary tract
Septicaemia
HIV

Metabolic / physiological
Organ failure (cardiac, pulmonary, renal, hepatic)
Electrolyte disturbance
Diabetic complications (hypo/hyperglycaemia, ketoacidosis)
Other endocrine disorder, e.g. thyroid or glucocorticoid abnormalities
Nutrition, e.g. vitamin deficiencies

Primary central nervous system disorders
Head injury
Cerebrovascular causes (stroke, subdural haematoma, transient ischaemic attack)
Epilepsy
Meningitis/encephalitis
Raised intracranial pressure

Other rare causes
Systemic lupus erythematosus
Porphyria
Heavy metal poisoning
Non-metastatic effect of carcinoma

---

pathogenic mechanism in delirium and, further, the reduction in cerebral-oxidative metabolism seen in delirium results in decreased synthesis of neurotransmitters, especially acetylcholine and noradrenaline. This partly explains why patients with dementia, especially Alzheimer's disease, are particularly prone to the development of delirium. Many other drugs may be associated with the development of delirium and the list in Table 11.3 is by no means comprehensive. A drug-induced cause should be considered in every case of delirium. Likewise, withdrawal from alcohol and from sedative hypnotic drugs are common causes of delirium and they should particularly be considered in patients who have been recently hospitalised and thus separated from their supplies of drugs and alcohol. Infections of all sorts are common precipitants of delirium. It is important to appreciate that even relatively innocuous and non-life-threatening infection, particularly in the elderly (especially those who are dementing), can precipitate delirium. Postoperative delirium, which occurs in 10–15% of surgical patients in later life, is particularly common in those who are on anticholinergic drugs or misuse alcohol. In an ever increasingly cost-sensitive NHS it should be pointed out that delirium considerably prolongs hospital stay.

Investigations

Physical examination and investigation of patients presenting with delirium is of paramount importance in identifying an underlying cause and guiding treatment. Taking an adequate history (which in this case invariably involves interviewing a third party) and examining the patient will guide the choice of investigations. In most cases full blood count, erythrocyte sedimentation rate and urea and electrolytes, liver function tests, thyroid function and blood glucose, urine analysis and culture of midstream urine and chest radiography will be appropriate. An electrocardiograph may also be useful and, particularly in cases where there are diagnostic doubts, an electroencephalogram will be helpful. If these initial investigations reveal no underlying cause for delirium it will be necessary to carry out further investigations. These will include CT, urine screen for illicit drugs, cardiac enzymes, blood cases, blood cultures, calcium, phosphate, vitamin B_{12} and folate. Occasionally even more rare disorders have to be considered and other investigation such as autoantibody screen, urinary porphyrins, syphilis serology and urine screen for heavy metals may have to be carried out. The possibility of HIV-related disease must be borne in mind, though screening for this disorder without a patient's consent can be problematic.

Pathogenesis

The pathophysiology of delirium has been concisely reviewed by Van der Mast (1996). As she points out, much light has been shed on the underlying pathophysiology by examining the main risk factors for delirium. These include old age, impaired cognitive function, severe physical illness, alcohol abuse, use of psychoactive medications, dehydration, infection, electrolyte disturbance and low plasma albumin. A reduction in cerebral-oxidative metabolism and neurotransmitter imbalance is present in delirium. The underlying causes for this include lack of oxygen, glucose and amino acids, vitamin deficiency, deficient synthesis and blockade of neurotransmitters, accumulations of toxins and false transmitters, altered cerebral blood flow, increased permeability of the blood–brain barrier and damage to the cell membranes. Deficits in the cholinergic system appear to underlie many of the symptoms in delirium. The cholinergic system is widely distributed throughout the brain and is involved in visual attention, memory and sleep, all of which can be disordered in delirium. It is likely, however, that other neurotransmitters play a role in delirium, with for example an excess of glutamate and dopamine contributing to the psychotic features of delirium (Gibson et al 1991). Further cholinergic overactivity may be related to some forms of delirium, particularly alcohol withdrawal. Van der Mast comments that, as many neurotransmitter systems are affected by the many different aetiologies in delirium, it may well be the case the more basic processes in neurones are affected, namely intracellular messenger systems involving G proteins, calcium, the phosphatidylinositol cascade, cyclic nucleotides and protein phosphorylation, which are of importance in synthesis and release of neurotransmitters.

Changes in the brain related to ageing, especially deterioration in cholinergic function, probably account for the increased sensitivity of the elderly to developing delirium.

Treatment

Three principles underlie the treatment of delirium. First, due attention must be paid to general and supportive measures; second, treatment should be aimed at identifying and treating the underlying condition causing the delirium; and, third, pharmacological interventions should be considered only when due attention has been paid to the first two principles. Good management of delirium involves close liaison between doctors, nurses and pharmacists, and indeed relatives and friends of the patient. Access to liaison psychiatry services is important, as liaison psychiatrists can give appropriate advice on investigation and management and also on the not infrequent problems of consent and possible use of the mental health acts.

The provision of adequate, trained nursing staff is crucial in patients with delirium. The patient should be nursed by as few nurses as possible and particular attention should be paid to the need to constantly orientate the patient and to carefully explain any examinations and procedures which need to be carried out. Attention to details such as this can often prevent behavioural disturbance from occurring. It should be ensured that the patient has adequate fluid and electrolyte balance and is adequately nourished. Attention should be paid to the environment in which the patient is nursed. Both over- and understimulation can make delirium worse. Where practical, the patient should be nursed in a quiet, adequately illuminated environment. The presence of a clock and some objects with which the patient is familiar can be of advantage. Care should be taken, as far as is possible, to exclude from the environment objects with which the patient can harm himself or others. Family members should be used, where possible, to reassure and orientate the patient.

Adequate history, examination and investigation will in most cases reveal the underlying cause of the cerebral dysfunction, which should be removed or treated as soon as possible. Knowledge of the underlying cause can also have a bearing on pharmacological treatment when this is necessary, for example many sedative hypnotic drugs cause respiratory depression and need to be used with care in certain patients. It is unfortunate that the sedative drugs with which many non-psychiatric junior doctors are most familiar are phenothiazines, including chlorpromazine and thioridazine. These drugs are often given inappropriately to patients with delirium. They are unsuitable for many such patients on account of their side-effect profiles, especially their anticholinergic side-effects. They can also cause postural hypotension, tachycardia and excessive sedation, all of which merely add to the morbidity (and sometimes mortality) of patients with delirium. In patients with alcohol- or benzodiazepine-induced delirium they can precipitate epileptic seizures. Most authors agree that the drug of choice for most delirious patients is haloperidol (Lipowski 1989, Taylor & Lewis 1993). It has the advantage of limited anticholinergic side-effects, a lower sedating potential and does not cause postural hypotension. Its main disadvantage is that it can cause extrapyramidal symptoms and it should therefore be given in as low a dose as possible (often 0.5 mg 2–3 times a day will suffice in the elderly). Haloperidol should be avoided in cases of benzodiazepine and alcohol withdrawal and also in hepatic failure. Benzodiazepines are the drugs of choice for the treatment of delirium due to withdrawal from alcohol and benzodiazepines. In hepatic failure, benzodiazepines with no active metabolites, e.g. lorazepam or oxazepam, are the drugs of choice.

In cases of severe emergency, for example when the patient is placing himself or others at serious risk, droperidol intravenously in doses of 5–15 mg (lower doses for the elderly) is probably the drug of choice.

Outcome

Delirium is usually a transient condition, resolving

Table 11.4 Causes of dementia
Alzheimer's disease
Vascular dementias
Lewy body dementia
Parkinson's disease
Frontal lobe dementias (including Pick's disease)
Huntington's disease
Prion-related disease (including Creutzfeldt–Jakob disease)
Head injury
Alcoholism
Wilson's disease
Aluminium poisoning (in renal dialysis)
Cerebral tumour
Endocrine disorders, e.g. hypothyroidism
General paralysis of the insane
Normal pressure hydrocephalus
Vitamin deficiencies

within days or weeks. There is no doubt, however, that in the elderly and those with serious underlying physical illness the mortality is greatly increased by the coexistence of delirium.

DEMENTIA

Dementia is a syndrome with a large number of underlying causes, some of which are listed in Table 11.4. It is a common syndrome, which increases with age but is not a part of normal ageing. Dementia is a progressive (though occasionally reversible) disorder, characterised by multiple cognitive deficits, including memory impairment, but also including other problems, i.e. difficulties in executive functioning, aphasia, apraxia and agnosia.

Estimates of the incidence and prevalence of dementia have been bedevilled by problems of diagnostic accuracy and reliability (Cooper 1991). However, field studies using operational criteria and standardised interview techniques estimate the prevalence of all dementias in the over 65s to be in the order of 5%. It is clear that prevalence increases with age above the age of 60 years, approximately doubling with each 5 years of age thereafter. Above the age of 85 years, around 20% of people suffer from dementia, highlighting the fact that even amongst very old people the majority do not have dementia.

Alzheimer's disease

Alzheimer's disease is the most common cause of

dementia. It was first described in 1907 by Alzheimer, who reported the case of a 51-year-old woman with memory loss, topographical disorientation, persecutory delusions, hallucinations, misidentifications and behavioural disturbance. The disorder described by Alzheimer has become an increasing public health problem in this and other countries, particularly as the population is ageing. Although the global population in both the developing world and the Western world is increasing, the increase in the elderly is disproportionately large.

Epidemiology

Estimates of incidence and prevalence of Alzheimer's disease have varied in published studies. Difficulties of diagnosis and assessment have already been commented on and other difficulties have involved the age, range and size of samples used in studies. More recent studies have attempted to minimise such difficulties, and to produce data which are likely to be more reliable. Rocca et al (1991) made use of the National Institute for Neurological and Communicative Disorders and Stroke and the Alzheimer's Disease and Related Disorders Association (NINCDS–ADRDA) operationalised criteria for Alzheimer's disease in a large epidemiological study. Prevalence rates (per 100 population) in this study were 0.3 in the age group 60–69 years, 3.2 in the age group 70–79 years, and 10.8 in the age group 80–89 years.

Reports of incidence, i.e. rates of occurrence of new cases, suggest rates of 1.9–2.6 per 1000 for men and 2.1–4.1 per 1000 for women aged above 60 years (Bickell & Cooper 1989). These incidence rates are for all causes of dementia. Incidence studies have suggested that presenile and senile Alzheimer's constitute a single disease, as studies have shown a unimodal rather than bimodal distribution in rates.

Most studies have shown that Alzheimer-type dementia (DAT) is more common in women.

Aetiology

A number of factors have been said to increase the risk of Alzheimer's disease. These include genetic factors, increasing age, Down's syndrome, sex, aluminium, head injury, viral infection, autoimmune processes and parental age, to name but a few. The association with increasing age is beyond dispute, and the excess of Alzheimer's disease in women already noted. Research in the aetiology of Alzheimer's disease has gathered considerable momentum in the last decade, largely due to advances in molecular biology, but also in the area of epidemiological studies looking at the risk factors.

Studies have demonstrated an aetiological connection between genetics and risk of Alzheimer's disease which is now beyond doubt. The relationship between other reputed risk factors and Alzheimer's remains less clear.

Genetics Alzheimer's disease is known to have a high prevalence is some families and the importance of genetic factors has been confirmed in twin studies (Deary & Whalley 1988). For many years genetic research in DAT was bedevilled by the same kind of problems of case definition already mentioned in relation to epidemiological research. A further problem is posed by the late age of onset of DAT, which means that many people potentially at risk will die from other causes before expressing the gene. It has been suggested (Burns et al 1995, Lovestone 1996b) that the observation that up to 50% of first-degree relatives who live to the age of 90 in some Alzheimer's families develop the disease is compatible with an autosomal dominant model, at least in these families. The picture, however, is almost certainly more complex than this. In recent years genetic research on DAT has focused on three chromosomes: 21, 14 and 19.

Chromosome 21 The observation that most older subjects with Down's syndrome develop Alzheimer's type pathology (Mann 1988) aroused interest in chromosome 21. Goate et al (1991) demonstrated an early-onset form of DAT was associated with a mutation in the amyloid precursor protein (APP) gene on chromosome 21. Further research has, however, made it clear that many families do not show linkage to the APP gene and that perhaps as few as 25% of cases are linked to this abnormality. It was, however, of considerable interest that the gene for amyloid precursor protein was linked to DAT in some cases, as APP is broken down to β-amyloid (β-A4) which is found in the senile plaques of DAT.

Chromosome 14 Schellenberg et al (1992) demonstrated that a number of early-onset cases of DAT were linked to markers on chromosome 14. Sherrington et al (1995) reported a missense mutation in a gene on chromosome 14 designated S182. This gene seems to be associated with an early-onset form of Alzheimer's disease. The gene codes for a membrane bound protein, the precise function of which remains unclear. Lovestone (1996b) has speculated that this gene may exert its effect by altering APP processing or affecting the interaction between APP and tau protein. Burns et al (1995) have suggested that as many as 75% of early onset cases of DAT may be linked to chromosome 14.

Chromosome 19 A gene on chromosome 19 seems to be linked to late-onset cases of DAT. This gene is the gene for apolipoprotein E (apo E). It exists in three isoforms in the population and one of these (ε4) has now been reported in many studies of late-onset DAT (see Lovestone 1996b for a summary). Lovestone has pointed out that the association with apo E may not be specific to Alzheimer's disease and may occur in Lewy body dementia, vascular dementias and Creutzfeldt–Jakob disease.

Very recently a similar gene to S182 on chromosome 14 has been described on chromosome 1 (Levy-Lahad et al 1995) in a cohort of Volga German families with early-onset autosomal dominant Alzheimer's disease. The reader is advised that the genetic and other aspects of the molecular biology of Alzheimer's disease is changing with such rapidity that it is virtually certain that by the time they read this there will have been other significant developments.

The identification of genes linked to development of DAT has already led to interest in and demand for genetic testing and screening. Genetic testing can either be diagnostic (to confirm diagnosis) or predictive (to test asymptomatic relatives). Diagnostic and predictive testing are already available in some centres, but as Burns et al (1995) have pointed out, the relatively late onset of the illness and lack of diagnostic accuracy make testing of families with DAT more hazardous than testing for other genetic disorders, e.g. cystic fibrosis. Lovestone (1996b), however, takes the view that screening for the APP mutation in chromosome 21 and the S182 gene on chromosome 14 may be of value, as the age of onset in affected families is younger and the virtually complete penetrance of these genes adds some reliability to risk assessment. Ethical dilemmas and difficulties in counselling have now been well discussed in relation to other dementias, e.g. Huntington's chorea, and there are now well-established internationally accepted procedures which should be followed (Simpson & Harding 1993).

Aluminium A number of pieces of evidence suggest an association between aluminium and Alzheimer's disease, though the nature of this remains unclear. Elevated aluminium levels have been demonstrated in the brain in Alzheimer's disease (Crapper et al 1976). Prolonged renal dialysis can result in a syndrome involving dementia with neurological abnormalities (Burks et al 1976). Such patients have an elevated aluminium content in the brain, especially the grey matter (McDermott et al 1978). Further, it is known that the senile plaques seen in the brains of patients with DAT contain aluminium (Candy et al 1986).

It has also been suggested that Alzheimer's disease could be treated with an aluminium chelating agent, desferrioxamine. These observations notwithstanding, there remains no convincing evidence that aluminium contributes to the development of DAT. Epidemiological studies trying, for example, to link levels of aluminium

in water to increased prevalence of Alzheimer's disease have produced ambiguous results.

Smoking There appears to be an inverse relationship between smoking and the prevalence of DAT. This has now been confirmed by a number of studies (e.g. Van Duijn & Hoffman 1991). Burns et al (1995) have suggested that it is possible that stimulation of nicotinic receptors is protective against DAT. It should be pointed out that smoking increases the risk of other dementias, e.g. vascular dementia, by contributing to hypertension and cardiovascular disease.

Other aetiological factors A number of other factors have been suggested to be of aetiological importance in Alzheimer's disease. There is evidence in animals that infection with viruses can cause amyloid deposition and plaque development. This, combined with the observation that herpes simplex virus 1 (HSV-1) has a predilection for brain areas which are particularly affected by DAT, has led to the notion that viruses may be of some importance. Although the role of viruses as putative aetiological agents in DAT has not yet been excluded, there is as yet no direct evidence that they contribute to the cause of DAT.

Similarly, autoimmune factors have been fairly extensively examined, but again, although some people with DAT appear to have antibodies against brain tissue, this does not appear to be a general finding and it has been suggested that this may be a consequence rather than a cause of the disease.

Repeated head trauma can cause a dementia syndrome (as in boxers' encephalopathy) (Casson et al 1984) and case reports have suggested that serious head injury may increase risk of DAT. Larger prospective studies following up patients with head injury have, however, produced negative findings.

More recently there has been interest in ascertaining whether people with poor education are at increased risk of developing DAT. Studies have been made difficult by the fact that tests for dementia rely on measurement of cognitive function, which is itself a function of premorbid educational level. Burns et al (1995) have reported that studies have shown a relationship between cognitive decline and neocortical synaptic density in DAT and also that there is some evidence that education can increase synaptic density. If confirmed, these observations may lend weight to the notion of 'intellectual reserve' in patients of higher education, which, as Burns has pointed out, raises as many political as scientific questions.

Pathology

Macroscopically the brain of patients with DAT may look normal, though more commonly widened sulci, increased size of the ventricles and atrophy, particularly of temporal, parietal and frontal lobes, may be visible. Microscopically the characteristic lesions of Alzheimer's disease are senile plaques and neurofibrillary tangles, which had been recognised even before the description by Alzheimer in 1907. The major lesions in Alzheimer's disease are senile plaques, which are widely distributed in the hippocampus and neocortex. Plaques have an amyloid core and contain paired helical filaments, which are composed of abnormally phosphorylated tau proteins. The core itself contains a protein, β-amyloid or β-A4, which is cleaved from a larger protein, amyloid precursor protein, (APP). It is known that β-A4 deposition occurs early in Alzheimer's disease.

The second major feature found histologically in DAT is the neurofibrillary tangle, which is also seen in Parkinson's disease, Down's syndrome and normal ageing. Tangles are intracellular inclusion bodies which contain paired helical filaments. Both plaques and tangles correlate with the severity of the clinical picture in DAT.

Neuronal loss also occurs in Alzheimer's disease, causing brain atrophy, with up to 10% of large neocorticol neurones being lost, particularly in the frontal and temporal lobes. Cholinergic neurones are affected, particularly in the basal nuclei, including the nucleus of Meynert. Noradrenergic and serotonergic nuclei are also involved.

More recently other abnormalities have been described in DAT, including the development of Hirano bodies, which are filamentous structures found in, or close to, pyramidal nerve cells, principally in the hippocampus (Hughes et al 1992). They are invariably accompanied by granulovascular degeneration, i.e. the appearance in pyramidal nerve cells of vacuoles containing dense granules. Lewy bodies have also been described in DAT, but are not specific to it. These are neuronal inclusion bodies, usually associated with severe neurone loss in Parkinson's disease.

Neurochemistry

The major neurochemical deficits in DAT have been described in the literature for many years now. Many systems are involved.

Abnormalities in cholinergic systems These were the first to be described in DAT. Choline acetyltransferase activity was found to be substantially reduced in patients with DAT (Davies & Maloney, 1976). Following this demonstration of loss of neurones in the nucleus of Meynert (the largest cluster of cholinergic nerve nuclei) and the medial septal nuclei serve to further emphasise the importance of the cholinergic system in DAT. There is also a deficiency in presynaptic

muscarinic receptors, whereas postsynaptic muscarinic receptors remain intact, a consideration which is likely to be important with respect to therapies directed at the enhancement of cholinergic function.

Noradrenaline and dopamine Dopamine hydroxylase activity has been shown to be reduced in DAT, which of course results in deficits in noradrenaline. These abnormalities have been described largely in patients with severe dementia and may occur later in the disease. The low level of dopamine observed in the thalamus, caudate and putamen may relate to parkinsonian symptoms, not uncommonly seen in patients with DAT.

Serotonin Low cortical levels of serotonin and its active metabolite 5-hydroxyindoleacetic acid (5-HIAA) have been demonstrated in patients with DAT, which probably relate to pathological changes in the basal nuclei. Furthermore 5-hydroxytryptamine 2 (5-HT$_2$) receptors are diminished in number in DAT.

Peptide and amino acid transmitters γ-Aminobutyric acid (GABA), an inhibitory neurotransmitter, is widely distributed throughout the brain. The activity of GABAergic neurones is reflected by glutamic acid decarboxylase (GAD) and abnormalities of this enzyme have been described in DAT, as have deficits in GABA itself, particularly in the temporal cortex. GABA receptors appear unaffected.

Glutamate is an excitatory amino acid transmitter. It has been hypothesised that loss of cortical pyramidal neurones, which use glutamate as a transmitter, is important in DAT. *N*-methyl-D-aspartate (NMDA) receptors are held to be markers of glutamate activity and changes in these receptors have been described in DAT (see Bowen & Procter 1991 for a review). Although the importance of neurotransmitter disturbances in DAT cannot be denied, and although these disturbances are key targets for replacement therapy, the fact that so many neurotransmitter deficits have been described in DAT makes it unlikely that any single replacement therapy will lead to global improvement in function.

Molecular biology

Research in the molecular biology of DAT in the last few years has been considerable. Burns et al (1995) and Lovestone (1996a) have recently summarised the major advances. Most work has focused on amyloid protein (found in the central core of senile plaques) and the tau protein (found in the paired helical filaments of neurofibrillary tangles).

Amyloid protein (β-amyloid or β-A4) Amyloid is a peptide 40 amino acids in length. It is derived from APP which lies across cell membranes. The precise function of APP is not known, but it may help regulate cell membrane stability, or indeed act as a receptor. Amyloid is also found in blood vessels, suggesting it may reach the brain via the vascular system. β-A4 peptide has been implicated in DAT for the following reasons:

- senile plaque density correlates with cognitive impairment
- β-A4 deposition occurs very early in DAT
- β-A4 deposition is relatively specific to DAT
- β-A4 is neurotoxic
- Mutations in amyloid precursor protein have been linked to early-onset familial DAT.

It is still not known in which way β-A4 metabolism is abnormal in DAT. It has been hypothesised that drugs which alter APP metabolism may slow down the deposition of β-A4 protein and, as secretory APP has been found in the cerebrospinal fluid of patients with DAT in high concentration and also at lower levels in asymptomatic carriers, this has raised hopes that such a drug may be able to slow down the progress of the disease

Tau protein Tau protein is found in the paired helical filaments of neurofibrillary tangles. Tau proteins are associated with microtubules in the CNS (Lovestone & Anderton 1992). Hanger et al (1991) demonstrated that the tau protein found in the brains of patients with DAT was abnormally phosphorylated and that this abnormally phosphorylated tau protein was not associated with microtubules. Microtubules are vital to normal neurotransport and therefore the abnormal tau found in paired helical filaments interferes with that process. Burns et al (1995) has speculated that abnormally phosphorylated tau has a specific biological marker, as the tau found in the brains of patients with DAT can be recognised by an antibody (called Alz 50). He has further noted that there are a number of tau kinases associated with paired helical filament tau and that there may be benefits in blocking the action of such

enzymes and therefore halting the abnormal phosphorylation of tau. Burns also suggests that an interplay of APP metabolism and abnormal phosphorylation of tau may result in the altered metabolism that causes DAT. This mechanism, known as the amyloid cascade, is illustrated in Figure 11.1. Lovestone (1996b) has suggested that as neurofibrillary tangles correlate with deterioration in DAT, even more than do senile plaques, more attention should perhaps be focused on tau protein. As further evidence of the importance of tau protein he highlights the fact that hyperphosphorylated tau seems fairly specific to DAT and is not, for example, found in Parkinson's disease or Lewy body disease.

Clinical features

It is important to note that the clinical features described here are not specific to Alzheimer's disease, many being found in other types of dementia, particularly those involving the cortex. The accuracy with which a particular clinical picture can be tied to a specific diagnosis is limited. Burns et al (1990a) reported an 88% accuracy for diagnosis of DAT, using NINCDS–ADRDA criteria based on later autopsy findings. All clinical descriptions emphasise global impairment of higher cortical functions, including memory, problem-solving abilities, motor skills, functions, social skills and emotional reactions. Most definitions used in clinical practice and in research emphasise the progressive, and generally irreversible, nature of the disorder. They also usually emphasise the fact that the clinical picture of dementia occurs in clear consciousness in order to distinguish it from delirium, though delirium can, and frequently does, punctuate the course of dementia and alterations in consciousness are seen in one kind of dementia (Lewy body disease).

The time from onset of clinical features to presentation to doctors varies considerably, and often depends on social factors, including the attitudes of the patient's

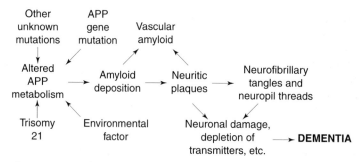

Fig. 11.1 Possible mechanisms by which a change in APP metabolism may lead to a dementia syndrome. (Source: Burns et al 1995.)

family and the patient's premorbid personality. Crises, for example wandering during the night or starting fires, still unfortunately dictate the time of referral in too many cases.

Cognitive impairment

Memory Loss of memory is generally the first clinical feature that comes to the notice of patients and their relatives. This is usually initially failure to learn newly presented information but later retrieval of information becomes impaired. Memory impairment may be reflected in repetitiveness of speech, in missing appointments, mislaying objects and burning meals. Topographical memory is also commonly affected. In the early stages this is usually confined to the environment away from the patient's home, but as the disease progresses it can occur in familiar environments. The evolution of memory impairments in Alzheimer's disease follows Ribot's law. Confabulation often occurs and this can either take the form of insertion of false memories or ectopic true memories from the past. In late stages of the illness, even long-term memory is affected. It is important to note that something which may be attributed to memory loss may be due to other factors; for example, failure to name people may be due to nominal dysphasia.

Language Dysphasia (aphasia – the two terms are used interchangeably) is common. It may manifest as impoverished speech, which may be diminished in quantity and range, but can progress as far as mutism in severe cases. Nominal dysphasia, with difficulty in naming objects, is a common early sign. Later both fluent and non-fluent dysphasias (described earlier in the chapter) and jargon dysphasia may occur. Fluent or receptive dysphasia is the most common language problem after nominal dysphasia and is severely disabling as the combination of memory loss and inability to comprehend is devastating. An important clinical point to note is that even in severe cases when language has disintegrated completely, patients may understand non-verbal communication, for example gestures and pictures. Failure to appreciate this can be very distressing, even for severely demented people.

Praxis Apraxia is the loss or diminished ability to perform coordinated motor tasks (assuming no neurological or other damage to the peripheral motor apparatus). It reflects dominant parietal lobe involvement in the dementing process. It is a major cause of loss of independence in patients, as it is reflected in inability to dress, wash, toilet and feed. Occasionally, and unwittingly, relatives add to the patient's distress by misinterpreting his inability to carry these acts out as laziness or as a lowering of standards, for example of hygiene. This is one area in which education of relatives is important.

Agnosia Failure to recognise sensory stimuli at a cortical level is a frequent part of the clinical picture. This may take the form of visual agnosia, as reflected in the functional misuse of every day objects, for example urinating in the sink, or prosopagnosia, the inability to recognise faces, even of familiar friends and relatives. It is important to recognise that agnosias can occur in all sensory modalities. Some demented patients may not, for example, recognise smells, including the smells of fires which they have accidentally and unknowingly started.

Other cognitive abnormalities Other abnormalities seen in dementia include left/right disorientation, dyscalculia, dysgraphia and finger agnosia. This combination comprises the so called Gerstmann's syndrome. Dyslexia has also been described in patients with dementia.

Personality and behavioural change Notwithstanding the devastating effects of the cognitive deficits described above, it is not infrequently the changes in personality and behaviour that the families of patients with dementia find most distressing. In assessing personality changes the clinician frequently relies heavily on the accounts of informants, usually close family members or friends. It is important to recognise that these accounts may be biased by the effects of illness and the stress this imposes on carers. It is often useful to have more detached information about a patient's premorbid personality, such as may be available from his general practitioner. Relatives vary in their description of personality and behavioural change. Some overemphasise unpleasant changes, while others deny any changes at all, even in the face of overwhelming evidence to the contrary. In some cases personality changes take the form of mere deficits. People may lose drive and initiative, they may become less decisive and more introverted, and the spectrum of emotions displayed may become narrowed, with loss of warmth and loss of sense of humour. Such patients often sit all day long in the same place, apparently doing very little. In presentations like this it is important to think of the possibility of depressive illness. In other patients changes in behaviour are reflected in overactivity and disinhibition. Social skills may be lost, they may become insensitive to others and exhibit loss of emotional control. They may be sexually disinhibited and display poor personal hygiene. Some patients manifest the so called 'catastrophic reaction', with outbursts of extreme emotion, either weeping or rage and aggression.

Behavioural change in dementia can take many forms. Patients may wander, even leaving their homes in the middle of the night. The catastrophic reaction and loss of emotional control described above may lead to shouting, screaming and aggressive behaviour.

Faecal smearing is sometimes seen. Although behavioural change may relate directly to personality changes, it is important to consider the possibility that some apparent behavioural problems may be related to the cognitive deficits already described, for example dyspraxia and agnosia.

Other mental state abnormalities A variety of other mental state abnormalities have been described in patients with dementia. In the case of patients with DAT these phenomena have been described in detail by Burns et al (1990b, 1990c). Burns notes that delusions occur in around 16% of patients with DAT. These are usually persecutory delusions or delusions of infidelity or theft. They are less systematised than delusions seen in schizophrenia and may be more transient. He notes the difficulty at times in distinguishing confabulations from delusions. Hallucinations occur in 10–15% of patients, with visual hallucinations being slightly more frequent than auditory hallucinations. Hallucinations in other sensory modalities have also been noted. Burns found an association between the presence of hallucinations and cognitive decline. Rubin et al (1988) described a number of misidentification problems, including inability to recognise one's own reflection and treating characters on television as if they existed in three-dimensional space. It should be noted that the sudden appearance of perceptual abnormalities should raise suspicions of a superimposed delirium.

Abnormalities of mood are also well described in patients with dementia, and indeed in the early stages depression is occasionally misdiagnosed as dementia. Mania is also occasionally seen in patients with dementia. It has been noted that depression appears to correlate with a lesser degree of cognitive impairment and may reflect retained insight in some cases.

Physical changes It is important for psychiatrists to remember that changes in the physical state add to the disability of patients with dementia. A large number of physical changes have been described in patients with Alzheimer's disease. These include weight loss, weakness, abnormalities of gait and loss of muscle bulk. Postmortem examinations of such patients reveal loss of weight of most internal organs. The most common cause of death in patients with DAT is bronchopneumonia. The reasons for these physical changes are poorly understood, but it has been suggested that DAT may be a systemic illness and not confined to the central nervous system. Alternatively the physical abnormalities may reflect loss of appetite, loss of ability to feed and poor self-care in advanced disease. Late in the disease process urinary and faecal incontinence occur. This may be due to direct neuronal degeneration in the brain, but may be secondary to cognitive abnormalities. When incontinence does occur it is important to rule out remediable underlying physical causes, for example urinary tract infection or impaction of faeces. Again, in end-stage disease there may be neurological signs, including return of primitive reflexes, tremor, myoclonus, extrapyramidal symptoms and epilepsy.

Tests of cognitive function

A large number of tests of cognitive function have been described, some brief and some more detailed and comprehensive. The Mini Mental State Examination (MMSE) (Folstein et al 1975) is probably most widely used. It is a 30 item test subject to some educational bias. A commonly used, more detailed and comprehensive schedule is the Cambridge Examination for Mental Disorders in the Elderly (CAMDEX) which has a cognitive subscale (CAMCOG) (Roth et al 1988). These more detailed tests are more suitable for research purposes than for routine clinical practice.

Investigations

At present the main purpose of investigating patients with DAT is clearly not to diagnose DAT but to exclude other reversible causes of dementia (discussed later). Although the EEG is usually abnormal in DAT, it is of little or no diagnostic value. With the improvement in both structural and functional brain imaging techniques in recent years these techniques have been applied to patients with dementia. CT is mainly used to exclude other treatable lesions. Burns (1991) has summarised the indications for CT in dementia. These include:

- Suspicion of underlying tumour (primary or secondary)
- Focal neurological signs
- Seizures
- Evidence of cerebral infarction
- Recent head injury
- Features suggestive of normal pressure hydrocephalus.

Between 5 and 10% of patients will have treatable lesions. Some patients with DAT have normal scans, and also some with atrophy on scan do not have dementia. The most common picture seen on CT scanning of patients with DAT is cortical atrophy and ventricular dilatation. MRI involves no radiation and has the advantage of providing images with better resolution and no bony artefact. There is prolongation in the T_1 relaxation time in both patients with DAT and multi-infarct dementia (MID) and the technique is therefore not good at distinguishing between the two. Functional magnetic resonance imaging (FMRI) is a more recently introduced technique, which is non-invasive and, unlike other methods of functional imaging such as SPECT and PET (Ch. 16), does not involve ionising radiation. It visualises activation of neuronal regions within the brain. At present it is a research technique and is not in general clinical use.

Functional brain imaging comprises single photon emission CT (SPECT or SPET) and positron emission tomography (PET). SPECT studies have demonstrated reduced cerebral blood in frontal and temporal regions in DAT (Peroni et al 1988). It has also been used to evaluate the relationship between specific brain areas and cognitive deficits (Burns et al 1989) and has demonstrated a relationship between amnesia and temporal hypofunction, aphasia and left hemispheric hypofunction and apraxia and posterior parietal hypofunction. PET assesses cerebral metabolism as opposed to blood flow. Its expense has dictated that its use so far has been as a research tool and it is not used in routine clinical practice. Temporoparietal deficits in glucose metabolism in DAT have been described by some workers.

Management

Most patients with DAT will sooner or later require an individually tailored package of care involving a multidisciplinary team. The organisation of the services required to deliver such care are described in Chapter 25. It should be clear to the reader that these social, behavioural and other non-pharmacological aspects of care are equally applicable to other dementias and not only to DAT. Among the techniques shown to be of benefit to patients are the following.

Reality orientation This can take place on either an individual or a group basis. Individual reality orientation depends on all those in regular contact with the demented person using every opportunity to provide orientating cues. These may include materials such as clocks, calendars, signposts and memory boards, but will also include verbal stimulation. Group reality orientation tends to occur in hospitals or day hospitals, with small groups of patients and a therapist, and involves discussing simple information and current affairs, and other materials chosen to provide stimulation and orientation.

Reminiscence therapy This, too, generally takes place in a small group. The group members are exposed to aids to reminiscence, including music, film, photographs and even foods, which may help them consider past experiences. Most patients and their carers enjoy reminiscence therapy and its principal effects are in improving mood.

Behavioural modification This is of value in dealing with difficult behaviours, including wandering, shouting, faecal smearing and aggressive behaviour and employs largely the principles of operant conditioning. A behavioural analysis is followed by a strategy rewarding desired behaviours and reducing undesired behaviours.

Drug treatments in dementia

Drugs for psychiatric symptoms and behavioural problems In general it is best to avoid drugs in DAT if at all possible. If they are required to treat psychiatric symptoms and behavioural problems they should be given short term. Some psychotropic drugs, particularly neuroleptics, make patients worse because of anticholinergic and extrapyramidal side-effects. Behavioural problems, including agitation and aggression, may need to be treated with drugs, but treatable underlying causes should be vigorously sought first, save in situations of real emergency. Sedative drugs are often requested for the treatment of nocturnal wandering. Where other efforts to deal with this fail, short acting benzodiazepines, preferably those with no active metabolite, e.g. temazepam or oxazepam, or chlormethiazole may be used. When more powerful medications are needed, thioridazine or haloperidol in small doses, preferably for as short a time as possible, should be tried.

Specific drugs for DAT Over the last few decades a variety of drugs, including vasodilators, dietary supplements and metabolic enhancers, have been used to treat patients with dementia. Results from using these agents have on the whole been disappointing. Newer approaches are based on the acquisition of the more detailed knowledge of the pathology and neurochemistry of DAT. Initial treatments were developed to enhance function in cholinergic systems. The first drug to be granted a licence (in the USA) for the treatment of DAT was Tetrahydroaminoacrodine (THA) or tacrine. Tacrine has in fact been around for decades and has been used as an opiate antagonist and antidelirium agent in the past. Burns et al (1995) have summarised the results of 10 trials of tacrine in patients with DAT, most of which (but not all) demonstrated some improvement in cognitive function. Unfortunately, many of these trials have also revealed significant side-effects, including gastrointestinal effects, aggression, irritability, skin rash and headaches. There is also concern that tacrine may cause liver damage in a significant number of patients. This appears to be dose dependent and reversible on cessation of the drug. The evidence from the trials is that tacrine may help some patients, but its use will be limited by its side-effects. More recently, a randomised controlled trial of a second cholinesterase inhibitor, donepezil, has been reported (Rogers & Friedhoff 1996). This drug has, at the time of writing, just been licensed in the UK, having already been available in the USA. The trials have demonstrated modest improvement or delay in deterioration in cognitive function, but with a better side-effect profile than is evident for tacrine. Kelly et al (1997) have highlighted some of the problems posed by successful drug treatments for DAT. Drugs are more likely to benefit patients early in the disease, when diagnosis may be difficult, and as these drugs are specific for DAT this is an important issue. They further point out that it is unclear what happens to patients when these drugs are stopped. The timing of discontinuation of drugs will be clinically and ethically challenging.

Finally, they highlight the issue of costs if drugs are provided to large numbers of patients. Though it has been argued that drug treatment for DAT will reduce the need for community support and possibly delay entry into institutions, this may simply increase burdens on families and shift some costs in the direction of primary care.

Other approaches to pharmacological treatment in Alzheimer's disease which are currently actively being investigated include:

- use of a group of benzoyl piperidine compounds known as ampokines, which upmodulate glutamate receptors
- use of neuronal protection agents, for example nerve growth factor (NGF)
- drugs which inhibit the processes involved in β-A4 production
- drugs which prevent the abnormal phosphorylation of tau protein. These approaches have recently been summarised by Fricker (1997).

Effect on carers

A crucial part of the management of DAT (and other dementias) is the provision of support for the families and other carers of suffers. There is now a considerable weight of literature on this subject (Morris & Morris 1993). Psychological problems in carers are common, with high rates of depressive illness. Behavioural problems, including aggression, wandering and urinary and faecal incontinence, seem to correlate highly with stress in carers, as does a poor premorbid relationship with the sufferer. Self-help organisations can provide an invaluable means of support for carers, for example the Alzheimer's Disease Society. Useful written advice can also be helpful (for example, Health Education Board for Scotland 1996).

Outcome

It has already been stated that DAT is a progressive dis-

ease which ends in death, usually by bronchopneumonia. Predicting survival times for individual subjects is, however, difficult. Early studies showed that admission to institutional care drastically reduced survival time, with 50% of patients being dead within 6 months. Survival times in institutions appear, however, to have increased, possibly due to increased standards of general and nursing care. Burns et al (1991) have documented characteristics of patients which predict reduced survival time. These include:

- younger age of onset
- aphasia
- the presence of psychotic symptoms
- male, sex
- poorer cognitive performance (at point of entry to the study).

It is well documented that mortality rates for patients with dementia are 3–5 times greater than those for age- and sex-matched controls.

Vascular dementias

Although dementia has been described after single large infarcts, cerebrovascular disease usually causes dementia by causing multifocal cerebral infarcts, hence the name multi-infarct dementia. MID is principally a disease of elderly people and accounts for around 15% of cases of dementia, making it second only to Alzheimer's disease as a cause, though some recent series have found Lewy body dementia to be as common, or even more common. It is more common in men, probably because more men suffer from hypertension and heart disease, two of the big risk factors for MID (Ueshima et al 1986). Hypertension is in fact *the* big risk factor for MID, with over 50% of patients giving a positive history for this disorder. Other risk factors essentially comprise the risk factors for stroke (Duthie & Glatt 1988), i.e. ischaemic heart disease, smoking, alcohol consumption and hyperlipidaemia. Many patients also give a history of peripheral vascular disease or transient ischaemic attacks.

Clinical features

Vascular dementias may present in a number of ways. As previously stated, they may present following a large stroke, but more commonly present as a slowly progressive disorder after small symptomatic infarcts or transient ischaemic attacks. Patchy deficits in intellect, often accompanied by focal neurological signs, are common. There may be evidence of systemic vascular disease and hypertension, for example carotid bruits, fundoscopic abnormalities and cardiomegaly. Mood disorders, especially depression, seem common

(Hasegawa et al 1986), occurring in up to a third of patients. Delusions and hallucinations seem more common than in DAT. Headaches, vertigo, tinnitus and loss of appetite are also common and in some cases symptoms and signs which are clearly related to lesion location may occur, for example urinary incontinence and return of grasp and sucking reflexes in frontal lobe lesions, Klüver–Bucy syndrome and memory loss in temporal lesions and Gerstmann's syndromes and dysphasias in parietal lobe lesions.

Binswanger's disease (progressive, subcortical vascular encephalopathy) is a severe arterosclerotic disorder of cerebral arteries affecting the subcortical areas. The age of onset is between 50 and 65 years and the disorder presents with dysphasia, hemianopias, hemiplegias and sensory disturbances. They usually have histories of very severe hypertension, systemic vascular disease and stroke. They gradually develop focal neurological signs, dementia and motor disturbance, often ending in pseudobulbar palsy. Kinkel et al (1985) reported that CT and MRI techniques are useful in the diagnosis of Binswanger's disease, revealing markedly enlarged ventricles and subcortical infarcts.

Differentiating vascular dementias from DAT is important, though often difficult and may have therapeutic implications. Table 11.5 provides a comparison of the clinical picture in vascular dementias and in DAT. Hachinski et al (1974) provided a scale which they claimed helped differentiate MID from DAT. It is not widely used and is thought to be of dubious value, particularly in cases where age of onset is greater.

CT and MRI

CT and MRI may demonstrate the presence of infarcts and haemorrhages. They provide, however, a far from perfect way of diagnosing vascular dementias. The diagnosis of small or very recent infarcts may be missed by CT. It has been suggested that the accuracy of CT is improved by repeating the scan a month or so after small strokes to improve visualisation of lesions.

MRI is an excellent method of displaying cerebral white matter. It may, however, reveal white matter lesions in patients who are not demented and white matter lesions per se do not imply a vascular cause for dementia. It is therefore not particularly helpful diagnostically.

Management of vascular dementias

The general management of vascular dementias is little different to that described for patients with DAT. Attention should be paid to treating underlying hypertension and heart disease. Though this will not reverse the dementing process it may slow down progression. Low-dose aspirin should be used as prophylaxis against further stroke and symptomatic treatment should be given for other problems such as headache and insomnia. As in DAT, it is important to treat comorbid depressive illness and other psychiatric syndromes.

Prognosis

Hasegawa et al (1980) demonstrated that patients with vascular dementias had a threefold increase in mortality when compared with non-demented controls. In the same study 93% of patients had died within the 5 year follow-up period. Factors associated with highest mortality included urinary incontinence, severity of dementia and being bedridden.

Frontal lobe dementias, including Pick's disease

The last decade has seen an upsurge in interest in frontal lobe dementias, triggered largely by the work of the Lund group in Sweden (Brun 1987). Prior to the work of this group, Pick's disease was regarded as the main dementing illness selectively involving frontal lobes. There has been debate about whether frontal lobe-type dementia is a variant of Pick's disease but most authors still regard them as distinct from one another.

Epidemiology and aetiology

Brun (1987) reported that 10% of a series of 158 cases of dementia going to autopsy had frontal lobe-type dementias, of which a quarter had Pick's disease and

Table 11.5 Differentiating Alzheimer's disease from vascular dementias	
Alzheimer's disease	Vascular dementia
More common in females	More common in males
Onset insidious	Onset may be sudden
Somatic complaints less common	Somatic complaints, e.g. headaches, dizziness
Focal neurological signs absent	Focal neurological signs
Fits and hypertension rare	Fits and hypertension common
Insight lost	Insight often retained
Mood flattened or euphoric	Affective symptoms common
Gradual progressive course	Stepwise course

the other three-quarters had dementia of frontal lobe type (DFT). Fifty per cent of the Lund sample had a family history in first-degree relatives, a finding confirmed by other studies.

Clinical features

A high proportion of cases of DFT are presenile, though the onset can be later. The onset is usually slow and involves changes in personality, behaviour, affect and language. Disinhibition, poor judgement, loss of social skills and lack of awareness are common, often combined with a shallow, labile and at times inappropriate affect. More rarely patients describe hyperalgesia or features of the Klüver–Bucy syndrome (hyperorality, visual agnosia and eating disturbances). Other clinical features described include obsessionality, rigidity and meticulous attention to the keeping of routines. Language abnormalities include loss of spontaneity of speech, reduction in output of language and echolalia, with progression to mutism later in the illness. In some patients memory is impaired, though this is usually less prominent than in Alzheimer-type dementia.

The differential diagnosis obviously includes Alzheimer-type dementia, cerebrovascular disease and frontal lobe tumours. CT and SPECT scanning may be helpful. Frontal lobe atrophy and occasionally temporal lobe atrophy are seen on CT. Selective reduction or absence of emission from frontal lobes has been reported (Deary & Whalley 1988).

Management and prognosis

Though no specific treatment exists for frontal lobe dementia, the general management is similar to that of Alzheimer's disease. In the study of Brun (1987), mean survival time was 8 years for DFT and 11 years for Pick's type dementia. The clinical course was usually one of slow deterioration, often ending in akinetic mutism.

Dementia associated with Parkinson's disease

Around 20–30% of those with Parkinson's disease develop a dementia. As Parkinson's disease is principally a disorder of old age, it is possible that some of these patients, in addition to suffering from the dementia associated with Parkinson's disease, may have other causes for dementia, for example Alzheimer's or cerebrovascular disease. Another source of difficulty in estimating the true prevalence of dementia in Parkinson's disease is that some patients with Alzheimer's disease develop extrapyramidal signs, and, further, the distinction between Parkinson's disease and Lewy body dementia is a matter of some debate and controversy. Brown & Marsden (1984) have suggested a figure of 10–15% may be more accurate for the prevalence of true Parkinson's disease-related dementia.

Clinical features

General slowing of comprehension, visuospatial impairment and problems with abstract reasoning are common cognitive deficits in patients with Parkinson's disease. Some memory impairment is seen, usually involving recent memory. Assessment of cognitive decline in Parkinson's disease is hampered by three things. firstly, depression complicates Parkinson's disease, and the accompanying psychomotor retardation with slowness in responding to questions and thinking may mimic dementia. Secondly, the clinical features of Parkinson's disease itself, especially bradykinesia, can mislead clinicians into misdiagnosing dementia. Finally, drug treatment of Parkinson's disease may also stimulate cognitive impairment. With regard to all of these, neuropsychological testing can be helpful in identifying those with true cognitive impairment.

Management

The approach to the patient with Parkinson's disease suffering from dementia follows the general principles already described in relation to Alzheimer's disease. It is important to note that drugs used to treat Parkinson's disease, even if they help with the motor symptoms of Parkinson's disease, do not help the dementia, though there is some evidence that monoamine oxidase B inhibitors, e.g. selegiline, may slow the progression of the dementia. Anticholinergic drugs should be avoided as they will exacerbate the cholinergic deficit which occurs in Parkinson's disease.

It is not yet known whether treatment with transplanted material (adrenal medulla or fetal brain) improves the cognitive decline associated with Parkinson's disease.

Dementia of Lewy body type (DLT)

It has been recognised in the last 10 years that there is a dementia associated with the presence of diffuse Lewy bodies in the cerebral cortex. Lennox et al (1989) have claimed that this is an underrecognised cause of dementia and that it is as common a cause as vascular disease. Recent autopsy studies estimate that 5–15% of all dementia sufferers have Lewy body disease. Lewy bodies are intracytoplasmic inclusion bodies which show a predilection for temporal lobe, cingulate gyrus and insular cortex in DLT. It has been noted that cortical Lewy bodies are found in Parkinson's disease but usually at lower densities than in DLT. Further, in DLT there is 40–60% loss of nigral dopaminergic neurones (as opposed to 80% or more in Parkinson's disease) (Perry et al 1990). The fact that senile plaques and neurofibrillary tangles are seen in DLT has led others to consider it to be a variant of Alzheimer's disease. DLT certainly shares clinical features with both Alzheimer's disease and Parkinson's disease and it has been suggested (Harrison & McKeith 1995) that DLT forms part of a spectrum of disorders, with pure Parkinson's disease at one end and pure Alzheimer's disease at the other end of the continuum.

Clinical features

The clinical presentation of DLT can vary considerably. Byrne et al (1989) reported on 15 cases, of whom six presented with dementia, six with parkinsonism and three with both. The disorder invariably does progress with dementia and a motor disorder indistinguishable from Parkinson's disease, with myoclonus. Clinical features of dementia are not dissimilar to those of DAT, but the mental state tends to fluctuate more. Visual hallucinations and alterations in consciousness may occur, as in delirium (Byrne et al 1989). Although the clinical distinction from DAT can be difficult, the combination of a cortical dementia with parkinsonism should alert clinicians to the possibility of DLT. Another clinical feature which may well help distinguish DLT from DAT is the observation that 50% of patients with DLT are very sensitive to treatment with neuroleptics, developing acute extrapyramidal symptoms and occasionally neuroleptic malignant syndrome (McKeith et al 1992b). This has led the Committee on Safety of Medicines to urge caution in the use of neuroleptics in patients with DLT. Atypical neuroleptics, for example risperidone, may be less likely to cause problems. The sensitivity to neuroleptics may be explicable by the fact that dopaminergic deficits in terms of number of neurones and dopamine levels have been described in DLT, as have deficits in choline acetyltransferase activity, which may have some relevance to treatment (see below).

The clinical course of DLT is usually more rapid than DAT, with most patients surviving 2–5 years.

Genetic studies have shown an increased frequency of the apolipoprotein E ϵ4 allele and decreased ϵ2 and ϵ3 frequency in DAT. Patients with DLT appear to have the increased ϵ4 frequency without the decreased ϵ2 frequency. It is suggested on this basis that DLT and DAT share a genetic risk factor (the ϵ4 apolipo protein, which is linked with β-amyloid and plaque formation), though difference in the frequency of ϵ2 allele leads to the differing propensity for tangle formation in DAT and DLT

Management

The parkinsonian features of DLT can be treated with antiparkinsonian drugs, though with the caution that these may exacerbate psychiatric symptoms. The balance between acceptable motor function and acceptable control of psychiatric symptoms, particularly psychotic symptoms, can be difficult to find. It has been previously noted that considerable caution has to be exercised in using antipsychotic drugs to control psychiatric symptoms in behavioural disturbance because of the sensitivity which many patients with DLT have to these drugs. Newer, atypic antipsychotics, e.g. risperidone, are to be preferred. Ondansetron, a 5-HT$_3$ receptor antagonist, is currently the subject of clinical trials in patients with DLT and it is hoped that it may be able to improve both cognitive and psychotic symptoms without worsening parkinsonism. Finally, the cholinergic deficits seen in DLT have led some to predict that drugs which facilitate cholinergic neurotransmission may improve cognitive function in DLT. Indeed, it has been reported (Levy et al 1994) that some good responders in trials of cholinergic agents, for example tacrine, have turned out to have Lewy body disease and not DAT.

Neuropsychiatric sequelae of acquired immune deficiency syndrome (AIDS)

The most common cause of AIDS is the human immunodeficiency virus type 1 (HIV-1). This is a virus of the genus *Lentivirus*, a group of viruses known to cause neurological disease in animals. Neuropsychiatric sequelae of infection with HIV-1 are common in humans: 50–70% of HIV-positive patients develop neurological signs or symptoms during the course of their disease (McGuire 1996). Neuropsychiatric sequelae of HIV infection occur in three ways:

- primary infection of the central nervous system by HIV-1 virus
- opportunistic infection
- tumours, e.g. intracranial lymphoma.

HIV-1 virus crosses the blood–brain barrier early in the disease, most likely at the point of the primary infection. There is a latency period of around 10 years before CNS complications are seen. Both opportunistic infection and primary HIV-related disease usually occurs in patients with CD4 lymphocyte (T helper cell) counts of less than 200×10^6, i.e. patients who are severely immunocompromised. Aseptic meningitis is the chief exception to this rule. Non-specific cerebrospinal fluid changes (raised protein, raised white cell count, raised IgG) are common in patients who are

HIV positive but are not usually associated with symptoms.

Psychiatric sequelae of HIV infection

A variety of psychiatric disorders and psychological problems have been described in relation to HIV infection (Maj 1990, Catalan et al 1995). Following a positive antibody test, anxiety and depression and adjustment disorders are not uncommon. Major affective disorders and psychotic illness are common in patients with AIDS and in some cases may reflect organic brain disease. The risk of suicide is increased. For a full account of these disorders and their management the reader is referred to the work of Catalan et al (1995). This section concentrates on AIDS-related-dementia.

AIDS dementia

Most HIV-positive patients do not develop AIDS dementia. McGuire (1996) has reported that a large number of studies suggest that asymptomatic seropositive individuals have no cognitive decline over time. Between 20 and 30% of patients do develop a dementia and in 6% dementia is the first AIDS defining illness. As there are around 18 million people infected with HIV-1 virus worldwide, it can, however, therefore be assumed that AIDS will lead to millions of new cases of dementia globally.

Clinical features   The dementia usually has an insidious onset and presents with apathy and social withdrawal. Impairment of memory, concentration and mental slowing are also common. Neurological signs include tremor, ataxia, increased reflexes, poor coordination and balance and dysarthria. As the disease progresses, psychomotor retardation becomes marked, memory deficits become more severe, there is loss of fine motor control, parkinsonian features and incontinence. The disease may end in a phase of akinetic mutism, with death usually occurring because of opportunistic infection. The mean survival time from diagnosis of dementia is 7 months (McGuire 1996).

Investigations   CSF total protein and IgG levels are increased. The CD4 count is invariably low. CT and MRI demonstrate cerebral atrophy with ventricular dilatation and widened sulci. MRI also shows focal increase in white matter signals. SPECT reveals increased glucose metabolism in thalamus and basal ganglia, and in late stages hypometabolism in cortical and subcortical grey matter is seen.

Differential diagnosis   The differential diagnosis of AIDS dementia is important as it includes some treatable disorders. In the early stages social withdraw-

al, apathy and poor concentration must be distinguished from depressive illness, which is common in patients with AIDS. Neuropsychological testing usually helps distinguish cognitive decline from depression. Delirium due to drug treatment, adrenal hypofunction, electrolyte imbalance and other metabolic problems must also be excluded. In addition, it is important to rule out other treatable central nervous system diseases, which are common in AIDS. The more common include:

- cryptococcosis
- tuberculosis
- syphilis
- toxoplasmosis
- cytomegalovirus (CMV) infection.

The less common include:

- herpes zoster infection
- herpes simplex infection
- lymphomatous meningitis
- aspergillosis
- primary lymphoma
- progressive multifocal leucoencephalopathy (PML).

For an account of the treatment of these disorders the reader is referred to McGuire (1996) and Harrison (1995).

Cryptococcosis is the most common of these disorders and presents as a meningoencephalitis with marked headache. Less than a third of patients, however, have neck stiffness and photophobia and a high degree of vigilance is therefore necessary. India ink stain examination of CSF demonstrates the presence of cryptococcus, and cryptococcal antigen is also found in the blood. Toxoplasmosis presents with confusion and headaches. Focal neurological signs usually develop rapidly, as can seizures. MRI or CT reveals multiple mass lesions with ring enhancement and oedema. Cytomegalovirus infection is difficult to diagnoses clinically. CT and MRI reveal ventriculitis and ependymitis. Culture of CSF for cytomegalovirus is normally negative and treatment usually has to be on the grounds of strong clinical suspicion. Herpes zoster and herpes simplex present with a picture of meningoencephalitis. Progressive multifocal leucoencephalopathy is caused by opportunistic viral infection of white matter leading to demyelination. MRI reveals areas of abnormal signal in white matter, with no mass effect.

Pathogenesis   The pathogenesis of AIDS dementia is poorly understood. The HIV-1 virus does not directly affect neurones, astrocytes and oligodendrocytes; macrophages and microglia are principally affected. The pathognomonic feature of HIV encephalitis is the multinucleated giant cell (macrophages packed with

HIV virions). Macrophages are able to resist the cyctotoxic effects of HIV virus and therefore maintain latent infection. They can carry infection from the periphery to the CNS and act as viral reservoirs in CNS. This has been described as the 'Trojan horse effect' by McGuire (1996).

AIDS dementia appears to involve a number of promoting and inducing factors (McGuire 1996), including:

- immune-mediated factors functioning as neurotoxins and causing indirect neural injury, e.g. tumour necrosis factor, enhancing HIV replication
- calcium-mediated neurotoxicity (HIV infection can overactivate receptors mediating calcium entry into neural cells)
- damage by viral proteins or by neurotoxins secreted by HIV-infected macrophages
- coinfection with other viruses, e.g. CMV
- strains of HIV -1 which may be particularly 'neurovirulent'.

Treatment It is important to rule out treatable infections and lymphoma (see above). There is no known treatment for AIDS dementia, though high-dose Zidovudine (AZT) may improve cognitive function in the short term.

Huntington's disease

Huntington's disease, also known as Huntington's chorea, was first described in Long Island in 1872 by George Huntington. It has a prevalence of around 5 per 100 000, with men and women being equally affected. It has been the focus of intensive research by molecular biologists in the last 15 years, since Gusella et al (1983) found a marker for Huntington's disease on chromosome 4, leading to the discovery of the gene 10 years later (Huntington's Disease Collaborative Research Group 1993).

Aetiology

Huntington's disease is inherited in an autosomal dominant manner, though occasionally sporadic cases occur. As indicated, the gene was located to chromosome 4 in 1983 and identified in 1993. The disease is related to a trinucleotide repeat mutation, which appears to account for all cases of the disorder. Recent work is shedding light upon the pathogenesis (Davies et al 1998, Martindale et al 1998).

Pathology and neurochemistry

The pathology is characterised by cortical atrophy, particularly prominent in frontal lobes and associated with ventricular dilatation. There is marked neuronal loss in the striatum, with atrophy of the head of caudate and putamen. Further neuronal loss is seen in the outer cortical laminae, again particularly prominent in the frontal lobes. Loss of striatal GABAergic neurones is seen.

Autopsy studies have revealed deficits in GABA on inhibitory neurotransmitters in the caudate, putamen and globus pallidus (Perry et 1973). Increased dopamine concentration in the basal ganglia has also been described and it is suggested that the imbalance between GABA and dopamine may lead to the abnormal movements seen in the disease.

Clinical features

Oliver (1970) noted that around 40% of patients who later developed Huntington's disease had prodromal behavioural disorders and suggested that this in itself may predict the development of the illness. These disorders included violence, aggressive behaviour, marital disharmony, sexual perversions and criminal behaviours. Depression, apathy and even psychotic symptoms have also been described in the prodromal period and are held by some to have predictive value in identifying those who will develop the disease. Other authors, for example Bolt (1970), have suggested that it is more common for behavioural and psychiatric disturbance to postdate the onset of chorea. A high suicide rate has been described, not only in those with the disease but also in the relatives, and schizophrenia has been observed to occur more frequently than would be expected in this population (Dewhurst & Oliver 1970).

Onset of the disease is usually in middle age, with a mean onset in the 40s, though occasional cases with onset during adolescence have been described and generally progress more rapidly. The diagnosis is not usually made until both movement disorder and cognitive impairment are present, though there can be a gap of years between the onset of neurological and psychiatric symptoms. Onset of the illness is usually insidious and may consist of abnormal movements, which some patients may attempt to cover up. Choreiform movements appear most commonly in head, neck and arms. Facial twitching is common. Later, athetoid movements of the limbs appear and speech and swallowing are affected. Rigidity and epilepsy may occur. It is usually later in the disease that dementia appears. This initially presents with mild memory difficulties, difficulties in organisation and planning, and difficulties in verbal skills. It is important to note that insight is often retained for some years and undoubtedly contributes to depression and suicide. Death usually occurs 10–15 years from onset of the disease.

Brain imaging

In established disease caudate atrophy may be seen on CT. PET studies have shown decreased glucose metabolism, which is evident even before the clinical onset of the disease. Reduced blood flow in the striatum has been demonstrated using SPECT.

Treatment

No treatment is known to halt the progress of the disease. Neuroleptics are invariably required to treat chorea, psychosis and behavioural disturbance. Tetrabenazine (in doses of 25–200 mg) has been said to be effective in the movement disorder, but the evidence for this is largely anecdotal. Depressive illness is treated in the usual way.

Genetic testing

Both diagnostic and predictive testing are now widely available. Prenatal testing and diagnosis is also an option (Adams et al 1993). The ability to test for presence of the Huntington's disease gene has raised concerns about both ethical and psychological consequences of testing. Wiggins et al (1992), in a study of the psychological health of participants in a programme of genetic testing, noted better than expected results both for those at increased and those at decreased risk of inheriting the gene for the disease. Ethical issues have surrounded the consequences of positive testing with regard to employment, personal insurance and relationships, and also around the issue of how to deal with families where some members wish to be tested and others do not (Harper 1993). There are now fairly widely accepted procedures guiding genetic counselling (Simpson & Harding 1993).

Wilson's disease (hepatolenticular degeneration)

Wilson's disease is a rare, inherited disorder principally affecting the liver and the CNS. It was first described by Wilson in 1912. The mode of inheritance is autosomal recessive. The disease is a disorder of copper metabolism, characterised by a low serum caeruloplasmin (a globulin which binds copper) and overabsorption of dietary copper. High levels of unbound copper result in its deposition in the liver, basal ganglia, cerebrum and eyes. More rarely the renal tubules and bones are affected.

The clinical features usually become obvious in childhood or adolescence, though occasionally later onset is seen. The disorder may present with liver disease, neurological disease or with both. Bearn (1972) has reported that about 20% of cases present psychiatrically. Clinical features attributable to the liver disease include jaundice, hepatosplenomegaly, ascites and haematemesis (from ruptured oesophageal varices). The neurological features are usually motor. Extrapyramidal rigidity, tremor and athetoid movements with dystonic posturing of the limbs is common. There may be a stiff, motionless facial expression. In those where neurological features predominate, misdiagnosis as conversion disorder is by no means uncommon. In some cases there are bulbar symptoms, including dysarthria and dysphagia. Epilepsy and alterations of consciousness have also been described.

The Kayser–Fleischer ring is a brown/green ring seen at the margin of the cornea. It may be visible to the naked eye, though in some cases it is only seen on slit-lamp examination.

CT reveals ventricular dilatation, cortical atrophy and enlargements of the cisterns around the brain. Hypodense areas are commonly seen in the basal ganglia.

Treatment is by means of chelating agents, of which the most commonly used is D-penicillamine. Most patients appear to benefit, at least in part, from treatment (Walshe 1968). Walshe has highlighted the importance of keeping people on a large enough dose for long enough to prevent relapse occurring. Some authorities recommend a strict low copper diet, though Walshe has suggested that this is unnecessary, though he does recommend excluding foods rich in copper, including nuts, liver, shellfish, chocolates, mushrooms, dried fruit and whisky. The neurological features respond better to treatment than the hepatic features.

The most common psychiatric symptoms seen in Wilson's disease are personality change, behavioural disturbance and dementia. The combination of the behavioural disturbance with neurological features is another pitfall which leads many to diagnose a conversion disorder in these patients. Some patients with Wilson's disease develop psychotic symptoms. In a proportion of the cases psychiatric symptoms may be present before there are any signs of neurological or hepatic disease (Walker 1969). The psychiatric symptoms respond partially to treatment with D-penicillamine, but respond less well than do the neurological features.

Alcoholic dementia

A dementia syndrome distinct from the Wernicke–Korsakoff syndrome (described below) occurs in patients who chronically misuse alcohol, and indeed is more common than the Wernicke–Korsakoff syndrome. It is a consequence of the neurotoxic effects of alcohol on the brain. Women are considerably more susceptible than men to the development of this syndrome and the elderly are also more vulnerable. Disorders of mood and psychotic symptoms, including visual or auditory hallucinations or delusions, are common, in addition to cognitive impairment characterised by poor memory, poor retention of newly presented information and disorientation. This disorder is usually slowly progressive.

Progressive supranuclear palsy (Steele–Richardson syndrome)

Progressive supranuclear palsy (Steele et al 1964, Steele 1972) is a degenerative disorder of the brainstem, cerebellum and basal ganglia. The onset is usually at over 50 years of age. It causes a subcortical dementia. Patients generally present with gait disturbance, including toppling over; paralysis of extraocular movements, dysarthria, neck dystonia and truncal dystonia follow. Pathologically, cell loss and gliosis are described in brainstem nuclei, basal ganglia and cerebellum. There is no known treatment.

Other causes of dementia

There are many other causes of dementia but they are not common. They include intracranial infections, endocrine disorders, vitamin deficiencies and other neurological disorders, e.g. multiple sclerosis. Although rare, it is important to bear these in mind as some may have treatment implications. Some are discussed later in the chapter in relation to their other psychiatric sequelae.

Reversible dementias

It is important to remember that a proportion of dementing illnesses may be caused by a treatable underlying disorder. Lishman (1987) concluded from studies of presenile patients that 5% had reversible causes for their dementia (excluding alcohol). In the elderly the numbers with a reversible cause were probably lower, none the less there is a need to be vigilant with regard to treatable underlying causes and to investigate patients thoroughly and appropriately before designating them untreatable. Table 11.6 lists the causes of reversible dementias as outlined by Lishman (1987). To these should now be added opportunistic infections accompanying AIDS. Lishman has pointed out that treatment does not always lead to full recovery in all cases, and that the term 'reversible' may therefore be slightly misleading.

Normal pressure hydrocephalus

Adams et al (1965) described a syndrome charac-

Table 11.6 Potentially reversible causes of dementia
Intracranial disorders
Tumours
Subdural haematoma
Normal pressure hydrocephalus
General paralysis of the insane (GPI)
Systemic disorders involving cerebral function
Anoxia (several underlying causes)
Hypoglycaemia
Myxoedema
Renal and hepatic disease
Vitamin deficiencies
Alcoholism
Poisoning (by drug or chemicals)
'Pseudodementia' secondary to psychiatric disorder, e.g. depression

terised by dementia, ataxia and urinary incontinence. Pneumoencephalography revealed enlarged ventricles and normal CSF pressure was demonstrated on lumbar puncture. So-called normal pressure hydrocephalus can occur in the course of Alzheimer's disease with the same symptoms, but there are patients with the syndrome who benefit from the insertion of shunts and who do not suffer from Alzheimer's disease.

A small number of patients with normal pressure hydrocephalus have had a preceding head injury, subarachnoid haemorrhage or infection with meningitis.

Onset of the disorder is usually in the 60s and 70s and this often leads to misdiagnosis as Alzheimer's disease. Early incontinence is the most helpful distinguishing clinical feature, as incontinence is usually a late clinical feature in Alzheimer's. Behavioural disturbance is uncommon in normal pressure hydrocephalus, as are psychotic symptoms.

Diagnosis

CT often reveals dilated ventricles, especially the third ventricle, and narrowing of the sulci at the vertex. The diagnostic accuracy of CT is, however, poor, with both false negatives and false positives occurring. Because of this, treatment is usually carried out on the grounds of clinical suspicion in patients with the previously described triad of symptoms.

Treatment

Treatment consists of surgical insertion of a shunt, usually between the lateral ventricles and the inferior vena cava. There is a not insignificant operative morbidity, most commonly caused by tearing of meningeal vesicles. Successful surgery usually leads to rapid improvement (within weeks) of the cognitive deficits and the incontinence. The gait abnormality may take longer to improve.

Prion body dementias

Prion protein is a normal brain protein, the function of which is unknown. Prion-related diseases occur when the protein undergoes a conformational change which render it insoluble (Fleminger & Curtis 1997). This insoluble form is metabolised less well than the normal form and therefore accumulates, causing cell death and other pathological changes, including spongiform changes, astrocyte proliferation and on occasion amyloid plaque deposition.

The diseases caused by prions are spongiform encephalopathies which are transmissible dementias. There are four forms of the disease in humans, all of which are rare. These are:

- Creutzfeldt–Jakob disease (CJD)
- Gerstmann–Straussler syndrome (GSS)
- kuru
- fatal familial insomnia (FFI).

With the exception of kuru a proportion of the other human prion diseases (10–15%) are inherited as autosomal dominant mutations. Kuru is found in the Fore tribe of Papua New Guinea and was caused by cannibalistic rituals, which no longer occur. Because of the long latency period of the disease (around 40 years), some cases continue to be seen.

Iatrogenic CJD can be transmitted via corneal grafting, the use of human cadaveric pituitary growth hormone and by handling CNS tissue at postmortem examination. Although rare, CJD is the most common of the human prion diseases and in its classic form results in a rapidly progressing degenerative disorder characterised by dementia, myoclonus, spasticity, extrapyramidal rigidity and choreoathetoid movements. As the disease progresses, dysarthria and dysphagia supervene and it invariably ends in akinetic mutism. Death usually occurs within 2 years. Variant forms described include the so-called Heidenhain form, in which cortical blindness is accompanied by extrapyramidal signs and myoclonus. In the ataxic form, cerebellar ataxia, abnormal and voluntary movements and myclonus are prominent. In common with the classic form, both of these usually end in akinetic mutism.

GSS presents as a progressive cerebellar ataxia with dementia. It has a longer clinical course than CJD (around 5 years). Similarly kuru presents with progressive cerebellar ataxia and dementia, often with accompanying mood and personality change. FFI classically presents with untreatable, intractable insomnia with motor symptoms. It is very rapidly progressive.

New variant CJD

In 1996 Will et al (1996) described 10 patients with an apparently new variant of CJD. Their presentation was unusual, with behavioural and psychiatric disturbance being prominent and with 9 of the 10 initially having been referred to a psychiatrist, either with suspected mood disorder or behavioural problems. None of these patients had risk factors in the form of iatrogenic exposure or prion protein mutations. All were under 40 years old at the age of onset. All had abnormal EEGs, but without showing classic CJD appearances. At autopsy all had a spongiform encephalopathy with plaques. Mallucci & Collinge (1997) have noted that the clinical picture was similar to that of kuru (with psychiatric disturbance and ataxia) and of iatrogenic CJD caused by contaminated growth hormone or gonadotrophin. This led them to suggest the route of entry of prions affects the resultant clinical syndromes. Of further interest is the observation (Collinge et al 1996) that all patients with new variant CJD described so far are homozygous for a polymorphism at codon 129 of prion protein. Both sporadic and iatrogenic CJD are known to occur mainly in individuals homozygous for this polymorphism.

The arrival of new variant CJD has led to renewed interest, and indeed some alarm that there is a new risk factor for CJD. Matthews (1990) suggested that an animal prion disease, bovine spongiform encephalopathy (BSE), found in cattle may be transmissible to man via infected meat. The arrival of the new variant, with its different pathology and clinical course, has once again raised the possibility that exposure to bovine prions has led to transmission of BSE to humans, presumably before the bovine offal ban of 1989. Assuming patients with new variant CJD were exposed to BSE in the mid-1980s, their incubation period would be 5–10 years.

By mid-1996 there had been 160 000 cases of BSE in the UK, though the long incubation period and under-reporting make it likely that as many as 1 million cattle may be infected (Harrison 1997). About half of these cattle entered the food chain before the offals ban of 1989, making it beyond dispute that humans were exposed to BSE through diet. After a period of debate about the evidence for and against transmission of BSE, to humans, Harrison (1997) now writes 'It appears likely that BSE has led to human prion disease.' The emergence of new variant CJD, the demonstration that BSE can cause plaque-type neuropathology in monkeys and the demonstration by Collinge et al (1996) that prion proteins in new variant CJD shared the same molecular signature of those seen in BSE-affected cows, has clearly tipped the balance of evidence in favour of the notion that BSE transmission to humans has caused new variant CJD. At the time of writing 15 new variant CJD cases have been identified. Harrison comments that because of the uncertainty about the length and variability of the incubation period it is difficult to predict how many will eventually suffer, with estimates varying from 80 to 80 000.

Whichever is the case, the new variant highlights the need for clinicians (and especially psychiatrists) to be vigilant in looking for behavioural and psychiatric abnormalities in younger people with cerebellar signs and cognitive impairment.

Diagnostic tests

Hsich et al (1996) have described a test involving detection of a marker in CSF which may allow CJD to be diagnosed before death. It remains to be thoroughly evaluated and it is clear that false positives may occur, for example due to cerebrovascular accident or viral encephalitis.

Amnestic syndrome

Amnestic syndrome refers to a disorder characterised by memory loss and resulting from a number of different aetiologies. These include primary cerebral disease, systemic medical disorders, substance misuse and drugs. Major aetiological factors are listed in Table 11.7.

Clinical features

The key clinical feature is impaired ability to learn new information. Recall of previously learned information and recall for past events are also impaired. These impairments are sufficient to interfere with social and occupational functioning. They will usually affect both verbal and visual memory. Immediate memory, for example as assessed by digit span, is often intact in patients with amnestic disorders.

In the early stages of the disorder confabulation is common, with patients recalling imaginary events in order to fill in gaps in their memory. This phenomenon usually gets less with the passage of time. Disorientation for time and place is common but disorientation for person exceedingly rare. Patients with this disorder frequently lack insight and this may interfere with relationships with others. Many patients display apathy and lack of interest in their surroundings. Although they are superficially agreeable and friendly, the range of emotional expression is shallow.

Table 11.7 Aetiology of amnestic disorders
Thiamine deficiency
Alcohol
Malnutrition
Malabsorption, e.g. after gastric surgery, small bowel disease
Severe protracted vomiting (rare)
Cerebral disease and injury
Closed head trauma
Cerebrovascular disease, especially posterior cerebral artery infarct
Herpes simplex encephalitis
Temporal lobe surgery
Penetrating missile wound
Focal tumours
Hypoxia
Toxins
Carbon monoxide
Lead
Organophosphate insecticides
Industrial solvents
Drugs
Anticonvulsants
Intrathecal methotrexate

Wernicke–Korsakoff's syndrome

Korsakoff (1889) was the first to publish reports of amnestic disorder. The causes were thiamine deficiency secondary to alcohol consumption, persistent vomiting and puerperal sepsis. Prior to this Wernicke (1881) had described a neurological disorder of acute onset in alcoholic patients. It was characterised by nystagmus, lateral rectus palsy, paralysis of conjugate gaze, ataxia, peripheral neuropathy and retinal haemorrhages. The patients also displayed clinical features of delirium. All Wernicke's patients died and at postmortem examination had haemorrhages in the grey matter surrounding the third and fourth ventricles of the brain. It has been recognised that the syndromes described by Wernicke and Korsakoff are in effect different stages of the same disease process. Many cases of the acute Wernicke syndrome (even some of those who are treated) progress into the Korsakoff syndrome, with enduring cognitive impairment. Victor et al (1971) suggested calling the syndrome the Wernicke–Korsakoff syndrome for this reason. Victor has reported that, even with treatment, a considerable number of patients go on to develop an enduring amnestic syndrome (84% of those who survive the acute encephalopathy). When Korsakoff's syndrome was established, complete recovery occurred in only a quarter, with no improvement in half and an incomplete recovery in the remaining quarter.

Further postmortem studies in patients with Wernicke's encephalopathy have revealed, in addition to the third and fourth ventricular grey matter haemorrhages described by Wernicke himself, that there are petechial haemorrhages in the mamillary bodies and inferior colliculi. Pratt et al (1985) have demonstrated that some patients with alcohol problems are unable to utilise thiamine normally, resulting in ineffective transketolase enzyme systems. This system is involved in brain glucose, metabolism and neurotransmitter formation. This appears to be partly genetically determined and may explain some individual differences in patients in their susceptibility to cerebral damage subsequent to alcohol abuse. Patients with Wernicke–Korsakoff's syndrome need to be treated promptly. In Victor's series there was a 17% death rate during the acute encephalopathy. Prompt treatment also reduces (though does not altogether prevent) subsequent cognitive impairment.

Treatment employs large doses of thiamine, 50 mg intravenously and 50 mg intramuscularly. The intramuscular dose is usually continued for a few days until the patient is eating a normal diet. Other B vitamins are given orally for up to 6 months. Two particular dangers attend the treatments of patients with severe thiamine deficiency. The first is of cardiovascular collapse and highlights the requirements for bed-rest in the acute stages. The second is that patients must be given thiamine and B vitamins before being given a carbohydrate load. In patients who are given carbohydrate, and in particular glucose, before being given adequate thiamine, their last reserves of B vitamins, and especially thiamine, may be depleted and this can precipitate Wernicke's encephalopathy where it was not present before; and where it was present it can be worsened.

Pathology

The pathological processes which underlie amnestic disorder involve medial temporal lobe structures, including mamillary bodies, hippocampus, fornix and amygdala. The pathology is usually bilateral but deficits may occur with unilateral lesions.

Brain imaging in amnestic disorder

MRI and CT reveal no specific or diagnostic features. Unsurprisingly, however, middle temporal lobe structural damage is common and this may be manifest in enlargement of the temporal horns or the third ventricle or in structural atrophy.

Differential diagnosis

It is important to differentiate amnestic disorder from dementia. The core feature of amnestic disorder is inability to learn and recall new information and to recall previously learned factual knowledge. In contrast to dementia this occurs in the absence of other cognitive deficits, for example aphasia, apraxia, agnosia and abnormalities of executive functioning. The other major differential diagnosis is from dissociative amnesia. Patients with dissociative amnesia usually display no deficits in new learning and in recalling new information. Their problem is an inability to recall previously learned information while functioning normally in the present day. Further, dissociative amnesia usually starts and ends abruptly and is associated with an awareness of having no memories at all for the duration of the amnesiac state. Dissociative amnesias are not infrequently accompanied by fugue states.

Course and outcome

The course and outcome of amnestic disorder depends on the underlying aetiology. This has already been discussed in relation to Wernicke–Korsakoff's syndrome. In other causes of thiamine deficiency, or where there is temporal lobe pathology or destruction by surgery, amnestic syndrome is virtually always persistent.

After head trauma, amnestic disorders can show improvement for up to 24 months. There is usually little further improvement after this time. Amnestic disorders caused by cerebral vascular aetiologies are often recurrent, with variable recovery between episodes.

Treatment

Treatment should be aimed, where possible, at the underlying cause, for example, thiamine deficiency in Wernicke–Korsakoff's syndrome, antiviral medication in herpes simplex, encephalitis or aspirin in cerebrovascular disease. No treatment clearly reverses memory deficits when they become established. In the most severe cases, when memory disturbance causes considerable impairment in social functioning, supervision and support with activities of daily living is necessary.

HEAD INJURY

Head trauma resulting in brain injury has a wide variety of psychiatric manifestations. It can lead to all the major syndromes described in this chapter, including delirium, dementia and amnestic disorder, as well as secondary psychiatric syndromes leading to mood disorder, personality change and psychotic symptoms.

Head injury is extremely common. One year prevalence figures are 10–15 per 100 000 for severe head injury, 15–20 per 100 000 for moderate head injury and 250–300 per 100 000 for mild head injury (Powell 1994). The age groups at highest risk for head injury are 15–29 years and over 65 years. Males are three times more likely than females to have a head injury and this difference is even more marked in the younger age group. The most common causes of head injury are road traffic accidents (50%), domestic and industrial accidents (30%), sports injuries (10–15%) and assaults (10%).

Although most head injuries are minor and most people recovery fully, health and social services have to cope with the annual addition of around 1000 severely disabled individuals as a result of head injury. The services for these individuals are largely held to be inadequate.

Classification

Head injury is usually described as open (penetrating) or closed. In open or penetrating injury, which is relatively rare, objects, for example bullets, fracture the skull and enter the brain, causing largely localised damage, though damage can also be caused by bone fragments being showered into the brain and (in the case of bullets) expansion of hot gases around the missile itself.

Closed injuries, which are more common, occur as a result of acceleration/deceleration or rotational injuries when the head collides with other objects, for example the windscreen of a car, the road or a large rock. It is these violent movements which cause the brain injury in closed head injury, rather than the presence of foreign bodies within the brain.

Pathogenesis

Brain injury is caused through a multiplicity of direct and indirect mechanisms. Direct mechanisms include contusions underlying the point of trauma, contusions opposite the point of trauma (contrecoup injury) and compression from skull fractures or haematomas. Indirect effects have been well described by Alexander (1982) and include diffuse impact damage (particularly to cerebral white matter, corpus callosum and rostral brainstem) and secondary cerebral and systemic processes (Table 11.8). In addition, some brain areas are particularly vulnerable to injury, independent of the site of impact. These include orbitofrontal, anterior temporal and frontal polar regions (Alexander 1982).

Holbourne (1943) was the first to describe the mech-

Table 11.8 Secondary cerebral and systemic insults contributing to brain injury

Cerebral	Systemic
Haematoma	Hypoxaemia
Raised intracranial pressure	Arterial hypotension
Seizures	Anaemia
Infection	Hypocarbia
Vasospasm	Hypercarbia
	Pyrexia
	Hyponatraemia
	Hypoglycaemia
	Hyperglycaemia

anism of brain injury. He concluded that the rotational movements of the head produced shearing of brain substance, and in particular blood vessels and nerve fibres. The damage thus caused is diffuse and extensive and is unrelated to the site of impact. In further studies (Strich 1956, 1961) reported white matter degeneration and hydrocephalus in postmortem studies of brain injury victims. She reported that the prominent histological feature of those surviving after initial injury was axonal retraction balls denoting severed nerve fibres, from which axoplasm had leaked. She further reported widespread cerebral white matter changes and changes in the long tracts of the brainstem, typical of wallerian degeneration. She concluded that the cause of this degeneration was shearing and tearing of nerve fibres at the moment of impact.

In penetrating head injuries, patients may be spared from the damage caused by indirect effects, despite direct damage. However, it should be noted that penetrating missile injuries disturb neuronal function through the effects of vibratory waves and this can lead to injury beyond the actual site of impact.

Course and outcome

Severity of head injury is commonly assessed using the Glasgow Coma Scale (GCS) (Table 11.9) (Teasdale & Jennett 1974). After injury, GCS scores are usually recorded serially, with a deteriorating score indicating potentially ominous complications.

Another way of assessing severity of injury is to measure post-traumatic amnesia (PTA). PTA is the period that elapses between the time of injury and the restoration of continuous memory for day-to-day events. It has been demonstrated to be clearly related to severity of injury. Russell (1932) produced the following scale:

PTA < 1 hour = mild injury

Table 11.9	Glasgow Coma Scale (GCS)		
Eye opening		*Verbal response*	
None	1	None	1
To pain	2	Incomprehensive	2
To speech	3	Inappropriate	3
Spontaneous	4	Confused	4
		Orientated	5
Motor response			
None	1	Mild injury	GCS 13–15
Extension	2	Moderate injury	GCS 9–12
Abnormal flexion	3	Severe injury	GCS 3–8
Withdrawal	4		
Localises pain	5		
Obeys commands	6		

PTA 1–24 hours = moderate injury
PTA 1–7 days = severe injury
PTA > 7 days = very severe injury

This is a generally reliable guide to severity of injury but it has limitations. For example, PTA increases with age for any given injury. Likewise, PTA is of less value in penetrating brain injury, when there may be considerable local damage but a fully conscious patient.

The majority of patients with minor injuries have a symptom cluster characterised by headaches, fatigue and dizziness with no neurological signs or intracranial complications. Some such persons have brief loss of consciousness, lasting a few minutes. It is not uncommon for such patients in the few weeks following injury to report, in addition to the aforementioned symptoms, sleep disturbance, tiredness and memory problems. A minority go on to develop postconcussional syndrome, which is described below.

Patients with moderate and severe injuries usually pass through several stages which are characterised by different symptoms. For the most severely head-injured patients the initial stage is one of coma. When consciousness is resumed, the patient is frequently delirious and PTA becomes evident. In addition, patients will manifest retrograde amnesia, which in moderate injuries usually last seconds to minutes, but for more severe injuries can cover intervals of days. The pattern of retrograde amnesia follows Ribot's law, which states that the most recent memories are the most susceptible to disruption, with recall of more remote memories being least affected. Resolution of retrograde amnesia follows the same law, with the period of memory loss shrinking backwards towards the accident, with more remote memories being recovered first.

Jennett & Bond (1975) have devised the Glasgow Outcome Scale to assess outcome of moderate to severe head injuries. It is recommended this is used 6 months postinjury. By this time the greater part of recovery has taken place, though some improvement continues to 12 months, and even beyond. The Glasgow Outcome Scale includes death and four categories of survival. These categories are:

- *Persistent vegetative state* This applies to the small group of patients who never recover consciousness after the initial brain trauma. Patients in this state have no evidence of cerebral cortical functioning, though a working brainstem allows vegetative functioning to be maintained. Such patients have sleep–wake cycles and may allow themselves to be fed, and occasionally move their limbs. This, however, does not imply meaningful cognitive activity and these actions are considered to be reflexive.
- *Severe disability* These patients are likely to be hospitalised. They have usually have a PTA of >24 hours. They not infrequently have serious physical and psychological deficits. They require supervision and support with activities of daily living and usually require hospitalisation and postacute rehabilitation.
- *Moderate disability* These patients have usually had an initial period of loss of consciousness, lasting from minutes to a few hours, and a period of PTA of up to 24 hours. They are independent, but remain disabled, often with physical, cognitive and behavioural problems resulting from their brain injury. When compared with their premorbid status they function poorly.
- *Good recovery* Patients with good recovery have had very brief periods of PTA (less than 1 hour). They may have mild cognitive deficits and neurological complications but are for the large part independent and physically and socially competent. They often return to full employment.

It has recently been suggested that blood alcohol level at the time of trauma affects recovery from severe closed head injury (Kaplan & Corrigan 1992). This interesting observation awaits further study. It has also been suggested that traumatic brain injury can lead to an increased risk of Alzheimer's disease (Graves et al 1990), though this has been contested by other workers (Breteler et al 1995).

Psychiatric syndromes following head injury

As previously stated, a variety of psychiatric syndromes and psychological problems may follow head-injury. It is particularly important that these are assessed in the light of some knowledge of the patient's premorbid personality. When compared with general population controls, head-injured patients manifest higher rates of pre-morbid psychiatric disturbance and personality problems. A large number of head injuries are related to the ingestion of alcohol. Patients with head injuries have increased rates of premorbid alcohol problems. Studies have also described increases in the premorbid incidence of antisocial personality traits in head injury patients, such persons being more likely than others to engage in high-risk behaviours. Other reasons for increased rates of premorbid psychiatric disorder include the suggestion that patients with psychosis and depression may be more likely to sustain head injuries when engaged in suicidal acts, e.g. high-speed road traffic accidents (Capruso & Levin, 1992). These factors highlight the importance of attempting to make an adequate assessment of premorbid personality and of taking a detailed past psychiatric history.

Cognitive disorders

There is little doubt that a wide range of cognitive functions may be impaired after a closed brain injury. Psychometric test batteries, e.g. the Halstead–Reitan and the Wechsler Adult Intelligence Scale, demonstrate clear abnormalities of memory, language and executive functioning, including planning, organising and sequencing. More specific tests, e.g. the Progressive Matrices Test and Mill Hill Scale, have been used to assess non-verbal and verbal IQ, respectively. These reveal that performance deficits are more prominent than verbal deficits in head-injured patients (Brooks & Aughton 1979). Most recovery of intelligence has occurred by 1 year after injury, with little change in levels of intelligence after this. Loss of short-term memory is usually the most persistent of the cognitive sequelae of head injury. This may take the form of transient or prolonged amnestic disorder, but most patients with severe post-traumatic memory deficits have more global cognitive impairment, often associated with language difficulties and neurological signs, e.g. hemiparesis. A dementing illness with progressive deficit has been described in association with multiple recurrent head trauma. This has been described as 'chronic traumatic encephalopathy' or 'boxers' encephalopathy', as it not infrequently occurs in boxers, particularly those nearing the end of their careers. The pattern of dementia is subcortical with parkinsonian features, as well as memory impairment.

Both fluent and non-fluent dysphasia, as well as nominal dysphasia, have been described in head-injured patients. In fluent dysphasia the problem is one of poor language comprehension, making paraphasic errors and using jargon. In non-fluent dysphasia the number of words used is reduced. In nominal dysphasia patients will have difficulties in naming objects and in word finding, despite intact comprehension and repetition abilities. The recovery of language after closed head injury appears to be sequential, with visual and auditory comprehension recovering first (the patient may, for example, understand gestures and spoken language) and reading, writing and oral expression recovering later (Najenson 1978).

Mood disorder

Organic affective syndromes have been described after brain injury. Eames (1997) cites good evidence for an increase in both depression and mania, particularly the latter (Verdoux & Bourgeois 1995). In most cases there is a gradual improvement in mood-related symptoms, though persisting depression and anxiety occur in up to 25% of patients (this is similar to the frequency of these disorders in populations with chronic general medical disorders). The development of major depressive illness usually occurs some months, or even years, after injury. Its aetiology has been debated, but it is probably wisest to see it as being multifactorial in origin, developing in the context of the multiple physical, psychological and social sequelae of brain-injury. There is no conclusive evidence that it is caused by brain damage per se. Although persisting depression and mania may require pharmacological intervention, brain-injured patients are especially vulnerable to the effects of psychotropic drugs. This is particularly true in the first few months after injury, where there is evidence that psychotropic drugs can adversely effect recovery in a way which persists to some extent in many patients (Goldstein 1993).

One disorder seen after brain injury, which can be confused with affective disorder, is 'the syndrome of pathological laughing and crying' or 'dysprosopeia' (Eames 1997). This appears to be related to bilateral hemispheric or bulbar lesions, though recently Zeilig et al (1996) have suggested a right hemispheric origin. This disorder seems to be associated with severity of head injury, though it can occur after more minor injuries. Eames has pointed out that it contributes considerably to morbidity of head-injured patients by interfering with interpersonal skills and day-to-day social interactions.

Personality changes

The majority of patients who survive severe head injury manifest changes in personality which result in behavioural deficits. In the long term these problems are often the major source of ongoing problems, both for the patient himself and for his family. Two main patterns have been observed. The first is characterised by lack of drive and volition, limited emotional reactivity, apathy and indifference. Such patients present a challenge to those attempting to rehabilitate them. They may respond poorly, or at best slowly, to standard behavioural techniques. This can be so severe that some have advocated the use of CNS stimulants, including amphetamine, to try and improve arousal and cooperation in such patients. By contrast, other patients are characterised by affective instability, outbursts of aggression or rage, poor social judgement, egocentricity, disinhibition and sexually inappropriate behaviour. Sometimes this may represent exaggeration of premorbid personality traits, but these features can without doubt be seen for the first time after an injury. Irritability, which is extremely common in brain-injured patients, can often underlie episodes of both physical and verbal aggression, especially in those with similar premorbid personality traits. Consideration should, however, be given to other possibilities. Where aggression and violence is unprovoked and sudden in onset, the so-called 'episodic dyscontrol syndrome' (Maletzky 1973) should be considered. In this syndrome the EEG is usually abnormal and a trial of carbamazepine is worthwhile. Finally, complex partial seizures can follow brain injury. Here again, EEG is a helpful investigation and carbamazepine the treatment of choice.

Sexual problems are common after head injury, and while the sexual activity of people who have experienced head injury can be increased or decreased, it is usually the former which brings them to medical attention. Inappropriate and disinhibited sexual behaviour can occur in both men and women, and is often exacerbated by a general lack of social skills, impatience and impulsivity. Although the mainstay of management of sexual problems is behavioural in severe cases, the use (in male patients) of cyproterone acetate, an antiandrogen, may need to be considered.

Substance abuse and criminality have also been described as complications of brain injury, though this again seems more common in people with problems in these areas premorbidly.

Psychotic syndromes

A number of authors have described psychotic syndromes after head trauma. Davison & Bagley (1969) claim that schizophrenia-like syndromes occur at a rate well above that expected. Psychotic symptoms may occur during the early recovery from a head injury, usually as a component of delirium, but are also described months to years after the original injury. It has been claimed that trauma leading to psychosis usually involves the temporal lobe (Cummings 1988) and also that post-traumatic psychoses are more common in

patients whose original CT scan indicated diffuse cerebral swelling and intracranial shift secondary to haematoma (Capruso & Levin, 1992). The most common symptoms described are persecutory delusions, which are often fragmentary and poorly systematised, in contrast to the delusions seen in schizophrenia. Syndromes indistinguishable from schizophrenia have, however, also been described in patients who have sustained a head injury. Hallucinations, other than during the period of delirium, seem to be less common and self-limiting. Persisting psychotic syndromes will require suitable drug therapy. In addition to the previously mentioned sensitivity of brain-damaged patients to psychotropic drugs, attention may also need to be paid to the seizure inducing capacity of many neuroleptics, which can be a problem in such patients.

Post-traumatic neurotic syndromes

Depression and anxiety are both very common after brain damage. Anxiety is often due to loss of self-confidence and is exacerbated by cognitive deficits, particularly if the patient is experiencing problems with memory and orientation. Some patients will experience panic attacks, particularly when alone in unfamiliar environments.

Adjustment disorder Some patients (and their families) have considerable difficulties in adjusting to loss of function (physical and mental), especially if this is accompanied by other psychological symptoms, including irritability and anxiety. Loss of work, with its financial consequences, the not infrequent legal entanglements and changes in family dynamics are other major stressors to which patients may have to adapt. Premorbid personality is an important influence on adaptability.

Dissociative and somatoform disorder Somatisation, the tendency for psychological distress to manifest itself in physical symptoms, is not uncommon after brain injury. It appears to be more common after mild to moderate injuries and less common after severe injuries. Patients may complain of persisting aches and pains, especially headaches, and may also exhibit neurological syndromes, either motor or sensory, and non-epileptic seizures. Neurological symptoms should be treated with caution, as they not infrequently coexist with organically determined disorders. Dissociative amnesia (i.e. the ability to recall important personal information) and dissociative fugue (sudden, unexpected travel away from one's home or one's customary place of daily activities, often associated with amnesia) have been described after head injury. In dissociative amnesia after head injury, in contrast to the amnestic disorder which can occur, the disturbance of recall is almost always anterograde, i.e. restricted to the period after the trauma. Care should be taken to distinguish dissociative fugues and amnesias from syndromes which are the direct physical consequence of the head injury. A particularly important differential diagnosis is that of complex partial seizures, during which wandering, with semipurposeful behaviour and subsequent amnesia, is characteristic. The EEG is a helpful investigation in such cases.

Obsessional symptoms Obsessive–compulsive symptoms after closed head injury have been well described (Kant et al 1996). In some patients they consist of a strong need for an ordered and structured existence, but in others full-blown obsessive–compulsive disorder is described.

Postconcussional syndrome

Postconcussional syndrome is the name given to a common disorder which emerges within days of (usually) mild head injury. The main symptoms are headache, fatigue, dizziness and reduced concentration. Other symptoms include mild cognitive impairment, sleep disturbance, irritability, anxiety and depressed mood. It is of interest that research criteria for this disorder have been included in Appendix B of DSM-IV in order to promote its further study. For most patients this is a self-limiting syndrome, lasting from weeks to months after injury. However, in a significant minority it becomes persistent. Rutherford et al (1977) have claimed that 15% of patients have symptoms 1 year after injury. When postconcussional symptoms persist beyond 3 months, clinicians should exclude the possibility of additional underlying brain pathology, for example subdural haematoma. In some patients persisting post-concussional headaches, and even post-traumatic migraine, can be disabling and require appropriate treatment. More severe secondary mood disorder can occur and require specific antidepressant treatment.

For some time now there has been considerable debate over the origins of postconcussional disorder. Miller (1961) claimed that it amounted to a 'litigation neurosis'. This has now been emphatically refuted. Fenton et al (1993) claim that there is now overwhelming evidence for the contribution of biological factors in the genesis of this syndrome. This includes evidence of diffuse axonal injury, small focal cerebral contusions and intracranial haematomas, labyrinthine injury and changes in cerebral circulation and brain electrical activity. This notwithstanding, Fenton and his colleagues have also demonstrated that psychosocial factors contribute to the formation and persistence of symptoms of postconcussional syndrome. In a study of 45 patients they demonstrated that chronic cases (more than 6 months duration) tended to be older, female and to have had more social difficulties premorbidly. This work highlights the need for a holistic view to be taken – of both aetiology and management of postconcussional syndrome.

Epilepsy

Post-traumatic epilepsy occurs in up to 5% of patients after closed head injury. The presence of seizures in the first 7 days after injury predicts future risk. Of those who do not have early seizures, only 3% subsequently have late epilepsy, whereas up to 30% of those with seizures in the first 7 days go on to late epilepsy, which usually develops within a year of injury. With penetrating head injury the incidence of epilepsy is higher; Lishman (1968) reported an incidence of 45%.

Intracranial haematoma

Both mild and severe head injuries can give rise to intracranial haematoma, which greatly increases morbidity. Subdural haematomas are more common in older patients. By contrast, extradural haematomas tend to occur in younger patients (Teasdale & Jennett 1981). Galbraith et al (1976) have pointed out that intracranial haematoma following trauma is frequently misdiagnosed and attributed, for example, to alcohol intoxication. In Galbraith's study 25% of intracranial haematomas were undiagnosed until postmortem examination. This highlights the need for considerable clinical vigilance in assessing patients with evidence of head injury who also smell of alcohol.

Chronic subdural haematoma often presents without a history of head injury or with a history of minor head injury. It tends to occur in older people and chronic alcohol misuse is a risk factor. Even when there is a history of injury, haematoma develops slowly, over weeks to months, and clinical manifestations may therefore be distant from the initial injury. Headaches, fluctuating conscious level and memory impairment are common symptoms. These are not invariable, though memory impairment is usually evident in long-standing cases. Most patients have neurological signs, usually spastic weakness and hyperreflexia, with an extensor plantar response. Dilated pupils and ptosis is a bad prognostic sign, indicating tentorial herniation of the temporal lobe.

CT will reveal the haematoma in most cases when skull radiographs and EEGs are unhelpful. A subdural haematoma should be drained surgically.

Physical sequelae of head injury

It is important for psychiatrists involved in the management of patients with head injury to appreciate that, although the majority of stress for patients and their families following head injury is caused by cognitive behavioural and emotional symptoms, physical symptoms can significantly add to these problems. After severe injury there may be motor problems affecting movement coordination and balance. Hemiplegia or hemiparesis may persist for some patients. Cerebellar damage will lead to problems with balance and coordination which can be exacerbated by damage to the vestibular system.

Dyspraxia may lead to problems with sequencing actions, which may affect feeding and dressing. Occasionally sensory loss occurs. This can take the form of loss of sensation for light touch or pain, but can also present as visual problems, including diplopia, difficulties in judging distances and visual field defects. Language problems caused by various dysphasias have already been discussed but occasionally the muscles required for articulation of speech are affected by cranial nerve damage and this can lead to dysarthria.

Incontinence of urine and faeces can occur. This may be due to the direct physical effects of the head injury, but may also occur in patients with personality change; it may be an attention-seeking manoeuvre.

Family reactions to head injury

Powell (1994) has highlighted the importance of recognising the stresses on families after head injury, making the point that 'there are not just head injured individuals but rather head injured families'. Family members experience depression and anxiety during the few years after head injury. Initial anxieties over whether or not their loved one will survive, and what deficits he will have, are often replaced by difficulties in coping, particularly with the severe emotional and behavioural problems that can follow head injury. Spouses may be trapped in a marriage in which their own emotional needs are unsatisfied. This is particularly true when there is great personality change, and one often hears people make comments such as 'He is not the man I used to be married to.' There is a high divorce rate in marriages in which one partner sustains a severe head injury. Children, too, experience emotional problems, again usually related to emotional and behavioural problems in a head-injured parent. These are often compounded by the fact that the other parent is so taken up with the care of the partner that the children's needs may be neglected, leading to behavioural disturbance in the children or impaired performance at school and work.

It cannot be overemphasised that families need considerable input after severe head injury. They will need support, education, specific advice and direction to the appropriate services which can offer them help.

Management

There is an increased body of research looking at pharmacological means of protecting the acutely damaged brain. Eames (1997), summarising this, says that no clear conclusions can yet be made. He does, however, highlight the fact that research based on the principle that neurotransmitter depletion occurs in traumatic brain injury has led to some successful treatment trials, for example of motivational disorders with bromocriptine, a dopamine agonist (Powell et al 1996), and chronic confusional states with physostigmine and lecithin (Eames & Sulton 1995). These pharmacological advances notwithstanding, it remains the case that for the bulk of patients surviving severe head injury the main approach to treatment is one of rehabilitation. Ideally this work should be carried out by a multidisciplinary team, not only including doctors and nurses, but equally importantly physiotherapists, clinical psychologists, occupational therapists, speech therapists and social workers. Powell (1994) has summarised the key attributes of good rehabilitation. These are:

- Accurate assessment and understanding of the patient's strengths and weakness (skills and deficits)
- Improving areas of weakness by planning work towards realistic goals: breaking these goals down to small, achievable steps
- Teaching, practising and learning those small steps
- Providing directed and limited stimulation to all senses
- Increasing motivation and offering encouragement
- Helping adjustment to limitations and increasing insight into them
- Helping patients manage impairment where recovery is unlikely by means of provision of aid and coping strategies and techniques.

Rehabilitation services in the UK are in short supply and unevenly distributed. The cumulative increase in numbers of patients requiring ongoing rehabilitation has clearly overstretched the availability of services. This has continued, despite arguments that rehabilitation makes sound financial sense, as increasing the patient's independence makes them less reliant on family, other carers or indeed the state. There is evidence for the effectiveness of rehabilitation (Anderson et al 1996, Eames et al 1996), though there is no doubt that many patients have continuing care needs and the majority of those with severe head injury are unable to return to work.

Medicolegal issues

Many patients with head injuries, particularly those resulting from accidents, are involved in claims for compensation after their accident. It is unfortunate that these proceedings often drag on for many years. Although Miller's view that many post-head injury neurotic symptoms were motivated by a desire for compensation has been refuted, there is no doubt that prolonged compensation cases can add to the stress which patients experience after head injuries. Patients are often required to attend for a considerable number of expert medical and professional reports from neurologists, surgeons, psychiatrists, psychologists and occupational therapists, to name but a few. Many patients find this difficult and anxiety provoking and the stress associated with this process may prolong symptoms for some patients. The standard medical and psychological advice is that such claims should be dealt with as quickly as possible. Unfortunately the workings of the legal system are such that this is rarely feasible.

Driving and head injury

Those who have had injuries which could affect their fitness to drive are legally obliged to inform the Driver Vehicle Licensing Centre (DVLC). In practice this includes any injury, the effects of which are likely to last for more than a few months, which includes most head injuries involving a hospital stay of more than a few days. The DVLC will then usually seek medical reports from a general practitioner and hospital consultant, on the basis of which they will make a decision about the patient's ability to drive. Patients who have had epileptic seizures will not be eligible to drive until they have gone 2 years without a seizure. In cases of doubt it is a wise precaution to ask for expert assessment at a disabled driving centre as many patients have subtle problems after head injury, e.g. poor concentration, slowed reaction time and perceptual, visual and memory problems that could affect their driving.

EPILEPSY AND PSYCHIATRIC DISORDER

Epilepsy is best seen as a symptom of cerebral disorder, which can arise from a number of underlying causes, rather than as a condition in its own right. The International League Against Epilepsy (ILAE 1989) has proposed a compound classification scheme, classifying epilepsy, firstly on the basis of seizure type, and secondly taking into account anatomical features, EEG findings, age of onset and aetiology. The widely used

---

Table 11.10 ILAE classification of seizure type

Partial seizures
Simple partial seizures
Complex partial seizures
Partial seizures evolving to secondarily generalised seizures

Generalised seizures
Absence seizures
Atypical absence seizures
Myoclonic seizures
Clonic seizures
Tonic seizures
Tonic–clonic (grand mal) seizures
Atonic seizures

Unclassified seizures

ILAE classification according to seizure type is illustrated in Table 11.10.

Partial seizures

In partial seizures, activity begins in a focal area of the cerebrum with the clinical features reflecting the affected brain area. It thus follows that symptoms which may occur are protean. The three main types are the following.

Simple partial seizures These usually have an abrupt onset and ending and last but a few seconds, with no loss of consciousness. Symptoms depend on site of discharge. When the frontal areas are involved this frequently includes jerking or spasticity of limbs. Sensory symptoms predominate in parietal lobe seizures and psychological symptoms in temporal lobe seizures. Simple partial seizures usually arise from a structural lesion, e.g. tumour, vascular lesions or developmental abnormalities. Simple partial seizures sometimes progress to become complex partial seizures.

Complex partial seizures These are the most common type of partial seizure. They most commonly arise in the temporal lobe, with the frontal lobe being the next most common site of origin. Although, classically, three features are described in complex partial seizures, not all patients exhibit all three. The first feature is the aura, which in temporal lobe seizures usually takes the form of a psychic symptom (e.g. intense fear, déjà vu, olfactory or gustatory hallucinations). This is often followed by a period of absence, amnesia, loss of consciousness and motor activity. The patient appears to stare blankly into space and to look vacant. Posturing of the limbs is common and a sign of contralateral seizure onset. Thirdly, complex partial seizures may be accompanied by automatism. This usually takes the form of a stereotyped piece of behaviour, for example lip-smacking, swallowing, aimless searching and occasional verbal expression. Confusion is common after a complex partial seizure. Frontal lobe complex partial seizures are more unusual in form and are often mistaken for hysteria or even deliberate feigning of illness. Phonation during seizures is more common in those of frontal origin, and unilateral frontal discharges can lead to bilateral motor symptoms, including flailing arms and bicycling movements of the legs.

Partial seizures evolving to secondarily generalised seizures Both simple and complex partial seizures can evolve to secondarily generalised seizures, which are usually tonic–clonic in type.

Generalised seizures

The most common type of generalised seizure is the tonic–clonic seizure. In these seizures there is loss of consciousness and a tonic phase during which there is sudden spasm of all the muscles of the body for several seconds. There may be tongue biting and loss of control of bladder and bowels, though Betts has pointed out that frequent faecal incontinence should lead to suspicion of a non-epileptic seizure (Betts & Kenwood 1992). There follows characteristic rhythmic jerking of the limbs and head (clonic phase) which usually lasts a few minutes. The patient may by cyanosed during the seizure and increased production of saliva can lead to an appearance of frothing at the mouth. It is common for the attack to end with a large intake of air, accompanied by coughing and choking in an effort to clear secretions. Confusion is common and many patients wish to sleep after attacks. Vomiting is an occasional accompaniment to tonic–clonic seizures. Pure tonic and pure clonic seizures usually occur in childhood and are usually briefer than full blown tonic–clonic seizures. In atonic attacks, which are also most common in childhood, sudden loss of consciousness is accompanied by sudden loss of muscle tone and falling to the ground.

Generalised absence attacks may be simple or complex. Simple attacks, known as petit mal, consists of loss of awareness of one's surrounding. The attack lasts a few seconds and consciousness is lost. The onset and offset are abrupt. Other signs include minor muscle tone changes, upward rolling of the eyes or increased blinking. These attacks may be easily provoked by hyperventilation and EEG reveals a 3 cycle per second spike wave activity. Complex absences are often symptomatic of underlying brain damage and are accompanied by evidence of other generalised epileptic activity, including myoclonic jerking, retropulsive attacks and atonic attacks.

Aetiology

This has recently been reviewed by Shorvon (1996). He points out that the range of causes is highly age dependent, with congenital and genetic causes predominating in children, tumours and substance misuse in young adults and cerebrovascular disease in the elderly. He also points out that in some parts of the world infectious causes are particularly common. It is by no means unusual for the cause in an individual to be multifactorial. Hauser & Kurland (1975) pointed out that in three-quarters of patients with epilepsy there is no evidence of an underlying pathological lesion. In their large series, of those with a known cause, birth injuries, congenital abnormalities, head injuries, infections, vascular lesions and cerebral tumour dominated. Less than 1% of epilepsy was caused by neurodegenerative disorder. Of those with complex partial seizures originating in the temporal lobe, around 50% show mesial temporal sclerosis. This may possibly be due to hypoxia caused by severe infantile convulsions.

Relationship of epilepsy and psychiatric disorder

Studies looking at the prevalence of psychiatric disorder in patients with epilepsy have generally found a raised prevalence, especially in those with chronic epilepsy (Levin et al 1988). This seems only to be marginal where epilepsy is well controlled (Jacoby 1992). It is important to be aware that patients with epilepsy have a number of handicaps directly related to the disorder itself, but also a number of psychosocial handicaps, including problematic attitudes in carers, peer group, teachers, potential employers and indeed the general public. These can lead to problems with self-esteem, dependency, lack of opportunity to develop social skills and depression. It is also important to bear in mind that many of the drugs used to treat epilepsy may lead to cognitive impairment and mood disorder. A useful classification of psychiatric disorders found in epilepsy is that of Fenton (1981), which is outlined in Table 11.11.

Psychiatric disorder due to underlying brain disease causing fits This may include a variety of mental handicap syndromes and organic brain syndromes in which fits may occur, e.g. Alzheimer's disease, multi-infarct dementia and focal brain disease.

Disorders associated with the seizures Irritability and dysphoric mood may occur for hours, or even days, before the onset of fits, but symptoms usually improve following the seizure itself. Psychic phenomena are particularly common in partial seizures of temporal lobe or limbic origin. Illusions and automatisms may occur

Table 11.11 Psychiatric disorders of epilepsy: classification

1. Disorders due to the brain disease causing the fits
2. Disorders time locked to the occurrence of seizures:
   Preictal: (Prodromal)
   Ictal: Complex partial seizures
   Absence status
   Complex partial status
   Postictal: Automatism
   Confusional/clouded states
3. Disorders unrelated in time to the seizure occurrence:
   Interictal
   Disorders of childhood and adolescence
   a. Neurotic, antisocial and mixed
   b. Childhood psychoses
   Disorders of adult life
   a. Personality disorder
   b. Personality change (from a 'normal' previous personality)
   c. Neuroses
   d. Behaviour disorder
   e. Sexual dysfunction
   f. Psychoses:
   Affective/schizoaffective
   Chronic schizophrenia-like
   g. Dementia

during seizures. Epileptic automatisms can vary, both from patient to patient and in the same individual from seizure to seizure. Diminished awareness and lack of responsiveness is common. In longer episodes stereotyped, repetitive movements, including swallowing or chewing, may occur. Sometimes more complex and pseudopurposeful behaviour is seen, for example removing clothes or wandering. Automatisms usually last a few minutes and virtually never longer than 1 hour. Serious violence during epileptic automatism is rare (Gunn & Fenton 1971).

Interictal disorders These are disorders which occur between attacks in the absence of seizures. There is often an assumption that the epilepsy contributes to the interictal psychiatric disorder, though there is no convincing evidence of a direct relationship between epilepsy and psychiatric disorder. Indirect associations do, however, occur. As Fenton (1981) has pointed out, the type of mental state and behavioural problems that occur do not differ significantly between psychiatric patients with and without epilepsy. These include neurotic disorder and conduct disorder in children and per-

sonality disorders (including organic personality changes, a consequence of the epilepsy, its treatment or its underlying cause) and neurotic and psychotic syndromes in adults.

Hoare (1984), in a study comparing epileptic and diabetic children, confirmed that the increased prevalence of psychiatric disorder in children with epilepsy is not simply due to the stress of coping with chronic illness, and probably arises for multiple reasons, including organic brain dysfunction, temporal lobe disorder and family influences.

The relationship between epilepsy and psychiatric syndromes in adults seems less clear. Hermann & Whitman (1984) have reported that the prevalence of minor psychiatric morbidity in patients with epilepsy is not significantly higher than in patients with chronic diseases not affecting the nervous system. Fenton has pointed out that the clinical features which patients with epilepsy develop are influenced by age, with children and adolescents presenting with behavioural difficulties and adults with mild affective symptoms. Some patients with temporal lobe epilepsy develop a paranoid psychosis resembling schizophrenia. The argument continues as to whether there is a specific association between temporal lobe epilepsy and schizophrenia. This is explained by those who support the association in terms of a common neurodevelopmental abnormality in the medial temporal lobe (Mendez et al 1993).

Suicide is more common in those with epilepsy than in the general population (Barraclough 1981). Personality disorder usually (unless due to focal brain lesions) reflects lifelong chronic illness, often accompanied by a history of behavioural problems in childhood. The 19th century concept of a specific epileptic personality, characterised by features such as slowness, religiosity, irritability and impulsivity, has now largely been abandoned.

Epilepsy, crime and violence

Though the prevalence of epilepsy amongst prison populations is higher than in the general population, crimes of violence are no more common among epileptics than other offenders (Gunn & Fenton 1969). There is no specific relationship between temporal lobe epilepsy and violence, though this has been suggested in some texts in the past. Gunn & Fenton give a number of possible explanations for the higher prevalence of epilepsy in offenders:

- Brain damage causing fits and antisocial behaviour
- Psychosocial problems in chronic epilepsy leading to stigmatisation and antisocial behaviour

- Deprived early environment contributing both to acquisition of brain damage and to learning an aggressive behavioural repertoire
- Brain damage and epilepsy resulting as a consequence of a patient's impulsive, disorganised lifestyle, including criminality.

Sexual problems in epilepsy

Loss of libido and sexual dysfunction are common, particularly in male patients with epilepsy. Their relationship is likely to be complex and to reflect a number of factors, including poor social skills in some restricted lifestyles, parental protection and side-effects of medication. The subject of sexual problems in epilepsy has been well reviewed by Toone (1986).

Differentiating epileptic and non-epileptic seizures

The psychiatrist is often called upon to give advice both on differential diagnosis and management of seizures that are thought to be non-epileptic in origin (formerly known as pseudoseizures). He should exercise great caution in doing so for a number of reasons. Firstly, non-epileptic seizures occur very commonly in patients who also experience epileptic seizures and it is therefore often unwise to become locked in an either/or debate. Secondly, as Betts & Kenwood (1992) have emphasised, distinguishing between epilepsy and non-epilepsy is difficult, takes considerable time and may be impossible. Assessment of EEG tracing rarely provides the last word in this respect. Betts & Kenwood emphasise the importance of observing as many seizures as possible, videotaping them where at all possible, and not diagnosing attacks as epileptic unless one is very confident that they are. For a full account of issues surrounding the investigation and differential diagnosis of non-epileptic attacks, the interested reader is referred to the work of Betts & Kenwood (1992). Fenton (1981) has pointed to clinical features which help distinguish non-epileptic seizures from epilepsy, though he cautions that few, if any, of these are absolute. Non-epileptic seizures are often more bizarre; seizures originating in the frontal lobe with the pattern of attack often varying from seizure to seizure may certainly provide a bizarre presentation. Non-epileptic seizures usually take the form of generalised convulsive episodes and are mistaken for tonic–clonic (grand mal) attacks. Generalised rigidity with arching of the back and random thrashing of the limbs often occurs. The movements often increase if an attempt is made to restrain the patient and this may occasionally precipitate violence. Movements in non-epileptic seizures contrast with the stereotype tonic–clonic movements seen in grand mal epilepsy. Other things which help distinguish between epilepsy and non-epileptic attacks include the fact that corneal reflexes are often lost during or after grand mal attacks and plantar reflexes may briefly be extensor. All these reflexes are unaltered in non-epileptic seizures. Incontinence and tongue biting are common in epilepsy but are rare in non-epileptic attacks. Serum prolactin is sharply raised after generalised tonic–clonic seizures but this information is less useful when differentiating frontal seizures from non-epileptic attacks. Multiple attacks in one day are a common feature of non-epileptic seizures but rare in true epilepsy. Speaking or shouting is much more common in non-epileptic attacks (though again be aware of frontal lobe attacks).

Principles of management

Psychiatrists are rarely involved in initiating drug management of epilepsy in the UK. It is, however, helpful to know that at present the drug of first choice for partial epilepsy is carbamazepine, and for generalised epilepsy sodium valproate. Carbamazepine is usually effective in patients with partial seizures and secondary generalisation. Polypharmacy should be avoided where at all possible. Particular problems occur in women taking the oral contraceptive pill in combination with those preparations which are enzyme inducing (carbamazepine, phenytoin). Likewise, anticonvulsants may cause fetal malformations, and valproate and phenytoin in particular are best avoided in women who may become pregnant.

The psychosocial handicaps of epilepsy have already been highlighted. It is important that patients are given information and education about their disorder. Anxiety management is often helpful for those who fear having fits in public, and counselling and education of patient's families are important in preventing overprotection and dependency occurring and adding to the handicap of the illness itself.

Treatment of coexisting interictal psychiatric disorder is broadly similar to that in patients without epilepsy. It should be noted, however, that many psychotropic drugs, both antidepressants and antipsychotics, can lower the seizure threshold and increase seizure frequency.

NEUROPSYCHIATRIC SEQUELAE OF NEUROLOGICAL AND OTHER GENERAL MEDICAL DISORDERS

This section describes the neuropsychiatric sequelae of some important neurological and general medical disorders. For a comprehensive account the reader is referred to Lishman (1987).

Cerebrovascular disorders

Stroke

Stroke is an acute neurological disorder resulting from cerebrovascular disease and lasting for more than 24 hours. It can be caused by cerebral infarction, intracerebral haemorrhage or subarachnoid haemorrhage. Cerebral infarction is by far the most common cause, accounting for 85% of all strokes (Brown 1996). The incidence of stroke is around 2 per 1000 of the population per year and it causes 12% of all deaths in the UK. It is therefore a disorder of considerable importance. The major risk factor for stroke is hypertension. Brown reports that the incidence of transient ischaemic attacks (TIAs) is about a quarter that of stroke, but points out that about 30% of these patients suffer a stroke within 5 years.

It has been recognised for decades that psychiatric disorder following stroke is by no means uncommon. Johnson (1991) has provided a thorough and erudite review of this literature. The literature is largely focused on poststroke mood disorder and Johnson has argued that this emphasis has led to neglect of other important psychiatric sequelae of stroke. This emphasis has probably occurred for a variety of reasons. Depression tends to arouse more concern in carers, and indeed in doctors, than do other psychiatric syndromes, for example anxiety. Further, nearly all the early studies of stroke were based on hospitalised populations, which would be biased towards more disabled patients. Johnson has highlighted a number of other factors accounting for the overemphasis on mood disorder, including the fact that these are common, and often treatment resistant in the elderly, and also the fact that depression in particular is simpler to measure than many other psychiatric disorders. Johnson has suggested that organic personality syndrome and anxiety disorders may also be common after strokes and there are some studies that suggest that this is true (Slater 1962, Robinson et al 1983), though few studies have looked for these disorders seriously. Johnson is particularly critical of the neglect of anxiety disorder, arguing that stroke has tended to be seen as a loss event and hence likely to produce depression, whereas for those who recover fully it is more likely to be a threatening event (due to fear of recurrence) and therefore to be associated with anxiety.

The literature on poststroke depression is now considerable. Figures for reported prevalence vary widely, probably due to use of a variety of assessment instruments and case identification criteria (House 1987). Prevalence rates for major depressive illness 6 months poststroke reported in the literature vary from 13 to 34%. Lower rates are reported in community-based studies (House 1988). As Johnson has highlighted, the significance of some of these prevalence figures is not clear, due to the failure of some studies to examine appropriate control groups. House suggests that the evidence from community-based studies is that, although there is an increased prevalence of depression after stroke, the difference when compared with age-matched controls is modest.

Another source of considerable debate in the literature concerns the aetiology of poststroke depression. Severity of cognitive impairment and lesion size all seem to correlate weakly with depression, though measures of cognitive impairment have been inadequate in most studies. Many authors have emphasised the importance of lesion location. Most studies which have looked at this have found an increase in poststroke depression with left hemisphere lesions, particularly where the lesion is close to the frontal pole. There are, however, some discrepant studies and many studies looking at lesion location have been carried out on small numbers of highly selected patients. With regard to the role of poststroke social functioning, it remains unclear whether impairment of social functioning is primary or secondary to depression. There are no good studies looking at the impact of life events other than the stroke itself, and surprisingly little data on past or family history of psychiatric disorder. In summary, although there is a large literature on psychiatric disorder after stroke, it has looked at mood disorder and depression particularly at the expense of other psychiatric disorders. Studies have been biased towards hospitalised, more disabled patients and have inadequately examined the importance of past and family psychiatric history, social circumstances and premorbid personality. Future studies should address these issues and further clarify the relationship between stroke and psychiatric disorder.

Subarachnoid haemorrhage

Around 8% of strokes are caused by subarachnoid haemorrhage, which can be caused by ruptured aneurysms, primary haemorrhages, angiomas or arteriovenous malformations.

In the clinical presentation, consciousness may or may not be lost. If not severe, occipital headache is common, with associated nausea and vomiting. There is usually photophobia and neck stiffness and there may be localising signs.

There is a high initial mortality, with 50% of patients

dying in the first few weeks. Of those who survive the first few weeks only a quarter survive 5 years, one-third of whom are disabled.

There is a high psychiatric morbidity. In the early stages, in those who do not lose consciousness, delirium is common. After recovery from the acute episode personality change is extremely common and there is measurable intellectual deterioration in 40%. This is severe in 10%. Those with middle cerebral artery bleeds seem particularly vulnerable to intellectual deterioration. Storey (1967) has reported some personality change in 41% of patients and has rated it as 'severe' in 4%. Frontal lobe-type personality changes are common after anterior communicating artery aneurysms. Storey also notes, however, that, for a significant minority of patients, friends and relatives report improvement in personality, often describing a mood of relaxed contentment. Other common symptoms include irritability and minor mood disorder. Lishman (1987) has reported that some patients are severely disabled by anxiety about having a further bleed.

Transient global amnesia

Although this syndrome was described some time ago in neurological texts, it was given its name by Fisher & Adams in 1965. It can occur in either sex but is slightly more common in males. The onset is in middle or late life and the clinical presentation is with abrupt onset of amnesia lasting several hours. There is a global loss of recent memory and impaired new learning but no other abnormalities of cognitive functioning. During episodes patients are alert and responsive, but usually bewildered. Compete recovery is the rule, but patients have amnesia for the episode itself. It is thought to be vascular in origin and there appears to be an association with migraine.

Multiple sclerosis

Multiple sclerosis (MS) is the most common cause of neurological disorder in young persons. It is an inflammatory, demyelinating disorder which can affect any part of the CNS. Many patients live for decades after the onset of the illness and its social and interpersonal consequences are therefore devastating.

There is considerable variation in its prevalence worldwide, with a higher prevalence in temperate zones. The prevalence in the UK is around 50 per 100 000, though in Orkney and Shetland the prevalence is 300 per 100 000. It is slightly more common in women.

The cause is unknown, though on balance it is thought that an environmental agent operates in genetically susceptible individuals (Thompson & McDonald 1996). Viruses are thought to be the most likely causative agents. Support for a genetic aetiology comes from twin studies in which the concordance rate is higher for monozygotic twins than dizygotic twins (30% versus 4%). An association with the HLA region of chromosome 6 has also been described.

The main pathological feature of MS is the presence of multiple demyelinating plaques with axonal preservation, gliosis and inflammation. The optic nerve, spinal cord and periventricular areas appear to be particularly vulnerable to these lesions. Immunological mechanisms appear to play a role in the pathogenesis of MS. This has been recently been reviewed by Thompson & McDonald (1996).

The clinical presentation of the disease is very varied. In the vast majority of patients there is a relapsing and remitting course, sometimes with full recovery between relapses. A small minority of patients develop progressive disability from the onset. The most common modes of presentation are optic neuritis, sensory and motor disturbances in the limbs, and brainstem or cerebellar symptoms, for example diplopia and ataxia. Other symptoms include pain (e.g. trigeminal neuralgia), seizures, bladder and bowel dysfunction, sexual dysfunction and disorders of swallowing. Psychiatric symptoms are common in MS and Skegg et al (1988) pointed out that it is not uncommonly misdiagnosed as a psychiatric disorder. Fleeting mood disorder is very common and at some point in the course of the illness up to 50% of patients suffer from a major depressive episode (Ron & Feinstein 1992). Ron & Feinstein have reported that depression is more common in MS than in other chronic disabling disease. The risk of suicide is increased. Some authors suggest that the depression seen in MS does not respond to standard medications, though the clinical experience of most people is that some patients do respond to standard treatment. The emphasis on euphoria in earlier texts seems ill founded. It occurs in around 10% of patients and correlates with severe cognitive impairment (Surridge 1969).

Cognitive impairment is common in MS. Occasionally a rapidly progressive dementia occurs. More usually deterioration is slow and subtle, with dementia not being obvious until late in the course of the illness. Personality change is an important problem which often adds to the burden of the disorder for carers.

The social and economic burden of this illness is considerable and usually has to be borne for many decades. In addition to the burden of the neurological symptoms themselves, personality change, cognitive impairment, mood disorders and sexual dysfunction can pose a great stress on the families and friends of sufferers.

Cerebral tumours

Cerebral tumours, both primary and secondary, commonly cause psychological symptoms. Lishman (1987) has reported that 50–80% of patients with cerebral tumours have psychological symptoms at some stage. Some tumours, for example frontal meningiomas, can produce considerable psychological symptoms, with minimal, or even absent, neurological signs.

The type and severity of symptoms depends on a number of factors, including the site of the tumour (see earlier), the presence of raised intracranial pressure, the rate of growth of the tumour and the patient's premorbid personality. Lishman has noted that brain tumours can present with virtually any kind of psychiatric disorder, including depression, schizophrenia, mania and neurotic symptoms. Cognitive impairment is also common, though focal cognitive deficits are more frequent than dementia.

It is important for psychiatrists to be alert to the possibility of underlying brain tumours, particularly in treatment-resistant patients or in patients with unexplained personality change.

Intracranial infections

A large number of intracranial infections, including tropical diseases such as malaria, can lead to cognitive impairment, most commonly presenting as delirium. This section considers disorders of most interest to psychiatrists practising in the UK.

Neurosyphilis

Although now very rare in the UK, neurosyphilis has been of considerable historical interest, not least because the discovery of its cause (*Treponema pallidum*) prompted research for organic causes of other psychiatric disorders.

There are three main forms which the disorder may take: generalised paralysis of the insane (GPI), tabes dorsalis and meningovascular syphilis. GPI is the most common and the most likely to lead to psychiatric presentations. The main psychiatric features of presentation are personality change, minor affective symptoms and a degree of social disinhibition and indiscretion. Cognitive impairment may occur. The grandiosity described in older textbooks is relatively rare, occurring in only about 10% of cases (Dewhurst 1969). The VDRL (Venereal Disease Reference Laboratory) test is positive in 75% and the TPHA (*Treponema pallidum* haemagglutination) and FTA (fluorescent treponemal antibody) tests are positive in about 95% of cases in both blood and CSF.

Injectable procaine penicillin is the treatment of choice for neurosyphilis. It may lead to improvement in some cases, but in others may merely prevent deterioration.

Encephalitis

Encephalitis may present as a primary viral disease or complicate bacterial meningitis, cerebral abscess or septicaemia. Herpes simplex virus is the most common cause. Other commonly implicated viruses are influenza, measles and rubella. Encephalitis rarely occurs after vaccination. It may present with headache, fever, vomiting and impaired consciousness. Seizures are common and the most common psychiatric syndrome seen is delirium. Herpes simplex virus may specifically damage the temporal lobes and cause amnestic syndrome. Following recovery from the acute episode a variety of psychiatric syndromes have been described (Lishman 1987). These include anxiety and depression, personality change and dementia.

Endocrine disorders

Hypothyroidism

This is a disorder resulting from low levels of circulating thyroxine (T_4) or tri-iodothyronine (T_3). The term 'myxoedema' alludes to the deposition of a mucopolysaccharide beneath the skin, resulting in nonpitting oedema.

It is a disorder of insidious onset. It is not infrequently misdiagnosed as depression or dementia. Despite the fact that every psychiatrist in training is made aware of the importance of this disorder in the differential diagnosis of psychiatric syndromes, cases are still missed and may be far advanced before treatment is given. In a psychiatric context it is important to bear in mind that 5% of patients taking lithium for 18 months or more will develop hypothyroidism, with females being at much greater risk (Jefferson 1979). Cold intolerance, lack of energy, slowness in thought and action, weight increase, hoarseness, dry rough skin, changes in hair texture, constipation and paraesthesia are all important clinical features. Serum T_4 is reduced and thyroid stimulating hormone (TSH) raised in primary hypothyroidism. Normochromic or macrocytic anaemia and raised ESR may be found.

Although slowness of thinking, reduced concentration, depression and dementia are the most frequently described psychiatric sequelae of untreated hypothyroidism, occasionally a more florid paranoid psychosis is seen, with hallucinations and delusions and features of delirium. This is the so-called 'myxoedema madness' described by Asher (1949).

In severe untreated hypothyroidism neurological complications are seen and, in addition to dementia, include epilepsy, transient ischaemic attacks, cerebellar ataxia and more rarely coma with hypothermia.

Treatment is often rewarding, even when evidence of dementia is present. An important point to remember in treatment is that the doses of thyroxine given should initially be low (50 μg) in view of the possibility of cardiac complications of hypothyroidism (i.e. angina or cardiac failure).

Hyperthyroidism (thyrotoxicosis)

The clinical features of this disorder arise from an excess of T_4 and/or T_3. Important clinical features include excessive sweating, increased appetite (with weight loss), anxiety, agitation, tiredness and eye signs (exophthalmos, lid retraction and lid lag). Helpful clinical signs include goitre, hot sweaty palms, tremor, tachycardia or atrial fibrillation.

It is not unusual for thyrotoxicosis to present with psychiatric symptoms, anxiety and lability of mood, with accompanying overactivity being common. Thyrotoxicosis is not infrequently mistaken for an anxiety disorder or agitated depression. Careful physical examination should reveal some or all of the signs mentioned above. The presence of an increased sleeping pulse rate (above 90 beats per minute) is a useful sign in distinguishing thyrotoxicosis from anxiety. Affective and schizophrenic psychoses have been described in patients with hyperthyroidism, but are probably non-specific. Delirium may accompany thyrotoxic crisis, though this presentation is now only rarely seen. Treatment of the underlying thyroid disease usually leads to improvement in the psychiatric symptoms.

Hyperparathyroidism

This disorder is usually caused by benign adenoma of the parathyroid glands. It should be suspected in patients presenting with psychiatric symptoms in the presence of thirst and polyuria. Depression, irritability and mild cognitive impairment are the most common psychiatric features of the disorder, but in more severe cases with higher serum calcium delirium may be seen. The psychiatric features usually resolve when the adenoma is removed.

Hypoparathyroidism

Although this may be an idiopathic disorder it most commonly occurs following thyroidectomy. In post-thyroidectomy cases the abrupt fall in serum calcium precipitates psychiatric disturbance. The presentation is one of delirium. In idiopathic disease the clinical features included tetany, cataracts and epilepsy and the main psychiatric features are depression and irritability, with cognitive impairment in more long standing disorder. In hypoparathyroidism the psychiatric features are related to the serum calcium level and usually resolve with treatment of the underlying disorder.

Cushing's syndrome

This syndrome is the result of excess gluococorticoid and the most common cause is prolonged treatment with prednisolone. Of the non-iatrogenic causes, pituitary adenomas are the most common, leading to pituitary-dependent Cushing's syndrome (Cushing's disease). Other causes include adrenal tumour and ectopic adrenocorticotrophic hormone (ACTH) syndrome secondary to carcinoma. Clinical features include a characteristic appearance, with moon face and so called 'buffalo' obesity, muscle weakness, striae on the abdomen and thighs, bruising, osteoporosis, reduced glucose tolerance, hypertension and (in women) amenorrhoea and hirstutism are common.

More than half of patients with Cushing's syndrome have psychiatric features, usually depression (Michael & Gibbons 1963). In a review of the literature Whybrow & Hurwitz (1976) noted that 35% of patients developed depression, 16% cognitive impairment, 9% psychosis and 4% euphoria. In a more recent study, Cohen (1980) suggested that 86% of patients had significant depression. When the syndrome is caused by exogenously administered corticosteriods the psychiatric features are rather different. Although depression does occur it is much less common. Psychotic symptoms, including hallucinations, delusions and disturbed behaviour, with or without impairment of consciousness, is more common, with frank mania being seen in some. Euphoria is also described in this group of patients.

As with other endocrine disorders the cornerstone of treatment is to treat the underlying disorder, which usually results in improvement of the psychiatric features, though in more severe cases patients may require treatment with psychotropic drugs as well.

In patients where psychiatric disorder is caused by prescribed corticosteroid drugs it may not always be possible to stop the drug without compromising the physical health of the patient. In these cases concurrent psychotropic drug use will have to be considered, and in the case of drug-induced mania lithium prophylaxis may be useful.

Addison's disease

This results from deficient production of corticosteroids by the adrenal gland. The onset is usually insidious. Weakness, fatigue, weight loss and gastrointestinal symptoms are prominent. Hyperpigmentation on exposed areas and skin creases is a useful clinical sign.

The main psychiatric features are apathy, lack of drive, depression and mild cognitive impairment. These nearly always respond to treatment of the underlying disorder.

Hypopituitarism

This usually results from pituitary tumours or surgical destruction of the pituitary gland. Lack of energy and drive, hair loss, impotence (in men) and amenorrhoea (in women) are common presenting features. Subsequently features of hypothyroidism may be seen. Psychiatric symptoms are very common (Vance 1994). These include depression, poor concentration and mild cognitive impairment. In more prolonged cases amnestic syndrome has been described and delirium may herald the onset of pituitary coma. Once again, treatment of the underlying disorder usually results in resolution of the psychiatric features.

Diabetes mellitus

Diabetes is a chronic, often lifelong endocrine disorder in which psychological factors are of crucial importance in influencing control of the disease and therefore in preventing complications. Mayou et al (1991) have reviewed the psychiatric aspects of this disorder. It can lead to a variety of forms of metabolic dysfunction which can present with mild confusion, delirium or coma. These include ketoacidosis, lactic acidosis and hypoglycaemia. More indirectly, diabetic complications, such as renal failure and arteriosclerosis, may result in cognitive impairment, which is not uncommonly seen in long standing diabetics. Recurrent hypoglycaemic attacks may produce similar cognitive impairment (Perlmutter et al 1984).

Vitamin deficiency

It has long been recognised that chronic malnutrition has a number of psychiatric sequelae. Such sequelae have most often been described in prisoners of war (Helweg-Larsen et al 1952). When vitamin deficiencies occur in adults they are usually reversible with refeeding, but infants and young children may be permanently cognitively impaired.

B vitamins seem to be the most important in this respect, particularly thiamine and nicotinic acid. Deficiency of vitamin B_{12} and folic acid is also important in relation to psychiatric syndromes.

Chronic thiamine deficiency usually presents with beriberi neuropathy, oedema and cardiac failure, with fatigue, weakness and depression often predating these physical features. Acute deficiency leads to Wernicke's encephalopathy, which has been described earlier. Nicotinic acid deficiency produces the syndrome of pellagra, with gastrointestinal disturbance, skin lesions and cognitive impairment. Occasionally in more acute depletion a picture of delirium may be seen.

Vitamin B_{12} deficiency gives rise to peripheral oedema and may be accompanied by acute degeneration of the spinal cord. Psychiatric syndromes include cognitive impairment, depression and occasionally paranoid psychosis. The cognitive impairment seems most specific to Vitamin B_{12} deficiency, with other psychiatric symptoms being seen in patients with other kinds of anaemia. Treatment of the vitamin B_{12} deficiency with hydroxocobalamin results in resolution of the psychiatric symptoms.

Porphyria

There are six porphyria syndromes in which increased intermittent excretion of porphyrins in the urine and faeces is seen. Three types may present with neuropsychiatric features and all of these are hepatic porphyrias with excess hepatic production of porphobilinogen. They are:

- acute intermittent porphyria (the most common)
- variegate porphyria
- hereditary coproporphyria.

These are inherited disorders (autosomal dominant) which present with neuropsychiatric, gastrointestinal and cardiovascular symptoms. They are often precipitated by the administration of drugs, including barbiturates (especially anaesthetic agents), sulphonamides, the contraceptive pill and griseofulvin. Fasting is also a common precipitant of acute attacks. Key clinical features include abdominal pain with vomiting, confusion, psychotic symptoms, tachycardia and hypertension. Neurological symptoms, including limb weakness or even paralysis, and cranial nerve signs may be seen. Schizophrenia and affective disorders have been reported in patients with acute intermittent porphyria and McAlpine & Hunter (1967) claim that the madness of King George III was caused by this disorder.

Connective tissue disorder

Psychiatric features are seen in a number of connective tissue disorders, but most commonly in systemic lupus erythematosus (SLE). Connective tissue disorders have to be considered in the differential diagnosis of a variety of syndromes in medicine, and psychiatric syndromes are no exception. The connective tissue disorders are multisystem disorders which are autoimmune in nature, though the aetiology is poorly understood.

Systemic lupus erythematosus

This disorder most commonly presents in young women. Fever, arthralgia, malaise and weight loss are the most common clinical features, with or without so called 'butterfly rash' on the face. Virtually every body system can be affected by the disease and neuropsychiatric features are described in up to 60% (Lishman 1987). Both delirium and chronic cognitive impairment are described, though personality change and mood disorders are also seen. This has recently been reviewed by Calbrese & Stern (1995). These authors have highlighted the fact that in some patients the corticosteroids used to treat the disorder may play a part in producing the psychiatric symptoms, though it is likely that arteritis and ischaemia are important contributors to central nervous system disease and hence to psychiatric symptoms.

Lyme disease

Lyme disease is caused by *Borrelia burgdorferi*, a tick-borne spirochaete. It is so called because it was first described in 1975 in Lyme, Connecticut. It is a syndrome which affects multiple different organs, with 15% of patients having neurological symptoms, with neuropsychiatric manifestations in some of these. Direct infection of the central nervous system leads to a meningoencephalitis with cranial nerve lesions and radiculopathy. Psychiatric features are usually non-specific, with fatigue and apathy being prominent. Its main relevance in psychiatric practice is in the liaison psychiatry setting, where it should be considered as an often overlooked potential cause of chronic fatigue syndrome. Diagnosis is made by demonstrating raised antibody titres to the infecting organism. Treatment is with penicillin, erythromycin or tetracycline.

Carbonmonoxide poisoning

The most common cause of carbonmonoxide poisoning nowadays is deliberate or accidental poisoning from car exhaust fumes. This may become less common with the advent of catalytic converters on exhausts. It may present as coma without any preceding delirium. Most cases are successfully resuscitated, though in a proportion prolonged coma and death occur. As the coma resolves, around a fifth of patients show prolonged delirium (Lishman 1987). Amnestic syndrome usually becomes apparent fairly quickly. Extrapyramidal fea-

tures are also common. Lishman reports that in most cases both neurological and psychological disturbances improve over weeks or months, even where there is early severe disability, though there is no doubt that a proportion of cases are left with a degree of cognitive impairment, which may be permanent (Smith & Brandon 1973).

One interesting clinical feature of carbonmonoxide poisoning is that in some cases there is a latent period between recovery from coma and the onset of neurological or psychiatric disorder. In this situation patients appear to have made a full recovery, but about 2 weeks later relapse with extrapyramidal symptoms and delirium. Even in these cases some patients go on to a virtually full recovery.

Non-metastatic manifestations of carcinoma

It has already been noted that primary or secondary brain tumours can present with virtually any psychiatric syndrome. It is also important for the psychiatrist to be aware that among the many non-metastatic syndromes related to cancer are some with neuropsychiatric symptoms. This may be more common with bronchogenic carcinomas, particularly those of the oat cell type. Delirium, often with accompanying neurological signs, has been described. More rarely, classical affective disorders and schizophrenia have been observed in advance of evidence of clear-cut delirium. In other cases memory loss and early dementia have been clearly described. In the absence of a history of head injury or family history of dementia, or any obvious cause for dementia, the possibility of underlying malignancy should be considered in patients with dementia and normal brain scans.

REFERENCES

Adam S, Wiggins S, Whyte P et al 1993 Five year study of prenatal testing for Huntington's disease: demand, attitudes and psychological assessment. Journal of Medical Genetics 30: 549–556

Adams R D, Fisher C M, Harim S, Ojemann R G, Sweet W H 1965 Symptomatic occult hydrocephalus with 'normal' cerebrospinal fluid pressure. A treatable syndrome. New England Journal of Medicine 273: 117–126

Alexander M P 1982 Traumatic brain injury. In: Benson D F, Blumer D (eds) Psychiatric aspects of neurological disease. Grune & Stratton, New York, vol II

Anderson S I, Wilson C L, McDowell I P et al 1996 Late rehabilitation for closed head injury: a follow up study of patients 1 year from time of discharge. Brain Injury 10: 115–124

APA 1994 Diagnostic and statistical manual of mental disorders, 4th edn. American Psychiatric Association, Washington, DC

Asher R 1949 Myxoedematous madness. British Medical Journal 2: 555–562

Barraclough B 1981 Suicide and epilepsy In: Reynolds E H, Trimble M R (eds) Epilepsy and psychiatry. Churchill Livingstone, Edinburgh

Bearn A G 1972 Wilson's disease. In: Stanbury J B, Wyngaarden J B, Fredrickson D S (eds) The metabolic basis of inherited disease, 3rd edn. McGraw-Hill, New York

Berrios G E 1995 Delirium and cognitive states. In: Berrios G, Porter R (eds) A history of clinical psychiatry. Athlone Press, London

Betts T, Kenwood C 1992 Patients with attack disorders. In: Practical psychiatry. Oxford Medical Publications, Oxford, pp 243–288

Bickel H, Cooper B 1989 Incidence of dementing illness amongst persons aged over 65 in an urban population. In: Cooper B, Helgason T (eds) Epidemiology and the prevention of mental disorder. Routledge, London

Blazer D G, Federspiel C F, Ray W A, Schaffner W 1983 The risk of anticholinergic toxicity in the elderly: a study of prescribing practices in two populations. Journal of Gerontology 38: 31–35

Bolt J M W 1970 Huntington's chorea in the west of Scotland. British Journal of Psychiatry 116: 259–270

Bowen D M, Procter A W 1991 The neurochemistry of the major dementias of old age and indications for future drug treatment. In: Jacoby R, Oppenheimer C (eds) Psychiatry in the elderly. Oxford Medical Publications, Oxford

Breteler M M, de Groot R R, Van Romunde L K, Hofman A 1995 Risk of dementia in patients with Parkinson's disease, epilepsy and severe head trauma: a register based follow up study. American Journal of Epidemiology 142: 1300–1305

Brooks D N, Aughton M E 1979 Psychological consequences of blunt head injury. International Rehabilitation Medicine 1: 160–165

Brown M M 1996 Cerebrovascular disease: Epidemiology, history, examination and differential diagnoses. Medicine 9: 35–46

Brown M M 1996 Cerebrovascular disease: epidemiology, history, examination and differential diagnosis. Medicine 25: 5, 35–41

Brown R G , Marsden C D 1984 How common is dementia in Parkinson's disease? Lancet ii: 1262–1265

Brun A 1987 Frontal lobe degeneration of the non-Alzheimer type I – neuropathology. Archives of Gerontology and Geriatrics 6: 193–208

Burks J S, Alfrey A C, Huddlestone J, Novenberg M D, Lewin E 1976 A fatal encephalopathy in chronic haemodialysis patients. Lancet i: 764–768

Burns A 1991 Electroencephalography and imaging In: Jacoby R, Oppenheimer C (eds) Psychiatry in the elderly. Oxford Medical Publications, Oxford

Burns A, Philpot M, Costa D C et al 1989 The investigations of Alzheimer's disease with SPET. Journal of Neurology, Neurosurgery and Psychiatry 52: 248–253

Burns A, Luthert P, Levy R, Jacoby R, Lantos P 1990a Accuracy of clinical diagnosis of Alzheimer's disease. British Medical Journal 301: 1026

Burns A, Jacoby R, Levy R 1990b Psychiatric phenomena in Alzheimer's disease II. Disorder of thought content. British Journal of Psychiatry 157: 72–76

Burns A, Jacoby R, Levy R 1990c Psychiatric phenomena in Alzheimer's disease III. Disorder of perception. British Journal of Psychiatry 157: 76–81

Burns A, Lewis G, Jacoby R, Levy R 1991 Survival in Alzheimer's disease. Psychological Medicine 21: 363–370

Burns A, Howard R, Pettit W 1995 Alzheimer's disease: a medical companion. Blackwell, Oxford

Byrne E J, Lennox G, Lowe J, Godwin-Austin R B 1989 Diffuse Lewy body disease: clinical features in 15 cases. Journal of Neurology, Neurosurgery and Psychiatry 52: 709–717

Calbrese L V, Stern T A 1995 Neuropsychiatric manifestations of systemic lupus erythematosus. Psychosomatics 36: 344–359

Candy J M, Oakley A E, Klinowski J et al 1986 Aluminosilicates and senile plaque formation in Alzheimer's disease. Lancet i: 354–357

Capruso D X, Lewin H S 1992 Cognitive impairment following closed head injury. Neurologic Clinics 10: 579–893

Casson I R, Siegel O, Sham R, Campbell E A, Tarlaum, di Domenico A 1984 Brain damage in modern boxers. Journal of the American Medical Association 251: 2663–2667

Catalan J, Klimes I, Bergess A 1995 Psychological medicine of HIV infection. Oxford University Press, Oxford

Chadwick J, Mann W N (trans) 1950 The medical works of Hippocrates. Blackwell, Oxford

Cohen S I 1980 Cushing's syndrome – a psychiatric study of 29 patients. British Journal of Psychiatry 136: 120–124

Collinge J, Beck J, Campbell T, Estibeiro K, Will R G 1996 Prion protein gene analysis in new variant cases of Creutzfeldt–Jakob disease. Lancet 348: 56

Cooper B 1991 Epidemiology of dementia In: Jacoby R, Oppenheimer C (eds) Psychiatry in the elderly. Oxford Medical Publications, Oxford

Crapper D R, Krishnan S S, Quittkat S 1976 Aluminium, neurofibrillary degeneration and Alzheimer's disease. Brain 99: 67–80

Cummings J L 1988 Organic psychosis. Psychosomatics 29: 16–26

Davies P, Maloney A J R 1976 Destruction of central cholinergic neurones in Alzheimer's disease. Lancet ii: 1403

Davies S W, Beardsall K, Turmaine M D, Figlia M, Aronin N, Bates G P 1988 Are neuronal intranuclear inclusions the common neuropathology of striplet-repeat disorders with polyglutamine-repeat expansions? Lancet 351: 131–133

Davison K, Bagley C R 1969 Schizophrenia like psychoses associated with organic disorders of the central nervous system: a review of the literature. In: Herrington R N (ed) Current problems in neuropsychiatry. British Journal of Psychiatry Special Publication no 4. Headley, Ashford, Kent

Deary I J, Whalley L J 1988 Recent research in causes of Alzheimer's disease. British Medical Journal 297: 807–810

Dewhurst K 1969 The neurosyphilitic psychoses of today. A survey of 91 cases. British Journal of Psychiatry 115: 31–38

Dewhurst K, Oliver J E, McKnight A L 1990 Socio-psychiatric consequences of Huntington's disease. British Journal of Psychiatry 116: 255–258

Duthie E H, Glatt S C 1988 Understanding and treating multi-infarct dementia. Clinics in Geriatric Medicine 4: 749–766

Eames P 1997 Traumatic brain injury. Current Opinion in Psychiatry 10: 49–52

Eames P, Sutton A 1995 Protracted post-traumatic confusional state treated with physostigmine. Brain Injury, 9: 729–734

Eames P, Cotterill G, Kneale T A, Storras A L, Yeomans P 1996 Outcome of intensive rehabilitation after severe brain injury: a long term follow up study. Brain Injury 10: 631–650

Fenton G W 1981 Psychiatric disorders of epilepsy: classification and phenomenology. In: Reynolds E G, Trimble M R (eds). Epilepsy and psychiatry. Churchill Livingstone, Edinburgh

Fenton G, McClelland R, Montgomery A et al 1993 The post concussional syndrome: social antecedents and psychological sequelae. British Journal of Psychiatry 162: 493–497

Fisher C, Adams R D 1965 Transient global amnesia. Acta Neurologica Scandinavica 40 (suppl 9)

Fleminger S, Curtis D 1997 Prion diseases. British Journal of Psychiatry 170: 103–105

Folstein M F, Folstein S W, McHugh P K 1975 Mini-mental state: a practical method of grading the cognitive state of patients for the clinician. Journal of Psychiatric Research 12: 189–198

Folstein M F, Bassett S S, Romanoski A J, Nestadt D 1991 The epidemiology of delirium in the community – the Eastern Baltimore Mental Health Survey. International Psychogeriatrics 5: 169–176

Fricker J 1997 From mechanisms to drugs in Alzheimer's disease. Lancet 349: 480

Galbraith S, Murray W R, Patel A R 1976 The relationship between alcohol and head injury and its effects on conscious level. British Journal of Surgery 63: 138–140

Geaney D P 1994 Single photon emission tomography. In: Burns A, Levy R (eds) Dementia. Chapman Hall, London, pp 437–456

Gibson G E, Blass J P, Huang H M, Freeman G B 1991 The cellular basis of delirium and its relevance to age related disorders including Alzheimer's disease. In: Miller M E, Lipowski Z J, Lebowitz B D (eds) Delirium – advances in research and clinical practice. International Psychogeriatrics 3: 373–395

Goate A, Chartier-Harlin M C, Mullan M et al 1991 Segregation of missense mutation in the amylkoid precursor protein gene with familial Alzheimer's disease. Nature 349: 704–706

Goldstein L B 1993 Prescribing of potentially harmful drugs to patients admitted to hospital after head injury. Journal of Neurology, Neurosurgery and Psychiatry 58: 753–755

Graves A B, White E, Koepsell T D et al 1990 The association between head trauma and Alzheimer's disease. American Journal of Epidemiology 131: 491–501

Gunn J, Fenton G W 1969 Epilepsy in prisons: a diagnostic survey. British Medical Journal 4: 326

Gunn J, Fenton G W 1971 Epilepsy, automatism and crime. Lancet i: 1173–1176

Gusella J F, Wexler N S, Conneally P et al 1983 A polymorphic DNA marker genetically linked to Huntington's disease.

Hachinski V C, Lassen N A, Marshall J 1974 Multi-infarct dementia. A cause of mental deterioration in the elderly. Lancet ii: 207–210

Hanger D P, Brion J P, Gallo J M et al 1991 Tau in Alzheimer's disease and Down's syndrome is insoluble and abnormally phosphorylated. Biochemistry Journal 275: 99–104

Harper P S 1993 Clinical consequences of isolating the gene for Huntington's disease. British Medical Journal 307: 397–398

Harrison M 1995 Neurological manifestations In: Adler M W (ed) ABC of AIDS, 3rd edn. BMJ Publishing, London

Harrison P 1993 Alzheimer's disease and chromosome 14. British Journal of Psychiatry 163: 2–5

Harrison P J 1997 BSE and human prion disease. British Journal of Psychiatry 170: 298–300

Harrison R W S, McKeith I G 1995 Senile dementia of Lewy Body type: a review of clinical and pathological features – implications for treatment. International Journal of Geriatric Psychiatry 10: 919–926

Hasegawa K, Homma A, Yook K M, Amamoto H, Sato H, Itami A 1980 A gerontopsychiatric five year follow up on age related dementia residing in the community. Japanese Journal of Geriatrics 17: 630–638

Hasegawa R, Homma A, Imai Y 1986 An epidemiological study of age related dementia in the community. International Journal of Geriatric Psychiatry 1: 45–55

Hauser W A, Kurland L T 1975 Epidemiology of epilepsy in Rochester, Minnesota 1935–67. Epilepsia 16: 1

Health Education Board for Scotland 1996 Coping with dementia – a handbook for carers. HEB, Edinburgh

Helweg-Larsen P, Hoffmeyer H, Kieler J et al 1952 Famine disease in German concentration camps: complications and sequelae. Acta Psychiatrica et Neurologica Scandinavica. Supplement 83: 1–460

Hermann B P, Whitman S 1984 Behaviour and personality correlates of epilepsy: a review, methodological critique and conceptual model. Psychological Bulletin 95: 451

Hoare P 1984 The development of psychiatric disorders among school children with epilepsy. Developmental Medicine and Neurology 26: 2

Hodgkinson H M 1973 Mental impairment in the elderly. Journal of the Royal College of Physicians of London 7: 305–317

Holbourne A H S 1943 Mechanics of head injury. Lancet ii: 438–441

House A 1987 Depression after stroke. British Medical Journal 294: 76–78

House A 1988 Mood disorders in the first six months after stroke. In: Murphy E, Parker S W (eds) Current approaches: affective disorders in the elderly. Duphar Laboratories, Southampton, pp 6–12

Hsich G, Kenney K, Gibbs C J, Leek H, Harrington M G 1996 The 14-3-3 brain protein in cerebrospinal fluid as a marker for transmissible spongiform encephalopathies. New England Journal of Medicine 335: 924–930

Hughes C, Berg L, Danzigger W 1992 Cytoskeletal abnormalities in Alzheimer's disease, Current opinion. In: Neurology and Neurosurgery 5: 883–888

Huntington's Disease Collaboration Research Group 1993 A novel gene containing a trinucleotide repeat that is expanded and unstable on Huntington's disease chromosomes. Cell 72: 971–983

ILAE 1989 Commission on classification and terminology of the international league against epilepsy. Proposal for classification of seizures and epileptic syndromes. Epilepsia 30: 389

Jacobs J W, Bernhard M R, Delgado A et al 1977 Screening for organic mental syndrome in the medically ill. Annals of Internal Medicine 86: 40–46

Jacoby A 1992 Epilepsy and the quality of everyday life. Social Science and Medicine 34: 657–666

Jefferson J W 1979 Lithium carbonate induced hypothyroidism – its many faces. Journal of the American Medical Association 242: 271–272

Jennett B, Bond M R 1975 Assessment of outcome after severe brain injury. A practical scale. Lancet i: 480–484

Johnson G A 1991 Research into psychiatric disorder after stroke. The need for further studies. Australian and New Zealand Journal of Psychiatry 25: 358–370

Jones P A, Andrews P D J, Midgley S et al 1994 Measuring the burden of secondary insults in head injured patients during intensive care. Journal of Neurosurgical Anaesthesiology 6: 4–14

Kant R, Smith-Seemiller L, Duffy J D 1996 Obsessive–compulsive disorder after closed head injury: review of literature and report of four cases. Brain Injury 10: 550–563

Kaplan C P, Corrigan J D 1992 Effect of blood alcohol level on recovery from severe closed head injury. Brain Injury 6: 337–349

Kelly C A, Harvey R J, Cayton H 1997 Drug treatment for Alzheimer's disease. British Medical Journal 314: 693–694

Kinkel W R, Jacobs L, Polachini I, Bates V, Hetner R R 1985 Subcortical arteriosclerotic encephalopathy (Binswanger's disease) – computed tomographic, nuclear magnetic resonance and clinical correlations. Archives of Neurology 42: 951–959

Kolb B, Whishaw I Q 1990 Fundamentals of human neuropsychology, 3rd edition. Freeman, New York

Korsakoff S S 1889 Etude médicopharmacolique sure une forme de malades de mémoire. Revue Philosophique 28: 501–530

Lennox G, Lowe J, Landon M, Byrne E J, Majer R J, Goodwin-Austin R B 1989 Diffuse Lewy body disease: correlative neuropathology using anti-ubiquitin immunocytochemistry. Journal of Neurology, Neurosurgery and Psychiatry 52: 1236–1247

Levin M 1956 Varieties of disorientation. Journal of Mental Science 102: 619–623

Levin R, Banks S, Berg B 1988 Psychosocial dimensions of epilepsy: a review of the literature. Epilepsia 29: 805–816

Levy R, Eagger S, Griffiths M et al 1994 Lewy bodies and response to tacrine in Alzheimer's disease. Lancet 343: 176

Levy-Lahad E, Wijsman E M, Nemens E et al 1995 A familial Alzheimer's disease locus on chromosome 1. Science 269: 970–973

Lipowski Z J 1989 Delirium in the elderly patient. New England Journal of Medicine 320: 578–582

Lishman W A 1968 Brain damage in relation to psychiatric disability after head injury. British Journal of Psychiatry 114: 374–416

Lishman W A 1987 Organic psychiatry, 2nd edn. Blackwell, Oxford

Lovestone S 1996a It takes tau to tangle. International Journal of Geriatric Psychiatry 11: 363–368

Lovestone S 1996b The genetics of Alzheimer's disease – new opportunities and new challenges. International Journal of Geriatric Psychiatry 11: 6491–6497

Lovestone S, Anderton 1992 Cytoskeletal abnormalities in Alzheimer's disease. Current Opinion in Neurology and Neurosurgery 5: 883–888

McAlpine I, Hunter R 1967 George the third and the mad business. Lane, London

McDermott J R, Smith A I, Ward M K, Parkinson I S, Kerr D N S 1978 Brain aluminium concentration in dialysis encephalopathy. Lancet i: 901–904

McGuire D 1996 Neurological aspects of AIDS. Medicine 24 (9): 131–133

McKeith I, Perry R H, Fairbairn A F, Jabeans S, Perry E K 1992a Operational criteria for senile dementia of Lewy body type (SDLT). Psychological Medicine 22: 911–922

McKeith I, Fairburn A, Perry R, Thompson P, Perry E 1992b Neuroleptic sensitivity in patients with senile dementia of Lewy body type. British Medical Journal 305: 673–678

Maj M 1990 Psychiatric aspects of HIV infection and AIDS. Psychological Medicine 20: 547–563

Maletzky B M 1973 The episodic dyscontrol syndrome. Diseases of the Nervous System 34: 178–185

Mallucci G R, Collinge J 1997 Neuropsychiatric presentations of prion disease. Current Opinion in Psychiatry 10: 59–62

Mann D M 1988 Alzheimer's disease and Down's syndrome. Histopathology 13: 125–137

Matthews W B 1990 Bovine spongiform encephalopathy. British Medical Journal 300: 412–413

Mayou R A, Peveler R, Davies B, Mann J, Fairburn C 1991 Psychiatric morbidity in young adults with insulin dependent diabetes mellitus. Psychological Medicine 21: 639–645

Mendez M F, Grav R, Doss R C, Taylor J L 1993 Schizophrenia in epilepsy: seizure and psychosis variables. Neurology 43: 1073–1077

Michael R P, Gibbons J L 1963 Interrelationships between the endocrine system and neuropsychiatry. International Review of Neurobiology 5: 243–302

Miller H 1961 Accident neurosis. British Medical Journal 1: 919–925, 992–998

Morris R, Morris L 1993 Psychosocial aspects of caring for people with dementia. In: Burns A (ed) Ageing and dementia; a methodological approach. Edward Arnold, London

Najenson T 1978 Recovery of communicative functions after prolonged traumatic coma. Scandinavian Journal of Rehabilitation Medicine 10: 15–23

Oliver J E 1970 Huntington's chorea in Northamptonshire. British Journal of Psychiatry 116: 241–253

Perani D, Di Piero V, Vallar G et al 1988 Technetium 99m HMPAO SPET study of regional cerebral perfusion in early Alzheimer's disease. Journal of Nuclear Medicine 29: 1507–1514

Perlmutter L C, Harami M R, Hodgeson-Harrington C et al 1984 Decreased cognitive functioning in ageing noninsulin dependent diabetic patients. American Journal of Medicine 77: 1043–1048

Perry R H, Irving D, Blessed G, Perry E K, Fairbairn A F 1990 Senile dementia of Lewy body type. A clinically and neuropathologically distinct type of Lewy body dementia in the elderly. Journal of Neurological Science 95: 115–139

Perry T L, Hansen S, Kloster M 1993 Huntington's chorea: deficiency of gamma-aminobutyric acid in brain. New England Journal of Medicine 288: 337–342

Powell J H, Al-Adwani S, Morgan J, Greenwood R J 1996 Motivational deficits after brain injury: effects of bromocriptine in 11 patients. Journal of Neurology, Neurosurgery and Psychiatry 60: 416–421

Powell T 1994 Head injury: a practical guide. Winslow Press

Pratt O G, Jeyasingham M, Shaw G R 1985 Transketolase variant enzymes and brain damage. Alcohol and Alcoholism 20: 223–232

Robinson R G, Kubos K L, Bookstarr L, Rao K, Price T R 1983 Mood changes in stroke patients: relationship to lesion location. Comprehensive Psychiatry 24: 555–566

Rocca A, Hofman A, Procter A W 1991 The neurochemistry of the major dementias of old age and indications for future drug treatment. In: Jacoby R, Oppenheimer C (eds) Psychiatry of the elderly. Oxford Medical Publications, Oxford

Rogers S Z, Friedhoff L T 1996 The efficacy and safety of donepezil in patients with Alzheimer's disease. Results of a US multicentre randomized, double blind, placebo controlled trial. Dementia 7: 293–303

Ron M A, Feinstein A 1992 Multiple sclerosis and the mind. Journal of Neurology, Neurosurgery and Psychiatry 55: 1–3

Roth M, Huppert F A, Tym E, Mountjoy C Q 1988 CAMDEX. The Cambridge examination for mental disorders of the elderly. Cambridge University Press, Cambridge

Rubin E H, Drevets W C, Burke W J 1988 The nature of psychotic symptoms in senile dementia of the Alzheimer type. Journal of Geriatric Psychiatry and Neurology 1: 16–20

Russell W R 1932 Discussion on the diagnosis and treatment of acute head injuries. Proceedings of the Royal Society of Medicine 25: 751–757

Rutherford W A, Merrett J D, McDonald J R 1977 Sequelae of concussion caused by minor head injuries. Lancet i: 1–4

Schellenberg G P, Bird T D, Wijsman E M et al 1992 Genetic linkage evidence for a familial Alzheimer's disease locus in chromosome 14. Science 258: 668–671

Sherrington R, Rogan E I, Liang Y et al 1995 Cloning of a gene bearing missense mutations in early onset familial Alzheimer's disease. Nature 375: 754–760

Shorvon S 1996 Epilepsy: cause, classification and diagnosis. Medicine 24(b): 60–64

Simpson S A, Harding A E 1993 Predictive testing for Huntington's disease: after the gene. The United Kingdom Huntington's Disease Predictive Consortium. Journal of Medical Genetics 30: 1036–1038

Skegg K, Corwin P A, Skegg D C 1988 How often is multiple sclerosis mistaken for psychiatric disorder? Psychological Medicine 18: 733–736

Slater E T O 1962 Psychological aspects. In: Modern views on stroke illness. Chest and Heart Association, London

Slater E, Beard A W, Glitheroe E 1963 The schizophrenia-like psychoses of epilepsy. British Journal of Psychiatry 109: 95–112

Smith J S, Brandon S 1973 Morbidity from acute carbon monoxide poisoning at 3 year follow up. British Medical Journal 1: 318–321

Steele J C 1972 Progressive supranuclear palsy. Brain 95: 693–704

Steele J C, Richardson J C, Olszewski J 1964 Progressive supranuclear palsy. Archives of Neurology 10: 333–359

Storey P B 1967 Psychiatric sequelae of subarachnoid haemorrhage. British Medical Journal 3: 261–266

Strich S J 1956 Diffuse degeneration of the cerebral white matter in severe dementia following head injury. Journal of Neurology, Neurosurgery and Psychiatry 19: 163–185

Strich S J 1961 Shearing of nerve fibres as a cause of brain damage due to head injury. A pathological study of twenty cases. Lancet ii: 443–448

Stuss D T, Benson D E 1983 Emotional concomitants of psychosurgery. In: Hellman K M, Satz P (eds) Neuropsychology of human emotion. Guildford Press, New York

Surridge D 1969 An investigation into some psychiatric aspects of multiple sclerosis. British Journal of Psychiatry 115: 749–764

Taylor D, Lewis S 1993 Delirium. Journal of Neurology, Neurosurgery and Psychiatry 56: 742–751

Teasdale G, Jennett B 1974 Assessment of coma and impaired consciousness. Lancet ii: 81–83

Teasdale G, Jennett B 1981 Management of head injuries. Contemporary neurology series. F A Davies, Philadelphia

Thompson A J, McDonald W I 1996 Multiple sclerosis. Medicine 24(6): 69–75

Toone B K 1986 Hyposexuality among male epileptic patients: clinical and hormonal correlates. In: Trimble M R, Boling T G (eds) Aspects of epilepsy and psychiatry. Wiley, Chichester

Ueshima H, Takako O, Asakura S 1986 Regional differences in stroke mortality and alcohol consumption in Japan. Stroke 7: 19–24

Vance M L 1994 Medical progress: hypopituitarism. New England Journal of Medicine 330: 1651–1662

Van der Mast R C 1996 Delirium: the underlying pathophysiological mechanisms and the need for clinical research. Journal of Psychosomatic Research 41(2): 109–113

Van Duijn C, Hoffman A 1991 Relation between nicotine intake and Alzheimer's disease. British Medical Journal 302: 149–154

Verdoux H, Bourgeois M 1995 Secondary mania caused by cerebral organic pathology. Annals of Medical Psychology (Paris) 153: 161–168

Victor M, Adams R D, Collins G H 1971 the Wernicke–Korsakoff syndrome. Blackwell, Oxford

Walker S 1969 The psychiatric presentation of Wilson's disease (hepatolenticular degeneration) with etiologic explanation. Behavioural Neuropsychiatry 1: 38–43

Walshe J M 1968 Some observations on the treatment of Wilson's disease with penicillamine. In: Bergsma D (ed) Wilson's disease. Birth defects original article series. National Foundation, New York, vol 4, no 2

Warshaw G A, Moore J T, Friedman S W 1982 Functional disability in the hospitalised elderly. JAMA 248: 847–850

Wernicke C 1881 Lehrbuch Gehirnkrankherten. Berlin, vol 1

WHO 1992 International classification of diseases and related health problems, 10th revision. World Health Organization, Geneva, vol 1, pp 311–387

Whybrow P C, Hurwitz T 1976 Psychological disturbances associated with endocrine disease and hormone therapy. In: Sachar E J (ed) Hormones, behaviour and psychopathology. Naren Press, New York

Wiggins S, Whyte P, Higgins M et al 1992 The psychological consequences of predictive testing for Huntington's disease. New England Journal of Medicine 327: 1401–1405

Will R G, Ironside J N, Zeidler M et al 1996 A new variant of Creutzfeldt–Jakob disease in the UK. Lancet 347: 921–925

Zeilig G, Drubach D A, Katz-Zeilig M, Karatinds J 1996 Pathological laughter and crying in patients with closed traumatic brain injury. Brain Injury 10: 591–597

12
Substance misuse

Malcom Bruce   Bruce Ritson

DEPENDENCE ON ALCOHOL AND OTHER DRUGS

It is hard to think of any country which does not rely on some drug or other to facilitate social relations, mark festivals or enhance religious rituals. In Britain, alcohol is the most widely used and misused drug, but other forms of drug misuse are not a new phenomenon in this country. A 19th century reporter visiting Aberdeenshire noted:

> Few people are aware to what a frightful excess the vice of opium eating has extended lately in this country and how rapidly it is increasing both in England and in Scotland. I could name one apothecary's shop where innumerable small packets, costing only a penny of this pernicious drug are prepared every night, and where a crowd of the wretched purchasers, many of them women, glide silently up to the counter, deposit the price, and without uttering a word, steal away like criminals, to plunge themselves into a temporary delirium, followed by those agonies of mind and body by which both are at last distorted and ruined (Geikie 1904).

In considering the consequences of drug use, it is helpful to differentiate between the pharmacology of the drug, the hazards inherent in the route of administration, the dose and frequency of use and the health and personality of the user. Finally, and perhaps more crucial, is consideration of the setting in which the drug is taken, the immediate surroundings, the presence of friends, their attitudes and expectations, the culture and folklore surrounding the drug as well as the legal sanctions on its use. Drugs regarded as hazardous and illegal in one culture or time in history have been condoned or even promoted in another.

Alcohol

Ethyl alcohol is a natural product of the breakdown of carbohydrates in plants. Its euphoriant and intoxicating properties have been known from prehistoric times and almost all cultures have had some experience of its use. Fermentation with yeast can achieve alcohol concentrations of approximately 10%. Higher strengths require distillation which is thought to have been discovered by the Persian chemist Rhases in AD 800. The word 'alcohol' is Arabic in origin.

Early Egyptian and Greek writings make several references to alcohol and distinguish between its beneficial effects in moderation and the problem of drunkenness, for which severe penalties were often prescribed, particularly when it occurred amongst the young. Hippocrates recognised many of the medical complications of excessive drinking and Seneca introduced the idea of loss of control and habituation. Throughout the 17th century in Britain drunkenness was widespread. In an effort to promote agriculture, positive incentives were given to produce cheap gin. This policy succeeded so completely that by 1736 consumption of spirits was approximately 1 gallon a head per annum. Gradually, by means of licensing and taxation, consumption was reduced, only to rise again during the 19th century. The chief opponent of drunkenness at that time was the Temperance Movement. Initially it advocated moderate consumption but later moved to champion total abstinence. At that time the prevailing view was that drunkenness was a vice or moral weakness. Some physicians, such as Benjamin Rush in the USA and Thomas Trotter in Scotland, pointed out both medical and psychological consequences of alcohol abuse, and moved toward the contemporary concept of alcohol addiction.

The Temperance Movement scored its greatest victory in the 18th Amendment of the US Constitution which prohibited the manufacture and sale of alcohol except for therapeutic or sacramental purposes. The Amendment was difficult to enforce and led to gangsterism. Because of these social consequences and lack of public support, it was repealed in 1933. (It is noteworthy that cirrhosis mortality declined during the years of prohibition.)

The Temperance Movement never attained the political strength in Britain which it enjoyed in the USA or some Scandinavian countries. None the less, it was a considerable force by the end of the 19th century and it facilitated the introduction of control measures which Lloyd George imposed during the First World War. The Government was deeply concerned at the drunkenness amongst munitions workers and introduced taxation and licensing controls in an effective attempt to limit consumption.

There is nothing fixed or unchanging about a nation's drug or alcohol usage. Habits have changed dramatically in Britain during the past century, most often in response to economic and social influences. 'Dry' generations are often followed by those that are relatively 'wet'. The consequences give rise to the reinstatement of controls and the cycle repeats itself. These cycles, which are evident in many countries, should be an encouragement to preventive strategies which might hope to influence the tide of change and fashion in the direction of harm reduction.

PREVENTION

In the past, primary prevention of both drug and alcohol misuse has focused principally on controlling availability, or strengthening the resistance of the individual by education and persuasion. The health and social costs of a substance are not necessarily reflected in the effort invested in education or control. Tobacco, which is the most damaging drug in health costs, is legally available and advertised in many countries.

This chapter will not be concerned with tobacco but it is important to recognise its addictive properties, damaging health consequences and the difficulty experienced by individuals in changing this habit once they have become addicted. The majority of smokers in their late teens wish they had never taken it up and find it very difficult to stop.

Prevention of alcohol misuse

For alcohol-related problems, prevention should be better than cure because the efficacy of treatment is uncertain and the problem is endemic in most industrialised countries. The mean per caput level of alcohol consumption in a population and the prevalence of heavy drinking are closely correlated ($r = 0.97$) (Rose & Day 1990). Thus a 10% decline in consumption would reduce the number of heavy drinkers by a similar percentage. While excessive drinkers experience many more alcohol-related problems than other drinkers,

their contribution to the level of alcohol-related harm in a community is lower than that arising from the much larger population of moderate and light drinkers. Focusing a preventive strategy only on those at 'high risk' would have less impact on the overall level of harm than would a population-based approach. This is termed *the preventive paradox* (Kreitman 1986). A population-based approach targeted at all drinkers with the goal of reducing overall per caput consumption is likely to be more effective but requires all drinkers to moderate their consumption.

Unfortunately, a population-based approach to prevention is often unpopular, possibly because in the public mind it is misleadingly linked to concepts of prohibition and interference with the liberty of the individual.

Prevention is most visibly effective when a specified effect can be traced to a cause which is readily amenable to influence. For example, the association between drink-driving and road accidents is clear-cut and the 1967 legislation imposing penalties on those driving with a raised blood alcohol level had an immediate effect in reducing the number of road fatalities by 15%, although the effect diminished as drivers began to realise that the risk of detection was low. There is evidence that the introduction of random breath testing would lead to a further decline in alcohol-related accidents.

Primary prevention

Primary prevention is aimed at reducing the prevalence of hazardous drinking, or in some cases the hazards of drinking (for example by separating drinking from driving) in the population. It relies on three strategies: control of availability, education about sensible use, and providing alternative pursuits (Table 12.1). These approaches are not mutually exclusive alternatives but are interdependent. For instance, it would be politically unwise to introduce controls which did not enjoy a measure of public acceptance, an aim which would have to be pursued first by an active public education programme. There is considerable scope for local action aimed, for instance, at licensing practices, road safety or providers of alternative leisure pursuits (Ritson 1995). In some cases the task is to separate drinking from certain contexts such as drinking and work, sport such as swimming, or driving.

Controls
Availability Prohibition is an extreme form of control. It proved effective in reducing mortality from liver cirrhosis in the USA in the 1920s, but these gains were outweighed by other social problems which arose. The limitations of prohibition and similar restrictive endeav-

Table 12.1 Primary prevention strategy

Strategy	Method	Aim
Controls	Fiscal Legislative	To reduce availability
Education	The general public Young people and at risk groups Key professionals; politicians	To foster moderate informed drinking and promote awareness of hazards
Provision of alternatives	Promoting alternative leisure activities; facilitating sensible drinking, for instance with meals; ensuring that inexpensive non- or low-alcohol beverages are readily available	To promote sensible drinking

ours include the public resentment which they may generate, difficulties with enforcement, loss of tax revenue (currently over £6000 million per annum in the UK), and the growth of smuggling and illicit production of what may prove to be lethal brews. Most countries now endeavour to control rather than prohibit availability. (An exception is within Islam where cultural tradition sustains prohibition.)

Legislation restricting times of sale and the number, type and location of licensed premises probably influences consumption, but the impact is hard to judge because such legislation is usually introduced at times when other attitudes are changing, making it difficult to pinpoint its effectiveness. Major restrictions on permitted hours in Britain were introduced by Lloyd George in 1915 in an effort to ensure that the workforce was sufficiently sober to meet the demands required by the war effort. Consumption dropped at that time and remained low for more than a decade. In the UK the control, and particularly enforcement, of licensing laws and permitted hours of opening is amenable to considerable local influence and can be seen as one example of the importance of local action in influencing the level of alcohol-related harm in a community. Other examples are bans on public drinking and restrictions on alcohol at sporting events, which have been shown to lead to an improvement in public order in the target areas.

Most countries impose a minimum age at which young people are allowed to drink in public. In the USA and Canada experience has shown that states or provinces which lowered the permitted age experienced a rise in motor accidents and drink-driving offences amongst the young. Young people are most frequently first introduced to alcohol at home by their parents.

Clandestine public drinking commonly starts before the permitted age.

Advertisers argue that they are simply concerned with promoting or sustaining brand loyalties amongst drinkers but research suggests that they also stimulate overall consumption (McGuiness 1980). The effect of advertising on alcohol consumption remains controversial. It is certainly a major investment: £160 million in the UK. Alcohol has been described as the 'supreme image product' (Clark 1988), promoting fantasies of social prestige, success and high-quality lifestyle. Sponsorship is another less direct form of advertising, often linked with sports teams or fixtures. The effects of advertising on the young is a particular concern and most counties have controls on advertising that specifically seek to attract youngsters or are placed near schools. In some communities there has been a total ban. In the UK cases of unethical alcohol advertising should be referred to the Advertising Standards Authority.

Price Over the past 300 years, alcohol consumption in Britain has shown marked fluctuations. Every time the price of alcohol relative to disposable income has fallen, as it has almost continuously since 1945, consumption has risen. While it is simplistic to consider price as the only important variable, an increase in the excise duty on alcohol is probably the most effective way of reducing the per caput consumption of the population. In 1981 an increase in the excise duty on beer and spirits caused their price to rise faster than the retail price index and average disposable incomes. These economic changes were associated in Edinburgh with a decline in alcohol consumption of 18% and a reduction in alcohol-related harm of 16%. Contrary to predictions, heavy drinkers and even dependent drinkers reported a disproportionate reduction in their consumption (Kendell et al 1983).

The health lobby is but one competing interest group in the debate about controlling the availability and consumption of alcohol. Other groups argue in favour of continuing growth in the alcohol market. There is, for instance, the employment argument (the drink trade in Britain employs 750 000); the desire to expand overseas trade (a viewpoint which ignores the probably harmful effect on health in developing countries); and the needs of the tourism and advertising industries. Very large tax increases result in a growth in home brewing or illicit production and smuggling. Some have argued that a ban on advertising would prompt and enable producers to lower prices or fund other means of promotion such as sponsorship.

Education   Education needs to take into account the medium, the audience and the message. In the past, education has often been woolly in focus and content, but even with carefully considered campaigns the lasting impact may be disappointingly small (Moskowitz 1989). Target groups include the general public or specific segments of the population, such as schoolchildren, the elderly or ethnic minorities, or particular high-risk groups, such as pregnant women, drivers or those in hazardous occupations. Education can also be aimed at opinion leaders in attempts to broaden their understanding of alcohol-related problems and also focused on professions such as nursing, medicine and social work.

Education in schools should recognise that in the UK there is evidence that children know about alcohol from the age of 6 years onwards and that their attitudes towards drinking change markedly and become more positive between 11 and 14 years, as the peer group begins to exert more influence than parents or teachers. The style and content of presentation should be consonant with the child's developmental stage. Information about the alcohol content of various alcoholic beverages, sensible drinking practices and safe limits for consumption are facts which should be part of every young person's knowledge of the world. Skill and confidence in coping with social pressures to drink should be part of education. Evidence shows that it is easier to improve knowledge than to influence attitudes, or particularly behaviour.

Public education can have a number of objectives. It can be concerned with informing the public about alcohol problems along with giving specific advice about where to seek help. Campaigns of this kind have not influenced drinking habits but have often produced an increase in utilisation of treatment and counselling facilities. Education at least signals awareness that alcohol is a legitimate cause for public concern. Wallack et al (1993) have pointed to the importance of influencing the media to ensure that health issues are given a fair hearing and presentation in public debate. Recently information has been disseminated about sensible drinking, along with booklets describing self-help strategies for limiting consumption. There are many other forms of population-based information policies, such as warning labels, interaction self-help computer games, or local health campaigns.

Provision of alternatives   Many communities are heavily dependent on drinking places as a principal source of entertainment. Clearly the pub has a significant social role in its neighbourhood but those concerned with planning should ensure that other leisure pursuits are encouraged and that other non-alcoholic beverages are readily available. The promotion of low-alcohol beers and wine has proved helpful. Alternative choices for relieving tension and facilitating social contacts can be taught – for instance, relaxation, meditation and social skills training. These alternative styles of coping could be explored within schools, if the curriculum were thoughtfully redrawn.

Secondary prevention

Secondary prevention aims to prevent the further progression of a condition by identifying and treating cases at an early stage. Symptom-free excessive drinkers see little reason to change their habits. However, a primary care worker, consulted perhaps for some other reason, can take the opportunity to educate and persuade him to cut down. The general practitioner, occupational health physician, social worker, nurse or health visitor are in a position to do this, provided they understand alcohol problems sufficiently.

There are a number of questionnaires available which facilitate early recognition of hazardous drinking (Babor et al 1986). Primary health care physicians can also use the mean corpuscular volume (MCV) and γ-glutamyltranspeptidase in screening, since about 60% of heavy drinkers will show an elevation on one or other test (Chick et al 1981).

A sensible policy which would immeasurably enhance recognition would be to follow the Royal College of Physicians (1987) recommendation that every person seen in general practice or in hospital should be asked about alcohol intake as a matter of routine, along with questions about smoking and medication and the answers recorded. Unfortunately these simple procedures are often overlooked in both medical and psychiatric practice.

A number of studies have shown that simple advice given by a suitably trained doctor or nurse can produce a significant decline in hazardous drinking, with demonstrable benefit to health. For example, Wallace et al (1988) randomly allocated heavy drinkers (men reporting drinking at least 35 units a week and women drinking at least 21 units) to a treatment or control group. Treatment involved simple advice from the general practitioner about reducing consumption and follow-up at 3-monthly intervals. After one year, 44% fewer men were drinking excessively in the treatment group compared with 26% fewer amongst controls, 48% fewer women were drinking heavily in treatment compared with 29% in controls. Chick et al (1985) demonstrated that a significant reduction in consumption followed one session of advice and counselling given by a trained nurse to male patients in a general hospital who had been identified as drinking in a hazardous way. Self-help manuals have proved effective as a further means of helping drinkers reduce their consumption (Miller & Taylor 1980).

Prevention of drug misuse

Reducing supply through customs and enforcement agencies is outwith the scope of this chapter. However, reducing demand through health promotion does justify elaboration. Current strategies in drug education can be divided into a number of categories.

- Providing information (whether 'scare' or 'balanced')
- Seeking to remedy supposed deficits of moral values or living skills
- Decision-making skills in the context of antidrug norms
- Providing alternatives to drug use through youth and community participation
- Harm minimisation of secondary prevention
- Peer lead approaches involving youth groups with facilitators

The first strategy, information-type programmes, may slow transitions to heavier or hazardous use but do not stop experimentations. As for the second strategy, there is no support from outcome studies in adopting a moral value or living skills approach to drug prevention. The third, resistance strategies, may reduce experimentation but it promotes a polarised community, and drug use in those that use tends to be more hazardous. Providing alternatives, the fourth strategy, appears ineffective, but if linked to broader community initiatives may prove useful. The fifth strategy, secondary prevention in the form of harm minimisation for those already using, has shown substantial benefits, elaborated further under Goals of Treatment. The final strategy requires further research, but early studies suggest a positive response (Dorn & Murji 1992).

Prevention is not only limited to stopping initial drug use but may also be related to detecting use at an earlier stage; this involves targeting, among others, parents to educate them about drugs and solvents so that the thresholds for detection in their children are lowered (Health Publications Unit 1993). In the USA, drug testing kits have been approved for sale and it may be that, in the future, parents or schools may do random testing to try and detect drug misuse. Hair analysis for drugs may have also produced a technological breakthrough or an ethical quagmire, depending on your point of view (Strang et al 1993).

Special circumstances are found in prison and the introduction of mandatory drug testing in British prisons in February 1995 to detect, deter and prevent drug use may be having unexpected results, such as the switching from cannabis to injectable, shorter acting drugs to avoid detection (Gore et al 1996). Attempts at lowering the thresholds of detection and early intervention and prevention of serious drug problems have also been attempted in the workplace. Staff training has been evaluated and shown to improve confidence and the ability of staff to deal with drug and alcohol problems and hence their willingness to intervene (Gossop & Birkin 1994). As for the legal – illegal axis of drug prevention, some view the relaxation in legal controls as being one way of trying to prevent much of the problems associated with psychoactive substances; this has been reviewed by Heath (1992) and others (for example, Stevenson 1994).

EPIDEMIOLOGY OF SUBSTANCE USE/MISUSE

Epidemiology of drinking and alcohol-related harm

The prevalence of alcohol-related problems in a population is linked to the alcohol consumption per person in that population. There is a high correlation between national consumption and cirrhosis mortality. Within countries, fluctuations in consumption over time are positively correlated with fluctuations in cirrhosis mortality (Skog 1980). Changes which increase consumption, such as price, enhanced availability, more advertising or sales outlets or greater social permissiveness, also contribute to rising problem rates. Of course, overall consumption is not the only influence: different styles of drinking are linked to different problems. In cultures where a bout pattern of drinking predominates there is a higher level of social harm than in areas where consumption is less episodic. Similarly, the Nordic countries, which have relatively low per caput consumption, have higher rates of acute alcohol poisoning than southern European countries.

Influences on consumption

Government revenue statistics are the usual source of information about overall national alcohol consumption. Revenue on beer and spirits has been collected in the UK since the 17th century. The lowest point in per caput consumption of all forms of alcohol for three centuries occurred in the 1930s. In common with many other countries, consumption of alcohol in the UK rose steadily from 1945 to 1980.

Since then consumption has increased only slightly in many countries, including the UK. In southern Europe wine consumption has declined by 42% in the past 30 years. This has been partially offset by the increased popularity of beer. Some have interpreted this as evidence of a homogenisation of drinking habits across Europe. Death rates from cirrhosis of the liver have fallen significantly in France and Italy over the same period of time (Gual & Colom 1997). In 1988 there were severe restrictions on official production and sales in Russia and consumption declined, but with the advent of free market competition the 1990s have seen a dramatic growth in alcohol use and alcohol-related problems.

In the UK beer and spirit consumption peaked in 1980 but wine consumption has almost quadrupled in the past 25 years. Increased advertising and marketing, increasing numbers of outlets, extension of licensing hours and falling relative price have been shown in Britain (McGuiness 1980) and in other countries to contribute to rises in consumption. It has been unusual for alcohol not to be served at both private and public functions. 'Going out for a drink' is England's most popular leisure activity, and the most common reason men give for drinking is that it is 'what their friends do when they get together' (Wilson 1980).

Drinking amongst women   This has increased greatly, particularly when the second half of the 20th century is compared to the 19th century. Changes in the woman's role, with the result that she enters more male environments and has more income, have contributed. Advertising directed specifically at women has possibly played a part too. There has been a gradual rise in the proportion of women drinking more than 14 units per week from 9% in 1984 to 11% in 1992. This pattern is seen in all age groups.

Regional differences within the UK   Surveys show that, although the mean consumption and the proportion of drinkers who are heavy drinkers is similar in England and Wales, Scotland and Northern Ireland, in Scotland drinking seems to be concentrated into fewer days of the week. Amongst males the highest weekly consumption is found in the north of England. In Northern Ireland the proportion of abstainers is much higher than elsewhere in the UK.

Ethnic and religious minorities   Islam, Hinduism, Sikhism, Seventh Day Adventism and the Baptist Church oppose or prohibit consumption of alcohol. The percentage drinking over 36 units/week among Afro-Caribbean men is about half the national average for men of comparable age and social status. Some heavy drinkers are to be found amongst Pakistanis and Indians, including some Muslims (Cochrane & Bal 1990).

Occupation   There are various reasons for the association of heavy drinking and certain occupations: availability of alcohol at work (e.g. the licensed trade); social expectations (e.g. the business lunch); separation from normal social and sexual relationships (e.g. seamen, servicemen). Men in the drinks industry have the highest average per person consumption, while the construction industry has the highest proportion of men who drink 'heavily' (over 50 units per week). The drinks industry tends to recruit men who are already heavy drinkers, to which an 'availability' factor is added. Freedom from supervision may contribute to the fact that doctors, lawyers and senior executives have an increased risk of being heavy consumers. The standardised mortality rate, which used to be 300 or more for cirrhosis amongst doctors, had reduced to 115 in the 1982–1983 mortality data (Chick 1992).

Prevalence of alcohol-related disorders

Attempts to estimate the prevalence of 'alcoholism' are misleading and epidemiologists now study the components of this conglomerate concept, for example breaking it down into identifiable components such as alcohol dependence and the adverse health and social consequences of drinking. Data on the prevalence of physical damage from alcohol are available in mortality records and hospital admissions statistics. Mortality from cirrhosis is greatest in the grape-growing countries of central and southern Europe where consumption is higher. The increase in cirrhosis deaths in the UK which has occurred since 1945 is accounted for by an increase in alcoholic cirrhosis (Saunders et al 1981). By 1980 a peak had been passed in the USA, Canada and Sweden and a decrease noticed, the reasons for which remain to be clarified (Smart & Mann 1991), but getting more alcoholics into treatment and into mutual help groups may be a factor. In Scotland the number of general hospital admissions in which alcohol was recorded as one of the diagnoses increased nearly fourfold between 1968 and 1978. The majority of studies show a dose–response relationship between alcohol consumption and hepatic cirrhosis.

In general hospitals 20–30% of all male admissions and 5–10% of female admissions are deemed to be 'problem drinkers', the rate varying with the catchment area of the hospital and, of course, with the definitions of 'problem drinker' (Chick 1987).

Alcohol disorders account for approximately one-fifth of psychiatric first admissions, but admission figures are influenced by availability of beds, and fashions in day and outpatient care versus inpatient care. This may be a partial explanation for the greater rate of alcoholism admissions in Scotland than in England, and a trend towards outpatient treatment and detoxification may have contributed to the fall in Scottish figures in the 1980s.

The general population survey permits a prevalence estimate that is not subject to the vagaries of hospital admission and referral policies or the defining processes of social agencies. However, the door-to-door interviewer has difficulty in finding the heavy drinker at home and, when found at home, he or she tends to underreport consumption and problems. The 1978 survey of England and Wales derived a point prevalence figure of 'problem drinking' of 5.3% in men and 1.6% in women.

Doorstep comments by refusers suggested that at least a further 0.77% might have been classified as problem drinkers (Wilson 1980). Estimates are very sensitive to alterations in the definition of a case, for example the number and severity of alcohol-related symptoms required to reach the criterion for inclusion, and whether or not past as well as present symptoms are counted. A survey of the prevalence of psychiatric morbidity in adults (aged 16–64 years) living in private households in the UK was conducted in 1993. The annual prevalence rate of symptoms of alcohol dependence was 4.7%. Men were three times more likely to be alcohol dependent than women. The prevalence was particularly high among young men. A remarkably similar prevalence was found in a comparable survey in the USA (Mason & Wilkinson 1996).

In North America DSM-III criteria have been applied in general population surveys. The St Louis sample revealed a lifetime prevalence of alcohol dependence of 16.1% for men and 3% for women. The same instrument (Diagnostic Interview Schedule, DIS) was translated for use in Korea and Taiwan where rates among men were 20% and 3%, respectively, perhaps reflecting the less severe oriental flushing reaction in Koreans compared with Taiwanese, as well as the high tolerance, indeed encouragement, of

drinking in males in South Korean society (Helzer et al 1990).

Level of consumption and adverse consequences

Community samples must be studied if estimates are to be made of the risk to health of drinking at particular levels. It has been shown for a particular district in France, by comparing what cirrhotics drink and what a sample from the rest of the population drinks, that the risk of cirrhosis increases logarithmically with increasing consumption, starting at 6 units per day in women and 8 units per day in men. At 12 units per day the risk in men is increased 14-fold. The risk for delirium tremens begins at 12 units per day. This research is based on what people admit to drinking. The risk of being admitted to a medical ward for a variety of diagnoses (gastrointestinal, liver, cardiovascular disorders, myocardial infarction) was shown in a sample of Scottish men to rise at 21 units per week (Chick et al 1986). Stroke death in Chicago begins to be linked with alcohol when consumption reached 42 units per week (Dyer et al 1980).

Estimates have been made of the contribution of alcohol to the death rate, using data from follow-up studies where self-reports of alcohol consumption were obtained at entry to the study. Anderson (1988) arrived at a figure for England and Wales, for ages 15–74 years, of 28 000 excess deaths. Those who drink 1–3 units of alcohol per day have a lower death rate than abstainers, but it is likely (though still debated) that this is due partly to the light drinkers being overrepresented among those whose lifestyle is healthy in other ways, and partly because abstainers often turn out to be abstaining because of pre-existing ill-health. None the less there does appear to be a U-shaped relationship between drinking alcohol and all-cause mortality. Mortality risk rises in men taking more than 3 units per day and women more than 2 units per day. Current evidence suggests that low to moderate consumption of alcohol may protect middle-aged men and postmenopausal women from developing coronary heart disease. The benefits for women need to be offset against the risk of breast cancer. In younger people, of course, any benefits are more than countered by the relationship between alcohol use and accidents, and suicide. (For a further discussion of this topic see report by the Royal Colleges of Physicians, Psychiatrists and General Practitioners, 1995).

It is clear that the risk of psychosocial harm also rises with increased consumption. It is also noteworthy that many of the social costs associated with drinking impinge principally, or even exclusively, on third parties such as the drinker's partner, pedestrians, bystanders or workmates. Social harm is also strongly influenced by pattern of drinking, with regular intoxication being particularly damaging. Room et al (1995) have shown that the frequency of having five drinks or more per occasion is at least as important as the overall intake in predicting alcohol-related personal and social problems.

Patterns of illegal drug use and their related problems

The majority of drug users are not known and, as the behaviour is illegal, they wish it to remain that way. Therefore, anonymity and confidentiality are essential in trying to access this hidden population. A well-designed and regular national illicit drug use survey in the UK taking into account these difficulties does not exist, although it has been proposed (Sutton & Maynard 1992). Assessing the pattern of drug use in Britain is therefore like putting together a jigsaw with most of the pieces missing. It is estimated that in any one year at least 3% of the adult population will take an illegal drug – some 1.4 million people (Institute for the Study of Drug Dependence, 1995). Most take cannabis, and most use it only occasionally. Population averages can be misleading when applied to young adults and schoolchildren. A longitudinal study of knowledge and experience of young people regarding drug misuse has been monitored every 5 years since 1969 in one English town. Over this period, the proportion of people who knew someone taking drugs increased from 15 to 65%, and the proportion who had been offered drugs increased from 5 to 45%. The major change occurred primarily between 1989 and 1994. Stimulants were more commonly mentioned than opiates (Wright & Pearl 1995). Cross-sectional studies across the UK have shown that, in pupils aged 15–16 years, at least 40% had used illicit drugs, mainly cannabis, at some time. Geographical variations also occur – for example levels of drug use are higher in Scotland (Miller & Plant 1996). In a cross-sectional study in Scotland which represented all local council areas and 189 different schools, with just under 10 000 young pupils aged between 11 and 17 years, participating, many of the findings by Miller & Plant (1996) were confirmed. Typically, cannabis use was reported most commonly in at least 40% of the group of 14–15- year-olds and then, in descending order, pain killers, solvents, amphetamine, magic mushrooms, LSD, tranquillisers, ecstasy, cocaine and heroin. Only 1.2% had tried heroin. In the 14-and 15-year-old group, 14% used drugs once a week or more, 15% once a month and 10% once a year (Fast Forward Positive Lifestyle 1996). Perhaps surprisingly, geographical dif-

ferences across Scotland showed that there was slightly higher experimentation with drug use in semirural areas than in urban areas. The evidence is for increasing use of 'soft' drugs, but the use of heroin seems to be fairly stable across Europe, with a typical lifetime risk of around 2% and a male:female ratio of 2:1 (Hartnoll 1994). Regular users of drugs may subsequently develop problems related to their drug use and may then present to the criminal justice system, the health service or other caring agencies outside the health service. Criminal statistics incorporate a variety of data on drugs, including the quantities and number of seizures by customs and by police, as well as a record of the number of offences against the Misuse of Drugs Act, 1971. Cannabis remains the most common drug seized, involving 80% of cases. Where there have been increases in most drug categories, the most marked increases have been in stimulants, such as 3,4-methylenedioxymethamphetamine (MDMA) and amphetamine. The purity of amphetamines remains stable at around 5% but heroin purity seems to be increasing to above 50%. Typical retail prices of drugs on the illicit market tend to be fairly stable, suggesting that the supply and demand match is relatively constant. Most police forces in Scotland have above UK average seizures per head of population (Home Office Statistical Bulletin 1995b).

Prior to May 1997 there was a statutory obligation for health service professionals to provide information to the Home Office Addicts Index about people who presented as being dependent on opiates and cocaine (details in the *British National Formulary* prior to June 1997). This Index used to provide some indication of addicts presenting to medical care but there was undoubtedly underreporting and its prime value was as an indicator of trends: the number of notifications to the Home Office in the last few years up to 1997 increased year on year by 15% (Home Office Statistical Bulletin 1995a). Prevalence tends to be higher in major cities, typically 2–3 times the national average. The highest published population rate is for Glasgow: 700–1200 per 100 000 in 1989 (Frischer 1992). Since 1990 the Home Office Addicts Index has been partially replaced by regional databases. These data confirm national trends and report other categories of drug use. The advantage of the regional databases is that non-NHS services are also encouraged to report, giving a broader indication of local trends. The methodological and practical issues concerned in accessing this hidden population of drug users not in contact with services have been explored by Griffiths and colleagues (1993). The 'capture, recapture technique' is explained and promoted by others as being the method for prevalence estimation when direct methods are not feasible (Domingo-Salvany et al

1995). The National Addiction Centre in London has also used a ratio estimation method for determining prevalence of cocaine use in the UK, suggesting that there may-be 1.6 times the number of heroin users, i.e. 116 000 cocaine users. (Gossop et al 1994). When looking at dependent drug use, there is a strong association with social deprivation – the most deprived areas having the highest rates of drug dependence (Domingo-Salvany et al 1993, Babor 1994).

Natural history of problem drinking

The problem drinker is not an individual irredeemably condemned to addiction; many people move into and out of problem drinking. Surveys record low rates of drinking problems after age 50 years. An Australian study, examining the ages of alcoholics known to agencies, concluded that the prevalence of alcoholism in the population diminishes more rapidly with age than can be accounted for by mortality and successful treatment. One-half to one-third of respondents in several large US surveys who reported a given 'problem' no longer reported that problem when reinterviewed 4 years later. Though some of these had developed a different alcohol-related problem instead, others had stopped or reduced their drinking. Positive changes in social circumstances such as job and personal relationships are important in the history of these recovered individuals (see Evaluation of Drug Treatments p. 361). In a Swedish general population cohort, reinterviewed after a 15 year interval, 41% of the 71 alcoholics identified originally and still alive were completely free of drinking problems (Ojesjo 1981). A similar proportion (45%) of 120 problem drinkers from the Boston inner-city sample (Vaillant et al 1985) followed during 20 years on average were no longer in difficulties. However, 10% had died and 40% continued to have drinking problems. At conscription to the Swedish armed forces, men who are drinking over 30 units per week have three and a half times the expected death rate in the coming 15 years (Andreasson et al 1988), which is similar to the excess rate shown by those who are discharged from hospital diagnosed as alcoholics.

Natural history of drug taking

The vast majority of non-regular drug users do not become regular users. Non-regular users tend to use to keep in with their friends and to 'act hard'. It is only when they begin to use drugs to forget about problems, or to avoid boredom, or primarily to get a good feeling, that they risk becoming regular users (Fast Forward Positive Lifestyle 1996). Natural history tends to vary with culture, social setting, drug and route of use. For heroin, in a community sample of London users, there was a move from smoking to injection, but this was not inevitable. The majority of smokers never moved to regular injecting, despite often using high doses for many years. Women were less likely to move to injecting – 16% of the sample smokers had previously been regular injectors and this is a less well-known natural progression (Griffiths et al 1994). Indeed, in the late 1990s, initiation is no longer by injecting but by smoking (Strang et al 1992). In a 22 year follow-up study of heroin addicts from a London clinic, the mortality rate was assessed at 2% annually, an excess mortality ratio of 12. No sex differences in mortality rates were demonstrated but the excess mortality was concentrated at younger ages. No prediction of survival could be made on the length of heroin use or age at intake into the study (Oppenheimer et al 1994). In those that survived, two-thirds were not using opiates and had not transferred their dependence on to other substances, such as alcohol, but there was a high incidence of smoking. They expect to find tobacco-related disease in future follow-ups (Tobutt et al 1996).

The natural history of cocaine remains uncertain. A longitudinal study in Canada on 100 adult users in the community in 1990, with 54 reinterviewed at 1 year, showed that the fear of adverse health, social and financial consequences cautioned users. Most had quit or reduced their use without professional help, suggesting that the natural history of cocaine use is a self-limiting phenomenon of relatively short duration (P. G. Erickson 1993, unpublished data). Others have suggested six career types: descending use; use reaching a peak and extinguishing; intermittent use; chaotic use but extinguishing over a period of time; stable regular use; and increasing chaotic use with increasing tolerance or increasing level of drug use. It was only the last group (10%) that had negative careers (J. Ditton 1993, unpublished data).

DEFINITIONS OF DEPENDENCE ON PSYCHOACTIVE SUBSTANCES

'Alcoholism' still has currency among many clinicians and therapists in the field and the term is still used at times in this chapter. Though imprecise, it carries the implication that the drinker is dependent and has incurred harm to himself or others.

The ICD-10 categorises the mental and behavioural disorders due to psychoactive substance use by drug types (Table 12.2). Within each drug category, there is then the possibility of a number of clinical conditions (where 'X' refers to the drug type) (Table 12.3).

The clinical condition F1X.2, dependence syn-

Table 12.2   Classification of mental and behavioural disorders due to psychoactive substance use

Code	Drug
F10	Alcohol
F11	Opioids
F12	Cannabinoids
F13	Sedative or hypnotics
F14	Cocaine
F15	Other stimulants, including caffeine
F16	Hallucinogens
F17	Tobacco
F18	Solvents
F19	Multiple drug use and other psychoactive substances

Table 12.3   Classification of clinical conditions due to psychoactive substance use

Code[a]	Clinical condition
F1X.0	Acute intoxication
F1X.1	Harmful use
F1X.2	Dependence syndrome
F1X.3	Withdrawal state
F1X.4	Withdrawal state with delirium
F1X.5	Psychotic disorder
F1X.6	Amnesic syndrome
F1X.7	Residual and late onset psychotic disorder
F1X.8	Other mental and behavioural disorders
F1X.9	Unspecified mental and behavioural disorders

[a] X refers to the drug type.

drome, has diagnostic guidelines based on the Edward & Gross paper on the alcohol dependence syndrome (1976). The diagnostic guidelines are:

- A strong desire or sense of compulsion to take the substance
- Difficulties in controlling substance-taking behaviour in terms of its onset, termination or level of use
- A physiological withdrawal state when the substance use has ceased or been reduced
- Evidence of tolerance
- Progressive neglect of alternative pleasures or interests

- Persistence with substance use despite clear evidence of overtly harmful consequences.

Narrowing of the personal repertoire of pattern of psychoactive substance use has also been described as a characteristic feature. There was a move to have tolerance and withdrawal as a mandatory requirement for the diagnosis of the dependence syndrome. This would be in keeping with the prominence that was historically given to 'dependence' and 'physical dependence'. However, studies have shown that tolerance and withdrawal do not emerge as superior to other dependence criteria on several indicators of concurrent and predicted validity, including severity (Carroll et al 1994a). The original dependence syndrome was developed on studies on alcohol dependence and there is only limited support for other individual drug classes – in the case of hallucinogens, none at all (Morgenstern et al 1994). In contrast to the ICD-10, the American diagnostic system DSM-IV has a measure of severity. The measure of severity correlates reasonably well with measures of quantity and frequency of drug use and associated problems. It may be useful in the future to incorporate this within the ICD-10 as severity is one of many factors that can influence outcome (Woody et al 1993). The ICD-10 diagnosis of harmful use has poor agreement with the DSM-IV category of abuse and future revisions may see changes in these definitions (Rapaport et al 1993, Rounsaville et al 1993).

COMORBIDITY

Drug use is a problem for 20–50% of the young mentally ill and leads to excess disability. Patients with psychotic disorders use stimulants, hallucinogens, cannabis and alcohol. Compared to psychotic patients with no comorbidity of substance misuse, they suffer more frequent and severe relapse, expect higher rates of rehospitalisation, and are considerably more difficult to engage in treatment (Nigam et al 1992). Treatment systems have been developed integrating both substance use and psychiatric illness within one comprehensive programme, emphasising continuous treatment teams which offer a form of logical management of behaviour shaping strategies, skills training techniques and assertive case management (Roberts et al 1992, Galanter et al 1994). The dual diagnosed patients are often characterised by high morbidity, poverty and social instability. The burden they place on clinical services by far exceeds what would be expected from the size of this patient group. The improvement in psychiatric illness by joint management of comorbid conditions is not limited to the psychotic disorders. An outcome study at 12 month follow-up showed that obsessive–compulsive disorder (OCD) patients with dual diagnosis who received treatment for their OCD and substance abuse stayed in treatment longer and showed greater reduction in severity of OCD symptoms and a higher overall abstinence (Fals-Stewart & Schafer 1992). Preliminary data from the MacArthur Violence Risk Assessment Study of 1000 discharged acute psychiatric patients found that drug or alcohol misuse, combined with mental disorder, could treble or quadruple the risk of violence, showing the need for integrated treatment programmes (News item 1996a).

AETIOLOGY OF ALCOHOL DEPENDENCE AND MISUSE

Availability of alcohol is a powerful determinant of level of consumption, and culture and tradition are potent influences on the pattern and context, but many other factors play a part in determining the individual development of harmful drinking and dependence. For some problem drinkers the causes are to be found principally in their environment, for others there is a major genetic contribution. Transmission may be of a greater propensity to dependence at a given dose, or a personality type (e.g. 'impulsive') that leads to a troublesome pattern of use; or a personality or constitution that leads to the individual obtaining particular rewards from drinking and/or an absence of undesirable effects. Genetic transmission of alcohol dependence may well involve a mixture of these processes.

On present evidence it seems likely that alcohol dependence is a phenomenon that has many forms which, though phenotypically similar, are genotypically different, some with a high environmental contribution, some with a fairly high environmental contribution, some with a high genetic contribution. There is good epidemiological evidence that heavy drinking runs in families (Marshall & Murray 1991). A summary of factors influencing an individual's disposition to use a drug or drink alcohol is shown in Figure 12.1.

Personality

Sufferers from alcohol-related problems who attend clinics contain a higher proportion of individuals with personality deviations and early family disturbance than is found in the general population. This is partly to be expected as clinics in UK tend to be based in psychiatric services and thus attract psychiatrically disturbed cases. In the general population, follow-up studies of young men show that the impulsive, rebellious, more extrovert individual is somewhat more at risk of developing alcoholism, particularly alcohol-related social problems. Childhood conduct disorder (itself related in general population studies, as well as in clinical work, to parental disharmony) also predicts alcohol-related problems, typically of early onset and linked to criminality. A debate developed in the 1980s about whether there is a type of male alcoholism, with early onset, severe problems especially social problems, a manner that is socially detached, distractible, confident and also linked to a similar pattern in the biological father ('type 2' – Cloninger 1987), which contrasts with a more dependent, anxious, rigid, less aggressive, more guilty alcoholic ('type 1') with either biological mother or father an alcoholic. Some have felt that type 2 is best seen as alcoholism secondary to antisocial personality (ASP) (Schuckit & Irwin 1989). ASP (with alcohol-related items excluded from the ASP algorithm) greatly increases the risk that a man or a woman will have an alcohol problem in longitudinal and cross-sectional community studies. However, most alcoholics have not had childhood conduct disorder. Having ASP and/or a family history of alcoholism in a large community study identified 48% of male alcoholics and 63% of female alcoholics (Lewis & Bucholz 1991). ASP (lifetime) in that study was diagnosed in 8.7% of the population.

Drake & Vaillant (1988), in a 33-year longitudinal study of 456 inner-city adolescent boys chosen as non-delinquent at that age, found that in this sample adolescent indicators of personality disorder were good predictors of adult personality disorder, but not alcoholism. Having an alcoholic father was the best predictor: 28% of sons developed alcoholism as opposed to 12% of sons of non-alcoholic fathers. Apart from the severe disturbance associated with childhood conduct disorders and parental drinking habits, community studies do not usually, especially in middle-class subjects, find evidence linking parenting styles to subsequent alcoholism (Vaillant 1983).

As well as antisocial personality disorder in the community, alcohol dependence is found to be associated with phobic disorder, anxiety disorder, other psychotropic substance misuse (notably tranquilliser dependence) and (especially in women) depression (for example, Lewis & Bucholz 1991).

Alcohol may be used to anaesthetise grief by the bereaved and may complicate pathological grief. Phobias, especially agoraphobia, are common in alcoholics attending psychiatric hospitals (Kushner et al 1990). Alcohol, because it is a short-acting sedative causing rebound arousal, may exacerbate or even precipitate anxiety states. However, the phobia in some instances clearly predates the alcohol dependence. Manic–depressive illness, including the manic phase, may result in drinking to the point of physical dependence.

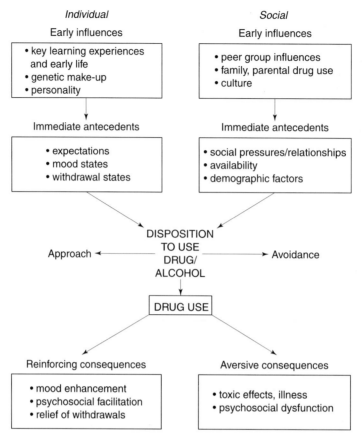

Individual

Early influences
- key learning experiences and early life
- genetic make-up
- personality

Immediate antecedents
- expectations
- mood states
- withdrawal states

Social

Early influences
- peer group influences
- family, parental drug use
- culture

Immediate antecedents
- social pressures/relationships
- availability
- demographic factors

Approach ← DISPOSITION TO USE DRUG/ ALCOHOL → Avoidance

DRUG USE

Reinforcing consequences
- mood enhancement
- psychosocial facilitation
- relief of withdrawals

Aversive consequences
- toxic effects, illness
- psychosocial dysfunction

Fig. 12.1   Factors influencing an individual's drug/alcohol use.

Psychological aspects of alcohol dependence in women

Women make up a third of alcoholics seen in psychiatric practice. There is often a male heavy drinker either in the family history, or the marriage. Women more often than men attribute the onset of problem drinking to a particular lifestress. However, community surveys have not shown either in Scotland or in North America that adverse life events predict whose drinking will increase during a follow-up period (Romelsjo et al 1991). Familial and interpersonal stress may precipitate a depressive episode. Depression in middle life following the departure of the children ('the empty nest'), or in the lonely spinster or widow, can lead to excessive drinking. Typically this is at home and secret, and associated with considerable shame and denial. She may have come to believe that it is only with alcohol that she can appear confident, make decisions and assert herself.

Childhood experience of sexual abuse, when asked for in a research interview, is more commonly reported in women alcoholics than in the general population. It is not yet known if it is more common than in other psychiatric disorders (Hurley 1991).

Female patients, whether presenting with dependence, psychiatric or medical complaints, often give a shorter history of excessive drinking than men and tend to report a lower intake of ethanol, even after correction for body weight. A given dose of ethanol per kilogram of body weight produces a higher peak blood level in a woman than a man. This may be due in part to the female body having a lower ratio of water to fat than the male body (alcohol dissolves more readily in water than in fat), and to lower activity of alcohol dehydrogenase in the gastric mucosa.

Role of marital relationships

In an alcoholic's marriage, hostility, mistrust and attempts by one partner to control the other are common. Communication may be poor. Women problem drinkers sometimes have husbands whose energies are all directed toward their work or their hobbies, or husbands who make them feel worthless. It is difficult to disentangle cause from effect, and adequate research, which would need to be longitudinal, has not yet been conducted. However, some marital problems undoubtedly improve when the drinking ceases.

AETIOLOGY OF DRUG USE

Factors vary, depending on what stage of drug use one is examining. Factors determining initiation of drug use vary with those influencing continuation of drug use, the move into dependent use, and the causes of relapse. The aetiology of relapse will be discussed later in the chapter.

Initiation of drug use

Mankind has used psychoactive drugs at all stages of history:

> Most men and women lead lives at worst, so painful, at the best, so monotonous, poor and limited, that the urge to escape, the longing to transcend themselves only for a few moments, is always and has been one of the principal appetites of the human soul (Huxley 1940).

Whether an individual will take a particular drug will depend on its availability, cost, legal status, alleged effects and, risks and, in some cases, the form of the drug. Why one particular individual will choose to use a drug alongside another who chooses not to, given the same situation, is more complex. Personality traits, such as rebelliousness and curiosity, are thought to contribute to drug experimentation, as is a wish to express independence or hostility. The wish to seek peer group approval may also contribute. Influences also occur in individuals from families and society and here, role models and group pressure may result in some individuals taking drugs, whereas others would not. In some instances, initiation of drug use is iatrogenic, for example in treatment of severe pain. It is in the initiation of drug use that the moral judgemental model is strongest. An assumption of freedom of choice lies behind all 'just say no' campaigns.

Continued use

The factors involved in the initiation of use may play greater or lesser importance in subsequent drug behaviour; however, additional factors come into play when people continue to take drugs. For an individual drug to be continued, it must give positive effects and minimal negative effects. These positive effects will be the beginning of the development of 'positive outcome expectancy', which later with continued reinforcement develops into craving. With use, the onset of classical conditioning and conditioned responses become more apparent, the pharmacology of the drug determining much of what users would then choose to do. On the individual level, continued use is associated with non-conformity generally. Genetic contributions to individual differences in sensitivity to drugs and their influencing behaviour are not fully developed, but will play a part in future understanding of the aetiology of why some people move from experimental to recreational and then dependent use (Morse et al 1995). Individual distress or unrecognised psychiatric illness can lead on to the search of self-medication and the short-term alleviation of symptoms by continued use.

Dependent use

Once the dependence syndrome has developed, tolerance and withdrawal symptoms are frequently a feature of the condition and the quality and severity of withdrawal is primarily determined by the substance of use. Avoidance of withdrawal then becomes a major factor in continued drug use. At the individual level, personality traits in people dependent on drugs, particularly heroin addicts, are certainly different from normal controls. There is an increased incidence of low self-esteem, submissiveness, dependence on others and a craving of approval, lack of self-confidence, a learnt helplessness, low expectations for the future, and a tendency to give up easily. However, is this a cause or an effect of the dependence syndrome? This has not been resolved by prospective studies. Much is said about individual denial of problems related to drug use, or at least a lack of awareness. Alternatively, dependent drug users may choose to continue using as the benefits of giving up are not outweighed by the advantages of continued use. An other theory for continued drug use in dependent users is that they have not developed the options of different coping mechanisms to deal with problems and that their use of drugs is their main coping mechanism. As mentioned above, classical conditioning and learning theory play an increasing role the longer the drug is used.

PSYCHOBIOLOGY OF ALCOHOL DEPENDENCE

Initiation and reinforcement

Initiation into drinking is influenced by the setting, the

company and expectations about the likely effects. All of these contribute to whether alcohol has a relaxing or euphoriant impact as much or more than its pharmacological action (Young et al 1990).

The consequences of drinking for the novice drinker may well have an effect on their subsequent drinking career. Individuals with high levels of anxiety will be conscious of alcohol's relaxing properties. Alcohol has a euphoriant effect for some individuals in some settings and this is a potent *reinforcer* of continued drinking. Genetic factors may make some individuals experience euphoria or tension reduction more intensely at this stage (Marshall & Murray 1991). It is also interesting that there is a greater concordance in drinking style in monozygotic than dizygotic twins, even allowing for the greater social closeness of the former (Heath & Martin 1988).

Orientals have varying degrees of acetaldehyde dehydrogenase deficiency, and the consequent 'flushing' reaction to alcohol is a deterrent to drinking for some (though alcohol dependence does develop in some Orientals despite flushing).

Sons of alcoholics, identified both from among sons of clinic attenders, in a general population cohort, and by questionnaire survey, for example in college students, have been compared with controls on numerous measures (Pihl et al 1990). In sons of alcoholics, alcohol has a greater dampening effect on the physiological correlates of stress than is seen in controls. Children of alcoholics of school age tend to be distractible, quick to resort to aggression and often in trouble with authority. These traits may, of course, also be contributed to by parental separation and neglect. There is debate about whether some of the *cognitive abnormalities* seen in alcoholics, such as rigidity of thought, poor abstracting and problem-solving and impaired self-regulation and planning memory, are also to be found more than expected in children of alcoholics.

A twin study did not find cognitive impairment (nor cortical atrophy) in the non-alcoholic monozygotic twins in discordant pairs, which also provides some evidence against the hypothesis that an inherited predisposing trait in alcoholism might be cognitive impairment. It points to aspects, at least, of cognitive impairment being a result rather than a precursor of the drinking (Gurling et al 1991).

Trait markers

A number of biological markers have been identified which may predict a vulnerability to developing alcohol-related problems. Mostly they have been observed in the detoxified alcoholic and in greater frequency in the offspring of alcoholics. They include reduced EEG α activity and reduced P300 wave amplitude. Autonomic responsiveness to stress has been shown to be greater in the sons of alcoholics.

A search is being made for *biochemical abnormalities* which occur in alcoholics and can also be demonstrated in their predrinking children. After drinking, alcohol levels of prolactin are lower in offspring with a family history of alcoholism than in controls. The rise in cortisol and adrenocorticotrophin (ACTH) after a drink of alcohol is less among those men with a family history than those without. It has been shown that young men with family histories of alcoholism have heightened sensitivity to pituitary β-endorphins. Analogous findings have been found in genetically predisposed animals. This is one of a number of illustrations of the way in which genetic predisposition may in a variety of subtle ways make individuals more at risk of drinking in a harmful way.

Tolerance and withdrawal

As drinking becomes a regular habit, many drinkers find that they have to take more to obtain the desired effect; this is evidence that tolerance is increasing and it may seem hard to cut down.

A behavioural explanation of tolerance and withdrawal is that an organism 'expects' the drug because it is confronted with signals that previously heralded the drug, 'drug compensatory conditional responses' act to cancel the effect of the drug, producing tolerance if the drug is administered, or a 'withdrawal' state if the drug is withheld. Thus animals may only display tolerance to alcohol in an environment where the alcohol was initially administered and not in a novel setting.

It seems probable that the development of neurophysiological tolerance is a key step along the way to establishing dependence. The understanding of the neurochemical basis of the actions of alcoholics is currently at an exciting and rapidly developing stage. This has occurred because new neuroimaging techniques – positron emission tomography (PET) and (single photon emission computed tomography (SPECT) – have enhanced the capacity to study and understanding the biological basis of dependence. Prior to these developments much of the research relied on animal studies.

Alcohol, in common with other neuroactive drugs, alters brain transmitter function. It has several actions on different brain sites, including dopamine release in the nucleus accumbens. When alcohol is stopped, dopamine release drops below normal, which may account for the depressed mood associated with early withdrawal. It is thought that overactivity of dopamine contributes to the excitability observed in delirium tremens. Alcohol also appears to act on γ-aminobutyric acid (GABA) and excitatory amino receptors.

There is evidence that endogenous opioid transmitters also play a part in the effects of alcohol. It has also been shown that relapse in dependent alcoholics can be mitigated by opiate antagonists (naltrexone, see p. 358). The activity of noradrenaline is decreased by opioids, and withdrawal symptoms are in part thought to be an expression of a rebound of noradrenaline activity.

Some mention should be made of calcium channels in this complex story. Calcium homeostasis is critical to all cells and several different calcium channels control the passage of this ion across cell membranes. Alcohol reduces entry through the channels. As a result they increase in number. One consequence of this is that calcium flux becomes excessive during withdrawal. Some speculate that this intense calcium flux contributes to neuronal death (Nutt 1996). The varied actions may account for the euphoriant and anxiety reducing properties of the drug.

The original demonstration that 'rum fits' and delirium tremens were withdrawal symptoms of alcohol dependence was made by Isbell et al (1955). In this experiment, recovered opiate addicts consumed between 1 and $1\frac{1}{2}$ bottles of spirits per day (250–370 g ethanol) for 7 weeks. On cessation all had withdrawal symptoms, and some had fits or delirium. Such a short history is unusual (not unknown) in clinical practice. Usually the tendency to drink such large amounts over successive days takes years to develop. Nevertheless, traces of withdrawal phenomenon (insomnia, restlessness, increased rapid eye movement (REM) sleep) occur even after single large doses of a sedative such as alcohol. Hangover is in part a mild withdrawal state.

Genetic differences in propensity to develop withdrawal symptoms has not been shown in humans, but has been in strains of animal bred as alcohol-preferring.

Relapse and reinstatement

Some clinicians believe that there is a protracted physiological withdrawal state which outlasts the visible tremor, tachycardia, sweating and anxiety of the initial 3–10 days. Cognitive deficits are still improving several months after abstinence, cerebral atrophy also resolves in some patients, and cerebral blood flow improves. During this time, abnormalities in EEG evoked response and sleep architecture, and complaints of insomnia, persist; patients complain of anxiety and depressive symptoms, diminishing proportionally with the length of abstinence; and there appears to be reduced suppression in the dexamethasone suppression test and blunted thyrotrophin response to thyrotrophin-releasing hormone (Garbutt 1991). The indications are that GABA receptors, their chloride channels, and perhaps upregulation of N-methyl-D-aspartate (NMDA)

receptors continue to be abnormal (For further discussion see Nutt 1996.)

During this time, some patients feel an urge to drink and they struggle with craving. There are of course psychological and social processes during this period, as well as neurochemical ones. These include a range of cues to drinking that have been learnt over the years. Such cues may be environmental: social situations; the pub or club; the wine shop by the bus stop; the chair in which the drinker customarily watches television. Cues may also be internal; for example, drinking may have become associated with feeling happy, sad, angry, tired, hungry, or all of these. Brain damage is likely to be important in impeding an alcoholic's intentions: thinking may have become inflexible and he or she is unable easily to plan ahead.

During these initial months some contend that further – even slight – use of alcohol may erode resolve about further consumption, and lead to relapse. Many alcoholism recovery programmes recommend absolute abstinence. After tolerance has been lost, five or six drinks may be sufficient to dissolve one's intention not to take a seventh. However, there seems no obvious reason why that should lead to a return in the next day or so to heavy harmful drinking, reinstatement of craving and withdrawal symptoms. There is no evidence that one drink sets off a neurophysiological tripwire, but disposition to drink in alcoholics (measured objectively as work done to obtain alcohol or speed of drinking under standard conditions) has been shown in laboratory settings to increase after as little as three large measures of spirits. Increased disposition to drink in abstinent alcoholics has also been demonstrated on the morning after a dose of alcohol. Thus, in alcohol-dependent individuals that have been abstinent for some time the pattern of response to renewed drinking is 'carried over' from their previous drinking period. Carry-over has been demonstrated in monkeys and in rats: physical dependence, (tendency to withdrawal phenomena) is more easily evoked in animals that have been previously made physically dependent, even after 37 days abstinence. 'Reinstatement' is also used to describe the carry-over phenomenon. It is interesting that prior severity of dependence in alcoholics may not predict relapse, but may predict severity of relapse.

As well as a learning theory/neurophysiological view of reinstatement a cognitive explanation has also been put forward. It is said that abstinent alcoholics who relapse on recommencing drinking do so because they believe, as a result of treatment or attendance at Alcoholics Anonymous, that one or two drinks necessarily leads to harmful drinking – 'the self-fulfilling prophecy'. Of course, having a drink can also be seen as a stimulus with a long-ingrained conditioned response –

taking another drink. This view has led some to advocate cue-exposure, including exposure to drinking environments, as a way of reducing severity of relapse. This approach is not yet proven as a treatment method (Drummond et al 1990).

Apart from the biological forces which may be operating, the alcoholic who has at one point decided to stop drinking experiences many mental processes which are completely conscious (well described by Ludwig 1988). Sometimes these are best seen as the mind's way of justifying an urge to drink, for example thinking 'one won't harm me' or 'I'm not an alcoholic actually'. Sometimes it will be a feeling – self pity, anger, guilt, frustration – which is followed by the thought 'a drink will get me over this'. By retraining their thinking alcoholics can free themselves, sometimes completely, from the mental processes that eventually lead to relapse (see below). Otherwise, rationalisation, distortion of reality (minimising the harm alcohol has done to him), projection (putting the blame on someone else), will allow the alcoholic to do what he wants (to drink alcohol) without a feeling of guilt or conflict.

PSYCHIATRIC COMPLICATIONS OF ALCOHOL ABUSE

Withdrawal states with delirium (F10.4)

The condition commonly known as delirium tremens is often taken as the hallmark of alcoholism but it is not common, being reported by only about 5% of patients attending alcoholic clinics. It occurs when an individual who is severely dependent on alcohol stops or reduces drinking.

The full syndrome is characterised by marked tremor of the limbs, body and tongue, restlessness, loss of contact with reality, clouding of consciousness, disorientation and illusions progressing to terrifying hallucinations which are most commonly visual, but may be auditory or tactile. Delusions, often of a paranoid kind, may also occur, often associated with the hallucinations. Fever, sweating and tachycardia are pronounced. The disturbance usually develops out of milder withdrawal symptoms one day after cessation of drinking and rarely persists for more than 4 days. Symptoms are often worse at night. There is a significant mortality (approximately 10%), partly because it often complicates other medical emergencies such as infections or injuries. The development of fever, dehydration and signs of shock are ominous prognostic signs. It is important to remember that concomitant infection, Wernicke's encephalopathy, metabolic disturbance, hypoglycaemia or head injury may complicate

the clinical features and prognosis. Withdrawal fits may occur at any time from the first to the 14th day (Isbell et al 1955).

Admission to hospital will usually be necessary. The patient's environment should be uncluttered and uniformly lit to avoid ambiguities. Parenteral multivitamin preparations (Parentrovite) may be given provided resuscitation equipment is available. Electrolytes and plasma glucose should be checked. An oral benzodiazepine, such as chlordiazepoxide, commencing at 100–150 mg/day and reducing after the second or third day, will usually be sufficient to contain the patient's agitation and can be stopped after a week. It is important that the dosage should be progressively reduced, and should not be continued after, at most, 14 days.

Psychotic disorder: alcoholic hallucinosis (F10.5)

In this condition hallucinations occur in clear consciousness. Sometimes these are a continuation of hallucinations first experienced during withdrawal from alcohol. However, hallucinations may also commence de novo in a patient who is still drinking. Usually these experiences are auditory and begin as fragmentary sounds. For example, a woman, of previous stable personality, who had begun drinking heavily in her job as a motor trade representative and hostess, was surprised to hear the clinking of glasses and sounds of merriment from a neighbour's flat. Though the flat was in fact empty most of the time, she began to believe that continuous parties were taking place and heard people coming to and fro with bottles.

In such cases the sounds gradually become formed and voices are heard, often making unpleasant remarks: 'She ought to be ashamed of herself', 'He's a lush', etc. The voices give commands to do things against the subject's will and persecutory delusions may develop. The experiences may be very compelling and distressing, occasionally resulting in violence or suicide.

In the two large published series of cases (Bendetti 1952, Victor & Hope 1958) only a few cases (5–10%) continued to have symptoms for 6 months or more if abstinence was maintained. Renewed drinking, however, tends to bring about a return of hallucinations.

Despite the close resemblance of the hallucinations to those of acute schizophrenia, only a few go on to show typical schizophrenic deterioration: four out of 76 in Victor & Hope's series and 13 out of 113 in Bendetti's series, but Cutting in a more recent series (1978) observed 19%. In distinguishing this condition from schizophrenia, it is noteworthy that in the initial presentation there is no disturbance of volition or experience of interference with thinking. Premorbid adjustment in the social and sexual spheres tends to be normal. A family history of schizophrenia is usually absent except in the cases where hallucinations persist and schizophrenic personality deterioration occurs. There is no close relationship with gross cognitive impairment.

Management commonly requires admission to hospital, withdrawal from alcohol and, if the hallucinations still continue, phenothiazines. It is usually possible to stop the phenothiazines after 2–3 months. Thereafter the patient usually has full insight into the illness and the experience may have been so frightening that he or she never drinks again.

The basis of alcohol hallucinosis is presumably subtle alcohol-induced damage or dysfunction, perhaps of the temporal lobes, though this has not been proven.

Pathological jealousy (Othello syndrome) (F10.5)

Firmly held delusions of infidelity are not uncommon in alcohol misuse. They may be precipitated by the patient's feeling of inadequacy stemming from alcohol-induced impotence and further aggravated by the spouse's growing indifference towards a drunken partner. The patient's accusations become repetitive, and aggressive demands for proof are reinforced by violence. No amount of contrary evidence will dispel the delusion and cases sometimes end tragically in assault or murder. Alcohol misuse is not the only cause of this syndrome (Ch. 15). Treatment is of the underlying condition. Sometimes the only feasible and safe solution is for the couple to separate permanently.

Depression

Symptoms of depression are common amongst excessive drinkers. This is understandable considering the lifestyle of dependent drinkers who frequently wake with a hangover facing a day overshadowed by the problems caused by their drinking. Biological changes induced by excessive drinking may also contribute to depressed mood.

Excessive drinking may mask the symptoms of depressive illness, an association more common in females. Menninger (1938) described alcoholism as chronic suicide, alcoholics being in his view depressive personalities who seek temporary oblivion in drinking. Alcohol also releases inhibitions which make it easier to express feelings of sadness and to give way to self-destructive impulses. It is therefore hardly surprising that alcohol figures so prominently in studies of para-suicide and successful suicide. Factors increasing risk are previous attempts, a history of depression and evident physical and social problems. If secondary diag-

noses of alcoholism are included the proportion of suicides affected range from 20% to 40%, or to 55% if only males are included (Duffy & Kreitman 1993).

The clinician should discriminate between those patients whose alcohol abuse is symptomatic of depression and the much larger number who have become depressed because of their drinking. In the latter, improvement usually follows cessation of drinking and appropriate therapy, whereas the former may require antidepressant medication, combined with a period of abstinence.

Nakamura et al (1983) studied 88 alcoholics in a treatment programme. Although 75% had depressive symptoms at the onset, only 5% had any after 4 weeks abstinence. Depression is a primary factor in a relatively small number of alcohol-dependent individuals. This is more commonly the case in women.

Cognitive impairment and brain damage

Some 50–60% of alcoholics attending psychiatrists perform worse on cognitive testing than would be predicted from their verbal intelligence, educational level and age. There is impairment of memory, visual more than verbal; narrowing and rigidity of thought processes, i.e. difficulty changing from one way of construing and categorising to another, difficulty learning new material and impairment of visuospatial and visuoperceptive skills. A variety of factors may contribute to cognitive impairment amongst excessive drinkers: the neurotoxic effect of alcohol; thiamine deficiency; repeated head injury; and the consequences of alcohol withdrawal fits. A spectrum of cognitive disabilities has been observed extending from mild impairment to end-stage alcoholic dementia. That some of these deficits might predate the heavy drinking has been discussed earlier.

Imaging techniques show cortical atrophy and ventricular enlargement in 50–70% of admissions for alcohol dependence. There are modest correlations between atrophy and cognitive impairment. Magnetic resonance imaging (MRI) relaxation time and brain density measured during computerised tomography (CT) are altered in proportion to lifetime consumption. The shrinkage is mainly in white matter. In liver cirrhosis hepatic encephalopathy is an additional factor.

Cognitive deficits often improve with long-term abstinence. Social functioning is of paramount importance and good outcome has been observed in abstinent alcoholics despite significant impairment on formal testing (Lennane 1988). It is prudent to give thiamine-containing vitamin supplements for at least 4 months. Small bowel malabsorption, in addition to poor intake and excessive utilisation, contributes to vitamin deficiency in alcoholics. Since this may take some weeks to recover, parenteral vitamins, despite their small risk of allergic reaction, are necessary initially.

The characteristic defects observable in psychometric testing are problems with abstracting ability so that patients have great difficulty in changing their mental set to cope with new challenges. Typically they perseverate long after it has become apparent that a novel approach is required. Verbal learning is also impaired, as is perceptual organisation. Patients often find it very difficult to judge objects in space. For example, a middle-aged man had worked for many years loading furniture vans. After a severe bout of delirium tremens he found he was never again able to regain his facility for placing objects in the van so that they were carefully and correctly stowed. Testing showed that he had severe visuospatial defects.

In many cases impaired memory and attention improves following withdrawal. Cognitive assessment is inappropriate during the first 3 weeks after withdrawal. The patient's neuropsychological state is too unstable during that period, and the presence of benzodiazepines will often further complicate the clinical picture. A great deal of improvement can be observed during the first 3 weeks and this continues gradually, up to a year after stopping.

Formal cognitive testing should therefore be postponed until the patient has been abstinent for at least 3 weeks and then monitored thereafter at 3-monthly intervals. The uses of testing include:

- Where there is clinical evidence of impairment and a more formal judgement is required. This is particularly helpful in assessing whether the patient is likely to be able to utilise certain cognitive behavioural techniques and make changes in his way of life.
- As a basis for feedback to the patient, who may need to know that drinking has affected his memory or intellectual powers. This often proves a powerful motivating influence.
- In monitoring progress, both for the clinician and patient.
- As a guide to employability and any hazards which may be experienced in particular occupations.

Testing will often reveal a decline in intellectual ability, poor performance on visuospatial tasks, and impaired planning and coordination ability. In common with all tests, the patient's attention and mood are confounding factors. It is surprising how well some individuals cope despite significant defects. More ecologically based tests are currently being explored which will provide a better measure of the patient's capabilities in tackling real-life situations.

PHYSICAL COMPLICATIONS OF EXCESSIVE DRINKING

Cancer (oesophageal and oropharyngeal), cardiovascular disease, cirrhosis, pancreatic and gastrointestinal disease, accidental death, suicide and greater vulnerability to infection such as tuberculosis, all contribute to the raised mortality amongst excessive drinkers.

Neurological complications

Wernicke's encephalopathy The triad of confusion, ataxia and ocular palsy was described by Wernicke in 1881. Patients dying of this condition show haemorrhages in the brainstem and hypothalamus. Identical lesions have been produced in thiamine-deficient animals. The condition responds to urgent treatment with intravenous thiamine and withdrawal of alcohol but even with such measures there is often a residual dementia or Korsakoff psychosis (Victor 1962). This condition is often overlooked and it is unwise to wait for the classical triad of symptoms before commencing therapy.

Disturbance of consciousness in the alcoholic must also raise the suspicion of traumatic subdural haematoma, though unilateral signs will then probably be present. Occasionally dementia is marked and accompanied initially by incontinence, generalised weakness, tremor persisting long after withdrawal from alcohol, slurred speech and ataxia. Alcoholic cerebellar degeneration presents as ataxia of stance and gait.

Polyneuropathy, contributed to by vitamin deficiency, is common in alcoholics in at least a mild form, with asymptomatic absence of the ankle jerks and calf tenderness. In the established condition the patient complains of muscular cramps and unpleasant paraesthesiae in the feet and calves and unsteadiness of gait. All forms of sensation are impaired in a stocking distribution. Flaccid weakness in the limbs may progress to wrist drop. The cranial nerves are spared. Incontinence, if admitted to, is usually not due to nerve damage but to intoxication to the point of stupor.

Alcoholic myopathy presents as chronic weakness with wasting, punctuated by exacerbation during bouts of drinking.

Korsakoff's psychosis This late consequence of alcoholism is characterised by impairment of short-term memory with a tendency to confabulate. Although these are the classic features which, along with peripheral neuropathy, first attracted the attention of the Russian pathologist Korsakoff to the condition, the defects are less clear-cut than at one time thought and a wide range of other memory and cognitive defects may also be present. Total recovery, even after abstinence and treatment with thiamine, is rare but gradual improvement is often observed over many months. Observed pathological changes are chiefly necrosis and gliosis in the mamillary bodies.

Gastrointestinal complications

Gastritis, presenting as upper abdominal pain and haematemesis, perhaps accompanied by acute gastric erosions, is common in those who drink excessively. Peptic ulcer, though it occurs in 10% of alcoholics, is as common in the general population so it is unlikely that alcohol is a cause. Alcohol nevertheless provokes the symptoms of an ulcer and probably delays healing. Severe diarrhoea sometimes occurs in excessive drinkers and small bowel damage leading to malabsorption exacerbates dietary vitamin deficiency. Chronic relapsing pancreatitis is characterised by recurring acute abdominal pain with inflammation, fibrosis and eventually calcification of the pancreas. It is usually associated with an alcohol intake of over 20 units per day. A protein-deficient diet and hyperlipidaemia are believed to contribute.

Deaths from cancer of the mouth, pharynx, oesophagus and liver are elevated in heavy drinkers. The risk is augmented further in those who also smoke. Some, but not all, studies have also found a relationship between alcohol and cancer of the pancreas, breast and rectum.

Alcohol and liver disease

Over 90% of ingested alcohol is converted by an obligatory oxidative process in the hepatocytes to acetaldehyde, thence to acetate and finally to carbon dioxide and water. The redox state of the cell is altered with wide-ranging potential effects on fat, carbohydrate and nitrogen metabolism. Fat deposition in liver cells (steatosis) almost invariably accompanies heavy drinking and may be present even though liver function tests are normal. Less fortunate drinkers go on to develop hepatitis or cirrhosis. Cirrhosis of the liver is nowadays amongst the five most common causes of death in those under 60 years of age in most industrial countries.

Liver injury is related to volume and duration of alcohol consumption and not to type of beverage. Cirrhosis can be induced in the individual who has drunk moderately for years and then rapidly escalates consumption for 1 or 2 years. Women may be more vulnerable than men and there are indications that progression to cirrhosis depends on immune responses and also, from studies of the human leucocyte antigen system, that heredity contributes.

Modern treatments, despite being expensive, do not appear to have been very successful in reversing the complications of cirrhosis (hepatic failure, variceal bleeding, ascites and primary liver cancer) and there have not been improvements in recent years in the survival of patients with alcoholic cirrhosis. About one-third of patients will still be alive after 5 years, though with abstinence the survival rate doubles, so that those with compensated cirrhosis at presentation have a 90% 5-year survival (Saunders et al 1981).

Death from variceal haemorrhage and hepatic or renal failure may also result from alcoholic hepatitis in the absence of cirrhosis.

Alcoholics who are candidates for liver transplantation are usually expected to demonstrate an ability to abstain and a commitment to maintaining this after surgery. Despite this, many will drink again, particularly after this period of intensive follow-up ends (Howard et al 1994). None the less, patients transplanted for alcoholic liver disease appear to have a better survival than those with viral hepatitis.

Metabolic complications

Life-threatening hypoglycaemia occasionally follows 6–8 hours after heavy alcohol consumption in previously fasting individuals. It may follow imperceptibly from alcoholic stupor. Treatment is urgent intravenous glucose. Insulin-dependent diabetics who ingest moderate to large amounts of alcohol with little carbohydrate may become hypoglycaemic, as may well-fed normal subjects who undertake vigorous exercise in the cold. Chronic alcoholics are prone to reactive hypoglycaemia following a carbohydrate-rich meal, perhaps related to their known accelerated gastric emptying.

A condition closely resembling Cushing's syndrome sometimes occurs in alcoholics. It remits spontaneously over 1–3 weeks.

Acute renal failure after a beer-drinking binge has been reported in Britain and several other countries.

Cardiovascular disease

There is evidence that drinking 1–3 units per day diminishes the risk of coronary disease, but heavier consumption is related to increased morbidity and mortality from this cause. Drinking more than 6 units per day is associated with rising blood pressure and an increased risk of cerebrovascular accidents.

Alcohol is a cause of supraventricular arrhythmias, and of cardiomyopathy leading to congestive cardiac failure. Arrhythmias are particularly prone to occur after bouts of excessive drinking, sometimes known as *holiday heart syndrome.*

Sexual impairment

High blood alcohol level impairs penile erection by a direct pharmacological effect. Heavy drinkers who repeatedly fail to maintain an erection become anxious about their sexual performance, which itself leads to further failure. Alcohol also has direct toxic effects on the Leydig cells of the testis, resulting in reduced testosterone production, impaired spermatogenesis, infertility and testicular atrophy. A significant improvement in sperm count and fertility was noted in a sample of men attending an infertility clinic when they reduced their alcohol intake.

Fetal alcohol syndrome

This syndrome has been observed in children born to mothers who have severe alcohol problems. It is characterised by developmental and growth retardation, and facial and neurological abnormalities. It may be that there are critical developmental stages when alcohol is most likely to do damage. It is also likely that other drugs used, particularly smoking (Plant 1987), are confounding factors.

Forrest et al (1991) could not detect any effect of moderate maternal consumption on the development of their offspring at 18 months and concluded that pregnant mothers could safely consume 70–85 g of alcohol per week. Health authorities now advise women either to abstain or confine their drinking during pregnancy to one or two drinks once or twice a week.

ALCOHOL-RELATED SOCIAL HARM

As alcohol comes to play an increasingly salient part in the drinker's life, he or she often experiences a number of distressing social consequences. Frequently these have their first impact on family and work. Most of the social disabilities which arise are easier to list than quantify. They include the following.

Disruption of family relationships

Alcohol misuse contributes to as many as one-third of divorces, and domestic suffering and violence are commonplace. The relatives of the problem drinker may pass through stages of anguish and frustration as they struggle, sometimes fruitlessly, to bring about change in the drinker. Disappointments may lead to depression in the parent, child or spouse, or to a numbed state in which the drinker is disowned. The children of problem drinkers are specifically at risk of developing behaviour problems and alcohol problems later in life. They often show a facade of premature adult responsibility, losing the experience of childhood in consequence. A fellowship of support groups formed for adult children of alcoholics has been prominent in the USA in recent years. Although there is little evidence to support the belief that they have a specific syndrome, many find help in such groups.

Economic factors

Alcohol is expensive and the family budget suffers accordingly. Earning power is usually reduced, which compounds the disability. Debts may accumulate. The quality of accommodation which the alcoholic can sustain may decline, leading to homelessness.

Employment problems

Alcoholic employees usually develop a poor work record, with frequent absences due to sickness, erratic time-keeping, low productivity and a greatly increased risk of accidents involving themselves and others. The cost of all this to the employer has prompted many companies to set up programmes to encourage employees with drinking problems to seek early treatment (see below).

Crime

As many as 60% of prisoners report significant alcohol problems. Heather (1981) found 15% of young offenders were physically dependent on alcohol and a further 48% had alcohol problems. Young offenders whose crimes are alcohol related have been shown to benefit from attendance at alcohol education courses designed to promote sensible drinking practices (Baldwin 1991).

Drink-driving offences are common amongst dependent drinkers. One in three of all drivers killed has more than the legal limit of alcohol in the blood. Offenders whose blood alcohol is found to be exceptionally high (over 150 mg/%), or who have previous drink-driving convictions, are particularly likely to be alcohol-dependent. Many drink-driving offenders have an elevated serum γ-glutamyltranspeptidase, indicating that they are regular heavy drinkers. Conversely, drink-driving offences are common in patients with other alcohol-related problems.

Drunkenness offences

The majority of men and women charged by the police with drunkenness offences have been shown to be alcohol-dependent, and 60% are homeless or living in hostels. The *Report on the Habitual Drunken Offender*

(Home Office 1974) recognised that processing these unfortunate people through the courts was wasteful, and even dangerous as alcoholics sometimes died in police custody. Concern about the revolving door for these habitual offenders passing in and out of the penal system gave rise to a number of alternative approaches. In some countries, such as Finland, parts of Canada and the USA, public drunkenness was decriminalised, while in Britain the approach has been to divert the habitual drunken offender out of the courts into a medicosocial system. The Criminal Justice Acts in both England and Wales and Scotland now allow the police to take an individual charged with simple drunkenness to a 'designated place' for detoxification and rehabilitation. Very few of these places exist in Britain and policy has moved away from detoxification toward police cautioning, which takes no account of rehabilitation. It has been shown in this population that severe withdrawal symptoms are surprisingly rare and that non-medical detoxification is often sufficient, providing nursing and medical help is available for the 5% who become seriously disturbed. An effective detoxification service can be used as an entrée to a more stable lifestyle (Orford & Wawman 1986).

VICIOUS CIRCLES

The problems discussed above may create a misleading sense of a number of discrete social, psychological or physical disabilities, whereas in most cases they are interrelated. It is helpful to think of a number of vicious circles which interconnect. For example, drinking debts may be the focus of domestic rows which provoke assault, arrest and marital breakdown. The problem drinker then finds himself or herself unemployed, divorced and living alone in a hostel with others who drink heavily, and so on.

RECOGNITION AND CLINICAL MANAGEMENT OF ALCOHOL-RELATED PROBLEMS

General principles

Identification and assessment

The clinical manifestations of alcohol misuse are many and varied. The sickness certificates of people eventually diagnosed as alcohol-dependent reveal, for example, anxiety states, depression, injuries, 'gastritis', 'debility'. The general practitioner may have been aware of frequent absences from work for minor symptoms, or

stress symptoms in other members of the family, but the contribution which alcohol makes to these symptoms has been overlooked or ignored. Patients rarely acknowledge alcohol as a problem at a first interview; they may not appreciate the contribution of their drinking to their malady or they may deny it because of shame, dislike or fear of being advised to abstain. They may be evasive because they are sensitised to criticism about their behaviour. Sometimes it is better to avoid focusing the whole interview on the drinking, taking instead a problem-orientated approach starting with questions about the reason for seeking help. With respect to the drinking, enquire about a recent period (for example, the past 7 days) by asking in detail about work, leisure activities, the company kept, and the amount and type of beverage consumed. Spirits, wines and beers should be enquired into separately. Reconstruct the cues which have been important triggers to drinking: the situations and moods that precipitate drinking; the benefits that the patient experienced from alcohol; what has helped to control drinking on occasions in the past.

The first principle for the clinician is therefore always to bear alcohol in mind as a possible cause of presenting symptoms and to ask some questions about alcohol use as part of routine case-taking. There is good evidence that this simple step is often overlooked in both hospital, psychiatric and general practice.

Basic questions should include:

1. How often do you take a drink?
2. On a day when you drink, how many drinks would you take? on a typical day? Multiplying (1) and (2) together gives a very rough estimate of number of units per week.
3. Have there been any days in the past month when you have had more than 10 units?
4. Have you had any problems from drinking in the past year?

These simple questions should be asked of all newly admitted and referred patients.

There are standard brief questionnaires which can be used in screening, such as AUDIT (Babor et al 1989) or the very brief, four question CAGE (Table 12.4)(Ewing 1984). The latter is more useful in identifying established serious drinking problems.

Severity of dependence is assessed as follows. Mildly dependent patients will regularly notice restlessness at certain times of the day or in certain situations and at these times wish to have alcohol or seek out their drinking companions. They may have tried to cut down, and have found it difficult. If they occasionally have very heavy sessions, they may relieve the next morning's hangover with a drink, but this will not be more than

Table 12.4   CAGE questionnaire

Have you ever felt you should *cut* down your drinking?

Have people *annoyed* you by criticising your drinking?

Have you ever felt bad or *guilty* about your drinking?

Have you ever had a drink first thing in the morning to steady your nerves and get rid of a hangover (*eye*-opener)?

once or twice a week at most. More severely dependent patients report that the restlessness they feel without a drink is noticeable at times to colleagues or family, or prevents them from getting on with other activities. They organise their day to ensure that they are able to have a drink at times when they predict they will need one, such as the salesman who plans his morning's calls so that he is with a customer who drinks at around 11.30 a.m. when he is beginning to feel tense. There may be times when the individual feels unable to think of anything but getting a drink. Morning nausea, sweating and relief drinking may be reported for periods of many days consecutively. Insomnia becomes frequent unless late evening intake relative to daytime drinking is very heavy. Wakefulness in the small hours of the night, like daytime tenseness and anxiety in the dependent drinker, can be, of course, an effect of a falling blood alcohol level. A widely used rating scale is the Severity of Alcohol Dependence Questionnaire (Stockwell et al 1979).

Adverse consequences in the areas of health, work, family, friends and the law should be explored.

An epileptic fit for the first time in an adult should raise the suspicion of alcohol dependence. A withdrawal fit may occur without other gross signs. Tremor of the outstretched fingers or tongue, injected conjunctivae and sclerae, stigmata of liver disease, excessive facial skin capillarisation, and alcohol on the breath are valuable clues.

The mean cell volume is raised (without anaemia) in 30–50% of patients, probably due to a direct toxic action of alcohol on the marrow. The γ-glutamyltranspeptidase and/or other liver enzymes are elevated in 60–70% of patients, due to enzyme induction and/or liver damage. A specimen for blood alcohol or a reading on a portable breathalyser may help. In a 70 kg man, 1 unit of alcohol produces a peak blood alcohol concentration of 15 mg% after about half an hour, and takes an hour to be metabolised. Cognitive testing, important in planning future treatment, should be left until the patient has been free of alcohol for 3 weeks (p. 47).

If possible, the spouse or other relatives should be interviewed, to add objectivity and to assess the quality of their relationship with the drinker. These relationships are important in predicting outcome. The spouse often feels angry and guilty and is reassured when these feelings are acknowledged and understood. At this stage avoid judging 'motivation'. A moment's introspection shows that our own motivation to change familiar habits varies greatly. Problem drinkers are no exception. On some occasions, they feel strongly motivated to change their way of life, perhaps to save their job or their marriage. On other occasions, the attraction of the pub, the relief from daily worries and the familiar comfort of that first drink are overwhelming. Clinicians have to work with fluctuating levels of motivation. Probably the psychiatrist's most important first step is to acquire the trust of the patient and to establish an atmosphere in which frankness prevails and confrontation is seen as caring. Patients will then be able to start making decisions about themselves and plan to change their way of life.

Early intervention

There is good evidence showing the benefits of intervention, including advice about 'sensible drinking' given at an early stage in the patient's drinking career when they are drinking in a hazardous way, or have first experienced evidence of alcohol problems. It is much better to help patients at this stage before they have developed more serious and intractable problems related to their drinking. In these circumstances, simple focused advice given in a primary health care or general hospital setting, can be very effective. Bien et al (1993) have shown that in seven out of eight randomised control trials in a variety of health care settings, significant reductions in alcohol use were shown after brief intervention. It is important to remember that these interventions were mostly made in individuals with alcohol-related problems and not in the kind of population commonly attending specialist clinics where severely dependent and psychologically disturbed patients are commonly seen.

Helping patients change their drinking habits

Helping patients change their habits often requires a considered and phased approach.

Exploit the moment of decision

At first a patient's decision to seek help is often fleeting and characterised by ambivalence about change. The clinician can help by clarifying reasons for changing, for example by drawing up a balance sheet of the benefits versus the harm of continuing to drink in this way. (This avoids a fruitless argument about whether or not he or she is 'an alcoholic'.) It is often helpful to explain the physiology of symptoms that may be due to physical dependence and the role of alcohol in other presenting symptoms, be it sleep disturbance, tension, depression or family disharmony. The status and role of a physician is a powerful persuasive force. Often patients respond to a more socratic, less directive, interview style which results in the patient arguing their own case for a change in drinking habits (Miller 1983). This approach is known as *motivational interviewing.*

Motivational interviewing

While a significant number of patients seen in primary health care and in hospital settings will respond to simple advice about changing their drinking habits, others will require considerable help in making a commitment to change. Motivational interviewing is a technique which helps patients reach their own decision about changing their habits. The majority of early intervention strategies are focused on returning to problem-free drinking rather than total abstinence. Bien et al (1993) summarised the essential components of brief intervention in the acronym FRAMES:

- *F*eedback about personal risk or impairment
- *R*esponsibility – emphasis on personal responsibility for change
- *A*dvice to cut down or, if indicated because of severe dependence or harm, to abstain
- *M*enu of alternative options for changing drinking pattern
- *E*mpathic interviewing
- *S*elf-efficacy; an interview style which enhances this.

Motivational interviewing arises from the concepts of Prochaska & Di Clemente (1992), although the approach can be traced to the dialogues of Socrates. They observed that patients came to see clinicians at different stages of readiness to make changes and that motivation was not a fixed and unchanging entity, but fluctuated from day to day and in different circumstances. (A moment's introspection will reveal the truth of this observation.) They divided patients into those who came at a precontemplative stage before they had even recognised that alcohol was contributing to their problems; and others at a contemplative stage where they were beginning to recognise that drinking was a problem but were ambivalent about making change. They also recognised a 'readiness for action' stage when they would be willing to accept positive advice for change. The circle was completed by a period of relapse

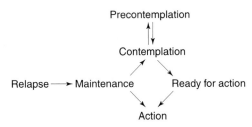

Fig. 12.2 Stages of change. (After Prochaska & Di Clemente 1992.)

or faltering of resolutions, requiring maintenance. The stages of change are summarised in the attached diagram (Fig. 12.2) and each has different implications for appropriate advice.

Other strategies for helping achieve change

Set goals Goals should be specific, attainable, short-term, immediately rewarding and ones which the patient defines. For example: no alcohol for 4 weeks; rewards – better physical health, better family atmosphere. Abstinence is often immediately rewarding and is an easier target for many than partial reduction of drinking. However, some see abstinence as totally inappropriate. For them a goal might be: reduce intake by half; or, reduce γ-glutamyltranspeptidase to below 50 units, when the reward is the satisfaction of watching this measure of liver function improve over the next 2–3 months.

Involve the family Family distress is common and advice on being firm with the drinker, not entering into fruitless struggles, but remaining caring and positive, is often beneficial. Without information from those near at hand, the clinician may not get the full picture from the patient. While the clinician's contact is only brief, the family usually has a lot of time in which to reinforce the strategies agreed at the time of the clinic visit.

Enhance self-esteem Often patients feel powerless to change their lives. The doctor should convey hope and encourage patients to believe in their own ability to change things. Help them to recognise their own strengths but also acknowledge that we all find it hard to change our habits.

Review impediments to change such as former cues and triggers to drinking. Such cues may be subjective, for instance the feelings of anxiety or depression which experience suggests will be relieved by a drink; or external, like the atmosphere among friends in the pub in which it is so tempting to accept just one pint. The barriers to change are varied (Table 12.5), which explains why a variety of therapeutic strategies are needed. Encourage substitute activities, alternatives to drinking. For some, physical dependence and the expe-

Table 12.5   Barriers to change
Dependence
Physical
Psychological
Stress
Intrapsychic
Interpersonal
Environment
Illness
Psychiatric
Physical
Influence of others
Stereotypes
Expectations

rience of withdrawal symptoms will be a significant impediment necessitating detoxification as the initial step.

Identify associated conditions   such as depressive illness or phobias, that might respond to specific treatment, but bear in mind that many will be secondary to the drinking.

Consider other agencies   such as voluntary councils on alcohol, which may provide a counselling service, or a social programme, such as Alcoholics Anonymous (see below), or hostels for recovering alcoholics.

Follow-up   Active follow-up is one of the ingredients of successful treatment. Relapse is common in the first 6–12 months after treatment. Brief but regular appointments help to remind the patient of goals; to give encouragement and praise; perhaps to repeat mean corpuscular volume or serum γ-glutamyltranspeptidase or breath alcohol measurements. It is important to be prepared to confront the patients when necessary and risk anger, while at the same time offering continued support. The spouse or partner should usually be encouraged to attend follow-up sessions. Relapse, if and when it occurs, should be viewed as an opportunity for further learning, not as an irrevocable catastrophe.

Close study of the precipitants of relapse shows that they have a lot in common across a range of addictions. Marlatt & Gordon (1984) analysed 311 relapses amongst patients with a variety of addictive behaviours (problem drinking, smoking, heroin addiction, gambling and overeating). They identified three high-risk situations which accounted for three-quarters of all relapses: negative emotional states, interpersonal conflicts and environmental triggers. Litman and colleagues (1983), in a study of 256 hospitalised alcoholics, found that unpleasant mood states, external events and euphoria, and lessened cognitive vigilance commonly presaged relapse. In therapy, the patient should learn to identify cues to relapse and develop strategies for handling them.

Faith and hope   Faith in the therapist, faith in the treatment, and the warmth, empathy and authenticity displayed by the therapist have often been termed non-specific ingredients of therapy but they have a major influence on efficacy.

In a 2 year follow-up study of outpatient treatment of problem drinkers, patients of low-empathy therapists were associated with the same or even a worse outcome compared with patients given a booklet only, while those of high-empathy therapists improved on the booklet-only outcome (Miller & Baca 1983). Non-specific factors in therapy need to be transformed into clearly defined specifics.

Medical aspects of treatment

Detoxification

Medication to minimise withdrawal symptoms makes stopping drinking easier. Hospital admission is only essential when delirium threatens or there is a history of fits. A long-acting benzodiazepine such as chlordiazepoxide (starting at 60–80 mg/day and reducing to nil over 5–7 days) is usually adequate for community detoxification. Larger doses may be needed in hospital to control agitation and offset the likelihood of confusional states. The final dose *should* be determined by regular clinical monitoring but the maximum dose should not exceed 400 mg chlordiazepoxide in 24 hours (CRAG/SCOTMEG 1994) It should not be continued for more than 10 days. If there is a history of fits, greater initial doses of the benzodiazepine should be given. In any circumstance the final dose should be determined by regular monitoring. Chlormethiazole is probably more addictive than long-term benzodiazepines. Alcohol–chlormethiazole interactions causing respiratory depression and even death have occurred. Chlorpromazine is less effective and may increase the risk of withdrawal fits.

When the patient is reasonably well-intentioned and there is someone at home, or a nurse or family doctor who can call, where there is no history of fits and no confusion, withdrawal can be undertaken at home (Stockwell 1987). The patient is best advised to take time off work, to rest, and to drink fruit juices and other soft drinks, but avoid large quantities of caffeine-containing tea and coffee. In more severe withdrawal it is sensible to check serum urea and electrolytes and aim to maintain an oral fluid intake of 2–2.5 litres daily.

In view of the frequency of cognitive impairment in heavy drinkers and its probable relation to vitamin depletion, vitamin supplements should be given in most patients, and, in patients in whom cognitive impairment or neuropathy is clinically demonstrable, for several months.

Alcohol sensiting agents

Disulfiram (Antabuse) and citrated calcium carbamide (Abstem) are alcohol sensitising deterrent drugs. Carbamide is available in the UK only on a 'named patient' basis. Both drugs interfere with the breakdown of alcohol and flood the system with acetaldehyde. Antabuse is a useful adjunct in the follow-up phase of treatment until a new lifestyle has developed. The disulfiram effect lasts for several days, whereas the effects of carbamide wear off after approximately 24 hours. Acetaldehyde is a toxic substance and produces an unpleasant reaction, with flushing, headache, nausea, tachycardia, laboured breathing and hypertension. On rare occasions the reaction may be life threatening, particularly in those who have cardiovascular disease.

Disulfiram should not be taken until the breath alcohol has returned to zero. The patient and his or her partner should be fully informed about the mode of action of the drug and its hazards. With the recommended dose of 200 mg daily, side-effects of disulfiram are uncommon, although tiredness and halitosis are sometimes noted. For these reasons some patients prefer to take the drug at night. Reversible neuropathies and confusional states have also been reported. It should not be given to patients with a history of recent heart disease or suicidal impulses, or those who take hypertensive drugs. It should also be treated with caution when there is very active liver disease. To ensure success, the patient will often agree to the nomination of a supervisor, for example the spouse, general practice, the clinic, or an occupational health nurse in cases with employment problems. The supervisor ensures that the compound is dispersed in water and swallowed. These measures improve compliance.

Other drug treatments

There has been understandable resistance to the use of psychotropic drugs in the treatment of alcohol problems because of the risk of precipitating a further addiction. Drugs which have specific effects on neurotransmitters have been shown to reduce alcohol consumption in animal experiments. Several studies have suggested that the frequency and severity of relapse can be reduced by use of the opiate antagonist naltrexone, particularly when combined with coping skills therapy (O'Malley et al 1992), and others have shown benefits from Acamprosate Calcium which is a GABA agonist

and glutamate antagonist (Whitworth et al 1996). These treatments are at a developmental stage but in some controlled studies appear to produce a modest but significant improvement in prognosis.

Antidepressants and other antipsychotic medications are of benefit to those problem drinkers who have associated psychiatric disorders, but it is important to keep in mind that most symptoms of anxiety and depression will clear after 2 or 3 weeks of abstinence without further drug therapy.

Social skills training

Many excessive drinkers are influenced by social cues and many report that they feel deficient in social skills. Refusing drinks, buying non-alcoholic drinks, applying for jobs, being firm with colleagues, expressing affection to loved ones and expressing annoyance without being insulting are some of the items of interpersonal behaviour that alcoholics find it useful to role-play in social skills training groups.

Group therapy

Participating in treatment in a group facilitates identification and enhances self-esteem. Fellow problem drinkers are quick to expose the rationalisations and self-deception of their peers, but often do so sympathetically and with great tolerance. If a member recommences drinking, it can be difficult to retain him in the group; but others will be able to empathise with his once again turning to alcohol as a response to, for example, rejection or disappointment.

Conjoint and family therapy

Cohesiveness of marriage and family life is a predictor of recovery (Orford & Edwards 1977). Bitterness, mistrust and fear in the spouse and children may take many months to subside even when the patient has achieved abstinence. Family interviews enable members to have their views heard, without the discussion spiralling into denials, accusations and counteraccusation. The patient can be helped to see that family members are bound to feel hesitant at first but that this need not imply that they do not care or appreciate the efforts that are being made. The man who has opted out of married and family life, or who has gradually been extruded because of his drinking, may suddenly want to resume his roles of husband and father, ignoring the fact that others in the family now have their own way of doing things (Chick & Chick 1992).

Other members of the family sometimes fear that the therapist is going to blame them for the patient's drink-

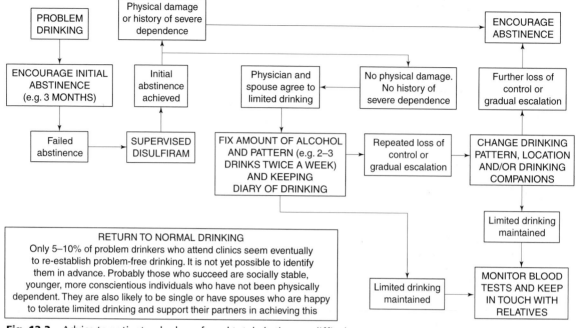

Fig. 12.3 Advice to patients who have found total abstinence difficult.

ing and so refuse to be involved in discussions. The psychiatrist's invitation to them might be 'to hear their views of how things have been, and to have their opinions on how X can best be helped'. Involving a partner or relative in therapy improves outcome and should be part of both assessment and treatment whenever possible (O'Farrell 1989).

To drink or not to drink

Abstinence is the safest goal, particularly for those who have sustained physical damage from alcohol or who have been physically dependent, and to patients aged 40 and over. However, in young people, particularly those who have not been severely physically dependent, return to limited drinking after a few month's abstinence is sometimes appropriate. Therapist and patient can work out appropriate strategies together (Fig. 12.3): stick to drinks that are low in alcohol (e.g. low strength beers rather than those that are extra strong); avoid buying rounds; intersperse drinks with non-alcoholic drinks; go to the pub at 9.30 p.m. instead of 7.00 p.m.; sip rather than gulp; no lunch-time drinking; eat while drinking; completely avoid situations or company where heavy drinking is likely; set a limit (e.g. never more than 6 units per day). Keeping a daily record of consumption can help monitor progress and review goals. Controlled studies on clinic attenders aimed at demonstrating the efficacy of controlled drinking

remain few and need replication (Heather & Robertson 1981).

Specialist services

Units for the treatment of alcohol problems

These units offer a specialised service in most regions of Britain. They have a responsibility for treatment, training and research and facilities of a similar kind are to be found in many parts of the industrial world. Traditionally they offered inpatient treatment of 6–8 weeks duration with an emphasis on group therapies. In recent years there has been a shift away from this devotion to inpatient treatment toward outpatient therapy combined with brief inpatient or day patient treatment. In response to evaluation studies which have cast doubts on the importance of very intensive forms of therapy, these units have become more flexible, offering a range of approaches, including behaviour therapy and marital and family therapy, as well as more familiar group and individual psychotherapy.

Glaser (1980) has criticised the tendency for specialist services to act as if the alcoholic population were homogeneous and to offer a single form of treatment for all. He has proposed a careful assessment of each patient's needs and the matching of these to a range of treatment options (US Department of Health and Human Services 1990).

Councils on alcohol and alcohol advice centres

Many developed countries now have counselling services separate from psychiatric or medical clinics. Problem drinkers or their families may initiate the contact and referrals will be accepted from doctors. In some countries drink-driving offenders will be directed by the court to seek help from these or other agencies. Other alcohol-related offences are commonplace and some courts have access to programmes which help offenders learn to drink sensibly and break the link between crime and alcohol.

Employment policies

Employers who are prepared to face the issue of drinking problems amongst their workforce may negotiate an *alcohol in employment* policy and arrange with their employees and trade union for those whose drinking is impairing performance to seek help at an early stage. Such firms usually realise the cost to the industry of absenteeism, accidents and inefficiency due to alcohol. When drinking has led to a breach of work regulations, the employee may be offered the opportunity of attending a treatment service rather than facing disciplinary proceedings. The outcome of problem drinkers identified and treated in the work context tends to be good.

Alcoholics Anonymous (AA)

Since the meeting of its two founder members, Dr Bob and Bill W. in Akron, Ohio, in 1935, AA has spread to most countries of the world. It grew particularly in the 1960s and 1970s in the USA and the UK, and is currently growing at a rate of 15% per annum. Members meet regularly and share a common faith that as alcoholics they are powerless where alcohol is concerned and that total abstinence is the only route to recovery.

The principles on which AA was founded are open self-scrutiny, the giving of aid to others, and fellowship. The AA programme offers hope and clear, simple advice (for example, avoid the first drink; attend meetings; take life one day at a time; 'stay sober for yourself', etc.). A prayer is said at every meeting: 'God give me the detachment to accept those things which I cannot alter; the courage to alter those things which I can alter; and the wisdom to distinguish the ones from the others'. However, each member may have his own conception of God and potential affiliates should not be put off by AA's spiritual language.

AA groups usually offer to meet a new affiliate personally and introduce him or her, though they will also make the new member welcome simply by attending the local meeting. Records are not kept and all members are anonymous but observation shows that AA helps large numbers of regular attenders (Robinson 1979). Those most likely to adhere to AA tend to have suffered much harm from their drinking, but this is by no means always the case. Al-Anon is a parallel organisation for the spouses of alcoholics, to whom it offers an opportunity for mutual support and understanding. Membership does not require the partner to attend AA or even admit he is an alcoholic. Affiliated to their organisation is Al-ateen for the teenage children of alcoholics. This offers them a chance to share some of the tensions and problems which they commonly experience.

Services for the homeless alcoholic

The homeless alcoholic usually finds abstinence unattainable unless he or she can be helped out of the 'skid row' environment of lodging houses or sleeping in the open. Hostels are an important part of rehabilitation. Most hostels for alcoholics require abstinence as a condition of residence, and they usually provide a therapeutic programme in which the residents help each other to find a new lifestyle. After a residence of up to 1 year, many find the transition to independent life extremely difficult and some areas provide half-way houses and supported accommodation as the next stage. In some cities there is accommodation for alcoholics who continue to drink. These so called 'damp houses' provide some shelter and support, hopefully on the way to longer term rehabilitation.

Hostels need not be the exclusive domain of the homeless. They are often valuable for alcoholics who live in unsatisfactory accommodation, or in a domestic setting which is so tense that a period of separation is a necessary prelude to a return to the family. Most hostels are managed by church or other voluntary organisations. In some cities they are also provided by the social work department.

CLINICAL RESPONSE TO DRUG-DEPENDENT PATIENTS

Assessment and management of clinical conditions associated with drug use

Every doctor is now likely to see patients who misuse drugs, be it in the accident and emergency department with acute intoxication, the general practitioner confronted with concerns around the harmful use of various substances, the obstetrician faced with a pregnant patient whose drug use has been disclosed because of concerns about the child, the police surgeon with a psychotic patient in the cells due to a drug-induced state, the house officer in the general hospital confronted with a patient undergoing withdrawal from drugs, the psychiatrist having to differentiate drug-induced psychopathology from other causes, or the specialist drug service trying to help patients with a dependence syndrome who have already failed to give up the substance by themselves. Prior to assessment, a low index of suspicion of drug misuse is required; early detection is preferable to the subsequent management of the dependence syndrome. Assessment is based on standard clinical skills of history, examination and investigation (Department of Health 1991). However, emphasis is given to:

- Drug use and previous treatment
- Areas of conflict: relationships, jobs, debt, the law
- Support structure
- Mental state
- Objective signs of withdrawal
- Needle marks
- Urine toxicology
- Comorbid, physical and mental conditions, e.g. the human immunodeficiency virus (HIV).

During the late 1980s and early 1990s, much of the funding and impetus for the setting up of services for drug use and its associated problems was motivated and driven by concerns around HIV. This is now becoming less of an issue among drug users as injecting declines and there is increased knowledge within the drug-using culture about the risks of spread of HIV and hepatitis B and C. This being said, knowledge in itself does not change behaviour and the incidence of sharing amongst those that inject continues to be high. As a result of this, detailed questioning may be required if injecting is practised.

Within each clinical condition induced by drug use, there are general principles of management. Specific drug and treatment options are discussed later in the chapter.

Acute intoxication (F1X.0)

This may require the medical or surgical management of injuries occurring secondary to the intoxication. It may also require observation of any head injuries. Life support may be required in the event of coma and, in some instances (e.g. opiates), antagonists may be available and given to reverse drug effects. Offensive or dangerous disinhibited behaviour may require containment until drug effects decline. Acute intoxication is a transient phenomenon and recovery is therefore complete.

Harmful use (F1X.1)

A patient may be recovered from intoxication or be pre-senting with some other medical condition and has raised drug use as a personal concern. Education is required about the dangers of drug use and the options available for changing that behaviour. Some patients may not see their drug use as a problem. The theory proposed by Prochaska & Di Clemente (1992) is a useful working model when helping patients. This model suggests at least four stages of change from precontemplation, contemplation, action and maintenance. If patients are experiencing harmful use but are in a precontemplative phase (i.e. do not recognise their drug problem), then efforts to encourage abstinence will fail. In this case, the process of motivational interviewing can be used to effect change towards awareness and a wish to move away from harmful drug use (Miller & Rollnick 1991).

Dependence syndrome (F1X.2)

Once this is developed, management will depend on the patient, drug and the patient's environment. If the patient is continuing to use (F1X.24), management is as outlined above for harmful use. Alternatively, if the patient is abstinent and in the community (F1X.20), then the focus should be on relapse prevention techniques, which are discussed later in the chapter. Other alternative categories within the dependence syndrome include the patient being abstinent but in a protected environment (F1X.21). These treatment settings may be divided into four groups: rehabilitation houses; religious units; community crisis rehabilitation units; and residential 12 step programmes. The essential elements of management within these units are to provide a safe drug-free environment, address pre-existing causes, solve current problems, and equip patients with greater personal resources for their discharge back to the community. Another category is when the patient is abstinent but receiving treatment with antagonist drugs (F1X.23) (e.g. opiate addicts receiving naltrexone). Management in this instance usually involves a partner supervising daily consumption at the start of a period of abstinence, and provides some chemical support while relapse prevention techniques are acquired. The final category is the patient in a clinically supervised maintenance or replacement regimen (controlled dependence) (F1X.22). In maintenance programmes chaotic illegal dependence is replaced with controlled legal dependence. Once established, then management is similar to those who are in protected environments. Two essential differences are that rehabilitation occurs within the patient's community rather than elsewhere, and that at a later stage in the recovery, usually once resocialisation has occurred, abstinence from drugs needs to be addressed.

Withdrawal state, with (F1X.3) or without delirium (F1X.4)

Withdrawal states may be managed by acute abstinence and symptomatic supportive measures or, more commonly, the initiation of substitute medication and then a graduated, more humane withdrawal over a period of time. The types of withdrawal and the drugs that may be used are discussed later under the individual drug types.

Psychotic disorder (F1X.5)

Drug-induced psychotic disorder requires the same management as any other psychotic disorder. It typically resolves at least partially within 1 month and fully within 6 months and, as long as the patient remains drug-free, is unlikely to reoccur.

Residual and late-onset psychotic disorders (F1X.7)

Here a variety of conditions may be present which have been caused by drug use but are now persisting despite termination of drug use. These conditions include flashback phenomena (F1X.70), personality or behavioural disorder (F1X.71), residual affective disorder (F1X.72), dementia (F1X.73), other persisting problems of impairment (F1X.74) and late-onset psychotic disorders (F1X.75). The management of these conditions is symptomatic.

Goals of treatment

The rationale for this heading may seem obscure because the goal of treatment is cure. However, cure has been associated with abstinence. An expectation of failure on the part of many in the medical profession when trying to achieve the goal of abstinence in drug users with a dependence syndrome has led to a sense of therapeutic nihilism. To avoid this in the future, it is important to elaborate on the goals of treatment. Most clinical conditions are self-limiting and only require supportive management. A few residual states exist where the management is no longer directed at drug use but at helping people live with their changed state. The difficulty comes when the clinician is confronted with people who continue to use drugs, or are dependent on drugs, and need help in moving from a lack of awareness of the problems that their drug use is causing them. The hierarchy of goals and harm reduction for intravenous drug users and others is as follows:

- The reduction of sharing of injecting equipment
- The reduction in injecting

- The reduction in street drug use
- Stabilisation on substitute prescribing
- Management of features associated with dependence syndrome
- Reduction in substitute prescribing
- Maintenance of abstinence from psychoactive drugs.

Health professionals are primarily focused on health issues. However, it needs to be accepted that in cost–benefit terms part of the motivation, as HIV becomes less of a driving force in establishing and maintaining services for drug users, will become drug-related crime and its prevention. It is estimated that the costs sustained by victims of drug-related crime by dependent heroin users alone is between £58 million and £864 million annually. The cost to the criminal justice system of dealing with drug users is similarly substantial, costing around £500 million per year (Hough 1996). Similar papers by UK political parties also support this view (Straw 1996). So far the rehabilitation of dependent drug users by the criminal justice system is less positive than that achieved by the health system. Diversion of resources from the criminal justice system into health care may become more important in the next decade.

Specific drugs and treatment options

Opiates

Acute intoxication with opiates can result in respiratory depression and sometimes death. This is not an uncommon event. A recent Australian study of heroin users indicated that two-thirds had had a drug overdose – a third within the past year (Darke et al 1995); others have reported lower incidence (Gossop et al 1996). Part of the reason for this may be that the purity of heroin may vary such that, when injecting, the exact dose being taken is unpredictable. Alternatively, a dose of drug that takes the user near to the edge of death contibutes to the euphoric effect. An increasing presentation of opiate intoxication is methadone overdose. The reasons for this are complex, but undoubtedly more users are presenting to services with methadone rather than heroin as their route into opiate dependence. Methadone overdose can be difficult to control and follows an unpredictable course in non-tolerant patients, who are at risk of sudden death (Cairns et al 1996, Hendra et al 1996). Clinical management of opiate overdose is along general guidelines. The opiate antagonist naloxone may be used in a dose of 0.4 mg i.v. to reverse respiratory depression, but as it is short-acting, and the overdose may be of a long-acting drug such as methadone, subsequent infusion may be required. Concern about the mortality associated with accidental opiate overdose has made some advocate the 'takehome' of naloxone by opiate addicts (Strang et al 1996a).

Patients with an opiate dependence syndrome traditionally constitute the bulk of specialist drug services' work. Their management depends on their current drug use. If still using, and not prepared to move towards abstinence from street drugs, then harm reduction strategies should be employed, as mentioned previously. Some may be abstinent and concentrating their therapy on relapse prevention techniques, as discussed later. Some may be abstinent, and supplementing their relapse prevention techniques with a trial of naltrexone at a dose of 50 mg per day. This is an opiate antagonist similar to naloxone but it can be administered orally and lasts for over 24 hours. A comprehensive review has been carried out by Gonzales & Brogden (1988). Most abstinent drug users, however, chose not to carry on with naltrexone. There has been some promising work using naltrexone as a condition of treatment for people who repeatedly offend to finance their drug habit. The best results with naltrexone treatment have been reported in studies with doctors who have developed a drug dependence syndrome on opiates (Washton et al 1984). A select group of patients may elect to go into drug-free rehabilitation programmes. Inpatient detoxification before transfer to a rehabilitation programme may improve retention rates as there is often a high drop-out if patients go direct to drug-free rehabilitation while still using. However, the majority of patients with opiate drug dependence syndrome tend to be managed, at least at some point, in a maintenance programme. This is probably the most evaluated treatment within this field and repeated reviews of the literature have confirmed that it retains people in treatment, reduces illicit drug use, reduces criminal activity, lowers risk of seroconversion for HIV, hepatitis B and hepatitis C, and improves resocialisation (Farrell et al 1994, Bertschy 1995). It needs to be remembered, however, that methadone itself is not the treatment: it must be given in conjunction with a full package of care (Hagman 1994). The research on maintenance prescribing is generally concerned with oral methadone. Dosages in the UK were primarily aimed at the minimum dose required to avoid withdrawal symptoms, but if the goal is the reduction of illicit drug use then a higher dose is usually needed. A typical dose may be in the region of 60 mg methadone mixture, 1 mg/1 ml per day. Doses of 50 mg and above have been associated with death in naive drug users. In addition, some substitute prescribing in Britain is of an injectable form, a practice which used to be exclusive to the UK. In a review of pharmacies in England and Wales it was found that 80% of methadone prescriptions were for liquid form, 11% for tablets, which are readily acknowledged as being easy to reconstitute for injection, and 10% for injectable ampoules. The recommendations in Scotland are that no injectable drugs should be prescribed. As for methadone tablets, there seems to be no indication for prescribing these in opiate dependence. Another difference between the UK and other countries is that more 'takehome' medication is prescribed in the UK, whereas in the USA and Australia the majority of medication is on a daily dispensing basis, often with supervised consumption at the point of collection. This does not seem to be the case in the UK, where nearly a third of all methadone dispensed is for weekly or fortnightly pick-up and a further third is for daily pick-up (Strang et al 1996b).

The withdrawal syndrome can be characterised by nausea, vomiting, muscle aches, lacrimation, rhinorrhoea, papillary dilatation, piloerection, sweating, diarrhoea, yawning, fever and insomnia. The severity and length of withdrawal is dependent on the drug of abuse, shorter acting drugs tending to have more severe withdrawal over shorter periods as compared with longer acting drugs, the effects of which are more protracted but less severe. Some describe withdrawal as a 'flu-like illness' but others demonstratively have a severe reaction. This may in part be due to expectation but is also contributed to by the level of tolerance and dependence on the drug. The withdrawal is managed with substitution of the opiate, usually with methadone, and a gradual reduction is then carried over a period of time. The shortest period advocated is 24 hours (Legarda & Gossop 1994). This needs to be carried out in an intensive care unit and involves naltrexone-induced withdrawal, with heavy sedation. More typical withdrawal periods are of 10–21 days on an inpatient basis, or longer for outpatient maintenance-to-abstinence programmes (Farrell 1994). Further symptomatic treatment can be given with the use of α_2-adrenergic agonists, such as clonidine and lofexidine but these drugs have no effect on the insomnia, craving and muscle aches associated with withdrawal. The medical management of opiate withdrawal is not complicated, other than in the very short procedures. The difficulty is in achieving continued abstinence, and this is discussed further below.

Stimulants

Intoxication with stimulants appears less common, possibly because of the loss of pleasurable effect at high doses and the fact that the mental state becomes associated with paranoia and psychosis and may end up with convulsions. Treatment is symptomatic along general guidelines. Patients with a stimulant dependence syndrome in the UK usually abuse amphetamines but occasionally may abuse cocaine, and in some areas 'crack' cocaine. If continuing to use, then harm reduction advice is essential, as with any other substance. However, based on the literature, treatment options are limited in that they are exclusively abstinence orientated, with the majority involving residential settings (Schuckit 1994). The main focus therefore is on relapse prevention, which is discussed later in this chapter. Various drugs have been suggested as being useful in the stimulant dependence syndrome, including bromocriptine, which theoretically should alleviate the hypothesised dopamine depletion of chronic stimulant abuse. Others drugs which boost dopamine activity include mazindol, flupenthixol and amantadine. Unfortunately, research results do not justify their use as part of a standard therapy for stimulant-dependent individuals. Antidepressant medication has been used in view of the mood swings experienced following stimulant abstinence. Again, while theoretically sound, the research does not provide relevant guidelines for day-to-day practice. As for maintenance prescribing or maintenance-to-abstinence prescribing for stimulant dependence syndrome, there are no randomised controlled trials published supporting this. However, some prescribing along these lines does occur in clinical practice within specialist drug units in the UK. More research needs to be done in this area before it can be advocated as a treatment. Stimulant withdrawal has been suggested by some to be a triphasic state with a 'crash', 'withdrawal' and 'extinction' phase. The crash typically occurs within 30 minutes and may last up to 40 hours. The withdrawal phase tends to peak at 2–4 days and various depressive symptoms last for several weeks after that, including hypersomnia, fatigue, anhedonia, sadness, suicidal ideation and general malaise (Lago & Kosten 1994). However, this description of stimulant withdrawal has not been repeated by others, who find a persistent, gradual improvement throughout the withdrawal period. There is no specific symptomatic treatment and the majority of stimulant users end their dependence without resorting to medical support.

Sedatives and hypnotics

Illicit use of drugs in this group is now restricted almost exclusively to benzodiazepines, although historically barbiturates have been important. The management of benzodiazepine acute intoxication is along general principles and the benzodiazepine antagonist flumazenil may be used to reverse the onset of respiratory depression and coma. This class of drugs is also commonly used in conjunction with others, particularly stimulants and alcohol. There is extensive, harmful use from these drugs, including increased risk behaviour amongst intravenous drug users (Strang et al 1994), an increased association with accidents (Currie et al 1995), aggression (Bond et al 1995), deterioration in performance (Kerr et al 1992), and amnesic effects, which can be used medically to good purpose as surgical premedication (Hindmarch et al 1993). Iatrogenic initiation of benzodiazepine dependence remains a concern (Surendrakumar et al 1992) despite the recommendations from the Committee of Safety of Medicines to limit treatment with benzodiazepines to short courses only (Committee on Safety of Medicines 1988). Medical negligence may be claimed in these cases and long-term use requires careful consideration (Hallstrom 1990). Numerically, iatrogenic benzodiazepine drug dependence is greater than high-dose illicit benzodiazepine drug dependence (usually in the context of polydrug use). The latter group pose a significant clinical challenge but have been studied the least. As to the former, clinical management has been reviewed (Higgitt et al 1985) and guidelines have been issued (Substance Abuse Committee of the Mental Health Foundation 1992). The best outcomes in this group are associated with younger patients, fewer withdrawal symptoms and, at 6 months after withdrawal, less personality disturbance and longer duration of use prior to withdrawal (Holton et al 1992). In high-dose illicit use management of a dependence syndrome may be different. One finding is that drug users prefer high dose short acting compounds and are more likely to seek these out (Griffiths & Wolf 1990). There is no research support for maintenance prescribing. However, based on the harm reduction philosophy, this has resulted in some substitute prescribing on a maintenance-to-abstinence basis being practised.

The withdrawal state has features which are clinically similar to, and sometimes indistinguishable from, anxiety states. Additional features include hypersensitivity in all senses, derealisation and depersonalisation. Late presentations of withdrawal include psychotic states and convulsions. The management of withdrawal involves substitute prescribing of a long acting benzodiazepine (e.g. diazepam). Gradual controlled withdrawal, with the cooperation of the patient, can then take place over a period of months. Rapid inpatient detoxification may be unsafe (Robertson & Bell 1993). Symptomatic treatment for associated features of withdrawal are managed as they arise and as outlined above for the treatment of iatrogenic dependence.

Hallucinogens

There is a large variety of hallucinogens that may be

used and could produce clinical conditions. These include psilocybin and mescaline (primarily found in fungicides), lysergic acid diethylamide (LSD) and MDMA and many other compounds with botanical origin (De Smet 1996). The main drugs used that sometimes present with clinical conditions are LSD and MDMA and these will be discussed further. Hallucinogenic intoxication usually only presents when there is a 'bad trip'. This is primarily dependent on the mental set and environmental setting of the user. If the user is not relaxed or is feeling under pressure of time, or has had a recent argument, or is holding major resentments, this may lead to a bad trip. In addition, solitary experimentation in an overstimulated environment can also precipitate bad experiences. These experiences usually wear off before medical intervention is sought. However, treatment should be directed at preventing patients from physically harming themselves, or others. Reducing external stimulation and focusing on a single individual, preferably a friend, may help the user calm down. The somatic (dizziness, paraesthesia, weakness and tremor), perceptual (altered reality) and psychic (labile mood, dreams, altered time sense and depersonalisation) symptoms may be so severe as to require neuroleptic medication, such as chlorpromazine. Some of the adverse reactions that occur after hallucinogenic use are not due, for example, to LSD but to contaminants, such as phencyclidine (PCP). There appears to be no significant dependence syndrome or withdrawal state for the hallucinogenic group. There is some concern over the hallucinogenic residual state of flashbacks which occurs in a small proportion. These may occur weeks or months after the original drug experience and need not necessarily be pleasant. Over time, their intensity, frequency and duration diminish (Frankel 1994). There is no evidence of any neurotoxic effects with LSD; however, this is not the case for MDMA.

Acute intoxication with MDMA can produce a syndrome similar to the serotoninergic syndrome and neuroleptic malignant syndrome (Demirkiran et al 1996). The management of these conditions is as for the management of the neuroleptic malignant syndrome. Harmful use of MDMA occurs as a result of tolerance, when users may increase the dose to get the original effect achieved and neurotoxicity may result. Subjects may take large doses (Green & Goodwin 1996). However, the significance of this in practical terms for users is challenged (Merrill 1996). The environment in the UK in which MDMA is used is associated with mortality not found elsewhere and extensive harm reduction advice is now available at these sites. The use of hallucinogenic drugs in neurochemical and psy-

chotherapeutic research disappeared during the 1970s and 1980s but is now re-emerging (Strassman 1995).

Cannabis

As with hallucinogens, the premorbid state and setting are influential in determining reactions to acute ingestion. In a dose–response manner, acute intoxication with cannabis can result in disturbances of perception and, in severe cases, psychotic states (Ghodse 1986, Thomas 1993). Treatment for these conditions remains along general guidelines with no specific separate indications. Cannabis dependence syndrome undoubtedly occurs in a small minority of users but treatment tends to be geared towards reduced consumption and abstinence; there have been no studies evaluating treatment. Withdrawal from cannabis is also reported for high-dose chronic users. Treatment is symptomatic. As for the long-term negative consequences for chronic users, little evidence has been found (Institute of Medicine 1982). That being said, marijuana smoke contains the same carcinogens as tobacco smoke, usually in somewhat higher concentration, and therefore long-term physical health may well be damaged. Recently, cannabis has been made available on prescription in two American states. This is for symptomatic treatment in conditions such as cancer, AIDS, anorexia, chronic pain, spasticity, coma, athritis and migraine (News item 1996b). However, the Federal Government in the USA remains concerned about this development (News item 1997).

Solvents

Acute intoxication with solvents can produce coma and death, and there are quite specific problems of sudden death with solvents, usually related to cardiac arrhythmia or vasovagal inhibition resulting in cardiac arrest. There seems to be no place for harm reduction in solvent misuse and the sole goal is one of abstinence. There is limited evidence that a dependence syndrome with specific withdrawal occurs. Residual states due to long-term use can occur as there is extensive multiple organ damage with protracted use. Treatment is symptomatic. The main focus for solvent use is prevention, early detection and abstinence (Advisory Council on the Misuse of Drugs 1995) .

RELAPSE PREVENTION

Once abstinent from the substance, the process of remaining drug-free can be described as relapse prevention. The theoretical psychological and psychobiological models are well developed (Connors et al 1996) but there has been limited outcome research to support the models with regards to addictions other than alcohol. Understanding the nature of relapse is fundamental to developing effective interventions for long-term management of substance misuse. Substance misuse needs to be seen as a chronic relapsing disorder. Progress in the area is hampered by definition of relapse itself. Reported outcomes between studies can vary depending on whether they report on a continuous basis along a dimension, or just for short periods repeatedly throughout that dimension. In addition, is relapse focused just on the substance misused or is there more of a comprehensive assessment of relapse, including other areas of physical, psychological and social functioning? What is the threshold at which a drug is being used, and what is the definition of a relapse? Does any use constitute a relapse or may it just been seen as a lapse which is rapidly followed by reinstatement of abstinence? The inclusion of assessments of whether there is transfer to another substance or behaviour of dependence and issues around verification and the importance placed on this is also undecided and makes across-study analysis difficult (Miller 1996). The continued development and harmonisation of accepted standards of outcome measures makes it more likely that in the future studies of individual groups can be generalised beyond the setting of the research. Miller and colleagues (1996) conducted an analysis of alcohol relapse that could be extended to other substances. In addition to pretreatment characteristics, they identified five theoretical areas causing potential relapse:

- Negative life events
- Cognitive appraisal, including self-efficacy, expectancy and motivation for change
- Client coping resources
- Craving experiences
- Affective/mood status.

The practical process of applying relapse prevention involves various key themes, outlined by Daley & Marlatt (1992):

- Help patients identify their high-risk relapse factors and develop strategies to deal with them
- Help patients understand relapse as a process and as an event
- Help patients understand and deal with substance cues as well as actual cravings
- Help patients understand and deal with social pressures to use drugs
- Help patients to develop a supportive relapse prevention network
- Help patients develop methods of coping with negative emotional states

- Help patients learn methods to cope with cognitive distortions
- Help patients work towards a balanced lifestyle
- Help patients develop a plan to interrupt a lapse or relapse.

Some specific work has been done with opiate addicts to assess whether they can predict their own relapse (Powell et al 1993). In this study, 43 opiate addicts who had undergone inpatient detoxification were followed up at 6 months. Those with lower self-esteem and higher positive expectancies were using less often. Latency to first lapse was longer in subjects with higher anxiety and neuroticism score. It is suggested that greater awareness of personal vulnerability may promote effective coping strategies. Experimental models have also been used with this population to examine mood effects (euphoria, depression, anxiety and anger). This showed that induced depression increased drug craving, and tended to increase opiate withdrawal symptoms. Other trends were also outlined and a suggestion was made that these may become a conditioned stimulus to trigger a relapse (Childress et al 1994). The role of attribution in abstinence, lapse and relapse has also been explored (Walton et al 1994).

A well-designed study, which should be replicated for other substances, was carried out by Carroll and colleagues (1994b). This study was a 1 year follow-up of 121 cocaine abusers who underwent two forms of psychotherapy, either relapse prevention or clinical management, and also were treated with either desipramine or placebo. Their analysis suggested a delayed improved response during follow-up in patients who received relapse prevention compared with supportive clinical management alone. They suggest that this reflects the subjects' implementation of generalisable coping skills conveyed through the relapse prevention treatment.

EVALUATION OF DRUG TREATMENTS

Of the various treatments discussed in this chapter, methadone maintenance has been more evaluated than any other. There is an extensive review of literature by Ward and colleagues (1992). In the United States in 1992, there were about 120 000 patients in treatment. In the UK and the rest of Europe, numbers are increasing. Research shows increased retention in treatment, reduction in crime by 50% year on year, reductions in illicit drug use, reductions in sharing and improvements in psychosocial functioning. Inpatient detoxification is also advocated in the UK and outcome studies do show abstinence rates near 50% at 6 month follow-ups (Johns 1994). As for other treatments in substance misuse, these show that not all treatments work on all patients. The attempts in alcohol research to match patients to particular treatments will no doubt be duplicated in other drugs. The management of abstinence and outcome studies related to relapse have been discussed above.

An evaluation of treatments in the opiate dependence syndrome is being carried out by the National Treatment Outcome Research Study (NTORS). This involves 1110 people who entered treatment in 1995: they were in either residential programmes, inpatient units, methadone maintenance or methadone reduction programmes. Preliminary findings have been published (National Treatment Outcome Research Study 1996). These show reductions in: heroin and other drug use; injecting; sharing injecting equipment; physical and psychological ill health; and criminal activity. However, the more important results addressing questions such as what the relationship is between client characteristics and treatment outcome or, what the relationship is between treatment structure, process and outcome, will follow in the coming years.

EVALUATION OF ALCOHOL TREATMENT

During the past 20 years there have been a large number of studies evaluating the effectiveness of treatment for alcoholism (Miller & Hester 1986, Saunders 1989). Most have shown that patient characteristics, particularly social and marital stability and, to a lesser extent, severity of dependence, are better predictors of outcome than specific features of therapy. Those features of therapy which have been shown to have some importance are: involvement of spouse; community reinforcement strategies; social skills training; and active follow-up. Specific approaches for which controlled studies have demonstrated efficacy are few. Disulfiram, when dispensed by a spouse as part of a contract, or by a clinic as part of an arrangement with the patient's employer, is of proven efficiency in maintaining abstinence for substantial periods (Azrin et al 1982, Chick et al 1992), reducing absenteeism at work (Robichaud et al 1979), and is also of proven value with socially deteriorated clients (Bourne et al 1966). Controlled studies of AA have not been conducted, but follow-up studies in the USA indicate strongly its efficacy. For example, Vaillant (1983) followed 100 patients at regular intervals for 8 years. Of the 39 men attaining stable abstinence, two-thirds did so through AA. In the same city, 120 problem drinkers identified in the community and not at clinics, and who were followed for between 10 and 30 years, yielded 34% who became stable abstainers. Of those, a third were regular AA attenders and

many had commenced abstinence through that route. Group treatment programmes teaching 'problem-solving' and 'social skills' (see above) proved effective in a controlled study (Chaney & O'Leary 1978) which has not yet been replicated.

There is considerable instability in the drinking status of samples of patients followed up in the first 2–4 years after commencing treatment (Polich et al 1981). Six studies are published where follow-up was at least 8 years and objective as well as subjective data are available on outcome. A fifth of subjects died (a mortality 2–3 times greater than expected). Of the survivors, half to two-thirds are still in some difficulty with their drinking. Of those who are well, most are abstainers. Some 5–10% have been drinking without problems for a year or more. Whether treatment improves on the natural history of the condition over such a timespan is impossible to evaluate (see above), because it is not possible or always ethical to withhold treatment. It is clear, however, from following problem drinkers identified in the community that many change their habits without professional help (Vaillant 1983).

In large samples of patients inpatient treatment has not shown clear advantages over outpatient treatment. There have even been difficulties in demonstrating superiority of standard treatments over very brief one-session interventions. Orford & Edwards (1977) randomly allocated 100 married male alcoholics to two treatment groups: one was offered intensive therapy, including admission to hospital when indicated; the other was assessed and given carefully chosen advice in a single session. The two groups were followed closely for 1 year. A total of 60% improved but no difference was found between the two groups, although 2 year follow-up suggested that severely dependent patients did better if given intensive treatment.

McLachlan & Stein (1982) compared day treatment with inpatient treatment and found no significant difference in outcome. More than a dozen controlled studies have examined the influence of duration and intensity of treatment on prognosis. With remarkable consistency these studies have failed to demonstrate any relationship (Institute of Medicine 1990). Chick et al (1988) compared very minimal treatment with a broad package of treatments, including for some inpatient and group therapy, along with a systematic follow-up for those patients who accepted it. This research showed that the stable abstinence rate was no higher after 2 years in the more intensively treated group; however, the intensive group had experienced less total problems related to their drinking than the advice-only group. Before concluding that there are no advantages inherent in more intensive treatment it is worth recording that relatively few studies have adequately characterised the clinic, and there are indications that more severely dependent patients do have a better outcome if offered somewhat more intensive treatment.

Such studies have cast doubt on the need for prolonged and expensive therapies for all alcoholics and have intensified the search for careful matching of patients and resources. Relatively little is yet known about optimal matching but alcoholics are not a homogeneous group and require a wide range of different rehabilitation strategies. A well designed matching project has shown the favourable outcome that can be achieved with well trained therapists but did not provide clear guidance on matching (Project MATCH Research Group 1997).

ORGANISATION OF SERVICES

Alcohol-related problems are extremely common and protean in their clinical manifestations. It is estimated that about one in 20 patients seen by a general practitioner will have an alcohol problem, and a further 10–20% will be drinking at amounts which increase their risk of future problems. In general medical wards approximately 20% of men and 12% of women will be found to be drinking at levels that are damaging to their health. Similar percentages have been identified in general psychiatric wards.

Alcohol-related problems vary enormously in character and severity; an appropriate community response requires a range of services that reflects this diversity. Emphasis should be placed on early recognition and help at primary level, for instance by general practitioners, occupational health services, general hospitals and courts.

The problem drinker experiences a series of crises. For example, Mr X regularly spent his wages on drinking with his friends. His wife was very distressed by this for a long time before she consulted the social work department about rent arrears and complained to the priest about her husband's behaviour. He was attending his general practitioner on account of recurrent gastritis, and repeated absences from work led to complaints from his supervisor. His daughter finally broke down at school and told the guidance teacher about the terrible conditions at home and help was obtained for the family.

This typical case illustrates the range of agencies encountered by the problem drinker. There is an opportunity for change inherent in each crisis, provided the problem is recognised and the primary-level agency has received adequate training and feels competent in coping with the problem and giving advice. The different layers of increasingly specialised intervention are illustrated in Table 12.6.

Table 12.6 Levels of intervention relevant to an effective response to alcohol problems

Level 1 The drinker, the family and friends
Level 2 Employers, work colleagues, police, bartenders, social welfare
Level 3 Primary health care, hospitals, social work, probation, counsellors
Level 4 Alcoholics anonymous, councils on alcohol, specialist alcohol treatment services

Level 1, awareness of hazardous drinking can lead to 'spontaneous' improvement – influenced by health promotion; level 2, although care is not a primary responsibility, these agencies are well placed to initiate an effective intervention; level 3, primary level caring agencies can be effective with sufficient training and support; level 4, specialist services.

Front-line services will require support from agencies, such as councils on alcohol, Alcoholics Anonymous and specialised treatment units. It is generally acknowledged that the majority of alcohol problems can be managed in the community, while a smaller number require some initial inpatient treatment or residential hostel care. Community alcohol teams have evolved as a means of providing support to the primary level and linkage with specialist resources (for discussion see Stockwell & Clement 1987). A comprehensive range of services will require planning coordination by health, social work and non-statutory sectors. Their joint plan for each district should be concerned with both prevention and treatment (Faculty of Public Health Medicine 1991, Ritson 1995).

There is evidence that only 10% of alcoholics are in contact with an appropriate agency, yet they are regularly in contact with other potential care-givers, as described above. The Department of Health and Social Security (1978) has recommended that 'treatment and care should be provided at a primary level' and identified the main tasks of the primary-level workers as:

- Recognising hazardous and harmful drinking, its causes and effects
- Having adequate knowledge of the help required by the problem drinker and the family
- Giving appropriate advice and help where necessary
- Knowing where and when to seek more specialist help
- Providing continuing care, support and follow-up.

Primary-level workers are often ill-equipped to provide this kind of service unless they receive adequate training and continuing support from a specialist team. The role of the specialist in alcohol problems increasingly involves providing this kind of support. He or she will work in a community alcohol team in which psychiatrist, social worker, nurse and psychologist combine to form a resource for the primary-level worker.

With specific reference to drugs there have been three recent documents dedicated, at least in part, to the organisation of services, one produced by the Advisory Council on the Misuse of Drugs (1993), the second set up by the Secretary of State for Scotland of a Ministerial Drugs Task Force (1994), and thirdly the English Task Force to Review Services for Drug Misusers (1996). The Task Force Reviewing Services made 12 recommendations that would greatly improve the effectiveness of drug services:

- A shared care model between specialist services and general practice. (Although the General Medical Services Committee has defined shared care arrangements with regard to treatment in drug dependence as non-core services. It seems that unless funding is available to support general practitioners in this extra work, resistance may occur regarding their involvement.)
- Opportunities should be made when drug misusers present to the criminal justice system. Treatment within the prison service and on release should be continuous with treatments in the community.
- Maintenance of syringe exchange facilities.
- Basic health checks for first point of contact with drug users.
- Hepatitis B vaccination being made available to injectors.
- Counselling and support services as co-components of treatment.
- Availability of: methadone reduction programmes; oral methadone maintenance programmes; residential rehabilitation programmes; specialist inpatient drug dependency units.
- A stop to the prescribing of methadone tablets to drug users.
- A limitation to the licence to prescribe injectable drugs to drug misusers.
- Maximum waiting times.
- Flexible opening times reflecting needs of drug users.
- Monitoring of key indicators of treatment organisations and outcomes.

The report by the Advisory Council on the Misuse of Drugs came up with 33 recommendations similar to those from the Task Force but, in addition, included a recommendation to expand outreach to try and contact hidden populations of drug users.

The Scottish Ministerial Drugs Task Force examined drug misuse and made recommendations, including in the area of services. It acknowledged the lack of expert advice on the effectiveness of provision, types or combination of types of service required to meet the needs of different drug users. It recommended the establishment of such expert advice.

It is clear that there are many similarities in the problems experienced by those who misuse alcohol or other drugs, and polydrug misuse is commonplace. This has led many authorities to plan a combined response to all forms of drug misuse, which has the benefit of sharing scarce specialist resources. None the less, differences in age, lifestyle and in the legal status of the drugs involved results in many agencies retaining some separation in the treatment systems for individuals who misuse alcohol or other drugs, while working closely together when this is advantageous.

REFERENCES

Advisory Council on the Misuse of Drugs 1993 Aids and drug misuse update. Department of Health, HMSO, London

Advisory Council on the Misuse of Drugs 1995 Volatile substance abuse. Home Office, HMSO, London

Anderson P 1988 Excess mortality associated with alcohol consumption. British Medical Journal 297: 824–826

Andreasson S, Alleback P, Romelsjo A 1988 Alcohol and mortality among young men: longitudinal study of Swedish conscripts. British Medical Journal 296: 1021–1025

Azrin N H, Sisson R W, Meyers R, Godley M 1982 Alcoholism treatments by disulfiram and community reinforcement therapy. Journal of Behaviour Therapy and Experimental Psychiatry 13: 105–112

Babor T 1994 Demography, epidemiology and psychopharmacology – making sense of the connections. Addiction 89: 1391–1396

Babor T F, Ritson E B, Hodgson R J 1986 Alcohol related problems in the primary health care setting: a review of early intervention strategies. British Journal of Addiction 81: 23–46

Babor T F, de la Fuente J R, Saunders J 1989 AUDIT: the alcohol use disorder identification test: guidelines for use in primary care. World Health Organization, Geneva

Baldwin S 1991 Alcohol education and young offenders. Springer, Berlin

Bendetti G 1952 Die Alkoholhalluzinosen. Thieme, Stuttgart

Bertschy G 1995 Methadone maintenance treatment: an update. European Archives of Psychiatry and Clinical Neuroscience 245: 114–124

Bien T H, Miller R W, Tonigan J S 1993 Brief intervention for alcohol problems: a review. Addiction 88: 315–336

Bond A J, Curran H V, Bruce M S, O'Sullivan G, Shine P 1995 Behavioural aggression in panic disorder after 8 weeks' treatment with alprazolam. Journal of Affective Disorders 35: 117–123

Bourne P G, Alford J A, Bowcock J Z 1966 Treatment of skid row alcoholics with disulfiram. Quarterly Journal of Studies on Alcohol 27: 42

Cairns A, Roberts I, Benbow E 1996 Characteristics of fatal methadone overdose in Manchester, 1985–1994. British Medical Journal 313: 264–265

Carroll K M, Rounsaville B J, Bryant K J 1994a Should tolerance and withdrawal be required for substance dependence disorders? Drug and Alcohol Dependence 36: 15–22

Carroll K M, Rounsaville B J, Nich C, Gordon L T, Wirtz P W, Gawin F 1994b. One-year follow-up of psychotherapy and pharmacotherapy for cocaine dependence. Delayed emergence of psychotherapy effects. Archives of General Psychiatry 51: 989–997

Chaney E F, O'Leary M R 1978 Skill training with alcoholics. Journal of Consulting and Clinical Psychology 46: 1092

Chick J 1987 Early intervention in the general hospital. In: Stockwell T, Clements S (eds) Helping the problem drinker. Croom Helm, London

Chick J 1992 Doctors with emotional problems: how can they be helped? In: Hawton K, Cowen P (eds) Dilemmas in the management of psychiatric patients. Oxford University Press, Oxford, vol 2

Chick J, Chick J 1992 Drinking problems: information and advice for the individual, family and friend, 2nd edn. MacDonald Optima Press, London

Chick J, Kreitman N, Plant M 1981 Mean cell volume and gamma glutamyl transpeptidase as markers of drinking in working men. Lancet i: 1249–1251

Chick J, Lloyd G, Crombie E 1985 Counselling problem drinkers in medical wards: a controlled study. British Medical Journal 290: 965–969

Chick J, Ritson B, Connaughton J et al 1988 Advice versus extended treatment for alcoholism; a controlled study. British Journal of Addiction 83: 159–170

Chick J, Gough K, Falkowski W et al 1992 Treatment of alcoholism. British Journal of Psychiatry 162: 84–89

Chick K, Duffy J, Lloyd G, Ritson B 1986 Medical admissions in men: the risk among drinkers. Lancet ii: 1380–1383

Childress A R, Ehrman R, McLellan A T, MacRae J, Natale M, O'Brien C P 1994 Can induced moods trigger drug-related responses in opiate abuse patients? Journal of Substance Abuse Treatment 11: 17–23

Clark E 1988 The want makers: lifting the lid off the world advertising industry. Hodder & Stoughton, London

Cloninger C R 1987 Neurogenetic adaptive mechanisms in alcoholism. Science 23: 410–415

Cochrane R, Bal S 1990 The drinking habits of Sikh, Hindu, Muslim and white men in the West Midlands: a community survey. British Journal of Addiction 85: 759–769

Committee on Safety of Medicines 1988 Benzodiazepine dependence and withdrawal symptoms. Current Problems 21

Connors G, Maisto S, Donovan D 1996 Conceptualisation of relapse: a summary of psychological and psychobiological models. Addictions 91 (suppl): S5–S14

CRAG/SCOTMEG 1994 The management of alcohol withdrawal and delirium tremens. Scottish Office, Edinburgh

Currie D, Hashemi K, Fothergill J, Findlay A, Harris A, Hindmarch I 1995 The use of anti depressants and benzodiazepines in the perpetrators and victims of accidents. Occupational Medicine 45: 323–325

Cutting J 1978. A reappraisal of alcoholic psychosis. Psychological Medicine 8: 285–296

Daley D, Marlatt G 1992 Relapse prevention: cognitive and behavioural intervention. In: Lowinson J, Ruiz P, Millman R (eds) Substance abuse: a comprehensive textbook, 2nd edn. Williams & Wilkins, Baltimore, pp 533–542

Darke S, Ross J, Hall W 1995 Overdose among heroin users in Sydney, Australia: 1. Prevalence and correlates of non-fatal overdose. Addiction 91: 405–411

Demirkiran M, Jankovic J, Dean J M 1996 Ecstasy intoxication: an overlap between serotonin syndrome and neuroleptic malignant syndrome. Clinical Neuropharmacology 19: 157–164

Department of Health and Social Security 1978 The pattern and range of services for problem drinkers. HMSO, London

De Smet P A 1996 Some ethnopharmacological notes on African hallucinogens. Journal of Ethnopharmacology 50: 141–146

Department of Health 1991 Drug misuse and dependence. Guidelines on clinical management. HMSO, London

Domingo-Salvany A, Hartnoll R L, Anto J M 1993 Opiate and cocaine consumers attending Barcelona emergency rooms: a one year survey (1989). Addiction 88: 1247–1256

Domingo-Salvany A, Hartnoll R L, Maguire A, Suelves J M, Anto J M 1995 Use of capture–recapture to estimate the prevalence of opiate addiction in Barcelona, Spain, 1989. American Journal of Epidemiology 141: 567–574

Dorn N, Murji K 1992 ISDD Research monograph 5. Drug Prevention: a review of the English language literature. ISDD, London

Drake R E, Vaillant G E 1988 Predicting alcoholism and personality disorder in a 33-year longitudinal study of children of alcoholics. British Journal of Addiction 83: 799–807

Drummond D C, Cooper T, Glautier S P 1990 Conditioned learning in alcohol dependence: implications for cue exposure treatment. British Journal of Addiction 85: 725–743

Duffy J, Kreitman N 1993. Risk factors for suicide and undetermined death among inpatient alcoholics in Scotland. Addiction 88: 757–766

Dyer A R, Stamler J, Oglesby P et al 1980 Alcohol consumption and 17-year mortality in the Chicago Western Electric Company study. Preventive Medicine 9: 78–90

Edwards G, Gross M 1976 Alcohol dependence: provisional description of a clinical syndrome. British Medical Journal 1: 1058–1061

Ewing J A 1984 Detecting alcoholism: the CAGE questionnaire. Journal of the American Medical Association 252: 1905–1907

Faculty of Public Health Medicine 1991. Alcohol and the public health: the prevention of harm related to the use of alcohol. Macmillan, London

Fals-Stewart W, Schafer J 1992 The treatment of substance abusers diagnosed with obsessive–compulsive disorder: an outcome study. Journal of Substance Abuse Treatment 9: 365–370

Farrell M 1994 Opiate withdrawal. Addiction 89: 1471–1475

Farrell M, Ward J, Mattick R et al 1994 Methadone maintenance treatment in opiate dependence: a review. British Medical Journal 309: 997–1001

Fast Forward Positive Lifestyle 1996 Scottish Schools Drug Survey 1996. Scotland Against Drugs, Readpath, Edinburgh

Forrest F, Floray C du V, Taylor D, McPherson F, Young J A 1991 Reported social alcohol consumption during pregnancy and infant development at 18 months. British Medical Journal 303: 22–25

Frankel F H 1994 The concept of flashbacks in historical perspective. International Journal of Clinical and Experimental Hypnosis 42: 321–336

Frischer M 1992 Estimated prevalence of injecting drug use in Glasgow. British Journal of Addiction 87: 235–243

Garbutt J C, Mayo J P, Gillette G M et al 1991 Dose–response studies with thyrotropin-releasing hormone (TRH) in abstinent male alcoholics: evidence for selective thyrotropin dysfunction? Journal of Studies on Alcohol 52: 275–280

Geikie A 1904 Scottish reminiscences. Maclehose, Glasgow

Ghodse H 1986 Cannabis psychosis. British Journal of Addiction 81: 473–478

Glaser F B 1980 Anybody got a match? Treatment research and the matching hypothesis. In: Edwards G, Grant M (eds) Alcoholism treatment in transition. Croom Helm, London

Gonzales J, Brogden R 1988 Naltrexone. A review of its pharmacodynamic and pharmacokinetic properties and therapeutic efficacy in the management of opioid dependence. Drugs 35: 192–213

Gore S, Bird A, Ross A 1996 Prison rights: mandatory drug tests and performance indicators for prisons. British Medical Journal 312: 1411–1413

Gossop M, Birkin R 1994 Training employment service staff to recognise and respond to clients with drug and alcohol problems. Addictive Behaviors 19: 127–134

Gossop M, Strang J, Griffiths P, Powis B, Taylor C 1994 A ratio estimation method for determining the prevalence of cocaine use. British Journal of Psychiatry 164: 676–679

Gossop M, Griffiths P, Powis B, Williamson S, Strang J 1996 Frequency of non fatal heroin overdose: survey of heroin users recruited in non-clinical settings. British Medical Journal 313: 402

Green A, Goodwin G 1996 Ecstasy in neurodegeneration. British Medical Journal 312: 1493

Griffiths P, Gossop M, Powis B, Strang J 1993 Reaching hidden populations of drug users by privileged access interviewers: methodological and practical issues. Addiction 88: 1617–1626

Griffiths P, Gossop M, Powis B, Strang J 1994 Transitions in patterns of heroin administration: a study of heroin chasers and heroin injectors. Addiction 89: 301–309

Griffiths R, Wolf B 1990 Relative abuse liability of different benzodiazepines in drug abusers. Journal of Clinical Psychopharmacology 10: 237–243

Gual A, Colom J 1997 Why has alcohol consumption declined in countries of southern Europe? Addiction 92 (suppl 1), S21–S31

Gurling H M D, Curtis D, Murray R 1991 Psychological deficit from a co-twin study. British Journal of Addiction 86: 51–155

Hagman G 1994 Methadone maintenance counselling. Definition, principles, components. Journal of Substance Abuse Treatment 11: 405–413

Hallstrom C 1990 Benzodiazepines and medical negligence. Hospital Update 1990 569–571

Hartnoll R 1994 Opiates: prevalence and demographic factors. Addiction 89: 1377–1383

Health Publications Unit 1993 Drugs and solvents, you and your child. DSS Distribution Centre, London

Heath A C, Martin N G 1988 Teenage alcohol use in the Australian twin register: genetic and social determinants of starting to drink. Alcoholism (clinical and experimental research) 12: 735–741

Heath D 1992 Prohibition or liberalisation of alcohol and drugs? A social, cultural perspective. Recent Developments in Alcoholism 10: 129–145

Heather N 1981 Relationship between delinquency and drunkenness among Scottish young offenders. British Journal of Addiction 16: 50–61

Heather N, Robertson I 1981 Controlled drinking. Methuen, London

Helzer J, Canino G, Yeh E-K et al 1990 Alcoholism –

N America and Asia. Archives of General Psychiatry 47: 313–319

Hendra T, Gerrish S, Forrest A 1996 Fatal methadone overdose; lesson of the week. British Medical Journal 313: 481–482

Higgitt A, Lader M, Fonagy P 1985 Clinical management of benzodiazepine dependence. British Medical Journal 291: 688–690

Hindmarch I, Sherwood N, Kerr J S 1993 Amnestic effects of triazolam and other hypnotics. Progress in Neuro-Psychopharmacology and Biological Psychiatry 17: 407–413

Holton A, Riley P, Tyrer P 1992 Factors predicting long-term outcome after chronic benzodiazepine therapy. Journal of Affective Disorders 24: 245–252

Home Office 1974 Report on the habitual drunken offender. HMSO, London

Home Office Statistical Bulletin 1995a Statistics of drug addicts notified to the Home Office, United Kingdom 1994. Research and Statistics Department, Home Office, Croydon

Home Office Statistical Bulletin 1995b Statistics of drugs seizures and offenders dealt with, United Kingdom, 1994. Research and Statistics Department, Home Office, Croydon

Hough M 1996 Drug misuse and the criminal justice system: a review of the literature, Drug prevention initiative paper 15. Home Office. HMSO, London

Howard L, Fahy T, Wong P, Sherman D, Gane E, Williams R 1994 Psychiatric outcome in alcoholic liver transplant patients. Quarterly Journal of Medicine 87: 731–736

Hurley D L 1991 Women, alcohol and incest: an analytical review. Journal of Studies on Alcohol 52: 253–268

Huxley A 1940 The doors of perception. Harper Collins, London

Institute of Medicine 1982 Marijuana and health. National Academy Press, Washington, DC

Institute of Medicine 1990 Prevention and treatment of alcohol problems? Research opportunities. National Academy Press, Washington, DC

Institute for the Study of Drug Dependence (ISDD) 1995 National audit of drug misuse in Britain 1994, College Hill Press, London

Isbell H, Fraser H F, Wikler D W et al 1955 An experimental study of the etiology of 'rum fits' and delirium tremens. Quarterly Journal of Studies on Alcohol 16: 1–23

Johns A 1994 Opiate treatments. Addiction 89: 1551–1558

Kendell R E, de Roumanie M, Ritson E B 1983 Effect of economic changes on Scottish drinking habits 1978–1982. British Journal of Addiction 78: 365–379

Kerr J S, Hindmarch I, Sherwood N 1992 Correlation between doses of oxazepam and their effects on performance of a standardised test battery. European Journal of Clinical Pharmacology 42: 507–510

Kreitman N 1986 Alcohol consumption and the preventive paradox. British Journal of Addiction 81: 353–363

Kushner M G, Sher K J, Beitman B D 1990 The relation between alcohol problems and anxiety disorders. American Journal of Psychiatry 147: 685–695

Lago J A, Kosten T R 1994 Stimulant withdrawal. Addiction 89: 1477–1481

Legarda J J, Gossop M 1994 A 24-h inpatient detoxification treatment for heroin addicts: a preliminary investigation. Drug and Alcohol Dependence 35: 91–93

Lennane K J 1988 Patient with alcohol related brain damage: therapy and outcome. Australian Drug and Alcohol Review 7: 89–92

Lewis C E, Bucholz K K 1991 Alcoholism, antisocial behaviour and family history. British Journal of Addiction 86: 177–194

Littman G, Stapleton J, Oppenheim A N et al 1983 Situations related to alcoholism relapse. British Journal of Addiction 78: 381

Ludwig A M 1988 Understanding the alcoholic's mind: the nature of craving and how to control it. Oxford University Press, Oxford

McGuiness I 1980 An econometric analysis of total demand for alcoholic beverages in the UK 1956–1975. Journal of Industrial Economics 29: 85

McLachlan J F C, Stein R L 1982. Evaluation of a day clinic for alcoholics. Journal of Studies on Alcohol 43: 262–272

Marlatt G A, Gordon J R 1984 Relapse prevention: maintenance strategies in addictive behaviour. Guildford Press, New York

Marshall E J, Murray R M 1991 Familial alcoholism: inheritance and initiation. British Medical Journal 303: 72–73

Mason P, Wilkinson G 1996 The prevalence of psychiatric morbidity. British Journal of Psychiatry 168: 1–3

Menninger K A 1938 Man against himself. Harcourt Brace, New York

Merrill J 1996 Advice is that 'less is more'. British Medical Journal 313: 423

Miller P, Plant M 1996 Drinking, smoking, and illicit drug use among 15 and 16 year olds in the United Kingdom. British Medical Journal 313: 394–397

Miller W 1983 Motivational interviewing with problem drinkers. Behaviour Psychotherapy 11: 147–172

Miller W 1996 What is a relapse? 50 ways to leave the wagon. Addiction 91 (suppl): S15–S27

Miller W R, Baca L 1983 Two year follow-up of bibliotherapy and therapist-directed controlled drinking training for problem drinkers. Behaviour Therapy 14: 441

Miller W R, Hester R K 1986 The effectiveness of alcoholism treatment methods, what research reveals. In Miller W R and Heather N (eds) Treating addictive behaviours: processes of change. Plenum, New York

Miller W, Rollnick S 1991 Motivational interviewing: preparing people to change addictive behaviour. Guildford Press, London

Miller W R, Taylor C A 1980 Relative effectiveness of bibliotherapy, individual and group self-control training in the treatment of problem drinkers. Addictive Behaviours 5: 13

Miller W, Westerberg V, Harris R, Tonigan J 1996 What predicts relapse? Prospective testing of antecedent models. Addiction 91 (suppl): S155–S172

Ministerial Drugs Task Force 1994 Drugs in Scotland: meeting the challenge. HMSO, London

Morgenstern J, Langenbucher J, Labouvie E W 1994 The generalizability of the dependence syndrome across substances: an examination of some properties of the proposed DSM-IV dependence criteria. Addiction 89: 1105–1113

Morse A C, Erwin V G, Jones B C 1995 Pharmacogenetics of cocaine: a critical review. Pharmacogenetics 5: 183–192

Moskowitz J M 1989 The primary prevention of alcohol problems: a critical review of the research literature. Journal of Studies on Alcohol 50: 54–88

Nakamura H, Overall J, Hollister L, Radcliffe E 1983 Factors affecting outcome of depressive symptoms in alcoholics. Alcoholism: Clinical and Experimental Research 7: 188–193

National Treatment Outcome Research Study 1996 Summary of the project, the clients and preliminary findings. Department of Health, HMSO, London

News item 1996a Violence may be predicted among psychiatric patients. British Medical Journal 313: 318

News item 1996b Two more USA states approve cannabis. British Medical Journal 313: 1224

News item 1997 Doctors penalised for prescribing cannabis. British Medical Journal 314: 92

Nigam R, Schottenfeld R, Kosten T R 1992 Treatment of dual diagnosis patients: a relapse prevention group approach. Journal of Substance Abuse Treatment 9: 305–309

Nutt D J 1996 Addiction: brain mechanisms and their implications for treatment. Lancet 347: 31–36

O'Farrell T J 1989 Marital and family therapy in alcoholism treatment. Journal of Substance Misuse Treatment 6: 23–29

Ojesjo 1981 Long-term outcome in alcohol abuse and alcoholism among males in the Lundby general population. British Journal of Addiction 76: 391–400

O'Malley S S, Jaffe A J, Chang G, Schottenfeld R S, Meyer R E, Rounsaville B. 1992 Naltrexone and coping skills therapy for alcohol dependence. Archives of General Psychiatry 49: 881–887

Oppenheimer E, Tobutt C, Taylor C, Andrew T 1994 Death and survival in a cohort of heroin addicts from London Clinics: a 22 year follow-up study. Addiction 89: 1299–1308

Orford J, Edwards G 1977 Alcoholism. Oxford University Press, London

Orford J, Wawman T 1986 Alcohol detoxification services: a review. Department of Health and Social Security, London

Pihl R, Paterson J, Finn P 1990 Inherited predisposition to alcoholism: characteristics of sons of male alcoholics. Journal of Abnormal Psychology 99: 271–301

Plant M 1987 Women, drinking and pregnancy. Tavistock, London

Polich J M, Armor D J, Braiker H 1981 The course of alcoholism four years after the treatment. Wiley, New York

Powell J, Dawe S, Richards D 1993 Can opiate addicts tell us about their relapse risk? Subjective predictors of clinical prognosis. Addictive Behaviors 18: 473–490

Prochaska J, Di Clemente C 1992 Stages of change in the modification of problem behaviours. In: Hersen M, Eisler R, Miller P (eds) Progress in behaviour modification. Sycamore Publications, Sycamore, IL, vol 23

Project MATCH Research Group 1997 Matching alcoholism treatments to client heterogeneity. Journal of Studies on Alcohol 58: 7–29

Rapaport M H, Tipp J E, Schuckit M A 1993 A comparison of ICD-10 and DSM-III-R criteria for substance abuse and dependence. American Journal of Drug and Alcohol Abuse 19: 143–151

Ritson B 1995 Community and municipal action on alcohol. WHO Euro no 63. World Health Organization, Copenhagen

Roberts L J, Shaner A, Eckman T A, Tucker D E, Vaccaro J V 1992 Effectively treating stimulant-abusing schizophrenics: mission impossible? New Directions for Mental Health Services 53: 55–65

Robertson M, Bell J 1993 Are rapid inpatient benzodiazepine detoxifications unsafe?. Medical Journal of Australia 158: 578–579

Robichaud C, Strickler D, Bigelow G, Liebson I 1979 Disulfiram maintenance alcoholism treatment: a 3-phase evaluation. Behaviour Research and Therapy 17: 618

Robinson D 1979 Talking out of alcoholism: the self help process of Alcoholics Anonymous. Croom Helm, London

Romelsjo A, Lazarus N B, Kaplan G A, Cohen R D 1991 The relationship between stressful life situations and changes in alcohol consumption. British Journal of Addiction 86: 157–169

Room R, Bondy A, Ferris J 1995 The risk of harm to oneself from drinking, Canada 1989. Addiction 90: 499–513

Rose G, Day S 1990 The population mean predicts the number of deviant individuals. British Medical Journal 301: 1031–1034

Rounsaville B J, Bryant K, Babor T, Kranzler H, Kadden R 1993 Cross system agreement for substance use disorders: DSM-III-R, DSM-IV and ICD-10. Addiction 88: 337–348

Royal College of Physicians 1987 A great and growing evil. Tavistock, London

Royal College of Physicians, Royal College of Psychiatrists, Royal College of General Practitioners 1995 Alcohol and the heart in perspective. London

Saunders J B 1989 The efficacy of treatment for drinking problems. International Review of Psychiatry 1: 121–138

Saunders J B, Walters J R F, Davies P, Paton A 1981 A 20-year prospective study of cirrhosis. British Medical Journal 282: 263–266

Schuckit M A 1994 The treatment of stimulant dependence. Addiction 89: 1559–1563

Schuckit M A, Irwin M 1989 An analysis of the clinical relevance of type 1 and type 2 alcoholics. British Journal of Addiction 84: 869–876

Skog O J 1980 Liver cirrhosis epidemiology: some methodological problems. British Journal of Addiction 74: 282–283

Smart R G, Mann R E 1991 Factors in recent reductions in liver cirrhosis deaths. Journal of Studies on Alcohol 52: 232–240

Stevenson R 1994 Winning the war on drugs – to legalise or not. Paper 124. Institute of Economic Affairs, London

Stockwell T 1987 The Exeter home detoxification projects. In: Stockwell T, Cleriene S (eds) Helping the problem drinker. Croom Helm, London

Stockwell T, Clement S (eds) 1987 Helping the problem drinker: new initiatives in community care. Croom Helm, London

Stockwell T, Hodgson R, Edwards G et al 1979 The development of a questionnaire to measure severity of alcohol dependence. British Journal of Addiction 73: 79–87

Strang J, Griffiths P, Powis B, Gossop M 1992 First use of heroin: changes in route of administration over time. British Medical Journal 304: 1222–1223

Strang J, Black J, Marsh A, Smith B 1993 Hair analysis for drugs: technological breakthrough or ethical quagmire? Addiction 88: 163–166. Comments: Addiction 1994 89: 295–300

Strang J, Griffiths P, Abbey J, Gossop M 1994 Survey of use of injected benzodiazepines among drug users in Britain. British Medical Journal 308: 1082

Strang J, Darke S, Hall W, Ali R 1996a Heroin overdose: the case for take-home naloxone. British Medical Journal 313: 1435

Strang J, Sheridan J, Barber N 1996b Prescribing injectable and oral methadone to opiate addicts: results from the 1995 national postal survey of community pharmacies in England and Wales. British Medical Journal 313: 270–272

Strassman R J 1995 Hallucinogenic drugs in psychiatric research and treatment. Perspectives and prospects. Journal of Nervous and Mental Disease 183: 127–138

Straw J 1996 Breaking the vicious cycle: Labour's proposals for tackling drug-related crime. Labour Party, London

Substance Abuse Committee of the Mental Health Foundation 1992 Guidelines for the prevention and treatment of benzodiazepine dependence. Mental Health Foundation, London

Surendrakumar D, Dunn M, Roberts C 1992 Hospital admission and the start of benzodiazepine use. British Medical Journal 304: 881

Sutton M, Maynard A 1992 Yartic occasional paper 3. What is the size and nature of the 'drug problem' in the United Kingdom? Centre for Health Economics, University of York, York

Task Force to Review Service for Drug Misusers 1996 Report of an independent review of drug treatment services in England. Department of Health, HMSO, London

Thomas H 1993 Psychiatric symptoms in cannabis users. British Journal of Psychiatry 163: 141–149

Tobutt C, Oppenheimer C, Laranjeira R 1996 Health of cohort of heroin addicts from London clinics: 22 year follow up. British Medical Journal 312: 1458

U S Department of Health and Human Services 1990 Alcohol and Health. DHHS, Rockville

Vaillant G E 1983 The natural history of alcoholism: causes, patterns and paths to recovery. Harvard University Press, Boston

Vaillant G E 1995 The natural history of alcoholism revisited. Harvard University Press, Cambridge, Massachusetts

Victor M 1962 Alcoholism. In: Baker A B (ed) Clinical neurology. Hoeber-Harper, New York, vol 2

Victor M, Hope J M 1958 The phenomenon of auditory hallucinations in chronic alcoholism. Journal of Nervous and Mental Disease 126: 452

Wallace P, Cutler S, Haines A 1988 Randomised controlled trial of general practitioners in patients with excessive alcohol consumption. British Medical Journal 297: 663–668

Wallack L, Dorfman L, Jernigan D, Themba M. 1993. Media advocacy and public health: power for prevention. Sage, Newbury Park

Walton M A, Castro F G, Barrington E H 1994 The role of attributions in abstinence, lapse, and relapse following substance abuse treatment. Addictive Behaviors 19: 319–331

Ward J, Mattrick R, Hall W 1992 Key issues in methadone maintenance treatment. New South Wales University Press, New South Wales, Australia

Washton A M, Potash A, Gold M 1984 Naltrexone in addictive business executives and physicians. Journal of Clinical Psychiatry 45: 39–41

Whitworth A B, Fischer F, Lesch O et al 1996 Comparison of Acamprosate and placebo in long-term treatment of alcohol dependence. Lancet 347: 1438–1442

Wilson P 1980 Drinking in England and Wales. HMSO, London

Woody G E, Cottler L B, Cacciola J 1993 Severity of dependence: data from the DSM-IV field trials. Addiction 88: 1573–1579

Wright J, Pearl L 1995 Knowledge and experience of young people regarding drug misuse 1969–1994. British Medical Journal 310: 20–24

Young R M, Oei T P S, Knight R G 1990 The tension reduction hypothesis revisited: an alcohol expectancy perspective. British Journal of Addiction 85: 31–40

13
Schizophrenia

Eve C. Johnstone

Schizophrenia is the heartland of psychiatry and the core of its clinical practice. Every layman knows that the term means 'split mind' and his concept of madness is largely based on the oddities and abnormalities of those who suffer from this enigmatic illness. Because it is a relatively common condition, which often cripples people in adolescence or early adult life, it probably causes more suffering and distress and blights more lives than any cancer; and because it cripples people in their youth without greatly reducing their life expectancy it represents a major burden for health services. In the USA its financial cost has been estimated as 2% of the gross national product (Gunderson & Mosher 1975).

HISTORICAL INTRODUCTION

Although brief descriptions of an illness with some resemblance to schizophrenia are to be found in the Hindu Ayurveda as long ago as 1400 BC, and in the writings of the Cappadocian physician Aretaeus in the 2nd century AD, recognisable descriptions of schizophrenia are historically considerably less common, in medical texts or literature generally, than those of melancholia or mania. The earliest unambiguous descriptions date only from the end of the 18th century, and it was a further 100 years before the syndrome was defined with any clarity. That crucial step was achieved by Emil Kraepelin, professor of psychiatry at the University of Munich, in the fifth (1896) edition of his *Psychiatrie, ein Lehrbuch für Studierende und Ärzte*. Throughout the 19th century psychiatrists had struggled, with scant success, to develop a satisfactory classification of insanity. In 1856 Morel had coined the term *démence précoce* to describe an adolescent patient, once bright and active, who had slowly lapsed into a state of silent withdrawal. In 1868 Kahlbaum had described the syndrome of *Katatonie* and 3 years later Hecker had described *Hebephrenie*. But it was Kraepelin who first succeeded in going beyond straightforward

clinical description by his division of the myriad and shifting forms of insanity into two great groupings on the basis of their long-term course. The first, which he called manic–depressive insanity, pursued a fluctuating course with frequent relapses but full recovery after each. The second, for which he used Morel's term dementia praecox, embraced Kahlbaum's catatonia, Hecker's hebephrenia and his own dementia paranoides and was a progressive disease which either pursued a steady downhill course to chronic invalidism or, if improvement did occur, resulted only in partial recovery. Initially, Kraepelin was criticised for introducing yet another classification without any aetiological or pathological basis, but it was not long before the force and utility of his unifying concepts impressed themselves on his contemporaries and they started to come into general use. In 1911, however, while acceptance of this new classification was still incomplete, the Swiss psychiatrist Eugen Bleuler published his *Dementia Praecox or the Group of Schizophrenias*, which was to be at least as influential as Kraepelin's *Lehrbuch*. Although Bleuler regarded himself as confirming and developing Kraepelin's concept of dementia praecox, in fact he changed it fundamentally, and it was his term *schizophrenia* which eventually won universal adoption. Kraepelin had assumed, in the tradition of Griesinger (1845) and other German academic psychiatrists, that dementia praecox was a disease of the brain. Bleuler, influenced by the writing of Sigmund Freud and the infant school of psychoanalysis, thought of schizophrenia, meaning 'split mind', because he believed that the disorder was due to a 'loosening of associations' between different psychic functions, affecting both the transition from one idea to the next in thought and speech and the coordination between emotional, volitional (conative) and intellectual (cognitive) processes in general. He also drew a distinction between the thought disorder, the blunting or incongruity of affect, the autism and the pervasive ambivalence of the disorder, which he regarded as the 'fundamental symptoms', and the more obvious hallucinations, delusions and catatonic phenomena which for him were accessory phenomena of less importance. This led him to conclude that schizophrenia could develop and be diagnosed in the absence of hallucinations and delusions, and so to add a fourth type, simple schizophrenia, to the hebephrenic, catatonic and paranoid forms recognised by Kraepelin.

Although Bleuler's term schizophrenia eventually displaced Kraepelin's dementia praecox and his assumptions about the nature of the disorder became very influential, particularly in the USA, Kraepelin's original concept remained dominant in many European centres. This failure to resolve the incompatibility of the kraepelinian and bleulerian approaches, together with the inherent ambiguities of each, resulted in considerable confusion and seriously hindered fruitful research for the next half century.

The crucial characteristic of Kraepelin's dementia praecox – what distinguished it from manic–depressive insanity – was its prognosis. The illness progressed to a state of permanent impairment, and if recovery did occur it was either temporary or incomplete. However, it soon came to be recognised that some patients with the typical clinical characteristics of the condition did recover, and remained well indefinitely without any detectable defect. Kraepelin himself eventually accepted that this occurred in 13% of his own cases. Unfortunately, the implications of this were never properly faced. Kraepelin and most of the contemporaries had assumed that dementia praecox was a 'disease entity' with its own characteristic symptomatology, aetiology, pathology and course. But the aetiology and neuropathology remained a mystery and here was evidence that the course was variable and inconstant. Understandably, the predominant reaction to this quandary was to assume that this variable prognosis was an artefact, occurring because patients with a superficially similar psychosis of good prognosis were being confused with those suffering from real dementia praecox schizophrenia. Determined efforts were therefore made to distinguish the two. In Europe the Norwegian psychiatrist Langfeldt sought to distinguish between schizophrenia and what he called schizophreniform psychosis on the basis of a detailed study of the symptomatology of the illness. He presented evidence to suggest that the two had quite different outcomes, and that electroconvulsive therapy (ECT) and insulin coma therapy were ineffective in schizophrenia itself (Langfeldt 1960). Although his methodology had clear limitations his claim was initially widely accepted because it was so welcome. In the USA similar efforts were made by clinical psychologists, and a series of rating scales – the Elgin, Phillips and Kantor Scales – were developed to discriminate between what they called process and non-process schizophrenia, mainly on the basis of the premorbid personality and psychosexual adjustment. Both Langfeldt and these American workers assumed that true process was endogenous and hereditary and that schizophreniform or non-process psychoses were psychogenic, but neither succeeded in demonstrating a clear demarcation between the two. The cardinal defect of Bleuler's concept of schizophrenia was its lack of clear boundaries. Although he provided little empirical evidence to justify his belief that his 'fundamental symptoms' were indeed fundamental, his assumptions were widely accepted, particularly in the USA, and as a result the diagnosis of schizophrenia came to be based on the presence of one or more of the so-called 'four As' (loosening of associations or thought disorder, blunting or incongruity of affect, autism and ambivalence), whether or not the patient was psychotic. Unfortunately, all four of these phenomena are intangible qualities which with a little imagination can be detected in most psychiatric patients and in some healthy people, particularly when under stress. Their use as diagnostic criteria therefore led to a marked expansion of the concept of schizophrenia, to the point at which it was degenerating into a vague synonym for severe mental illness. Indeed, in the 1950s in the USA patients were diagnosed as having schizophrenia without having any characteristic features at all. An example of this diagnostic practice is the concept of 'pseudoneurotic schizophrenia' (Hoch & Polatin, 1949), where patients had a wide range of neurotic symptoms, such as phobias, obsessions and depersonalisation, often associated with severe anxiety and attacks of psychotic disturbance lasting days, hours or perhaps only minutes.

Between 1920 and 1960 the confusion increased steadily. With the partial exception of French psychiatry, which pursed its own traditions untroubled by outside influences, the term 'schizophrenia' was used throughout the world, but in a bewildering variety of different ways which were rarely made explicit. Some authorities, like Kleist and Leonhard in Germany and Langfeldt in Norway, insisted that the term should be restricted to illnesses resulting in permanent damage to the personality; others were prepared to use it freely regardless of outcome. Some psychiatrists would only make the diagnosis in adolescents or young adults; others were willing to do so at any age. Some insisted on the presence of certain key symptoms; others were prepared to make a confident diagnosis on the basis of indefinable subjective impressions, the so-called 'praecox feeling'. In the USA Bleuler's views predominated, largely because his concept of schizophrenia as a psychological, and possibly psychogenic, disorder was readily compatible with the prevailing psychoanalytic

Table 13.1   Kurt Schneider's 'symptoms of the first rank'

1. Auditory hallucinations taking any one of three specific forms:
   a. Voices repeating the subject's thoughts out loud (Gedankenlautwerden or écho de la pensée), or anticipating his thoughts
   b. Two or more hallucinatory voices discussing the subject, or arguing about him, referring to him in the third person
   c. Voices commenting on the subject's thoughts or behaviour, often as a running commentary
2. The sensation of alien thoughts being put into the subject's mind by some external agency, or of his own thoughts being taken away (thought insertion or withdrawal)
3. The sensation that the subject's thinking is no longer confined within his own mind, but is instead shared by, or accessible to, others (thought broadcasting)
4. The sensation of feelings, impulses or acts being experienced or carried out under external control, so that the patient feels as if he were being hypnotised, or had become a robot
5. The experience of being a passive and reluctant recipient of bodily sensation imposed by some external agency
6. Delusional perception – a delusion arising fully fledged on the basis of a genuine perception which others would regard as commonplace and unrelated

orientation. The overuse of the term was therefore most marked in that country. In most of Europe, on the other hand, Kraepelin's concepts still held sway. In most of the German-speaking world schizophrenia was regarded as an endogenous and hereditary psychosis and the diagnosis was restricted to patients exhibiting certain cardinal symptoms, mainly hallucinations and delusions of particular kinds. Kleist in Frankfurt and Leonhard in Berlin developed very detailed classifications of different forms of schizophrenia, mainly on the basis of a meticulous study of the chronic stage of the illness. Of greater influence, however, were the teachings of Kurt Schneider, who focused attention on the earlier acute stage of the illness and described a number of 'symptoms of the first rank' (Table 13.1) which he considered to be diagnostic of schizophrenia in the absence of overt brain disease (Schneider 1959).

Many of these hallucinations and delusions can be interpreted as the result of a failure to distinguish between ideas and impulses arising in the patient's own mind and perceptions arising in the external world, a so-called 'loss of ego boundaries'. However, they had no particular theoretical significance for Schneider himself; he regarded them simply as convenient diagnostic aids that were pathognomonic of schizophrenia in the absence of brain disease. He accepted that some patients with otherwise typical schizophrenic illnesses never exhibited any of these symptoms, and that all of them could occur at times in epileptic and other organic psychoses, but he regarded them none the less as sufficiently characteristic to be worth distinguishing from what he called 'second rank' symptoms like perplexity, emotional blunting and hallucinations and delusions of other kinds.

DEFINITIONS

The confusion caused by the unresolved differences between Kraepelin's and Bleuler's concepts of schizophrenia, and the subsequent development of other differences in usage as well, have already been mentioned. These differences were at their worst in the 1950s and the best known and most extensively studied were Anglo-American. Spurred by the observation that the first-admission rate for schizophrenia was considerably higher in the USA than in England and Wales, and that for manic–depressive illnesses the difference was the other way about, detailed studies were mounted of series of consecutive admissions to mental hospitals in the two countries, using identical interviewing methods and diagnostic criteria (Cooper et al 1972). These comparisons showed that the symptoms of patients admitted to public mental hospitals in New York and London were virtually identical, but the proportion of patients given a diagnosis of schizophrenia was nearly twice as high in New York as in London because the New York psychiatrists' concept of schizophrenia embraced many patients who in London would have been regarded as suffering from depressive or manic psychoses, or even from neurotic illnesses or personality disorders. Shortly after this the International Pilot Study of Schizophrenia confirmed that psychiatrists in Washington – and also, for rather different reasons, in Moscow – had a considerably broader concept of schizophrenia than their counterparts in the other seven countries involved, namely Colombia, Czechoslovakia, Denmark, India, Nigeria, Taiwan and the UK (WHO 1973).

Increasing awareness of the scale and consequences of international differences of this kind, and of the low reliability of psychiatric diagnoses generally, led in the 1970s to a widespread realisation that key terms like schizophrenia must be operationally defined in order to make it quite clear what criteria had to be satisfied to establish the diagnosis. Because schizophrenia, like most other psychiatric disorders, is still recognised by its syndrome and its aetiology is still obscure, this means that it must be defined either by the presence of particular symptoms or combinations of symptoms, or by its course, or by some combination of the two. In the last 20 years many different operational definitions of schizophrenia have been proposed and this has inevitably led to comparisons of their relative merits. High reliability and a reasonable concordance with traditional usage are obviously important qualities, but not sufficient by themselves. What we are really trying to do when faced with a choice between alternative definitions is to decide which is likely to be more useful in predicting response to treatment or long-term course, or which is likely to correspond most closely with the putative biological abnormality underlying the disorder. Because the syndrome of schizophrenia appears to merge into neighbouring syndromes, because we have not yet identified the underlying biological abnormality, and because political considerations are also involved, there is not yet any single agreed definition, or any immediate prospect of a consensus. Areas of agreement are emerging all the same. Bleuler's fundamental symptoms, and thought disorder in particular, have lost their former influence, mainly because they are too intangible, and therefore incapable of being reliably identified. Schneider's first-rank symptoms are still influential in Britain and Germany, partly because their presence can be reliably rated, but several studies have demonstrated that they have little significance for long-term prognosis. The presence of first-rank symptoms in the acute illness does not predict either incomplete recovery or the development of a schizophrenic defect state (Kendell et al 1979) and it is not uncommon for these symptoms to develop in the course of, what are in other respects typical, manic illnesses (Brockington et al 1980). In fact, it is increasingly apparent that none of the symptoms of the acute illness is as good a predictor of the long-term course as the duration and mode of onset. If the initial illness starts insidiously and lasts for several months a poor long-term prognosis is much more likely than if it starts acutely in response to obvious stress and lasts only a few weeks, regardless of the detailed symptomatology.

Currently, the most widely used definitions of schizophrenia, at least for research purposes, are the St Louis criteria (Feighner et al 1972), the Research Diagnostic Criteria (RDC) (Spitzer et al 1975) and the American Psychiatric Association's DSM-IV (APA 1994) criteria, and ICD-10 (WHO 1992). They all require clear evidence of psychosis, currently or in the past, and all but the Feighner criteria specify particular kinds of hallucinatory experience or delusional ideation. All four stipulate that affective symptoms must not be prominent and

all require a minimum duration of illness, but this is only 2 weeks for the RDC definition, 1 month for ICD-10 and 6 months for Feighner.

It is, of course, very confusing for everyone, not merely for students, to have several alternative definitions of a single disorder, particularly when it is commonplace for a patient to fulfil one set of criteria but not others. Under present circumstances, however, for the reasons described above, this is inevitable; and it is better for differences of this kind to be overt than to be concealed and unsuspected. The existence of a number of alternative definitions also helps to emphasise that all definitions are arbitrary, justified only their usefulness, and liable to be altered or supplanted. The St Louis and DSM-IV definitions, which require a 6 month symptom duration, are the most restrictive but have the merit of defining a group of patients with a poor long-term prognosis akin to Kraepelin's original dementia praecox. The schneiderian concept of schizophrenia and the criteria incorporated in the computer program, Catego, derived from it (Wing et al 1974) are broader, and because no account is taken either of symptom duration or of the presence of affective symptoms the outcome is more variable in both the short and the long term.

CLINICAL PRESENTATION AND SYMPTOMATOLOGY

It follows from what has been said above about the definition of schizophrenia that the symptoms and other characteristics of the condition will vary somewhat, according to the way in which the syndrome is defined. There is, none the less, a core group of patients who fulfil most definitions, and international comparisons using films or videotapes of diagnostic interviews confirm that psychiatrists throughout the world will confidently identify these as schizophrenics.

The premorbid personality

Although schizophrenia can develop in personalities of all kinds, some adults with schizophrenia were odd as children. Observations in support of this view have been made since the time of Kraepelin and Bleuler and the premorbid personality traits most often described are those of solitariness and coldness of affect. Some are noted to have been inclined to suspiciousness or to have abnormal speech patterns. These are often called schizoid/schizotypal traits. The relationship of such premorbid traits to the development of schizophrenia has not been easy to determine. In a review of early German studies of premorbid personality in schizophrenia, Cutting (1985) concluded that the schizoid trait complex was described in 25% of schizophrenic patients and other personality variants – for example, paranoid in a further 15%. In a study of 73 patients with either schizophrenia or affective psychosis, Foerster et al (1991) found an excess of schizoid/schizotypal traits and poor premorbid social adjustment in schizophrenic males as compared with affectively ill males but no differences between the diagnostic groups in the female patients. Such retrospective data confirm the existence of unusual personality characteristics prior to the onset of schizophrenic illness but offer no information as to whether such traits occur more often in those destined to develop schizophrenia than in their peers who will remain well, and they do not allow us to determine whether the schizoid/schizotypal trait complex is a risk factor which contributes independently to the disease or is in fact a preclinical manifestation of the disorder itself. Prospective data were however provided by a study by Done et al (1994) of adults who had participated in the national 1958 birth cohort study and had thus been assessed in terms of social behaviour at the ages of 7 and 11 years. Those who went on to develop schizophrenia in adult life were compared with those who developed other psychiatric disorders and those who remained well. At 7 and 11 years preschizophrenic boys showed significantly more anxiety for acceptance, hostility and inconsequential behaviour than those who would remain well, and at 11 years preschizophrenic girls were significantly more withdrawn than those who did not become mentally ill. Those destined to develop affective psychosis in later life differed little from normal controls. Clearly, therefore, many years before illness develops, there are significant excesses of abnormal social behaviour in children destined to develop schizophrenia in adult life. None the less, by no means all who go on to develop schizophrenia have been considered to be abnormal in any way and some have shown very high levels of social, academic and occupational functioning (for examples, see Johnstone 1994).

The acute illness

Although schizophrenia can occur at any age from 7 to 70 the onset is usually in adolescence or early adult life. Often it develops insidiously. A youth whose previous behaviour has been unremarkable slowly becomes more withdrawn and introverted. He may acquire a new interest in religion, psychology or the occult and drift away from his friends. He also loses his drive and determination and may fail to complete a university degree or an apprenticeship which had previously seemed well within his grasp. His parents may be worried by his fail-

ures, his apparent lack of interest in achievement and his progressive estrangement from them but they do not suspect that he is ill until one day, months or even years later, it suddenly becomes apparent that he is entertaining delusional ideas, or hearing voices. In other cases the onset is acute. Sometimes in the aftermath of some obvious stress, perhaps being spurned by a girlfriend or failing an exam, or while in the unfamiliar environment of a foreign country, the subject becomes obviously and sometimes floridly ill over the course of a few days. He becomes convinced that he is being watched or followed, may attach great significance to the colours of clothes or postage stamps, talk of Martians, laser beams or hypnosis, or suddenly be found, mute and inaccessible, kneeling on the floor.

The delusions of the acute illness are very variable in type and even more so in their detailed content. Delusions of reference and persecutory, grandiose, religious and hypochondriacal ideas of various kinds are all common but most characteristic are a variety of *passivity phenomena*. The subject feels that he is no longer in control of his own thoughts, feelings or will and that he is being influenced or controlled by some mysterious, alien force. Thoughts which are not his own are put into his mind (*thought insertion*), or his own thoughts are taken away (*thought withdrawal*) or somehow have become accessible to other people (*thought broadcasting*). Or he may be convinced that someone is trying to hypnotise him or impose their will on his. The subject's interpretation of these phenomena, which lie beyond the bounds of normal experience, depends on his cultural background. Our forefathers attributed them to God or the Devil; some people from other cultures attribute them to spirits or witchcraft; and the inhabitants of modern industrial countries attribute them to electricity, X-rays, television, laser beams and satellites. In short, the subject endeavours to make an unintelligible experience intelligible by attributing it to some powerful, invisible force with which he is conversant but does not fully understand.

The hallucinations are equally varied and may involve any of the five senses. Auditory hallucinations in the form of voices are the most common, however, and the visual, olfactory, gustatory and tactile hallucinations are all uncommon in the absence of hallucinatory voices. Although Schneider and others have drawn attention to particular types of hallucinatory voices that are characteristic of schizophrenia (Table 13.1), it is commonplace for schizophrenics to hear voices talking to them as well as about them, and the content is very variable. Indeed, from a diagnostic point of view the duration is probably more important than the detailed perceptual characteristics or the content, because hallucinatory voices do not often continue all day long, week after week, in other psychoses. Traditionally, psychiatrists have distinguished between true hallucinations, which have all the characteristics of normal perceptions and are therefore treated as genuine, and pseudohallucinations, which are sufficiently different for the subject to realise that he is 'hearing voices'. Although the distinction may have considerably practical significance – a man who hears a voice threatening to murder him behaves very differently from a man who realises he is hearing things – it rarely has much diagnostic significance. Indeed schizophrenic hallucinations frequently have a quality intermediate between that of a genuine auditory perception and a thought. Although the subject speaks spontaneously of a 'voice' he will often admit on questioning that he does not really hear it out loud or with his ears. It is in the mind, a 'silent voice', which none the less is insistent, troublesome and sometimes frightening. Often, too, the subject has difficulty describing what it says. Doubtless this is often due to embarrassment, or reluctance to divulge what the subject suspects his questioner will regard as evidence of insanity, but it does sometimes seem that the patient has genuine difficulty in describing the content of the hallucination, perhaps because the normal link between perception and memory is only partly established.

The patient's affect during the acute illness is as variable as his thought content but is nearly always disturbed in some way. Perplexity is a common and characteristic feature of acute schizophrenic illnesses. The subject suspects that something strange is going on around him but is not sure what, and ideas may come and go in rapid succession as he seeks to integrate his changing perceptions and affective state with his premorbid experience (*delusional mood*). At other times the subject may be depressed, elated or angry and it is sometimes difficult to tell whether the content of the delusions and hallucinatory voices is derived from the prevailing mood or vice versa. The most characteristic emotional abnormality, however, is either a general flattening or blunting of all affective responses, or incongruity. The former refers to a loss of the ability to feel, or at least to express, any deep or profound emotion, and a matching inability to evoke a sympathetic response in other people. The latter refers to a mismatch between the subject's emotional responses and the setting or the topic of conversation – silly giggling while important or distressing events are taking place being the most common example. Sometimes the patient knows that this is happening and may be able to explain that the emotion that he expresses is quite different from that which he feels.

Finally, the patient's global behaviour is affected. Again the nature of the change is variable but characteristically involves withdrawal from contact with and interest in other people, and actions which seem bizarre or inexplicable to the onlooker. Occasionally, the patient displays the particular behavioural abnormalities of Kahlbaum's catatonia, becoming mute, or stuporose, or adopting strange postures, sometimes for hours on end. Catatonic phenomena of this kind used to be common and figured prominently in Kraepelin's original descriptions of dementia praecox. Indeed, for an earlier generation of psychiatrists it was an important part of the clinical examination of any psychotic patient to determine which of a variety of other catatonic behaviours they exhibited, including automatic obedience (a wooden, robot-like response to all requests or commands, however silly or pointless), negativism (a similarly wooden response, but the opposite of that required by the request) and waxy flexibility (a curious disturbance of muscle tone in which the patient's limbs could be moved only slowly into new positions, but would then remain exactly as placed for minutes on end). Catatonic phenomena of this kind are rarely seen nowadays in industrialised countries. The reason why this should be so is a mystery, but it serves to emphasise that the clinical features of the illness are not inherent and predetermined but are partly the result of the subject's background and expectations. The behavioural abnormalities prior to first admission for schizophrenia were studied in over 250 cases (Johnstone et al 1986). In addition to bizarre non-understandable behaviour such as that described, behaviour damaging to property or potentially threatening to the life of the patient, or indeed to that of others, occurred in at least 25% of patients.

The chronic stage

Sooner or later the hallucinations and delusions of the acute illness become less. Often they disappear completely, and if they do persist for months or years on end their influence on the patient's behaviour usually wanes. Unfortunately, the disappearance of hallucinations and delusions does not always betoken recovery, even temporarily. Recovery may be, and often is, complete after one or two short-lived episodes of illness. But the more episodes a patient has had, and the more insidiously developing and longer lasting these have been, the more likely it is that some residual damage will remain. This 'defect state' is much less conspicuous than the florid symptoms of the acute illness and may not be apparent at all to those who did not know the patient well before his illness. But in the long run it is a far more serious handicap. In its mildest form it involves nothing more than a subtle loss of vivacity, enthusiasm and emotional responsiveness. More commonly, however, the patient's drive and determination are affected. He becomes apathetic, no longer strives, no longer cares. At the same time, and perhaps fundamentally for the same reason, he loses interest in other people. He talks much less ('paucity of speech') and his capacity to form enduring emotional relationships is greatly reduced. He is no longer capable of falling in love or even developing new friendships, and if unmarried is likely to remain so. It is this apathy and emotional blunting which make schizophrenia the terrible illness it is, because there are permanent changes in the personality which handicap the subject in every sphere – his ability to get and keep a job, to be an effective husband, wife or parent, to achieve anything, to fully enjoy anything.

Most patients with chronic schizophrenia have recurrent psychotic episodes with hallucinations and delusions, usually taking much the same form on each occasion, or faded remnants of earlier delusional systems, as well as this characteristic apathy and emotional blunting. Depression is also a common and important feature of chronic schizophrenia. Indeed, ICD-10 recognises postschizophrenic depression as a distinct subtype of schizophrenia (F20.4). Some patients become depressed in the immediate aftermath of their original psychotic episode, others make an apparently full recovery only to return weeks or months later with widespread depressive symptoms. It is sometimes suggested that this lowering of mood is induced by antipsychotics, but there is no convincing evidence from controlled trials that this is so. More likely, it is partly inherent in schizophrenia and partly an understandable psychological reaction to its dire effects and implications. Although the depression of chronic schizophrenia is rarely as severe, or accompanied by such a widespread disturbance of sleep, appetite and concentration as primary depressive disorders often are, it is none the less an important cause of suffering and disability. Furthermore it is often treatable (see below). Many schizophrenics, at least in the early stages of their illness, are well able to appreciate that it has deprived them of their capacity to enjoy or feel deeply about anything. Self-harm is common – 32% of a sample of 532 individuals with schizophrenia had harmed themselves at least once (Johnstone et al 1991), and some 10% die by suicide, usually in the early years of the illness (Miles 1977).

Frank Fish, and indeed Hughlings Jackson in the 19th century, used to distinguish between positive and negative symptoms, the former being based on some active disturbance of cerebral function, the latter reflecting a reduction or loss of normal function. Crow (1980) developed these concepts in relation to schizophrenia in proposing that there are two pathological processes in the disorder which can occur either separately or together in an individual case. Crow's type I syndrome is characterised by positive symptoms (delusions, hallucinations and thought disorder) and tends to be acute, while the type II syndrome is characterised by negative symptoms (affective flattening, apathy and poverty of speech) and is usually chronic. Problems with this formulation include the question of whether it is the type of symptomatology or the chronicity that is the important factor, and the issue of whether thought disorder should be considered as a positive or a negative symptom. Liddle (1987) then developed these issues further by examining the pattern of correlation between schizophrenic symptoms in a group of patients with illnesses of similar chronicity and found that the symptoms segregated into not two but three distinguishable syndromes: psychomotor poverty (poverty of speech, flatness of affect, decreased spontaneous movement); disorganisation (disorder of form of thought and inappropriate affect); and reality distortion (delusions and hallucinations). This pattern of segregation into three syndromes has been replicated in other studies employing factor analysis of schizophrenic symptoms (for example, Pantelis et al 1991), including a large study of patients with illnesses of variable chronicity (Johnstone & Frith 1996). The work has further been developed by neuropsychological studies (Liddle & Morris 1991) which show that each syndrome is characterised by a specific pattern of test performance, and by studies of regional cerebral blood flow using position emission tomography (Liddle et al 1992) which showed that the different syndromes were associated with altered perfusion in different sites in the brain.

In his original monograph Bleuler had maintained that intelligence, and cognitive function in general, was unimpaired in schizophrenia and this view was generally accepted until recently. It was well known, of course, that many schizophrenics performed poorly on formal tests of intelligence. But it was assumed that this could usually be explained as a secondary consequence of apathy, or of the subject's preoccupation with hallucinatory experiences or delusional ideas. There was no doubt too that chronic schizophrenia was compatible, at least in some people, with high intellectual achievement, and that some of the patients who scored badly on an intelligence test on one occasion performed far better on retesting. This view was challenged by the demonstration by computerised tomography (CT) that many chronic schizophrenics had abnormally large lateral ventricles (Johnstone et al 1976), for if schizophrenia was accompanied by some form of atrophic cerebral pathology, cognitive decline was to be expected. Members of the same Medical Research Council research group at Northwick Park quickly showed that many chronic schizophrenics were disoriented in time and did not even know how old they were (Crow & Stevens 1978) and, when the cognitive abilities of chronic schizophrenics were examined in detail, evidence of widespread impairments was soon found. They have since been extensively studied (for example, McKenna et al 1990, Shallice et al 1991, Frith 1992).

Thought disorder

Thought disorder is a characteristic feature of schizophrenia. This rather unsatisfactory term has traditionally been applied to a variety of ill-defined abnormalities of the subject's speech and writing which are assumed – and it is an assumption – to be secondary to a more fundamental disturbance of thinking. (The term 'formal thought disorder' is sometimes used to emphasise that it is an abnormality of the form rather than of the content of speech, i.e. thought disorder does not embrace delusional ideation.) These abnormalities were first noted by Hecker in 1871 ('a peculiar departure from normal logical sentence structure, with frequent changes in direction that may or may not lose the train of thought'), and then by Kraepelin, but they were studied and described in much more detail by Bleuler who regarded them as a direct consequence of the 'loosening of associations' which he assumed to be the fundamental deficit of schizophrenia. It is therefore to Bleuler that we owe the long-lived assumption that thought disorder was of cardinal importance, aetiologically and diagnostically, and that it was exhibited by all schizophrenics and by no one else. These were unfortunate assumptions for several reasons. No one has ever succeeded in producing a satisfactory definition of the term thought disorder, or in identifying any fundamental psychological or linguistic deficit capable of accounting for the various observable abnormalities of schizophrenic speech. Worse still, few of the abnormalities Bleuler and his successors identified have proved to be specific to schizophrenia, and none to be manifested by more than a proportion of patients with what in other respects are typical schizophrenic illnesses. Indeed, large studies of the symptomatology of schizophrenia (for example, Owens & Johnstone 1980, Johnstone et al 1991) show them to be rare in comparison to delusions and hallucinations.

The most obvious abnormality in the early stages of the illness is the subject's inability to give a straight answer to any but the simplest of questions, so that the interviewer suddenly realises, after talking to his patient for 5 or 10 minutes, that he has not yet learned anything useful. Usually none of the patient's statements or replies has been obviously nonsensical or bizarre, but

almost every one has been vague or irrelevant, and as a result little useful information has been transmitted. This abnormality is sometimes (for example, Wing et al 1974) referred to as poverty of content of thought. Metaphorical terms like 'derailment' and 'Knight's move thinking' have been coined to describe the sudden changes of topic sometimes observed in schizophrenic speech but gross abnormalities of this kind are comparatively rare, at least in the acute illness. More commonly there is a gradual slippage in which a sequence of minor shifts eventually produces a major change of theme. Rochester had drawn attention to another important cause of the listener's difficulty in comprehension – the subject's failure to provide normal cohesive links between one sentence and the next, with the result that the listener is uncertain which of several previously mentioned nouns subsequent pronouns refer to. The problem is often compounded by the subject's preoccupation with abstruse themes and also by his failure to appreciate his listener's difficulties. Quite unlike the aphasic, who is usually distressed by his inability to make his meaning clear, the schizophrenic either fails to appreciate his listener's difficulties or is indifferent to them.

It is sometimes said that thought disorder involves the semantic content rather than the syntactic structure of speech and that the latter remains intact until a very late stage. This is not so. It has been demonstrated by detailed linguistic analysis that the syntactic structure of schizophrenics' speech is quite different from both that of manic and of normal controls (Morice & Ingram 1982), and also that these abnormalities progress with the passage of time. Schizophrenic speech may be harder to comprehend in the acute illness, partly because the patient is often excited and preoccupied with abstruse themes and delusional ideas. Its structure is more abnormal in the chronic stage. Sentence structure becomes more primitive, with fewer and less deeply embedded subordinate clauses, and grammatical errors of varied kinds become more frequent. Above all, the total quantity of speech is reduced.

Bleuler and Kretschmer regarded thought disorder as a result of a generalised 'dissociation' of psychic functions. Subsequently, Babcock suggested that it was simply due to a slowing of all intellectual processes, but later work showed that, although schizophrenics were indeed slower than normals, so too were depressives and psychotics in general. In the 1940s Cameron suggested that 'over-inclusiveness' was the fundamental disability, by which he meant an inability to maintain conceptual boundaries because of a failure to exclude irrelevant associations. This has some empirical support from object sorting tests, and has interesting parallels with the psychophysiological evidence that schizophrenics have difficulty discriminating between relevant and irrelevant sensory information. Both, in other words, might be due to the breakdown of some hypothetical filtering or attentional focusing mechanism. In the 1960s it was claimed, through never fully confirmed, that schizophrenic speech tended to be less 'redundant' than normal speech, so that, if every fourth or fifth word was deleted (the Cloze technique), naive readers were less successful at guessing the identity of the missing words. It is established, however, that schizophrenics tend to use a more restricted range of words, and hence to have a lower 'type:token ratio' than normal people, and that this tendency to repetition applies to syllables as well as to words and phrases, indicating that the cause is something more fundamental than simply having a limited vocabulary. Bannister has also shown that, in terms of Kelly's personal construct theory, schizophrenics' constructs are less stable and more idiosyncratic than those of other people.

Unfortunately, none of these observations has yet proved to be of much practical use and none of these various hypotheses has illuminated the fundamental nature of thought disorder. At present it seems that, however thought disorder is defined, a significant proportion of schizophrenics do not exhibit the phenomenon at all. Worse still, it is also exhibited by patients with other psychiatric disorder, particularly mania, and by several revered dramatists and poets. For this reason, interest in thought disorder has waned in the last 20 years and its diagnostic importance has been downgraded. Andreasen (1979) attempted to define 20 of the terms most widely used to describe different facets of thought disorder, including derailment, tangentiality, clanging and illogicality. She succeeded in demonstrating that most of these terms can be defined and rated with reasonable reliability, and showed which were relatively specific to schizophrenia and which equally or more common in mania. She also suggested replacing the term thought disorder with the less ambiguous but more cumbersome phrase 'disorders of thought, language and communication'. These are valuable achievements, but a more radical approach is needed. Seventy years of research into thought disorder has achieved little, not because Bleuler was wrong in believing that there was something very odd about the speech of many schizophrenics, but because that research was conducted, often without adequate controls, by psychiatrists and psychologists who knew nothing of linguistics. It remains to be seen whether modern linguistic analysis will be any more successful, but future research is more likely to illuminate the fundamental nature of thought disorder if it is based on linguistic concepts like cohesion, lexical density

and dysfluency rather than on ancient clinical metaphors like derailment.

Varieties of schizophrenia

Kraepelin recognised three varieties of schizophrenia – hebephrenic, catatonic and paranoid – and Bleuler added a fourth – simple schizophrenia. Bleuler also said that, although he assumed schizophrenia to be a group of allied conditions rather than a single disease, he regarded these subdivisions as purely provisional, like a classification of tuberculosis into cases with and without haemoptysis, or with and without amyloidosis. It is ironical, therefore, that his four varieties have figured in most classifications of schizophrenia ever since. Although several additional varieties have often been added to them, no schema which attempted to supplant them has ever won more than local acceptance. The expansion of the concept of schizophrenia which took place in the 1940s and 1950s was partly due to the emergence of a series of new concepts, like residual schizophrenia, latent schizophrenia, schizoaffective psychosis (Kasanin 1933), which were added to the original four and had the effect of bringing new types of patients under the schizophrenic rubric.

The new (10th) revision of the ICD (WHO 1992) recognises seven varieties: Bleuler's original four (paranoid, hebephrenic, catatonic and simple) plus undifferentiated schizophrenia, residual schizophrenia and postschizophrenic depression. Schizoaffective states are classified separately from both schizophrenic and affective disorders. Schizotypal disorder, 'a disorder characterised by eccentric behaviour and anomalies of thinking and affect which resemble those seen in schizophrenia, though no definite and characteristic schizophrenic anomalies have occurred at any stage', is now included. Although schizotypal disorder does sometimes evolve into overt schizophrenia it is usually a stable and enduring personality disorder which is relatively common in the close relatives of schizophrenics and assumed to be part of the genetic 'spectrum' of schizophrenia (Kendler et al 1991).

In day-to-day clinical practice most British psychiatrists content themselves with a plain diagnosis of schizophrenia and only use the subcategories for the minority of patients whose symptomatology corresponds closely to one of the subcategory stereotypes. If the illness starts early and insidiously and is dominated by thought disorder and disturbance of affect it is called hebephrenic; if motor abnormalities like posturing or stupor are present it is called catatonic; if hallucinations and delusions are prominent and the personality relatively well preserved it is called paranoid; if progressive deterioration and increasing eccentricity develop in the absence of overt psychotic symptoms it is called simple; and if the original psychotic symptoms have died away, leaving only the apathy, emotional blunting and eccentricity of the defect state, it is called residual. Although the hebephrenic and catatonic forms tend to have the worst prognosis and the paranoid form the best, there are no consistent differences in response to treatment or prognosis between the various categories and patients may show the characteristic symptoms of different varieties at different stages in their careers. Nor is there convincing evidence from family studies that the different varieties 'breed true'. Partly for these reasons contemporary interest is focused primarily on how schizophrenia should best be defined rather than on how it should be subdivided. The current American classification (DSM-IV), (APA 1994), for example, recognises only five varieties – disorganised (hebephrenic), catatonic, paranoid, undifferentiated and residual – and emphasises that the distinction between them is based only on 'the predominant clinical picture that occasioned the most recent evaluation or admission to clinical care' and may therefore change over time.

EPIDEMIOLOGY

In most of the industrial countries in which population surveys have been carried out the lifetime risk of schizophrenia is about 1% and the incidence is of the order of 15 new cases per 100 000 population per annum. In the American Epidemiologic Catchment Area (ECA) survey, for example, which was based on over 18 000 interviews with random population samples in five sites, the lifetime risk for schizophrenia using DSM-III criteria was 1.3% (Regier et al 1988). Studies in Africa and Asia are less numerous and have tended to produce somewhat lower estimates. The International Pilot Study of Schizophrenia established that substantial numbers of schizophrenics were admitted to psychiatric hospitals in all the countries involved (Colombia, Czechoslovakia, Denmark, India, Nigeria, Russia, Taiwan, the UK and the USA) and that their symptoms were remarkably similar in all nine, despite major differences in language, religion, culture and degree of urbanisation (WHO 1973). The main findings of an even larger cross-cultural comparison by the World Health Organization, based on nearly 1400 patients from 12 centres in 10 countries, have been reported since then (Sartorius et al 1986). This study attempted to identify all schizophrenics making a first contact with any treatment agency, including religious institutions and traditional healers, within a defined geographical area, and so was able to generate incidence or inception

rates. Although affective symptoms (mainly depressive) were more common in the industrial countries, and visual and auditory hallucinations and catatonic symptoms more common in the developing countries, the core symptoms of schizophrenia were again remarkably similar in all centres. So too were the inception rates, and also the reasons for admission or referral. When the same operational definition (Catego class S+, which effectively identifies patients with schneiderian first-rank symptoms) was applied in all centres the inception rate ranged only from seven per 100 000 population per year in Aarhus (Denmark) to 14 in Nottingham, with both the urban and rural areas in Chandigarh (India), Dublin, Honolulu, Moscow and Nagasaki in between. This suggests rather strongly that the incidence of schizophrenia is fairly stable across a wide range of cultures, climates and ethnic groupings. Although Torrey (1987) has argued that there may be a 10-fold variation in prevalence from one geographical area to another, with the highest rates in the Arctic and the lowest in the tropics, there appears to be far less variation in the incidence of schizophrenia than for most other common diseases, apart from mental handicap and epilepsy.

It used to be assumed, mainly on the strength of the historical studies of Goldhamer & Marshall (1953) in Massachusetts and Astrup & Odegaard (1960) in Norway, that the incidence of schizophrenia had not changed since the first decades of the 19th century despite the profound social and cultural changes that have taken place since that time. Recently, however, Hare (1988) has marshalled a mass of historical data to support the view that schizophrenia either arose de novo, or at least became much more common, towards the end of the 18th century, and that its prevalence increased steadily for the next 100 years. It is also generally accepted that the presentation of the illness has changed, at least in Europe and North America, since the beginning of the 20th century, the hebephrenic and catatonic forms having become much less common and the paranoid form considerably more common since Kraepelin and Bleuler wrote their classical descriptions. These changes have been accompanied by a gradual improvement in prognosis and a rise in the average age of onset. There have also been several reports of declining hospital first-admission rates for schizophrenia in industrial countries in the last 25 years. Eagles & Whalley (1985) drew attention to a 40% fall in the first-admission rate in Scotland between 1969 and 1978, and similar declines have since been reported in Denmark, England and New Zealand. Although the consistency of these reports is impressive it seems likely that the observed decline is due either to changing diagnostic criteria or to an increasing reluctance to admit schizophrenics to hospital, or some combination of the two (Kendell et al 1993).

The onset of the disease is characteristically between the ages of 15 and 45 years, but it may be before puberty, or delayed until the seventh or eighth decades. Although schizophrenia is equally common in men and women, male schizophrenics are consistently admitted to hospital 4 or 5 years earlier than females, and this appears to reflect a genuine and unexplained difference in the age of onset in the two sexes (Häfner et al 1989). The incidence is considerably higher in the unmarried than the married in both sexes and both also have a considerably reduced fertility (see below).

The first-admission rate for schizophrenia is generally higher in urban than in rural areas, and much higher from the central areas of large cities then from the surrounding suburbs. Faris & Dunham (1939) first drew attention to this striking phenomenon in Chicago and it has since been confirmed in several other American and European cities. The highest admission rates are consistently from the poor working class areas adjacent to the business district and the railway stations and the lowest rates from the middle-class suburbs. This geographical gradient is accompanied by an equally impressive social class gradient, the admission rate of social classes IV and V (unskilled and semiskilled manual workers) being consistently higher than that of other occupational groupings. These findings were originally regarded as evidence that being brought up in a working class family, or in the central slum areas of a big city, created a predisposition to develop schizophrenia, and indeed a recent study of Swedish conscripts found a raised incidence of schizophrenia in those with an urban upbringing (Lewis et al 1992). Even so, it is generally believed that both phenomena are mainly due to selective migration and that the excess of schizophrenic admissions from city centres is largely due to the high admission rate of people who have moved there relatively recently, into bedsitters, hostels or lodging houses. Similarly, Goldberg & Morrison (1963) were able to show, by examining the birth certificates of a series of 672 young male schizophrenics, that although they themselves were predominantly from social classes IV and V, their fathers' social class had not differed from that of the general population, and that the disparity between the two was due to a 'downward drift' of the sons a few months or years before their admission to hospital. The young man, for example, who had started at university or became apprenticed had drifted away before finishing and was working as a labourer (and probably living in lodgings as well) at the time he was eventually admitted to hospital.

Migration has also long been associated with an increased risk of schizophrenic breakdown. Odegaard (1932) found the Norwegians who had emigrated to Minnesota had a higher risk of schizophrenic breakdown than those who had remained in Norway, and Malzberg & Lee (1956) showed that immigrants to New York had a much higher hospital admission rate than native born Americans, with their children halfway between. More recently, Cochrane (1977) has shown that most immigrant groups to England and Wales, particularly West Indians, Asians and Poles, have higher hospital admission rates for schizophrenia than the English and the Scots. Similar findings have been reported from other countries but the relationship is not invariable. Jaco (1960), for example, failed to find any increased risk of schizophrenia in Spanish-speaking immigrants to Texas. At times the cause of this increased risk has had considerable political as well as scientific significance, with the host country or community being tempted to attribute the phenomenon to a selective migration of unstable undesirables, and the immigrants themselves and their fellow-countrymen back home attributing it to the stresses of living in a foreign and sometimes hostile land. In reality, it is not yet firmly established that the incidence of schizophrenia is increased in immigrants. Most studies have been based on hospital admissions, and psychiatrically disturbed immigrants are more likely to be admitted to mental hospitals than other people. Once admitted they are also at greater risk of being labelled as schizophrenic, particularly if their behaviour is unusual and the examining doctor has difficulty communicating with them. Moreover, most comparisons between immigrant and native populations have not matched the two for age, a crucial omission because most immigrants are young adults and schizophrenia is a disease of young adults.

It has recently been reported that the Afro-Caribbean populations of several English cities have extremely high hospital admission rates for schizophrenia, perhaps 10 times as high as that of their white neighbours (McGovern & Cope 1987, Harrison et al 1988). Although it seems unlikely that differences of this magnitude could be generated by racial biasing of diagnostic criteria, inaccurate demographic assumptions (there were no questions about ethnicity in the 1981 census) or ethnic differences in contact rates with psychiatric services, these findings, which are largely generated by people born in the UK rather than first-generation immigrants, are bound to be controversial and politically sensitive until rigorously designed epidemiological comparisons have been carried out. No adequate explanation for this very high hospital admission rate has yet been offered, partly because at present it is unclear whether Afro-Caribbeans have a similarly high incidence of schizophrenia in the Caribbean. The widespread use of cannabis may be a partial explanation.

The fertility of schizophrenics has been studied many times and there is general agreement that they marry less often than other people, remain childless more often even when they do marry, and have fewer children than other people in or out of wedlock. In the past this was usually attributed to their confinement in sexually segregated asylums. However, it is now apparent that their fertility is low even before admission to hospital, and studies carried out in the 1960s and 1970s after the introduction of 'open door' policies confirm that, despite the increased opportunities for marrying and conceiving thus provided, schizophrenics still have far fewer children than other people.

Schizophrenics also have a raised mortality. Studies in Europe and North America suggest that their relative risk of death is increased twofold and most of this increased risk is accounted for by the first few years after diagnosis or hospital admission. Although this raised mortality is shared by other forms of mental illness, there have been repeated claims of associations, both positive and negative, between schizophrenia and other physical illnesses (Baldwin 1979). The only one of these relationships that seems well established at the present time is a negative, and as yet unexplained, association between schizophrenia and rheumatoid arthritis. Despite many conflicting claims it is not established that schizophrenics are either more or less likely to develop cancers in general, or any particular form of cancer, than other people. Nor is the claimed association between schizophrenia and coeliac disease supported by convincing evidence.

One of the most important reasons for studying the epidemiology of a disease is to obtain clues to its aetiology. At one time the striking relationships found between schizophrenia and the central areas of big cities, low social class, being unmarried and being a migrant all seemed capable of providing that vital clue. But the relationship with migration is still in doubt and the other three have turned out to be consequences rather than causes of the disorder. There is, however, one important relationship which is safe from this risk and must have some aetiological significance: the relationship between schizophrenia and season of birth. It has been found in virtually every country in the temperate latitudes of the northern hemisphere that schizophrenic first admissions are more likely to have been born in the early months of the year than the rest of the population, and correspondingly less likely to have been born in July to September. This relationship is not shared by other diagnostic categories and, although the excess of births in January to March is only about 8%, it is consistent and highly significant statistically (Bradbury & Miller 1985). In Australia and South Africa the excess of births is in July to September (i.e. the winter months, as in Europe). Preliminary evidence also indicates that the siblings of schizophrenics show the same distribution of birth dates as the general population and that the excess of winter births of schizophrenics is greater the colder the winter. This suggests that the incidence of schizophrenia is influenced by some widely distributed seasonal variable, probably infective or dietary, acting either in utero or in the early months of life. Intrauterine viral infection is one such possibility, for many viral infections have a well-defined seasonal variation, and rubella demonstrates that an inconspicuous infection in a young woman may cause permanent damage to the fetal nervous system if she is pregnant at the time. There have been several reports in recent years, from Finland, Denmark, England and Scotland, that fluctuations in the birth dates of schizophrenics can be related to fluctuations in the incidence of influenza 2 or 3 months beforehand (for example, see Sham et al 1992), suggesting that damage to the fetus in the sixth or seventh month of pregnancy may be aetiologically important. Another issue of interest is severe maternal food deprivation during pregnancy. This is of course by no means rare but is often associated with civil disorganisation and a failure of collection of organised records such as registration of births. In northern Holland, at the end of the Second World War during the winter of 1944–1945 the entire population was severely deprived of food. The deprivation was relatively circumscribed in time and organised record keeping was maintained. An increased rate of schizophrenia was found in the daughters of women who suffered severe food deprivation during the first trimester of pregnancy (Susser & Lin 1992). Until the mechanism involved is established, however, the meaning of these potentially important findings will remain unclear.

AETIOLOGY

The causes of schizophrenia are not fully understood. None the less, a number of factors are now known to be relevant to the aetiology – and we have moved a very long way from the position outlined by Kraepelin in 1919: 'the causes of dementia praecox are at the present time still mapped in impenetrable darkness'. Indeed the current position has been described in optimistic terms by Weinberger (1995) '20 years ago, the principal challenge for schizophrenia research was to gather objective scientific evidence that would implicate the brain. This challenge no longer exists.' He is probably right but it has been so rewarding for those investigating the biological basis of schizophrenia to be able to say that there is good evidence that this dreadful disease is associated with identifiable lesions which will one day

Table 13.2 Biological factors relevant to the aetiology of schizophrenia

- Familiality of the disorder
- Occurrence of 'schizophrenic-like' psychoses
- Pharmacological mechanism of antipsychotic drugs
- Miscellaneous effects relating to pregnancy and birth complications
- Brain changes demonstrable by structural imaging
- Changes in regional cerebral blood flow (in relation to neuropsychological test performed) demonstrated by functional imaging

Table 13.3 Nature of organic diagnoses in Northwick Park study of first schizophrenic episodes (Johnstone et al 1987)

Organic diagnosis	No. of cases
Alcohol excess/withdrawal	3
Drug abuse/withdrawal	2
Syphilis	3
Carcinoma of the lung	1
Autoimmune multisystem disease (systemic lupus erythematosus)	1
Thyrotoxicosis	1
Cerebrovascular accident	1
Sarcoidosis	2
Cerebral cysticercosis with secondary epilepsy	1

yield to investigation that it has not always been easy to see that the next challenge must be addressed. Efforts must now be directed to exploring the mechanisms by which the factors known to be relevant to the aetiology allow the demonstrated lesions to produce the clinical features of schizophrenia.

Biological factors

The biological factors known to be relevant to the aetiology of schizophrenia may conveniently be considered under the headings listed in Table 13.2.

Familiality

It has long been known that schizophrenia is a disorder with a familial tendency. This suggests that genetic factors are likely to be important, but of course disorders can be familial because family members share the same disadvantaged environment – for example, tuberculosis where infection can spread from one family member to another and rickets where relatives are likely to share the same poor diet and living conditions. As far as schizophrenia is concerned the matter of whether the relevant factor was shared genetic material or shared environment was elegantly clarified by the adoption studies of Kety et al (1975), who found high rates of schizophrenia in the biological relatives of schizophrenics who had been adopted away at birth and high rates of the later development of schizophrenia in children of schizophrenic mothers who had been adopted away at birth. Clearly it is shared genetic material that is relevant and further details of genetic studies in this area are described in Chapter 7.

'Schizophrenic-like' psychoses

In the great majority of schizophrenic patients the ill-

ness develops in the absence of demonstrable organic disease. None the less, certain organic diseases, which could not result from any of the social and environmental disadvantages secondary to the disorder, occur in association with schizophrenia more often than would be expected by chance (Davison & Bagley 1969). The conditions are many and varied so that it is difficult to see any common path by which they could all come to produce the same clinical picture, although there is some tendency for them to affect the temporal lobes of the brain. When the occurrence of these conditions was studied in relation to a large defined cohort of first schizophrenic episodes (Johnstone et al 1987), underlying organic disease of at least possible aetiological significance was found in 15 of 268 cases (6%) (Table 13.3). The worrying possibility that other organic cases are missed is obvious but this cohort was followed up for a further 5 years and no additional relevant illnesses were known to develop. Clarification of the mechanism by which those conditions produce schizophrenic-like psychoses is likely to illuminate our understanding of the pathogenesis of the generality of schizophrenia.

Antipsychotic drugs

Chlorpromazine was introduced into psychiatric practice by Delay & Deniker in 1952 and by the early 1960s it was clear that phenothiazines relieved schizophrenic symptoms and were not simply supersedatives. A large number of other antipsychotic agents were introduced and it became evident that they all shared the property of blockade of D_2 dopamine receptors and that their antipsychotic efficacy was proportional to their ability to block these receptors. By the early 1970s a number of pieces of evidence led to the conclusion that antischizophrenic drugs acted by blocking D_2 receptors. Although there was no evidence of an excess of dopaminegic transmission in schizophrenia, the fact that reduction in such transmission by antipsychotic drugs was consistently effective in controlling the disorder was considered very much suggestive of the possibility that dopaminagic transmission must have some central role in the underlying mechanisms of schizophrenia. The evidence for this position has been made much less clear by the demonstration that clozapine (a weak D_2 antagonist with a wide range of other pharmacological effects) is in some circumstances of greater efficacy against psychotic symptoms than traditional antipsychotics which are much more effective D_2 blockers. The conclusion is that D_2 blockade and some other pharmacological mechanism is more effective in antipsychotic terms than D_2 blockade alone. Intensive investigation of the possible additional mechanisms is being conducted at present and when replicable results have been established they may lead to the production of more effective treatments as well as to greater understanding of antipsychotic mechanisms. In the meantime the relatively consistent relationships between antipsychotic effects and pharmacological mechanisms provide evidence for the importance of neurotransmission in schizophrenia, although we are less certain about the type of neurotransmission that is involved than we thought we were some years ago.

Pregnancy and birth complications

This evidence includes the well-documented tendency for individuals who later develop schizophrenia to have been born in the winter months of the year, and the possible effects of maternal influenza or food deprivation in pregnancy described above. In addition a number of studies have examined the frequency of perinatal and birth complications in individuals who go on to develop schizophrenia in comparison with controls. These studies have variable findings (McNeil 1987, Done et al 1991) and are not always easy to interpret because many of them are retrospective but there certainly is some evidence that birth complications are associated with the later development of schizophrenia.

Brain changes

Pneumoencephalographic studies of schizophrenia conducted since the 1920s have indicated that there is a degree of ventricular enlargement and a reduction of brain tissue but they were difficult to interpret because of the problems of conducting this investigation in control subjects. The introduction of non-invasive imaging (CT and later magnetic resonance imaging (MRI)) allowed controlled studies to be carried out and the finding of enlarged ventricular spaces in schizophrenia (Johnstone et al 1976) has been widely replicated. Later studies have suggested cerebral cortical volumes (Harvey et al 1993, Zipursky et al 1994) are reduced and some have indicated particular involvement of temporal lobe structures (Shenton et al 1992). These findings have stimulated a resurgence of interest in the neuropathological work in schizophrenia which was first conducted in the early part of this century. Recent work has indicated that the brains of patients with schizophrenia are smaller and lighter and that they have an excess non-specific focal pathology (Jellinger 1985, Bruton et al 1990). Subtle cytoarchitectural abnormalities in the hippocampus and in the cerebral cortex in schizophrenia have been found by a variety of writers (Kovelman & Schiebel 1984, Jacob & Beckman 1986, Benes et al 1986, Pakkenberg 1990, Conrad et al 1991). These findings have been interpreted as indicating that schizophrenia may be a disorder of neurodevelopment (Murray & Lewis 1987, Falkai & Bogerts 1995, Weinberger 1995).

Changes in regional cerebral blood flow

In 1974, Ingvar & Franzen demonstrated that patients with schizophrenia had relatively reduced cerebral blood flow in the frontal lobes. This 'hypofrontality' was confirmed in some subsequent studies but not in others. More recently studies comparing activity during performance of a specific neuropsychogical test and that in a reference condition have been conducted (neuropsychological challenge studies). A variety of studies have been carried out and, taken together, they may be interpreted as indicating imbalances between neuronal activity at diverse interconnected brain sites rather than abnormal function at a single location. There is a difficulty in activating various regions and this has been interpreted as indicating that in schizophrenia there is a disturbed connectivity between cerebral areas (Friston & Frith 1995).

These various biological factors are described in more detail in Chapter 16.

Social factors

Although the twin and adoption studies described in Chapter 7 prove beyond reasonable doubt that schizophrenia is genetically transmitted, this evidence also established that environmental influences must play a major role as well, for estimates of the concordance rate in monozygotic twins derived from whole populations are consistently less than 50%. In other words, someone whose genetically identical twin develops schizophrenia has less than a 50:50 chance of doing the same, and whether or not he does so must depend on his past or present environment.

In the last 40 years the possibility that pathological relationships or patterns of communication within the nuclear family may lead, at least in genetically vulnerable children, to the eventual development of schizophrenia has received a great deal of attention, particularly in the USA. In the 1940s Freda Fromm-Reichmann coined the phrase 'schizophrenogenic mother' and later workers supported the concept, with claims that the mothers of schizophrenics were both overprotective and hostile to their children. A few years later Bateson at Palo Alto (Bateson et al 1956) suggested that schizophrenia was produced by the constant reception of incongruent messages from a key relative – to take a trite example, the verbal message 'You know that Mummy loves you' accompanied by non-verbal behaviour implying something quite different – and this 'double-bind hypothesis' remained in vogue for a decade or more. Shortly afterwards, Lidz and his colleagues at Yale carried out a series of intensive studies of 17 upper middle-class families with what they regarded as schizophrenic children. They described several highly abnormal relationships within these families which differed with the sex of the schizophrenic child and which they suggested were associated with the development of schizophrenia in this son or daughter (Lidz et al 1965). Their work aroused great interest and their terms 'marital schism' and 'marital skew' obtained the same wide currency at Bateson's 'double-bind'. Unfortunately, these studies all had serious methodological defects and owed their influence more to their catch phrases and the prevailing climate of opinion than to objective evidence. They were not conducted blind, had no adequate control groups, involved a very diffuse concept of schizophrenia and were retrospective, so that it was difficult to tell which of the observed abnormalities had preceded the onset of schizophrenia in the child, and might therefore have some aetiological significance, and which were merely reactions to the child's illness.

Alongside these global studies of parental personalities and family interactions a series of more limited and better designed studies of communication patterns in schizophrenic and non-schizophrenic families was carried out. The most influential of these were by Singer & Wynne (1965) who gave Rorschach tests to the parents of schizophrenics and claimed that they consistently produced more deviant responses (i.e. that they were more 'thought disordered') than control parents. However, when Hirsch & Leff (1975) repeated this work they were unable to confirm Wynne's findings. Although there was a significant difference between the average deviance scores of the parents of schizophrenics

and the parents of neurotic controls, the overlap was considerable and the higher deviance scores of the former were entirely due to the fact that they spoke at greater length, i.e. there was no difference in the rate at which the two groups made deviant responses.

What then survives from all this? There is some evidence that the parents of schizophrenics are emotionally disturbed more often than the parents of normal children and that more of the mothers have schizoid personality traits. Moreover, it is claimed that the parents of schizophrenics seem to be in conflict with one another more often than the parents of other psychiatric patients, and the mothers more concerned about and protective towards their children. These unfortunate people do of course have a very great deal to worry them. It could be claimed that there was scope in all this for baneful influence on the preschizophrenic child, but as yet there is no convincing evidence that any of these influences do in fact contribute to the development of schizophrenia. Furthermore, all the well-substantiated parental abnormalities are easily explicable in genetic terms, and none is invariably present.

Events in the weeks or months immediately prior to the onset of illness have received less attention than the events of childhood but there is some evidence that they may be important. Steinberg & Durrell (1968) showed in the 1960s that the schizophrenic breakdown rate of recruits to the US army was much higher in their first month of military service than at any time in the next 2 years, suggesting that the transition from civilian life to recruiting barracks was contributing to the genesis of these illnesses. The effect was the same in volunteers as in enlisted men and they were able to produce fairly convincing evidence that the illnesses presenting in the first month of service were indeed new and not merely newly detected. Further evidence was provided by Brown & Birley (1968), who obtained detailed information about the events of the previous 12 weeks from 50 patients with schizophrenic illnesses of recent onset and 400 controls from the same neighbourhood. They found that the schizophrenics had experienced significantly more life events than the controls in the 3 weeks immediately prior to the onset of illness, but only in those 3 weeks. The difference between schizophrenics and controls remained, even when all events which might have been a consequence of incipient illness (i.e. losing a job by being sacked as opposed to the closure of the firm) were eliminated. It has to be borne in mind, however, that the concept of schizophrenia employed in both these studies was a broad one. In Brown & Birley's study, 24 patients were only 'probably schizophrenic' and, furthermore, only 24 of the 50 were first admissions.

More attention has been paid to the determinants of

relapse in those who have already had one episode of schizophrenia, mainly because the comparatively high probability of a further episode makes it feasible to mount prospective studies. Brown et al (1972) showed that the relapse rate over the next 12 months in young men who had just recovered from a first episode of schizophrenia was far higher (58% versus 16%) in those who returned to live with a relative, usually a parent or wife, who was prone to make critical comments about them than in those who lived with a relative who was more tolerant and accepting. Moreover, the ill-effects of what the authors called 'high expressed emotion' or high EE were mitigated to some extent if the patient was receiving antipsychotic drugs, and also if patient and relative were in contact with one another for less than 35 hours a week, i.e. social withdrawal seemed to be protective. These findings have been confirmed by Vaughn & Leff (1976) and Vaughn et al (1984) in California, and since that time have been widely although not invariably replicated (Bebbington & Kuipers 1994). A combination of the results of 25 studies of expressed emotion involving 1246 cases showed a relapse rate for high EE cases of 50% compared with 21% in low EE cases (Bebbington et al 1995). This result is overwhelmingly significant ($P < 0.00001$). The origins of the behaviour measured by EE are uncertain. It is possible that the EE measure is predictive at least in part because relatives respond in a particular way to sufferers whose illness in any case has a poor prognosis. There is evidence that at least some components of high EE are associated with a variety of abnormalities in the patient (Miklowitz et al 1983, Mavreas et al 1992). Birchwood & Smith (1987) argue that high EE develops over time as part of the coping style of relatives in response to the difficulty of living with someone with schizophrenia. The fact that high EE is less evident in relatives of first-episode patients than in those with subsequent admissions is used in support of this argument.

Psychological theories

Innumerable psychological theories of both the aetiology and the pathogenesis of schizophrenia have been proposed in the past. Many were derived from psychoanalysis, others from behavioural or cognitive psychology. Apart from the defective filter theory of sensory overload, few were backed by any substantial empirical data and most are now of only historical interest. Recently, however, some new and more promising hypotheses have been propounded.

Frith (1992) has suggested that it is possible to explain the symptoms and signs of schizophrenia in terms of abnormalities of three main cognitive processes:

Table 13.4 Three principal abnormalities of cognitive process which underlie schizophrenia (Frith 1992)	
• Inability to generate willed action	Poverty of action Perseveration Inappropriate action (distractibility, disorganised action)
• Inability to monitor willed action	Delusions of passivity Certain auditory hallucinations Thought insertion
• Inability to monitor the beliefs and intentions of others	Delusions of reference Paranoid delusions Third-person hallucinations Certain kinds of incoherence

- Negative symptoms and some inappropriate behaviours, e.g. perseverations, may be considered as the result of inability to generate spontaneous (willed) actions.
- Some positive symptoms, e.g. passivity experiences, auditory and somatic hallucinations, may be considered the result of a lack of awareness of the prior intention that accompanies a deliberate act. Being unaware of their own intentions, patients will experience their own actions, thoughts and subvocal (and perhaps vocal) speech as resulting from some source other than themselves.
- Delusions of persecution and reference may be understood as the result of an inability to correctly infer the intentions of other people. Similarly their inferences about what other people are thinking may be incorrectly perceived as information coming from an external source. This could provide an explanation for third person auditory hallucinations.

In terms of this theory schizophrenia may be explained as a defect of the mechanism (referred to as 'meta representation') which enables us to be aware of our goals and our intentions and to infer the beliefs and intentions of others (Table 13.4).

Frith has gone on to develop this work in relation to changes in regional cerebral blood flow (demonstrated by functional brain imaging) in response to provocative neuropsychological tests. This has led him to suggest that the failure of some schizophrenic patients to distinguish between their own actions and intentions and internal events may be due to a functional disconnection between frontal brain areas concerned with action and more posterior areas concerned with perception (Frith 1996). Much of this is of course speculation but the possibility of testing the components of the theory against demonstrable physiological changes (i.e. changes in regional blood flow) means that specific hypotheses derived from it will be able to be formally tested.

Animal models of serious mental disorders have obvious problems and are less fashionable than they were at one time. Latent inhibition has however continued to be studied. It is a phenomenon, readily demonstrable in animals and man, whereby repeated exposure to a stimulus without consequence retards subsequent conditioning to that stimulus. (For example, a rat repeatedly exposed to a particular odour will take longer to learn the significance of that odour if the odour is subsequently paired with a rewarding or punishing stimulus.) It has recently been shown that, although schizophrenics in remission display latent inhibition in the same way as normal controls, acutely ill schizophrenics do not (Baruch et al 1988). Quite apart from the intrinsic interest of a simple and widely applicable paradigm in which schizophrenics perform better than normals, latent inhibition is known to be abolished in rats by amphetamine, and to be strengthened by antipsychotics. It has the makings, therefore, of a promising animal model of schizophrenia, and the potential to link the neurochemical dopamine hypothesis with the cognitive evidence that schizophrenics are unable to filter out, or ignore, irrelevant sensory information. As will be seen in the section on treatment however, there are increasing problems for the dopamine hypothesis.

Summary

The most plausible synthesis of the genetic, neuropathological and epidemiological evidence described above and in Chapters 6 and 7 is that schizophrenia is a neurodevelopmental disorder, as Weinberger (1995) has suggested. The architecture of the hippocampus and other temporal lobe structures, and the connections between these and the frontal lobes, are abnormal in at least a substantial proportion of schizophrenics. These abnormalities may either be genetically determined or produced by injury to the developing brain (mediated perhaps by disruption of the normal sequence of neuronal migrations), either in utero or at the time of birth. This would account for the enlarged lateral ventricles of schizophrenics, the changes in their brains found at postmortem examination and the subtle intellectual and social disabilities of schizophrenic children before the overt onset of their illness.

The 20–30 year delay before the onset of the psychosis could be explained in maturational terms.

Myelination and synaptic pruning are not complete in the frontal lobes until or after puberty, and it has been shown that the behaviour of infant monkeys with surgical lesions of their dorsolateral prefrontal cortex does not become overtly abnormal until they are adult (Weinberger 1987). A model of this kind could explain many of the best established facts about schizophrenia. There are, of course, major speculative elements in the model but it does at least provide, almost for the first time, a plausible conceptual framework to guide future research.

COURSE AND PROGNOSIS

Although Kraepelin's original concept of dementia praecox was founded on the belief that such illnesses all progressed to a state of global deterioration, or at least resulted in permanent damage to the personality, the outcome of schizophrenic illnesses, as Kraepelin himself eventually came to realise, is in fact very variable, however the syndrome is defined. Some resolve completely, with or without treatment, and never recur. Some recur repeatedly with full recovery every time. Others recur repeatedly but recovery is incomplete; that is, there is a persistent defect state that characteristically becomes more pronounced after each successive relapse. Finally, some illnesses pursue a progressive downhill course from the beginning. The relative frequency of these different outcomes depends a great deal on how schizophrenia is defined. If it is defined in such a way as to exclude those with prominent affective symptoms, the proportion of patients making a full recovery is reduced; and if the diagnosis is also restricted, as it is by the Feighner and DSM-IV definitions, to patients with a 6 month history, the proportion recovering without permanent defect is reduced still further.

The matter of predicting the type of course that the illness of individual patients will take is naturally an issue of clinical importance. Schofield et al (1954) and Vaillant (1964), in the days before operational definitions for schizophrenia were used, defined factors predictive of outcome. To some extent these were of features less than central to the disorder. Vaillant's seven items predictive of good outcome were: acute onset; a stressful precipitating event; family history of depressive illness; no family history of schizophrenia; absence of schizoid traits in the premorbid personality; confusion or perplexity; prominent affective symptoms. The development of more closely defined criteria for schizophrenia might have been expected to improve the prediction of outcome but this hope has not really been realised. Studies have been conducted in which more and less restrictive criteria for the diagnoses have been applied to groups of patients who were then followed up for periods of years (for example, Hawk et al (1975, Kendell et al 1979). On the whole the criteria were not very successful in identifying groups of patients with a poor outcome, and in general what success there was lay in defining symptomatic rather than social outcome. Many studies of outcome have been published over the years. Mayer-Gross in 1932 published a 16 year follow-up of 294 cases. Many of these studies class patients in simple categories of outcome such as 'recovered', 'improved' and 'not improved' (for review, see Johnstone 1990). Interpretation of even such simple terms can vary: some classing patients as recovered when their delusions, although present, are not readily revealed, and others classing such individuals as having continuing symptoms. Among the more optimistic of relatively recent studies is that of Harding et al (1987), where 82 patients fulfilling DSM-III criteria and referred to a rehabilitation programme in 1955–1960 were followed up in 1980–1982. No more than a few symptoms were found in two-thirds of the patients and 40% had been employed in the previous year. A detailed study of 532 patients discharged from inpatient care in a London borough between 1975 and 1985 and followed up between 1987 and 1990 was conducted by Johnstone et al (1991) and produced rather less reassuring findings. The mean number of admissions required during the follow-up period was 5.4, and on average patients spent 14 months out of 10 years as inpatients. The heterogeneity of outcome of schizophrenia was very evident in this study and, while there were some striking successes, unemployment, social difficulties and a restricted lifestyle were common and many patients had continuing symptoms.

Outcome seems to be determined more by the circumstances under which the illness develops and the premorbid personality than by the symptomatology of the illness itself. Illnesses that develop acutely in response to stress have a much better prognosis than those that develop insidiously for no apparent reason. And if the patient has prominent schizoid personality traits, particularly if he is also young, of low intelligence and has a poor work record, the outlook is much bleaker than if he is married, more mature and with a more normal personality. Several studies have also reported a worse prognosis, at least where hospital discharge rates are concerned, in men than in women. Social considerations are partly responsible for this difference. In many societies women lead rather more protected lives than men. They are more likely to possess the basic housekeeping skills needed for survival outside hospital, and also pose less threat of violence to others. But the fact

that women also have a later age of onset than men suggests that there are intrinsic differences in the nature of the illness between the sexes.

Illnesses, of course, do not have an outcome in vacuo, or even a natural history. Outcome is always affected for good or ill by treatment and other environmental influences, and there is little doubt that the outcome of schizophrenia has improved considerably in the last 50 years. Follow-up studies conducted in the 1920s and 1930s, before any effective treatments were available, only reported full recovery in about 12% of patients, and at least 70% were either unimproved or dead at the time of assessment (Stalker 1939). Since the 1950s all comparable follow-up studies have shown much better results. Wing's (1966) 5 year follow-up of 111 schizophrenic first admissions to three mental hospitals in southern England is as representative as any. Only 7% of these patients remained in hospital as long as 2 years, only 28% spent any part of the last 2 years in hospital, and at the time of final follow-up 63% of the men were employed and 69% of the women were either employed or successfully running a household. To what extent this improvement was due to the phenothiazine drugs introduced in 1953 and to what extent it was due to the changes in the milieu of mental hospitals and in public attitudes to mental illness taking place simultaneously is difficult to determine, but the combination certainly produced a substantial change. In most industrial countries the number of mental hospital beds fell by at least 50% between 1950 and 1990, and although financial and political considerations played an important role in many places, the major cause of this massive reduction was the changed outlook and management of schizophrenia. There is little doubt, though, that the effects of antipsychotics on the long-term prognosis of schizophrenia are less impressive than the short-term effects. Although contemporary patients spend less time in hospital than their predecessors, and are far less likely to end their days as permanent hospital invalids, a disturbingly high proportion still remain chronically handicapped by defect states or recurring hallucinations and delusions and still require repeated admissions to hospital despite long-term drug therapy.

The follow-up studies described so far were all carried out in the industrialised countries of western Europe and North America. There is, however, fairly substantial evidence that the prognosis of schizophrenia is considerably better in so-called underdeveloped countries, despite their meagre psychiatric services. The most important evidence to this effect comes from the International Pilot Study of Schizophrenia. In that study a large series of psychotic patients, the majority of whom were schizophrenics, were studied in nine different centres in different parts of the world. The same structured interviewing methods were used in all nine centres and the patients were reinterviewed at 2 years and 5 years, again using the same methods and criteria throughout. Quite unexpectedly, the average outcome was considerably better in the underdeveloped countries (Colombia, India and Nigeria) than in the industrialised countries (Czechoslovakia, Denmark, the UK, the USA and Russia) (Sartorius et al 1977). The difference did not lie in the proportion of patients pursuing a steady downhill course (pattern D); this was much the same throughout. It lay in the proportion suffering recurrent relapses. Despite the much more extensive follow-up treatment available in the industrial countries, a high proportion of their patients had further psychotic episodes, whereas Colombian, Nigerian and Indian patients did not. The same finding had emerged from an earlier comparison of the outcome of schizophrenia in London and Mauritius. Although careful comparisons of the initial symptomatology and other characteristics of the patients from the nine study centres did not reveal any important differences between them, the possibility that these differences in outcome were due to unrecognised differences in the types of patients admitted to hospital in the nine centres can obviously not be excluded. Certainly people with acute behavioural disturbances are more likely to come to medical attention in settings where psychiatric services are novel and thinly spread than are those with insidiously developing disorders that do not cause the same alarm; and the former are, of course, likely to have a better prognosis than the latter. Partly to elucidate these intriguing differences in outcome the WHO mounted a further international comparison, involving 12 centres in 10 countries, known as the Determinants of Outcome of Severe Mental Disorders Programme. The preliminary results of this major study confirm that, at follow-up 2 years after their initial inception into treatment, schizophrenic illnesses have a better prognosis in developing than in developed countries (Sartorius et al 1986). Part, but only part, of this difference is attributable to a higher proportion of illnesses in the developed countries having a relatively insidious onset. It seems likely, therefore, that there is something about the social organisation of contemporary industrial societies, or their family structure or attitude to mental illness, which has a deleterious effect on the course of schizophrenic disorders.

Schizophrenia used to be regarded as a steadily progressive disease with a poor prognosis. It is now clear that this is not so, or perhaps no longer so. Not only is the long-term prognosis rather better than we used to believe, the course of the illness is very variable, and its outcome worse in industrial than in developing countries, and probably worse in urban than in rural areas within industrial countries. Indeed a recent comparison has shown that the functioning of schizophrenic patients in the rural district of Nithsdale in Scotland was higher than that of similar patients from South London (McCreadie et al 1997). To what extent this is due to the much higher use of the psychiatric services by the Nithsdale population is a matter for speculation. On the whole patients do not deteriorate further after the first 5–10 years, and even chronic patients may show surprising changes, either improvement or deterioration, after many years of apparent stability. These facts are difficult to reconcile with the idea that schizophrenia is a steadily progressive brain disease; they force us to consider aetiological hypotheses of quite different kinds. Schizophrenia also seems to have a better prognosis now than it had at the beginning of the 20th century and, at least in industrial countries, its clinical presentation has changed. The catatonic and hebephrenic forms have become much less frequent, and paranoid forms more frequent. These changes and differences are usually attributed to advances in treatment and to the pathoplastic effects of cultural differences and social changes. It is possible, however, that they are actually due to a slowly progressive change in the nature of the disease, as occurred with general paresis during the 19th century and with scarlet fever in the 20th.

If such a change has indeed taken place, it is likely to be due to some change in the environmental factors contributing to the aetiology of the condition.

TREATMENT

Physical methods

Before the 1930s there was no effective treatment for any of the so-called functional psychoses and the prime function of mental hospitals was to keep their patients in tolerable comfort and physical health in the hope that spontaneous remission would take place. Regimens were essentially custodial, with whatever occupational, recreational and spiritual accompaniments local custom and resources allowed. The introduction of Sakel's insulin therapy in 1933, Moniz's prefrontal leucotomy and von Meduna's convulsive therapy in 1935 and Cerletti's ECT in 1938, and the possibilities of cure which these dramatic new therapies seemed to offer, had a profound effect on the atmosphere and morale of mental hospitals throughout the world. ECT and insulin coma therapy were both widely used throughout the 1940s and thousands of patients were enthusiastically subjected to prefrontal leucotomy. The discovery of the tranquillising effects of chlorpromazine by

Charpentier & Laborit in the 1950s had an even more profound effect, and within a few years of the introduction of these new phenothiazine drugs the insulin coma regimen and leucotomy both passed into a rapid decline. ECT remained in widespread use much longer, but mainly in combination with phenothiazines, or as a second-line treatment for patients who had failed to respond to these drugs.

Antipsychotic drugs such as phenothiazines, butyrophenones and thioxanthenes were initially used in schizophrenia for the purpose of treating the positive symptoms of acute episodes. In the 1960s several large-scale trials demonstrated that these drugs were highly effective in combating such symptoms and were not merely supersedatives (Hollister et al 1960, National Institute of Mental Health 1964). None the less, about 30% of patients show only limited effects in such trials (Davis 1976) and about 7% of cases do not appear to show any response at all, even to prolonged treatment (Tuma & May 1979, Macmillan et al 1986). The management of the positive symptoms of acute episodes is only one aspect of the management of schizophrenia and it is not difficult to make the case that the reduction of relapse rates and the treatment of the negative symptoms of the defect state are at least as important. Many studies have focused upon the role of antipsychotic drugs in reducing schizophrenic relapse. Benefits of both oral (Leff & Wing 1971) and depot medication (Hirsch et al 1973) have been clearly demonstrated and, in reviewing 24 controlled studies, Davis (1976) concluded that the evidence for the efficacy of maintenance antipsychotic treatment is overwhelming. The drugs do not, however, abolish the tendency to relapse. In a 2 year follow-up study of oral antipsychotics versus placebo, rates of schizophrenic relapse in placebo-treated patients were 80%, whereas those of patients on active antipsychotics were 48% (Hogarty et al 1974). To exclude the possibility that the substantial relapse rate in those prescribed active antipsychotics was due to poor compliance, Hogarty et al (1979) conducted a further study comparing maintenance prophylaxis with oral and with depot antipsychotics. There was no difference between the 2 groups and the 2 year relapse rate remained substantial. Clearly significant benefits of antipsychotic medication have therefore been demonstrated in the treatment of acute episodes and in the reduction of relapse rates. There is however no drug treatment that can reliably be recommended as relieving negative symptoms in the same way that traditional antipsychotic agents relieve positive symptoms. The effect of these drugs on negative symptoms is uncertain. Controlled trials have yielded conflicting evidence. Antipsychotics have been said to improve (Goldberg et al 1965, Meltzer 1985), to have no effect

upon (Angrist et al 1980) or to exacerbate (Marder et al 1984, Hogarty et al 1988) negative symptoms. The general conclusion can only be that these symptoms are not overwhelmingly affected by antipsychotic agents.

The results of these clinical trials provide the basis of a rational prescribing policy. Acute schizophrenic illnesses should almost invariably be treated with antipsychotic agents and it is probably wise to try to keep most patients on a maintenance dose for a year or two thereafter, even if their recovery is complete and rapid. With so many similar preparations to choose from, the choice of drug is largely a matter of personal preference and relative costs. Many psychiatrists will use chlorpromazine in the acute phase, and if the patient is overactive or frightened its sedative effects are valuable. However, the hypotensive effects of chlorpromazine (and of thioridazine) may be dangerous in the elderly or in patients with a history of heart disease and in them a drug like trifluoperazine or droperidol is preferable. Usually the drug can be given orally but intramuscular injection may be necessary initially if the patient is aggressive or refusing to take tablets, and liquid medication is preferable if there are doubts about compliance.

Partly because of individual differences in absorption and metabolism, the dose required to bring psychotic symptoms under control varies considerably from one patient to another, in chlorpromazine equivalents from 150 mg/day to as much as 1000 mg/day. Baldessarini et al (1988) reviewed all published comparisons of different neuroleptic dosages in the treatment of schizophrenia. They concluded that, in the acute illness, moderate doses (chlorpromazine 300–600 mg/day, or equivalent doses of other antipsychotics) are most effective, and that quite low doses (chlorpromazine 50–100 mg/day or equivalent) often provide adequate maintenance therapy. They also suggest that if a patient does not respond to moderate doses of antipsychotics it is as logical to decrease the dose as to increase it.

Because they also affect the dopamine receptors of the nigrostriatal system, all conventional antipsychotics tend to produce troublesome extrapyramidal side-effects, and the liability of any individual drug to do so is, with one or two exceptions, proportional to its potency as an antipsychotic agent. For this reason some clinicians prescribe antiparkinsonian drugs routinely whenever they want to use more than a small dose of an antipsychotic. This is not good practice, for a variety of reasons. Akathisia and parkinsonism are the most common and troublesome extrapyramidal side-effects and there is little evidence that the routine prescribing of antiparkinsonian drugs reduces them to any worthwhile extent (for example, see Mindham et al 1972). There is also some evidence that the use of these drugs may impair the efficacy of antipsychotics, particularly in controlling positive symptoms (for example, see Singh et al 1987), and increase the incidence of tardive dyskinesia; and because they have mild stimulant properties some patients abuse them or become dependent. In general, therefore, antiparkinsonian drugs should only be used if the patient actually develops troublesome akathisia or parkinsonism and it is not feasible to reduce the dose of antipsychotic. And even if this is necessary, and successful, an attempt should be made to withdraw the antiparkinsonian agent after a couple of months because it will often be possible to do so without the extrapyramidal symptoms returning.

The case for giving antipsychotic drugs to chronic schizophrenics year in, year out is much less compelling than the case for using them during acute episodes or exacerbations. The disadvantage of doing so are also substantial. Many patients are seriously distressed by chronic akathisia or muscular rigidity, and others who are fortunate enough not to suffer in this way are understandably reluctant to continue 'taking drugs' indefinitely. There is also the long-term risk of tardive dyskinesia to consider. Certainly, it is well established that indistinguishable involuntary movements are not uncommon in elderly schizophrenics who have never received antipsychotics of any kind (for example, see Owens et al 1982), and that persistent chewing movements and other dyskinesias were observed in chronic schizophrenics long before antipsychotics existed (Farran-Ridge 1926). It is also important to realise that stopping patients' maintenance medication may, paradoxically, result in their receiving an increased rather than a decreased total dose over the next year or two, because they relapse and then require a substantially larger dose to bring their hallucinations or other symptoms back under control (Johnson et al 1983). Only rarely is it appropriate to give patients two or more different antipsychotics simultaneously. Sometimes there are good reasons for temporarily increasing the effective dose in a patient on an injectable depot preparation by giving a second drug orally as well; and some patients cannot tolerate an adequate dose of one drug because of its hypotensive or sedative effects, or an adequate dose of another because of its extrapyramidal effects, but can tolerate a mixture of the two. But most polypharmacy is simply a public display of pharmacological ignorance.

Patients with schizophrenia are often unreliable at taking tablets once their acute symptoms have subsided and they have left hospital. There are several reasons for this. They may not accept that they have been ill in the first place, and, even if they do, may not accept that there is any risk of the illness recurring. And the drugs often cause akathisia and other unpleasant side-effects which are more obvious than their antipsychotic effect. For these reasons 'depot' preparations capable of producing adequate serum levels when administered at intervals of 2 weeks or more have been developed. Most of these preparations, like fluphenazine decanoate (Modecate) and flupenthixol decanoate (Depixol), are phenothiazines or thioxanthenes esterified with a long-chain fatty acid from which they are slowly released in vivo. The introduction of these injectable depot preparations 20 years ago was hailed as a great advance and they are now very widely used, often with special clinics and elaborate follow-up arrangements to ensure that patients do not miss their regular injection every 2, 3 or 4 weeks. Probably they are a significant advance, but it is important not to forget that no trial comparing long-term relapse rates on daily tablets and fortnightly injections has demonstrated any clear advantage for the latter (for example, see Falloon et al 1978).

Concern about the extrapyramidal side-effects of antipsychotics has led in recent years to several attempts to maintain chronic patients on very small doses of antipsychotics, or to give these drugs only at the first sign of impending relapse. The results have been disappointing. Johnson et al (1987), for example, found that if chronic schizophrenics who were well controlled on relatively low doses of Depixol (up to 40 mg i.m. fortnightly) were transferred double-blind to half that dose, their relapse rate over the next 3 years was significantly increased. Jolley et al (1990) were more ambitious. They attempted to maintain schizophrenic outpatients in stable remission off all medication, but to ensure that they received oral haloperidol at the first signs of relapse by warning both patients and their relatives what those signs were likely to be and providing both monthly follow-up appointments and a 24 hour telephone contact. Unfortunately, the experiment failed, partly because only 50% of the relapses were preceded by any prodromal symptoms at all; and, although the drug-free patients had fewer extrapyramidal symptoms than their controls, this was not accompanied by any improvement in social functioning.

From the 1970s until the early 1980s the psychopharmacology of acute schizophrenia was dominated by the idea of the relevance of dopamine receptor blockade. This situation changed with the comeback of the 'atypical' antipsychotic clozapine. The concept of 'atypicality' with reference to antipsychotic drugs was derived from the idea that the antipsychotic and extrapyramidal effects of such drugs are linked, so that in order for a drug to be an effective antipsychotic it must necessarily produce extrapyramidal side-effects in patients. Clozapine produces minimal extrapyramidal effects. It was introduced in the 1970s but withdrawn from use in the USA, Great Britain and much of continental Europe after it was shown to be associated with agranulocytosis in a small percentage of cases. In 1988 Kane et al reported a large multicentre trial in the USA concerning 268 patients with chronic schizophrenia who had failed to respond to at least three different antipsychotics and also to a 6 week trial of haloperidol 60 mg/day. In this situation clozapine (in doses of up to 900 mg/day) was found to be more effective than chlorpromazine in doses up to 1800 mg/day; in a 6 week double-blind comparison 30% of clozapine versus 4% chlorpromazine patients achieved preset standards of improvement. Clozapine has a wider ranging pharmacological profile than most traditional antipychotics. It has a relatively modest affinity for D_1 and D_2 receptors and effects upon many other neurotransmitter receptors, including other dopamine receptor subtypes, serotonin and α-adrenergic receptors (Kane & McGlashan 1995). Which of these effects is relevant for the enhanced antipsychotic efficacy is not established at the present time. Furthermore, the mechanism whereby antipsychotic drugs are able to exhibit 'atypicality' (i.e. a low propensity to induce extrapyramidal side-effects with or without greater efficacy to alleviate the symptoms of schizophrenia) is unknown (Waddington 1995). The established value of clozapine lies in its enhanced antipsychotic activity in treatment-resistant cases and in its low liability to produce extrapyramidal side-effects. Evidence that it has additional benefits in other situations in the treatment of schizophrenia is so far lacking (Owens 1996). The disadvantages of clozapine are its very high cost and the fact that frequent neutrophil counts are necessary in order to detect incipient marrow depression and to prevent deaths from agranulocytosis. Other 'atypical' antipsychotics, such as risperidone, zotepine, sertindole and olanzapine, have been introduced. They appear to have advantages as far as side-effects are concerned but whether or not their antipsychotic activity is as much enhanced as is that of clozapine is yet to be clearly established. They do not share the problem of agranulocytosis, and thus the requirement for frequent neutrophil counts, but some of them are closer in price to clozapine than to the traditional antipsychotics.

Although antipsychotics have been the mainstay of the treatment of acute schizophrenia for the past 40 years, ECT and analytically oriented psychotherapy have been extensively used in some centres, though less so now than in the past. The results of May's (1968) trial in California indicated quite unequivocally that psychodynamic psychotherapy was valueless in the active phase of the illness. The only detectable effects, whether psychotherapy was given alone or in combination with a phenothiazine, were on the duration and cost of hospital treatment, both of which were substan-

tially increased. Patients treated with ECT fared significantly better, though less well than those receiving phenothiazines. Two more recent English trials of ECT, both comparing real and dummy ECT under double-blind conditions, found it to have genuinely beneficial effects in acute schizophrenia, though these were no longer detectable 3 or 4 months later (Taylor & Fleminger 1980, Brandon et al 1985). For this reason the only strong indications for using ECT in the treatment of schizophrenia nowadays are schizoaffective illnesses (whose relationship to schizophrenia is uncertain) and rare cases of catatonic stupor.

Tricyclic and other antidepressants are frequently given to schizophrenics in an attempt to relieve their associated depressive symptoms. The apathy and flattening of affect of the schizophrenic defect state can superficially resemble depression but, in addition to this, the occurrence of depressive symptoms in schizophrenic patients when they are not actively psychotic has increasingly been reported (McGlashan & Carpenter 1976, Hirsch et al 1989). The value of adjunctive antidepressant treatment both on an acute (Siris et al 1987) and on a maintenance basis (Siris et al 1994) has been clearly demonstrated.

Social and psychological measures

Although in the short run antipsychotics have a much more dramatic effect on the symptoms of schizophrenia than any other therapeutic measure, there is a great deal more to the treatment of the disorder than prescribing antipsychotic agents. There is abundant evidence that the course of schizophrenic illnesses and the resulting social handicaps can be affected, for good or ill, by the patient's social environment, and it has been known for 30 years that many of the most obvious behavioural abnormalities of chronic schizophrenics, like posturing and talking to themselves, are not intrinsic or inevitable, but are to a considerable extent the product of a monotonous, unstimulating environment. This was well illustrated by Wing & Brown's (1961) comparison of three mental hospitals in southern England. In their hospital C, patients had few if any personal possessions, little liberty, spent much of the time unoccupied in the wards, and were generally treated as 'inmates', whereas in hospital A they had their own clothes and other personal possessions, spent most of the day actively employed and generally lived as free and normal a life as possible. The incidence of social withdrawal (underactivity, lack of conversation, neglect of hygiene and personal appearance) and socially embarrassing behaviour (incontinence, mannerisms, purposeless overactivity, threats of violence, talking to self) was higher in hospital C than it was in A (B was intermediate in all respects), despite the fact that their patients' initial type and severity of illness appeared to have been the same, and there were no important differences in the prescribing and discharge policies of the two hospitals.

Too much stimulation, or stimulation of the wrong kind, can also be harmful. There is, for example, the evidence that schizophrenic illnesses may be precipitated by events in the previous few weeks, pleasant and unpleasant, which disrupt the subject's normal lifestyle (Brown & Birley 1968). There is also the evidence that returning to live with a critical or hostile relative after a schizophrenic illness greatly increases the relapse rate over the next 12 months (Vaughn & Leff 1976, Parker & Hadzi-Pavlovic 1990). The overall management of schizophrenia is based, therefore, on an attempt to avoid both extremes. To this end, attempts are made to get the patient out of hospital and into an occupation and a domestic setting in which they have some real but limited responsibilities, in which they have a daily routine which is ordered and predictable without being too monotonous, and in which they are protected from emotional demands they cannot meet. It is often easier said than done.

For the last 40 years, partly because of the realisation that mental hospitals themselves could have profoundly harmful effects on their patients if they stayed too long, and partly for straightforward financial reasons, intensive efforts have been made to discharge schizophrenics as soon as their psychotic symptoms have resolved and to keep them 'in the community' as much as possible thereafter. To be successful, or for the patient to be better off, such a policy requires the provision of a range of hostels, day centres, 'half-way houses' and sheltered workshops in the community. Unfortunately, these facilities have not yet materialised in anything like adequate numbers. For this reason many psychiatrists (though not hospital managers) are increasingly questioning whether early discharge is always in the patient's interests, and whether mental hospitals have not been too eager to discard their traditional 'asylum' role. A back bedroom can be just as deprived and harmful an environment as a back ward, and a park bench even more so. Discharging patients from hospital when adequate community facilities are not available may also place a heavy burden on relatives, a burden which psychiatrists and social workers do not fully comprehend and often do little to relieve (National Schizophrenia Fellowship 1974).

Although some patients have a home and a job to return to, or succeed in obtaining accommodation and employment without the aid of any formal rehabilitative measures, others are too badly handicapped by the effects of illness on their drive, initiative and demeanour, by the social stigma of having been mentally ill, and often too by their previous lack of education and marketable skills, to be capable of obtaining a job without assistance. In the past it was one of the primary functions of rehabilitation programmes to help people who had had schizophrenic illnesses to obtain suitable paid employment subsequently. However, in the last decade or so this has become increasingly difficult, partly because the general level of unemployment has risen, and partly because fundamental industrial changes have resulted in a substantial reduction in the need for unskilled or semiskilled workers. As a result, rehabilitation programmes are increasingly geared to help patients with defect states or recurring psychotic episodes to cook and shop for themselves, to obtain temporary or unpaid employment and to use their leisure time productively.

Some people with schizophrenia have become homeless by the time they are first admitted to hospital; others become so later on after a series of further relapses and readmissions. Accommodation has to be found for most such patients if they are ever to leave hospital and many of them are unable to cope in ordinary rented accommodation even if landladies can be persuaded to take them. So other types of accommodation geared to their needs have to be provided. In the past, hostels were often provided by psychiatric hospitals themselves, either on the hospital site or elsewhere, and supervised to varying extents by nurses. Now hostels, group homes, flats and bed-sitters reserved for former psychiatric patients are increasingly provided by local authority social work departments and voluntary organisations. The amount and quality of supervision provided is very variable, but the greater quantity and variety of protected housing available increases the likelihood that individual patients will eventually find a suitable niche. The fact that insufficient amounts of suitable supported accommodation are currently available is made very clear in the recent report of the King's Fund London Commission (King's Fund 1997).

A more difficult situation arises when the patient is living with a relative, usually a spouse or parent, who is willing to have him back, but it becomes clear while the patient is in hospital that this relative cannot accept and adapt to the change that has come over him and remains angry, frightened and critical. There are various ways of trying to deal with this potentially hazardous situation. It may be possible to arrange for the patient to move into a hostel instead of returning home; but suitable accommodation is not always available, and even if it is it may be impossible to persuade either the patient or the relative that this is preferable to returning home. Indeed, it is often the mothers who are most critical of their schizophrenic son's or daughter's behaviour who are least willing to be parted from them.

An alternative strategy in such circumstance is to mitigate the ill-effects of the relative's emotional involvement by reducing the time the two spend in one another's company. A full-time job is, of course, the best way of doing this, but, if this is impossible, regular attendance at a day hospital or day centre of some kind may achieve the same ends.

A further preventive strategy is to try to alter the attitudes and behaviour of the relatives, and various forms of family therapy to this end have been developed in the last two decades. Several small-scale but important clinical trials have now been reported. In the first, 24 schizophrenics who were all living in a 'high expressed emotion' environment, and therefore at high risk of relapse, were randomly allocated either to routine outpatient care or to receive a special package of social interventions consisting of factual talks to their relatives about schizophrenia, fortnightly group meetings for the relatives designed to help them share experience, discharge emotions and learn new coping techniques, and regular family therapy sessions in the patient's home designed to lower expressed emotion and face-to-face contact (Leff et al 1982). All 24 patients received depot antipsychotics throughout. After 9 months the relapse rate was 50% in the controls but only 9% in the treatment group ($P = 0.40$) and the only patients in the treatment group to relapse were the two in whom no reduction in expressed emotion or face-to-face contact was achieved. The results of this trial therefore adds to the evidence that high expressed emotion does provoke relapse and that reduced face-to-face contact is protective. They do not, of course, reveal which elements of the treatment package were most important.

A more recent trial by Tarrier et al (1989) in Salford has confirmed that the relapse rate in schizophrenics living with 'high expressed emotion' relatives can be reduced to that of schizophrenics living with 'low expressed emotion' relatives if the key relatives are given about a dozen sessions of information and advice about schizophrenia, coping with stress and coping with the patient's frustrating behaviour. It seems clear, therefore, that there needs to be a substantial shift in emphasis in the management of schizophrenia, with far more attention being given to patients' families than in the past.

The effect of social casework on the patients themselves in their postpsychotic, posthospital phase of the illness had previously been explored in a large American trial (Goldberg et al 1977). Four hundred newly discharged schizophrenics were randomly allocated to one of four groups and followed up for 2 years. The first group received maintenance chlorpromazine plus what the authors called 'major role therapy' (a combination of intensive psychoanalytically oriented social casework and vocational rehabilitation); a second group received maintenance chlorpromazine but only minimal contacts with a social worker; a third group received placebo tablets and 'major role therapy'; and a fourth group received placebo tablets and minimal social contacts. As expected, the relapse rate was much lower in patients on maintenance chlorpromazine than in those on placebo (48% versus 80%). Overall, 'major role therapy' had no effect on the relapse rate. But more detailed analysis showed that in patients who might have been expected to have a good prognosis the relapse rate was reduced by this treatment, and in those who might have been expected to have a relatively poor prognosis the relapse rate was increased. In other words, as other trials of the efficacy of psychotherapy have demonstrated in other settings, some patients benefited but others were harmed and the two tended to cancel each other out. What the mechanism of harm is we can only speculate, but it is easy to imagine how an intensive relationship with a keen social worker might create something akin to a 'high expressed emotion' situation. The moral is clear. Would-be psychotherapeutic relationships and other emotional pressures may be positively harmful to those who have recently had a schizophrenic illness, and so should only be offered if it is quite clear that the patients are capable of responding. Emotional withdrawal is not merely a symptom; it is also a valuable protective strategy.

Related disorders

Disorders 'related' to schizophrenia include a variety of conditions, described by a wide range of terms, which share some of the features of schizophrenia, but not all. In general they tend to be characterised by acute psychotic symptoms but they do not have the chronicity, the lack of a mood-related component or perhaps the poor prognosis.

As noted above, the range of disorders which have been given the diagnosis of schizophrenia has at times been very wide, and whether or not a psychotic episode will fulfil current criteria for schizophrenia depends very much upon the operational definition used. Definitions like that in DSM-IV in which a 6 month duration is an obligatory necessity exclude many first-episode cases, and using DSM-IV cases with a duration of at least 1 month and less than 6 months would be classed as schizophreniform disorder (APA 1994). Following Kraepelin's separation of dementia praecox and manic–depressive disorder, it was recognised (Bleuler 1911, Kasanin 1933) that a not inconsiderable proportion of patients with functional psychotic illness fit neatly into neither category, having features considered typical of both. The term schizoaffective psychosis (introduced by Kasanin in 1933) is often used to describe such cases. It is however rarely clearly defined and formal study has shown the level of agreement between various definitions of schizoaffective psychosis and of related terms is low (Brockington & Leff 1979).

The term 'schizophrenia-like' disorder is used in ICD-10 (WHO 1992) to refer to conditions with features of schizophrenia but which are due to brain damage and dysfunction and to physical disease. This is not intended to mean the subtle abnormalities which modern techniques, such as imaging, can show to be present in schizophrenia but refers to primary cerebral disease or to systemic disease affecting the brain secondarily. Sometimes such disorders are referred to as the 'secondary schizophrenias' (Lewis 1995). They are uncommon but, as noted earlier in this chapter, in addition to their practical importance in the individual cases where they occur, they are of theoretical importance as they may shed light upon the causation of the generality of schizophrenia.

For many years there has been reference in the literature to the concept of psychoses which are too brief or insufficiently severe to qualify for criteria for schizophrenia and where the illness does not appear to be affective. The diagnostic classifications bouffée délirante (Legrain 1886), reactive psychosis (Wimmer 1916), cycloid psychosis (Leonhard 1939), like the IDC-10 terms (WHO 1992) psychogenic paranoid psychosis, schizophrenic reaction and DSM-IV's brief psychotic disorder (APA 1994), are used to describe syndromes which are assumed to have a more favourable outcome than schizophrenia. Stromgren (1989) has however suggested that 'reactive psychosis' always has a better prognosis than manic–depressive psychosis (and by implication than schizophrenia) and that the appropriate treatment is psychotherapeutic. Much of this literature is descriptive, but evidence of the better prognosis of short-lived psychoses with features of schizophrenia was shown in 1996 by Johnstone et al. Patients with illnesses which did not fulfil operational criteria for schizophrenia were followed up after 2 years and compared with those who did. 'Partial' illnesses (i.e. those where the delusions did not appear to be held with full conviction) had a prognosis very similar to that of typical schizophrenic illness, but 'transient' illnesses (those where symptomatology was short-lived), although clearly recurrent, had a good outcome in terms of social variables and symptomatology. It does therefore appear that there is a group of psychotic illnesses with clinical features which at first glance are typical of schizophrenia but which are short lived and do not seem to be associated with residual symptomatology or social decline.

REFERENCES

Andreasen N C 1979 Thought, language and communication disorders. Archives of General Psychiatry 36: 1315–1321, 1325–1330

Angrist B, Rotrosen J, Gershon S 1980 Differential affects of amphetamine and antipsychotics on negative vs positive symptoms in schizophrenia. Psychopharmacology 72: 17–19

APA 1994 Diagnostic and statistical manual of mental disorders, 4th edn. American Psychiatric Association, Washington, DC

Astrup C, Odegaard Ø 1960 The influence of hospital facilities and other local factors upon admission to psychiatric hospitals. Acta Psychiatrica et Neurologica Scandinavica 35: 289–301

Baldessarini R J, Cohen B M, Teicher M H 1988 Significance of neuroleptic dose and plasma level in the pharmacological treatment of psychoses. Archives of General Psychiatry 45: 79–91

Baldwin J A 1979 Schizophrenia and physical disease. Psychological Medicine 9: 611–618

Baruch I, Hemsley D R, Gray J A 1988 Differential performance of acute and chronic schizophrenics in a latent inhibition task. Journal of Nervous and Mental Disease 176: 598–606

Bateson G, Jackson D D, Haley J, Weakland J H 1956 Toward a theory of schizophrenia. Behavioral Science 1: 251–264

Bebbington P E, Kuipers L 1994 The predictive utility of expressed emotion in schizophrenia. Psychological Medicine 24: 707–718

Bebbington P E, Bowen J, Hirsch S R, Kuipers E A 1995 Schizophrenia and psychosocial stresses. In: Hirsch S R, Weinberger D R (eds) Schizophrenia. Blackwell, London, pp 587–604

Benes F M, Davidson J, Bird E D 1986 Quantitative cytoarchitectural studies of the cerebral cortex of schizophrenia. Archives of General Psychiatry 43: 31–35

Birchwood M, Smith J 1987 Schizophrenia in the family. In: Orford J (ed) Coping with disorder in the family. Croom Helm, London

Bleuler E 1911 Dementia praecox or the group of schizophrenias. Zinkin J (trans) 1950. International University Press, New York

Bleuler M 1972 Die schizophrenen Geistesstörungen im Lichte langjähriger Kranken- und Familiengeschichten. Thieme, Stuttgart

Bradbury T N, Miller G A 1985 Season of birth in schizophrenia: a review of evidence, methodology and etiology. Psychological Bulletin 98: 569–594

Brendon S, Cowley P, McDonald C, Neville P, Palmer R, Wellstead Eason 1985 Leicester ECT trial: results in schizophrenia. British Journal of Psychiatry 146: 177–183

Brockington I F, Leff J P 1979 Schizoaffective psychosis: definitions and incidence. Psychological Medicine 9: 91–99

Brockington I F, Wainwright S, Kendell R E 1980 Manic patients with schizophrenic or paranoid symptoms. Psychological Medicine 10: 73–83

Brown G W, Birley J L T 1968 Crises and life changes and the onset of schizophrenia. Journal of Health and Social Behaviour 9: 203–214

Brown G W, Birley J L T, Wing J K 1972 Influence of family life on the course of schizophrenic disorders: a replication. British Journal of Psychiatry 121: 241–258

Bruton C J, Crow T J, Frith C D, Johnstone E C, Owens D G C, Robertson G W 1990 Schizophrenia and the brain: a prospective clinical neuropathological study. Psychological Medicine 20: 285–304

Cochrane R 1977 Mental illness in immigrants to England and Wales: an analysis of mental hospital admissions, 1971. Social Psychiatry 12: 25–35

Conrad A J, Abebe T, Austin R, Forsythe S, Scheibel A B 1991 Hippocampal pyramidal cell disarray in schizophrenia as a bilateral phenomenon. Archives of General Psychiatry 48: 413–417

Cooper J E, Kendell R E, Gurland B J, Sharpe L, Copeland J R M, Simon R 1972 Psychiatric diagnosis in New York and London. Maudsley monograph 20. Oxford University Press, London

Crow T J 1980 Molecular pathology of schizophrenia: more than one disease process? British Medical Journal 280: 66–68

Crow T J, Stevens M 1978 Age disorientation in chronic schizophrenia: the nature of the cognitive deficit. British Journal of Psychiatry 133: 137–142

Cutting J 1985 The psychology of schizophrenia. Churchill Livingstone, Edinburgh

Davis J M 1976 Recent developments in the drug treatment of schizophrenia. American Journal of Psychiatry 133: 208–214

Davison K, Bagley C R 1969 Schizophrenia-like psychoses associated with organic disorders of the nervous system: a review of the literature. In: Herrington R N (ed) Current problems in neuropsychiatry. Headley, Ashford, Kent.

Delay J, Deniker P 1952 Le traitement des psychoses par une méthode neurolytique derivée de l'hiberno therapie. In: Cossea J (ed) Congrés de medicines alienistes et neurologistes de France. Masson, Paris, pp 497–502

Done D T, Johnstone E C, Frith D C, Golding J, Shepherd P M, Crow T J 1991 Complications of pregnancy and delivery in relation to psychosis in adult life. Data from the British perinatal mortality survey sample. British Medical Journal 302: 1576–1580

Done D J, Crow T J, Johnstone E C, Sacker A 1994 Childhood antecedents of schizophrenia and affective illness: social adjustment at ages 7 and 11. British Medical Journal 309: 699–703

Eagles J M, Whalley L J 1985 Decline in the diagnosis of schizophrenia among first admissions to Scottish mental hospitals from 1969–78. British Journal of Psychiatry 146: 151–154

Falkai P, Bogerts B 1995 The neuropathology of schizophrenia. In: Hirsch S R, Weinberger D R (eds) Schizophrenia. Blackwell, London, pp 477–493

Falloon I, Watt D C, Shepherd M 1978 A comparative controlled trial of pimozide and fluphenazine decanoate in the continuation therapy of schizophrenia. Psychological Medicine 8: 59–70

Faris R, Dunham W 1939 (reprinted 1960) Mental disorders in urban areas. Hafner, New York

Farran-Ridge C 1926 Dementia praecox and epidemic encephalitis. Journal of Mental Science 72: 513–523

Feighner J P, Robins E, Guze S B, Woodruff R A, Winokur G, Munoz R 1972 Diagnostic criteria for use in psychiatric research. Archives of General Psychiatry 26: 57–63

Foerster A, Lewis S, Owen M, Murray R 1991 Premorbid adjustment and personality in psychosis: effects of sex and diagnosis. British Journal of Psychiatry 158: 171–176

Friston K J, Frith C D 1995 Schizophrenia: a disconnection syndrome. Clinical Neurosciences 3: 88–97

Frith C D 1992 The cognitive neuropsychology of schizophrenia. Erlbaum, Hove

Frith C D 1996 Neuropsychology of schizophrenia. In: Johnstone E C (ed) Biological psychiatry. British Medical Bulletin 52: 618–626

Goldberg E M, Morrison S L 1963 Schizophrenia and social class. British Journal of Psychiatry 109: 785–802

Goldberg S C, Klerman G L, Cole J O 1965 Changes in schizophrenic psychopathology and ward behaviour as a function of phenothiazine treatment. British Journal of Psychiatry III: 120–133

Goldberg S C, Schooler N R, Hogarty G E, Roper M 1977 Prediction of relapse in schizophrenic outpatients treated by drug and sociotherapy. Archives of General Psychiatry 34: 171–184

Goldhamer H, Marshall A 1953 Psychosis and civilisation. Free Press, Illinois

Griesinger W 1845 Die Pathologie und Therapie der psychische Krankheiten. A Krabbe, Stuttgart

Gunderson J G, Mosher L R 1975 The cost of schizophrenia. American Journal of Psychiatry 132: 901–906

Häfner H, Riecher A, Maurer K, Löffler W, Munk-Jørgensen P, Strömgren E 1989 How does gender influence age at first hospitalisation for schizophrenia? Psychologicial Medicine 19: 903–918

Harding C M, Brooks G W, Ashikaga T, Strauss J S, Breier A 1987 The Vermont longitudinal study of persons with severe mental illness. American Journal of Psychiatry 144: 718–726, 727–735

Hare E H 1988 Schizophrenia as a recent disease. British Journal of Psychiatry 153: 521–531

Harrison G, Owens D, Holton A, Neilson D, Boot D 1988 A prospective study of severe mental disorder in Afro-Caribbean patients. Psychological Medicine 18: 643–657

Harvey I, Ron M A, Du Boulay G, Wicks S W, Lewis S W, Murray R M 1993 Reduction of cortical volume in schizophrenia on magnetic resonance imaging. Psychological Medicine 23: 591–604

Hawk A B, Carpenter W T, Strauss J S 1975 Diagnostic criteria and five year outcome in schizophrenia. Archives of General Psychiatry 32: 343–347

Hirsch S R, Leff J P 1975 Abnormalities in parents of schizophrenics. Maudsley monograph 22. Oxford University Press, London

Hirsch S R, Gairid R, Rhode P D, Stevens B C, Wing J K 1973 Outpatient maintenance of chronic schizophrenic patients with long acting fluphenazine: double blind placebo controlled trial. British Medical Journal 1: 633–637

Hirsch S R, Jolley A G, Barnes T R E et al 1989 Dysphoric and depressive symptoms in chronic schizophrenia. Schizophrenia Research 2: 259–264

Hoch P, Polatin P 1949 Pseudoneurotic forms of schizophrenia. Psychiatry Quarterly 23: 248–256

Hogarty G E, Goldberg S C, Schooler S, Ulrich R F 1974 Collaborative study group. Drugs and sociotherapy in the aftercare of schizophrenic patients II. Two year relapse rates. Archives of General Psychiatry 31: 603–608

Hogarty G E, Schooler N R, Ulrich T, Mussare F, Fesso P, Hesson E 1979 Fluphenazine and social therapy in the aftercare of schizophrenic patients. Archives of General Psychiatry 36: 1283–1294

Hogarty G E, McEvoy J P, Munetz H 1988 Dose of fluphenazine, familial expressed emotion and outcome in schizophrenia. Archives of General Psychiatry 45: 797–805

Hollister L E, Trauts L, Prusmack J T 1960 Use of

thioridazine for intensive treatment of schizophrenia refractory to other tranquillizing drugs. Journal of Neuropsychiatry 1: 200–204

Ingvar D H, Franzen G 1974 Abnormalities of cerebral blood flow distribution in patients with chronic schizophrenia. Acta Psychiatrica Scandinavica 50: 425–462

Jakob H, Beckmann H 1986 Prenatal development disturbances in the limbic allocortex in schizophrenics. Journal of Neural Transmission 65: 303–326

Jellinger K 1985 Neuromorphological background of pathochemical studies in major psychoses. In: Beckman H, Riederer P (eds) Pathochemical markers in major psychoses. Springer, Heidelberg, pp 1–23

Johnson D A W, Pasterski G, Ludlow J M, Street K, Taylor R D W 1983 The discontinuance of maintenance neuroleptic therapy in chronic schizophrenic patients: drug and social consequences. Acta Psychiatrica Scandinavica 67: 339–352

Johnson D A W, Ludlow J M, Street K, Taylor R D W 1987 Double-blind comparison of half-dose and standard-dose flupenthixol decanoate in the maintenance treatment of stabilised out-patients with schizophrenia. British Journal of Psychiatry 151: 634–638

Johnstone E C 1990 What is crucial for the long term outcome of schizophrenia? In: Hafner H, Gattaz W F (eds) Search for the causes of schizophrenia. Springer, Berlin, vol II

Johnstone E C 1994 Questions and answers derived from the large clinical studies. In: Searching for the causes of schizophrenia. Oxford University Press, Oxford

Johnstone E C, Frith C D 1996 Validation of three dimensions of schizophrenic symptoms in a large unselected sample of patients. Psychological Medicine 26: 669–679

Johnstone E C, Crow T J, Frith C D et al 1976 Cerebral ventricular size and cognitive impairment in chronic schizophrenia. Lancet ii: 924–926

Johnstone E C, Crow T J, Johnson A L, Macmillan J F 1986 The Northwick Park study of first episodes of schizophrenia. Presentation of the illness and problems relating to admission. British Journal of Psychiatry 148: 115–120

Johnstone E C, Macmillan J F, Crow T J 1987 The occurrence of organic disease of possible or probable organic aetiological significance in a population of 268 cases of first episode schizophrenia. Psychological Medicine 17: 371–379

Johnstone E C, Frith C D, Leary J, Owens D G C, Wilkins S, Hershon H I 1991 Disabilities and circumstances of schizophrenic patients – a follow-up study (1). Background, method and general description of the sample. British Journal of Psychiatry 159 (suppl 13): 7–12

Johnstone E C, Connelly J, Frith C D, Lambert H T, Owens G D C 1996 The nature of 'transient' and 'partial' psychoses: findings from the Northwick Park 'functional' psychoses study. Psychological Medicine 26: 361–369

Jolley A G, Hirsch S R, Morrison E, McRink A, Wilson L 1990 Trial of brief intermittent neuroleptic prophylaxis for selected schizophrenic outpatients: clinical and social outcome at two years. British Medical Journal 301: 837–842

Kane J M, McGlashan T H 1995 Treatment of schizophrenia. Lancet 346: 820–825

Kane J, Honigfield G, Singer J et al 1988 Clozapine for the treatment-resistant schizophrenic. Archives of General Psychiatry 45: 789–796

Kasanin J 1933 The acute schizoaffective psychoses. American Journal of Psychiatry 90: 97–126

Kendell R E, Brockington I F, Leff J P 1979 Prognostic implications of six alternative definitions of schizophrenia. Archives of General Psychiatry 36: 25–34

Kendell R E, Malcolm D E, Adams W 1993 The problem of detecting changes in the incidence of schizophrenia. British Journal of Psychiatry 162: 212–218

Kendler K S, Ochs A L, Gorman A H et al 1991 The structure of schizotypy: a pilot multitrait twin study. Psychiatry Research 36: 19–36

Kety S S, Rosenthal D, Wender P I L, Schulsinger F, Jacobson B 1975 Mental illness in the biologic and adoptive families of adopted individuals who became schizophrenic: a preliminary report based on psychiatric interviews. In: Fieve R R, Rosenthal D, Brill H (eds) Genetic research in psychiatry. Johns Hopkins University Press, Baltimore

King's Fund 1997 London's mental health. King's Fund, London

Kovelman J A, Schiebel A B 1984 A neurohistological correlate of schizophrenia. Biological Psychiatry 19: 1601–1621

Kraepelin E 1896 Psychiatrie, ein Lehrbuch für Studierende und Ärzte, 5th edn. Barth, Leipzig

Kraepelin E 1919 Dementia praecox. Barclay R M (trans), Robertson G M (ed), facsimile edition published 1971 by Krieger, New York

Langfeldt G 1960 Diagnosis and prognosis of schizophrenia. Proceedings of the Royal Society of Medicine 53: 1047–1052

Leff J P, Wing J K 1971 Trial of maintenance therapy in schizophrenia. British Medical Journal 3: 599–604

Leff J, Kuipers L, Berkowitz R, Eberlein-Vries R, Sturgeon D 1982 A controlled trial of social intervention in the families of schizophrenic patients. British Journal of Psychiatry 141: 121–134

Legrain M 1886 Du délire chez les dégénérés. Deshaye & Lecrosnier, Paris

Leonhard K 1939 Aufteilung der endogenen Psychosen (Classification of endogenous psychoses), 2nd edn. Akademie, Berlin

Lewis G, David A, Andréasson S, Allebeck P 1992 Schizophrenia and city life. Lancet 340: 137–140

Lewis S W 1995 The secondary schizophrenias. In: Hirsch S R, Weinberger D R (eds) Schizophrenia. Blackwell, London

Liddle P F 1987 The symptoms of chronic schizophrenia: a re-examination of the positive–negative dichotomy. British Journal of Psychiatry 151: 145–151

Liddle P F, Morris D L 1991 Schizophrenic syndromes and frontal lobe performance. British Journal of Psychiatry 158: 340–345

Liddle P F, Friston K J, Frith C D, Jones T, Hirsch S R, Frackowick R S J 1992 Problems of cerebral blood flow in schizophrenia. British Journal of Psychiatry 160: 179–186

Lidz T, Fleck S, Cornelison A R 1965 Schizophrenia and the family. International Universities Press, New York

McCreadie R G, Leese, M, Tilak-Singh D, Loftus L, MacEwan T, Thornicroft G (1997) Nithsdale, Nunhead and Norwood: similarities and differences in prevalence of schizophrenias and utilisation of services in urban and rural areas. British Journal of Psychiatry 170: 31–36

McGlashan T H, Carpenter W T 1976 Post psychotic depression in schizophrenia. Archives of General Psychiatry 33: 231–239

McGovern, D, Cope R V 1987 First psychiatric admission rates of first and second generation Afro-Caribbeans. Social Psychiatry 22: 139–149

McKenna P J, Tamlyn D, Lund C E, Mortimer A M, Hammond S, Baddeley A D 1990 Amnesic syndrome in schizophrenia. Psychological Medicine 20: 967–972

Macmillan J F, Crow T J, Johnston A L, Johnstone E C 1986 The Northwick Park study of first episodes of schizophrenia II. Short term outcome in trial entrants and trial eligible patients. British Journal of Psychiatry 148: 128–133

McNeil T F 1987 Perinatal influenza in the development of schizophrenia. In: Helmchen H, Henn F A (eds) Biological perspectives in schizophrenia. Wiley, Chichester

Malzberg B, Lee E S 1956 Migration and mental disease: a study of first admission to hospitals for mental disease, New York, 1939–1941. Social Science Research Council, New York

Marder S R, Van Putten T, Mintz J et al 1984 Costs and benefits of two doses of fluphenazine. Archives of General Psychiatry 41: 1025–1029

Mavreas V G, Tomarqs V, Karydi V, Economom M, Stefaris C 1992 Expressed emotion in families of chronic schizophrenics and its association with clinical measures. Social Psychiatry and Psychiatric Epidemiology 27: 4–9

May P R A 1968 Treatment of schizophrenia. Science House, New York

Mayer-Gross W 1932 Prognosis of schizophrenia. Handbuch Gersteskrank 9: 534–536

Meltzer H Y 1985 Dopamine and negative symptoms in schizophrenia: critique of the Type I–II hynothesis. In: Controversies in schizophrenia – changes and circumstances. Guildford, New York

Miklowitz D J, Goldstein M J, Falloon I R H 1983 Premorbid and symptomatic characteristics of schizophrenics from families with high and low levels of expressed emotion. Journal of Abnormal Psychology 3: 359–367

Miles C P 1977 Conditions predisposing to suicide: a review. Journal of Nervous and Mental Disease 164: 231–246

Mindham R H S, Gaind R, Anstee B H, Rimmer L 1972 Comparison of amantadine, orphenadrine and placebo in the control of phenothiazine induced parkinsonism. Psychological Medicine 2: 406–413

Morice R D, Ingram J C L 1982 Language analysis in schizophrenia: diagnostic implications. Australian and New Zealand Journal of Psychiatry 16: 11–21

Murray R M, Lewis S W 1987 Is schizophrenia a neurodevelopmental disorder? British Medical Journal 295: 681–682

National Institute of Mental Health, Psychopharmacology Service Center Collaborative Study Group 1964 Phenothiazine treatment of acute schizophrenia. Archives of General Psychiatry 10: 246–261

National Schizophrenia Fellowship 1974 Living with schizophrenia – by the relatives. National Schizophrenia Fellowship, Surrey

Odegaard Ø 1932 Emigration and insanity: a study of mental disease among Norwegian-born population in Minnesota. Acta Psychiatrica et Neurologica Scandinavica. Supplementum 4

Owens D G C 1996 Adverse effects of antipsychotic agents: do newer agents offer advantages? Drugs 51: 895–930

Owens D G C, Johnstone E C 1980 The disabilities of chronic schizophrenia: their nature and factors contributing to their development. British Journal of Psychiatry 136: 384–395

Owens D G C, Johnstone E C, Frith D D 1982 Spontaneous involuntary disorders of movement. Archives of General Psychiatry 39: 452–461

Pakkenberg B 1990 Pronounced reduction of total neuron numbers in mediodorsal thalamic nucleus and nucleus accumbens in schizophrenics. Archives of General Psychiatry 47: 1023–1028

Pantelis C, Harvey C, Taylor J et al 1991 The Camden schizophrenia surveys: symptoms and syndromes in schizophrenia. Biological Psychiatry 29 (suppl): 464S

Parker G, Hadzi-Pavlovic D 1990 Expressed emotion as a predictor of schizophrenic relapse: an analysis of aggregated data. Psychological Medicine 20: 951–965

Regier D A, Boyd J H, Burke J D et al 1988 One-month prevalance of mental disorders in the United States. Archives of General Psychiatry 45: 977–986

Sartorius N, Jablensky A, Shapiro R 1977 Two-year follow-up of the patients included in the WHO international pilot study of schizophrenia. Psychological Medicine 7: 529–541

Sartorius N, Jablensky A, Korten A et al 1986 Early manifestations and first contact incidence of schizophrenia in different cultures. Psychological Medicine 16: 909–928

Schneider K 1959 Klinische Psychopathologie. Hamilton M W (trans). Grune & Stratton, New York

Schofield W, Hathaway S R, Hastings D W, Bell D M 1954 Prognostic factors in schizophrenia. Journal of Consulting Psychology 18: 155–166

Shallice T, Burgers P, Frith C D 1991 Can the neuropsychological case study approach be applied to schizophrenia. Psychological Medicine 21: 661–673

Sham P C, O'Callaghan E, Takei N et al 1992 Schizophrenia following pre-natal exposure to influenza epidemics between 1939 and 1960. British Journal of Psychiatry 160: 461–466

Shenton M E, Kikinis R, Jolesz F A et al 1992 Abnormalities of the left temporal lobe and thought disorder in schizophrenia. New England Journal of Medicine 327: 604–612

Singer M T, Wynne L D 1965 Thought disorder and family relations of schizophrenics. Archives of General Psychiatry 12: 187–212

Singh M M, Kay S R, Opler L A 1987 Anticholinergic-neuroleptic antagonism in terms of positive and negative symptoms of schizophrenia: implications for psychological subtyping. Psychological Medicine 17: 39–48

Siris S G, Morgan V, Fagerstrom R, Fifkin A, Cooper T B 1987 Adjunctive imipramine in the treatment of post psychotic depression: a controlled trial. Archives of General Psychiatry 44: 533–539

Siris S G, Bermanzohm P C, Mason S E, Shuwall M A 1994 Maintenance imipramine therapy for secondary depression in schizophrenia. Archives of General Psychiatry 51: 109–115

Spitzer R, Endicott J, Robins E 1975 Research diagnostic criteria. Instrument 58. New York State Psychiatric Institute, New York

Stalker H 1939 The prognosis in schizophrenia. Journal of Mental Science 85: 1224–1240

Steinberg H R, Durrell J 1968 A stressful social situation as a precipitant of schizophrenic symptoms: an epidemiological study. British Journal of Psychiatry 114: 1097–1105

Stromgren E 1989 The development of the concept of reactive psychoses. British Journal of Psychiatry 154 (suppl 4): 47–50

Susser E S, Lin S P 1992 Schizophrenia after prenatal exposure to the Dutch hunger winter of 1944–1945. Archives of General Psychiatry 49: 983–988

Tarrier N, Barrowclough C, Vaughn C et al 1989 Community management of schizophrenia. British Journal of Psychiatry 154: 625–628

Taylor P, Fleminger J J 1980 ECT for schizophrenia. Lancet: 1380–1382

Torrey E F 1987 Prevalence studies in schizophrenia. British Journal of Psychiatry 150: 598–608

Tuma A H, May P R A 1979 And if that doesn't work what next? A study of treatment failures in schizophrenia. Journal of Nervous and Mental Disease 167: 566–571

Vaillant G E 1964 Prospective prediction of schizophrenic remission. Archives of General Psychiatry 11: 509–518

Vaughn C E, Leff J P 1976 Influence of family and social factors on the course of psychiatric illness. British Journal of Psychiatry 129: 125–137

Vaughn C E, Snyder K S, Jones S et al 1984 Family factors in schizophrenic relapse. Archives of General Psychiatry 41: 1169–1177

Waddington J L 1995 The clinical pharmacology of antipsychotic drugs in schizophrenia. In: Hirsch S R, Weinberger D R (eds) Schizophrenia. Blackwell, Oxford, pp 341–357

Weinberger D R 1987 Implications of normal brain development for the pathogenesis of schizophrenia. Archives of General Psychiatry 44: 660–669

Weinberger D R 1995 From neuropathology to neurodevelopment. Lancet 346: 552–557

WHO 1973 Report of the International Pilot Study of Schizophrenia. World Health Organization, Geneva

WHO 1992 The ICD-10 classification of mental and behavioural disorders: clinical descriptions and diagnostic guidelines. World Health Organization, Geneva

Wimmer A 1916 Psykogene sindssygdoms former. In: Wimmer A (ed) St Hans Hospital 1816–1915. Gad, Copenhagen, pp 85–216

Wing J K 1966 Five year outcome in early schizophrenia. Proceedings of the Royal Society of Medicine 59: 17–18

Wing J K, Brown G W 1961 Social treatment of chronic schizophrenia: a comparative survey of three mental hospitals. Journal of Mental Science 107: 847–861

Wing J K, Cooper J E, Sartorius N 1974 Description and classification of psychiatric symptoms. Cambridge University Press, Cambridge

Zipursky R B, Marsh L, Lim K O et al 1994 Volumetric assessment of temporal lobe structures in schizophrenia. Biological Psychiatry 35: 501–516

14
Mood disorder

Guy Goodwin

INTRODUCTION

Mood disorder is the term now widely applied to a range of conditions in which the most prominent symptom is elevation or depression of mood. It is used synonymously with affective disorder. The most extreme forms of elation (mania) or depression (melancholia) have been recognised since the writings of Hippocrates. There is continuing uncertainty about how to subclassify the less severe syndromes of mood disorder. Understanding of mood disorder is also coloured by the experience and perception of normal mood both by patients and health care workers. Normal mood necessarily has an uncertain boundary with minor illnesses.

NORMAL MOOD

A moment's introspection will tell us that we use the word mood to describe pervasive feelings that are in part purely psychical but also have a powerfully physical component. When we feel happy we tend to have positive thoughts, feel more energetic, physically comfortable and lighter in limb. In the opposite state we are more prone to pessimistic and negative ideas, may feel literal physical discomfort and find action more effortful. What is perhaps most characteristic about mood is that it captures the character of any transient state of consciousness. Since it can dramatically change, what has the most power to change it? This can obviously be answered easily, if anecdotally: events, relationships, music, alcohol. There is no shortage of ordinary experience, therefore, that informs both our prejudices and our expectations of theories of mood.

The most influential contemporary psychological approach to mood has been cognitive. It supposes that a critical part of what determines mood tone is thinking and reflection. Beliefs and assumptions will clearly influence how we think. Abnormal beliefs or habits of thought could then provide an explanation for why optimistic or depressive interpretations might be made of events or experience. The extension of this view, usually attributed to Beck (Beck 1976), would place 'cognitive distortions' at the heart of mood disorder. Efforts to treat depression have been devised that are intended to change the beliefs of individuals with depressive illness. Notice that this view of mood disorder lends itself to an exclusively mentalistic view of mood. The Cartesian split between mind and body tends to make us think of 'mental illness' as not physical. The simplest cognitive account of mood perpetuates this. The prominence given to beliefs allows little credible room for biological mechanisms because, while we know that beliefs must be a product of brain function, they are so high level as to make the point academic.

Nevertheless, the broad alternative to a cognitive formulation of mood is a more biological one. Where cognitive psychology correctly emphasises the potential for thoughts to influence mood, more biological theories emphasise the potential for mood to induce particular patterns of thought. The widespread use of alcohol and stimulant drugs is informal testimony to the power of brain chemistry to influence human experience and behaviour through broadly mood-related mechanisms. In addition, the idea that 'stress' can influence body and brain states is also an old one. The relevance of this to our understanding of clinical states and their treatment will emerge below. However, the parallel strands provided by cognitive mechanisms on the one hand, and biological on the other, do not offer mutually exclusive alternatives: they demand some form of unification. William James famously proposed that emotion rested on the perception of the peripheral autonomic/somatic response to any emotion-provoking stimulus, although he also allowed that the efferent outflow might itself contribute feedback to the percept. This essentially placed peripheral bodily structures in series with brain regions mediating emotional experience. It predicted the abolition or at least modification of normal emotion by, for example, spinal transection, and the induction of strong emotion by peripheral autonomic agents such as adrenaline. The idea appears to have been widely discounted after an influential critique by Cannon (Cannon 1927). However, that the balance of autonomic and motor input/output may modify emotional experience still seems likely in view of the prominence of adverse visceral and muscular sensation in mood disorder. The evaluation of afferent information probably requires a particular central set or context which may easily be thought of as having either or both a cognitive and a neurochemical component. A direct experimental confirmation of the interaction between cognitive input and drug-induced autonomic changes was provided by Schachter (Schachter 1966). Hence a strong interoceptive stimulus must be interpreted in an emotional context derived from other mainly cognitive clues. This seemed best to reflect anxious or angry responding and is close to or identical with contemporary ideas about the evolution of panic anxiety from the misinterpretation of interoceptive cues (Ch. 17).

Emotion emerges from such analyses as something of a by-product. However, the history of human folly, and human triumph, suggests that it may influence our reason in most potent ways. Damasio has re-established this precedence experimentally rather than experientially by showing that somatic and autonomic factors are critical to normal *cognitive* performance in the domains of planning and judgement, not just in domains that are conventionally emotion laden. He has developed his arguments from the observation that brain lesions in critical areas produce impairments of on-line decision making and processing of emotion. These areas are the ventromedial prefrontal cortex, the amygdala and the somatosensory cortex in the right hemisphere. The relevance of these arguments to the neurobiology of mood disorder will be developed below. The ideas are extremely important for psychiatry generally in embracing a unitary approach to the mind–body problem and Damasio's book *Descartes' Error* should be required reading for all disciplines working with mentally ill patients (Damasio 1994).

MOOD DISORDER: AN ILLNESS OR A WEAKNESS?

The idea that we give meaning to ourselves and our experiences in part by interpreting the mood states that they provoke or recall is a powerful one. It means that subjective psychology and philosophy can accommodate disorders of mood into normalising views of human experience. It can give rise to the view that depressive illness does not in some sense exist. The argument behind this is usually that the concept of depressive illness is 'not scientific' because it is based

on arbitrary diagnostic criteria, or cannot be shown to be an illness in the way that, say, bacterial endocarditis can. Instead, the argument tends to go, it should be viewed as an existential struggle against despair. This point of view is put most uncompromisingly in books for popular consumption. The manner in which authors such as Dorothy Rowe or Peter Breggin set out to convince is to demand premature certainties of psychiatry. The scientific need to embrace hypotheses provisionally and cautiously can then be taken as proof of the discipline's failure and, further, as license for an author's personal agenda to be imposed instead. It is one of the more curious aspects of human psychology that unfounded intuitive certainty, like fundamentalism in its many forms, exercises a greater attraction for a significant section of the population than the reliable methods of scientific inquiry. Perhaps emotion intrudes into its own interpretation. This chapter will be written from the point of view that mood can show extreme manifestations, like other natural biological phenomena such as the level of blood pressure or blood sugar. It would be nonsense to dismiss descriptions of hypertension or diabetes by referring to the normality of having a blood pressure or a blood sugar level. By the same token, extremes of mood cause 'disease' in the people who suffer from them. Psychiatry aspires to bring the methods of science to bear on the problem: there have been some successes. However, in clinical circumstances psychiatrists and psychologists have to make what can be a difficult distinction between the two domains of normal experience and mood disorder. They have a boundary and at this boundary distinctions are difficult. Clinically the best guide to where one lies is in the realm of the phenomena we call symptoms and it is to these that we will turn first in outlining a disease-orientated understanding of mood disorder.

SYMPTOMS AND DIAGNOSIS OF MOOD DISORDER

Operational diagnosis of psychiatric disorder has been the major advance in psychiatry within the last 35 years. It seeks simply to identify the pattern of symptoms that most reliably characterises a given illness. It makes no claims about aetiology but, instead, makes possible the fundamental scientific activity of classification and, thereby, communication about similar patients. Clinicians can share experience and base their observations of treatment interventions on a sound footing. The identification of symptoms is however an arbitrary process and is based upon a judgement of severity, duration and, in some cases, quality of experience. Case identification can be made by self-rating or

Table 14.1 Criteria for major depressive episode (DSM-IV)

Five (or more) of the following symptoms have been present during the same 2 week period and represent a change from previous functioning; at least one of the symptoms is either (1) depressed mood or (2) loss of interest or pleasure.

Note: Do not include symptoms that are clearly due to a general medical condition, or mood-incongruent delusions or hallucinations.

1. Depressed mood most of the day, nearly every day, as indicated by either subjective report (e.g. feels sad or empty) or observation made by others (e.g. appears tearful). Note: In children and adolescents, can be irritable mood
2. Markedly diminished interest or pleasure in all, or almost all, activities most of the day, nearly every day (as indicated by either subjective account or observation made by others)
3. Significant weight loss when not dieting or weight gain (e.g. a change of more than 5% of body weight in a month), or decrease or increase in appetite nearly every day. In children, consider failure to make expected weight gains
4. Insomnia or hypersomnia nearly every day
5. Psychomotor agitation or retardation nearly every day (observable by others, not merely subjective feelings of restlessness or being slowed down)
6. Fatigue or loss of energy nearly every day
7. Feelings of worthlessness or excessive or inappropriate guilt (which may be delusional) nearly every day (not merely self-reproach or guilt about being sick)
8. Diminished ability to think or concentrate, or indecisiveness, nearly every day (either by subjective account or as observed by others)
9. Recurrent thoughts of death (not just fear of dying), recurrent suicidal ideation without a specific plan, or a suicide attempt or a specific plan for committing suicide

describe a loss of interest and pleasure in life. Suicidal thoughts and in some cases specific plans are quite common. While these symptoms may often be seen as the core of depressive illness, such experience is described by a range of people in unhappy situations, with unhappy backgrounds or with abnormal personalities. For that reason the additional symptoms necessary for a diagnosis of depressive illness are critical and must always be sought and identified with confidence. In clinical practice, diagnosis may rely particularly on evidence of impaired social, occupational or other function together with additional symptoms. If operational criteria are used, five symptoms from Table 14.1 are necessary for a diagnosis of major depression according to DSM-IV (APA 1994): comparable rules apply for a depressive episode (F32) in ICD-10 (WHO 1992). This is a relatively undemanding threshold and, as will be obvious on a moment's reflection, could include patients with a range and diversity of symptoms. Indeed two patients may score their five symptoms from entirely different parts of the alternatives shown in Table 14.1. This remains an unsatisfactory but unresolved paradox at the heart of diagnosis and classification of mood disorder.

Specimen cases

These illustrate contrasting types of clinical syndrome. They were chosen both to be males although either could have been female. The emphasis is on presentation and symptoms. The features that contribute to diagnosis are emboldened.

*A 48-year-old self-employed businessman presented with a **5 week** history of increasing **loss of interest** and **impairment of concentration**. In the preceding 4 months he had experienced problems following the death of a close friend who was also a business colleague. This had resulted in unexpected company debts, increased pressures of work and concerns about the security of his colleague's family.*

*In the last **2 weeks** he was **unable to work at all** and spent much of the time at home pacing up and down and **unable to make decisions**. He became increasingly **convinced that his business was going to fail and that he was probably already bankrupt**. His **sleep was grossly disturbed** and he had **impaired appetite** and **no sexual interest**. There was some **diurnal variation** of mood such that he tended to be more withdrawn and quiet in the early part of the day. He frequently expressed concern that the **problems were of his own making** and his life was a failure. On direct questioning he volunteered that he*

observer-rating methods. Observer-rating relies upon the interview of the patient by another person, usually a psychiatrist and tends to be regarded as more reliable than self-rating. The use of operational criteria strengthens the reliability of a conventional clinical interview. The symptoms that comprise a diagnosis of major depression are shown in Table 14.1. Notice that the symptoms have to be present for at least 2 weeks, although in practice they may often have been present for longer before a patient consults the doctor. The subjective experience of patients commonly leads them to describe their mood as depressed or negative and/or to had **had thoughts of ending his life by jumping from a bridge** close to his house.

What is striking is the extreme contrast between the patient when well and the state of depression. This man has markedly endogenous features (see below) despite an obvious precipitant and he poses a suicide risk. His beliefs about being bankrupt were almost delusional. Note that he did not complain specifically of being depressed but of his loss of interest and the capacity to solve problems. Paradoxically, therefore, he has a severe illness but the diagnosis could be missed if one has an approach to depressive mood disorder based on 'understandability' and experience of our everyday manageable misery. As William Styron (Styron 1990) pinpointed 'Depression ... used to be termed melancholia ... "Melancholia" would still appear to be a far more apt and evocative word for the blacker forms of the disorder, but it was usurped by a noun with a bland tonality and lacking any magisterial presence, used indifferently to describe an economic decline or a rut in the ground, a true wimp of a word.'

A 20-year-old male university student presented complaining of increasing worries about work. He dated these difficulties to a change in tutor who had been appreciably more aggressive in handling his written work. This had also activated resentments about coming to this particular university to please his parents. He described **crying virtually every day** for the last **3 weeks** and that his head felt 'about to burst'. He had **withdrawn from social activity** and was avoiding lectures. His anxiety was greatest in relation to work-related situations but he could **no longer concentrate** at all on reading. He was **low in spirits** and often ruminated about the probability of his failure and his lack of any subsequent prospects. He could see no future for himself and had thoughts of impulsively **taking an overdose** of paracetamol. He found such thoughts frightening but was concerned that he might nevertheless act on them. He described **sleeping for longer than usual** with occasional wakenings and bad dreams. His sleep however was unsatisfying and he felt **tired all the time**. Food consumption was normal but he had **no interest in sex**.

This is a man with prominent subjective distress who will be much more easily identified and may be more likely to seek help. The irony here is that, while he has a diagnosis of major depression (see the marked symptoms), the prominence of his anxiety symptoms may result in an explanation based on his 'personality' or the 'stress' of his academic schedule. The essence of an operational approach is that it identifies the relevant pattern of symptoms. This discipline is essential to clinical assessment before one addresses the more obvious psychosocial issues that seem to have precipitated illnesses of the sort described here. Nevertheless, the description of both these cases as major depression clearly misses something else, which is that they may represent different types of illness.

Subclassification of major depression is primarily to identify the more severe sort of disorder (as in the first case above) which is known as melancholia (DSM-IV) or somatic syndrome (ICD-10). The important additional symptoms include complete loss of pleasure in virtually all activities, lack of reactivity, a distinct almost painful quality to the depressed mood, motor slowing, agitation, marked disturbance of sleep and appetite and diurnal variations of symptoms. Guilt may be excessive or even psychotic. The patient is more likely to require inpatient admission. Melancholia is often diagnosed when there is a previous history of similar episodes responsive to treatment and showing full recovery (recurrent mood disorder). There is commonly a family history of mood disorder. An understanding of where the pressure for this sort of division of mood disorder originates can best be appreciated by a brief survey of the history of diagnosis in this area (a fuller account is given by Parker and colleagues (Parker & Hadzi-Pavlovic 1996)).

Severe depression has always been seen as the preserve of psychiatrists. Psychotic depression may result in a patient becoming virtually immobile, mute, indifferent or negative towards food and fluids and incontinent. The severity of these illnesses was well recognised in the 19th century, as was their tendency to show recovery. It is worth remembering however that patients might in some cases require 2 or 3 years in hospital, during much of which time they might require tube feeding to support their normal physiology (in depressive stupor). There was an associated acute mortality. When a classification of psychiatric disorder was being developed, these patients were placed in the general framework of manic–depressive psychosis: this of course was Kraepelin's contribution to the subdivision of psychosis in general. Patients with severe depression may show both delusions and hallucinations, although they are mood congruent. In other words, the delusions will have a deeply depressive colouring: the patient is bankrupt, he has a malignancy, infection or infestation, he is evil, can harm others, etc. Hallucinations will be accusing and derogatory. This territory of mood disorder was (and remains) very different from that inhabited by relatively minor cases of mood disorder seen in the community. Minor cases were initially seen as essentially the preserve of doctors offering supportive psychological treatment. The extension of psychiatric boundaries from the gates of the lunatic asylum to the greener pastures of primary care resulted in broadening of the umbrella under which mood states could be encompassed. However, the historical dichotomy between very severe illnesses (endogenous, psychotic) and less severe illnesses (reactive, neurotic) became controversial. There was a seminal debate between what can be described as the Newcastle School (Carney et al 1965), which claimed that suitable statistical treatment of symptom profiles resulted in a bimodal distribution of cases, and the Maudsley School, which denied that such operations were effective or that, when they were, they were influenced by the preconceptions of the doctors making the ratings (Lewis 1934, Kendell 1968). Broadly speaking, the Maudsley view prevailed and major depression came to be seen as displaying a continuum of symptoms from psychotic to neurotic.

It is probably correct that patients in general cannot be readily dichotomised on the basis of interviews that seek subjective phenomena as the criteria for diagnosis. However, an interesting alternative approach has been developed within the last few years by Parker and colleagues. This has sought to base classification upon what they describe as a sign- rather than a symptom-based typology. In other words, they suggest that to observe particular signs in patients is more discriminating than eliciting the common subjective clinical symp-

toms. The reason for this is made obvious in Table 14.2, which shows the relative frequency of signs and symptoms in psychotic, endogenous and neurotic cases with major depression. A symptom such as suicidal ideation is common in all groups. Thus it is a good identifier for major depression but a poor discriminator between the putative subtypes. By contrast, a sign such as slowing of speech rate is very unusual in neurotic depression but occurs in almost 30% of endogenous cases. Accordingly, it would be a poor item for diagnosis of major depression but a good discriminator between endogenous/psychotic and neurotic cases. Identification of a group of signs contributing this pattern of difference made possible the construction of an endogenicity measure (the CORE). It shows a bimodal distribution across the patient population where symptom scores (and the Hamilton rating scale) do not (Fig. 14.1). The existence of such bimodality is what much of the preceding debate had been about. A re-analysis of Lewis' own data (Parker & Hadzi-Pavlovic 1993) gave the same result! In addition, entirely objective tests of psychomotor speed give a bimodal result (Parker & Hadzi-Pavlovic 1996). This is the revised basis for thinking of mood disorder as having two somewhat separate incarnations as melancholic or non-melancholic illnesses. That the separation may nevertheless be largely an effect of severity of illness is suggested by analysis of the genetics of melancholic depression, albeit defined primarily by symptoms

Table 14.2 Percentage of patients with particular selected signs and symptoms rated as present in each of three diagnostic subgroups of major depression

Clinical feature	Percentage affirming feature			
	Psychotic (n=73)	Endogenous (n=140)	Neurotic (n=200)	Odds ratio
Signs				
Non-reactivity	96	84	33	14.6***
Delay in responding verbally	64	39	4	22.1***
Poverty of associations	84	61	10	20.8***
Delay in motor activity	44	29	1	103.8***
Slowing of speech rate	36	27	2	28.2***
Symptoms				
Appetite loss	83	82	57	3.4***
Weight loss	78	69	45	3.1***
Indecisive	82	93	83	1.6
Unpleasant thoughts	94	82	84	1.2
Suicidal thoughts	71	62	76	0.6
Loss of interest in pleasurable activities	96	96	88	2.1
Energy worse in morning	42	60	43	1.5

Odds ratio comparing psychotic + endogenous depressed with neurotic depressed *** P<0.001.

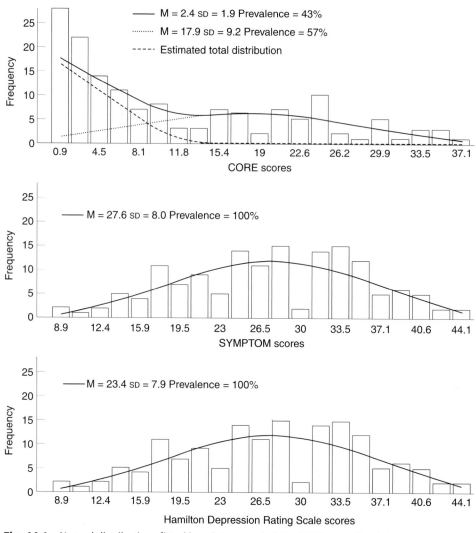

Fig. 14.1 Normal distributions fitted by mixture analysis to CORE scores (top), SYMPTOM scores (middle) and Hamilton scores (bottom). Number of distributions plotted determined by significance test.

rather than signs (Kendler 1997). Only a molecular genetic account is likely eventually to clarify the true relationship between the phenotypes.

Although there is a general belief that DSM-IV and ICD-10, in their slightly different ways, are no better than provisional classifications, there is no consensus on how they could be improved. Indeed, they are the only consensus. The terminology is outlined in Table 14.3. Alternative classifications are of limited interest. For example, the distinction between primary and secondary depression is one that has found some favour in the USA (Winokur 1990). Secondary depressions are defined as being preceded by another psychiatric illness (alcohol dependence, eating disorder, anxiety disorder)

or accompanying a serious physical illness. Primary depressions may only be preceded chronologically by mania. Like other diagnostic schema this is an attempt to isolate a core depressive syndrome and separate it from the many other cases where the diagnosis of depression is complicated by a variety of other features. The primary advantage of this classification has been assumed to be that it will identify a subgroup of patients with a specific (genetic) aetiology: in fact, it performed poorly in a twin study to estimate heritability for different definitions of illness (Kendler et al 1992). The classification seems unlikely to be adopted for clinical purposes as it has little to contribute to prognosis and treatment.

Tables 14.3 Classification of depressive disorders	
DSM-IV	ICD-10
Major depressive episode Mild Moderate Severe Severe with psychosis	*Depressive episode* Mild Moderate Severe Severe with psychosis
	Other depressive *episodes* Atypical depression
Major depressive *disorder recurrent*	*Recurrent depressive* *disorders* Currently mild Currently moderate Currently severe Currently severe with psychosis In remission
Dysthymic disorder	*Persistent mood* *disorders* Cyclothymia Dysthymia
Depressive disorders not *otherwise specified* Recurrent brief depression	*Other mood disorders* Recurrent brief description
Hypomanic episode *Manic episode* Mild Moderate Severe Severe with psychosis	*Manic episode* Hypomania Mania Mania with psychosis
Bipolar I and bipolar *II disorder* Current (or most recent episode) Hypomanic Manic[*] Depressed Mixed[*] *Cyclothymia*	*Bipolar affective* *disorder* Currently hypomanic Currently manic Currently depressed Currently mixed In remission
*Excludes bipolar II.	

Atypical depression

The use of this term has varied over the years but has increasingly converged on a presentation where there are reversed biological symptoms (increased eating and sleeping) and unusual reactivity of mood. There may also be a characterological sensitivity to personal rejection. Indeed the apparent prominence of personality difficulties may serve to distract the clinician from iden-

tifying the major depressive episode. It is claimed that the response to monoamine oxidase inhibitors (MAOIs) is better than to tricyclic antidepressants (Quitkin et al 1988, 1989). A subclassification of depressive syndromes on the basis of likely therapeutic response retains an important potential value for clinical practice. The differential effect of phenelzine relative to imipramine is also seen at drug withdrawal after 6 months. Phenelzine-treated atypicals were much more likely to relapse if it was discontinued compared with those treated with imipramine (Stewart et al 1997).

Brief recurrent depression

The existence of short episodes of severe but transient depression of mood lasting 2–7 days recurring frequently is not a new finding (Paskind 1929). However, recurrent brief depression was first formally described for community samples by Angst and colleagues (Angst et al 1990). There may be an important relationship with similarly short periods of anxiety (Angst & Wicki 1992) and with the risk of deliberate self-harm (Angst & Hochstrasser 1994). The comorbidity with major depression (and dysthymia) is striking and serially patients may show conversion from major depression to recurrent brief depression and vice versa (Angst 1996). Recurrent brief depression is a category in ICD-10 (F38.10) but the concept has been slow to be adopted in the USA (Keller et al 1995). Treatment trials have been disappointing (Montgomery et al 1994). The area is likely to remain important because, together with the problem of residual symptoms, a shift to longer term treatment in mood disorder will raise the importance of longer term outcomes, both in the domains of symptoms and of personal or social function.

Minor depression, dysthymia and depressive personality

Minor depressive states still present a diagnostic muddle. Efforts to wring meaningful classifications out of minor symptoms, present to a greater or lesser degree either with more obvious temperamental abnormality or with more prominent anxiety symptoms, remain of dubious clinical value. Symptoms that are both milder and are present for longer periods of time have attracted attention recently. DSM-IV includes a category of mood disorder described as dysthymia where fewer depressive symptoms are present for over 2 years. As well as the symptoms contributing to a diagnosis of major depression, there are symptoms such as feelings of pessimism, low self-esteem, low energy, irritability and decreased productivity. In the past these clinical cases would have been largely subsumed under the notion of neurasthenia or depressive personality (Hirschfeld 1994) but interest in them has been provoked by the reports of responsiveness to drug treatment (Baldwin et al 1995; Thase et al 1996). This is of particular relevance given the availability of drugs of greater specificity and therefore of lower side-effect profile than tricyclic antidepressants and old-style MAOIs. The diagnosis is sometimes made in patients with superimposed major depression.

The status of depressive personality disorder is uncertain. Personality disorder must be present from adolescence, invariant, more or less, throughout life. Akiskal has argued that temperament is critical to understanding the spectrum of chronic affective disorder (Akiskal 1983), and this has echoes of the emphasis of an earlier generation of clinicians on illnesses as reactions by personality types (Slater & Roth 1969). Certainly, the stability of measures of personality such as neuroticism (N) is well established across the life-span by very large studies (Costa & McCrae 1994) and the disposition in high N subjects to react negatively appears to have validity in acute experimental studies (Larsen & Ketelaar 1989). What makes the notion of depressive personality disorder difficult is the addition of yet another arbitrary threshold for 'diagnosis'. Personality dimensions par excellence seem to require continua not categories. It seems quite likely that diagnosis of discrete syndromes would in general be enriched by systematic measures of personality. This is no less true in states where euphoria may alternate with depression, as will be described below.

Mania

The development of manic states is a feature of those mood disorders described as bipolar or manic–depressive. Association of manic states with depressive states serially in the same individuals was a key observation of Kraepelin. The symptoms of mania are characterised by disinhibition of psychomotor function. Patients are more active, experience pressure of thought and may show flight of ideas as thoughts crowd in faster than the patient can speak. Projects get started and not finished. They frequently attribute an increased importance and meaning to their thoughts and plans. The emotional rapport is often infectiously euphoric but opposition may be met with irritability and even violence. The presentation may be frankly psychotic and delusions are typically grandiose in content. In the most severe illnesses, patients may also experience hallucinations of the sort usually associated with schizophrenia. Distinction between psychotic and non-psychotic mania is an arbitrary one. However, patients generally show impaired judgement in manic states. In their

---

Table 14.4 Criteria for manic episode (DSM-IV)
A. A distinct period of abnormally and persistently elevated, expansive, or irritable mood, lasting at least I week (or any duration if hospitalisation is necessary)
B. During the period of mood disturbance, three (or more) of the following symptoms have persisted (four if the mood is only irritable) and have been present to a significant degree: 1. Inflated self-esteem or grandiosity 2. Decreased need for sleep (e.g. feels rested after only 3 hours of sleep) 3. More talkative than usual or pressure to keep talking 4. Flight of ideas or subjective experience that thoughts are racing 5. Distractibility (i.e. attention too easily drawn to unimportant or irrelevant external stimuli) 6. Increase in goal-directed activity (either socially, at work or school, or sexually) or psychomotor agitation 7. Excessive involvement in pleasurable activities that have a high potential for painful consequences (e.g. engaging in unrestrained buying sprees, sexual indiscretions or foolish business investments)
C. The symptoms do not meet criteria for a Mixed Episode.
D. The mood disturbance is sufficiently severe to cause marked impairment in occupational functioning or in usual social activities or relationships with others, or to necessitate hospitalisation to prevent harm to self or others, or there are psychotic features
E. The symptoms are not due to the direct physiological effects of a substance (e.g. a drug of abuse, a medication, or other treatment) or a general medical condition (e.g. hyperthyroidism)

---

expansive state of mind they may spend large amounts of money, indulge in risky or undesirable sexual activity which they subsequently regret and may be extremely difficult with the people around them. Dangerous driving is a particular hazard and patients with a history of severe mania are required to notify the licensing authorities and are disqualified from driving for 6 months after a severe episode. Since patients may have a good deal to lose by exposing people in the family, and particularly at work, to their behaviour when manic, it would be wrong to see the boundary between psychotic and non-psychotic mania as a particularly critical one in terms of management. Patients also show prominent sleep disturbance, commonly going for days without feeling the need for sleep, the sleep deprivation probably thereby contributing to their irritability and erratic behaviour. The diagnostic criteria for mania are shown in Table 14.4. Unipolar recurrent mania is unusual but has been described. However, more common is a lifetime history of mood disorder characterised by episodes of mania and depression.

Hypomania is the term that describes states of euphoria and overactivity short of mania. Subjectively, patients tend to feel unusually well and energetic. Their capacity to work and be creative may be genuinely increased but the limits over which they may slip to become judgement impaired are always uncertain. Subjective accounts capture the experience very graphically. It is a particular problem that hypomania is usually, perhaps understandably, viewed very positively by patients (Jamison 1995). Poor compliance with drug treatment and the denial of more severe disturbance is often related to the wish to experience hypomania in its least troubled forms. Unfortunately, hypomania, like mania, is also associated with depressive swings.

The depressive states of bipolar disorder are indistinguishable from those of severe unipolar depression. The only difference emerging from modern comparisons has been shorter episodes and more agitation in the melancholic forms of bipolar depression (Mitchell et al 1992). This may reflect the underlying neurobiology that underpins the manic upswing. In addition, mixed states may be seen where symptoms of mania and depression may be comingled or alternate over short periods of time.

In recent years, there has been increasing interest in the occurrence of hypomania in association with recurrent major depression (bipolar II disorder in DSM-IV). This may, in over 10% of cases, be succeeded by the development of a frank manic episode. However, more important conceptually is the idea that bipolarity in its minor or temperamental forms is much more common than is currently appreciated. Cyclothymia also identifies a subsyndromal predisposition to cyclical mood change. The most persuasive proponent of the importance of subsyndromal mood disorder is, again, Akiskal (Akiskal & Akiskal 1988). The dilemma, as ever with DSM-type classification, is where to draw the line around a syndrome of a particular severity and finite duration and where we should be seeking to capture the quantitative and qualitative range of individual temperament. However, there is the further problem that while premorbid personality measures of subjects with a subsequent unipolar course show high neuroticism, bipolars are normal (Clayton et al 1994). Retrospective measures of temperament may be influenced by a recent illness: the so-called scar effect on personality. The issue awaits resolution and is not simply academic if mood stabilising drugs are a better choice in patients with minor bipolar disorders than antidepressants alone.

CLASSIFICATION OF MOOD DISORDER BY CLINICAL COURSE

Mood disorders tend to recover but to recur. Kraepelin placed a central emphasis on recovery between episodes in his great division between schizophrenia and manic–depressive psychosis. Unipolar depression describes patients having recurrent depressive episodes (and includes perhaps 5% of patients who will subsequently be found to be bipolar) and the term bipolar disorder is reserved for patients with a history of mania. Unipolar mania is sufficiently unusual to be ignored. The bipolar/unipolar distinction was proposed by Leonhard and popularised in the English language literature by Perris and others. However, it was intended to apply to recurrent endogenous illness so the extension of the term unipolar to all cases of major depression is arbitrary. The unipolar/bipolar division is clinically useful because it appears to have implications for treatment. The contemporary classification of mood disorders in DSM-IV and ICD-10 is shown in Table 14.3.

Seasonal affective disorder

Mood has a seasonal variation within the normal population. Seasonal affective disorder (SAD) was a term introduced to describe patients who answered newspaper advertisements designed to recruit people who thought they had a seasonal mood disorder. It turned out that they tended to describe rather consistent atypical symptoms: hypersomnia, hyperphagia, tiredness and low mood in winter (but the syndrome does not include rejection sensitivity) (Rosenthal et al 1984). It was initially claimed that the condition was responsive to bright light therapy in the early morning and this was attributed to a physiological resetting of the photoperiod (perhaps involving melatonin). This turns out to have been a beautiful hypothesis rather spoiled by the facts. It has proved difficult to show any benefit in SAD of bright light over dim light (Levitt et al 1994) or of early morning exposure compared to midday (Jacobsen et al 1987, Lafer et al 1994) or increased sensitivity to light in the suppression of melatonin (Murphy et al 1993). Furthermore community studies do not support the notion of a specific syndrome, although there is some seasonality of mood disorder in general, as long recognised (Wicki et al 1992). The status of SAD and light therapy accordingly remains unclear. Patients with winter episodes of major depression are best treated conventionally.

EPIDEMIOLOGY OF THE DEPRESSIVE DISORDERS

Our knowledge of the incidence and prevalence of mood disorders comes from detailed structured interviews of representative population samples. This is a relatively recent innovation (Ch. 6) so that our understanding of the extent of mood disorder is better now than it has ever been. However, there are difficulties. Population studies immediately throw up a boundary problem. There appears to be a more or less continuous variation between the well and the ill with regard to subjective distress, identification of particular symptoms or groups of symptoms, duration and degree of impairment. Where one sets the threshold for defining a case of depression therefore determines what actual percentage value one obtains for incidence and prevalence. In the epidemiological catchment area (ECA) programme in the USA, representative samples of more than 18 000 adults aged 18 years or over were interviewed in five representative centres (Regier et al 1988). The lifetime prevalence for all DSM-III affective disorders was between 6.1% and 9.5%. Major depression was the most common diagnosis, showing a lifetime prevalence in women between 4.9% and 8.7% and for men of 2.3% to 4.4%. These studies have now been extended multinationally (Weissman et al 1996). The lifetime rates for major depression varied across countries, ranging from 1.5 cases per 100 adults in Taiwan to 19.0 cases per 100 adults in Beirut. The annual rates ranged from 0.8% in Taiwan to 5.8% in New Zealand. The mean age at onset showed less variation (range 24.8–34.8 years). There was an increased risk of comorbidity with substance abuse and anxiety disorders. Individuals who were separated or divorced had significantly higher rates of major depression in most of the countries, and the risk was somewhat greater for divorced or separated men than women in most countries. The rates of major depression are usually higher for women than men. As a rule the multiplier is approximately ×2 and appears at puberty (Angold & Worthman 1993). The cause of this female excess is a source of controversy. At least in part, it could be an artefact. Men may be less likely to admit to having depressive symptoms and more likely to forget previous symptoms that they have experienced (Angst & Dobler-Mikola 1984). However, a genuinely higher prevalence of depressive disorder in women is still widely accepted. The relative contribution of psychological, social and biological influences to the sex difference is not understood. The potential explanatory factors include psychological attributes (temperament, personality and attributional/coping styles) and the experience of psychosocial adversity, as the need for social support seems stronger in women. Menstruation, childbirth and child-rearing may also increase the risk of depression. The possible biological underpinnings of such differential mechanisms will be considered with other aspects of the neurobiology. Whatever the mechanism, the consequences of mood disorder may be worse in men even when symptoms are mild, with increased premature mortality described in the Stirling County cohort (see below).

Major depression overlaps critically with dysthymia. A survey of five American communities showed that dysthymia affected approximately 3% of the adult population (Weissman et al 1988). It had a high comorbidity with other psychiatric disorders, particularly major depression; only about 25–30% of cases occur over a lifetime in the absence of other psychiatric disorders. Although the onset and highest risk for more severe mood disorder was young adulthood, a residual state of dysthymia occurs typically in middle and old age.

Because of the potentially uncertain boundary between chronic symptoms and mood disorder reaching criteria for major depression, cross-sectional epidemiological studies risk confounding incidence with recurrence. A longitudinal investigation of psychiatric epidemiology in a general population – the Stirling County study (Murphy et al 1989) – has suggested that the incidence of depression and anxiety disorders is low relative to prevalence because these disorders have long durations. In an average year approximately nine adults among 1000 experienced a first-ever episode of one of these disorders. This work highlights the difficulty of interpreting retrospective accounts of symptoms. Recovery to some criterion may distort a true picture of long-term symptoms and difficulties, the severity of which waxes and wanes. This affects the vexed question of whether the incidence of mood disorder is rising.

Are we in an age of melancholia?

Recent epidemiological studies have suggested that the risk of major depression has been increasing in recent decades. In 1985, the results of interviews with 2289 relatives of 523 probands with affective disorder in the USA were published (Klerman et al 1985). It was observed that the lifetime occurrence of depression was higher in younger relatives than older relatives: the opposite of what would be expected if risk had remained constant. When the relationship between decade of birth and risk of illness by age was analysed, the effect was even more striking. For women born after 1950, the risk of major depression appears to be almost 70% by age 30! This appears to represent a major shift forward in the age of onset and the lifetime risk. All these relatives necessarily had an increased risk of mood disorder compared with the general population but the same pattern has been observed in the ECA population study (Klerman 1988, Klerman & Weissman 1989). Indeed there is also prospective longitudinal evidence favouring a trend to earlier onset of depression from the Stirling County study (Murphy 1994). Simple memory artefacts in older subjects, while they must occur along with other biases, appear not to be a full explanation for the cross-sectional findings (Warshaw et al 1991). Interpretation should remain cautious because the same pattern of increasing risk in recent birth cohorts is seen for mania (Lasch et al 1990), which appears much more epidemiologically stable (see below). What such findings actually imply, if correct, can only be guessed at. Social changes could be exercising strong and changing influences on the risk for depression of Western populations but, specifying how, for example, family relationships or the frequency of life events has changed over the last century will not be feasible. It also seems improbable that the social change should have been so consistently for the worse. For the moment, we have no way of knowing whether these findings represent an accurate basis for predicting further growth in the burden of disability imposed on societies by mood disorder in the coming decades. It is safe to predict a growth on the basis of improved detection of cases.

EPIDEMIOLOGY OF BIPOLAR DISORDER

The lifetime rates for bipolar I disorder are much lower and more consistent across countries (0.3/100 in Taiwan to 1.5/100 in New Zealand), the sex ratio is more equal and the onset age is earlier than for major depression. It is of particular interest that female sufferers have proportionately fewer manic episodes. It is increasingly claimed that the onset of bipolar disorder may often be in the teenage years when the diagnosis may be missed: this is an age for which systematic epidemiological studies are not available. In addition, bipolar disorder may develop in children referred with attention deficit hyperactivity disorder. The unipolar–bipolar conversion rate is of the order of 5%. New onsets may increase in the elderly (Eagles & Whalley 1985). The very stability of its demographic characteristics favour a primarily biological explanation for the causes of bipolar I illness. As already indicated, bipolar II disorder is of emerging interest. It appears likely to be more common than bipolar I disorder (Simpson et al 1993) and must often be misclassified as unipolar depression.

AETIOLOGY OF MOOD DISORDER

Our understanding of the aetiology of mood disorder is developing rapidly on the basis of critical scientific inquiry. It is important not least for the emphasis properly placed on alternative modes of treatment. More biologically determined conditions appear more likely to require medicines. More psychosocial causes of mood disorder may more plausibly prompt psychological interventions.

Individual cases of unipolar depression often appear to have understandable antecedents (life events or difficulties) which precipitate an illness. The extent to which such events independently and literally *cause* a depressive illness is always more questionable. The majority of individuals appear to negotiate the same losses and disappointments without decompensating and becoming ill: they cope. The failure to cope appears to be strongly determined by vulnerability factors which may in some cases be largely genetic, and in others the consequences of adverse early environmental experience. Recovery may be spontaneous or promoted by drug or psychological intervention. The aetiology of individual cases is always more speculative than that of experimental cohorts but it is worthy of formulation both as an exercise for the clinician but also as a help for the patient. Interpersonal psychotherapy (IPT) (Klerman et al 1984) has as its central ingredients clear identification of symptoms, diagnosis and formulation of causal factors. Improved objective understanding of aetiology can be used constructively by patients in managing their illnesses. Self-management of mood disorder is likely to assume increasing importance as patients become better informed about what is known of their conditions.

Studies of the inheritance of mood disorder

Family studies

As has been noticed in the preceding section, affective disorder is more common in the relatives of identified probands with affective disorder than in the general population. The highest risks are seen with the most severe illnesses. This is illustrated in Figure 14.2, which shows the relative risks of different sorts of affective disorder for the first-degree relatives of normal controls, patients with unipolar disorder, bipolar disorder and schizoaffective disorder. The striking conclusion is that the risk of unipolar illness is about constant in the relatives of patients with these illnesses (around 20%). However, there is an increased risk of bipolar and schizoaffective disorder, respectively, in the relatives of patients with these illnesses in the index proband.

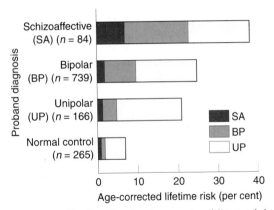

Fig. 14.2 Affective disorders in parents, siblings, adult offspring of probands, Bethesda, USA

These findings are compatible with the view that the more severe the illness in an index case, the greater the risk of a severe illness in first-degree relatives. Clearly average risks of this sort may respectively underestimate or overestimate the risks in a single family. For example, the family of Vincent van Gogh, who had a severe mood disorder and, of course, committed suicide, had above average rates of severe psychiatric disorder (Jamison & Wyatt 1992). Such observations do not of course prove a genetic cause: families might influence the risks of mood disorder by their interactions and behaviour. Proof requires twin studies, where a discrepancy is sought between the concordance for monozygotic or genetically identical twins and dizygotic twins who should show simply the first-degree risks shown by other siblings. Such studies have been conducted classically on twin series from hospital registers but more recently also upon large community samples of twins. We now know a great deal about the relationship between genetic risk, environmental or familial influences and mood disorder.

The genetic basis is strongest for bipolar disorder where almost 60% of identical twins will develop the same bipolar illness as cotwins in monozygotic samples, compared with something of the order of 14% in dizygotic pairs. Severe unipolar illness shows similarly high concordance for hospital samples. For example, probands with major depressive disorder ascertained via the Maudsley Hospital Twin Register showed proband-wise concordance of 46% in monozygotic ($n = 68$) and 20% in dizygotic ($n = 109$) twins. There was no evidence of a sex difference in heritability or of shared environmental effects. A duration of longest episode of less than 13 months, multiple episodes, and an endogenous rather than neurotic pattern of symptoms tended to predict a higher monozygotic:dizygotic

concordance ratio (McGuffin et al 1996). Heritability was between 48% and 75%.

The links between genetic, temperamental and other risk factors and major depression have been forged most significantly by the ground breaking work of Kendler's group at the Medical College of Virginia. They originally interviewed a large sample of female–female twin pairs and used nine definitions of major depression, producing lifetime prevalence rates from 12% to 33% (Kendler et al 1992). For seven of the definitions, the estimated heritability of liability ranged from 33% to 45%. For the two definitions that included only primary cases of depression, the heritability was lower (21% to 24%). The critical conclusions were that the tendency for depression to aggregate in families results largely from shared genetic and not from shared environmental factors and the magnitude of genetic influence was similar in broadly and narrowly defined forms of major depression. Most environmental experiences of causative importance for depression are those not shared by members of an adult twin pair (i.e. more likely to be individual events rather than shared environmental factors) (Kendler et al 1992). Genetic factors are apparently shared between major depression and generalized anxiety disorder. Whether a vulnerable woman develops major depression or generalized anxiety disorder is a result of her individual environmental experiences (Kendler 1996). The essential conclusion is that major depression in community samples is a markedly, but by no means overwhelmingly, genetic condition. Genetic explanations that ignore environment are likely to be partial. However, environmental explanations that ignore genetics will equally be misleading.

Of the genetic liability to major depression, 55% appeared to be shared with the personality trait, neuroticism or N. A value for N 1 SD above the mean increased the risk of major depression within the next year by 100–130%. In fact, Kendler's group developed an exploratory but comprehensive model that accounted for 50% of the variance in the liability to major depression in a 1 year follow-up. Stressful life events, genetic factors, a previous depressive episode and N emerged as the best predictors of a subsequent depressive episode (Kendler et al 1993b).

The heritability of neurotic traits has also emerged from smaller studies. A genetic analysis was conducted on trait neuroticism and symptoms of anxiety and depression in 462 mixed-sex twin pairs from the Australian Twin Registry interviewed five times at regular intervals (Andrews et al 1990). When the lifetime history of these subjects was determined, rates of diagnosable disorder were low and the study lacked the power to detect a genetic pattern. However, there was substantial genetic involvement in the average level of neuroticism and current symptoms. Neither genes nor the shared environment of the twins was a significant cause of lability in these measures, which was primarily affected by adverse life events.

The co-occurrence of mood disorder with alcohol and illicit substance abuse / dependence

The association between alcohol misuse and mood disorder is both clinically and theoretically important. There were significant genetic correlations (from +0.4 to +0.6) between major depression and alcoholism in women, which were higher using narrower criteria for alcoholism (Kendler et al 1993a). Thus, comorbidity in women appears to result largely from genetic factors that influence the risk to both disorders. Other genetic factors exist that independently influence the liability to mood disorder without influencing the risk for alcoholism, and vice versa. Cigarette smoking is also weakly related to the risk of mood disorder: twin analysis suggests that it results solely from genes that predispose to both conditions (Kendler et al 1993d). It is tempting to speculate that abnormal function in reward mechanisms may underpin these associations.

Molecular genetic findings in mood disorder

The molecular genetic approach promises to give us clues to the underlying biochemistry of mood disorder (Ch. 7). The inheritance of mood disorder is unlikely to be due to the gene mutations that underlie the best known (but much rarer) genetic diseases such as Huntington's chorea or the larger deletions of genetic material that underlie many severe congenital diseases, in most cases leading to mental handicap. These are genetic mistakes which can express their consequences independent of environmental influence. More common diseases are likely to be related to the presence of what are called polymorphisms. These are different forms of normal genes (or alleles) present at different rates in the population, whose variation may be benign under most circumstances but still increases the risk of a disorder via dysfunction of the physiology that they control.

The role of putative loci can be established by linkage or allelic association studies. The best known linkage study was of a large Old Order Amish pedigree which was originally believed to show linkage of bipolar affective disorder to markers on chromosome 11 (Egeland et al 1987). Unfortunately this proved to be the first of several (false) positive studies announcing the linkage of the major psychiatric disorders to loci that could not

subsequently be confirmed (Kelsoe et al 1989; Pauls et al 1991). The effort has, however, continued with renewed caution in accepting initial positives. There have been further putative reports of linkage of bipolar disorder to chromosome 4 (Blackwood et al 1996), chromosome 18 (Berrettini et al 1994; Freimer et al 1996) and chromosomes 6, 13 and 15 (Ginns et al 1996). Single studies of this sort need to be adequately powered or to be collaborative so that findings from many centres using comparable methods can be combined. The preliminary results of a major American initiative are appearing and suggest loci on chromosomes 1, 6, 7, 10, 16 and 22 (Nurnberger et al 1997). These effects appear worryingly small and it remains to be seen how many of these findings will prove to be, first, replicated and, second, sufficiently localising to identify the relevant gene involved. If the function of the gene is known, the progress is likely to be straightforward. If it is not, then efforts to determine the function of individual genes are extremely complicated and a long time is likely to elapse between the identification of the site and an understanding of why it is important.

It is now quite easy to genotype large numbers of patients and controls and to determine whether or not particular alleles are present in excess in patient populations. In consequence, allelic association studies of so-called 'candidate' genes are proliferating. Findings from the gene coding for the serotonin transporter protein (SERT) have attracted particular attention because of the importance of the serotonin transporter as a singular site of action for antidepressants such as fluoxetine and the other selective serotonin reuptake inhibitors (SSRIs) (see below). The first report of this sort described an association between the rare allele of a variable number tandem repeat sequence in an intron of the SERT and mood disorder (both unipolar and bipolar patients) (Battersby et al 1996; Ogilvie et al 1996). This association could represent a type 1 error, a direct effect of the allele on the function of the gene or linkage disequilibrium with a site close by of more direct relevance to the actual effect. The latter possibility is raised by the finding that another allele has been associated with bipolar disorder (Collier et al 1996). What is undeniably interesting is to implicate a gene that is coding for a protein critical to the action of antidepressants. Nevertheless, the significance of all these findings is tempered by the small size of the effects. This means that the contribution of these genes to the total risk of mood disorder may be quite low. It is also still possible that particular drugs may be differentially effective in individuals carrying particular polymorphisms; there are some preliminary examples of this demonstrated in psychiatry.

The significance of advances in this area will be to confirm the role of particular neurotransmitters and their receptors for mood disorder. There is also the potential to identify entirely new receptor mechanisms or pathways which may become a target of yet more effective and more focused treatments. At present we have no way of knowing whether the total risk is contributed by a few factors of relatively large effect or whether only factors of small effect predominate. This will be of considerable importance to whether genetics makes any impact at all in shaping our approach to treatment of mood disorder. If all the genes discovered are in fact of small effect, it is possible that genetics will offer no logical way to increase the effectiveness of our existing drug treatments. The contribution of genetics may then be to justify efforts to improve psychosocial treatments!

Environmental risk factors for affective disorder

While genetic factors determine the major risk of bipolar and severe unipolar disorder, there is an appreciable environmental contribution to the timing of severe illnesses and the incidence of less severe depressive illness. We have already noticed the variation in incidence of major depression between different societies and apparent increases in its frequency over time which seem to imply a major cultural effect on its expression. Kendler's exploratory attempt to weight the contributions of multiple factors to the onset of depression in the community is an important framework for starting to understand the role of 'social' factors as independent variables (Kendler et al 1993b). The studies that have hitherto attracted most attention in 'social psychiatry' have not controlled for the effects of genes. Surveys of inner-city populations of working-class and single mothers have indicated that adverse experiences in childhood and adolescence (involving parental indifference, and sexual and physical abuse) considerably raise the risk of both depression and anxiety conditions (with the exception of mild agoraphobia and simple phobia) in adult life (Brown & Harris 1993, Brown et al 1993). Given a strong prevailing bias to construe minor psychiatric disorder in these terms, the idea that vulnerability to depression is a socially determined risk has enjoyed easy acceptance. However, there is a quantitative balance between what is genetic and what is purely social. In a sense, what is left after the appropriate genetically controlled experiments have been done could be regarded as the 'environmental variance'. However, this must also contain error and chance. The problem is an intriguing one and is perhaps best illuminated by the example of 'independent life events'.

Life events emerged strongly from Kendler's studies as predictors of the onset of major depression. In the best known social studies, the impact of specific life events has been judged with a strong emphasis on their context (Brown 1993). This means that life events are not judged as simple objective setbacks, such as the loss of a spouse or parent, but instead are given a weighting which relates to the closeness of the lost relative and the impact upon the individual patient. While this clearly has clinical meaning, it risks incorporating factors that are equally to do with personality and, potentially, genetic endowment. It inevitably confounds these factors, while attributing to them an independent status. Despite this, the important social findings such as the differential effects of threat and loss events (to produce anxiety or depression) have been strengthened by genetically controlled studies. The less rigorous methodology has also suggested a useful difference between first episodes and recurrences in more endogenous cases, with life events playing a part in the former, but not to the same extent in the latter conditions (Brown et al 1994). However, the new genetic findings suggest that genes contribute significantly to the vulnerability that is sometimes regarded as entirely social in origin (Kendler et al 1993c) and even to the exposure to life events. The 'heritability of life events' had been highlighted in other studies (McGuffin et al 1988, Thapar & McGuffin 1996). In Kendler's community sample, genetic liability to major depression was associated with a significantly increased risk of assault, serious marital problems, divorce/breakup, job loss, serious illness, major financial problems and trouble getting along with relatives/friends. The effect was not due to events occurring during depressive episodes (Kendler & Karkowski-Shuman 1997). About 10% of the total genetic liability to major depression may be mediated by genetically determined life events. In other words, certain traits appear to predispose individuals to select high-risk environments.

The significance of genes for social activity remains controversial. However, if we concede that socialisation has been a critical evolutionary development for the human species, it is difficult to argue that genes will have had no impact on behaviour and predispositions within it. The precise pattern and interaction of genes with early experience of loss and adversity that can predispose to depression is uncertain. Kendler's model lacked the power to distinguish between various pathways to vulnerability (Kendler et al 1993b). To take a specific example, the idea that early loss may have important long-term consequences for individual psychopathology is an old one. It is the sort of concrete idea that appealed to Freud, for example. However, actually proving a specific association with depression has proved much harder. Early loss appears to make individuals more likely to seek help for all sorts of medical ailments. Case series of almost any diagnosis will then show an excess of parental death.

The relationship between lack of adequate parental care in early life and an increased risk of depression is more convincing. Abuse and neglect are, however, highly non-specific factors which increase the risk of psychiatric disorder generally, and reflect gross disruption of the nurturing process. It is more difficult to decide whether more subtle disturbance of the parent–child relationship contributes as much as is popularly believed to the development of adult psychopathology. Adult reports of childhood difficulties can be systematised with the Parental Bonding Instrument (Parker 1983, Parker 1986, Parker & Barnett 1988). It identifies two dimensions: caring/non-caring and protective/overprotective. Non-caring and overprotective parental styles are associated with mood disorder in later life, but most strikingly with non-melancholic disorder (Parker et al 1987, 1995). There are non-causal explanations of this association: current depression might influence judgement of parental characteristics, reported parental characteristics may simply be wrong and those with a depressive predisposition might elicit less parental care and greater overprotection. The first two explanations appear to be excluded by appropriate experiments (Parker 1981). However, the determinants of parenting are obviously complicated and a recent examination of the same measures in twins suggested that parental warmth was influenced by personality factors in both parents and children, while authoritarianism was related to educational and religious background (Kendler et al 1997a).

Recovery and improvement, when compared with conditions not changing, has been claimed to be associated with a prior positive event (Brown et al 1992). Such events were characterised by one or more of three dimensions: the 'anchoring' dimension involved increased security; 'fresh-start', increased hope arising from a lessening of a difficulty or deprivation; and 'relief', the amelioration of a difficulty not involving any sense of a fresh start. Events characterised by anchoring were more often associated with recovery or improvement in anxiety, and those characterised as fresh-start were associated with recovery or improvement in depression. Recovery or improvement in both disorders was more likely to be associated with both anchoring and fresh-start events. The effects of improved mood per se on the social measures could not be clearly differentiated and these ideas remain highly provisional. Again, genes play a part. In a twin design, the four variables that influenced the time to recovery from depressive episodes were financial difficulties, obses-

sive–compulsive symptoms, severe life events and genetic risk (Kendler et al 1997b). All depressive episodes meeting symptomatic DSM-IIIR criteria were divided into early (5–28 days) and late (> 28 days) phases. Cases with more chronic depression showed an effect of personality, financial problems and genetic risk as predictors of slow time to recovery, suggesting different processes in recovery from brief versus prolonged depressions.

Bipolar disorder

The effects of life events on the recurrence or onset of bipolar disorder have received much less attention than for non-endogenous major depression. There appears to be a small excess of life events in advance of manic recurrence in bipolar illness (Hunt et al 1992a). The best known example of a life event precipitating mania is childbirth, where 1 in 500 mothers may develop a psychosis within 3 weeks of delivery, which is usually manic in form (Kendell et al 1987). Manic illness appears not to occur in any particular season but bipolar depression may be more common in the autumn (Silverstone et al 1995). Perhaps 10% of patients appear to manifest an individual seasonality (Hunt et al 1992b): this can be clinically useful in advising patients on self-management.

Drugs and hormones

Depressive symptoms are strongly associated with the withdrawal of alcohol and stimulants like amphetamine or MDMA (ecstasy) (Peroutka et al 1988). Ecstasy has relatively selective effects on the serotonergic system and it is tempting to suppose that these effects are generally related to serotonergic projections because specific depletion of these neurones produces depressive symptoms (see below). Since these are non-prescribed drugs, some uncertainty surrounds the effects. A more specific problem is posed by corticosteroids which appear to increase the risk of affective disturbance and, in particular, of mania or hypomania, in relation to dose. Almost 3% of patients treated with a high dose of steroid may develop a clinically significant disorder of mood and this is by far the highest sort of risk known for an exogenous stimulus (Boston Collaborative Drug Surveillance Program 1972). Recent controlled studies have confirmed high rates of subclinical mood elevation after 1 week of steroid administration (Naber et al 1996). Chronic exposure to corticosteroids, as in Cushing's syndrome, tends to be associated with depression of mood (see below). There are many anecdotal claims associating specific drug classes with effects on mood, but only calcium channel blockers and digoxin have been associated with depression by replicated, well-conducted studies (Patten & Love 1997). β-Adrenoceptor blockers and thiazide diuretics probably do not have important effects on mood.

Physical illness

Physical illness increases the risk of developing depressive illness (see also Ch. 27). While this may be understandable in the sense that the threat of a severe illness to an individual may provide a very powerful and pervasive negative context to his life, it nevertheless merits treatment. There are some specific associations which may turn out to be of particular aetiological interest and will be described here.

Depressive illness and stroke

It has been suggested that depression is common after stroke and that the particular site of the brain insult may influence the risk of subsequent mood disorder. Thus, as well as a non-specific risk from the severe illness there may be a specific neuropsychiatric impact, depending on the localisation of the lesion. The original studies concentrated on selected groups of patients requiring hospital admission and longer term care. They suggested an association between depression and left frontal pole regions, and euphoria and right hemisphere lesions (Robinson et al 1983). This is of some interest given the neuroimaging findings implicating left frontal cortex in mood disorder (Ch. 15). Even in an unselected series of patients recruited from the community, in the 12 months after the stroke emotionalism was 10–20% and there was again an association with left-sided anterior lesions (House et al 1989), but there was a smaller number of cases of major depression. However, subsequently, the same study was summarised much more negatively as showing low rates of mood disorder and no evidence for localising lesions (House et al 1990). A comparably negative study has been reported using a similar patient sample (Burvill et al 1996). Clearly rates of depression vary between series (Andersen et al 1994) and are likely to be influenced by a range of general risk factors for depression that may often swamp the effects of the site of lesion (Burvill et al 1997). The question of whether, in an appropriate case–control series, there are nested associations between lesion location and risk of depression remains of neurobiological interest. For example, lesions in the region of the left basal ganglia have been suggested to be more specifically associated with depression (Herrmann et al 1995).

Whatever the aetiology, depression is also of appreciable practical importance for the management of stroke patients (Robinson 1997). Drug treatment of poststroke depression has been subjected to a number of small controlled trials. The evidence is that antidepressants are effective, although some tricyclic drugs may be prone to produce confusion (Robinson et al 1995).

Heart disease

Findings in patients with myocardial infarction (MI) with depressive symptoms are surprising and interesting. Several studies have now described an association between short-term mortality following MI and the presence of significant depressive symptoms. For example, 222 patients were interviewed between 5 and 15 days following the MI and were followed up for 6 months (Frasure-Smith et al 1993). Depression was a significant and independent predictor of mortality from cardiac causes (95% CI 4.61 to 6.87). The effect was confirmed at 18 months (Frasure-Smith et al 1995). Traditionally, it might be supposed that depressive symptoms after MI would be reactive. In fact, there is evolving evidence that depressive symptoms can predict an elevated risk of MI many years before it occurs (Barefoot & Schroll 1996) and/or in the few weeks before an acute admission (Carney et al 1990). A follow-up of the Baltimore cohort of the epidemiologic catchment area study showed that, compared with respondents with no history of dysphoria, the odds ratio for MI associated with a history of dysphoria was 2.07 (95% CI 1.16 to 3.71), and with a history of major depressive episode was 4.54 (95% CI 1.65 to 12.44), independent of coronary risk factors (Pratt et al 1996). A recurrence detectable in the coronary care unit may carry a particularly poor prognosis (Lesperance et al 1996). Patients with severe affective disorder have long been known to have an increased mortality from cardiovascular causes and the association between the two is of considerable evolving interest. If the most common cause of death is cardiac arrhythmia, as seems likely (Frasure-Smith et al 1995), the relation between autonomic function and the neurobiology of mood will be of renewed interest.

NEUROBIOLOGY

There are no even partly satisfactory animal models of mood disorder but there is a highly relevant emerging literature on the understanding of emotion in animals. Behaviour theory was erected on the idea of primary reinforcing stimuli, positive ones such as taste and smell increasing associated responses, negative ones such as pain producing avoidant responses. Secondary associations are postulated to grow out of the pairing of primary reinforcers with a particular context. The complex emotional associations we experience with social situations, specific people and events could clearly be elaborated upon a basic theory of this sort. Intriguingly we increasingly understand where the neural processing must be occurring. It appears to be in inferior frontal cortex. Primary reinforcing stimuli such as taste and smell are modalities whose representation in secondary sensory areas is directly within this cortical region (Rolls 1990). Visual input is from much more highly elaborated representations that have already been processed through a number of cortical association areas. Are we in a position to say whether a lesion in inferior frontal areas renders people incapable of experiencing emotion? The answer is, probably, yes: the experience of emotion is different in such individuals (Rolls et al 1994) and the failure of their on-line monitoring of interoceptive bodily feelings seems to deprive them of 'gut feelings' that are essential for normal cognition (Damasio et al 1990, Bechara et al 1996). The question of pathological depression or elation of mood is more difficult since 'normal emotion' usually refers to anxiety. However, imaging studies have tended to localise the critical areas for mood change in mesial frontal cortex (Goodwin 1996).

The understanding of mood *disorder* in terms of neurobiology remains tentative while we have limited animal models. The identification of trait neuroticism as a risk factor with a significant heritability should be understandable in biological terms. Gray explicitly proposed that it might reflect an enhanced sensitivity of a 'behavioural inhibitory system' to negative experiences (Gray 1982), which echoes Eysenck's own approach to understanding neuroticism in man. Experimentally, high N individuals show a greater sensitivity to negative mood induction, while high E (extraversion) is associated independently with a greater sensitivity to positive mood induction (Larsen & Ketelaar 1989, 1991; Watson et al 1994). Why some depressive states persist and seem to become metastable is not understood. How cognitive information is processed may be important (Carr et al 1991, Dritschel & Teasdale 1991). The differences in cognitive function between individuals may be manifestations of different neuronal connectivity. Alternatively, there may be local properties of the brain areas directly involved in subserving mood that decide mood stability. For example, it has been claimed recently that a lobule of inferior frontal cortex, thought to be a critical node for the integration of mood, is atrophic in major depressive illness (Drevets et al 1997). Other abnormalities in brain structure might influence inferior frontal cortex through diffuse failures in afferent input. Severe mood disorder tends to be associated with ventricular enlargement and sulcal prominence (Elkis et al 1995). First episodes of severe depression occur more frequently with increasing age and tend to be more refractory to treatment (Ch. 25). Such illnesses are associated with evidence of structural abnormality in the brain (Soares & Mann 1997) and cognitive impairment (Abas et al 1990, Beats et al 1996). Therefore, imaging suggests that something is permanently wrong in the brains of patients with particularly intractable mood disorder. Indeed this finding may be linked to poor outcome (Hickie et al 1995). This emphasises the need to ground explanations of illness in a unitary appreciation of psychological and biological variables. Structural brain abnormality is not of course an explanation for the more familiar illnesses that do show recovery.

Most of what we know, or think we know, about the neurobiology of mood disorder is based on the modulation of mood by drug treatments. In other words the reversibility of mood disorder has seemed to require a neurochemical rather than a structural basis. It has given rise to what is generally called the monoamine hypothesis of affective disorders. Drugs such as reserpine can induce a depressed mood, whereas amphetamine and, particularly, ecstasy can induce euphoria, overactivity and excitement. Because these drugs modulate the levels and release of monoamines in the brain this provides prima facie evidence of their relevance to the normal regulation of mood and possibly to the mechanisms of mood disorder. The monoamines concerned are noradrenaline, dopamine, 5-hydroxytryptamine (5-HT, serotonin) and acetylcholine. Cells containing these chemicals are present in neurones whose cell bodies are in the brainstem and midbrain. They project diffusely into forebrain areas where they appear to regulate global behavioural states or functions such as the sleep–wake cycle, appetite, motivation, motor activity, aggressiveness, sexual responsiveness and aspects of learning and memory. The evidence for involvement in these integrated behavioural responses is derived from animal experimentation, but it will be immediately obvious that these functions echo elements of psychiatric symptomatology described in depression. The first generation of drugs discovered to treat mood disorder also have their primary actions on monoamines. Monoamine oxidase inhibitors (MAOIs) inhibit the breakdown of monoamines via the enzyme monoamine oxidase which exists in two forms: the A form catalyses the breakdown of noradrenaline and 5-HT and the B form that of dopamine (and 5-HT). The original MAOIs were non-selective between the A and B form and irreversible in their action. Subsequently, drugs more selective for monoamine oxidase A and showing reversibility (e.g. brofaromine, moclobemide) have been shown to be effective antidepressants.

The other mechanism for antidepressant action is via the inhibition of monoamine reuptake. The tricyclic antidepressants appear primarily to act in this way, inhibiting the reuptake of both noradrenaline and 5-HT (but not dopamine at clinical doses). Their antidepressant actions were discovered initially by accident through the clinical investigation of the drug imipramine (Kuhn 1958). This led to the discovery that imipramine and the other tricyclics inhibit the reuptake of monoamines. Reuptake was recognised as a novel means of terminating neurotransmitter action both in the periphery and in the brain. Blockade of these receptors prolongs transmitter availability.

The most important development since then has been that of genuinely selective inhibitors of the reuptake of 5-HT. These drugs, called the SSRIs, have been shown to be effective antidepressants at doses where their action must be essentially on a single receptor. This is an exceedingly important theoretical and practical observation. It means that a highly complex disease can be treated by a drug acting at a single receptor in the brain. This is in itself a powerful argument that reduced serotonergic function is a central abnormality in mood disorder and that its correction leads to clinical response. Other evidence supports the proposition that 5-HT is unusually and specifically involved in mood disorder. The evidence for this is based on a number of different lines of enquiry. It will serve as the introduction to a neuroscience literature which is too large to survey here comprehensively. However, the fundamental weakness of the monoamine theory is its failure to take account of what is most puzzling and important about mood disorder: its poor outcome in a significant number of severe cases.

CSF metabolites

The monoamines are metabolised by relatively simple pathways that give rise to a small range of metabolites. These can readily be measured in cerebrospinal fluid (CSF) and allow rough estimates of transmitter turnover. In general these have revealed small and not always consistent differences in neurotransmitter metabolism in patients compared with controls. The National Institute of Mental Health (NIMH) study showed a tendency for increased levels of metabolites of noradrenaline and dopamine in the manic state compared with controls, and a relative depression of levels in the depressed state, particularly in dopamine turnover (Koslow et al 1983). The findings for 5-HT suggest increases in the manic state, particularly in women, and did not show significant decreases in depression. Reduced 5-HT metabolite level (and, hence, turnover) has been described in a variety of other studies. Most consistently this has implicated violent acts either towards the patients themselves (Traskman et al 1981) or others (Virkkunen et al 1994). The association between violent and impulsive behaviour and reduced 5-HT function also emerges from studies of non-human primates (Mehlman et al 1994). A series of patients undergoing neurosurgery for depression, from whom CSF was obtained, also had depressed 5-HT metabolites (Francis et al 1993). Even if the results had been consistent it would have been difficult to distinguish between different possible causes because the physiology of people who are significantly sleep disturbed or who have lost weight may be different from that of normal controls but may be only indirectly related to disturbance of mood.

Tryptophan depletion

Perhaps the most convincing evidence that 5-HT is involved in mood disorder comes from depletion of its amino acid precursor tryptophan. Tryptophan, both in peripheral blood and in brain, can be driven to very low levels by loading with large neutral amino acids which both compete with it for access to the brain amino acid transporter and increase the metabolism of all large neutral amino acids peripherally. The consequence is reduced synthesis and release of 5-HT. Tryptophan depletion might be expected to uncover vulnerability to depressive symptoms normally gated by 5-HT neurotransmission. That it does so is very important confirmation of the 5-HT hypothesis. Tryptophan depletion produces reductions in mood in females, not males (Ellenbogen et al 1996), which may parallel both the vulnerability of women in general to mood disorder and the greater vulnerability of the serotonergic system to dietary perturbation (Goodwin et al 1987). There is a similar effect in males with a family history of mood disorder (Benkelfat et al 1994). However, much more striking is that, in patients who have recovered from a depressive episode during treatment with a 5-HT selective reuptake inhibitor, tryptophan depletion produces a transient but clear-cut return of severe symptoms (Delgado et al 1990, 1991). Patients treated with an inhibitor of noradrenaline reuptake, such as desipramine, do not appear to show the effect. This finding has now been extended to patients with a history of recurrent major depression who are euthymic but off all medication (Smith et al 1997). These findings directly implicate 5-HT specifically in the mechanism involved in the development of mood disorder. What is particularly intriguing is that prominent objective symptoms of retardation and cognitive distortion return in both a stereotyped and severe way, reflecting symptoms when previously ill. By contrast, suicidal thoughts and other cognitive measures usually sensitive to self-rating do not. The apparent immediacy of the link between neurotransmitter function and symptoms may be the reason why the most vulnerable groups need long-term treatment with antidepressant drugs to remain well.

Hypercortisolaemia

It is well established that patients with major depression have a raised cortisol output and that this tends to normalise on recovery. The most significant effect appears to be an elevation of the usual nadir in the evening, although total cortisol levels are increased generally. The meaning of this phenomenon is still highly uncertain. An attempt was made to develop a test for severe depression based on the suppression of endogenous cortisol secretion by dexamethasone (the dexamethasone suppression test or DST). Suppression occurs when the sensitivity of the normal glucocorticoid receptor-mediated inhibitory feedback to the hypothalamus is present: non-suppression of endogenous cortisol occurs, for example, in Cushing's disease. It implies either reduced feedback and/or enhanced central drive to release cortisol. The initial findings were that the 1 mg DST showed high specificity (96%) and sensitivity (67%) for melancholia (Carroll et al 1981). This result has proved difficult to replicate. The high specificity was only established against normal controls and is clearly much less when other patient groups are included (Berger et al 1984). Non-suppression reflects hypercortisolaemia and there is quite a strong association between hypercortisolaemia and psychotic illness in general, particularly psychotic mania (Christie et al 1986). It is also possible that some patients show DST non-suppression as a result of weight loss (Mullen et al 1986), or because of altered metabolism of dexamethasone (Holsboer et al 1986).

In some respects the cortisol story has been too quickly devalued because of its failure to tie in with conventional ideas about how mood disorder should be diagnosed. Instead it should perhaps have been regarded as a phenomenon to be explained rather in the way that we may regard retardation, itself not specific to depression. Hypercortisolaemia certainly occurs and is both easy and objective to measure. This is of course less true of other symptoms that we identify as part of the depressive syndrome. In addition, relatively impaired glucocorticoid feedback has been described in the relatives of patients with mood disorder (Holsboer et al 1995). It appears that increased cortisol production is associated both with an increased release of hypothalamic β-endorphin (Goodwin et al 1993) and probably a pulsatile increase in adrenocorticotrophin (ACTH). However, in addition there appears to be peripheral hypertrophy of the adrenal glands which results in a measurable increase in size on magnetic resonance imaging (MRI) and an enhanced response to a given dose of corticotrophin (Gerken & Holsboer 1986). Like the hypercortisolaemia itself, the MRI change is reversible on recovery (Rubin et al 1995).

What remains unclear is whether cortisol actually contributes to the clinical picture by a direct action on the brain. This is of interest because of the association between exogenous cortisol administration and affective symptoms. It has led to efforts to treat mood disorder by inhibition of cortisol synthesis with metyrapone: preliminary results suggest this may be effective (O'Dwyer et al 1995, Thakore & Dinan 1995). This has led to the speculation that excessive cortisol secretion can produce depressive symptoms, as, indeed, seems to occur in Cushing's disease (Loosen 1994). Cortisol could of course be a plausible mediator between a variety of stresses and the biological components of mood disorder (Stokes 1995). Thus, the onset of depressive symptoms and their diurnal change could be accounted for by altered diurnal modulation of cortisol secretion. This concept of 'cortisol toxicity' remains to be convincingly tested. If this were indeed the explanation for mood disorders, in general, antagonists of cortisol's action should be extremely effective antidepressants. This appears inherently implausible but is clearly worth excluding. The other contradictory aspect of these findings is that when depressed patients are given large doses of cortisol, they tend to show acute mood enhancement (Goodwin et al 1992). This could lead to a mirror image hypothesis that actually cortisol is a euphoriant (or antidepressant) and therefore the hypercortisolaemia is an effort to mount an antidepressant action via the stress regulating mechanisms of the brain. An additional complication is that cortisol is believed to act on two receptors in the brain (the glucocorticoid and mineralocorticoid receptors) which may have opposed actions (DeKloet et al 1997). There is accordingly scope for opposing hypotheses of glucocorticoid action. Furthermore there is some emerging evidence that patients with early experience of abuse and neglect and individuals with post-traumatic stress disorder may show hypocortisolaemia. The future development of this field requires the elucidation of the psychotropic effects of cortisol itself upon the brains of patients who are potential hyper-or hyposecretors. The lumping together of depressions with different aetiology may explain our failure to find consistency hitherto. Given that hypercortisolaemia remains one of the more robust biological findings in mood disorder, we will have to return to it eventually for our understanding of the neurobiology to be complete.

Other endocrine abnormalities

There is also persistent interest in the role of the thyroid axis in mood disorder. There are abnormalities of the thyrotrophin (TSH) response to thyrotrophin-releasing hormone (TRH). The TSH secretion that results is impaired in some patients with depressive illness but this effect is poorly understood and has few accepted clinical associations. The use of thyroid hormones in treatment is sufficiently interesting to suggest that there is more to be learned than we know currently about this endocrine axis. There is certainly evidence that thyrotropin has important interactions with transmitter systems within the brain, and whether these are abnormally regulated in mood disorder remains unknown.

Sleep disturbance

Sleep is disturbed in depression in a variety of ways. The most typical, early morning waking, is by no means the only pattern that is seen, and trouble getting to sleep, frequent wakings and unsatisfactorily prolonged sleep are also common. Like other biological manifestations of the disorder, the extent to which sleep is simply a consequence of depression or contributes to its biology is tantalisingly uncertain. In favour of the latter view, patients even with severe depression may respond to sleep deprivation with a transient increase in mood. This occurs in patients refractory to other forms of treatment but has a limited value because the effect is rarely sustained and the consequences of chronic sleep deprivation are too difficult to make it a practical alternative. The fundamental involvement of the sleep–wake cycle in mood disorder is however interesting in view of the rhythmicity seen in bipolar disorder in particular and the possibility that some of the mechanisms that are involved may overlap and have a common biology. EEG recording either in a sleep laboratory or using ambulant methods has allowed the characterisation of the sleep disturbances in mood disorder (Berger & Riemann 1993). In melancholia the most characteristic effects are a reduction in the total length of slow-wave sleep and a shortened latency to the appearance of rapid eye movement or REM (dreaming) sleep. REM induction has been claimed to represent a cholinergic mechanism that may be abnormal in depression (Giles et al 1988, Berger & Riemann 1993), although its fundamental involve-

ment in mood disorder is made less likely by the observation that REM changes can be mimicked by sleep restriction (Mullen et al 1986).

General problems with biological investigations of mood disorder

There are rather few measures of physiological, neuropharmacological, neuroanatomical or biochemical abnormality in the brain or blood or urine of subjects that could not be made the subject of a study that contrasts patients with mood disorder with normal controls. Attention has been focused here on those areas that have been most interesting. However, the acute disturbances of physiology and behaviour that are seen in severe depression are such that almost no aspect of the performance of an organism is likely to be entirely untouched by the state of depression. This implies that any of the changes that have been seen may be epiphenomena of the physiology that is so obviously disturbed in depression and mania (Mullen et al 1986, Goodwin et al 1987). What would be much more interesting is an abnormality that is demonstrably present in the euthymic condition. There is probably an increasing realisation of this and a move therefore to studying patients who are at high risk of mood disorder but are well. Such studies must also recognise our improved understanding of aetiology. Abnormalities in vulnerable subjects when compared to low-risk individuals are much more potentially interesting and much more potentially relevant to the development of new interventions.

EFFECT OF BRAIN AGEING

Age is an important risk factor for the development of severe mood disorder. This is true of both mania and depression (Eagles & Whalley 1985, Young & Klerman 1992) and may provide additional clues to the pathophysiology of mood disorder at the level of regional connectivity and in relation to specific markers. Normal ageing is accompanied by a decline in a variety of indices of monoamine function, including presynaptic markers of 5-HT innervation. There is some evidence for reduced binding at these sites post mortem in depression (Perry et al 1983) and suicide (Mann et al 1996). Whether a reduced serotonergic innovation is the critical change that increases the vulnerability to mood disorder of patients with advancing years is not yet established. Postmortem studies in elderly depressed patients appear likely to have more potential validity than the (much more numerous) reports on schizophrenia: a definitive study is awaited.

TREATMENT OF DEPRESSION: PRIMARY CARE

If patients are reluctant to seek treatment and the detection of depressive illness in primary care is as low as it appears to be, then the majority of episodes of depression receive no treatment at all. Most placebo-controlled trials of antidepressant treatment are accordingly most relevant to patients seen in primary care. There tends to be a high placebo response rate (40%). The choice of effective drugs that we now have available is quite large. In addition we have at least two classes of psychological treatment which also have efficacy relevant to treatment in primary care: cognitive behaviour therapy (CBT) and interpersonal psychotherapy (IPT) and the related method of problem solving. At present we really have no way of deciding which should be regarded as best practice. There are a number of issues, which include relative efficacy, adverse effects, subsequent risk of recurrence, costs both direct and indirect, and last, but not least, acceptability to patients. Really large comparative trials will be required to decide what the strategy should be for treatment of depressive illness in primary care. At present, the most likely choice is between one of the antidepressant drugs.

Reuptake inhibitors

Tricyclic drugs and the newer, more selective compounds (selective serotonin reuptake inhibitors or SSRIs) act primarily to block active transport of neurotransmitters back into neurones (Ch. 4). The older compounds (amitriptyline, imipramine, chlomipramine) are still widely used and, if anything, are more effective than the newer drugs in patients with severe illness (Anderson & Tomenson 1994). Quantitative reviews comparing the actions of the tricyclic drugs with the newer compounds suggest equality of efficacy in less severe illness (Song et al 1993). This has formed the basis for advice to general practitioners favouring tricyclics, heavily influenced by their cheapness. The major problem with the tricyclics is the need to employ doses of 150 mg at night or higher (correspondingly lower in older patients). At such therapeutic levels there are commonly important side-effects. These are due to actions at cholinergic receptors (dry mouth, sweating, mild tachycardia), histamine receptors (sedation, weight gain), serotonergic receptors (weight gain, disturbed sexual function). Amitriptyline tends to have more actions of this sort, imipramine (and especially desipramine) rather less. However, the sedative action is sometimes valued by patients who are having difficulty sleeping or who have marked anxiety symptoms. These side-effects are usually, however, a disadvantage and a reason why patients may discontinue treatment (Anderson et al 1994, Maddox et al 1994). Taken with their greater danger in overdose, there is an argument that newer compounds should be employed because of their greater acceptability. In principle, more patients will be treated effectively with a drug that they will take than with one that they will not. While this is a compelling argument in theory, it requires more information from pragmatic clinical trials of adequate power. The alternative newer compounds are as follows.

SSRIs (selective serotonin reuptake inhibitors)

These drugs work at a single receptor and their adverse effects are accordingly related to the central therapeutic action of the drug. They are not however free of side-effects, which include nausea and even vomiting (tending to diminish with time), orgasmic impotence, which is a major problem in long-term use for some patients (albeit a possible advantage for male patients with premature ejaculation), and sleep disturbance. The SSRIs available in the UK are fluvoxamine, fluoxetine, paroxetine, sertraline and citalopram. While pharmacologically similar they are not identical and some patients experience idiosyncratic reactions to one of the drugs that they do not experience on others (for example, marked agitation). The use of the SSRIs has increased dramatically since their introduction. What is interesting is that most of this increase in prescribing appears to be additional to, not just instead of, tricyclic prescribing. This may reflect the greater acceptability of SSRIs. They are also easier to prescribe because of their simple dosing requirements.

Receptor antagonists

Other drugs increase the availability of monoamines (specifically 5-HT and noradrenaline) by mechanisms other than reuptake inhibition (Davis & Wilde 1996). The most widely prescribed include mianserin and its successor mirtazapine. Compounds such as trazodone may also fall into this category.

Reversible inhibitors of monoamine oxidase

The conventional MAOIs (see below) would rarely be considered first-line treatments in primary care but their successors are reversible compounds which require fewer dietary precautions, are safer in overdose and carry a lower risk of interactions with tyramine-containing foodstuffs. Moclobemide may, accordingly, be an adequate antidepressant for use in primary care.

Its relative advantages are not yet established. Particular caution is required if patients are prescribed moclobemide and an SSRI sequentially. There is then the risk of a combined overdose which can produce a very dangerous toxic serotonin behavioural syndrome with hyperthermia (Neuvonen et al 1993). The MAOIs and SSRIs (and clomipramine) should never be used together because they can produce related effects at therapeutic doses.

TREATMENT OF DEPRESSION: SECONDARY CARE

Tricyclic antidepressants

Tricyclic drugs remain an important and useful class of drugs for treatment of severe depression in secondary care. As already indicated, the main problem is the need to treat with doses which almost inevitably incur adverse effects, although most patients are prepared to persevere with treatment because of the severity of their mood disturbance. The apparent advantages of tricyclic drugs over newer compounds are most clearly seen in older inpatients where clomipramine has been shown to be superior to citalopram and paroxetine (Gram 1986, Anderson et al 1990, Anderson & Tomenson 1994). This is a theoretically important finding if it reflects the action of clomipramine on both noradrenergic and serotonergic reuptake sites to facilitate transmission in both pathways. Venlafaxine is a compound which inhibits reuptake in vitro at both sites but has few other actions. It shows the predicted superiority to fluoxetine in at least one trial in inpatients (Clerc et al 1994): milnacipram has the same sort of profile. The selectivity of these drugs with a double action (including mirtazapine) should confer advantages compared with tricyclics in the treatment of patients in secondary and tertiary care.

Monoamine oxidase inhibitors

Patients who fail to respond to tricyclic drugs may respond to monoamine oxidase inhibitors. The previous reputation of these compounds for lack of efficacy resulted from the use of too small a dose in influential trials (Medical Research Council 1965). A drug such as phenelzine should be given at doses above 45 mg daily. The major disadvantage with the MAOIs is the requirement for strict dietary avoidance of fermentation products to prevent the so-called cheese reaction (the ingestion of tyramine-containing foods that are toxic in the presence of complete and irreversible monoamine inhibition). They may also produce postural hyperten-

sion at relatively low doses. Severe cases of mood disorder merit a trial of an MAOI where tricyclics have failed.

Electroconvulsive therapy

ECT is an important treatment for severe depression. The indications are usually psychotic or endogenous features and, commonly, the failure of drug treatment. In addition, ECT is indicated in emergencies where depressed patients are refusing food and drink, on the basis of extreme retardation or nihilism. ECT is now always administered under general anaesthesia with a neuromuscular blocking agent 2 or 3 times per week. Its unpleasantness is about the same as going to the dentist. The effectiveness of ECT is well supported by clinical trials and there are no established long-term adverse sequelae. Despite this, the rate of administration clearly varies a good deal from region to region and consultant to consultant, probably reflecting the ebb and flow of opinion about its use, which has long been controversial. The Royal College of Psychiatrists produces regular guidelines to regulate practice and maintain standards. Unless contraindicated by confusion, bilateral ECT is preferable and seizure duration should be monitored as greater than 20 s to ensure optimal efficacy. The number of administrations required varies a good deal but is usually between 4 and 6 treatments. The earliest changes occur in feeding and locomotion and the response rate under naturalistic conditions should be about 80%. The problem is sometimes maintaining improvement in patients who may be relatively refractory to drug treatments.

Combination treatments

Patients seen by psychiatrists are much more likely to have a poor outcome or fail to respond at all to first-line treatments than those seen in primary care. Their management is therefore empirically based upon the use of logical drug combinations. The discussion of the pharmacology of this approach is beyond the scope of this chapter, and experience and considerable care are probably required to avoid problems. That said, the most important options are the following.

Augmentation with lithium The addition of lithium to either tricyclic antidepressants, SSRIs or MAOIs appears to be associated with an acute antidepressant effect in up to 50% of patients otherwise refractory to monotherapy. This is a relatively simple drug combination but there is uncertainty about its longer term benefits. Use of lithium increases the complexity and difficulty for the patient because of the need for continuing plasma monitoring.

Addition of tryptophan It was probably the first application of rational psychopharmacology to add tryptophan in the treatment of patients refractory to MAOIs (Coppen et al 1963). It may also be a useful adjunct to treatment with clomipramine and there are advocates for the addition of both tryptophan and lithium to either an MAOI or clomipramine in the treatment of the most severely refractory patients. The withdrawal of tryptophan (because of fears about impurities) produced relapse in the patients treated long term with these combinations (Ferrier et al 1990).

Thyroid augmentation There is evidence to support the augmentation of antidepressant treatment with tri-iodothyronine (T_3) (Joffe et al 1993, Aronson et al 1996).

In general this is an area of considerable uncertainty and efforts to trial different combination treatments, preferably combined with newer compounds of dual action, are probably necessary.

STRATEGIES OF MANAGEMENT IN MAINTENANCE AND CONTINUATION TREATMENT

In primary care, the primary objective is to treat, be it with drugs or psychological methods, to a good short-term outcome over about 6 months. At that point treatment is usually withdrawn: many patients will have only a single episode of mood disorder. We are very unsure whether active treatment affects the long-term outcome of mood disorder in individual patients. Since many patients must be untreated, the natural course of illness in younger patients may be spontaneous recovery. It seems reasonable to assume that more decisive treatment is necessary with later onset or with chronic or repeated illnesses. The evidence for this however remains circumstantial.

Patients referred to psychiatrists tend by definition to have more severe illnesses either in relation to the severity of symptoms, their duration or their tendency to recur. The strategy for treating most patients with mood disorder seen in secondary and tertiary care should be, first, to get effective acute treatment using the necessary strategies outlined above, and then to continue with an acceptable maintenance treatment for a further period of time. How long that should be remains controversial. In cases of severe illness the risk of chronicity and recurrence are so great that the objective of treatment should probably be long term (i.e. indefinitely). At present this is a difficult conclusion for many doctors and patients themselves to accept. The evidence is however that with each recurrence the risk of a further subsequent illness is increased and the time at which it will occur tends to advance.

There is evidence that long-term treatment with lithium is effective in treating unipolar disorder (Souza & Goodwin 1991). This is a logical continuation treatment for patients who have required lithium augmentation in the acute phase of their illness but seems not to be very commonly considered because there is no particular evidence of an advantage over the use of long-term reuptake inhibitors. There have been good long-term studies demonstrating the efficacy of imipramine up to 5 years in patients showing recurrent unipolar depression (Kupfer et al 1992). Continuation treatment for up to 2 years has been examined for the SSRIs.

THE PLACE OF PSYCHOLOGICAL TREATMENTS

The idea that a psychological treatment might be as effective as a drug treatment in acute illness and offer greater protection from recurrence is an attractive one (Andrews 1996). Maintaining recovery is an important objective of effective psychological treatments for panic disorder or eating disorders. Trials in primary care have tended to suggest a particular benefit from CBT in depression (Blackburn et al 1981, 1986), although most such patients recover, however treated (Scott & Freeman 1992).

For more severe depressive illness, however, there is reasonable evidence from a large NIMH multicentre trial (Elkin et al 1995) that cognitive therapy is not particularly effective in the acute treatment phase. Indeed ITP was probably superior. Although the original analysis of this study was probably inadequate, reanalysis has not changed the conclusions, much as it has served to sharpen the debate. The tentative finding that patients failing CBT respond to imipramine (Stewart et al 1993) underlines the conclusion that severe depressive illness is best treated with an effective antidepressant. The issue, which remains uncertain, is whether, nevertheless, CBT may improve the long-term outcome. This can only be answered by a trial of cognitive therapy specifically directed at the prevention of relapse or recurrence. The difficulty with cognitive therapy is that it is complicated and requires extensive training. Interpersonal psychotherapy (Klerman et al 1984) and its close relation, problem-solving psychotherapy, is easier to teach and because it focuses almost exclusively on relationships is a more generic approach to the problems of patients of all sorts. In relative terms it remains neglected compared with CBT but merits much more attention than it has so far received.

TREATMENT OF MANIA

Mania is often an indication for admission to a specialised psychiatric unit. Detention under the appropriate section of the Mental Health Act may also be necessary because of the loss of judgement and insight associated with severe upswings in mood. In the past, severe manic states were associated with increased mortality as a result of exhaustion, dehydration and hyperthermia. Although modern practice has reduced this particular risk considerably, it needs to be remembered, together with the potential for suicide, although this is rarely an important risk in uncomplicated mania. Admission allows the supervision and titration of adequate drug treatment and a well-run ward is an important component of treatment.

Drug treatment

The objectives are to control behaviour, to terminate the episode and to prevent early recurrence. Dopamine receptor antagonists (major tranquillisers or neuroleptics) are the first-line drugs in acute severe mania. The dose must be established empirically by giving repeated small doses of the chosen compound until an adequate effect is established. The urgency of this titration clearly depends upon the patient. Where there is a fear of violence or conflict it is easy to get drawn into using high doses of neuroleptics. However, it is probably wrong to think too readily of neuroleptics as achieving 'tranquillisation'. The most beneficial effects of neuroleptics may relate to psychomotor slowing and antipsychotic effects. Sedation by neuroleptics may require very high doses and this is increasingly realised to be undesirable and potentially dangerous. The difficulty with neuroleptics resides in their actions on myocardial transmission and the risk of sudden death. There is therefore contemporary interest in developing alternative regimens which depend upon a neuroleptic in low to moderate doses combined with more explicitly sedative compounds such as lorazepam or clonazepam. The advantage of benzodiazepines is their remarkable safety at high doses. No individual drug or class of neuroleptics has been shown to have particular advantages for mania. Indeed the number of trials in mania is nothing like the number in schizophrenia. We await clear evidence of the utility of atypical neuroleptics in the treatment of acute mania. Freedom from extrapyramidal effects

is an important apparent advantage of such drugs (e.g. olanzapine). The usual duration of treatment is dictated by the time of remission of symptoms. Depressive symptoms may develop and require treatment in their own right. In fact the resolving phase of an acute manic disturbance is often difficult to treat and patients are frequently discharged from hospital before they are completely well. Recovery usually takes approximately 6 months.

Lithium is itself effective in acute mania and is advocated especially in the USA (see below). It is not sedative and does not reach adequate intracellular concentrations quickly when given in conventional doses of 800–1600 mg daily. It should be chosen only after careful medical screening. A plasma concentration of about 1 mmol/l, i.e. the upper end of the therapeutic range (or higher), is said to be superior in acute illness. Careful monitoring of plasma concentrations is essential. Concurrent use of a dopamine blocker is often necessary but must be cautious (see description of neurotoxic effects below).

Carbamazepine and sodium valproate are not usually used in acute treatment of mania, although valproate has actually been shown to be as effective as lithium in these circumstances (Bowden et al 1994). Valproate is certainly a useful alternative and may be the preferred choice when rapid cyclical mood changes or mixed mania (combining manic and depressive features during the course of the day) are prominent. Any sedative drug may be useful in refractory mania and there is anecdotal experience to support the use of barbiturates, high-potency benzodiazepines as described and even paraldehyde. Whether any of these drugs influence the course of the underlying disorder is uncertain and they are often used together with neuroleptics. ECT can be very useful in refractory mania and there is also evidence for a paradoxical tranquillising effect of amphetamine. Finally, verapamil and other calcium antagonists may have antimanic actions, the pharmacological basis for which is poorly understood. It is important to understand that alternatives to neuroleptics remain in the absence of a therapeutic response to conventional management.

We are entering the age of clinical guidelines. Treatment of mania is regarded by American authorities as revolving round the choice of a mood stabiliser as primary treatment (lithium or an anticonvulsant) and necessary 'adjunctive' treatments (neuroleptics and benzodiazepines). To describe a neuroleptic as a first-line drug (as above) would then be to fail to treat the disorder. Caution appears necessary in accepting the distinction between moodstabilisers and adjunctive treatments. This may be more a linguistic convention than an empirical difference.

Prevention of recurrence

Lithium

The role of lithium in the prophylaxis of bipolar disorder is well known, and its use can transform an individual's life. The usual indications for starting treatment in otherwise uncomplicated cases are two illnesses within 2 years or three illnesses in 5 years. Given an early onset, a strong family history, and severe disorder, the destructive potential of bipolar illness justifies prophylactic treatment after the first episode. In practice, however, the resistance of the patient or the family to an indefinite course of drug treatment before the illness has shown evidence of recurrence may limit the clinician's actions. In any case, on average, recurrence with subsequent illnesses is the rule rather than the exception.

Baseline investigation of renal and thyroid function and an electrocardiograph are required before starting lithium. It can usually be prescribed as a single dose at night. The unusually low therapeutic index requires monitoring of plasma concentration. Blood should be regularly sampled 12 hours after the last dose; a concentration of 0.5–1.0 mmol/l is usually effective. Plasma concentrations over 1.10 mmol/l or certainly 1.20 mmol/l are predictive of toxicity. Recommendations about how frequently levels should be checked vary enormously: once the level is stable, every 3 months is probably prudent. Concentrations at the lower end of the range are usually adequate for prophylaxis.

The most common side-effects are tremor, polyuria and weight gain. It is worth lowering the dose to try to reduce these symptoms, as all may affect compliance. If necessary, tremor can be treated with a beta blocker and polyuria with amiloride. The introduction of any diuretic requires careful monitoring of the plasma lithium concentration. Neurotoxicity is an important but rare complication. It can develop insidiously, sometimes after a dose increase, sometimes at notionally 'therapeutic' levels, sometimes in conjunction with other drugs, especially neuroleptics, sometimes in association with intercurrent illness or other brain pathology (Kemperman & Tulner 1990, Bell et al 1993). The resulting encephalopathy has no defining features and may be reversible. However, the most characteristic bad neurological outcome is a cerebellar syndrome.

Manic illness following discontinuation of lithium in bipolar patients is a particular problem. Suppes and colleagues reviewed 14 studies involving 25 patients with bipolar disorder, and found that more than 50% of new episodes of illness occurred within 10 weeks of stopping treatment (Suppes et al 1991). The length of treatment preceding discontinuation varied widely, but averaged about 30 months. This risk means that pro-phylactic treatment with lithium must continue for longer than 2 years because premature withdrawal may bring forward the time of the next recurrence of mania (Goodwin 1994). A long period of mood stability while taking lithium is not a guarantee of stability on its withdrawal. In addition, anecdotal evidence suggests that recurrent mania after withdrawal may be refractory to subsequent treatment (Post et al 1992). For these reasons, indefinite maintenance treatment with lithium is often recommended.

Alternatives to lithium prophylaxis

If there is no clinical benefit from lithium prophylaxis, the first alternative is carbamazepine, either alone or in combination with lithium. Despite initial scepticism, the use of carbamazepine in bipolar disorder has increased and is supported by limited clinical trials. A low initial dose of 100–200 mg at night should be given. The optimal dosage, usually 400–600 mg daily, must be established empirically, as for the treatment of epilepsy. Dosage should be titrated slowly to allow adaptation to the unwanted sedative effects, and the maximum recommended is 1.6 g daily. Plasma concentration measurements establish primarily that the patient is taking the tablets, and are no guide to clinical effect. Adverse effects include sedation and rashes, especially if lithium has been used. Other anticonvulsants, specifically sodium valproate and lamotrigine, may also be worth trying alone or in combination with lithium or each other, but they are unlicensed for mania in the UK at present.

The second major alternative to lithium is the use of neuroleptics, either alone or together with lithium. The evidence supporting such a strategy is based on anecdote and clinical audit. Depot neuroleptics have the advantage of ensuring compliance. The disadvantages of neuroleptics relate primarily to their extrapyramidal effects, which may be more likely to occur in patients with affective illness. Some patients taking lithium have regular (e.g. seasonal) manic upswings that can be managed by giving oral chlorpromazine for a few weeks as an outpatient. It is advisable to provide an advance supply of the drug for this purpose to responsible patients.

Finally, it should be remembered that antidepressants may precipitate and even exacerbate mania. Their use in patients with bipolar illness during depressive episodes requires care.

COURSE AND OUTCOME OF MOOD DISORDERS

It is appropriate, and necessarily humbling, to return to

a consideration of the course and outcome of mood disorder after reviewing our current treatment options. The seriousness of mood disorder is still something that needs formally to be reaffirmed for the medical profession and public alike, and there remain many problems in the delivery of the treatments we have, before we achieve their known limitations (Hirschfeld et al 1997). It is an irony of the mood disorders that the most severe episodes of mania and psychotic depression have in some senses the best short-term outcome. Patients have a high probability of short-term recovery but the near certainty of subsequent recurrence with or without treatment. How the outcome should be represented for the whole spectrum of mood disorder remains uncertain.

Approximately half of all incident cases of major depression in the community will not have a subsequent episode. The mean time to recurrence with the second episode is about 15 years, and to the third episode about 10 years. However, this sort of retrospective reporting is subject to obvious biases. The longer-term prospective studies are only now becoming available (Murphy, 1994).

The best-known follow-up studies have been based on inpatient cohorts. For example, a 40 year follow-up of a cohort of patients admitted to the Iowa Psychopathic Hospital between 1934 and 1945 allowed the contrast to be drawn between the mood disorders and schizophrenia. Depressive disorders generally had a better outcome than schizophrenia but the general conclusion from studies of this sort is that the outcome is not particularly good. This is perhaps underlined by detailed follow-up studies of more recent cohorts. Lee & Murray showed that only 11 of 89 patients first seen in the sixties after admission to the Maudsley Hospital had a good outcome (Lee & Murray 1988). Twenty-five had an extremely poor outcome. This finding was echoed by a very similar study from Australia (Kiloh et al 1988). The Maudsley depressives showed the worst outcome for those who had the most psychotic or endogenous symptoms at the index admission.

The outcome in severe mood disorder is similar in bipolar and unipolar samples. For example, in a recent 27 year prospective study of 186 unipolar depressives and 220 bipolars, there was a progression from unipolar depression, schizodepression, pure affective bipolar disorder to schizobipolar disorder showing a systematic decrease in age of onset and length of episode. When compared to unipolar disorders, the bipolars showed more frequent but shorter episodes. The only difference in course between schizoaffective subjects and those with pure affective disorder was a greater frequency in episodes requiring hospitalization among schizoaffectives (Angst & Preisig 1995a). Eleven per cent of the sample had committed suicide and the risk was associated with clinical severity and onset prior to the age of 60. Late onset of affective illness was associated with chronicity (10–19% of cases) and recovery was more frequent among unipolar than among bipolar patients. The 5 year remission rates (26% in unipolars, 16% in bipolars) were independent of the number of episodes (Angst & Preisig 1995b).

Mortality

Patients with mood disorder have a reduced life expectancy (Black et al 1987). This is true for all severities of illness. The primary causes in younger age groups are cardiovascular disease and suicide. A recent naturalistic retrospective 17 year follow-up of 472 bipolar patients showed greater mortality from suicide and cardiovascular and respiratory causes compared with the general population (Sharma & Markar 1994). The deceased were more likely to have been unmarried, showed greater frequency and duration of admissions, a shorter follow-up period and were less likely to have received lithium treatment. The suicides were significantly younger at onset and death than the index and control groups, and suicide was uncommon where follow-up extended over 10 years.

Suicide

Depressive illness is often characterised by bleak and persistent thoughts of suicide. Only rarely are such thoughts the logical conclusion of an autonomous person performing some existential calculus. On recovery they usually disappear completely. It is not surprising, therefore, that depressive illness is the most common single antecedent to suicide, and suicide is the most common cause of death in affective disorder. Social 'explanations' for suicide rates can seem blind to the concept of depressive illness even though the social factors that are invoked to account for changes in suicide rates may operate in large part through the agency of affective disorder. The association is also poorly understood by the public and the media, who almost invariably report celebrity suicides as unaccountable and mysterious. Improved public understanding of the relationship between the risks of suicide and the prevalence of mental illness is desirable simply to reduce the reluctance of some individuals to seek help. In the UK, voluntary organisations have tended to take the lead in popularising a psychosocial interpretation of suicide and parasuicide. While appropriate to the latter phenomenon, it may simultaneously do disservice to the former.

The broad issue of suicide is covered in Chapter 26,

in which it is emphasised that there are no psychological or biological measures that can be used to estimate the risk of subsequent suicide in an individual being treated for depression. However, since psychiatric referrals with depression collectively represent an identified group at high risk of suicide, general improvement in their care would be as appropriately targeted as any. That could mean clearer adherence to the principles of treatment outlined above. It is reasonable to ask whether prophylactic treatment reduces mortality. At present the most positive findings come from specialised lithium clinics where suicide rates may actually appear lower than expected (Coppen et al 1991, Ahrens et al 1995, Muller-Oerlinghausen et al 1996). The obvious difficulty is that such clinics will tend to select patients with the best compliance, best insight, and, one might suggest, the best likely outcome. Furthermore, prophylactic lithium treatment is often not offered until patients have survived the interval of highest apparent risk in any case.

EVIDENCE-BASED MENTAL HEALTH

The challenge in devising treatments in future will be to improve the basis on which we currently make clinical decisions. This involves the collation of the trials that already exist to form meta-analyses that can better inform choices between different drug treatments. It also means providing up-to-date guidelines and quantitative reviews to all clinicians via advanced communication links. If you have a problem deciding what to do in a clinical setting you should be able to click on to an appropriate body of evidence immediately from the computer at your elbow.

While the use of evidence, rather than authority and opinion, is a traditional strength of medical practice, the explosion of information taking place in recent decades requires novel solutions to avoid information overload. Evidence-based medicine is an approach to teaching and learning designed to allow continuous updating of a clinician's knowledge and understanding. It grew out of the teaching innovations at McMaster University in Canada (Sackett et al 1997). It places a premium upon understanding the statistical meaning of evidence and its critical appraisal. The explicit introduction of this way of thinking into psychiatry is an important contemporary development which should have an impact in all treatment modalities. It encourages clinicians to ask critical questions about their practice. The development of this approach can best be appreciated by looking at the work of the Evidence Based Mental Health Unit and the Cochrane Collaboration in Oxford. Interested readers may access materials via appropriate web sites (for links, contact http://www.psychiatry.ox.ac.uk/).

CONCLUSION

The challenge of the mood disorders lies in their apparently rising incidence and prevalence, the realisation that long-term disability and even mortality is likely to be increasingly evident, and the need for better delivery of more effective treatments. Against these challenges can be set our improving understanding of aetiology and the likely development of novel treatments. That we have a capacity, albeit finite, to treat mood disorder is one of its recurring clinical rewards.

REFERENCES

Abas M A, Sahakian B J, Levy R 1990 Neuropsychological deficits and CT scan changes in elderly depressives. Psychological Medicine 20: 507–520

Ahrens B, Muller-Oerlinghausen B, Schou M et al 1995 Excess cardiovascular and suicide mortality of affective-disorders may be reduced by lithium prophylaxis. Journal of Affective Disorders 33: 67–75

Akiskal H 1983 Dysthymic disorder: psychopathology of proposed chronic depressive sub-types. American Journal of Psychiatry 140: 11–20

Akiskal H S, Akiskal K 1988 Reassessing the prevalence of bipolar disorders: clinical significance and artistic creativity. Psychiatrie et Psychobiologie 3: 29s–36s

Andersen G, Vestergaard K, Riis J O, Lauritzen L 1994 Incidence of post-stroke depression during the first year in a large unselected stroke population determined using a valid standardized rating scale. Acta Psychiatrica Scandinavica 90: 190–195

Anderson B, Brosen K, Christensen P et al 1990 Paroxetine: a selective serotonin reuptake inhibitor showing better tolerance, but weaker antidepressant effect than clomipramine in a controlled multicenter study. Journal of Affective Disorders 18: 289–299

Anderson I M, Tomenson B M 1994 The efficacy of selective serotonin re-uptake inhibitors in depression: a meta-analysis of studies against tricyclic antidepressants. Journal of Psychopharmacology 8: 238–249

Andrews G 1996 Talk that works: the rise of cognitive behaviour therapy. British Medical Journal 313: 1501–1502

Andrews G, Stewart G, Allen R, Henderson A S 1990 The genetics of six neurotic disorders: a twin study. Journal of Affective Disorders 19: 23–29

Angold A, Worthman C W 1993 Puberty onset of gender differences in rates of depression: a developmental, epidemiologic and neuroendocrine perspective. Journal of Affective Disorders 29: 145–158

Angst J 1996 Comorbidity of mood disorders: a longitudinal prospective study. British Journal of Psychiatry 168: 31–37

Angst J, Dobler-Mikola A 1984 The Zurich study III. Diagnosis of depression. European Archives of Psychiatry and Neurological Sciences 234: 30–37

Angst J, Hochstrasser B 1994 Recurrent brief depression: the Zurich study. Journal of Clinical Psychiatry 55: 3–9

Angst J, Preisig M 1995a Course of a clinical cohort of unipolar, bipolar and schizoaffective patients. Results of a prospective study from 1959 to 1985. Schweizer Archiv für Neurologie und Psychiatrie 146: 5–16

Angst J, Preisig M 1995b Outcome of a clinical cohort of unipolar, bipolar and schizoaffective patients. Results of a prospective study from 1959 to 1985. Schweizer Archiv für Neurologie und Psychiatrie 146: 17–23

Angst J, Wicki W 1992 The Zurich study XIII. Recurrent brief anxiety. European Archives of Psychiatry and Clinical Neuroscience 241: 296–300

Angst J, Merikangas K, Scheidegger P, Wicki W 1990 Recurrent brief depression: a new subtype of affective disorder. Journal of Affective Disorders 19: 87–98

APA 1994 Diagnostic and statistical manual of mental disorders, 4th edn. American Psychiatric Association, Washington, DC

Aronson R, Offman H J, Joffe R T, Naylor C D 1996 Tri-iodothyronine augmentation in the treatment of refractory depression: a meta-analysis. Archives of General Psychiatry 53: 842–848

Baldwin D, Rudge S, Thomas S 1995 Dysthymia. Options in pharmacotherapy. CNS Drugs 4: 422–431

Barefoot J C, Schroll M 1996 Symptoms of depression, acute myocardial infarction, and total mortality in a community sample. Circulation 93: 1976–1980

Battersby S, Ogilvie A D, Smith C A D et al 1996 Structure of a variable number tandem repeat of the serotonin transporter gene and association with affective disorder. Psychiatric Genetics 6: 177–181

Beats B C, Sahakian B J, Levy R 1996 Cognitive performance in tests sensitive to frontal lobe dysfunction in the elderly depressed. Psychological Medicine 26: 591–603

Bechara A, Tranel D, Damasio H, Damasio A R 1996 Failure to respond autonomically to anticipated future outcomes following damage to prefrontal cortex. Cerebral Cortex 6: 215–225

Beck A T 1976 Cognitive therapy and the emotional disorders. New American Library, New York

Bell A J, Cole A, Eccleston D, Ferrier I N 1993 Lithium neurotoxicity at normal therapeutic levels. British Journal of Psychiatry 162: 689–692

Benkelfat C, Ellenbogen M A, Dean P, Palmour R M, Young S N 1994 Mood-lowering effect of tryptophan depletion: enhanced susceptibility in young men at genetic risk for major affective disorders. Archives of General Psychiatry 51: 687–697

Berger M, Riemann D 1993 REM sleep in depression – an overview. Journal of Sleep Research 2: 211–223

Berger M, Pirke K M, Doerr P, Krieg J C, von Zerssen D 1984 The limited utility of the dexamethasone suppression test for the diagnostic process in psychiatry. British Journal of Psychiatry 145: 372–382

Berrettini W H, Ferraro T N, Goldin L R et al 1994 Chromosome 18 DNA markers and manic–depressive illness: evidence for a susceptibility gene. Proceedings of the National Academy of Sciences of the USA 91: 5918–5921

Black D W, Winokur G, Nasrallah A 1987 Is death from natural causes still excessive in psychiatric patients? A follow-up of 1593 patients with major affective disorder. Journal of Nervous and Mental Disease 175: 674–680

Blackburn I M, Bishop S, Glen A I M, Whalley L J & Christie J E 1981 The efficacy of cognitive therapy in depression: a treatment trial using cognitive therapy and pharmacotherapy, each alone and in combination. British Journal of Psychiatry 139: 181–189

Blackburn I M, Eunson K M, Bishop S 1986 A two-year naturalistic follow-up of depressed patients treated with cognitive therapy, pharmacotherapy and a combination of both. Journal of Affective Disorders 10: 67–75

Blackwood D H R, He L, Morris S W et al 1996 A locus for bipolar affective disorder on chromosome 4p. Nature Genetics 12: 427–430

Boston Collaborative Drug Surveillance Program 1972 Acute adverse reactions to prednisone in relation to dosage. Clinical Pharmacology and Therapy 13: 694–698

Bowden C L, Brugger A M, Swann A C et al 1994 Efficacy of divalproex vs lithium and placebo in the treatment of mania. Journal of the American Medical Association 271: 918–924

Brown G W 1993 Life events and affective disorder: replications and limitations. Psychosomatic Medicine 55: 248–259

Brown G W, Harris T O 1993 Aetiology of anxiety and depressive disorders in an inner-city population: 1. Early adversity. Psychological Medicine 23: 143–154

Brown G W, Lemyre L, Bifulco A 1992 Social factors and recovery from anxiety and depressive disorders. A test of specificity. British Journal of Psychiatry 161: 44–54

Brown G W, Harris T O, Eales M J 1993 Aetiology of anxiety and depressive disorders in an inner-city population: 2. Comorbidity and adversity. Psychological Medicine 23: 155–165

Brown G W, Harris T O, Hepworth C 1994 Life events and endogenous depression: a puzzle reexamined. Archives of General Psychiatry 51: 525–534

Burvill P W, Johnson G A, Chakera T M H, Stewart Wynne E G, Anderson C S, Jamrozik K D 1996 The place of site of lesion in the aetiology of post-stroke depression. Cerebrovascular Diseases 6: 208–215

Burvill P, Johnson G, Jamrozik K, Anderson C, Stewart Wynne E 1997 Risk factors for post-stroke depression. International Journal of Geriatric Psychiatry 12: 219–226

Cannon W J 1927 The James–Lange theory of emotions. American Journal of Psychology 39: 115–124

Carney M W P, Roth M, Garside R F 1965 The diagnosis of depressive syndromes and the prediction of ECT response. British Journal of Psychiatry 111: 659–674

Carney R M, Freedland K E, Jaffe A S 1990 Insomnia and depression prior to myocardial infarction. Psychosomatic Medicine 52: 603–609

Carr S J, Teasdale J D, Broadbent D 1991 Effects of induced elated and depressed mood on self-focused attention. British Journal of Clinical Psychology 30: 273–275

Carroll B J, Feinberg M, Greden J F 1981 A specific laboratory test for the diagnosis of melancholia. Archives of General Psychiatry 38: 15–22

Christie J E, Whalley L J, Dick H, Blackwood D H R, Blackburn I M, Fink G 1986 Raised plasma cortisol concentrations a feature of drug-free psychotics and not specific for depression. British Journal of Psychiatry 148: 58–65

Clayton P J, Ernst C, Angst J 1994 Premorbid personality traits of men who develop unipolar or bipolar disorders. European Archives of Psychiatry and Clinical Neuroscience 243: 340–346

Clerc G E, Ruimy P, Verdeau Pailles J 1994 A double-blind comparison of venlafaxine and fluoxetine in patients hospitalized for major depression and melancholia. International Clinical Psychopharmacology 9: 139–143

Collier D A, Arranz M J, Sham P et al 1996 The serotonin transporter is a potential susceptibility factor for bipolar affective disorder. NeuroReport 7: 1675–1679

Coppen A, Shaw D M, Farrell J P 1963 The potentiation of the antidepressive action of a monoamine-oxidase inhibitor by tryptophan. Lancet i: 79–81

Coppen A, Standish-Barry H, Bailey J, Houston G, Silcocks P, Hermon C 1991 Does lithium reduce the mortality of recurrent mood disorders? Journal of Affective Disorders 23: 1–7

Costa P T J, McCrae R R 1994 Stability and change in personality from adolescence through adulthood. In: Halverson CF Jr, Kohnstamm G, Martin R P (eds) The developing structure of temperament and personality from infancy to adulthood. Lawrence Erlbaum Associates Inc, Hillsdale, New Jersey, Chapter 7: 139–150

Damasio A R 1994 Descartes' error. Emotion, reason and the human brain. Picador, London

Damasio A R, Tranel D, Damasio H 1990 Individuals with sociopathic behavior caused by frontal damage fail to respond autonomically to social stimuli. Behavioural Brain Research 41: 81–94

Davis R, Wilde M I 1996 Mirtazapine. A review of its pharmacology and therapeutic potential in the management of major depression. CNS Drugs 5: 389–402

DeKloet E R, Vreugdenhil E, Oitzl M S, Joels M 1997 Glucocorticoid feedback resistance. Trends in Endocrinology and Metabolism 8: 26–33

Delgado P L, Charney D S, Price L H, Aghajanian G K, Landis H, Heninger G R 1990 Serotonin function and the mechanism of antidepressant action: reversal of antidepressant-induced remission by rapid depletion of plasma tryptophan. Archives of General Psychiatry 47: 411–418

Delgado P L, Price L H, Miller H L et al 1991 Rapid serotonin depletion as a provocative challenge test for patients with major depression: relevance to antidepressant action and the neurobiology of depression. Psychopharmacology Bulletin 27: 321–330

Drevets W C, Price J L, Simpson Jr J R et al 1997 Subgenual prefrontal cortex abnormalities in mood disorders. Nature 386: 824–827

Dritschel B H, Teasdale J D 1991 Individual differences in affect-related cognitive operations elicited by experimental stimuli. British Journal of Clinical Psychology 30: 151–160

Eagles J M, Whalley L J 1985 Ageing and affective disorders: the age at first onset of affective disorders in Scotland, 1969–1978. British Journal of Psychiatry 147: 180–187

Egeland J A, Gerhard D S, Pauls D L et al 1987 Bipolar affective disorders linked to DNA markers on chromosome 11. Nature 325: 783–787

Elkin I, Gibbons R D, Shea M T et al 1995 Initial severity and differential treatment outcome in the National Institute of Mental Health treatment of depression collaborative research program. Journal of Consulting and Clinical Psychology 63: 841–847

Elkis H, Friedman L, Wise A, Meltzer H Y 1995 Meta-analysis of studies of ventricular enlargement and cortical sulcal prominence in mood disorders. Archives of General Psychiatry 52: 735–746

Ellenbogen M A, Young S N, Dean P, Palmour R N, Benkelfat C 1996 Mood response to acute tryptophan depletion in healthy volunteers: Sex differences and temporal stability. Neuropsychopharmacology 15: 465–474

Ferrier I N, Eccleston D, Moore P B, Wood K A 1990 Relapse in chronic depressives on withdrawal of L-tryptophan. Lancet 336: 380–381

Francis P T, Pangalos M N, Stephens P H et al 1993 Antemortem measurements of neurotransmission – possible implications for pharmacotherapy of Alzheimer's disease and depression. Journal of Neurology, Neurosurgery and Psychiatry 56: 80–84

Frasure-Smith N, Lesperance F, Talajic M 1993 Depression following myocardial infarction: impact on 6-month survival. Journal of the American Medical Association 270: 1819–1825

Frasure-Smith N, Lesperance F, Talajic M 1995 Depression and 18-month prognosis after myocardial infarction. Circulation 91: 999–1005

Freimer N B, Reus V I, Escamilla M A et al 1996 Genetic mapping using haplotype, association and linkage methods suggests a locus for severe bipolar disorder (BPI) at 18q22–q23. Nature Genetics 12: 436–441

Gerken A, Holsboer F 1986 Cortisol and corticosterone response after syn-corticotropin in relationship to dexamethasone suppressibility of cortisol. Psychoneuroendocrinology 11: 185–194

Giles D E, Biggs M M, Rush A J, Roffwarg H P 1988 Risk factors in families of unipolar depression. I. Psychiatric illness and reduced REM latency. Journal of Affective Disorders 14: 51–59

Ginns E I, Ott J, Egeland J A et al 1996 A genome-wide search for chromosomal loci linked to bipolar affective disorder in the Old Order Amish. Nature Genetics 12: 431–435

Goodwin G M 1994 Recurrence of mania after lithium withdrawal. British Journal of Psychiatry 164: 149–152

Goodwin G M 1996 Functional imaging, affective disorder and dementia. British Medical Bulletin 52: 495–512

Goodwin G M, Fairburn C G, Cowen P J 1987 The effects of dieting and weight loss on neuroendocrine responses to tryptophan, clonidine, and apomorphine in volunteers. Important implications for neuroendocrine investigations in depression. Archives of General Psychiatry 44: 952–957

Goodwin G M, Muir W J, Seckl J R et al 1992 The effects of cortisol infusion upon hormone secretion from the anterior pituitary and subjective mood in depressive illness and in controls. Journal of Affective Disorders 26: 73–83

Goodwin G M, Austin M P, Curran S M et al 1993 The elevation of plasma beta-endorphin levels in major depression. Journal of Affective Disorders 29: 281–289

Gram L F 1986 Citalopram: clinical effect profile in comparison with clomipramine. A controlled multicenter study. Psychopharmacology 90: 131–138

Gray J A 1982 The neuropsychology of anxiety. Oxford University Press. Oxford

Herrmann M, Bartels C, Schumacher M, Wallesch C W 1995 Poststroke depression: is there a pathoanatomic correlate for depression in the postacute stage of stroke? Stroke 26: 850–856

Hickie I, Scott E, Mitchell P, Wilhelm K, Austin M P, Bennett B 1995 Subcortical hyperintensities on magnetic-resonance-imaging – clinical correlates and prognostic significance in patients with severe depression. Biological Psychiatry 37: 151–160

Hirschfeld R M A 1994 Major depression, dysthymia and depressive personality disorder. British Journal of Psychiatry 165: 23–30

Hirschfeld R M A, Keller M B, Panico S et al 1997 The National Depressive and Manic-Depressive Association consensus statement on the undertreatment of depression.

Journal of the American Medical Association 277: 333–340

Holsboer F, Wiedemann K, Boll E 1986 Shortened dexamethasone half-life in depressed dexamethasone nonsuppressors. Archives of General Psychiatry 43: 813–815

Holsboer F, Lauer C J, Schreiber W, Krieg J C 1995 Altered hypothalamic–pituitary–adrenocortical regulation in healthy-subjects at high familial risk for affective-disorders. Neuroendocrinology 62: 340–347

House A, Dennis M, Molyneux A, Warlow C, Hawton K 1989 Emotionalism after stroke. British Medical Journal 298: 991–994

House A, Dennis M, Warlow C, Hawton K, Molyneux A 1990 Mood disorders after stroke and their relation to lesion location: a CT scan study. Brain 113: 1113–1129

Hunt N, Bruce Jones W, Silverstone T 1992a Life events and relapse in bipolar affective disorder. Journal of Affective Disorders 25: 13–20

Hunt N, Sayer H, Silverstone T 1992b Season and manic relapse. Acta Psychiatrica Scandinavica 85: 123–126

Jacobsen F M, Wehr T A, Skwerer R A, Sack D A, Rosenthal N E 1987 Morning versus midday phototherapy of seasonal affective disorder. American Journal of Psychiatry 144: 1301–1305

Jamison K R 1995 Manic–depressive illness and creativity. Scientific American 272: 62–67

Jamison K R, Wyatt R J 1992 van Gogh,Vincent: illness. British Medical Journal 304: 577–577

Joffe R T, Singer W, Levitt A J, MacDonald C 1993 A placebo-controlled comparison of lithium and tri-iodothyronine augmentation of tricyclic antidepressants in unipolar refractory depression. Archives of General Psychiatry 50: 387–393

Keller M B, Klein D N, Hirschfeld R M A et al 1995 Results of the DSM-IV mood disorders field trial. American Journal of Psychiatry 152: 843–849

Kelsoe J R, Ginns E I, Egeland J A et al 1989 Re-evaluation of the linkage relationship between chromosome-11p loci and the gene for bipolar affective-disorder in the Old Order Amish. Nature 342: 238–243

Kemperman C J F, Tulner D M 1990 Neurotoxicity of lithium. Lithium 1: 195–202

Kendell R E 1968 The classification of depressive illness. Maudsley monograph. Oxford University Press, Oxford

Kendell R E, Chalmers J C, Platz C 1987 Epidemiology of puerperal psychoses. British Journal of Psychiatry 150: 662–673

Kendler K S 1996 Major depression and generalised anxiety disorder. Same genes, (partly) different environments – revisited. British Journal of Psychiatry 168: 68–75

Kendler K S 1997 The diagnostic validity of melancholic major depression in a population-based sample of female twins. Archives of General Psychiatry 54: 299–304

Kendler K S, Karkowski-Shuman L 1997 Stressful life events and genetic liability to major depression: genetic control of exposure to the environment? Psychological Medicine 27: 539–547

Kendler K S, Neale M C, Kessler R C, Heath A C, Eaves L J 1992 A population-based twin study of major depression in women: the impact of varying definitions of illness. Archives of General Psychiatry 49: 257–266

Kendler K S, Heath A C, Neale M C, Kessler R C, Eaves L J 1993a Alcoholism and major depression in women: a twin study of the causes of comorbidity. Archives of General Psychiatry 50: 690–698

Kendler K S, Kessler R C, Neale M C, Heath A C, Eaves L J 1993b The prediction of major depression in women: toward an integrated etiologic model. American Journal of Psychiatry 150: 1139–1148

Kendler K S, Neale M, Kessler R, Heath A, Eaves L 1993c A twin study of recent life events and difficulties. Archives of General Psychiatry 50: 789–796

Kendler K S, Neale M C, MacLean C J, Heath A C, Eaves L J, Kessler R C 1993d Smoking and major depression: a causal analysis. Archives of General Psychiatry 50: 36–43

Kendler K S, Sham P C, MacLean C J 1997a The determinants of parenting: an epidemiological, multi-informant, retrospective study. Psychological Medicine 27: 549–563

Kendler K S, Walters E E, Kessler R C 1997b The prediction of length of major depressive episodes: results from an epidemiological sample of female twins. Psychological Medicine 27: 107–117

Kiloh L G, Andrews G, Neilson M 1988 The long-term outcome of depressive illness. British Journal of Psychiatry 153: 752–757

Klerman G L 1988 The current age of youthful melancholia – evidence for increase in depression among adolescents and young adults. British Journal of Psychiatry 152: 4–14

Klerman G L, Weissman M M 1989 Increasing rates of depression. Journal of the American Medical Association 261: 2229–2235

Klerman G L, Weissman M M, Rounsaville B J, Chevron E S 1984 Interpersonal psychotherapy of depression. Aronson, London

Klerman G L, Lavori P W, Rice J et al 1985 Birth-cohort trends in rates of major depressive disorder among relatives of patients with affective-disorder. Archives of General Psychiatry 42: 689–693

Koslow S H, Maas J W, Bowden C L et al 1983 CSF and urinary biogenic amines and metabolites in depression and mania. A controlled, univariate analysis. Archives of General Psychiatry 40: 999–1010

Kuhn R 1958 The treatment of depressive states with G22355 (imipramine hydrochloride). American Journal of Psychiatry 115: 459–464

Kupfer D J, Frank E, Perel J M et al 1992 Five-year outcome for maintenance therapies in recurrent depression. Archives of General Psychiatry 49: 769–773

Lafer B, Sachs G S, Labbate L A, Thibault A, Rosenbaum J F 1994 Phototherapy for seasonal affective disorder: a blind comparison of three different schedules. American Journal of Psychiatry 151: 1081–1083

Larsen R J, Ketelaar T 1989 Extraversion, neuroticism and susceptibility to positive and negative mood induction procedures. Personality and individual differences 10: 1221–1228

Larsen R J, Ketelaar T 1991 Personality and susceptibility to positive and negative emotional states. Journal of Personality and Social Psychology 61: 132–140

Lasch K, Weissman M, Wickramaratne P, Livingston-Bruce M 1990 Birth-cohort changes in the rates of mania. Psychiatry Research 33: 31–37

Lee A S, Murray R M 1988 The long-term outcome of Maudsley depressives. British Journal of Psychiatry 153: 741–751

Lesperance F, Frasure-Smith N, Talajic M, Cameron O 1996 Major depression before and after myocardial infarction: its nature and consequences. Psychosomatic Medicine 58: 99–112

Levitt A J, Joffe R T, King E 1994 Dim versus bright red (light-emitting diode) light in the treatment of seasonal affective disorder. Acta Psychiatrica Scandinavica 89: 341–345

Lewis A J 1934 Melancholia: a clinical survey of depressive states. Journal of Mental Science 80: 277–378

Loosen P T 1994 Cushing's syndrome and depression. Endocrinologist 4: 373–382

Maddox J C, Levi M, Thompson C 1994 The compliance with antidepressants in general practice. Journal of Psychopharmacology 8: 48–53

McGuffin P, Katz R, Bebbington P 1988 The Camberwell Collaborative Depression Study. III. Depression and adversity in the relatives of depressed probands. British Journal of Psychiatry 152: 775–782

McGuffin P, Katz R, Watkins S, Rutherford J 1996 A hospital-based twin register of the heritability of DSM-IV unipolar depression. Archives of General Psychiatry 53: 129–136

Mann J J, Henteleff R A, Lagattuta T F, Perper J A, Li S, Arango V 1996 Lower ³H-paroxetine binding in cerebral cortex of suicide victims is partly due to fewer high affinity, non-transporter sites. Journal of Neural Transmission 103: 1337–1350

Medical Research Council 1965 Clinical trial of the treatment of depressive illness. British Medical Journal 1: 881–886

Mehlman P T, Higley J D, Faucher I et al 1994 Low CSF 5-HIAA concentrations and severe aggression and impaired impulse control in nonhuman primates. American Journal of Psychiatry 151: 1485–1491

Mitchell P, Parker G, Jamieson K et al 1992 Are there any differences between bipolar and unipolar melancholia? Journal of Affective Disorders 25: 97–105

Montgomery D B, Roberts A, Green M, Bullock T, Baldwin D, Montgomery S A 1994 Lack of efficacy of fluoxetine in recurrent brief depression and suicidal attempts. European Archives of Psychiatry and Clinical Neuroscience 244: 211–215

Mullen P E, Linsell C R, Parker D 1986 Influence of sleep disruption and calorie restriction on biological markers for depression. Lancet ii: 1051–1054

Muller-Oerlinghausen B, Wolf T, Ahrens B et al 1996 Mortality of patients who dropped out from regular lithium prophylaxis – a collaborative study by the international group for the study of lithium-treated patients (IGSLI). Acta Psychiatrica Scandinavica 94: 344–347

Murphy D G M, Murphy D M, Abbas M et al 1993 Seasonal affective disorder: response to light as measured by electroencephalogram, melatonin suppression, and cerebral blood flow. British Journal of Psychiatry 163: 327–331

Murphy J M 1994 The Stirling County study: then and now. International Review of Psychiatry 6: 329–348

Murphy J M, Sobol A M, Olivier D C, Monson R R, Leighton A H, Pratt L A 1989 Prodromes of depression and anxiety. The Stirling County study. British Journal of Psychiatry 155: 490–495

Naber D, Sand P, Heigl B 1996 Psychopathological and neuropsychological effects of 8-days' corticosteroid treatment. A prospective study. Psychoneuroendocrinology 21: 25–31

Neuvonen P J, Pohjola Sintonen S, Tacke U, Vuori E 1993 Five fatal cases of serotonin syndrome after moclobemide–citalopram or moclobemide–clomipramine overdoses. Lancet 342: 1419

Nurnberger Jr J, DePaulo J R, Gershon E S et al 1997 Genomic survey of bipolar illness in the NIMH genetics initiative pedigrees: a preliminary report. American Journal of Medical Genetics – Neuropsychiatric Genetics 74: 227–237

O'Dwyer A M, Lightman S L, Marks M N, Checkley S A 1995 Treatment of major depression with metyrapone and hydrocortisone. Journal of Affective Disorders 33: 123–128

Ogilvie A D, Battersby S, Bubb V J et al 1996 Polymorphism in serotonin transporter gene associated with susceptibility to major depression. Lancet 347: 731–733

Parker G 1981 Parental reports of depressives. An investigation of several explanations. Journal of Affective Disorders 3: 131–140

Parker G 1983 Parental 'affectionless control' as an antecedent to adult depression. A risk factor delineated. Archives of General Psychiatry 40: 956–960

Parker G 1986 Validating an experiential measure of parental style: the use of a twin sample. Acta Psychiatrica Scandinavica 73: 22–27

Parker G, Barnett B 1988 Perceptions of parenting in childhood and social support in adulthood. American Journal of Psychiatry 145: 479–482

Parker G, Hadzi-Pavlovic D 1993 Old data, new interpretation: a re-analysis of Sir Aubrey Lewis' MD thesis. Psychological Medicine 23: 859–870

Parker G, Hadzi-Pavlovic D 1996 Melancholia: a disorder of movement and mood. Cambridge University Press, Cambridge

Parker G, Kiloh L, Hayward L 1987 Parental representations of neurotic and endogenous depressives. Journal of Affective Disorders 13: 75–82

Parker G, Hadzi-Pavlovic D, Greenwald S, Weissman M 1995 Low parental care as a risk factor to lifetime depression in a community sample. Journal of Affective Disorders 33: 173–180

Paskind H A 1929 Brief attacks of manic–depressive depressions. Archives of Neurology 22: 123–134

Patten S B, Love E J 1997 Drug-induced depression. Psychotherapy and Psychosomatics 66: 63–73

Pauls D L, Gerhard D S, Lacy L G et al 1991 Linkage of bipolar affective disorders to markers on chromosome 11p is excluded in a second lateral extension of Amish pedigree 110. Genomics 11: 730–736

Peroutka S J, Newman H, Harris H 1988 Subjective effects of 3,4-methylenedioxymethamphetamine in recreational users. Neuropsychopharmacology 1: 273–277

Perry E K, Marshall E F, Blessed G, Tomlinson B E, Perry R H 1983 Decreased imipramine binding in the brains of patients with depressive illness. British Journal of Psychiatry 142: 188–192

Post R M, Leverich G S, Altshuler L, Mikalauskas K 1992 Lithium-discontinuation-induced refractoriness: preliminary observations. American Journal of Psychiatry 149: 1727–1729

Pratt L A, Ford D E, Crum R M, Armenian H K, Gallo J J, Eaten W W 1996 Depression, psychotropic medication, and risk of myocardial infarction – prospective data from the Baltimore ECA follow-up. Circulation 94: 3123–3129

Quitkin F M, Stewart J W, McGrath P J et al 1988 Phenelzine versus imipramine in the treatment of probable atypical depression: defining syndrome boundaries of selective MAOI responders. American Journal of Psychiatry 145: 306–311

Quitkin F M, McGrath P J, Stewart J W et al 1989 Phenelzine and imipramine in mood reactive depressives. Further delineation of the syndrome of atypical depression. Archives of General Psychiatry 46: 787–793

Regier D A, Boyd J H, Burke Jr J D et al 1988 One-month prevalence of mental disorders in the United States, based on five epidemiologic catchment area sites. Archives of General Psychiatry 45: 977–986

Robinson R G 1997 Neuropsychiatric consequences of stroke. Annual Review of Medicine 48: 217–229

Robinson R G, Starr L B, Kubos K L, Price T R 1983 A two-year longitudinal study of post-stroke mood disorders: findings during the initial evaluation. Stroke 14: 736–741

Robinson R G, De Carvalho M L, Paradiso S 1995 Post-stroke psychiatric problems. Diagnosis, pathophysiology and drug treatment options. CNS Drugs 3: 436–447

Rolls E T 1990 A theory of emotion and its application to understanding the neural basis of emotion. Cognition and Emotion 4: 161–190

Rolls E T, Hornak J, Wade D, McGrath J 1994 Emotion-related learning in patients with social and emotional changes associated with frontal lobe damage. Journal of Neurology, Neurosurgery, and Psychiatry 57: 1518–1524

Rosenthal N E, Sack D A, Gillin J C et al 1984 Seasonal affective disorder. A description of the syndrome and preliminary findings with light therapy. Archives of General Psychiatry 41: 72–80

Rubin R T, Phillips J J, Sadow T F, McCracken J T 1995 Adrenal-gland volume in major depression – increase during the depressive episode and decrease with successful treatment. Archives of General Psychiatry 52: 213–218

Sackett D L, Richardson W S, Rosenberg W, Haynes R B 1997 Evidence based medicine. Churchill Livingstone, Edinburgh

Schachter S 1966 The interaction of cognitive and physiological determinants of emotional state. In: Spielberger C D (ed) Anxiety and behaviour. Academic Press, London, p. 193

Scott A I F, Freeman C P L 1992 Edinburgh primary care depression study: treatment outcome, patient satisfaction, and cost after 16 weeks. British Medical Journal 304: 883–887

Sharma R, Markar H R 1994 Mortality in affective-disorder. Journal of Affective Disorders 31: 91–96

Silverstone T, Romans S, Hunt N, McPherson H 1995 Is there a seasonal pattern of relapse in bipolar affective disorders? A dual northern and southern hemisphere cohort study. British Journal of Psychiatry 167: 58–60

Simpson S G, Folstein S E, Meyers D A, McMahon F J, Brusco D M, DePaulo J R Jr 1993 Bipolar II: The most common bipolar phenotype? American Journal of Psychiatry 150: 901–903

Slater E, Roth M 1969 Mayer–Gross, Slater and Roth's clinical psychiatry, 3rd edn. Baillière Tindall, London

Smith K A, Fairburn C G, Cowen P J 1997 Relapse of depression after rapid depletion of tryptophan. Lancet 349: 915–919

Soares J C, Mann J J 1997 The anatomy of mood disorders – review of structural neuroimaging studies. Biological Psychiatry 41: 86–106

Song F, Freemantle N, Sheldon T A et al 1993 Selective serotonin reuptake inhibitors: meta-analysis of efficacy and acceptability. British Medical Journal 306: 683–687

Souza F G M, Goodwin G M 1991 Lithium treatment and prophylaxis in unipolar depression: a meta-analysis. British Journal of Psychiatry 158: 666–675

Stewart J W, Mercier M A, Agosti V, Guardino M, Quitkin F M 1993 Imipramine is effective after unsuccessful cognitive therapy: sequential use of cognitive therapy and imipramine in depressed outpatients. Journal of Clinical Psychopharmacology 13: 114–119

Stewart J W, Tricamo E, McGrath P J, Quitkin F M 1997 Prophylactic efficacy of phenelzine and imipramine in chronic atypical depression: likelihood of recurrence on discontinuation after 6 months' remission. American Journal of Psychiatry 154: 31–36

Stokes P E 1995 The potential role of excessive cortisol induced by HPA hyperfunction in the pathogenesis of depression. European Neuropsychopharmacology 5: 77–82

Styron W 1990 Darkness visible. Cape, London

Suppes T, Baldessarini R J, Faedda G L, Tohen M 1991 Risk of recurrence following discontinuation of lithium treatment in bipolar disorder. Archives of General Psychiatry 48: 1082–1088

Thakore J H, Dinan T G 1995 Cortisol synthesis inhibition: a new treatment strategy for the clinical and endocrine manifestations of depression. Biological Psychiatry 37: 364–368

Thapar A, McGuffin P 1996 Genetic influences on life events in childhood. Psychological Medicine 26: 813–820

Thase M E, Fava M, Halbreich U et al 1996 A placebo-controlled, randomized clinical trial comparing sertraline and imipramine for the treatment of dysthymia. Archives of General Psychiatry 53: 777–784

Traskman L, Asberg M, Bertilsson L, Sjostrand L 1981 Monoamine metabolites in CSF and suicidal behavior. Archives of General Psychiatry 38: 631–636

Virkkunen M, Rawlings R, Tokola R et al 1994 CSF biochemistries, glucose metabolism, and diurnal activity rhythms in alcoholic, violent offenders, fire setters, and healthy volunteers. Archives of General Psychiatry 51: 20–27

Warshaw M G, Klerman G L, Lavori P W 1991 Are secular trends in major depression an artifact of recall. Journal of Psychiatric Research 25: 141–151

Watson D, Clark L A, Harkness A R 1994 Structures of personality and their relevance to psychopathology. Journal of Abnormal Psychology 103: 18–31

Weissman M M, Leaf P J, Livingston Bruce M, Florio L 1988 The epidemiology of dysthymia in five communities: rates, risks, comorbidity, and treatment. American Journal of Psychiatry 145: 815–819

Weissman M M, Bland R C, Canino G J et al 1996 Cross-national epidemiology of major depression and bipolar disorder. Journal of the American Medical Association 276: 293–299

WHO 1992 International statistical classification of diseases and related health problems, 10th revision. World Health Organization, Geneva

Wicki W, Angst J, Merikangas K R 1992 The Zurich Study. XIV. Epidemiology of seasonal depression. European Archives of Psychiatry and Clinical Neuroscience 241: 301–306

Winokur G 1990 The concept of secondary depression and its relationship to comorbidity. Psychiatric Clinics of North America 13: 567–583

Young R C, Klerman G L 1992 Mania in late life – focus on age at onset. American Journal of Psychiatry 149: 867–876

15
Paranoid disorder and related syndromes

Lindsay D. G. Thomson

INTRODUCTION

Between the great temples in modern psychiatry of schizophrenia and affective disorders lies the roadside shrine of paranoid disorder and its related syndromes, considered unworthy of a vast number of research pilgrims but none the less forming a significant part of clinical practice. Opinion on the very existence of these disorders as entities independent from schizophrenia and manic depression has varied over the last one 100 years and confusion has arisen over the wide number of terms coined to describe them. 'Paranoia' has been used to describe both a symptom and a diagnosis, from general suspiciousness to a form of psychosis or a personality disorder. The spectrum of disorders involving paranoia is shown in Table 15.1. The adjective 'paranoid' is often employed to refer to persecutory ideas rather than the more accurate meaning, arising from the German, of delusions relating to the individual (delusions of reference, grandiose or persecutory delusions). Many different labels, reflecting many diverse psychiatric traditions, have been used to describe paranoid disorders.

This chapter examines the history of the concept of paranoia and relates this to the modern diagnoses of persistent delusional disorders, acute and transient delusional disorders and induced delusional disorder. In so doing, an attempt is made to place the varying labels within a modern diagnostic framework. Different terms often describe the same condition. This may lead to considerable confusion, as in the case of delusional disorder – erotomanic type, which is also known as erotomania or de Clérambault's syndrome. While it is preferred to use ICD-10 (WHO 1992) or DSM-IV (APA 1994) terminology in everyday practice, it is inevitable that older names will be encountered and practitioners must be aware of their meaning. This chapter follows the format of ICD-10, and other terms are discussed under the relevant ICD-10 heading, although those employed by no means represent an exhaustive historical list.

Schizoaffective disorder is described in Chapter 13 and paranoid personality disorder in Chapter 21.

HISTORY

Paranoia, arising from the ancient Greek for madness, is a term causing much academic discourse throughout the history of psychiatry. Schifferdecker & Peters (1995) examined in detail the origin of this concept. Johann Christian August Heinroth is credited with the first use of the term in his *Handbook of Disorders in the Life of the Soul*, published in 1818. He described paranoia, or *Verruckheit*, as 'unfreedom of spirit with exaltation of the faculty of thought; perversion of concepts, but undisturbed perceptions.' He therefore outlined a disorder of thought rather than a disorder of perception.

In France, Pinel's concept of *manie sans délire* referring to patients 'whose reason seemed to have suffered no injury, yet were gripped by frenzies, as though only their will had weakened' was extended by his student Esquirol who described monomania as a disorder of the will and ideas. The concept of monomania was used in Germany via Heinroth's intervention and subsumed into the concept of paranoia.

Table 15.1	The Paranoid Spectrum

Organic disorders
Schizophrenia (paranoid)
Schizoaffective disorder
Schizotypal disorder
Bipolar disorder
Persistent delusional disorders (paranoid psychoses)
Acute and transient psychotic disorders
Induced delusional disorder
Paranoid personality disorder

In the 1840s Griesinger moved psychiatric thinking away from a psychogenic to an organic basis but he never used the concept of paranoia. Karl Ludwig Kahlbaum (1828–1899) in his classification of mental illness returned to the term paranoia (for disorders with delusions as a primary feature) as a subgroup of partial disorders involving a disturbance of the intellect and described three types: *paranoia ascensa*, in which the patient claims to be someone or something else; *paranoia descensa*, in which the patient feels possessed; and *immota*, which is a paranoia including oversensitivity to stimuli and hallucinations.

In 1865 Ludwig Snell combined Heinroth's concept of paranoia and Esquirol's concept of monomania to describe a disorder in which the individual continued to function in terms of everyday activities but was absorbed by delusional ideas. Griesinger in 1868 described delusional systems which were often persecutory or grandiose. In 1869 Krafft-Ebing drew near to the modern idea of paranoia when he used the term to represent mental disorders whose presentations were based on delusional ideas unrelated to an affective illness and with preservation of the intellect. Kraepelin in his writing between 1883 and 1915 differentiated between dementia praecox, later to be known as schizophrenia, manic depression and paranoia defined as a 'chronic development of a persistent delusional system with normal presence of mind'.

In the first half of this century psychiatric thinking moved away from the idea that paranoia was a diagnosis in its own right. Hermann Krüger in 1917 used the concept of paranoia to describe paranoid schizophrenia, although in 1920 Bleuler distinguished this from schizophrenia and used it to describe a reactive psychosis. Kolle in 1931 studied 66 patients and concluded that paranoia was a subtype of schizophrenia. Kurt Schneider in 1949 subsumed paranoia into schizophrenia and viewed delusional systems without deterioration of personality and functioning as a subtype of schizophrenia.

Paranoia was dissociated once more from schizophrenia in modern diagnostic classifications and in ICD-9 was defined as 'a rare chronic psychosis in which logically constructed systematised delusions have developed gradually without concomitant hallucinations or the schizophrenic type of disordered thinking'. In ICD-10 the term 'persistent delusional disorders' is used. The debate continues as to whether paranoia as defined by Kraeplin exists, and if it does whether or not it is a subtype of schizophrenia. Winokur (1977) found only 29 patients out of a study of 21 000 casenotes fulfilled his definition of delusional disorder of non-bizarre delusions developing before the age of 60 in the absence of hallucinations, flattened or inappropriate affect, organic brain disease or symptoms of depression or mania. In a literature review on the nosologic validity of paranoia, Kendler (1980) recognised the methodological limitations of some studies but concluded that delusional disorder was distinct from schizophrenia. This view was supported by the finding that the risk of developing schizophrenia or schizoid/schizotypal personality disorder was raised in the first-degree relatives of patients with schizophrenia but not in patients with delusional disorder (Kendler & Hayes 1981, Kendler et al 1985).

The relative infrequency with which the diagnosis of delusional disorder is made stems from a number of factors in addition to its low prevalence. Firstly, these patients do not view themselves as ill and often continue to function relatively normally, thereby failing to come to psychiatric attention. Secondly, if they do seek medical help they do so on the basis of their delusional beliefs and therefore present to other specialities, such as dermatology or plastic surgery, rather than to psychiatrists. Finally, if they do present to a psychiatrist they may be misdiagnosed as schizophrenic if the diagnosis of delusional disorder is not considered.

PERSISTENT DELUSIONAL DISORDERS

Presentation

The essence of a delusional disorder is the presence of a non-bizarre delusion or delusional system (Table 15.2). The delusions are non-bizarre in that they have some understandable foothold in reality and are in keeping with cultural norms – for example, being poisoned by avaricious relatives, deceived by a partner's unfaithfulness or believing oneself to be loved by a famous person. The nature of the delusions is a key factor in distinguishing the disorder from schizophrenia. There must be no evidence of an organic mental disorder or of inducement by drugs or alcohol, and the criteria for

Table 15.2 Persistent delusional disorders
Non-bizarre delusions / delusional system
Preservation of social functioning (common)
Hallucinations, if present, intermittent or content related to delusions
No persistent depressive symptoms
Not secondary to organic disorders, substance misuse or schizophrenia

schizophrenia must not be fulfilled. Where depressive symptoms are present these are intermittent and the delusional beliefs persist in their absence. Hallucinations may occur but again are usually intermittent. DSM-IV allows persistent hallucinations if they are related to the delusional belief – for example, that one is rotting and emits a foul odour. In DSM-IV the delusions must be present for at least 1 month and in ICD-10 for 3 months. In addition, DSM-IV adds the criteria that social functioning and behaviour are not markedly abnormal other than that arising directly from the delusions. Often patients may appear entirely normal until the subject of their delusional beliefs is raised. Sometimes the impact of the delusional beliefs may be such that the individual is disabled – for example, being unable to leave home for fear of kidnap or assault.

The beliefs develop into an encapsulated, consistent delusional system which is often chronic. The individual usually continues to function well and the delusional intensity of the beliefs may vary. The patient lacks insight into his condition. Manschreck (1996) described the general characteristic features of paranoia as 'anger, irritability, attention to small details, guardedness, evasiveness, litigiousness, hostility, secretiveness, humourlessness, self-righteousness, hypersensitivity, sullenness, and suspiciousness'.

There are various subtypes of delusional disorder occurring with different frequencies. Opjordsmoen & Retterstøl (1991) in a study of 72 patients found that 41 had persecutory delusions, 14 delusions of jealousy, 6 self-referential delusions, 5 hypochondriacal, 2 grandiose, 2 erotomanic and 2 others. It is the content of the delusions that determines the subtype.

Aetiology

It has been debated whether delusional disorder is a distinct diagnostic entity, a subtype of schizophrenia or a subtype of bipolar disorder (Kendler 1980). Unlike schizophrenia, delusional disorder has not been shown to have a clear genetic basis. Almost twice the usual population incidence of schizophrenia in first-degree relatives of individuals with delusional disorder has been shown in some studies (Kolle 1931) but not in others, and such a finding has been made for other disorders, such as obsessive–compulsive disorder, which are not viewed as a variant of schizophrenia. Indeed this evidence can be considered part of a general family tendency towards psychopathology in patients with delusional disorder. This idea is further supported by the work of Munro & Mok (1995) who found 20% of family members of delusional disorder probands had psychopathology. Most of the evidence indicates that delusional disorder is a diagnosis in its own right and

not a subtype of schizophrenia. Kendler & Hays (1981) found that the prevalence of schizophrenia was significantly lower in first- and second-degree relatives of delusional disorder probands (0.6%) than in the first- and second-degree relatives of patients with schizophrenia (3.8%). No difference was found in the rates of affective disorder, antisocial personality disorder, anxiety or obsessive–compulsive disorder between relatives of both groups. Feelings of inferiority were more commonly encountered in relatives of delusional disorder probands than schizophrenic probands. Paranoid personality traits were found to be increased in first-degree relatives of delusional disorder probands compared with controls (Kendler et al 1985), as was delusional disorder (Manschreck 1996).

Some patients with delusional disorder have been shown to have had avoidant and paranoid premorbid personality traits (Opjordsmoen 1988). They were often oversensitive, with what Kretschmer described as a sensitive personality (*sensitive Beziehungswahn*); sometimes had a physical abnormality such as a cleft palate; and were frequently socially displaced, coming from a different racial or socioeconomic background than their neighbours. Precipitating factors such as social isolation were often identifiable in delusional disorder. Eitinger (1960), in a study of mental disease among refugees in Norway, found that delusional disorder was much more likely to occur in an immigrant population.

It has been suggested that delusional disorder is caused by defective social vigilance mechanisms and responses. These vigilance mechanisms are said to assess and react to the social environment and external events in the way that the body's physiological mechanisms assess and react to the physical environment. They are programmed responses to certain situations. This theory is supported by the consistent themes found in delusional disorder – for example, jealousy; the continuum that can be shown between a frank delusional idea and an overvalued idea; and the limited response by patients with delusional disorder to conventional neuroleptics. It has been postulated that suspicion and anxiety carry a selective advantage in evolutionary terms, but when misapplied or inappropriately regulated on account of adaptive hypersensitivity or situational unfamiliarity may result in delusional disorder (Schlager 1995).

The later age of onset of delusional disorder in comparison to schizophrenia means that the lower socioeconomic origins and educational attainment of these patients cannot be explained by a downward social shift caused by the illness, as occurs with schizophrenia. This would support the case initially put by Kraepelin that delusional disorder is the result of 'the influence of the stimulus of life'.

Deafness is a well-recognised predisposing factor to delusional disorder, probably due to secondary social isolation. Acquired deafness is more likely to lead to delusional disorder than congenital deafness, and tinnitus may contribute to the production or maintenance of auditory hallucinations (Cooper et al 1974), as may hyperacusis (Munro 1991). The vast majority of deaf people do not however develop paranoid ideation (Corbin & Eastwood 1986).

Isolation, whether arising from deafness, language or social barriers, imprisonment or immigration, may lead to feelings of insecurity which, in combination with an oversensitive personality and low self-esteem, may then be projected outwards to the surroundings, resulting in misinterpretations and paranoid delusions. This phenomenon is seen in prisons where the effect of a stressful environment on vulnerable individuals with low self-esteem and often with a history of substance abuse can lead to the development of a paranoid disorder, acute or persistent.

Organic factors such as head injury have been implicated (Munro 1991) in the development of delusional disorder. The occurrence of delusions in organic disorders, particularly temporal lobe epilepsy, extrapyramidal disease and other subcortical disorders, suggests that they may be the result of dysfunction of particular brain regions (McAllister 1992) and Cummings (1992) theorised that this was caused by limbic dysfunction involving the caudate nuclei and temporal lobes.

Epidemiology

Typically delusional disorder presents in the middle to late years of life. The male:female prevalence rates are equal; although the results of some studies have suggested a female preponderance, these may be explained by the subtype of delusional disorder examined. For example, delusional jealousy is more common in men and erotomania in women. Sufferers are more likely to have a lower socioeconomic origin and educational attainment than the general population. It is increased in immigrant populations. More marry than in a schizophrenic population but divorce or widowhood are common. The prevalence of delusional disorder has been estimated at less than 30 per 100 000 population (Schlager 1995). The incidence of delusional disorder resulting in psychiatric admission has been estimated to be 1–3 per 100 000 population per year (Kendler 1982).

Course and prognosis

Opjordsmoen (1988) found after 22–39 years that delusions had faded in 61%, were unchanged in 17%

and were worse in 17% of delusional disorders. There was a full recovery in 37%, a mild defect in 32%, moderate impairment in 10% and severe impairment in 22%. The outcome was better in reactive (clear precipitant) delusional disorder than non-reactive delusional disorder, which in turn had a better prognosis than schizophrenia. Over 27 years it was found that the jealous subtype of delusional disorder had a better outcome than the other subtypes and these patients were more likely to be in employment and to have social contacts (Opjordsmoen & Retterstøl 1991). The jealous subtype was over 6 years older at first admission, had experienced symptoms for over 1 year longer and had more psychosocial stressors than the persecutory subtype. Being married was associated with a better prognosis. Symptoms lasting longer than 6 months before commencement of treatment had a worse outcome. The course of the disorder is variable by both subtype and individual patient. The disorder can become chronic and it may follow a remitting relapsing course. Between 3 and 22% of patients with delusional disorder develop schizophrenia (Kendler 1980).

Differential diagnosis

Paranoid delusions of whatever form, whether persecutory, litigious, grandiose, self-referential, hypochondriacal, jealous or erotomanic, have little diagnostic value, as such delusions can be symptomatic of a number of different disorders. They can occur in organic disorders, such as an acute confusional state, where the patient is unable to interpret their surroundings and interactions with others correctly and may become very suspicious and disruptive; in dementia, where paranoid delusions may occur prior to any cognitive impairment; or in delirium tremens. They can be induced by alcohol or drug abuse; or by over-the-counter preparations such as antihistamines, or prescribed drugs such as steroids. They can be found in schizophrenia or affective disorders. A potential organic basis must be thoroughly investigated and the use of illicit substances and alcohol explored. In schizophrenia, the delusional beliefs tend to be bizarre and there may be deteriorated behaviour, negative symptoms, thought disorder or persistent auditory hallucinations. In affective disorder there is a temporal relationship between the affective symptoms and the delusional beliefs. A persistent low mood with biological symptoms, such as early morning wakening, loss of appetite and poor concentration, and the belief that the individual was dying would be consistent with a diagnosis of depression. It should be noted however, that mild depressive symptoms are relatively common in delusional disorder as a response to the paranoid beliefs.

Paranoid delusions of a grandiose nature, such as being of royal birth or of having great wealth, can occur in mania. Acute and transient psychotic disorder can be differentiated from delusional disorder by its development to a full psychotic disorder within a 2 week period and its resolution within 3 months. In induced delusional disorder the symptoms arise within the confines of a close relationship, in which two or more parties share the same delusions which resolve upon separation from the primary psychotic source. Hypochondriasis, body dysmorphic disorder and obsessive–compulsive disorder are all differentiated from delusional disorder by the lower intensity with which the individual holds his beliefs and by the greater degree of insight with which he recognises that the beliefs may not be accurate – for example, by acknowledging that he may not be dying of a serious disease or by noting that the shape of his ears would be viewed as normal by other people. In paranoid personality disorder the beliefs are not of delusional intensity.

Management

The first stage in the management of these disorders is a full assessment, including a thorough investigation of possible underlying causes, information gathering from all available sources, and a risk assessment focusing upon the potential for aggression arising from the delusional beliefs. Treat any underlying condition. Once a diagnosis of delusional disorder has been established, management involving both psychotherapeutic and pharmacological interventions can be initiated. This is often difficult in this group of patients because of their general suspiciousness and lack of insight, often leading to a poor doctor–patient relationship and to non-compliance. At times inpatient care and the use of mental health legislation will be required. Separation of the patient from the focus of the delusions can assist greatly.

Approach the patient in a relaxed, friendly, interested and professional manner. Do not collude or immediately challenge his delusional beliefs. Be reassuring and empathic – for example, commenting on how frightening or troublesome a specific delusion must be. Inform and educate the patient about his diagnosis and acknowledge that you may have to agree to differ over the cause of his symptoms. Be overtly pragmatic in your treatment strategies and discuss ways of helping him with his problems. For example: does he need a hearing test; would he like to attend a day hospital for some company or a community psychiatric nurse to visit; and will he try medication to see if this will reduce his distressing thoughts? Specific psychotherapeutic treatments have been suggested, including cognitive therapy with reality testing and direct challenging of delusional beliefs.

Neuroleptic medication is the mainstay of treatment, in particular pimozide, but evidence regarding the efficacy of pharmacological interventions is limited. The newer antipsychotic drugs have not been assessed for these disorders. Munro & Mok (1995) reviewed 1000 articles published after 1961 on delusional disorder and used only cases fulfilling DSM-IV criteria. They commented on methodological problems, noting that the quality of the articles was variable, basic information was often missing, that because pimozide in practice had become the drug of choice for these disorders its success might be due to its use as a first-line treatment, and that a comparison of one drug with a collection of others may hide the efficacy of another medication. Furthermore, they noted that non-compliance was common in this disorder, adding further methodological problems. Of 209 cases studied 52.6% were said to have made a recovery defined as 'a return to full function, with total or near-total remission of symptoms'; 28.2% had made a partial recovery; and 19.2% had shown no improvement. In patients receiving pimozide 68.5% recovered and 22.4% showed a partial recovery but for those receiving other neuroleptics the rates were 22.6% and 45.3% respectively. No difference in recovery rates was found between the various subtypes of delusional disorder, although most of the patients studied had somatic delusional disorder. Munro has found that over a tenth of successfully treated patients develop a postpsychotic depressive disorder and require treatment with an antidepressant.

There are reports on the successful use of antidepressants, in particular selective serotonin reuptake inhibitors (SSRIs), in the treatment of delusional disorder (Manschreck 1996). Mood stabilising drugs have also been utilised but there is little evidence of a role for electroconvulsive therapy (ECT).

Subtypes of delusional disorder (Table 15.3)

Persecutory delusional disorder

This is the classic form of the disorder, in which the patient has delusional beliefs that she, or someone close to her, is at the centre of a conspiracy to harm or cheat her, damage her reputation, or block her plans or goals. She considers herself to be the victim of a plot and everyday actions by others can be viewed as offensive and incorporated into the delusional system. The perceived injustice may lead to legal action (see litigious delusional disorder), anger or aggression against her alleged persecutors.

Table 15.3 Persistent delusional disorders: subtypes and related disorders

Persecutory
Litigious – querulous paranoia
Self-referential
Grandiose
Hypochondriacal (somatic) – monosymptomatic hypochondriacal psychosis, dysmorphophobia, Cotard's syndrome
Jealous – delusional jealousy, Othello syndrome
Erotomanic – erotomania, de Clérambault's syndrome

A 59-year-old woman believed that her neighbours were breaking into her house and stealing her belongings while she was out or asleep. She set up an elaborate security system involving lots of sticky tape, string and pots and pans to detect intruders. As medical staff became involved with her, she extended her delusional system so that the psychiatrists and her neighbours were plotting to take her into hospital in order to rob her house.

Litigious delusional disorder

The litigious or querulous paranoid holds the belief that he has been wronged and pursues justice with vigour and determination. He attempts to achieve justice from his perceived wrongdoer by endless complaints or litigation, the original point of which may be lost in the process. He may insist on representing himself in court and pursue litigation to his financial and social detriment. Querulous paranoia was first described by Krafft-Ebing in 1879. Litigious delusional disorder is a subtype in ICD-10 but is subsumed under the heading of persecutory delusional disorder in DSM-IV. The condition may more often present to legal or statutory agencies than to psychiatrists.

Goldstein (1995) describes three types of litigious paranoids: the paranoid complaining witness whose version of events is based on delusional material; the hypercompetent litigant who has legal knowledge and who may prefer to represent himself in the belief that he can do it better or that the legal profession is involved in his persecution; and the paranoid litigant in matrimonial proceedings whose delusional beliefs lead to legal battles alleging actions such as infidelity, physical abuse or child sexual abuse. Astrup (1984) found querulent paranoia was a rare condition, representing only 0.7% of all functional psychoses in a study of 2107 patients. He described many of the premorbid

personalities as assertive in this subtype, rather than sensitive.

A 54-year-old man believed that he had been cheated out of his birthright to nine titles such as Duke of X and Lord of Y. He explained that there was a conspiracy to prevent him from claiming his titles by the law courts. He had pursued numerous legal actions and had copious handwritten documents regarding his case. He finally came to psychiatric attention when he wrote threatening letters to court officers.

Self-referential delusional disorder

This arises from delusions of reference in which the patient believes that topics or people on the radio or television or in the newspaper refer to him or have particular meaning for him. He believes that others notice and discuss him in detail.

A 44-year-old, single, former bus driver had been made redundant 3 years previously at the same time as new neighbours had moved in next door. He became convinced that he was being accused by his neighbours of sexually abusing their daughters, aged 9 and 6, and that this was the subject of hidden references in the local newspaper and on the television. The media had carried items about child sexual abuse. He had only ever exchanged brief words with his neighbours and there was no evidence of any sexually inappropriate behaviour. The issue came to psychiatric attention via the police after he began to vehemently protest his innocence to his neighbours.

Grandiose delusional disorder

In this subtype the patient is convinced that she has great status, power, talent or wisdom. She may view herself as a powerful politician, scientific genius, great artist or brilliant businessperson. She may believe that she has a special relationship with an influential person, such as the prime minister, or have religious delusions – for example, that she is the Virgin Mary. She may preach in the street or join cults.

A 42-year-old woman believed that she was a great artist in the genre of Van Gogh. She produced numerous paintings in a variety of lurid colours, generally of flowers or fruit, in a rather child-like style. She distributed her paintings with benevolence to every carer or psychiatric institution she came in contact with. She spent considerable sums of money on canvas and oil paints and in attendance at art exhibitions, where she would harangue the upper echelons of the art world for its failure to recognise her talent.

Hypochondriacal or somatic delusional disorder

In this subtype the individual believes that he suffers from a physical illness or has an abnormal physical feature. Three disorders are described under this heading: while monosymptomatic hypochondriacal psychosis can be subsumed under hypochondriacal delusional disorder, dysmorphophobia is not always present with delusional intensity, and Cotard's syndrome occurs in depression as well as in delusional disorder.

Monosymptomatic hypochondriacal psychosis

This is characterised by a single delusional belief about health or bodily function. Munro (1988) identified three types of somatic disorder: olfactory-type, involving a delusion of extreme halitosis or body odour; body dysmorphic-type, involving a delusion of a physical defect; and infestation-type, in which the individual believes he is infested by parasites or insects. It occurs as a disorder in its own right, independent of schizophrenia or affective disorder. The term was popularised by Munro in 1980 in a description of 50 such cases. It can afflict those who are more self-conscious, particularly at times of psychosocial stress. Initially patients are more likely to present to their general practitioners or other specialists, such as dermatologists, rather than to a psychiatrist. The symptom has often been present for many years before a psychiatrist is consulted. The patient may give a stereotyped description of his complaint which he pursues energetically in the belief that there is a physical cause for his symptoms. His personality is usually well preserved, although his life may be adversely affected. He may be anxious and over alert, show anger and suspiciousness, feel dejection and shame, and avoid social contact. The onset is insidious in over 60% of cases (Munro 1988). Approximately one-third have some form of psychiatric history, usually with personality problems or substance abuse. The disorder tends to run a chronic course and pimozide has been reported to be of some benefit (Munro 1988, Osman 1991).

A 49-year-old man complained that something was dripping from his canine teeth. The onset was insidious and the delusion had been present for approximately 5 years. He ceased to care for himself and gave up work as a gardener. He would continually ask people to look in his mouth and see what was dripping from his teeth. He was admitted after his son became so exasperated that he punched

him in the mouth. He was treated unsuccessfully with pimozide.

Dysmorphophobia – delusional and non-delusional

This is a disorder, also known as body dysmorphic disorder, which presents as a preoccupation with a presumed defect in appearance. Typically, it involves some imagined or slight abnormality of the head, such as protruding ears, a large nose, hair or skin imperfections, but can feature any body part. Often the preoccupation represents an overvalued idea and is considered to be a hypochondriacal disorder but it can be held with delusional intensity and be associated with a complete lack of insight. Delusional dysmorphophobia is coded under other persistent delusional disorders in ICD-10. The individual thinks of herself as ugly and spends a considerable amount of time ruminating on her problem, grooming, mirror checking and seeking reassurance about her defect. She may try to hide it by the use of makeup, or in men by growing facial hair, and in some cases, resort to dermatological treatments or cosmetic surgery to improve the supposed defect. Such treatments are rarely of benefit and may themselves lead to further preoccupations and repeat surgery.

The disorder often commences in adolescence and is long lasting, although the severity of the preoccupation may vary over time. It causes considerable distress both by the primary effect of the preoccupation itself and also by its secondary effects in terms of social withdrawal and isolation. It can be a diagnosis in its own right, or be associated with, for example, a delusional disorder, a major depressive episode, an obsessive–compulsive disorder or a social phobia. Phillips et al (1994) have compared cases of delusional and non-delusional body dysmorphic disorder. They found little difference between the groups in terms of demographics, phenomenology, course, associated features, comorbidity and treatment response and concluded that there was a psychotic subtype that overlaps with, and may be the same as, hypochondriacal-type delusional disorder. A study of delusional and non-delusional body dysmorphic disorder found that both groups responded to serotonin reuptake inhibitors (McElroy et al 1993), while neither showed a good response to neuroleptics. It has also been shown that the patients in the delusional group score more highly in terms of obsessional ideas than those in the non-delusional group, suggesting that the delusional subtype is simply a more extreme form of the illness.

A 44-year-old woman presented to a plastic surgeon complaining that her ears stuck out. There was indeed a slight protrusion of the ears and surgery resulted in a technically satisfactory result. However, at follow-up she stated that her ears were still poking out. When it was put to her that they appeared normal she became verbally aggressive and complained that the surgeon was useless and had failed in the initial surgery. She cried and stated that nothing was right in her life and that since the failure of the surgery she was unable to go to work because everyone was laughing at her ears. She pleaded with the surgeon to help her but no amount or reassurance would convince her that her ears were normal. She was persuaded to see a liaison psychiatrist who diagnosed a delusional disorder.

Cotard's syndrome In 1880 Jules Cotard described the case of a 43-year-old woman which he thought exemplified a new type of depression. She believed that she had 'no brain, nerves, chest, or entrails, and was just skin and bone', that 'neither God or the devil existed', and that she did not need to eat because 'she was eternal and would live forever'. For many years debate has ranged as to whether Cotard's syndrome, or *délire de négation*, represents a diagnosis in its own right, or is instead a syndrome common to a number of different diseases, including depression and organic conditions. Berrios & Luque (1995) analysed 100 cases of Cotard's syndrome and divided them into three groups: psychotic depression; Cotard type 1, comprising patients who had no depression or other disease and appeared to have features consistent with a delusional disorder; and Cotard type II, comprising patients who displayed depression, anxiety and auditory hallucinations and fell in-between the other two groups. Eighty-nine per cent of patients had depressive symptoms but the presence of Cotard's syndrome was not found to relate to the degree of depression.

Delusional jealousy

In delusional jealousy, also known as morbid jealousy or the Othello syndrome, the patient is convinced that his partner is being unfaithful. In the Shakespearean tragedy *Othello* (1604) the title character strangles his wife, Desdemona, in a fit of rage, having been persuaded of her infidelity. Shepherd (1961) described the relationship between morbid jealousy and both mental illness and domestic violence. The distinction between morbid jealousy and normal jealousy can be unclear because they coexist on a continuum, with delusional jealousy at one extreme. Morbid jealousy can be a symptom of a number of disease processes, including schizophrenia, alcohol dependence, paranoid personality disorder and delusional disorder – jealous type. It is

recognised that jealousy is common, as indeed is adultery. Mullen & Martin (1994) in a community study of jealousy found that all 58% of the responders to a postal questionnaire had experienced jealousy at some point in their lives. Jealousy is both a cry for idealised love and an attempt to control the object of that love. During the Renaissance jealousy was viewed as a passion and defending one's honour was seen as socially correct behaviour. In the 20th century jealousy is considered to be undesirable and unhealthy, revealing underlying immaturity and insecurity. Overt jealousy is unacceptable and considered to require treatment.

Typically the sufferer is over 40 years of age and may have become increasingly suspicious before developing frank delusions. There is often no psychiatric history. The patient may dwell on past events suggestive of infidelity, may follow his partner, prevent her from going out, search her belongings for evidence of unfaithfulness and accuse her of having an affair. Mullen & Martin (1994) found that jealous men experienced increased anxiety and depressive symptoms and attempted to ignore and avoid their jealous beliefs, whereas jealous women tended to suffer from low self-esteem, and were younger, often less than 30 years old, at the time of presentation. The women were more likely to attempt to make themselves more attractive, to show distress, and to confront their partners about their beliefs of infidelity.

A variety of aetiological factors has been suggested, including low self-esteem, inadequacy, poor sexual performance, passive premorbid personality and excessive dependence on the partner. Jealousy is thought to have an evolutionary basis by which males protect their rights to females and thereby further their reproductive potential, and females protect the stable environment required for the rearing of children. Sociocultural norms play a role in a perceived threat to a relationship. Alcohol is a commonly associated feature and, in a study of 207 patients with alcohol dependence, 71 (34%) were found to suffer from morbid jealousy, 20 only when intoxicated, and 51 even when sober (Michael et al 1995).

Delusional jealousy often leads to contact with forensic psychiatry services due to the actual or perceived threat of violence. Mowat (1966) in a study of morbidly jealous murderers found 4.5 years between the onset of the disorder and the murder. This timescale was shorter if the jealousy was associated with depression or alcohol abuse. Most of the victims were wives. The delusions of infidelity often remained after the homicide. The diagnosis was of a delusional disorder in 7 cases, schizophrenia in 13, alcohol in 8, depression in 8, organic in 2 and 2 unspecified.

Treatment plans are dependent on the underlying

disorder. Marital therapy and cognitive therapy are used. Geographical separation of patient and victim can result in a reduction of the intensity of the delusional ideas and reduce the risk of aggression to the victim. Neuroleptic medication, such as pimozide, is used, as are selective serotonin reuptake inhibitor antidepressants. Cases secondary to a psychotic, rather than neurotic, illness have a better prognosis. Avoidance of alcohol and drugs, where they are identified precipitants, is important. It is essential to warn the victim of the jealousy about the potential risk of violence and to counsel her about the warning signs of increasing threats.

A 29-year-old man asked to see a psychiatrist while on remand in prison on a charge of assaulting his wife. For 3 years he had believed that she was having an affair and had stopped her from going out with female friends, searched through her possessions for evidence and constantly pushed her to admit to adultery. He had a 10 year history of alcohol bingeing. The day after consuming a considerable quantity of alcohol and while nursing a hangover he attacked his wife for no reason he could express. In prison he was remorseful and anxious that his absence from home would allow his wife to be unfaithful. At interview there was no evidence of a psychotic or affective illness. His ideas regarding infidelity at that stage were overvalued rather than delusional. He was strongly advised to abstain from alcohol abuse and informed of agencies to assist in this on his release. The issue of his jealousy and its relationship to his aggression and alcohol abuse was explained. With his permission his wife was interviewed. She confirmed his account and said that he had been aggressive on several occasions. She had considered leaving him but was frightened this would provoke further violence. She was given the same information as her husband and advised that morbid jealousy was associated with violence. On his return to court he was fined and went home.

Erotomania

This disorder of delusional loving focuses on the unfounded belief that the patient is loved from afar by another person. The syndrome bears the alternative name of *de Clérambault*, who gave the definitive description published in 1942. The object of this belief is usually of higher status and may be famous, wealthy, or in a professional relationship with the sufferer. He is usually married or unavailable. Actors, singers and doctors are all potential targets, although in some cases it can be a complete stranger. It may commence with a chance meeting, into which the patient reads additional meaning, or they may never have met. She becomes convinced that the individual is in love with her and will only be happy when they are together. She believes that he initiated the relationship and sometimes may reject his advance in her delusional thoughts but more often she falls in love with him. She may follow, telephone, write to and generally harass her target. Stalking has become a subject of media interest and can be secondary to erotomania. She may visit his home and allege marital infidelity to his wife. She develops a delusional system by which every encounter, be it in person or via television or cinema, has special meaning with regards to their affair. She believes that he communicates with her by covert methods. The continual rejection may initially be seen as a test of their love but may eventually lead to anger and aggression. Menzies et al (1995) studied erotomanic delusional disorder and dangerous behaviour and found it to be rare and related to a history of antisocial personality disorder and multiple delusional objects. The police are commonly involved as the victim attempts to ward off unwelcome advances.

Erotomania can present as a form of delusional disorder or as a symptom of other disorders such as schizophrenia or mania. A variety of aetiological theories have been proposed (Segal 1989). These include sexual frustration; the delusion of love as compensation for an otherwise disappointing and isolated life; a defence against heterosexual urges, aggression and low self-esteem; and the fulfilment of unmet narcissistic needs.

Erotomania has been reported for both sexes, but is more common among women. The sufferers are usually socially isolated, withdrawn, without a sexual relationship and in menial jobs. The syndrome is often chronic, although the intensity of the delusions may vary. Geographical separation is thought to be the best treatment to date, in combination with neuroleptic medication. ECT has been recommended if there is an underlying affective illness. Occasionally the syndrome is said to have vanished after confrontation of the delusional ideas but usually any form of therapeutic work is met with a blanket insistence of the veracity of their love and the intervention of psychiatrists is viewed as a further test of that love.

A 27-year-old woman followed a pop star on tour to Scotland where she threatened to harm his children if he did not publicly admit his love for her. She had been pursuing him for 3 years. After her arrest she was found to exhibit many of the classic symptoms of erotomania.

Delusional disorder – unspecified type

This subtype is used if the character of the delusions is unclear, if it does not fit into one of the above categories, or if a combination of subtypes is present.

Related paranoid disorders

Delusional misidentification syndromes

These are symptoms as opposed to diagnoses. They are always part of an underlying illness – commonly schizophrenia, organic, delusional or affective disorders. General features include symptom selectivity to one or a few persons, places or objects; involvement of a person with whom there is a special relationship such as a mother; behaviour displaying dual and dissociated thinking, for example believing that a nurse is a former boyfriend but relating to him as a member of the nursing staff; the presence of derealisation, depersonalisation, *déja vu* or *jamais vu*; and the description of some dissimilarities between the original and the double, such as the amputee who knows her double has all her limbs. These syndromes were extensively reviewed by Ellis et al (1993).

Capgras delusion   Described by Joseph Capgras and his assistant Reboul-Lachaux in 1923, the syndrome was called *illusion de sosies* (double). The patient believes that others, commonly relatives, have been replaced by identical or near identical impostors. The patient may be experiencing derealisation, have been separated from the 'impostor' for some time or believe that he is behaving differently towards her, for example by ignoring her. The condition has also been described in which animals or objects have been exchanged. It can be associated with dangerousness such as aggressive behaviour towards the supposed impostor.

Fregoli delusion   The term *illusion de Fregoli* was coined by Courbon and Fail in 1927 and used to describe the belief that an individual, usually unknown to the patient, contains within him someone with whom the patient is familiar. Often this disguised person will be following or persecuting the patient in some way. Fregoli was a well-known Italian actor and mimic. It has also been described for possessions as well as people.

Intermetamorphosis delusion   Courbon & Tusques in 1932 described the delusion in which the patient believes that she can see others change into someone else. The transformation is of both external appearance and internal personality and is usually temporary.

Subjective doubles delusion   Christodoulou in 1978 described the scenario in which the patient believes that her double is in existence and functioning independently.

Other forms of delusional misidentification syndromes have been described: in the autoscopic type the patient sees a double of herself projected on to a person or object nearby; in the reverse subjective double syndrome the patient believes that she is an impostor or in the process of being physically or psychologically replaced; and in reverse Fregoli syndrome there is the delusion that others have completely misidentified the patient.

The aetiology of these symptoms lies with the underlying disorder but both psychodynamic and organic explanations have been advanced as possible common causations, either alone or in combination (Markova & Berrios, 1994). These syndromes have been considered to be on the extreme of a continuum of every day misidentifications arising because of intense focusing on a particular detail; to be the result of the role of beliefs and emotion on perception, particularly in vulnerable personalities; to occur in the presence of disorders of mood, judgement and coenaesthesia in combination with imagination; and to arise from defence mechanisms such as projection, splitting of internalised object representation or regression with loss of identity and flawed attempts at reconstruction. Organic explanations include right hemisphere dysfunction, right and left hemisphere disconnection, anterior cortical atrophy, temporal lobe pathology and right hemisphere and bifrontal dysfunction. Cognitive neurophysiological tests have shown impaired facial recognition and information processing in some patients.

In a study of 195 consecutive admissions with a functional psychosis 4.1% were found to have a delusional misidentification syndrome: 6 Capgras, 1 subjective doubles and 1 Capgras plus subjective doubles. Six cases had schizophrenia, 1 manic depression and 1 drug abuse (Kirov et al 1994). A prevalence of 3.1% in a psychotic population has been reported (Joseph 1994). Over 90% had schizophrenia.

Treatment is directed at the underlying cause. Oral antipsychotic medication is most frequently used but ECT, anticonvulsants and lithium are also employed.

Paraphrenia

The terms paraphrenia or late paraphrenia are included under persistent delusional disorders in ICD-10. Paraphrenia was originally used by Kraepelin in 1920 to describe patients with paranoid delusions and prominent auditory hallucinations arising in middle age, without negative symptoms of schizophrenia. Late paraphrenia was described for cases of late-onset paranoid delusions not secondary to an acute confusional state, dementia or affective disorder. Howard et al (1994) in a study of late paraphrenia, onset after 60 years of age, found that

61.4% had schizophrenia, 30.7% delusional disorder and 7.9% schizoaffective disorder using ICD-10 classification. Howard's group also found (Howard et al 1997) that first-degree relatives of probands with late paraphrenia had the same lifetime risk of developing schizophrenia as a control group, but an increased risk of affective disorder, and concluded that late-onset non-affective psychosis was not linked genetically with schizophrenia. He proposed that late paraphrenia was caused by subtle brain degeneration in those with a genetic loading for affective disorder.

ACUTE AND TRANSIENT PSYCHOTIC DISORDERS

There has long been a recognition of the existence of paranoid illnesses of acute onset and short duration, often secondary to traumatic life events, although different schools of psychiatry have pursued varying concepts. In 1848 Esquirol coined the French term monomania to describe a delusional psychosis characterised by its sudden onset, brief duration and good prognosis. Magnan in 1893 used the expression *bouffée délirante* to describe an acute-onset psychosis. Prior to World War I, Jaspers classified reactive states. In Scandinavia the diagnosis of reactive psychoses was popularised by the work of Wimmer and Faergeman in the early and middle parts of this century, referring to a psychosis precipitated by major life events. In the USA the concept of hysterical psychosis gained credence in the 1960s.

As before, this section will use ICD-10 with information on such historical terms included within the modern terminologies.

Presentation

The acute and transient psychotic disorders develop full-blown symptomatology within a 2 week period (Table 15.4). The symptoms are wide ranging and include perplexity, inattention, thought disorder, delusions or hallucinations. DSM-IV uses the terms brief psychotic disorder for similar presentations lasting between 1 day and 1 month, with or without a known psychosocial precipitant, or schizophreniform psychosis for schizophrenia-like symptoms lasting between 1 and 6 months.

Aetiology

There is dubiety about the nosological validity of these diagnoses and research into their aetiology has therefore been limited. They may be precipitated by an acute

Table 15.4   Acute and transient psychotic disorders
Sudden onset Variable symptomatology – perplexity, inattention, thought disorder, delusions or hallucinations A precipitating factor may be identifiable Resolves within 3 months Not secondary to organic disorders, substance misuse or affective illnesses

stressor such as bereavement, marriage, unemployment, imprisonment, accident or childbirth. Migration and isolation secondary to a language or cultural barrier are known to be causal factors in some cases.

Epidemiology

These disorders have been associated with pre-existing paranoid, borderline and histrionic personality disorders. They are more prevalent in developing nations where there is a strong cultural emphasis on tradition (Jilek & Jilek-Aall 1970). The true prevalence of these disorders is difficult to assess as consistent criteria for diagnosis have not always been applied and because different countries have had varying traditions in the use of these terms. Allodi (1982) reviewed admissions to mental hospitals with a diagnosis of reactive psychosis in selected countries. The prevalence varied between 1% in Chile, 11% in England and 34% in Senegal.

Course and prognosis

By definition the course is brief. It is recognised that clinicians may make an initial diagnosis of an acute and transient disorder that may require revision with the passage of time as the disorder develops. Resolution of symptoms can take place within days, weeks or up to 3 months. The prognosis is said to be better the shorter the interval is between the onset of symptoms and the full-blown disorder. Johnstone et al (1996) found a better prognosis in cases of transient psychoses in terms of social outcome and symptomatology, although relapse was common. Patients with these disorders have increased mortality rates, in particular from suicide.

Differential diagnosis

The differential diagnosis includes organic disorders such as dementia or delirium where perplexity and impairment of attention and concentration may be marked; mania and depression with delusions of guilt and persecution; drug or alcohol problems (although substance abuse does not preclude a diagnosis of an

Table 15.5 Acute and transient psychotic disorders: subtypes and related disorders
Acute polymorphic psychotic disorder, with or without symptoms of schizophrenia – cycloid psychosis, *bouffée délirante* Acute schizophrenia-like psychotic disorder Other acute predominantly delusional psychotic disorders – psychogenic or reactive psychoses, hysterical psychosis, the Ganser syndrome

acute and transient disorder); personality disorder; culture-specific disorders; factitious disorder; and malingering. In the presence of schizophrenic symptoms these must not last longer than 1 month if the diagnostic criteria are to be fulfilled.

Management

Suggested management strategies involve full assessment, support, nursing care, assistance with any identified psychosocial stressors and short-term neuroleptic medication for symptomatic relief. Antidepressants and mood stabilisers to prevent relapse have also been used.

Subtypes of acute and transient disorders
(Table 15.5)

Acute polymorphic psychotic disorder with or without symptoms of schizophrenia

This disorder incorporates cycloid psychosis and the French concept of *bouffée délirante*. There is an acute onset and a rapidly changing clinical picture ranging from the depths of despair to the heights of ecstasy in the presence of fluctuating forms of delusion and hallucination. There is often no obvious precipitant, although sociocultural factors may be responsible. Most cases resolve quickly. There may be positive, negative or catatonic symptoms of schizophrenia and this distinction is made in ICD-10. If schizophrenic symptoms are present for more than 1 month the diagnosis should be changed to schizophrenia; otherwise the general symptoms can last for up to 3 months without a change in diagnosis.

Cycloid psychosis Perris (1974) described 60 cases of cycloid psychosis in a publication dedicated to Dr Karl Leonhard, the founder of this concept. He defined an acute psychosis characterised by the presence of two of the following symptoms: perplexity or confusion; delusions of reference, influence or persecution and/or hallucinations not syntonic with mood; hypo- or hyperkinesia; episodes of ecstasy; and pananx-

iety. It was more common in females and in the age range 15–50 years. The short-term outcome was good. An identifiable stressor was present in only one-third of cases. Twenty per cent of parents and 9% of siblings had had a similar illness, suggesting that this is a unique clinical syndrome. Relapse was common, with an interval between episodes on average of approximately 4 years, although this tended to shorten with repeated episodes. If untreated this increased to a mean of 4.5 episodes within a 10 year period. Perris (1978) demonstrated that the relapse rate could be reduced by lithium, supporting the theory that this condition may be a variant of bipolar disorder.

Bouffée délirante Magnan's term *bouffée délirante*, meaning a puff of madness, has been used to describe an acute-onset psychosis encompassing a wide variety of delusional beliefs and emotional states. At times the patient is totally consumed by her delusions and on other occasions she is able to stand back from them. It usually resolves completely within a few weeks but may be a precursor to schizophrenia. Allodi (1982) reviewed this concept, translated as 'acute paranoid reaction', and stressed the importance of arriving at the correct diagnosis to avoid long-term medication. He highlighted the aeteological role of sociocultural factors, particularly migration and language barriers. He found that 1.3% of all first admissions with psychosis to all psychiatric hospitals in Canada in 1969 had a diagnosis of *bouffée délirante*.

Acute schizophrenia-like disorder

This disorder, which can also be termed brief schizophreniform psychosis or schizophrenic reaction, lacks the emotional highs and lows and rapidly changing clinical picture of acute polymorphic psychotic disorder. It has an acute onset and schizophrenic symptoms but lasts for less than 1 month.

Other acute predominantly delusional psychotic disorders

This subtype lacks the affective and symptom variability of acute polymorphic psychotic disorder and the schizophrenic symptoms of acute schizophrenia-like psychotic disorder but has psychotic symptoms, delusions and hallucinations, almost continually present following an acute onset.

Psychogenic or reactive psychoses Incorporated under this most unimaginative of titles of other acute, predominantly delusional, psychotic disorders is the Scandinavian concept of psychogenic or reactive psychoses. It is empirically appealing to believe that psychosis can arise in an individual, vulnerable on account of constitutional makeup or experiential learning, in response to psychosocial stressors. *Stromgren* (1974) described precipitants: social disasters such as unemployment; family conflicts; isolation; inner conflicts, for example with the conscience; and impersonal events such as catastrophes and war. A psychotic reaction to war was said not to require predisposing constitutional traits. Different presentations of psychogenic psychoses were seen: emotional reactions in 65% of cases, disorders of consciousness in 15% and paranoid types in 20%. The paranoid type had the worst prognosis and disorders of consciousness the best.

This diagnosis is widely made in Scandinavia, sometimes in the absence of an identifiable stressor, but the reliability and validity of this diagnosis is in doubt because of a high frequency of subsequent changes in diagnosis and wide variations in its prevalence. In patients hospitalised with psychosis, Frey (1968) found a prevalence of psychogenic psychosis of 30–40% in Norway, 15–20% in Denmark and 5% in Sweden. In first admissions with a functional psychosis Retterstøl (1987) found that a diagnosis of psychogenic psychosis was made in 50% of cases in Denmark, 40% in Norway and 10% in Sweden. This is partly explained by the Swedish emphasis on organic and personality factors and the Danish focus on social and psychological variables (Stromgren 1974). Jorgensen & Jensen (1988), in an attempt to address the issue of diagnostic validity, set strict criteria: psychotic disorder including delusions lasting more than a few hours and preceded by a stressful life event or an exacerbation of one within the last 3 months; full remission within 3 months; exclusion of organic and affective disorders and first-rank schizophrenic symptoms and severe blunting of affect. Eighty-eight consecutive admissions (excluding organic disorders, substance withdrawal and severe mental retardation) were found to have a functional psychosis with paranoid symptoms, and 13 initially fulfilled the criteria for reactive delusional psychosis; 3 were subsequently reclassified as their illness lasted more than 3 months. Four of the remaining 10 were psychotic at 2 year follow up. Stromgren (1989) defends the concept of psychogenic psychosis on the grounds that research has shown them to be different nosologically from other major psychoses; that their prognosis is good; and that appropriate treatment is with supportive psychotherapy plus, where necessary, with short-term use of medication.

Hysterical psychosis The term hysterical psychosis does not appear in current classifications of disease. It has been used to describe psychotic reactions without features of schizophrenia or manic depression. Hirsch & Hollender (1969) defined the concept as a sudden, brief psychosis, often precipitated by a life event, with delusions, hallucinations, depersonalisation, grossly unusual behaviour and agitation. They described three types of hysterical psychosis: culturally sanctioned behaviour (abnormal actions and beliefs, but these are in keeping with cultural norms – not psychotic); appropriation of psychotic behaviour (conversion process); and true psychosis. The last has been explained psychoanalytically as a failure of repression when faced with acute stress in a vulnerable ego, such as is present in histrionic personality disorder. In the USA hysterical psychosis gained currency as the diagnostic label for reactive psychoses (Allodi 1982).

Ganser syndrome A possible subtype of hysterical psychosis is the Ganser syndrome, first described in 1898. It is characterised by approximate answers (*Vorbeireden*) in which the patient gives a ludicrous reply that at the same time indicates understanding of the question, such as 'how many legs has a horse?' – answer 'three'. Other features can include disorientation, clouding of consciousness, hallucinations, motor disturbances, and anxiety or apathy. Throughout the episode the patient continues to carry out activities of daily living. There is usually a sudden resolution with amnesia for that period. It was originally described in three prisoners awaiting execution. Proposed underlying mechanisms include a hysterical conversion syndrome, organic confusion, psychosis or malingering.

Other acute and transient psychotic disorders

This is a catch-all category for acute psychotic disorders not classifiable elsewhere, for example because delusions and hallucinations are present for a short period only.

Acute and transient psychosis, unspecified

This category is for the conceptually or motivationally challenged psychiatrist unable to further define an acute and transient psychotic disorder. It includes (brief) reactive psychosis not otherwise specified.

INDUCED DELUSIONAL DISORDER

This diagnosis, also known as *folie à deux*, is made when delusions are jointly held by two or more people living together in a close relationship while remaining somewhat isolated from the outside world (Table 15.6). The delusions are usually paranoid or grandiose. The dominant partner has a delusional system, most commonly as part of a schizophrenic illness or a delusional disorder, but it can have an affective or organic basis, and induces the delusional beliefs in the passive recipient.

Table 15.6   Induced delusional disorder
Shared delusional system by two or more people in a close relationship Dominant individual induces delusions in submissive recipient Recipient characteristics – submissive, dependent, isolated, less intelligent and educated than partner, sometimes with a physical disability or sensory impairment Main treatment by separation

Table 15.7 Induced psychosis: subtypes	
Folie imposée	Primary psychotic illness in one adopted by another
Folie simultanée	Primary psychotic illness in both with identical delusions
Folie communiquée	Primary psychotic illness in both developing at different times. Delusional material may be shared and can be initiated by either patient
Folie induite	Pre-existing primary psychosis with the addition of a fellow patient's delusional material

The recipient is usually a submissive, dependent personality, reclusive or suspicious, possibly with depression, physical disability or sensory impairment. She often has a lower IQ and educational attainment level than her psychotic counterpart (Howard 1994). It is a rare disorder and the prevalence is unknown. The delusions are perpetuated by the support of another believing person. It has long been recognised. William Harvey in 1651 described it in two sisters with delusional beliefs about a pregnancy. More than two people, or even families may be involved: *folie à trois* or *folie à famille*.

Psychodynamic and learning theories have been advanced as explanations for this. It can occur because of fear of losing an important relationship in an otherwise isolated person with little scope for reality testing. Psychodynamically it has been postulated that the passive acceptor has repressed oedipal fantasies that are released by the psychotic partner, causing identification of the dominant partner with a parent. Using learning theory it has been proposed that the recipient learns to think psychotically.

A review of the literature (Silveira & Seeman 1995) found that the sex distribution was equal, as was the age distribution between young and old; 90% were couples, siblings or parent–child relationships; comorbid dementia, depression and mental retardation were common; hallucinations were common and over two-thirds were socially isolated.

Subtypes of induced psychosis

See Table 15.7 (Gralnick 1942).

Management

Treatment is by separation of the passive and dominant partners. Separation only leads to complete resolution of symptoms in 40% of cases in the recipient. She may also require psychotherapy, as giving up the delusional beliefs represents a rejection of the relationship. ECT and neuroleptics should not be used in the passive partner in *folie imposée*. The active partner will require treatment of the underlying condition.

A 75-year-old former army sergeant believed that a terrorist organisation was planning to kill ex-British soldiers and their families. His wife was 72 and a retired school dinner lady. She had always taken a submissive role to her husband who was prone to bully her. They had one son who had emigrated to Australia. The husband bombarded his wife with 'evidence' of his beliefs from the newspapers and television and insisted they take elaborate security precautions. Their trips outwith the home were brief for fear of attack. They came to medical attention after she fell and fractured her hip. Both shared the delusional ideas but she gradually recovered and began to voice them with much less certainty while in hospital. He was unable to cope at home alone and it became apparent that he had cognitive deficits and was in the early stages of dementia.

REFERENCES

Allodi F 1982 Acute paranoid reaction (*bouffée délirante*) in Canada. Canadian Journal of Psychiatry 27: 366–373

APA 1994 Diagnostic and statistical manual of mental disorders, 4th edn. American Psychiatric Association, Washington, DC

Astrup C 1984 Querulent paranoia: a follow-up. Neuropsychobiology 11: 149–154

Berrios G E, Luque R 1995 Cotard's syndrome: analysis of 100 cases. Acta Psychiatrica Scandinavica 91: 185–188

Cooper A F, Curry A R, Kay D W K, Garside R F, Roth M 1974 Hearing loss in paranoid and affective psychoses of the elderly. Lancet ii: 851–857

Corbin S, Eastwood M 1986 Sensory deficits and mental disorders of old age: causal or coincidental associations? Psychological Medicine 16: 251–256

Cummings J L 1992 Psychosis in neurologic disease: neurobiology and pathogenesis. Neuropsychiatry, Neuropsychology and Behavioural Neurology 5: 144–150

Eitinger L 1960 The symptomatology of mental disease among refugees in Norway. Journal of Mental Science 106: 947–966

Ellis H D, Luaute J-P, Retterstøl N 1993 The delusional misidentification syndromes. Psychopathology: proceedings of the conference on delusional misidentification syndromes, pp 113–268

Frey T S 1968 On reactive psychosis. Acta Psychiatrica Scandinavica. Supplementum 203: 9–12

Goldstein R L 1995 Paranoids in the legal system. Psychiatric Clinics of North America 18: 303–315

Gralnick A 1942 Folie à deux: the psychosis of association. Psychiatry Quarterly 16: 230–263

Hirsch S J, Hollender M H 1969 Hysterical psychosis: clarification of the concept. American Journal of Psychiatry 125(7): 81–87

Howard R 1994 Induced psychosis. British Journal of Hospital Medicine 51: 304–307

Howard R, Almeida O, Levy R 1994 Phenomenology, demography and diagnosis in late paraphrenia. Psychological Medicine 24: 397–410

Howard R, Graham C, Sham P et al 1997 A controlled family study of late-onset non-affective psychosis (late paraphrenia). British Journal of Psychiatry 170: 511–514

Jilek W, Jilek-Aall L 1970 Transient psychoses in Africans. Psychiatric Clinics 3: 337–364

Johnstone E, Connelly J, Firth C, Lambert M, Owens D 1996 The nature of 'transient' and 'partial' psychoses: findings from the Northwick Park 'functional' psychosis study. Psychological Medicine 26: 361–369

Jorgensen P, Jensen J 1988 An attempt to operationalise reactive delusional psychosis. Acta Psychiatrica Scandinavica 78: 627–631

Joseph A B 1994 Observations on the epidemiology of the delusional misidentification syndromes in the Boston Metropolitan Area: April 1983–June 1984. Psychopathology 27: 150–153

Kendler K 1980 The nosologic validity of paranoia (simple delusional disorder). Archives of General Psychiatry 37: 699–706

Kendler K 1982 Demography of paranoid psychosis (delusional disorder). Archives of General Psychiatry 39: 890–902

Kendler K, Hays P 1981 Paranoid psychosis (delusional disorder) and schizophrenia. Archives of General Psychiatry 38: 547–551

Kendler K S, Masterson C, Davis K L 1985 Psychiatric illness in first degree relatives of patients with paranoid psychosis, schizophrenia and medical illness. British Journal of Psychiatry 147: 524–531

Kirov G, Jones P, Lewis A W 1994 Prevalence of delusional misidentification syndromes. Psychopathology 27: 148–149

Kolle K 1931 Die primare Verruckheit (Primary paranoia). Thieme, Leipzig

McAllister T 1992 Neuropsychiatric aspects of delusions. Psychiatric Annals 22: 269–277

McElroy S L, Phillips K A, Keck P E, Hudson J I, Pope H G 1993 Body dysmorphic disorder: does it have a psychotic subtype? Journal of Clinical Psychiatry 54: 389–395

Manschreck T C 1996 Delusional disorder: the recognition and management of paranoia. Journal of Clinical Psychiatry 57(suppl 3): 32–38

Markova I S, Berrios G E 1994 Delusional misidentifications: facts and fancies. Psychopathology 27: 136–143

Menzies P, Fedoroff J, Green C, Isaacson K 1995 Prediction of dangerous behaviour in male erotomania. British Journal of Psychiatry 166: 529–536

Michael A, Mirza S, Mirza K A, Babu V S, Vithayathil E 1995 Morbid jealousy in alcoholism. British Journal of Psychiatry 167: 668–672

Mowat R 1966 Morbid jealousy and murder: a psychiatric study of morbidly jealous murderers at Broadmoor. Tavistock, London

Mullen P E, Martin J 1994 Jealousy: a community study. British Journal of Psychiatry 14: 35–43

Munro A 1980 Monosymptomatic hypochondriacal psychosis. British Journal of Hospital Medicine 24: 34–38

Munro A 1988 Monosymptomatic hypochondriacal psychosis. British Journal of Psychiatry 153(suppl 2): 37–40

Munro A 1991 Phenomenological aspects of monodelusional disorders. British Journal of Psychiatry 159: 62–64

Munro A, Mok H 1995 An overview of treatment in paranoia/delusional disorder. Canadian Journal of Psychiatry 40: 616–622

Opjordsmoen S 1988 Long-term course and outcome in delusional disorder. Acta Psychiatrica Scandinavica 78: 576–586

Opjordsmoen S, Retterstøl N 1991 Delusional disorder: the predictive validity of the concept. Acta Psychiatrica Scandinavica 84: 250–254

Osman A 1991 Monosymptomatic hypochondriacal psychosis in developing countries. British Journal of Psychiatry 159: 428–431

Perris C 1974 A study of cycloid psychoses. Acta Psychiatrica Scandinavica. Supplementum 253

Perris C 1978 Morbidity suppressive effect of lithium carbonate in cycloid psychosis. Archives of General Psychiatry 35: 328–331

Phillips K A, McElroy S L, Keck P E, Hudson J I, Pope H G 1994 A comparison of delusional and nondelusional body dysmorphic disorder in 100 cases. Psychopharmacology Bulletin 30: 179–186

Retterstøl N 1987 Present state of reactive psychoses in Scandinavia. Psychopathology 20: 68–71

Schifferdecker M, Peters U 1995 The origin of the concept of paranoia. Psychiatric Clinics of North America 18: 231–249

Schlager D 1995 Evolutionary perspectives on paranoid disorder. Psychiatric Clinics of North America 18: 263–279

Segal J 1989 Erotomania revisited: from Kraepelin to DSM-III-R. American Journal of Psychiatry 146: 1261–1266

Shepherd M 1961 Morbid jealousy: some clinical and social aspects of a psychiatric symptom. Journal of Mental Science 107: 607–753

Silveira J M, Seeman M V 1995 Shared psychotic disorder: a critical review of the literature. Canadian Journal of Psychiatry 40: 389–395

Stromgren E 1974 Psychogenic psychoses. In: Hirsch S, Shepherd M (eds) Themes and variations in European psychiatry. Wright, Bristol

Stromgren E 1989 The development of the concept of reactive psychoses. British Journal of Psychiatry 154 (suppl 4): 47–50

WHO 1992 The ICD-10 classification of mental and behavioural disorders: clinical descriptions and diagnostic guidelines. World Health Organization, Geneva

Winokur G 1977 Delusional disorder (paranoia). Comprehensive Psychiatry 18: 511

16

Neuroimaging

K. P. Ebmeier

INTRODUCTION

Most internal organs are readily accessible to external examination. They can be scrutinised endoscopically or biopsied in vivo without any loss of function. One major exception is the central nervous system. Highly sensitive to even very localised disruption, it is completely shielded by bone. It can only be directly examined after major trauma with destruction of the skull or spine. For a long time, knowledge of brain function was, therefore, restricted to information derived from invasive experimental or accidental lesion studies (Phelps 1898, Penfield & Rasmussen 1950, Damasio et al 1994). Technical developments within the last 50 years have allowed us to construct images or maps of the brain without disrupting its surrounding tissues and without interfering substantially with its function. A great variety of such techniques is now available, from X-ray-based computerised tomography (CT), to radioligand-generated positron emission tomography (PET) or single photon emission (computerised) tomography (SPE(C)T), images generated by magnetic-resonance (MRI), maps computed from the intrinsic electrical or magnetic activity of the brain, electro-encephalography (EEG) or magnetoencephalography (MEG), to maps of motor or sensory cortex generated by transcranial magnetic stimulation (TMS). This chapter aims to give a concise description of these techniques and to summarise results relevant to psychiatry. Well-established findings of clinical importance will be reported in the chapters focusing on separate illnesses, so that the emphasis here will be on the scope and the potential of imaging techniques to clarify the aetiology and to help with the diagnosis and the treatment of mental illness.

X-RAY COMPUTERISED TOMOGRAPHY

X-rays pass through the body and generate shadow images on sensitive film on the opposite side of the patient. X-ray absorption increases with electron density. This is related to the atomic number of the elements involved; in human bodies the calcium of bones and teeth give by far the strongest absorption. In a plain skull X-ray, it, is, therefore, mainly bony structures that can be evaluated: sella erosion may be a pointer towards pituitary pathology; calcification of soft tissue the hall-mark of previus trauma or tumour. Specialist invasive techniques, such as air ventriculograms, during which cerebrospinal fluid is removed from the ventricles by cisternal puncture, have been used in the past to examine ventricular changes in patients. Such studies were the first to suggest ventricular dilatation in schizophrenia (Jacobi & Winkler 1927, Huber 1957). The availability of increasing computing power and appropriate backprojection algorithms allowed for the integration of a series of X-ray images taken from different angles into a three-dimensional 'electron density map' of the head, a CT-tomogram. CT technology allows for a spatial resolution in the milimetre range, using a relatively small radiation dose of 1.8 mSv (plain skull X-ray, 0.1 mSv; [^{99m}Tc]HMPAO SPECT scan, 4.7 mSv). However, electron density differences in normal and abnormal soft tissue are very small, only a few per cent, so that there are limitations to the clinical utility of CT. Occasionally, contrast enhancement with an iodine-containing intravenous compound increases vascular signal or demonstrates a local breakdown of the blood–brain barrier due to trauma or tumour. Soft-tissue calcification, for example of the basal ganglia, can be detected with relative ease. White matter translucencies have been used to diagnose Binswanger's disease, a cause of dementia particularly associated with hypertension. Cortical atrophy and ventricular dilatation occur in senile dementia, but overlap with the appearance in healthy control populations. Earlier reports of ventricular dilatation could be confirmed with CT in schizophrenia (Johnstone et al 1976). The large number of reported studies makes it possible to detect secular trends; ventricular abnormalities appear reduced with time, mainly due to the increasingly large ventri-

447

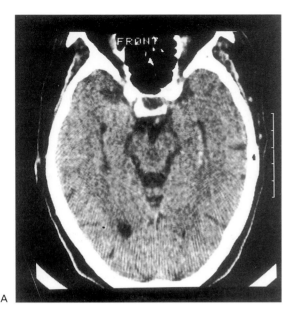 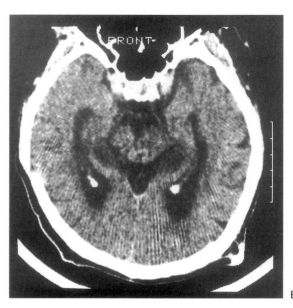

A   B

Fig. 16.1   Modified head orientation in the CT scanner makes it possible to scan the temporal lobes along their long axis. The hippocampus is now exposed in its longitudinal orientation and its thickness can be measured. Normal control and Alzheimer scan. (Courtesy of Professor D. Smith, Oxford.)

cles of (possibly better matched) controls in later studies (van Horn & McManus 1992). Meta-analysis can combine any number of results and allows us to test hypotheses about the homogeneity of patient groups in different studies. For example, the ventricle:brain ratio, a measure of relative ventricular size, is not bimodally distributed in schizophrenia, contradicting the hypothesis that ventricular abnormalties occur only in a discrete subgroup of patients (Daniel et al 1992).

A modified head orientation in the CT scanner makes it possible to scan the temporal lobes along their long axis. The hippocampus is now exposed in its longitudinal orientation and its thickness can be measured (Fig. 16.1). Hippocampal thickness is clearly decreased in patients with Alzheimer's disease, and moreover appears associated in time wiith cognitive deterioration (Jobst et al 1994).

MAGNETIC RESONANCE IMAGING

Principles of MRI

The principles of magnetic resonance imaging are quite different from those of the X-ray or radioligand-based imaging modes. Magnetic resonance occurs as the result of radiofrequency (rf) signals, used to disturb certain atomic nuclei that have previously been aligned within a static magnetic field. They precess (like spin-

ning tops) around the field with a certain frequency, the Larmor frequency, which is directly proportional to the strength of the static magnetic field. The localisation of signals within the scanner depends on this relationship. After the rf pulse, magnetic field gradients are superimposed in three dimensions, so that signals can be spatially encoded. The signal strength for different resonance frequencies can, therefore, be translated into signal intensity at spatial coordinates, thus creating the MR image. MR images are composed of one, or a mixture of three measures: proton density, the longitudinal T_1 and the transverse $T_2^\star$ relaxation time. Proton density mainly refers to the density of protons in free water which are able to resonate. T_1 reflects the rate at which nuclei realign with the static magnetic field (spin–lattice relation), whereas $T_2^\star$ is affected by factors, such as field inhomogeneities, which bring nuclei out of phase with each other (spin–spin relaxation) and reduce the overall signal. Further signal reduction occurs as the result of diffusion of free nuclei. By reversing the spin dephasing during the imaging sequence (spin–echo), the field inhomogeneities can be neutralised and the signal enhanced.

Principles of MRS

Following the same physical principles, variations of the static magnetic field due to shielding effects within mol-

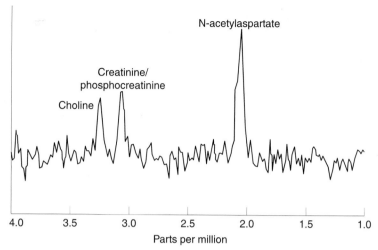

Fig. 16.2 The power in different resonance frequency bands is quantified, in order to measure the concentration of different molecular groups. Water supressed H+-spectrum. (Courtesy of Dr. I. Marshall, Edinburgh.)

ecules result in slightly differing reasonance frequencies for the same nucleus, e.g. H+, and can be used to quantify the relative contributions of different molecular groups. This method is called magnetic resonance spectroscopy (MRS), because the power in different resonance frequency bands is quantified, in order to measure the concentration of different molecular groups (Fig. 16.2). In vitro, MRS has long been used as a powerful method of analytical chemistry. In vivo sampling of brain volumes as small as 1 cm^3 (1 mL) in 6 minutes is now feasible, making functional chemical analysis of living brain tissue possible. While this may be practicable in cooperative healthy volunteers, the method has obvious limitations in psychiatric patients. Table 16.1 lists some of the more commonly used nuclei for MRS and their biological significance. In order to supply specific information about brain chemistry, nuclei have to have an unpaired proton, and be a component of biologically important molecules (^{31}P, ^{1}H) or be of intrinsic interest as elements (^{7}Li, ^{23}Na). Nuclei used to label molecules of interest are rare or absent in the brain, such as ^{19}F, or are a rare isotope of a more common element (^{13}C). Occasionally, the signal from the most abundant and uninformative molecule needs to be removed by technical means in order to measure the concentration of rarer, more interesting molecules (proton MRS with suppressed water signal).

Principles of fMRI

Traditional MRI acquisition sequences require a large number of rf pulses and well over 1 minute to spatially encode a whole brain. By using rf pulses at angles lower than the usual 90° to the static field (fast low-angle shot, FLASH), imaging time can be reduced to less than a second per slice. Recent technical advances allow for a further reduction in scanning time to about 50 ms by encoding a slice after only one rf signal (echo-planar imaging, EPI). FLASH and EPI are thus good candidates for the study of brain functions in the 100 ms to 1 second range, such as the performance of cognitive tasks.

The magnetic properties of intravascular contrast media can be exploited to track blood flow and volume during different functional states of the brain. Paramagnetic substances create magnetic field gradients around blood vessels which interfere with the MRI signal (T_2^*). The resulting change in image contrast is proportional to the concentration of the contrast agent and can therefore be used to compute regional blood volume (for a more detailed description, see Cohen & Bookheimer 1994, Turner & Jezzard 1994, Le Bihan & Karni 1995). Both perfusion and blood volume are known to change in a region-specific way with activation tasks. As paramagnetic contrast agents exogenous substances can be used, such as gadolinium diethylenetriaminepentaacetic acid (Gd-DTPA) (Table 16.2). Gd-DTPA has been used for some time as an intravascular MRI contrast agent that does not cross the blood–brain barrier, similar to iodinated contrast agents in CT. It is thus able to delineate areas of breakdown in the blood–brain barrier. Perfusion imaging with Gd-DTPA requires a new injection for each new study, after waiting for the elimination of any previously inject-

Table 16.1	Nuclei commonly used in MRS
Nucleus	Biologically significant molecules
^{13}C	[^{13}C]-glucose and other labels
^{19}F	^{19}F-labelled drugs, [^{19}F]-deoxyglucose
^{1}H	Glutamate, lactate, N-acetylaspartate, choline, creatinine
^{7}Li	For in vivo lithium measurement in the brain
^{23}Na	Intra- and extracellualr Na
^{31}P	Energy metabolism: ATP/ADP, membrane metabolism: phosphomono/diester, phosphocreatinine

Table 16.2	Methods of fMRI		
Method change	MRI/Functional measure	Signal during visual activation
Gd-DTPA injection	T_2*/blood volume, venous > arterial	40–50%
BOLD	T_2*/perfusion, venous > arterial	2–3% (1.5 tesla) 15% (4 tesla)
Arterial spin tagging, EPISTAR	T_1/perfusion, arterial > venous	1–2%[a]
Combination of flow sensitive and insensitive sequences	T_1/perfusion, arterial > venous	Not known
[a]Kwong et al (1992).			

ed Gd-DTPA. This limits repeatability and increases the potential toxicity of the contrast agent. More conveniently, endogenous protons can be magnetically tagged in arteries upstream to (Turner & Jezzard 1994) or even inside (Ye et al 1996) the imaging plane to measure blood flow. This former inflow method has two disadvantages. First, tagged protons relax magnetically over the unknown distance travelled in arteries from the tagging to the imaging plane. This introduces measurement error. Second, magnetisation transfer can cause image artefacts.

The most commonly used fMRI method is based on the observation that functional activation results in an increase in cerebral cortical blood flow that is in excess of oxygen extraction. The result is a local and temporary increase in oxyhaemoglobin. The differences in the magnetic properties of oxy- and deoxyhaemoglobin can be used to compute images of regional functional activation patterns (blood oxygen level dependent, BOLD). Deoxyhaemoglobin is more paramagnetic than oxyhaemoglobin, and therefore acts like Gd-DTPA as an intravascular paramagnetic contrast agent. In fact, changes in T_2* are proportional to changes in blood oxygenation (Turner & Jezzard 1994).

The first clinical studies using fMRI methods are now appearing in the medical literature, and some knowledge of possible methodological issues is neccessary to appreciate their significance and validity. Head movement, both during scan acquisition and in-between repeated scans, can be a problem. Sophisticated methods of realignment are essential for spatially accurate mapping of effects. The magnitude of the activation effect (signal to noise) is usually related to magnetic susceptibility and increases with the strength of the static magnetic field (Table 16.2). Most published studies report results acquired with field strengths of 1.5 tesla and above. The relative contribution of blood arterial oxygenation, blood volume, blood flow, haematocrit,

tissue oxygen uptake and perhaps blood flow velocity has not yet been established, although blood flow appears to dominate (Turner & Jezzard 1994). While the BOLD signal mainly comes from the venous system, it is not yet clear which level of the vascular tree contributes most to the signal. There are suggestions that spin–echo sequences are better able to extract the signal from the proximity of smaller vessels, because the image is mainly affected by diffusion – an effect that is greatest if the diffusion distance is relatively large compared with vessel size (Cohen & Bookheimer 1994).

Structual MRI: use in psychiatry

Structural MRI has gained widespread clinical acceptance, partially replacing X-ray CT for a number of reasons (Table 16.3). MRI is optimal in detecting structural variations. Fortunately, and partially by definition, psychiatric disorders are not usually associated with gross structural changes. On the other hand, cerebral atrophy occurs in a proportion of the elderly, which makes it a rather non-specific finding. In Alzheimer's disease and amnesia, temporal lobe structures are more likely to show sepcific tissue loss, related to memory impairment, as already suggested by CT (De Leon et al 1989, Press et al l989, Scheltens et al 1992). Reductions in temporal lobe volume have been reported for patients with schizophrenia in the majority of studies (see Ebmeier 1995, for a review). Moreover, a novel more sensitive and objective voxel-based method of image analysis (see below) has suggested an

Table 16.3	Comparing MRI with X-ray CT	
	MRI	X-ray CT
Bone signal	Virtually absent, marrow visible	Strongest signal
Soft-tissue contrast	100–200%	1–10%
Repeated examination	Not limited	Limited by radiation dose
Resolution	< 1 mm	> 1 mm
Posterior fossa	Well visualised	Partially obscured
Plane of acquisition	Any orientation	Positioning plane

association between reality distortion, i.e. delusions and hallucinations, and left superior temporal lobe grey matter density (Wright et al 1995). Temporal lobe changes have also been described in conditions associated with high stress (and cortisol) levels, such as depression and post-traumatic stress disorder (Axelson et al 1993, Bremner et al 1995), but the evidence for any causal connection is not conclusive. Similarly, frontal abnormalities, which were originally found during functional imaging and suggested by neuropsychological examination, have been described for MRI in schizophrenia and depression, but so far with limited evidence (Andreasen et al 1990, Coffey et al 1993, Soares & Mann 1997).

The high soft-tissue contrast achievable with MRI has made it the ideal instrument for investigating vascular changes, such as strokes and white matter hyperintensities. Both types of changes can be found in vascular dementia. White matter hyperintensities are also observed in Alzheimer's disease (Ebmeier et al 1987), in depression, particularly if late in onset (O'Brien et al 1996), and in old age, where they appear to be associated with impairment of more complex mental processing and disruption of EEG coherence between different cortical regions (Schmidt et al 1993, Leuchter et al 1994).

MRS: use in psychiatry

The clinical application of MRS in psychiatry is still very much in the experimental stage. In schizophrenia, frontal decreases in phosphomonoesters and increases in phosphodiesters have been reported repeatedly, a finding that is interpreted as evidence of membrane catabolism, or frontal pruning in adolescence (recently reviewed in Ebmeier 1995). Some studies have also

implicated the temporal lobes (Maier et al 1995, Fukuzako et al 1996, Maier & Ron 1996, Yurgelun-Todd et al 1996a). Whereas most studies have so far been limited to the examination of a single brain region, introducing a certain bias towards the regions examined, multislice whole brain MRS has recently confirmed the limitation of abnormalities to frontal and temporal brain areas (Bertolino et al 1996). Research in affective disorder has been lagging behind to some extent, but there is now evidence for abnormalities in high-energy phosphate metabolism and membrane breakdown in the basal ganglia (Kato et al 1996, Moore et al 1997). Lithium-MRS has been used to monitor brain lithium levels as a validation for 12 hour serum estimates (Jensen et al 1996). Finally, respiratory alkalosis during panic hyperventilation can be demonstrated in the brain using ^{31}P-MRS (Shiori et al 1996).

Functional MRI: use in psychiatry

Presently, the main research interest in the field of fMRI lies in the analysis of normal cognitive processes. However, some studies have been conducted in psychiatric patients. The logistics of scanning still require a high level of cooperation in subjects, so that a selection bias towards less disturbed patients is likely. Nevertheless, abnormalities during motor (Wenz et al 1994, Schroder et al 1995), visual (Renshaw et al 1994) and psychological (Yurgelun-Todd et al 1996b) activation procedures have been reported in schizophrenic patients. Emotionally laden stimuli, i.e. pictures of faces expressing a certain affect, appear to affect bilateral amygdala activity in a transient manner (Grodd et al 1995, Breiter et al 1996a). Finally, replicating studies with other imaging modalities (see below), activation in medial orbitofrontal, lateral frontal, anterior temporal, anterior cingulate and insular cortex, as well as caudate, lenticulate and amygdala, was observed in patients with obsessive–compulsive disorder during a specfic anxiety-provoking condition (Breiter et al 1996b).

POSITRON AND SINGLE PHOTON EMISSION TOMOGRAPHY

Just as three-dimensional brain images can be computed from transmission scans, as in X-ray CT, such images can be derived from γ rays that are emitted by isotopes inside the brain. Two different principles are used to localise the source of radiation. Single photon emission computerised tomography (SPECT) uses collimators, i.e. filters that are placed in front of the photon detectors and only let single photons arriving from a certain direction pass. Collimators absorb all other

Table 16.4   Comparing PET with SPECT

	PET	SPECT
Radiation energy	High (511 keV)	Lower (75–160 keV)
Radiation half-life	Short (^{15}O, 2 min; ^{11}C, 20 min; ^{18}F, 110 min)	Intermediate (^{99m}Tc, 6 h; ^{123}I, 13 h)
Scan sensitivity	High (< nanogram)	Lower (> nanogram)
Running cost	High (cyclotron, radiochemist)	Low (hospital radiopharmacy)
Quantifiable	Yes	Not all tracers
Repeatable	Up to 12 times in the same session	Up to twice in the same session
Scattered photons	Do not produce coincidence events	Have to be removed wth an energy filter
Attenuation correction	Empirical after transmission scan	A priori, based on homogenous model of the brain
Maximum resolution	Limited by distance between positron emitter and annihilation with electron	Limited by Compton scatter and collimator performance

radiation, thus focusing the 'view' of the detector. The principle of positron emission tomography (PET) is that an emitted positron reacts with an electron within a few millimetres of its place of origin. This reaction generates two photons with a well-defined enegry (511 keV) which move away in opposite directions. If two detectors within a detector ring are able to identify such 'coincident' photons, their source of origin must be on a straight line between those two detectors. Thus multiple emission events during SPECT and PET can be used to compute a density map of the radioactive tracer in different parts of the brain. Many differences between SPECT and PET come from the shorter half-lives of positron emitters that make the production of tracer near the scanner a necessity (Table 16.4). Other differences derive from the physical principles for localising the sources of radiation. During collimation much of the activity emitted is absorbed and is lost as information that could be used for the construction of the final image. This reduces the sensitivity of SPECT in comparison with PET. Compton scatter of photons in SPECT results in a reduction of photon energy and a change of direction of flight. If the filtering of lower energy photons is incomplete, a blurring of the image results, and spatial resolution is reduced. Compton scatter during a PET scan results in the loss of a coincidence signal, the single photon is ignored and does not add noise to the image. The likelihood of scatter or absorption increases with the distance of the tracer molecule from the detector (attenuation). Attenuation correction in SPECT is usually carried out mathematically, assuming a homogenous attenuation within an ellipsoid

brain. In PET, transmission scans are usually carried out before the emission scan, in which an external radiation source is used like an X-ray tube to produce an image of the electron density of the brain. Attenuation can therefore be corrected empirically. This increases the accuracy of local activity estimates.

γ Emitters, such as ^{123}I (iodine) and ^{99m}Tc (technetium), or positron emitters, such as ^{11}C (carbon), ^{15}O (oxygen) or ^{18}F (fluorine), can be incorporated into tracer molecules that distribute across the brain in a biologically significant way. Tracers may be distributed with regional cerebral blood flow, such as [^{15}O]-H_2O, [^{11}C]-butamol, [^{18}F]-fluoromethane, ^{133}Xe, [^{123}I]-IMP, [^{99m}Tc]-HMPAO or [^{99m}Tc]-L, L-ECD. Others distribute in proportion with regional glucose uptake into brain cells ([^{18}F]-deoxyglucose, [^{11}C]-glucose), or are taken up as precursors of neurotransmitters ([^{18}F]-DOPA), and as specific receptor ligands ([^{123}I]-iodobenzamide, [^{123}I]-iomazenil, [^{123}I]-β-CIT, [^{11}C]-ketanserin, [^{11}C]-raclopride, [^{11}C]-methyl-spiperone, [^{11}C]-deprenyl, [^{18}F]-flumazenil).

Imaging brain function

Brain cells rely on glucose as their substrate for energy metabolism. At rest, 40% of the energy requirement is due to axonal transport, synthesis of macromolecules, etc., a further 30% to synaptic transmission, and 30% to other ion flux and transport (Astrup et al 1981). During functional activation (and inhibition), most additional energy requirements are due to the restitution of ion gradients across depolarised synaptic membranes in neuropil (Herscovitch 1994). Glucose is metabolised both aerobically to CO_2 and anaerobically to pyruvate. Glucose uptake into both pathways can be measured with [18F]-deoxyglucose (FDG), which shows greater local activation effects than aerobic glucose metabolism measured with [11C]-glucose. Deoxyglucose (DG) is taken up into neurones, phosphorylated to DG-6-phosphate in the hexokinase reaction and trapped, because the further metabolic path usually followed by glucose is blocked. Sokoloff et al (1977) have proposed a three-compartment model to compute glucose uptake from:

- Plasma glucose concentration
- Plasma [14C]-DG activity
- [14C]-DG activity determined by autoradiography in rat brain 45 minutes after tracer injection
- [14C]-DG uptake into tissue up to this time
- The so-called 'lumped constant' which accounts for the difference in transport across the blood–brain barrier and phosphorylation between glucose and DG (Herscovitch 1994).

Because of the longer image acquisition process in PET compared with autoradiography, dephosphorylation may play a more important role, so that Sokoloff's model has to be augmented by an appropriate term for the dissociation of DG-6-phosphate. To quantify glucose uptake using FDG, a series of arterial blood samples or arterialised venous blood (hand heated to over 40°) are required in addition to the brain image acquired 30 minutes after injection. Because of the integration of brain activity over a long time, FDG is suitable for resting diagnostic examinations, but not particularly useful for functional activation studies. Very few physiological or psychological activation procedures can be sustained over this time without habituation or fluctuation in performance levels.

Regional cerebral blood flow (rCBF) responds to local requirements for substrate, so that under most conditions it follows the distribution of FDG (Fox et al 1988). Importantly, oxygen uptake measured with $^{15}O_2$-PET does not change substantially during sensory activation (5%, Fox & Raichle 1986, Fox et al 1988) and is, therefore, not a useful tracer for functional neuroimaging. The most commonly used PET tracer for the measurement of rCBF is ^{15}O-labelled water given as a bolus or infusion. An alternative tracer is $C^{15}O_2$, which is inhaled by the subject, catalysed by carbonic anhydrase to $H_2^{15}O$ in the lung and distributed throughout the body. A number of quantitative models have been employed to measure rCBF. The steady-state model has been used extensively in the past. It is suitable for scanners that operate best at low radioactive count levels and requires the inhalation of $C^{15}O_2$ over

10 minutes until blood radioactivity levels become constant. Its disadvantage is the non-linear relationship between measured and real rCBF at higher flow levels, which increases the measurement error in the higher rCBF range. The PET/autoradiographic method, which is used by most contemporary research, requires PET scanners capable of operating at higher radioactivity count rates after a bolus injection of $H_2^{15}O$. It integrates brain activity over time and requires the serial measurement of radioactivity in the arterial system (input curve). Variable time delays between activity in peripheral arteries and brain activity are a source of error, and limited diffusibility of water into brain tissue results in an underestimation of rCBF (Herscovitch 1994). Alternative tracers that provide more accurate rCBF estimates are available ([11C]-butamol, [18F]-fluoromethane), but have not found widespread use.

^{133}Xe is an inert gas that can be inhaled or injected and quickly distributes through brain tissues. On removing the supply of ^{133}Xe, the tracer is washed out from the brain in proportion to rCBF. Successive modifications of the technique and the underlying quantitation models have allowed for a reduction of inhalation time from 5–10 minutes to 1–2 minutes and the recording of the tracer clearance from 20–40 minutes to 2.5 minutes. Unfortunately, the low energy radiation of ^{133}Xe results in significant absorption and attenuation. It has been estimated that almost half of 'white matter' counts come from scattered grey matter photons, thus seriously limiting the information to be gleaned from ^{133}Xe scans about central brain areas (Sharp 1994). For this reason, ^{133}Xe has been limited to a few centres, mainly interested in functional cortical activation, often in an experimental context. For clinical brain SPECT, ^{123}I-labelled N-isopropyl-p-iodoamphetamine (IMP, Spectamine®) [99mTc]-d,l-hexamethylpropyleneamine oxim (HMPAO, exametazime, Ceretec™) and [99mTc]-ethylcysteinate dimer (L,L-ECD, bicisate, Neurolite™) are routinely used (Fig. 16.3). IMP is nearly completely extracted on first pass through the brain after intravenous injection and trapped, possibly due to pH shifts, amine metabolism and non-specific binding to amine binding sites (Morgan & Costa 1993). After 5 minutes, the brain distribution remains stable for about 1 hour and resembles closely the rCBF pattern at the time of injection. After this, washout from different brain regions starts to vary, so that the later activity patterns differ from perfusion images. The other disadvantage of IMP relates to the labelling with ^{123}I, a process that is only possible at certain specialised centres and which makes the production and distribution of the tracer relatively costly. Newer lipophilic tracers can be labelled with ^{99m}Tc, an isotope readily available from most radiopharmacies.

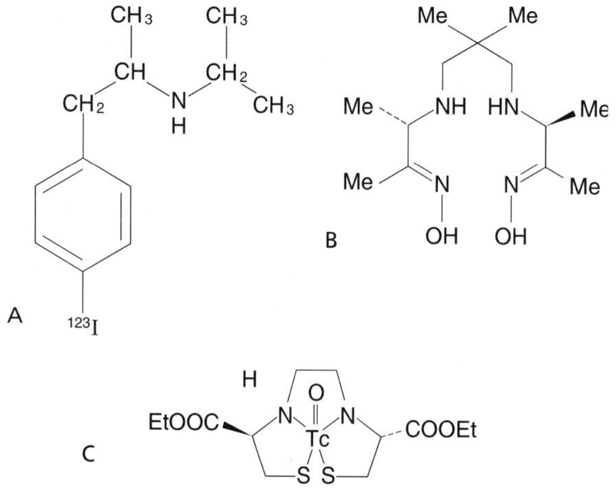

Fig. 16.3 **A** N-isopropyl-p-iodoamphetamine (IMP, Spectamine®), **B** d,l-hexamethylpropyleneamine oxim (HMPAO, exametazime, Ceretec™) and **C** ethylcysteinate dimer (L,L-ECD, bicisate, Neurolite™) – perfusion tracers for SPECT.

[^{99m}Tc]-HMPAO is retained in brain cells after conversion to a hydrophilic form, possibly by glutathione (Jalinous et al 1985), or, as recently published, depending on the redox equilibrium of the cell (Jacquier-Sarlin et al 1996b). [^{99m}Tc]-ECD is trapped in the brain depending on cytosolic esterase activity (Jacquier-Sarlin et al 1996a). After intravenous injection of HMPAO and ECD, both tracers are taken up on first pass through the brain, without noticeable redistribution over time. There is some evidence that the uptake may differ between HMPAO and ECD. The contrast between brain and soft tissues, between grey and white matter (Leveille et al 1992) and between Alzheimer disease lesions and normal tissue (van Dyck et al 1996) may be higher for ECD. Its rapid blood clearance gives a better dosimetry (Holman et al 1989, Leveille et al 1989).

Several tracers can thus be used to map functional activity in the brain. The main practical differences between these tracers relate to their resolution in space and time and to logistic issues of scan acquisition and compliance, particularly in psychiatric patients (Table 16.5).

PET and SPECT: use in psychiatry

If a theme from the functional imaging literature has gained general currency, it is the so called hypofrontality of schizophrenia. Since the original description by Ingvar and Franzen (1974) it has been found mainly in chronically ill, medicated patients, some of whom show poor performance on suspected frontal lobe performance tests (reviewed in Ebmeier 1995). There is some agreement that neuroleptic medication reduces frontal cortex and increases basal ganglia metabolism (Wiesel 1992). Investigations in unmedicated actively psychotic patients have, therefore, rather shown increases in lateral prefrontal cortex, sometimes associated with medial frontal (anterior cingulate) reduction in activity (Wiesel et al 1987, Ebmeier et al 1993). An important factor affecting brain activity patterns in patients is the task performed during tracer uptake. Most studies employing tasks have shown 'activation hypofrontality', which is associated with poor performance of the task by the patients. This finding is not surprising and teaches us more about the localisation of brain structures recruited during the task than about schizophrenia per se. Resting studies, particularly in patients whose 'mental set' is determined by continuous psychotic experiences, may be more suitable for picking up some of the variability related to mental state, and may therefore be useful in 'localising' the anatomy underlying psychiatric syndromes (Liddle et al 1992, Ebmeier et al 1993). More recently, studies have followed up this theme by examining the functional anatomy of hallucinations and other psychotic phenomena in repeat measures designs, relying on patients' self-reporting of symptoms (McGuire et al 1995, David et al 1996). In summary, the notion of hypofrontality in schizophrenia is much more differentiated today, requiring the consideration of medication state, cognitive demand and present symptom pattern. In accordance with MRI findings, some PET and SPECT studies have found temporal lobe abnormalities (see Ebmeier 1995).

Table 16.5	Comparing tracers used in PET and SPECT		
Functional tracer	Time window (min)	Resolution (mm)	Scan acquisition
Xenon SPECT	>2.5	>10	During tracer washout
IMP/HMPAO/ECD SPECT	1–2	>7	Hours after tracer injection
H$_2$O PET	1–2	>4	During tracer injection
FDG PET	30	>3	30 minutes after tracer injection

Depression is the reversible psychiatric illness par excellence. It should, therefore, be expected that most abnormalities discovered during the illness will normalise on recovery. A general consensus appears to be emerging that frontal portions of the brain, including anterior temporal lobes, and basal ganglia are underactive during the depressive episode (Goodwin 1996, Ketter et al 1996). This may exclude medial frontal structures, which in some studies appear to be activated in proportion with biological symptom severity (Austin et al 1992, Ebmeier et al 1997). While medial limbic structures, including the basal ganglia appear to normalise on recovery, dorsolateral prefrontal cortex may continue to show reduced activity in some patients (Goodwin et al 1993, Bench et al 1995, Bonne et al 1996). In repeat measures studies that examine the same patients within a short period during more or less depressed mood states, there appears to be an increased activity in orbitofrontal and limbic cortex during the more depressed state (reviewed in Ebert & Ebmeier 1996).

A consistent finding in obsessional disorder is symptom-related orbitofrontal and paralimbic overactivity that normalises as symptoms are alleviated (Lucey et al 1995, Baxter et al 1996, Cottraux et al 1996). Results are sufficiently consistent to allow first attempts at hypotheses about the neural circuits involved in obsessional symptoms. Changes in cortico-striatal-thalamic circuits with disinhibition of a loop including the orbitofrontal cortex have been suggested (cf. Ch. 17). Global brain metabolism appears to rise initially with increasing anxiety, but decreases if anxiety passes a certain intensity. It thus provides an explanation for the Yerkes–Dodson law linking anxiety and performance, which posits an inverted U-shaped relationship between the two (Gur et al 1987). Regional brain activity in anxiety and post-traumatic stress disorders regularly appears to involve sensory association cortex, probably related to anxious imagery (O'Carroll et al 1993, Fredrikson et al 1995, Rauch et al 1995, Fischer et al 1996, Wik et al 1996). Patients with anorexia nervosa show reduced metabolism, mainly in frontal and parietal cortex, that may be associated with cerebral atrophy (Delvenne et al 1995, Herholz 1996).

SPECT or PET are considered a useful adjunct to the differential diagnosis of Alzheimer's disease which is characterised by a regional reduction of blood flow in parietotemporal cortex (Altrocchi et al 1996). Such a perfusion pattern is thought to be of diagnostic value (Claus et al 1994), differentiating Alzheimer's disease from other conditions with a similar presentation, such as major depression (Upadhyaya 1990, Curran 1993, Sackeim et al 1993). Vascular dementia is often characterised on MRI only by non-specific white matter changes. Focal cortical hypoperfusion helps to confirm the diagnosis (Loeb 1995). The correlation of clinical SPECT diagnosis with postmortem findings can be impressive (92%), compared with clinical diagnosis (74.1%), when comparing Alzheimer's disease with non-Alzheimer dementias (Read et al 1995). However, SPECT does not distinguish between dementia in Parkinson's disease and Alzheimer's disease. The sensitivity of perfusion imaging to the detection early Alzheimer's disease and the specificity for the differential diagnosis with vascular dementia may be limited, so that some authors have questioned the usefulness of SPECT in this context (Mielke et al 1994, Van Gool et al 1995, Bergman et al 1997). Reduced hippocampal perfusion imaged with high-resolution SPECT appears to be a good marker for organic memory impairment, independent of the aetiology (Ohnishi et al 1995).

In vivo binding studies

Autoradiographic studies have greatly enhanced our knowledge of the topography of receptors in the brain, but postmortem studies in animals and humans have only limited relevance to brain changes associated with the aetiology of mental illness. In particular, treatment-free or naive patients hardly ever come to autopsy now, so that changes observed post mortem may be secondary to previous medication. Fortunately, the sensitivity and spatial resolution of PET and SPECT allow for the measurement and localisation of neurotransmitter receptors in vivo. Table 16.6 gives a summary of some of the ligands used in receptor imaging.

Table 16.6	Some ligands used in receptor imaging
Ligand	**Receptor site**
[^{123}I]iomazenil	Benzodiazepine receptor
[^{123}I]IBZM	Dopamine D2/3 receptor
[^{123}I]B-CIT	Serotonin and dopamine transporter
[^{123}I]QNB	Muscarinic receptor
[^{18}F]flumazenil	Benzodiazepine receptor
[^{11}C]SCH23390/39166	Dopamine D1/5 receptor
[^{11}C]raclopride	Dopamine D2/3 receptor
[^{11}C]N-methyl-spiperone	Dopamine D2/3/4 receptor
[^{11}C]nomifensine	Dopamine transporter
[^{11}C]ketanserin	5-HT$_2$ receptor
[^{11}C]nicotine	Nicotinic receptor
[^{11}C]scopolamine	Muscarinic receptor
[^{11}C]deprenyl	Monoaminoxidase B
[^{18}F]6-fluorodopa	Presynaptic dopamine terminal

In receptor ligands, carbon atoms can be replaced by ^{11}C without changing the pharmacological properties of the original compound. The larger ^{123}I iodine atom used to label SPECT ligands is more likely to change the binding properties of the drug, so that development of SPECT ligands has been slower than that of PET ligands. Central to the function of a good radioligand is its high binding affinity to the target receptor. Initial radioligand distribution is somewhat determined by regional ligand delivery, that is rCBF. Regional washout is inversely related to receptor binding affinity, it is fastest in regions with much non-specific binding and few receptors. Insufficient binding affinity of the radioligand to the receptor in question results in small specific to non-specific binding ratios, i.e. low signal to noise ratio. High affinity allows us to use tracer doses of the ligand (<0.001 mg), which have no pharmacological effect and entail exposure to only small amounts of radioactive label. Drug binding at therapeutic doses can still be examined by displacing labelled tracer with the cold drug. These methods have been employed extensively in the evaluation of antipsychotic drugs (Farde 1996). While the examination of drug-naive schizophrenic patients with [^{11}C]-raclopride has been disappointing, showing no relative increases, the tracer has been successfully used to determine receptor occupancy with cold antipsychotic drugs required for therapeutic dose levels (70–80%) and doses causing extrapyramidal side effects (>80%). Similary, [^{11}C]-SCH39166, a selective D_1 receptor antagonist, was used to demonstrate uptake into the brain and adequate receptor occupancy in treated patients, who nevertheless did not show any symptomatic response to D_1 blockade. A more positive example of the potential of PET to predict pharmacological characteristics is the 5-hydroxytryptamine (5-HT_{2A}) binding of clozapine, that is very similar to that of risperidone, and may provide a paradigm for the identification of further antipsychotics with a similar activity profile on negative symptoms of schizophrenia (Farde 1996). While PET ligands are easier to generate than SPECT ligands, occasionally the addition of ^{123}I to the original drug molecule increases its receptor binding affinity, as in the case of iomazenil, which has an affinity an order of magnitude greater than its PET equivalent flumazenil (Johnson et al 1990).

Receptor imaging in depressed patients with the D1/2 receptor ligand [132]I-iodobenzamide (IBZM), suggests that dopaminergic transmission is reduced in depression, possibly in proportion to psychomotor retardation (D'haenen & Bossuyt 1994, Shah et al 1997). In Giles de la Tourette syndrome, first results suggest a reduction in dopamine reuptake sites (Malison et al 1995), but postsynaptic receptor numbers seem to be normal in unmedicated patients (George et al 1994, Turjanski et al 1994).

Methods of quantitative scan analysis

In clinical practice, images are interpreted by an experienced examiner, who evaluates the patient scan, based on personal experience and textbook examples of known abnormalities. Most often abnormalities can be described as 'lesions', i.e. discontinuities in the scan appearance. 'Functional' psychiatric illness is characterised and defined by the absence of gross brain lesions, so the clinical assessment of images will not be sensitive enough to describe abnormalities. Quantitative methods of assessment are necessary. One such method is called the region of interest (ROI) method, because the examiner places regions over the scan in order to measure the average image intensity within this region. It is important that the regions are fitted in a reliable manner, best as an ensemble, so that results are as replicable and as unbiased as possible. The ROI method is best suited to situations where a clear hypothesis exists as to the location of the expected activation or the group effect. Effects that are small in spatial extent, as compared with the ROI, or effects that straddle several ROIs can easily go undetected. During ROI analysis different brains are compared by fitting templates in shape and size, so that ROI measures refer to equivalent brain areas. As an alternative, the brain images themselves can be transformed in shape and size until they fit into a standard coordinate space (Friston et al 1995a). Such a spatial transformation brings equivalent portions of different brains into the same co-ordinate space, so that images can be compared point by point (pixel by pixel, or voxel by voxel). Usually images are processed further to remove unnecessary noise. Images are filtered until variability in gyral anatomy disappears, and the effect of global activity, which is often of little relevance, is removed statistically (Friston et al 1995b). The probability of generating significant results by chance increases with the number of statistical tests, so that after 100 tests five results are expected by chance with a $P<0.05$. A voxel-based analysis clearly has to make allowances for this. From initial rather simple methods using χ^2 tests for the number of actually computed and expected significant results, statistical parametric mapping (SPM) has graduated to relatively complex statistical procedures taking into account the overall volume examined, the smoothness of the data, the peak effects and the volume of the brain showing a group or activation effect (Friston et al 1994). The result of this procedure is a statistical parametric map, which is a three-dimensional representation of the brain areas with significant effects (Fig. 16.4). This method

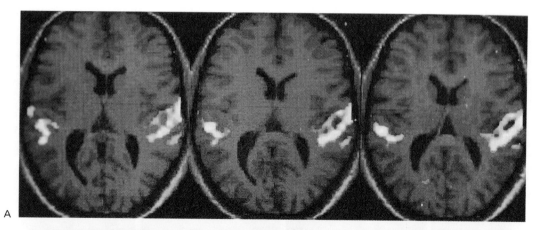

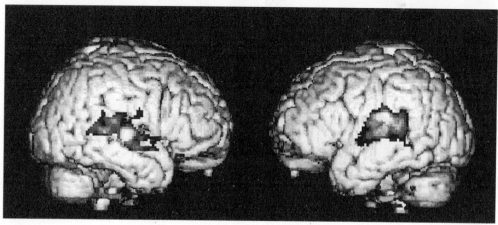

Fig. 16.4 Statistical parametric map based on auditory activation during functional MRI. **A** Transverse slices; **B** projection on to brain surface. (Courtesy of Dr G. Rees and Professor C. Frith, Wellcome Department of Cognitive Neurology, London.)

has a number of advantages over ROI methods. It is objective, because the spatial transformation and statistical analysis of images is fully automated. This makes the procedure much faster and less dependent on the employment and potential bias of skilled raters. SPM-based methods can be used without a prior hypothesis, because activation or group effects are displayed where they occur, disregarding any anatomical or preconceived boundary. It is ideal for examining the interaction between different brain regions, a phenomenon that can be expected as the result of distributed neural networks underlying brain functions. SPM can be applied to PET (Liddle et al 1992), SPECT (Ebmeier et al 1997) and functional MRI. It has also been used to analyse structural MRI, where, after segmentation of images into grey and white matter, a regional reduction of compartmental matter density can be determined (Wright et al 1995). Functional images usually have a poorer resolution than MRI. In order to identify

anatomical landmarks more accurately, whether for ROI analysis or spatial transformation, functional images are often coregistered, i.e. superimposed, with the corresponding structural scan (Fig. 16.5).

EEG AND MEG MAPPING

It is possible to record the intrinsic electrical activity of the brain by electrodes on its surface during neurosurgery or by needle electrodes, such as sphenoidal electrodes which are inserted into the vicinity of the brain structure of interest. More commonly, however, brain electrical and magnetic activity is recorded from the surface of the scalp. The psychiatrist and EEG pioneer Hans Berger realised very early that cognitive activity was reflected in fluctuations of EEG activity, for example in the α frequency band (Gevins et al 1995). But before topographical information about the

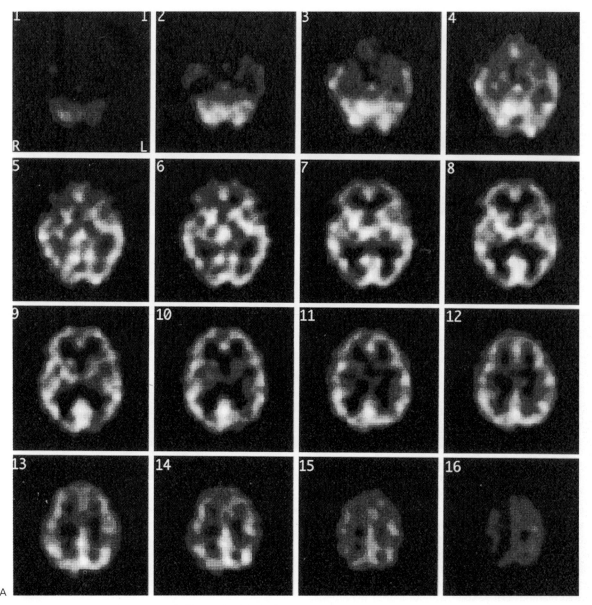

Fig. 16.5 In order to identify anatomical landmarks more accurately, whether for ROI analysis or spatial transformation, functional images (in this example SPECT, **A** are often coregistered, i.e. superimposed, with the corresponding structural scan (MRI, **B**).

'responsible' EEG generators could become available, more technical and theoretical developments had to take place. The traditional array of 19 EEG channels results in an interelectrode distance of approximately 6 cm, a distance sufficient for clinical neurological use to assess gross brain abnormality, but inadequate for the more refined study of cognitive brain function (Gevins et al 1995). Only with 100 or more electrodes does the distance between detectors approach the theoretical limit of resolution on the scalp (2.5 cm), which is given by the spread of the electromagnetic field between a point source on the cortex and the scalp. The choice of the reference in EEG (an electrical potential has to be measured between two electrodes!) is crucial and can systematically affect regional results. An improvement on using a linked-ear, a nose, or a body

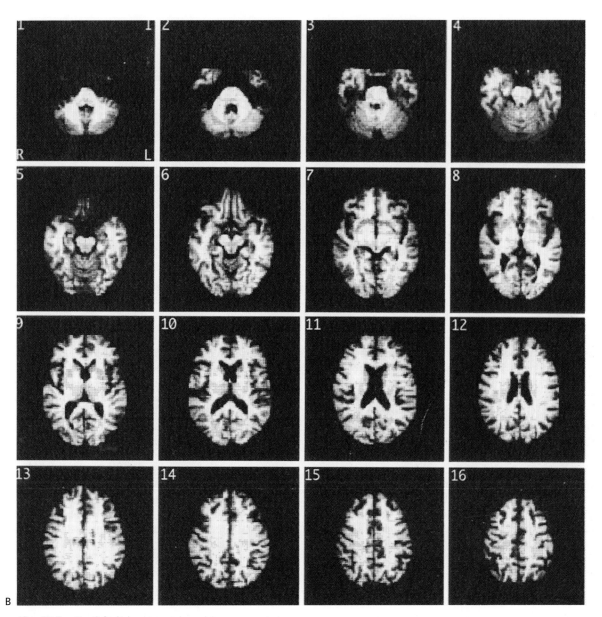

Fig. 16.5 *Cont'd*

reference which can be contaminated by regional neural or muscular potentials, is to compare each electrode with its adjacent partners. The second spatial derivative of the potential at each electrode site is called the Laplacian derivation. It reduces the impact of signals common to the local group of electrodes, and enhances the local cortical potential over the target electrode, thus increasing signal to noise ratio. If the actual distances and spatial orientations between electrodes are measured and taken into account, a more sophisticated

Laplacian derivation based on three-dimensional spline functions can further enhance the spatial resoluton of the EEG map (Gevins et al 1995). From scalp and skull thickness at each electrode site, measured on MRI scans, local conductivity can be estimated. This 'finite element deblurring' is a further method of sharpening the electrical potential map measured on the scalp surface. In contrast to electric fields which are affected by the conductivity of the soft tissues of the skull and the scalp, the spread of magnetic fields is unimpaired – the

Table 16.7 Comparing EEG with MEG

	EEG	MEG
Principle	Electrical potential difference between two surface electrodes	Reference free magnetic field at a single location
Instrumentation	Conventional electrodes	Superconducting quantum interference devices (SQUIDs)
Electrostatic shielding required	Minimal	Important
Multiple detector array (*n*>100)	Routine	Recent development
Effect of soft tissue	Affected by skull/scalp conductivity	None
Optimal orientation of dipole source	Perpendicular to surface	Tangential to surface
Head immobilised	No	Yes
Cost	Relatively small	Expensive

Partially adapted from Wikswo et al (1993).

tissues overlying the cortex are magnetically transparent. The development of so-called superconducting quantum interference devices (SQUIDs) in the 1980s made it possible to record the tiny magnetic fields generated by neurones. Some fundamental differences between EEG and MEG are listed in Table 16.7.

While the methodological improvements described above have enhanced the spatial resolution of EEG-based methods to match those available from MEG (Wikswo et al 1993), both techniques suffer from their inability to locate the source of electromagnetic activity in three-dimensional space. The so-called inverse problem, i.e. the derivation of underlying spatial dipoles which generate the observable surface maps, is mathematically ill conditioned: any of a large number of dipoles or dipole combination can account for the observed EEG/MEG map, so that external restrictions have to be imposed in order to decide which dipole model is correct. These restrictions can come from a prior knowledge of the localisation of relevant neural structures, from other functional imaging techniques, such as PET, SPECT or fMRI, or they may just be imposed by the desire for the most parsimonious explanation. But is the simple assumption true that surface activity derives from one, or at least a small number of, neural generators? We know that for simple sensory function this may be correct, but more complex cognitive processes are probably associated with the activation of connected and distributed neural networks, so that parsimony may not be the best guide. EEG and MEG maps are acquired over time, so that neural connectivity can be examined by relating the time courses

of activities over different regions to each other using statistical techniques, such as spectral coherence, correlation, covariance or different methods of statistical regression (Gevins et al 1995). Apart from analysing the EEG/MEG over a given time epoch with the subject at rest or performing a task, it is also possible to time lock a series of measurements, either in relation to a sensory stimulus or a motor response, thus generating phasic-evoked or event-related potentials. Such an association between specific, experimentally determined behaviour and brain events can help further to localise brain function in the space and time domains. Gevins et al (1995) give a number of examples for employing sophisticated EEG mapping techniques to spatial and verbal memory tasks and the interested reader is advised to consult this paper. Already, simple lateralising examinations of EEG frequency spectra have suggested that left frontal activation (α reduction) is associated with positive affect, right activation with negative affect (Ahern & Schwartz 1985, Davidson 1992, Fox et al 1992). The combination of EEG/MEG with a tomographic functional imaging technique (such as PET or SPECT) in a clinical context (Szelies et al 1994) is just beginning and promises to combine high quality information in the time and space domains (cf. Fig. 16.6).

TRANSCRANIAL MAGNETIC STIMULATION

Just as skull and scalp are 'transparent' to SQUIDs

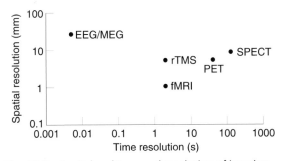

Fig. 16.6 Spatial and temporal resolution of imaging methods.

recording cortical electromagnetic activity, they also do not impede the transcranial application of magnetic fields from the outside to the brain. The principle of TMS is the rapid discharge of electricity through a coil that is placed over the head of the subject. The changing electric field in the coil is associated with a magnetic field. This magnetic field penetrates to the cortex underlying the coil and induces electric currents in nerve cells, which lead to functional activation (Barker 1985). TMS has been used since the mid-1980s to examine motor and sensory cortex function. For example, central conduction time can be computed by comparing the time from TMS of the motor strip to motor response with the motor conduction time from the cervical plexus (again stimulated magnetically). TMS is able to map cortical function with a resolution of a few millimetres. Not only can the optimal stimulation site for a specific motor response be localised, but plasticity during learning and exercise can be determined, both in terms of a change in shape and size of the cortical field involved and the magnitude of the evoked response (Pascual-Leone et al 1994, Samii et al 1996). An important difference of TMS to the previous imaging methods, which at best document an association between brain and behaviour, is that TMS, if properly controlled experimentally, actually demonstrates a causal connection between local stimulation and functional response. Paired stimuli can be used to examine habituation and amplification phenomena. Repeated TMS (rTMS), at frequencies between 5 and 20 Hz, has been shown to have direct enhancing and suppressing (quenching) effects on brain activity. rTMS over relevant frontal areas has, for example, been shown to disrupt learning (Pascual-Leone & Hallett 1994). Finally, effects of localised rTMS on mood and immune responses have been demonstrated, which only hint at the range of possible clinical and research applications in the future (George et al 1996).

REFERENCES

Ahern G L, Schwartz G E 1985 Differential lateralization for positive and negative emotion in the human brain: EEG spectralanalysis. Neuropsychologia 23: 745–755

Altrocchi P H, Brin M, Ferguson J H et al 1996 Assessment of brain SPECT – report of the therapeutics and technology-assessment subcommittee of the American Academy of Neurology. Neurology 46: 278–285

Andreasen N C, Ehrhardt J C, Swayze V W et al 1990 Magnetic resonance imaging of the brain in schizophrenia. Archives of General Psychiatry 47: 35–44

Astrup J, Sorensen P M, Sorensen H R 1981 Oxygen and glucose consumption related to Na^+-K^+ transport in canine brain. Stroke 12: 726–730

Austin M-P, Dougall N, Ross M et al 1992 Single photon emission tomography with ^{99m}Tc-exametazime in major depression and the pattern of brain activity underlying the psychotic/neurotic continuum. Journal of Affective Disorders 26: 31–44

Axelson D A, Doraiswamy P M, McDonald W M et al 1993 Hypercortisolemia and hippocampal changes in depression. Psychiatry Research 47: 163–173

Barker A T, Jalinous R, Freeston I L 1985 Non-invasive magnetic stimulation of the human motor cortex. Lancet i: 1106–1107

Baxter L R, Saxena S, Brodie A L et al 1996 Brain mediation of obsessive–compulsive disorder symptoms: evidence from functional brain imaging studies in the human and non-human primate. Seminars in Clinical Neuropsychiatry 1: 32–47

Bench C J, Frackowiak R S J, Dolan R J 1995 Changes in regional cerebral blood flow on recovery from depression. Psychological Medicine 25: 247–261

Bergman H, Chertkow H, Wolfson C et al 1997 HM-PAO SPECT brain scanning in the diagnosis of Alzheimer's disease. Journal of the American Geriatric Society 45: 15–20

Bertolino A, Nawroz S, Mattay V S et al 1996 Regionally specific pattern of neurochemical pathology in schizophrenia as assessed by multislice proton magnetic resonance spectroscopic imaging. American Journal of Psychiatry 153: 1554–1563

Bonne O, Krausz Y, Shapira B et al 1996 Increased cerebral blood flow in depressed patients responding to electroconvulsive therapy. Journal of Nuclear Medicine 37: 1075–1080

Breiter H C, Etcoff N L, Whalen P J et al 1996a Response and habituation of the human amygdala during visual processing of facial expression. Neuron 17: 875–887

Breiter H C, Rauch S L, Kwong K K et al 1996b Functional magnetic resonance imaging of symptom provocation in obsessive–compulsive disorder. Archives of General Psychiatry 53: 595–606

Bremner J D, Randall P, Scott T M et al 1995 MRI-based measurement of hippocampal volume in patients with combat related post-traumatic stress disorder. American Journal of Psychiatry 152: 973–981

Claus J J, Van Harskamp F, Breteler M M B et al 1994 The diagnostic value of SPECT with Tc-99m HMPAO in Alzheimer's disease – a population-based study. Neurology 44: 454–461

Coffey C E, Wilkinson W E, Weiner R D et al 1993 Quantitative cerebral anatomy in depression. Archives of General Psychiatry 50: 7–16

Cohen M S, Bookheimer S Y 1994 Localisation of brain function using magnetic resonance imaging. Trends in Neurosciences 17: 268–277

Cottraux J, Gerard D, Cinotti et al 1996 A controlled positron emission tomography study of obsessive and neutral auditory-stimulation in obsessive–compulsive disorder with checking rituals. Psychiatry Research 60: 101–112

Curran S M, Murray C M, Van Beck M et al 1993 A single photon emission computerised tomography study of regional brain function in elderly patients with major depression and with Alzheimer-type dementia. British Journal of Psychiatry 163: 155–165

Damasio H, Grabowski T, Frank R, Galaburda A M, Damasio A R 1994 The return of Phineas Gage: clues about the brain from the skull of a famous patient. Science 264: 1102–1105

Daniel D G, Goldberg T E, Gibbons R D, Weinberger D R 1992 Lack of a biomodal distribution of ventricular size in schizophrenia – a gaussian meta-analysis. Biological Psychiatry 30: 887–903

David A S, Woodruff P W R, Howard R et al 1996 Auditory hallucinations inhibit exogenous activation of auditory association cortex. Neuroreport 7: 932–936

Davidson R J 1992 Anterior cerebral asymmetry and the nature of emotion. Brain and Cognition 20: 125–151

De Leon M J, George A E, Stylopoulos L A, Smith G, Miller D C 1989 Early marker for Alzheimer's disease: the atrophic hippocampus. Lancet ii: 672–673

Delvenne V, Lotstra F, Goldman S et al 1995 Brain hypometabolism of glucose in anorexia-nervosa – a PET scan study. Biological Psychiatry 37: 61–169

D'haenen H A, Bossuyt A 1994 Dopamine D_2 receptors in depression measured with single photon emission computed tomography. Biological Psychiatry 35: 128–132

Ebert D, Ebmeier K P 1996 The role of the cingulate gyrus in depression: from functional anatomy to neurochemistry. Biological Psychiatry 39: 1044–1050

Ebmeier K P 1995 Brain imaging and schizophrenia. In: Den Boer J A, Westenberg H G M, van Praag H M (eds) Advances in the neurobiology of schizophrenia. Wiley, Chichester, pp 131–155

Ebmeier K P, Besson J A O, Crawford J R et al 1987 Nuclear magnetic resonance imaging and single photon emission tomography with radio-iodine labelled compounds in the diagnosis of dementia. Acta Psychiatrica Scandinavica 75: 549–556

Ebmeier K P, Blackwood D H R, Murray C et al 1993 Single photon emission computed tomography with ^{99m}Tc-exametazime in unmedicated schizophrenic patients. Biological Psychiatry 33: 487–495

Ebmeier K P, Cavanagh J T O, Moffoot A P R Glabus M F, O'Carroll R E, Goodwin G M 1997 Cerebral perfusion correlates of depressed mood. British Journal of Psychiatry 170: 77–81

Farde L 1996 The advantage of using positron emission tomography in drug research. Trends in Neurosciences 19: 211–214

Fischer H, Wik G, Fredrikson M 1996 Functional neuroanatomy of robbery re-experience: affective memories studied with PET. NeuroReport 7: 2081–2086

Fox N A Bell M A, Jones N A 1992 Individual differences in respone to stress and cerebral asymmetry. Developmental Neuropsychology 8: 161–184

Fox P T, Raichle M E 1986 Focal physiological uncoupling of cerebral blood flow and oxidative metabolism during somatosensory stimulation in human subjects. Proceedings of the National Academy of Sciences of the USA 83: 1140–1144

Fox P T, Raichle M E, Mintum M A, Dence D 1988 Nonoxidative glucose consumption during focal physiologic neural activity. Science 241: 462–464

Fredrikson M, Wik G, Annas P, Ericson K, Stone-Elander S 1995 Functional neuroanatomy of visually elicited simple phobic fear – additional data and theoretical-analysis. Psychophysiology 32: 43–48

Friston K J, Worsley K J, Frackowiak R S J, Mazziotta J C, Evans A C 1994 Assessing the significance of focal activations using their spatial extent. Human Brain Mapping 1: 214–220

Friston K J, Ashburner J, Frith C D, Poline J B, Heather J D, Frackowiak R S J 1995a Spatial registration and normalization of images. Human Brain Mapping 2: 165–189

Friston K J, Holmes A P, Worsley K J, Poline J-P, Frith C D, Frackowiak R S J 1995b Statistical parametric maps in functional imaging: a general linear approach. Human Brain Mapping 2: 189–210

Fukuzako H, Fukuzako T, Takeuchi K et al 1996 Phosphorus magnetic resonance spectroscopy in schizophrenia – correlation between membrane phospholipid metabolism in the temporal lobe and positive symptoms. Progress in Neuro-Psychopharmacology and Biological Psychiatry 20: 629–640

George M S, Robertson M M, Costa D C et al 1994 Dopamine-receptor availability in Tourette's syndrome. Psychiatry Research 55: 193–203

George M S, Wassermann E M, Post R M 1996 Transcranial magnetic stimulation – a neuropsychiatric tool for the 21st century. Journal of Neuropsychiatry and Clinical Neurosciences 8: 373–382

Gevins A, Leong H, Smith M E, Le J, Du R 1995 Mapping cognitive brain function with modern high-resolution electroencephalography. Trends in Neurosciences 18: 429–436

Goodwin G M 1996 Functional imaging, affective disorder and dementia. British Medical Bulletin 52: 495–512

Goodwin G M, Austin M-P, Dougall N et al 1993 State changes in brain activity shown by the uptake of ^{99m}Tc-exametazime with single photon emission tomography in major depression before and after treatment. Journal of Affective Disorders 29: 243–253

Grodd W, Schneider F, Klose U, Nagele T 1995 Functional magnetic resonance imaging of psychological functions with experimentally-induced emotion. Radiologe 35: 283–289

Gur R C, Gur R E, Resnick S M, Skolnick B E, Alavi A, Reivich M 1987 The effect of anxiety on cortical cerebral blood flow and metabolism. Journal of Cerebral Blood Flow and Metabolism 7: 173–177

Herholz K 1996 Neuroimaging in anorexia-nervosa. Psychiatry Research 62: 105–110

Herscovitch P 1994 Radiotracer techniques for functional neuroimaging with positron emission tomography. In: Thatcher R W, Hallett M, Zeffiro T, John E R, Huerta M (eds) Functional neuroimaging: technical foundations. Academic Press, San Diego, pp 29–46

Holman B L, Hellman R S, Goldsmith S J et al 1989 Biodistribution, dosimetry, and clinical evaluation of technetium-99m ethyl cysteinate dimer in normal subjects and in patients with chronic cerebral infarction. Journal of Nuclear Medicine 30: 1018–1024

Huber G 1957 Pneumenzephalographische und

psychopathologische Bilder bei endogenen Psychosen. Monographien aus dem Gesamtgebiete der Neurologie und Psychiatrie. Springer, Berlin

Ingvar D H, Franzen G 1974 Abnormalities of cerebral blood flow distribution in patients with chronic schizophrenia. Acta Psychiatrica Scandinavica 50: 425–462

Jacobi W, Winkler H 1927 Encephalographische Studien an Chronischen Schizophrenen. Archiv für Psychiatrie und Nervenkrankheiten 81: 299–332

Jacquier-Sarlin M R, Polla B S, Slosman D O 1996a Cellular basis of ECD brain retention. Journal of Nuclear Medicine 37: 1694–1697

Jacquier-Sarlin M R, Polla B S, Slosman D O 1996b Oxidoreductive state; the major determinant for cellular retention of 99mTc-HMPAO. Journal of Nuclear Medicine 37: 1413–1416

Jalinous R, Freeston I L, Neirinckx R D et al 1985 The retention mechanism of technetium-99m HMPAO: intracellular reaction with glutathione. Journal of Cerebral Blood Flow and Metabolism 8: S4–12

Jensen H V, Plenge P, Stensgaard A, Mellerup E T, Thomsen C A, Henriksen O 1996 12 hour brain lithium concentration in lithium maintenance treatment of manic depressive disorder – daily versus alternate-day dosing schedule. Psychopharmacology 124: 275–278

Jobst K A, Smith A D, Szatmari M 1994 Rapidly progressing atrophy of medial temporal lobe in Alzheimer's disease. Lancet 343: 829–830

Johnson E W, Woods S W, Zoghbi S, McBride B J, Baldwin R M, Innis R B 1990 Receptor binding characterization of the benzodiazepine radioligand [123]Ro 16-0154: Potential probe for SPECT brain imaging. Life Sciences 47: 1535–1546

Johnstone E C, Crow T J, Firth C D, Husband J, Kreel L 1976 Cerebral ventricular size and cognitive impairment in chronic schizophrenia. Lancet ii: 924–926

Kato T, Hamakawa H, Shioiri T et al 1996 Choline-containing compounds detected by proton magnetic resonance spectroscopy in the basal ganglia in bipolar disorder. Journal of Psychiatry and Neuroscience 21: 248–254

Ketter T A, George M S, Kimbrell T A, Benson B E, Post R M 1996 Functional brain imaging, limbic function, and affective disorders. Neuroscientist 2: 55–65

Kwong K K, Belliveau J W, Chesler D A et al 1992 Dynamic magnetic resonance imaging of human brain activity during primary sensory stimulation. Proceedings of the National Academy of Sciences of the USA 89: 5675–5679

Le Bihan D, Karni A 1995 Applications of magnetic resonance imaging to the study of human brain function. Current Opinion in Neurobiology 5: 231–237

Leuchter A F, Dunkin J J, Lufkin R B, Anzai Y, Cook I A, Newton T F 1994 Effect of white matter disease on functional connections in the ageing brain. Journal of Neurology, Neurosurgery and Psychiatry 57: 1347–1354

Leveille J, Demonceau G, Deroo M et al 1989 Characterization of technetium-99m-l, l-ECD for brain perfusion imaging, part 2: biodistribution and brain imaging in humans. Journal of Nuclear Medicine 30: 1902–1910

Leveille J, Demonceau G, Walovitch R C 1992 Intrasubject comparison between technetium-99m-ECD and technetium-99m-HMPAO in healthy human subjects. Journal of Nuclear Medicine 33: 480–484

Liddle P F, Friston K J, Frith C D, Hirsch S R, Jones T,

Frackowiak R S J 1992 Patterns of cerebral blood flow in schizophrenia. British Journal of Psychiatry 160: 179–186

Loeb C 1995 Dementia due to lacunar infarctions – a misnomer or a clinical entity. European Neurology 35: 187–192

Lucey J V, Costa D C, Blanes T et al 1995 Regional cerebral blood-flow in obsessive–compulsive disordered patients at rest – differential correlates with obsessive–compulsive and anxious-avoidant dimensions. British Journal of Psychiatry 167: 629–634

McGuire P K, Silbersweig D A, Wright I et al 1995 Abnormal monitoring of inner speech – a physiological basis for auditory hallucinations. Lancet 346: 596–600

Maier M, Ron M A 1996 Hippocampal age-related changes in schizophrenia – a proton magnetic resonance spectroscopy study. Schizophrenia Research 22: 5–17

Maier M, Ron M A, Barker G J, Tofts P S 1995 Proton magnetic resonance spectroscopy – an in vivo method of estimating hippocampal neuronal depletion in schizophrenia. Psychological Medicine 25: 1201–1209

Malison R T, McDougle C J, Vandyck C H 1995 [I-123]-Beta-CIT SPECT imaging of striatal dopamine transporter binding in Tourette's disorder. American Journal of Psychiatry 152: 1359–1361

Mielke R, Pietrzyk U, Jacobs A et al 1994 HMPAO SPET and EDG PET in Alzheimer's disease and vascular dementia: comparison of perfusion and metabolic pattern. European Journal of Nuclear Medicine 21: 1052–1060

Moore C M, Christensen J D, Lafer B, Fava M, Renshaw P F 1997 Lower levels of nucleoside triphosphate in the basal ganglia of depressed subjects: a phosphorous-31 magnetic resonance spectroscopy study. American Journal of Psychiatry 154: 116–118

Morgan G F, Costa D C 1993 Radiopharmaceuticals for conventional blood brain barrier and perfusion studies. In: Costa D C, Morgan G F, Lassen N A (eds) New trends in nuclear neurology and psychiatry. Libbey, London, p. 76ff

O'Brien J, Desmond P, Ames D, Schweitzer I, Harrigan S, Tress B 1996 Magnetic resonance imaging study of white matter lesions in depression and Alzheimer's disease. British Journal of Psychiatry 168: 477–485

O'Carroll R E, Moffoot A P R, Van Beck M et al 1993 Anxiety and the brain: the effect of anxiety induction on regional brain function as measured using single photon emission tomography (SPET). Journal of Affective Disorders 28: 203–210

Ohnishi T, Hoshi H, Nagamachi S et al 1995 High-resolution SPECT to assess hippocampal perfusion in neuropsychiatric diseases. Journal of Nuclear Medicine 36: 1163–1169

Pascual-Leone A, Hallett M 1994 Induction of errors in a delayed response task by repetitive transcranial magnetic stimulation of the dorsolateral prefrontal cortex. NeuroReport 5: 2517–2520

Pascual-Leone A, Grafman J, Hallett M 1994 Modulation of cortical motor output maps during development of implicit and explicit knowledge. Science 263: 1287–1289

Penfield W, Rasmussen T 1950 The cerebral cortex of man: a clinical study of localization of function. Macmillan, New York

Phelps C 1898 Traumatic injuries of the brain and its membranes. Kimpton, London

Press G A, Amaral D G, Squire L R 1989 Hippocampal abnormalities in amnesic patients revealed by high-resolution magnetic resonance imaging. Nature 341: 54–57

Rauch S L, Savage C R, Alpert N M et al 1995 A positron

emission tomographic study of simple phobic symptom provocation. Archives of General Psychiatry 52: 20–28

Rauch S L, Vanderkolk B A, Fisler R E et al 1996 A symptom provocation study of posttraumatic-stress-disorder using positron emission tomography and script-driven imagery. Archives of General Psychiatry 53: 380–387

Read S L, Miller B L, Mena I, Kim R, Itabashi H, Darby A 1995 SPECT in dementia – clinical and pathological correlation. Journal of the American Geriatric Society 43: 1243–1247

Renshaw P F, Yurgelun-Todd D A, Cohen B M 1994 Greater hemodynamic response to photic stimulation in schizophrenic patients – an echo planar MRI study. American Journal of Psychiatry 151: 1493–1495

Sackeim H A, Prohovnik I, Moeller J R, Mayeux R, Stern Y, Devanand D P 1993 Regional cerebral blood flow in mood disorders 2. Comparison of major depression and Alzheimer's disease. Journal of Nuclear Medicine 7: 1090–1101

Samii A, Wassermann E M, Ikoma K et al 1996 Decreased postexercise facilitation of motor evoked potentials in patients with chronic fatigue syndrome or depression. Neurology 6: 1410–1414

Scheltens P, Leys D, Barkhof F et al 1992 Atrophy of medial temporal lobes on MRI in 'probable' Alzheimer's disease and normal ageing: diagnostic value and neuropsychological correlates. Journal of Neurology, Neurosurgery and Psychiatry 55: 967–972

Schmidt R, Fazekas F, Offenbacher H et al 1993 Neuropsychologic correlates of MRI white matter hyperintensities: a study of 150 normal volunteers. Neurology 43: 2490–2494

Schroder J, Wenz F, Schad L R, Baudendistel K, Knopp M V 1995 Sensorimotor cortex and supplementary motor area changes in schizophrenia – a study with functional magnetic resonance imaging. British Journal of Psychiatry 167: 197–201

Shah P J, Ogilvie A, Goodwin G M, Ebmeier K P 1997 Clinical and psychometric correlates of dompamine D_2 binding in depression. Psychological Medicine 27: 1247–1256

Sharp P F 1994 The measurement of blood flow in humans using radioactive tracers. Physiological Measurement 15: 339–379

Shiori T, Kato T, Murashita J, Hamakawa, H, Inubushi T, Takahashi S 1996 High energy phosphate metabolism in the frontal lobes of patients with panic disorder detected by phase-encoded P-31-MRS. Biological Psychiatry 40: 785–793

Soares J C, Mann J J 1997 The anatomy of mood disorder – review of structural neuroimaging studies. Biological Psychiatry 41: 86–106

Sokoloff L, Reivich M, Kennedy C et al 1977 The [^{14}C] deoxyglucose method for the measurement of local cerebral glucose utilization: theory, procedure, and normal values in the conscious and anesthetized albino rat. Journal of Neurochemistry 28: 897–916

Szelies B, Mielke B, Herholz K, Heiss W-D 1994 Quantitative topographical EEG compared to FDG PET for classification of vascular and degenerative dementia. Electroencephalography and Clinical Neurophysiology 91: 131–139

Turjanski N, Sawle G V, Playford E D et al 1994 PET studies of the presynaptic and postsynaptic dopaminergic system in Tourette's syndrome. Journal of Neurology, Neurosurgery and Psychiatry 57: 688–692

Turner R, Jezzard P 1994 Magnetic resonance studies of brain functional activation using echo-planar imaging. In: Thatcher R W, Hallet M, Zeffiro T, John E R, Huerta M (eds) Functional neuroimaging: technical foundations. Academic Press, San Diego, pp 69–78

Upadhyaya A K, Abou-Saleh M T, Wilson K, Grime S J, Critchley M 1990 A study of depression in old age using single-photon emission computerised tomography. British Journal of Psychiatry 157: 76–81

van Dyck C H, Lin C H, Smith E O et al 1996 Comparison of technetium-99m-HMPAO and technetium-99m-ECD cerebral SPECT images in Alzheimer's disease. Journal of Nuclear Medicine: 37: 1749–1755

Van Gool W A, Walstra G J M, Teunisse S, Van der Zant F M, Weinstein H C, Van Royen E A 1995 Diagnosing Alzheimer's disease in elderly, mildly demented patients – the impact of routine single photon emission computed tomography. Journal of Neurology 242: 401–405

Van Horn J D, McManus I C 1992 Ventricular enlargement in schizophrenia. A meta-analysis of studies of the ventricle: brain ratio (VBR). British Journal of Psychiatry 160: 687–697

Wenz F, Schad L R, Knopp M V et al 1994 Functional magnetic resonance imaging at 1.5-T – activation pattern in schizophrenic patients receiving neuroleptic medication. Magnetic Resonance Imaging 12: 975–982

Wiesel F A 1992 Regional glucose metabolism in schizophrenic patients before and during neuroleptic treatment. Progress in Neuro-Psychopharmacology and Biological Psychiatry 16: 871–881

Wiesel F A, Wik G, Sjögren I, Blomqvist G, Greitz T, Stone-Elander S 1987 Regional brain glucose metabolism in drug free schizophrenic patients and clinical correlates. Acta Psychiatrica Scandinavica 76: 628–641

Wik G, Fredrikson M, Fischer H 1996 Cerebral correlates of anticipated fear: a PET study of specific phobia. International Journal of Neuroscience 87: 267–276

Wikswo J P, Gevins A, Williamson S J 1993 The future of EEG and MEG. Encephalography and Clinical Neurophysiology 98: 1–9

Wright I C, McGuire P K, Poline J-B et al 1995 A voxel-based method for the statistical analysis of gray and white matter density applied in schizophrenia. Neuroimage 2: 244–252

Ye F Q, Pekar J J, Jezzard P et al 1996 Perfusion imaging of the human brain at 1.5 T using a single-shot EPI spin tagging approach. Magnetic Resonance Imaging 36: 219–224

Yurgelun-Todd D A, Renshaw P F, Gruber S A, Ed M, Waternaux C, Cohen B M 1996a Proton magnetic resonance spectroscopy of the temporal lobes in schizophrenics and normal controls. Schizophrenia Research 19: 55–59

Yurgelun-Todd D A, Waternaux C M, Cohen B M, Gruber S A, English C D, Renshaw P F 1996b Functional magnetic resonance imaging of schizophrenic patients and comparison subjects during word production. American Journal of Psychiatry 153: 200–205

17

Neurotic disorders

C. P. L. Freeman

INTRODUCTION

We have decided to retain the term neurosis in the 6th edition. There is still no other term which adequately covers the conditions grouped here. Whether they should still be grouped together will be discussed later.

The term neurosis was introduced by the Edinburgh physician William Cullen in 1769. By neurosis he meant 'disorders of sense and motion' caused by a 'general affectation of the nervous system'. He included a wide range of conditions in which he felt there was some pathological deficiency in the nervous system but in which fever was absent, so that – as well as hysteria, hypochondriasis, melancholia and palpitations – epilepsy, mania, chorea, asthenia and diabetes were included.

Cullen was a classifier and subdivider of the first order. Some 60 years later Benjamin Rush mocked Cullen's penchant for useless subdivisions. He described 18 'species' of phobia including rum phobia ('a very rare disease'), want phobia ('confined chiefly to the elderly') and church phobia ('endemic in the city of Philadelphia'). Rush's comments are in quotes (Rush 1812). One hundred years later the concept had been refined so that by the end of the 19th century it had come to mean psychiatric disorders which were neither organic nor psychotic.

We owe to Freud the term *psychoneurosis*. He used it to mean three specific syndromes: anxiety hysteria (now called phobic anxiety); obsessive–compulsive neurosis and hysteria proper. He distinguished the 'psychoneuroses' from the 'actual' neuroses which were neurasthenia and anxiety neurosis. He saw the actual neuroses as being predominantly physical and chemical in nature and not due to underlying conflict. In contrast he saw the psychoneuroses as resulting from unconscious conflicts, either between opposing wishes or between wishes and prohibitions. He saw such conflicts leading to unconscious perception of anticipated danger which evokes defence mechanisms that become manifest as personality disturbances or symptoms or both. Freud used the term neurosis in at least two ways. Firstly to indicate an aetiological process, viz. unconscious conflict around anxiety and leading to maladaptive use of defence mechanisms that result in symptom formation; and secondly as a descriptive term to indicate a painful symptom in an individual with intact reality testing.

As the 20th century progressed, the use of the term widened again so that, if many current definitions of neurosis were taken literally, all forms of non-psychotic non-organic distress would be included. For example, the World Health Organization (WHO 1974) international glossary definition is as follows:

Mental disorders without any demonstrable organic basis in which the patient may have considerable insight and has unimpaired reality testing in that he usually does not confuse his morbid subjective experiences and fantasies with external reality. Behaviour may be greatly affected, although usually remaining within socially acceptable limits, but personality is not disorganised. The principal manifestations include excessive anxiety, hysterical symptoms, phobias, obsessional and compulsive symptoms and depression.

In this chapter the term neurosis is used in three distinct but related ways:

- As a global term to indicate all non-psychotic syndromes. The use here is synonymous with the term minor psychiatric morbidity and it is in this sense that the term has been used in most epidemiological research. The majority of such disorders are states of depression or anxiety or a mixture of the two. They have been called dysthymic states by some authors, but the term dysthymic disorder now has a more precise meaning in both DSM-IV and ICD-10.
- As a term to indicate specific neurotic disorders such as anxiety, depressive, obsessional and phobic neuroses.
- As a term to describe assumed underlying mental

mechanisms, so-called neurotic processes leading to the production of defence mechanisms.

The American (DSM-III; APA 1980) definition of neurotic disorders was as follows and encompassed the use of neurosis in the first and second sense above:

A symptom or group of symptoms that is distressing to the individual, or recognised by him/her as unacceptable and alien (egodystonic). Reality testing is grossly intact, behaviour does not actively violate gross social norms though functioning may be markedly impaired. The disturbance is relatively enduring or recurrent and is not noted to be a transitory reaction to stressors. There is no demonstrable organic aetiology or factor.

What is clear is that definitions which stress only the minor, transitory or minimally incapacitating nature of neurotic disorder cannot encompass all types of neuroses, for example the crippling nature of severe obsessional states, or the lifelong pattern of disability in somatisation disorder, or the poor response to treatment that many neurotic disorders show. In contrast, many psychoses are brief and respond dramatically to treatment.

Neurosis: should we retain the term?

DSM-IV (APA 1994) does not mention the term at all, whereas ICD-10 (WHO 1992) still retains the term for occasional use, viz. F40-48 'Neurotic, stress related and somotaform disorders'. The terms psychogenic and psychosomatic have also been dropped. The three main justifications for discarding the term are:

- That it groups together conditions which could be classified better in other ways
- That it involves aetiological assumptions which are unjustified
- That it is a redundant adjective, which we can do without.

The first argument is illustrated by the reclassification of minor depressive disorders or 'neurotic depressions'. In both DSM-IV and ICD-10 these are now grouped with other affective (mood) disorders. Rather than just reduce the types of neuroses by one, DSM-IV has tried to find new homes for all the other 'neurotic disorders' and in doing so has created as many problems as it has solved. Obsessional states are classified as a type of anxiety disorder, and depersonalisation syndromes are included under dissociative disorders. ICD-10, on the other hand, retains the general class of neurotic disorders.

The second argument is that the term neurosis is a confusing one and one with multiple meanings. It is used to refer to specific syndromes, to a variety of psychopathological processes and to a general class of non-psychotic non-organic psychological disorders. Gelder (1986) suggested that this problem can be solved by a more exact use of terms such as neurotic process and neurotic mechanism to distinguish these concepts from neurotic disorders.

The third argument is that the term is redundant. Adding the term neurosis to anxiety disorder or obsessional disorder adds nothing to the meaning, and the concept of a broad grouping of neurotic disorders is so vague that it is not worth using.

The most cogent reasons for retaining the term relate to this last point. Although there have been advances in the classification of neurotic disorders, such as separate recognition of panic disorder and somatisation disorder, there are still many cases which do not fit neatly into any existing category. There are patients who exhibit mixtures of anxiety, depressive, hypochondriacal and obsessional symptoms without any one cluster appearing to dominate. No satisfactory term for this group has emerged, though minor psychiatric disorder, subclinical neurosis and minor affective disorder have been suggested.

The recent UK household survey of psychiatric morbidity (Jenkins et al 1997) found that 'non specific neurotic disorder' was by far the most common syndrome.

It is unlikely that all these conditions represent variants of affective disorder, and the term minor is misleading, as some are serious and disabling. Until this problem is resolved it seems sensible to retain the term neurosis, or preferably neurotic disorder, to embrace this whole class of disorders. Without such a term there is a danger such patients will be classified as having personality disorder, with all the problems and confusion the term brings with it. A second weaker argument has been proposed by Sims (1985). He suggests that the shared clinical features, and to some extent the common methods of treatment, justify retention of the term. Although this is partly true, features such as bodily symptoms without organic cause and anxiety are not exclusive to the neuroses and frequently occur in other non-neurotic conditions.

In this chapter the term neurosis has been retained in the sense that it is used by ICD-10, though, as already mentioned, other uses of the term are not ignored.

NEUROSIS AS MINOR PSYCHIATRIC MORBIDITY

This section deals with investigations which have regarded neurosis as a global concept synonymous with minor psychiatric morbidity. Most studies of the nature and causes of neurosis have considered it in a global sense rather than describing individual clinical syndromes, so factors in the aetiology of neurosis are conveniently described here.

Epidemiology of neurosis

Figures for the prevalence, incidence and lifetime risk of neurotic disorder are virtually meaningless unless one has some idea of the criteria that were used for case identification. Two extreme examples will serve to illustrate the problem. The mid-town Manhattan survey (Srole et al 1962), in which a random sample of New Yorkers were asked by non-medical interviewers about the presence of psychiatric symptoms, found them to be present in 81.5% of that population. However, Fremming (1951), studying a Danish population and using a clinical interview, found a lifetime prevalence of only 1.3% for men and 3.7% for women. Clearly, with such disparity, widely differing concepts of mental illness of minor psychiatric morbidity are being used. One major advance has been the introduction of standardised interviews with clearly stated diagnostic criteria. With the aid of such instruments it is possible to produce some sort of definition of what is a psychiatric case. Unfortunately the border between a case and a non-case is blurred and most researchers have had to introduce some intermediate concept such as a probable case, borderline or threshold category, or subclinical disturbance. Despite the imprecise and vague nature of such terms there is considerable agreement amongst researchers that such subclinical disturbance consists

largely of symptoms such as fatigue, irritability, insomnia and dysthymia. Table 17.1 shows the results of five studies and gives percentage figures for definite and probable cases combined. Four of the studies used the Present State Examination (PSE) and are therefore roughly comparable. Figures are given for all psychiatric morbidity and for depressive illness alone. In all studies psychotic disorders formed a very small proportion of cases and therefore these figures can be regarded as representing the prevalence of minor psychiatric morbidity. We see that depression and depressive symptoms form a large part of the total in all studies. There is a marked sex difference in all studies in which both sexes have been examined, females outnumbering males in a ratio of between 3:2 and 2:1. It will be noted that, in the four studies which used the PSE, depression forms a greater part of the total psychiatric morbidity than in the American study which used the Schedule for Affective Disorders and Schizophrenia (SADS, Endicott & Spitzer 1978). This is in part because the PSE tends to group together cases which show both anxiety and depression and call them depression, and in part because the PSE does not regard alcoholism, organic states or personality disorders as psychiatric illness, whereas when the SADS is used, approximately 25% of diagnoses are either alcoholism or drug abuse. Table 17.2 summarises the major recent studies and the instruments used. Strictly speaking, studies which report results in terms of point prevalence, 1 month period prevalence and 1 year period prevalence cannot be compared. However, differences due to such factors are probably small when compared with the variability in case-finding techniques between studies. We can see

Table 17.1 Prevalence of all psychiatric disorder and of depressive illness and depressive symptoms in the general population. Results from five surveys.

Reference	Place	Method	Period	Depression (%)			All psychiatric morbidity (%)		
				Male	Female	Total	Male	Female	Total
Weissman et al (1978)	New Haven CT1975–1976	SADS +RDC	Point	6	7	7	16	19	18
Wing (1979)	Camberwell	PSE-10	1 month	5	7	6	6	12	9
Orley & Wing (1979)	Ugandan villages	PSE-10	1 month	14	23	18	19	29	24
Brown & Harris (1978)	Camberwell	PSE	1 year	—	15	—	—	17	—
Brown et al (1977)	North Uist, Outer Hebrides	PSE	1 year	—	8	—	—	12	—

Prevalence expressed as whole number percentages for clarity.

Table 17.2	Instruments used for classification and diagnosis in 'third generation' comorbidity studies	
Instrument (Study)	Description	Comments
SADS (Endicott & Spitzer 1978)	Includes diagnoses of alcohol and drug abuse	Used in New Haven studies (Weissman & Myers 1978)
PSE (Wing 1974)	Classification of a limited number of ICD categories, mainly functional psychosis and affective disorders	Threshold lower than DSM-IIIR or DSM-IV therefore ICD prevalences greater
PSE 10 – SCAN (Wing 1990)	Classification according to DSM-IIIR, DSM-IV, ICD-10	Administered usually by non-lay interviewers
DIS (Robins 1981)	DSM-III and DSM-IIIR categories	Uses lay interviewers; used in ECA study
CIDI (Robins 1981)	Largely based on DIS; includes some psychotic and neurotic items from PSE	Lay interviewers
UM – CIDI		Used in US National Comorbidity Survey
CIS (Laws 1992)		Used in UK National Pychiatric Morbidity Study

CIDI, Composite International Diagnostic Instrument; CIS, Clinical Interview Schedule; DIS, Diagnostic Interview Schedule; PSE, Present State Examination; SCAN, Schedules for Clinical Assessment in Neuropsychiatry; SADS, Schedule for Affective Disorders and Schizophrenia; UM-CIDI, University of Michigan version of CIDI.

that, as well as marked sex differences, there appears to be greater morbidity in an urban (Camberwell) than a rural (North Uist) setting and that the figures for the Ugandan villages are staggeringly high and that much of this is due to depressive disorders.

Table 17.3 gives the results of five large community studies which have used mainly the General Health Questionnaire (GHQ) as a screen and then confirmed cases with the PSE.

It would appear that, using the criteria of these investigators, between 17 and 24% of a Western population can be said to be a psychiatric case or a borderline case at any one point in time.

Two other studies are worthy of note. Hagnell

Table 17.3	Two-stage prevalence studies – 1981-1987						
Area	Reference	Size of study	Screening instrument	Case confirmation	Prevalence		Total
					(Male	Female)	
Spain (rural)	Vasquez-Barquero et al (1981)	1156	GHQ-60	CIS	19.1	28.3	23.8
Australia (urban)	Henderson et al (1979)	756	GHQ-30	PSE	7.1	11.1	9.0
England (urban)	Bebbington et al (1981)	800	PSE-40	PSE	6.1	14.9	10.9
Holland (urban)	Hodiamont et al (1987)	3282	GHQ-60	PSE	7.2	7.5	7.3
Spain (rural)	Vasquez-Barquero et al (1987)	1232	GHQ-60	PSE	8.1	20.6	14.7

GHQ, General Health Questionnaire; PSE, Present State Examination.

Table 17.4 ECA study sample characteristics

	New Haven	Baltimore	St Louis
Survey date	1980–1981	1981	1981–1982
Sample population size	298 000	175 000	277 000
Sample age range (years)	18+	18+	18+
Completed interviews	3058	3481	3004
Completed rate (%)	75.3	78	79.1

From Myers et al (1984)

(1966), studying a Swedish population, found a lifetime expectancy rate for neurosis alone of 13% (7.5% for males and 17% for females). Very similar figures were found by Helgason (1964), who intensively studied a cohort of 5395 Icelanders born between 1895 and 1897 and followed up over 60 years. He found a lifetime risk for neurosis of 8% for males and 16% for females.

Community studies looking at point prevalence rates on a single day (Finlay-Jones & Burvill 1977), using the GHQ as a screening measure and defining a case as anyone scoring 12 or more on that questionnaire, have shown point prevalence rates of 13.5% for men and 18.7% for women. The lowest rates were in the married and the highest in the widowed, with the single, the separated and the divorced in between. Rates in social classes I and II were 50% of those in social class V.

The Epidemiologic Catchment Area (ECA) study

The ECA programme was a massive collaborative study designed to apply common diagnostic and health utilisation instruments at 6 month intervals to large general population samples in the USA. It included both people at home and those in institutions. Lifetime and 6 month prevalence rates are available for 15 DSM-III diagnoses. Estimates have been derived from responses to the Diagnostic Interview Schedule (DIS), an instrument constructed to provide lifetime DSM-III, Research Diagnostic Criteria and Feighner diagnoses (Robins et al 1984). The total sample size was over 15 000, with over 3000 interviewed in each of the five sites. Details are given in Table 17.4. The five areas were New Haven (Connecticut), Baltimore, St Louis, Los Angeles and North Carolina.

Six month prevalence rates These are detailed in Table 17.5 and will be discussed more fully under the sections on each specific diagnosis.

The most common disorder in the three communities studies were phobia, alcohol abuse and/or dependence, dysthymia and major depression. The most common diagnoses for women were phobias and major depression, whereas for men the main disorder was alcohol abuse and/or dependence. In no site was the total rate of disorders higher in women than in men. This contrasts with previous findings and probably reflects the fact that earlier studies neglected to enquire systematically about male-predominant diagnoses such as alcoholism, drug dependence and antisocial personality.

Table 17.5 Six month and lifetime prevalence rates (%) from the ECA study

	6 month prevalence			Total lifetime prevalence
	Men	Women	Total	
Panic disorder	0.6	1.0	0.8	1.4
Obsessive–compulsive	1.2	1.9	1.6	2.5
Somatisation disorder	0	0.2	0.1	0.1
Simple phobia	4.3	9.4	7.0	—
Social phobia	1.3	2.0	1.7	—
Agoraphobia	1.8	5.4	3.8	—
Total phobia[a]	4.9	11.1	8.2	13.5
Total for any DSM-III diagnosis	17.7	18.3	18.1	32.6

[a]Subjects may have more than one phobic diagnosis.
From Myers et al (1984) and Robins et al (1984).

Lifetime prevalence The most striking finding and one that was replicated in all five sites was that most disorders have their peak occurrence in the 25–44-year-old age group. Panic disorder, obsessive–compulsive disorder, agoraphobia and simple phobias all showed a drop in prevalence over the age of 45 years. It is not yet clear what the explanation is for this finding. It may be due to an absence of affected older people because of death, emigration or institutionalisation or due to older persons forgetting their symptoms or being less willing to disclose them. There is also the possibility that there has been a true historical increase in neurotic disorders over the last 50 years. If so, then the current generation of 44 years of age and under will report even higher lifetime rates as they age.

Surprisingly, racial differences were small and non-significant. For most disorders in all five sites, rates were no higher in blacks than non-blacks. Rates were higher in blacks for simple phobias in two of the five sites. For psychiatric disorders as a whole, an inner-city environment was associated with higher lifetime rates, but this did not apply to any of the neurotic disorders studied. In fact the rate for panic disorder was significantly higher in a rural setting. In general, higher levels of education were associated with lower levels of disorder but this was most marked for non-neurotic disorders.

The National Psychiatric Morbidity Household Survey (NPMS)

This is the largest study carried out in the UK and the results are just being published (Jenkins et al 1997).

The sampling frame was approximately 13 000 adults, of whom 79.4% were successfully interviewed ($n = 10\,108$). The instrument used was the Clinical Interview Schedule (CIS-R) (see Table 17.2). One adult (age 16–44) in each household was interviewed at home by an experienced Office of Population Censuses and Surveys Interviewer. ICD-10 diagnosis were determined by using an explicit hierarchy. Depressive episode trumps obsessive–compulsive disorder and panic, which trump generalised anxiety disorder and social phobia, all of which trump specific phobic. Rates for both hierarchical symptoms have been published. The study was carried out in England, Scotland and Wales.

Neurotic symptoms The threshold scale for the CIS-R is 12 and 16% of the sample scored 12 or above. Details of 14 neurotic symptoms are given in Table 17.6. All symptoms are common in women, with fatigue being the most common. Surprising findings are the low rates of physical health worries and of phobias.

Neurotic disorder The CIS-R gives prevalences covering a 1 week period so comparisons are complex; details are given in Tables 17.7 and 17.8. The overall prevalence of any neurotic disorder is 19.5%, with non-specific neurotic disorder (synonymous with ICD-10 mixed anxiety depressive disorder) the most common, generalised anxiety disorder is next and then depressive episode. Depressive episode included all ICD-10 codes F32 to F32.2. Because diagnoses were determined on a hierarchical basis, data on comorbidity is lost and lower prevalence rates are reported.

The National Comorbidity Survey (USA)

This study, the NCS, was a congressionally mandated survey to study the comorbidity of substance use disor-

Table 17.6   Prevalence of neurotic symptoms in the UK from the National Psychiatric Morbidity Household Survey (NPMS) 1997

Symptom	Male %	Female %
Fatigue	20	33
Sleep problems	20	20
Irritability	18	21
Worry	16	24
Depression	8	12
Depressive ideas	7	12
Anxiety	8	12
Obsessions	7	13
Lost concentration	6	10
Somatic symptoms	5	10
Compulsions	5	8
Phobias	3	7
Physical health worries	4	5
Panic	2	3

Table 17.7   Prevalence of neurotic disorders in the UK from the National Psychiatric Morbidity Household Survey (NPMS) 1997

Diagnostic category	Women %	Men %	All %
Non-specific neurotic disorder	9.9	5.4	7.7
Generalised anxiety disorder	3.4	2.8	3.1
Depressive episodes	2.5	1.7	2.1
All phobias	1.4	0.7	1.1
Obsessive–compulsive disorder	1.5	0.9	1.2
Panic disorder	0.9	0.8	0.8
Any neurotic disorder	19.5	17.3	16.0

These are 1 week prevalence figures. Non-specific neurotic disorder corresponds to the ICD-10 mixed anxiety depressive category.

Table 17.8 The 1 week prevalence of neurotic disorders by gender and age: from the National Psychiatric Household Morbidity Survey (NPMS) 1997

Group	n	Prevalence %
Male	4859	12.3
Female	4933	19.5
Age (years)		
16–24	1871	15.0
25–39	496	16.6
40–54	2878	17.0
55–64	1547	13.7

ders and non-substance psychotic disorders in the USA. It was designed to build on the data produced by the ECA study, over which it has several advances. It generated DSM-IIIR rather than DSM-III diagnoses. It allows some comparisons between DSM-IV and ICD-10. It was designed to generate both prevalence and incidence figures and risk factors for disorders. It was a national study carried out in 48 of the 52 states. Details of this study are given in Table 17.9. I will report on some of the other findings in the next sections.

As already mentioned, comparisons with the UK NPMS are difficult. As well as taking into account 1 week versus 12 months prevalence the individual disorder prevalences in this study markedly exceed the prevalence of having any disorders. This indicates considerable comorbidity. If all lifetimes prevalences are summed the total is 102%. This means that of the 40% of the US population who have a mental disorder at some point in their life, the mean number of disorders they suffer from is actually 2.1.

The sampling frame was persons aged 15–54, the sample 8098 and the response rate 82.6%. The survey was carried out between 1990 and 1992 and publications began appearing in 1994 (Kessler et al 1994, Wittchen et al 1994). The instrument used was the UM-C1D1 (see Table 17.2) but diagnosis of schizophrenia and other non-affective psychoses were established by clinical reinterviews. Table 17.9 gives lifetime and 12 month rates from this study.

Neurosis in general practice

Shepherd et al (1966) found that 8.9% of patients on a general practitioner's list consulted in 1 year with a diagnosis of neurosis (11.7% for women and 5.6% for men), and that neuroses formed 63% of all psychiatric cases seen in general practice, whereas psychoses and character disorders formed only 4% each. This is in contrast to the approximate figures for outpatient referrals where neuroses account for 40%, character disorders 35% and psychoses 25%. Cooper (1972) studied eight general practices in the London area and found that depression and anxiety neuroses accounted for approximately 80% of all psychiatric cases. Most showed a mixed picture, and specific neurotic syndromes such as phobias, obsessions and hypochondriases were rare, accounting for only 2.8% of cases.

Outcome

In a study of non-psychotic illness presenting to general practitioners Mann et al (1981) found that after 1 year 24% had improved, 52% showed a variable course through the year and 25% a chronic course. Good out-

Table 17.9 The National Comorbidity Study (USA): lifetime and 12 month prevalence of DSM-IIIR disorders

Disorder	Male		Female	
	Lifetime (%)	12 months (%)	Lifetime (%)	12 months (%)
Anxiety disorders				
Panic disorder	2.0	1.3	5.0	3.2
Agoraphobia without panic disorder	3.5	1.7	7.0	3.8
Social phobia	11.1	6.6	15.5	9.1
Simple phobia	6.7	4.4	15.7	13.2
Generalised anxiety disorder	3.6	2.0	6.6	4.3
Any anxiety disorder	19.2	4.4	15.7	13.2
Other disorders (for comparison)				
Major depressive disorder	12.7	7.7	21.3	12.9
Non-affective psychosis	0.6	0.5	0.8	0.6
Any disorder	48.7	27.7	47.3	31.2

come was associated primarily with the patient having a stable, supportive family life. Being younger, male, without physical illness and not receiving psychotropic medication were also significant factors.

A chronic course was associated with being older, having more psychiatric disturbance at onset, having concomitant physical illness and receiving psychotropic medication. Social measures and severity of illness rather than type of neurosis or personality assessment appeared to be the most effective means of predicting outcome. A study by Huxley et al (1979) of psychiatric outpatient practice showed similar percentage figures for improvement and also found the best predictor of final outcome to be the initial severity of a neurotic illness rather than any particular diagnosis.

Life events

It may seem self-evident that major happenings in a person's life, especially stressful events and losses, will predispose them to neurotic illness. In fact this area has only been looked at in a systematic way over the past 25 years and it has proved exceedingly difficult to define causal relationships between life events and the onset of illness.

Much of the work has been on depressed patients, particularly depressed women. Life events, usually loss events, have been shown to cluster before the onset of depressive episodes. Occurrences such as increasing arguments with a spouse, marital separation, starting a new type of work, departure from home of a family member, severe illness and illness or death of a family member are classed as life events. The sociologist George Brown has proposed that three factors operate: what he call *vulnerability factors, long-term difficulties* and *provoking agents*. He has isolated four such influences. Three of them are long-term difficulties: having three or more children who are under the age of 14 years; being unemployed; and lacking an intimate or confiding relationship with a spouse or boyfriend. The fourth is a vulnerability factor: loss of the mother before the age of 11 years. Such long-term difficulties and vulnerability factors do not in themselves cause depression but make the onset of a depressive episode more likely in the presence of a provoking factor, particularly a life event causing loss.

Life event research is difficult and requires meticulous methodology. It is often hard to define a clear-cut onset of a neurotic episode or a well-defined exacerbation. So far most research has been retrospective and therefore subject to errors of omission, distortion and falsification. It is also difficult to decide whether events that do occur are independent of the patient's mental condition or related to it in some way. In other words,

are events causes or consequences of illness? For example, if an executive loses his job and then becomes depressed, what is the direction of causality? Did losing his job precipitate a depression or did the insidious onset of depressive symptoms cause him to function poorly at work, resulting in his dismissal? In much of Brown's work, events are only counted if they are clearly independent of the illness.

Cooper & Sylph (1973) looked at the relationship of life events to the onset of new episodes of neurotic illness in general practice. They found an increase in the total number of events in the 3 months prior to onset when cases were compared with controls, with a marked tendency for events to cluster in the weeks immediately prior to consultation. The type of event reported also differed between the two – cases reporting more unexpected crises and more failures to attain life goals. Only a quarter of cases reported no events at all.

It may be that, whereas major events or multiple events can provoke neurotic illness in previously stable individuals, minor events have a small contributory effect which becomes decisive only when the risk of breakdown is already great because of lack of social supports, personality variables or both. It is still to be established whether life events precipitate the onset of illness or precipitate the decision to seek medical help. What evidence there is suggests the former.

Much of the criticism of life event research has been directed towards the methodology involved. What is perhaps more important to the clinician is the power of life events to precipitate illness. Though 85% of depressions are preceded by life events, there is a sizeable minority where no events are detected. Conversely, the majority of events (90%) are not followed by illness. The term *relative risk* of an event (the rate of disease among those exposed to the event in question divided by the rate amongst those not exposed) is a measure of the power of the event to cause illness. Using this index and counting any exit event in the previous 6 months, Paykel (1978) found increased relative risks of 6.5 for depressive illness, 6.7 for attempted suicide and 3.9 for schizophrenia. Brown's most recent work (Brown et al 1993) has shown that a severe event involving loss is more often involved in depression, whereas an event involving danger triggers an anxiety disorder. Interestingly, he has also shown that both childhood adversity and adult lifetime adversity play a crucial role in depressive disorders but only childhood adversity plays a role in anxiety. When he looked at comorbidity he found that anxiety beginning later in a continuing depressive disorder was rare but onsets of depression in continuing anxiety disorders as mixed anxiety/depressive disorders was common.

(The role of life events and other stresses in the genetics of depressive illnesses is discussed in more detail in Chapter 14.)

Socioeconomic status

Most studies show a definite association of low social class and psychological disturbance and this holds whether the studies have been done in the community, general practice, patients referred to psychiatrists or patients admitted. In Brown's original study (Brown & Harris 1978) there was a four times greater rate of caseness amongst working-class women compared with middle-class women (23% versus 6%). In a similar Edinburgh study these social class differences only appeared for working-class women who had children (Surtees et al 1983). However, not all studies have shown this. Bebbington et al (1981) in their study in Camberwell found a non-significant difference between middle- and working-class women (11.1% versus 17.5%, respectively).

The NCS study (Kessler et al 1994) showed that rates of all disorders declined with increasing income and education and that this effect is more powerful for anxiety than for depressive disorders.

Social relationships

In a series of papers from Australia, Scott Henderson has looked at the interplay between social relationships and neurotic illness. He has produced evidence that a lack of social relationships is associated with neurotic illness and that the former probably produces the latter. It may not be the lack of such relationships that is aetiologically important, however, so much as the way they are perceived by the individual. In other words, those who view their relationships as inadequate have an increased risk of developing neurotic symptoms under conditions of adversity. Neurotic symptoms then emerge in individuals who consider themselves deficient in care, support or concern from those around them. In this sense neurotic symptoms can be seen as care-eliciting behaviour.

Housing

Several studies have shown a relationship between housing and psychiatric morbidity. As early as 1957, when the rehousing of families due to slum clearance was just beginning, it was shown that there were higher rates of 'neurosis' and of psychiatric admissions among adults living in high-rise flats when they were compared with those still living in traditional houses on the same estate. Other studies have shown similar findings and

confirmed that it appears to be the stress of living in such buildings rather than moving to them that contributes to psychiatric disorder. Studies in Newcastle and Northern Ireland (Byrne et al 1986, Blackman et al 1989) have confirmed the relationship but shown that there is probably an interaction between area of residence and type of residence. In other words, there is an additive effect of type of housing, quality of housing and the facilities and general environment of a housing estate. Platt et al (1991) studied a group of 1220 households, in Edinburgh, Glasgow and London, and housing conditions were the most powerful predictor of GHQ caseness. The families all came from areas of public housing where families with young children predominated. Despite the fact that the study was on a fairly homogeneous population, social and economic factors were still powerful predictors of psychiatric caseness. Women living in poor housing conditions (damp and mouldy dwellings), living on very low incomes, being unemployed themselves or living in a household where no one was employed, and bringing up children without the support of a partner all had higher risks of psychological disturbance.

Marriage and family

The prevalence of psychiatric disorders in both the husband and wife is greater than would be expected by chance. Most of this morbidity is neurotic illness and/or personality disorders. This could be because neurotics selectively marry other neurotics, but studies which have looked at the length of marriage and the time of onset of neurotic symptoms in the spouses of neurotic patients have found that a more important explanation is that neurotic illness in one partner creates stresses under which the spouse sooner or later breaks down. If assortative mating of neurotic individuals was the explanation for the excess of neurotic marriages, it would be expected that the recently married would show the same or greater concordance for neurosis as more long-standing marriages. This is not the case. The longer a marriage continues the more likely it is for both rather than one partner to be neurotic.

Male patients have sick wives more often than females patients have sick husbands, though it is not simply that marriage is a protective factor for men and a vulnerability factor for women. Neurotic couples spend more time alone together, are less socially integrated and have more conflict over roles than non-neurotic couples. All these factors may contribute to the onset of neurosis in the spouse.

Recently Weich et al 1997 found that social factors are most important in maintaining a disorder rather than triggering it. The most important factor was low household income, but not having a partner was independently associated with maintenance. No effects were found for ethnicity, number of children, education or occupational status.

Employment versus non-employment

There is now a confirmed relationship between unemployment and psychiatric status which applies for both men and women. Although most studies have concentrated on the unemployment status of men, there is a relationship between rates of attempted suicide and of completed suicide and unemployment in both men and women. The Edinburgh study (Surtees et al 1983) did find a relationship between psychiatric disorder and employment status for women but other studies have not found a striking relationship between paid employment and mental health for women. It is likely there is a complex interaction between many factors and that employment for women, particularly women with young children, may bring benefits in terms of social contact, extra money, variety of lifestyle and feelings of personal identity, but these may only be important if such factors are not met within their domestic role.

Culture and race

Many of the factors discussed above may not translate to different cultures. Most of the studies have been carried out not just in western but in northern European populations. One of the studies summarised in Table 17.3 carried out in rural Spain (Vasquez-Barquero et al 1987) did not show any relationship between psychiatric morbidity and unemployment, low social class or child care, though it continued to find much higher rates among women than men. It also found different patterns of symptom presentation, with much higher rates of phobic disorders and, for women, a reversal of the usually found excess of depressive as opposed to anxiety symptoms. Similar cultural variations in the ratio between presentation of depression versus anxiety have been found in another study which compared Greeks, Greek-Cypriots living in the UK and Londoners (Mavreas & Bevington 1987). It may be that cultural factors are the most powerful factors in determining which vulnerability and which stress factors increase the risk of minor psychiatric morbidity.

The NCS study in the USA (Kessler et al 1994) had some surprising results. Blacks in USA had significantly lower prevalences of affective disorder, substance use disorders and overall lifetime comorbidity. There were no disorders where either lifetime or current prevalence were significantly higher in blacks than for whites. These effects are not explained by controlling income and education. The same study found no black/white differences in the rates of anxiety disorder. In contrast the earlier ECA study had found twice the lifetime prevalence of simple phobia and agoraphobia in blacks. In contrast, the NCS found that when Hispanic and non-Hispanic whites were compared, rates were consistently higher in Hispanics except for rates of anxiety disorders.

Age

It is a commonly held view that prevalence rates increase with increasing age. However, several large studies have found quite a different pattern, with the highest prevalences in the 25–34 year age group (Wells et al 1989, Wittchen et al 1992, Kessler et al 1994). This is true for both lifetime and 12 month prevalence rates. Although age-related differences in willingness to report symptoms, forgetfulness, differential mortality and selection bias associated with age may contribute to these findings, there is increasing evidence from these studies that 'neurotic' disorders are becoming common.

Mortality

Neurosis does not cause death, but those with neuroses do appear to die prematurely. Hospitalised neurotics have about 1.5 times the risk of death of normal controls (Sims 1978). This is partly due to suicide, and partly to accidental death (which may not always be accidental). Alcoholism and drug abuse account for other deaths. Whether a neurotic mental state can precipitate a potentially fatal physical illness is still uncertain. It is possible, though, that the association of the 'type A' behaviour pattern and coronary artery disease may be an example of this. Type A behaviour is characterised by striving, an intense commitment to vocational goals, impatience and ambition. More relaxed people who do not display these goals are labelled as type B. A recent study followed up 3302 patients from Stockholm County, Sweden. These patients had all been discharged with a diagnosis of anxiety disorder between 1973 and 1986 (Allgulander & Lavori 1991). They found a definite excess mortality with a ratio of observed:expected deaths among men of 2.21 and among women of 2.45. This excess was nearly all due to suicide. Lower rates of death from other causes such as malignancy and cardiovascular disorders were found but this may have been because of the strong influence of premature death by unnatural causes and the relatively short follow-up period. An interesting subsidiary finding of the study was the lack of any influence of drug treatment. Within the sample just over 500 patients had been treated in units with an express policy of not prescribing anxiolytic drugs. They were compared with a similar-sized group who were treated in units with a more positive attitude and practice of anxiolytic drug therapy. No differences in mortality were found. The authors concluded that the risk of suicide for patients with anxiety disorders severe enough to warrant admission may be as high as patients with depressive illness who require inpatient care.

Physiological factors

It is well established that increase in heart rate, increase in forearm blood flow, decrease in finger pulse volume, decrease in salivation and augmentation of sweat gland and electromyogram (EMG) activity are physiological responses associated with arousal. The electroencephalogram (EEG) shows a more alert pattern, with diminished α and increased β activity. These changes occur in aroused individuals whether or not arousal is accompanied by anxiety and there are no physiological changes which are pathognomonic of anxiety. One possible exception is the different pattern of habituation of the galvanic skin response (GSR) to a standard stimulus in patients with thyrotoxicosis and with anxiety states. Both groups are aroused but the thyrotoxic group show a normal habituation pattern, whereas in anxiety states increased arousal is associated with decreased habituation. It has also been shown that an intravenous infusion of sodium lactate produces attacks of panic much more frequently in patients with a diagnosis of anxiety disorder than in controls. Infusions of glucose or normal saline do not have this effect. (This phenomenon is discussed more fully under the heading 'Panic disorder'.)

Childhood behaviour and adult neurosis

The relationship between behaviours in childhood and neurotic illness in adult life has been reviewed by Rutter (1972). He concluded that, although there was some continuity between child and adult neurosis, most neurotic children become normal adults and most neurotic adults develop their neurosis in adult life. Most of the evidence of a positive relationship comes from retrospective assessments of adult neurotic populations, and even when these are compared with carefully matched controls the possibility of retrospective distortion makes firm conclusions difficult to draw. Robins (1966) followed up a group of 5000 child psychiatric patients for a 30 year period and compared them with a matched control group of 100 normal children. She found that most of the children who were referred for neurotic problems did not suffer from neurosis as adults and that those adults who did show neurotic symptoms were just

as likely to have been in the control group as children as in the child psychiatric clinic group. Mellsop (1972) followed up a group of 3000 children who had presented to an Australian child psychiatric clinic 20 years earlier. He found that child psychiatric patients were three times as likely as controls to receive psychiatric treatment as adults but that there was little correlation between particular symptom patterns in childhood and adult life.

One interesting and consistent finding is that, whereas in adults there is a preponderance of females with neurosis, in children there is an excess of boys. This change in sex distribution takes place during adolescence. Its significance is not clear. It may be that adult female neurotics are more likely to seek and accept treatment from doctors than their male counterparts, or that neurotic symptoms evaporate during adolescence in males, or that males cope with stresses and anxieties with different behaviours such as alcohol and drug abuse in adult life. The so-called 'neurotic traits' of childhood, such as thumb sucking, nail biting, food fads, stammering and bed wetting, seem to have little association with either childhood or adult neurosis. These are all quite common phenomena and are usually not indicative of maladjustment or psychiatric disorder.

So far only the relationship between child and adult neurosis has been considered. Very little is known about other childhood behaviours or personality traits in children that may be associated with adult neurosis, and there is a need for prospective developmental studies continuing into adult life. One exception to this is a small study by Wolff & Chick (1980) who followed up a group of 22 young men diagnosed in childhood as having schizoid personalities. Ten years later, 18 out of 22 were still diagnosed as schizoid, compared with only one out of 22 controls. Clearly, there was still something distinctive about these formerly diagnosed schizoid individuals despite the vicissitudes of the intervening years from childhood to adulthood. Studies which have looked at non-neurotic adult populations who are high achievers, such as top-grade jet fighter pilots, show that there is an excess of first-born children, and that such people tend to have had unusually close father–son relationships.

SPECIFIC NEUROTIC SYNDROMES

Classification: ICD-10 and DSM-IV

ICD-10 represents a considerable change from ICD-9. Unlike DSM-IV the term neurosis is retained but only to cover the whole group of syndromes, viz. 'neurotic, stress-related and somatisation disorders'. Individual syndromes are referred to as disorder, so generalised anxiety neurosis became generalised anxiety disorder. Several new terms are introduced, most derived from DSM-III; these include panic disorder and somatisation disorder. The term neurasthenia is retained but it is recognised that in many, if not most, countries such cases would be diagnosed as depressive or anxiety disorder.

Table 17.10 compares the classification of pathological anxiety as described by ICD-10 and DSM-IV. There seems to be agreement that panic disorder justifies separate status but ICD-10 has not taken the view that panic disorder should take precedence in a hierarchical sense over agoraphobia and that the latter should become a subtype of panic disorder. ICD-10 keeps obsessive–compulsive disorder as a separate category of neurosis but DSM-IV includes it under the anxiety disorders. A new category of organic anxiety syndrome has also been included in DSM-IV. Organic factors include such stimulants as amphetamine-containing products and caffeine. This parallels the similar category in DSM-IV of organic affective syndrome.

Both ICD-10 and DSM-IV include the category of generalised anxiety disorder. This is a residual category for patients with anxiety symptoms but no panic or agoraphobic symptoms. The DSM-IV criteria are stricter than those of DSM-III and of DSM-IIIR.

Panic disorders

This syndrome was first given separate status by DSM-III, and ICD-10 also has a separate category of panic disorder subtitled 'episodic anxiety'. The decision is still a controversial one and the boundaries between panic disorder and generalised anxiety disorder and panic disorder and agoraphobia are by no means clear.

Clinical picture

The essential features are recurrent attacks of severe anxiety (panic) which are not restricted to any particular situation or set of circumstances and are therefore unpredictable. The dominant symptoms vary from individual to individual, but include the sudden onset of palpitations, sweating, trembling and feelings of unreality (depersonalisation and/or derealisation). There is almost always a secondary fear of dying, losing control or going mad. Typically, individual attacks last only for a few minutes, though they may last longer.

A common complication is the development of anticipatory fear of helplessness or loss of control during a panic attack, so that the individual may become reluctant to be alone or in public places away from home. Similarly, a panic attack occurring in a specific situation – e.g. on a bus – may lead to the development of a specific phobia of that setting. Panic disorder may in this way result in the development of agoraphobia or specific phobias.

When taking the history it is important to ask about subthreshold or limited symptom panic attacks. As well as full-blown episodes, patients may have near-panic attacks which do not quite meet the full criteria but may still be markedly handicapping and lead to definite avoidance.

Table 17.10	Anxiety disorder as classified by ICD-10 and DSM-IV			
	ICD-10		**DSM-IV**	
F40.0	Agoraphobia without panic			
	with panic	300.01	Panic disorder without agoraphobia	
		300.21	Panic disorder with agoraphobia	
		300.22	Agoraphobia without panic	
F41	Panic disorder (classified under other anxiety disorder)			
F40.1	Social phobia	300.29	Social phobia	
F40.2	Specific phobia	300.25	Specific phobia	
F41.1	Generalised anxiety disorder	300.02	Generalised anxiety disorder	
F41.2	Mixed anxiety and depressive disorder	293.01	Anxiety disorder due to medical condition	
F41.3	Other mixed anxiety disorders	291.292	Substance abuse anxiety disorder	
F41.9	Anxiety disorder NOS	300.03	OCD, 309.81 PTSD and 308.3 acute stress disorder also included	

NOS, not otherwise specified; OCD, obsessive–compulsive disorder; PTSD, post-traumatic stress disorder.

Why some patients have one limited symptom attack and then develop severe phobic avoidance, while others can have repeated severe spontaneous attacks and continue to function, remains unexplained.

Garssen et al (1996) monitored a total of 1276 panic attacks in 94 patients. They identified four types of attack: situational expected and unexpected, non-situational expected and unexpected. Surprisingly 50% of attacks were situational and expected whereas only 17% were the typical spontaneous (non-situational and unexpected) attacks which are emphasised as characteristic in much panic disorder literature. They also commented on the frequency and severity of preattack symptomatology weakening the concept of the suddenness of the onset of panic attacks.

Agoraphobia without panic disorders In a detailed examination of a cohort of such cases, Goisman et al (1995) found the majority of sufferers did have limited symptom attacks, and/or situational panic attacks, and nearly all had catastrophic cognitions which were very similar to subjects with full panic disorder.

Diagnostic guidelines

DSM-IV requires the occurrence of at least three panic attacks within a 3 week period, in circumstances where there is no objective danger, whereas ICD-10 requires 'several' severe attacks of autonomic anxiety in a period of about a month. The same clinical picture occurring during marked physical exertion or during a life-threatening situation is not regarded as a panic attack. There is also a requirement that the individual must be relatively free of anxiety between attacks, though phobic avoidance secondary to the attacks may be quite marked. If the patient has extensive depressive symptomatology around the time the attacks start, or if there is a history of recurrent depressive disorder, then it is likely that the panic attacks are symptomatic of a depressive illness and this diagnosis should take precedence.

Epidemiology

Figures from the ECA study show consistent findings across the five sites, with a 6 month prevalence of DSM-III panic disorder of between 0.6 and 1.0 per 100 of the population. The rates are slightly higher in women, and there is no strong relationship with race, education or age. The age range 25–44 years was the highest period of risk and the rates were generally lower in persons over the age of 65 years. These findings support earlier data. The 1975 New Haven study found a current prevalence rate for panic disorder of 0.4 per 100. In this study 17% of the subjects with panic disorder had at some time in

their life had a diagnosis of some other anxiety disorder. The New Haven study also showed that only about one-quarter of subjects with any current anxiety disorder had received treatment specifically for that disorder in the past year, though in fact they were high utilisers of health facilities for non-psychiatric reasons. In particular, subjects with panic disorders were the highest users of psychotropic drugs, especially minor tranquillisers. The 1979 National Survey of Psychotherapeutic Drug Use (Uhlenhuth et al 1983) used different diagnostic groupings and agoraphobia and panic were considered together. Annual prevalence rates were 0.5 per 100 for males and 1.8 per 100 for females, giving a total of 1.2%. Again, use of antianxiety agents was highest in the agoraphobic-panic group.

Weissman et al (1997) examined lifetime prevalence rates for panic disorder from community studies in 10 countries around the world. Rates were reasonably consistent, from 1.4% in Edmonton, Canada to 2.9% in Florence, Italy. Taiwan, with a very low rate of 0.4%, was an outlier but rates of most psychiatric disorders are significantly lower in Taiwan.

Goldstein et al (1997) looked at familial aggregation in panic disorder comparing early (before age 20) and late (after age 20) onset. There was a much greater tendency for early onset panic disorder to run in families, with a 17-fold increase in first-degree relatives. This compared with a sixfold increase in late onset cases.

Family studies

There is increasing evidence of a familial transmission of panic disorder. Crowe et al (1983) found a morbidity risk for panic disorder in the first-degree relatives of panic disorder patients of 17.3% definite and an additional 7.4% probable. These rates were significantly higher than control relatives at 1.8 and 0.4%. The risk of panic disorder was twice as high in female as in male subjects. The rate of generalised anxiety disorder was the same in both groups of families and no other psychiatric disorders were increased in the families of patients with panic disorder. These findings are from a family study and represent an unselected population, suggesting that the sex ratio is characteristic of the disorder and not a result of selection bias. The finding of no excess of relatives with generalised anxiety disorder, alcoholism or primary depression supports the separation of panic from other disorders by DSM-IV and ICD-10.

Biological aspects

Since 1967 it has been known that the intravenous infusion of 0.5 mol/l sodium lactate induces clinical panic attacks in some individuals. Recently there has been renewed interest in this area because of the finding that patients with panic disorder, but not normal controls, become panicky with sodium lactate infusion. The mechanism of this effect is unclear. It has been suggested that it may be secondary to hypocalcaemia, the induction of metabolic alkalosis, peripheral catecholamine release and/or central noradrenergic stimulation. It has also recently been demonstrated that breathing carbon dioxide produces panic in clinically vulnerable patients and does so with about the same frequency as sodium lactate. Both lactate and carbon dioxide increase cerebral blood flow and it has been postulated that there may be a hypersensitivity of the 'suffocation alarm mechanism' to rising levels of carbon dioxide and that central chemoreceptor hypersensitivity may explain panic induced both by carbon dioxide and by lactate (Fig. 17.1). At present there is no definitive hypothesis for this phenomenon but it seems more likely that it is a centrally induced experience rather than one due to peripheral catecholamine effects, depression of ionised calcium or induction of metabolic alkalosis.

Clinically, the importance of this phenomenon is that it provides further evidence of a biological susceptibility to panic attacks in some individuals.

Reiman and his group in St Louis, using positron emission tomography (PET), have found abnormalities in the right parahippocampal area of panic disorder patients vulnerable to lactate-induced panic. They have observed asymmetry in blood flow, blood volume and oxygen metabolism suggestive of abnormal increases in the right side. These are the first documented brain changes in such patients. They may represent an increase in neuronal activity or a relative or absolute increase in permeability of the blood–brain barrier in that area. The changes were observed in the basal non-panic state. The parahippocampal area receives input from all sensory modalities and has efferent connections to the septum, amygdala, hypothalamus and brainstem. These connections suggest that it functions to integrate sensory information and could initiate complex behavioural responses, especially those of a defensive nature (Reiman et al 1986).

Ambulatory monitoring of patients with panic disorder has shown that panic attacks are accompanied by an abrupt increase in heart rate of approximately 40 beats per minute and that these changes begin 4–5 minutes after the onset of a panic attack and last about 20 minutes.

Klein (1993) has postulated a broader theory than just carbon dioxide hypersensitivity and suggests that many asphyxia-relevant cues may trigger panic and that many clinical observations can be explained by such a theory. Dyspnoea is a central feature of panic but not of

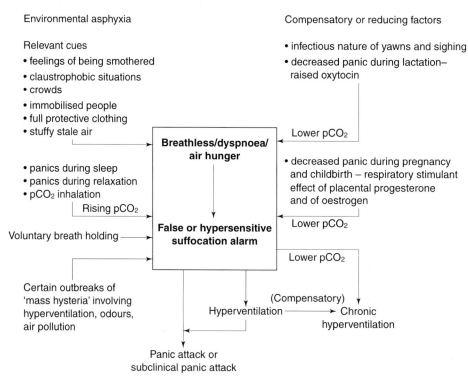

Fig. 17.1 Central role of suffocation alarm in panic attacks.

a fearful reaction to danger or of generalised anxiety disorder. Breathlessness is seen as a preliminary phase of panic, initiating hyperventilation rather than being caused by it, such as panic attacks occurring during sleep or relaxation, the increase in panic attacks in late luteal phase dysphonic disorder and the decrease of panic attacks during pregnancy, delivery and lactation.

Neurotransmitters

Functioning of the noradrenergic, serotonergic and γ-aminobutyric acid (GABAergic) systems have all been found in panic disorder. Some studies have implicated α_2-adrenoreceptor function. Serotonergic reuptake blockers such as fluvoxamine and fluoxetine appear to be effective antipanic agents, whereas serotonin (5-HT) receptor agonists such as ritanserin are ineffective or may even exacerbate panic symptoms. It has also been found that there is enhanced nocturnal production of melatonin in panic patients and that this disappears with antipanic drug treatment. 5-HT is the direct precursor of melatonin and this study provides further evidence of the role of 5-HT in panic. At present it is difficult to see how all the above biological and neuroendorine abnormalities are linked; many changes have been found but there is no coherent neurobiological view of panic disorder.

Treatment

Drug treatment A similar confusion is mirrored in the treatment for panic disorder. Many drugs with quite different properties all appear to be effective antipanic agents.

Benzodiazepines do reduce the frequency of panic attacks but they have to be given in relatively high doses. Clinically they appear to work quite quickly, reducing the frequency of attacks within a week. Alprazolam has developed a reputation as an antipanic drug, particularly in the USA, but there is no reason to suppose that it has a more powerful antipanic action than other benzodiazepines given in high dosage. Given that these drugs appear only to suppress panic attacks, and therefore need to be given over long periods, the risk of dependency is high and benzodiazepine drug treatment is not the treatment of choice.

Antidepressants Imipramine, phenelzine and clomipramine have all been shown to be effective in the treatment of panic disorder. At present it is not possible to say which, if any, of these drugs is superior, or that they have any differential effects on the syndrome. The largest study, by Klein et al (1980), compared imipramine with placebo, and in addition all patients received either behaviour therapy or supportive thera-

py. Imipramine was significantly better than placebo in blocking recurrence of panic attacks and the addition of either form of psychotherapy to imipramine significantly reduced the avoidance behaviour associated with the anticipation of panic.

Selective serotonin reuptake inhibitors (SSRIs) are effective in panic disorder. Several different drugs in this group have been shown to be effective and as yet there is little to choose between them. They are probably better tolerated than tricyclic antidepressants but, as with all drug treatments, the evidence appears to be that panic attacks are reduced or suppressed while the drug is being taken but return when the drugs are discontinued. What evidence there is suggests that antidepressant drugs should be given in full antidepressant doses, that their antipanic effects develop over 2–3 weeks and that the effects are independent of initial levels of depression. With regard to SSRI drugs there is some evidence of a biphasic response, with the panic attacks and background anxiety somewhat increasing in the first week of treatment before subsequent reduction.

Psychological treatment The key ingredient to psychological treatment is exposure, particularly if the panic is situational and/or includes phobic avoidance. Many patients are helped by breathing exercises and can easily learn to control the hyperventilation which is associated with most panic attacks. Cognitive therapy appears to be effective with the patient being taught the bodily sensations associated with panic attacks. The cognitive theory of panic predicts that panic disorder patients are more likely to interpret bodily sensations in a catastrophic fashion and that this interpretation leads to anxiety, which leads to further somatic symptoms. The patient then gets into a downward spiral of increasing panic. If the patient can learn to recognise the early signs of a panic attack and to reassign these symptoms to a less stressful cause then panic attacks may be aborted.

Generalised anxiety disorder (GAD)

Now that both DSM-IV and ICD-10 have separated panic disorders from anxiety states, generalised anxiety disorder has become a residual category containing patients who have anxiety symptoms without panic attacks, agoraphobia or other marked phobic symptoms. What used to be called anxiety neurosis has now become a much narrower concept. Much of the research in this area carried out before 1980 relates to the older, wider definition and studies of patients with anxiety states or anxiety neurosis, which included patients with panic attacks and significant phobic symptoms. Even before DSM-III, most classifications separated anxiety neurosis from phobias despite the large areas of overlap. The majority of patients with phobias have some degree of generalised anxiety and many with anxiety states find that their anxiety wells up into panic attacks from time to time. The biggest area of overlap would appear to be with agoraphobia, which seems in many respects identical to anxiety neurosis, and the term phobic anxiety neurosis has been proposed as an alternative to agoraphobia. The rest of the phobias are sufficiently distinct on clinical, prognostic and therapeutic grounds to justify separate diagnostic categories.

The second problem is the relationship between normal and abnormal anxiety. Anxiety disorder is not synonymous with anxiousness, which is a symptom rather than a syndrome. Anxiety symptoms and attacks can occur as a part of any psychiatric illness. It is only when they occur in the absence of other significant psychiatric symptoms that a diagnosis of anxiety disorder should be made. The third problem is the differentiation of anxiety states from minor depressive disorders and this is dealt with later in this chapter.

In 1869 an American physician, Beard, described the condition of *neurasthenia* or nervous exhaustion. It was a global term probably more inclusive than our present concept of anxiety neurosis. We owe the latter term to Freud (1894a; *Angstneurose*), who separated the syndrome of anxiety neurosis from neurasthenia in a description which has stood the test of time.

With the advent of DSM-IIIR in 1987, generalised anxiety disorder was no longer considered a residual diagnostic category. The central feature is excessive and/or unrealistic worry in areas unrelated to another Axis I disorder. Recent conceptualisations of GAD have referred to it as the 'basic anxiety disorder' because of its defining feature, namely worry or 'anxious expectation' and hyperarousal, because these reflect the basic processes of anxiety; thus one might expect to find the features of GAD in all anxiety disorders and perhaps in many mood disorders as well.

In general, GAD is associated with an earlier and more gradual age of onset than most other anxiety disorders (Brown et al 1994). This has led to the view that GAD may be conceptualised as a personality or characterological disorder which serves as a vulnerability factor for a wide range of subsequent emotional disorders. Although this gradual early onset is the most common presentation, there are a distinct subgroup with an adult onset often after a stressful life event.

Kendler et al (1992) in a large female twin pair study concluded that GAD was a modestly familial disorder; they calculated the heritability to be around 30%.

Several studies have compared the nature of worry in patients with GAD with that in non-anxious comparison groups. The differences appeared to be not in the content of the worry but in the controllability and pervasiveness of the thoughts, and that, compared with patients with other anxiety disorders, such as social phobia or panic disorder, GAD patients report worrying excessively over minor matters.

Perhaps the most interesting development has been the determination of a group of somatic symptoms associated with GAD that appear to be different to those present in other anxiety disorders. These are a group of somatic symptoms relating to motor tension, vigilance and scanning, such as restlessness, feeling keyed up and on edge, being easily fatigued, one's mind going blank, irritability and muscle tension. This has led to the diagnostic criteria in DSM-IV being much reduced so that three from six symptoms are required rather than the original six from 18 of DSM-IIIR.

The frequency with which different symptoms occur in anxiety states is listed in Table 17.11. Points worthy of note are the large and varied number of somatic symptoms and the frequency of symptoms such as chest pain, nausea/vomiting and loss of weight.

Symptom pattern

To some extent this appears to depend on where and by whom such patients are seen. The classic study of Wheeler et al (1950) using specific diagnostic criteria was carried out in a cardiologist's private practice. Only 18% of patients in that study had consulted a psychiatrist. Not surprisingly, very high rates of cardiovascular symptoms were reported. Wheeler also found that the course was usually chronic and that other psychiatric syndromes did not appear when patients were followed up. Anxiety neurotics who present to psychiatrists may be atypical. Such a group was described by Woodruff et al (1972). They found that less than half their patients had an uncomplicated anxiety neurosis and suggested that other problems, particularly secondary depression and the development of alcohol dependency, were important in bringing patients with anxiety neuroses to a psychiatrist.

Mitral valve prolapse

A number of studies have shown that up to a third of patients with anxiety disorders have structural and functional mitral valve lesions. This has led to the suggestion that this physical finding may be of aetiological importance in the development of anxiety disorders and that palpitations induced by mitral valve prolapse might lead to panic attacks. However, when a group of unselected patients with mitral valve prolapse is examined, one finds no excess of patients with anxiety symptoms. Mazza et al (1986), in a controlled study, found no dif-

Table 17.11 Symptoms of anxiety

Symptom	Psychological anxiety states (%)	Normal controls %	Symptom	Mixed anxiety states (%)	Normal controls (%)	Symptoms	Somatic anxiety states (%)	Nomal controls (%)
Attacks of nervousness	88	15	Fatigue, tiredness	75	22	Palpitations	73	17
			Restlessness	71	23			
Persisting nervousness	80	16	Irritability	69	9	Headaches	69	37
Poor concentration	54	12	Dyspnoea, choking sensations	64	14	Muscle aches, tensions	68	23
Fear of nervous breakdown	43	6	Insomnia, abdominal pain, discomfort	64	14	Sweating, flushing, chilly sensations	68	17
Fear of death or dying	42	11	Chest pain, discomfort	62	14	Dizziness, vertigo	63	10
			Fainting light-headedness	62	9	Paraesthesias	62	22
			Weakness, loss of libido	52	14	Trembling, shaking, nausea, vomiting	53	12
						Tinnitus	50	13
						Dry mouth	44	9
						Loss of weight	41	6
						Urinary frequency	42	12
						Blurred vision	40	7

Modified from Noyes et al (1980).

ference between valve prolapse patients and controls with respect to anxiety symptoms. They suggest that if any hypothesis is tenable it is that there is a group of patients suffering from anxiety disorders who develop prolapse because of the increased demands placed on their cardiovascular systems by anxiety.

Diagnostic criteria

DSM-IV requires persistent anxiety of at least 1 month's duration and at least three symptoms from a group of four categories, which are broadly labelled motor tension, autonomic hyperactivity, apprehensive expectation and problems with vigilance and scanning. ICD-10 is very similar but stipulates that symptoms should have been present on most days for several weeks on end. In DSM-IV symptoms have to be present for 6 months and at least three from a six item list of commonly associated symptoms have to be present. Finally, GAD is no longer a residual category. Patients with simple and social phobias frequently do not have generalised anxiety: but when they do, recognition of an associated GAD may have important treatment implications. Under DSM-IV it is possible to make concurrent diagnoses of phobic disorder and GAD.

Tyrer's (1984) review of the classification of anxiety suggests that a formal category of mixed states with both anxiety symptoms and other neurotic symptoms should be introduced, as anxiety–phobic states, anxiety–depression and anxiety–depersonalisation all occur commonly. Barlow et al (1986) have provided some support for this view. On examining a cohort of 108 anxiety disorder patients, they found that nearly all met the vague criteria for GAD as well as meeting criteria for panic disorder or agoraphobia, and that a group of GAD patients could not be distinguished by severity or chronicity. They suggest that the nature of the anticipatory anxiety is crucial. In other words, what are the patients worrying about? If they are worrying about their next panic attack or social encounter then this generalised anxiety can be seen as part of the panic disorder or social phobia. If, however, the focus of their apprehensive expectation is multiple life circumstances, then a separate diagnosis of GAD may be considered. They suggest that there is a group of chronic worriers who worry about all sorts of past and future events and that these events may be quite unrelated to the primary diagnosis of panic or phobic disorder. Such patients would warrant the additional diagnosis of GAD.

Differential diagnosis

Physical illnesses which produce similar symptoms include thyroid disease (particularly hyperthyroidism), parathyroid disease, phaeochromocytoma, and cardiac conditions such as angina pectoris, paroxysmal atrial tachycardia and mitral valve prolapse. This last may affect up to 5% of the population but is easily diagnosed by auscultation and ultrasound scan.

Outcome of anxiety disorders

Noyes et al (1980) followed up a group of patients with a diagnosis of 'anxiety neurosis' over a period of 6 years. They found that the diagnosis remained relatively stable and that the most common change in diagnosis was to alcoholism. About 50% of subjects had brief secondary episodes of depression. At follow-up 12% were completely symptom-free, 17% had mild symptoms with no real impairment, 39% had mild symptoms, 22% had moderate impairment and 9% had severe impairment. Thus, approximately 68% were mildly impaired or not impaired at all. Factors which predicted poor outcome were increasing age, long duration of illness so far, and lower social class.

Ronalds et al (1997) followed up a group of primary care attenders in a naturalistic study, and found that approximately half had improved at 6 month follow-up and that there were no differences between primarily depressed and primarily anxious subjects. The best predictor of outcome was a reduction in social difficulties. Other factors related to outcome were the quality of close relationships and the initial chronicity and severity of the disorder. In a longer follow-up study Ormel et al (1993) followed up primary care cases at 1 and 3.5 years. They found that, at 1 year, fewer than a third of patients with a definite disorder had recovered. Again there was no difference between anxiety and depressive disorders but there was a low rate of recovery in those with mixed anxiety depression (16%). At the second follow-up period, at 3.5 years, an additional 15% had fully recovered.

Syndromes related to anxiety disorders

Table 17.12 lists a large group of disorders, all of which are closely related to or part of anxiety disorders. There is no justification for any of these clusters of symptoms being regarded as a separate diagnostic category. A full discussion of each is beyond the scope of this book.

There has been considerable interest recently in the hyperventilation syndrome (HVS) and a good review is provided by Garssen & Rijken (1986). Respiration is characterised by an irregular sighing pattern or by rapid, shallow regular breathing. High-thoracic rather than diaphragmatic breathing is common. The syndrome is of interest because it can be provoked by voluntary respiration and because specific breathing regulation and relaxation exercises have been developed to control it.

Phobic disorders

These are a group of disorders in which anxiety is evoked only, or predominantly, in certain well-defined situations which are not inherently dangerous. Phobic anxiety is indistinguishable subjectively and physiologically from other types of anxiety and may vary in severity from mild unease to terror.

Marks (1969) gives the following classification of adult fears:
1. Normal fears
2. Abnormal fears (phobias)
   a. *Phobias of external stimuli*
      (i) Agoraphobia

Table 17.12 Syndromes synonymous with or closely related to anxiety disorders

Syndrome	Investigator
Neurasthenia	Beard (1869)
Cardiac neurosis	
Neurosis of the heart	William Osler
Irritable heart	'Da Costa (1871)'
Da Costa syndrome	
Soldier's heart (men)	Lewis
Effort syndrome (women)	Wood (1941)
Mitral valve prolapse syndrome	Wooley
Neurocirculatory asthenia	Friedländer (1918)
Disorderly action of the heart	
Hyperdynamic β-adrenergic circulatory state	Frolich (1966)
Hyperventilation syndrome (HVS)	Burns & Howell (1969)
Irritable bowel syndrome	
Irritable colon	Liss (1973)

(ii) Social phobias
(iii) Animal phobias
(iv) Miscellaneous specific phobias
 b. *Phobias of internal stimuli*
(v) Illness phobias (much overlap with hypochondriasis)
(vi) Obsessive phobias (usually classified with obsessional neurosis).

Normal fears occur in most young children and in many adults in some form. Mild fears of heights, lifts, darkness, aeroplanes, spiders, moths, mice, etc. are within cultural norms and do not usually lead to total avoidance of such objects. When fears become sufficiently intense to handicap the individual in his everyday life, then they can be said to amount to phobias.

Phobias can therefore be defined by the following four criteria:

• A fear out of proportion to the objective risks of the situation.
• The fear cannot be reasoned or explained away.
• The fear is beyond voluntary control.
• The fear leads to avoidance of the feared situation.

Phobic disorders range from isolated fears in otherwise completely healthy persons to extensive fears occurring in the presence of other psychiatric symptoms. Phobias can also be symptoms of other psychiatric disorders and when this is the case (e.g. in depressions) treatment is usually that of the underlying disorder.

Epidemiology

Phobic disorders are not commonly seen in psychiatric practice. They account for only about 3% of psychiatric outpatient referrals and Agras et al (1969) found a total prevalence of all sorts of phobias of 7.7% of the population. Only 2% of those were considered to be severely disabling, giving a 1 year period prevalence of 0.22%. In that North American community sample, the most common fears were of illness or injury, storms, animal phobias and agoraphobia, in that order. In a community survey from Zurich, Angst et al (1982) found a 1 year prevalence of all phobias, including agoraphobia of 3.0%. The ECA study found much higher rates, however. Details are given in Table 17.13. The much higher rates for Baltimore are probably due to a longer list of specific phobias being asked about in this centre.

Agoraphobia (synonym: phobic anxiety state, phobic anxiety depersonalisation)

Agoraphobia (literally fear of market places) is a misleading term. Although fear of open spaces is common

Table 17.13 Rates of phobia by sex in three sites of the ECA study (6 month prevalence)

Site	Men	Women	Total
Social phobia[a]			
Baltimore	1.7	2.6	2.2
St Louis	0.9	1.5	1.2
Simple phobia			
New Haven	3.2	6.0	4.7
Baltimore	7.3	15.7	11.8
St Louis	2.3	6.5	4.5
Agoraphobia			
New Haven	1.1	4.2	2.8
Baltimore	3.4	7.8	5.8
St Louis	0.9	4.3	2.7
Total phobia			
New Haven	3.4	8.0	5.9
Baltimore	8.5	17.5	13.4
St Louis	2.8	7.7	5.4

[a]Data not collected on social phobia for New Haven.

in this syndrome, the central features of the disorder are multiple phobic symptoms and a generalised high level of anxiety. There is considerable overlap with anxiety neurosis and some authors have suggested that the two syndromes should be combined. Pragmatically, a diagnosis of anxiety neurosis is made when symptoms of generalised or free-floating anxiety appear to predominate over phobic symptoms, and a diagnosis of phobic anxiety state when the converse is true.

The main fears are of open spaces, closed spaces, shopping, crowds, travelling on buses or trains and of social situations. In clinical practice it is more common than all other phobias put together. Women comprise 75% of sufferers, the symptoms usually developing between the late teens and the mid-30s. There is often much generalisation from specific phobias to other situations. Associated symptoms such as dizziness, depersonalisation, panic attacks and depression are common. Sufferers tend to be somewhat introverted and score highly on neuroticism questionnaires. The condition is probably much more common than the frequency of clinical presentation would suggest, many sufferers not reaching treatment. Agras et al (1969) found the prevalence to be 6.3 per 1000 of the population.

There is little evidence of specific precipitating factors, though in retrospect most patients can recall some incident which they feel may have triggered their symptoms. The onset of symptoms often seems to coincide with life changes which required the assumption of adult responsibilities, such as leaving home, marriage, the birth of a child or the loss of a close maternal relationship. Such individuals tends to have exhibited marked dependency traits before the onset of symptoms. Symptoms fluctuate markedly and the course is usually prolonged. Bluglass et al (1977) found that one-third of their patients could vary within a month from being virtually housebound to being able to move around with only minimal discomfort. This study compared married agoraphobics with normal controls on a large number of measures and, surprisingly, found that they were strikingly similar in terms of domestic organisation, social relationships and symptomatology in children and husbands. On one important point agoraphobics did differ – they had a history of having more unstable home backgrounds.

Noyes et al (1986) compared the first-degree relatives of agoraphobics and panic disorder patients. The risk of panic attacks in relatives was roughly equal – 19.9% in the agoraphobic and 19.2% in the panic disorder relatives – suggestive of a common fundamental disturbance in the two disorders. There was an increased risk of agoraphobia in the relatives of agoraphobic patients but not in the relatives of panic disorder patients. This finding is consistent with the view that agoraphobia is a more severe form of panic disorder. This has been incorporated in DSM-IV where agoraphobia has been downgraded as a separate category and panic disorder is qualified as uncomplicated or complicated by limited or extensive phobic avoidance.

ICD-10 retains separate categories for agoraphobia and panic disorder.

Figure 17.2 is a flow chart for the diagnosis of phobic disorders based on avoidance.

Animal phobias

These are the rarest variety of phobia in clinical practice (though not, of course, in the general population) and the most clearly defined in their presentation. Women comprise 95% of complainants and the phobias are isolated with little generalisation. There are few other symptoms, no generalised anxiety and sufferers are not neurotic as measured by personality tests. Adult animal phobics appear to be childhood animal phobics who for some reason have not lost their fears as they grew up. Interestingly, animal phobias in children occur equally in the sexes, boys apparently losing their fears around puberty, whereas a few girls seem to maintain theirs. Despite their chronicity, animal phobias respond well to systematic desensitisation.

Social phobias

These consist of a diffuse group of fears of meeting people or of eating, drinking, blushing or behaving oddly in public. Whereas agoraphobics who are afraid of crowds are usually afraid of the mass of people around them, social phobics are more afraid of personal interactions

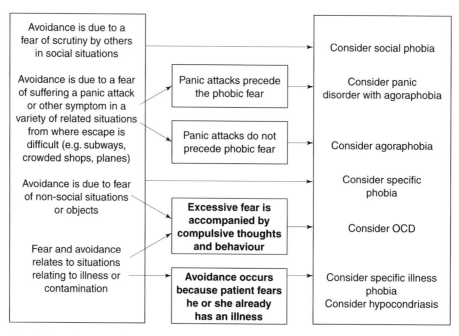

Fig. 17.2 Diagnosis of patients experiencing phobic avoidance.

in a social setting. The core features appears to be a fear of seeming ridiculous to others. Social phobics can often cope well with shopping, or travelling on buses or trains, provided they are on their own and do not meet someone they know. Unlike most other phobias the sex ratio is equal. There are usually few associated symptoms but sufferers score as neurotic and somewhat introverted on personality measures. Marked anticipatory anxiety often occurs, to the extent that performance may be impaired, thus providing apparent justification for the phobic avoidance. The onset is usually in the teens or early adulthood and rarely after the age of 30 years. The course is a continuous one and abuse of alcohol or anxiolytic drugs is a common complication. Lifetime and 12 month prevalence rates are given in Table 17.9.

The term primary social phobia is sometimes used to indicate patients who have the disorder in the absence of any other psychiatric condition. When social phobia is secondary, it is nearly always secondary to a depressive illness. Studies have shown that 20–40% of patients who develop a major depressive disorder develop some degree of social phobia while they are depressed and that these symptoms may persist long after the depressive symptoms have resolved. Secondary social phobia may be missed unless it is specifically asked about and this underlines the importance of asking about social functioning at follow-up after depressive illness.

It has been suggested that the term social phobia should be restricted to specific social fears of speaking, eating or performing in public and not include more general forms of social anxiety such as fears of initiating conversations or going to parties, this latter group being classified separately as avoidant personality disorder. At present, there is no empirical evidence for this distinction and it seems unwise to label such socially fearful patients as personality disordered. It is important to differentiate social phobia from paranoid ideation. The social phobic realises that his concerns are exaggerated and does not feel persecuted. A comprehensive review is provided by Liebowitz et al (1985).

DSM-IV subdivides social phobia into generalised and discrete (focal social phobia). This is a useful distinction and some of the differences are shown in Table 17.14. Those with focal social phobias tend to start very suddenly in the teenage years, rather than showing a gradual onset since childhood. They also have fewer associated problems such as depression or body dysmorphic disorder.

Interest in social phobia has increased over the last few years because of new drug treatments. In a study by Liebowitz et al (1988) it was suggested that phenelzine was a more effective drug treatment than the beta blocker atenolol or placebo. Gelernter et al (1991) showed cognitive behaviour therapy, phenelzine and alprazolam were all more effective than a pill placebo plus exposure treatment. Both these studies were short-term and longer-term follow-up results have not been published to date.

The largest drug study to date is of moclobemide (International Multicentre Clinical Trial Group on Moclobemide in Social Phobia 1997). Five hundred and seventy-eight patients were randomly allocated to placebo, 300 mg or 600 mg per day. Both doses were significantly better than placebo. Adverse events, except for insomnia, were not dose related, nor were there significant drug–placebo differences. Positive results in smaller studies have also been shown for sertraline and fluoxetine.

Social phobia versus social anxiety In an interesting study Stein et al 1994 conducted a telephone survey of social anxiety amongst 526 Canadian residents. They found public speaking to a large audience was the most frequently feared situation (55%), followed by speaking to a small group of familiar people (25%), dealing with people in authority (23%), attending social gatherings (14.5%), speaking to strangers or meeting new people (13.7%) and eating (7.1%) or writing (5.1%) in front of

Table 17.14 Generalised versus non-generalised social phobia		
Variable	Generalised	Non-generalised (focal or disparate)
Age at onset (years)	11	17
Marital status (% single)	64	37
Social disability	High	Low
Situation	Interactional and performance	Only performance
Comorbidity	Major depression (atypical!), alcoholism	Panic disorder
Familial	Yes	Yes

others. They then systematically modified the threshold for caseness and excluded subjects with pure public speaking phobia. The rate of 'social anxiety syndrome' in the community varied from 1.9 to 18.7%, depending on how the threshold was set. When it was set at the criteria for DSM-IIIR, the prevalence was 7.1%. Not surprisingly they concluded that the prevalence of 'social phobia' depends heavily on where the diagnostic threshold is set and that, if DSM-IIIR criteria had been applied in earlier studies, the documented prevalences of social phobia would be several times as high as currently accepted rates. They also demonstrated that social anxiety is common in the community.

Miscellaneous specific phobias

These are a group of monosymptomatic fears of specific situations such as heights, air travel, thunderstorms, darkness, etc. They can occur at any time of life. About 5% of adults have a specific fear of going to the dentist which is severe enough for them to avoid dental treatment. Other specific fears include fear of vomiting, of incontinence or of defecation. Sufferers who come to treatment are predominantly female and the course is usually continuous. There are few associated symptoms and low levels of general anxiety. Response to treatment is usually good but desensitisation may need to be prolonged.

Phobias of internal stimuli

In both illness phobias and obsessive phobias, the feared situation is internal and there is no external setting which has to be avoided to reduce anxiety. It is therefore doubtful whether this is an appropriate use of the term phobia, and illness phobias are described under hypochondriasis, and obsessive phobias under obsessional neurosis.

Aetiology

Phobias occur to certain stimuli much more frequently than to others and the age of onset varies with different types of fears. Infants are not born with fears but acquire them. These facts suggest that, at least for some phobias, humans have innate tendencies to form fearful links with some objects or situations, like snakes, spiders, the dark, and being alone or in an enclosed space, and that there may be critical times when these links are forged. It has also been suggested that these fears may have been acquired by natural selection, i.e. that they were advantageous to our distant ancestors. Little is known about why childhood fears become fixed in some people and progress into adulthood.

Natural history

Agras et al (1972) looked at the response of phobias to treatment. They found that childhood phobias were invariably improved 5 years later (40% were symptom-free and 60% improved). In adults, however, 37% were worse, 20% unchanged and 37% improved 5 years later. For childhood fears, then, the prognosis is good. For adults without treatment the prognosis appears poor and the majority of fears remain static or get worse. This is one of the few studies which has found a substantial proportion of those with a neurotic syndrome getting worse with time.

Relationship between anxiety and depression

Anxiety and depression commonly occur together and in community studies such mixed syndromes appear to be the most common type of psychiatric disorder. We must first consider whether anxiety and depression as normal human moods can be distinguished from each other. There are four basic propositions that are fundamental to an understanding of anxiety and depression as clinical symptoms:

- The fundamental or basic emotions, such as happiness, sadness, anger and fear, are differentiated psychobiological states consisting of subjective mood, psychophysiological (neuromuscular and autonomic) and behavioural components.
- Combinations and patterns of fundamental or basic emotions may occur to form stable complexes similarly distinguished from each other by mood, physiological and behavioural components.
- Normal, anxious and depressive states are differentiated complexes of fundamental emotions in which the predominant basic emotions are fear and sadness, respectively.
- Clinically, anxious and depressive symptom patterns are similar to the corresponding states in normals but are greater in intensity and more prolonged, and may in some instances have qualitatively different patterning. Simply stated, the major component of clinical anxiety is the fundamental emotion of fear, whereas the major component of depression is the fundamental emotion of sadness. However, anxiety is more than just fear, and depression is more than just sadness.

At the level of disorder at which many patients are seen in general practice it may be impossible to distinguish between anxiety and depressive disorders, either because the patient complains of both emotions equally, or because there are so few other associated symptoms that it is impossible to make a syndrome diagnosis at all.

As with the distinction between neurotic and psychotic depressions, psychiatrists can be divided into two conflicting camps on the basis of their views about the distinction between anxiety and depressive states. The separatists believe that anxiety and depressive disorders are basically discrete conditions, whereas the dimensionalists consider that no true separation exists and that a continuum from anxiety through mixed states to depression is a better working model. The validity of each view can be assessed by looking at three areas.

Clinical features

The Newcastle group headed by Roth published a series of papers supporting the view that there is a definite distinction between anxiety states and depressive disorders (Roth et al 1972). They concluded that the two syndromes could be separated on the basis of clinical features, past history and personality. Unfortunately, these studies added little weight to the separatist argument. All the patients studied were inpatients, and therefore not typical patients in whom mixed states are said to be common, and the bias of the observers towards a separatist view may have affected the recording of clinical data. Prusoff & Klerman (1974) used a self-report symptoms checklist to study female outpatients diagnosed as suffering either from anxiety neurosis or neurotic depressions. They found a large overlap of 25–40% between the two groups. They also found that depressed patients scored as more disturbed on all the subscales used except that measuring somatic symptoms. Thus, depressed patients scored themselves as more anxious than patients diagnosed as having anxiety neuroses. However, within the groups, depressed patients scored themselves as more depressed than anxious and anxious patients scored themselves as more anxious than depressed. A number of other studies have found similar extensive overlaps.

Outcome studies

The Newcastle group followed up their patients and found that those with an original diagnosis of anxiety neurosis had more persistent symptoms, particularly of anxiety, and a generally poor outcome. However, Clancy et al (1978) followed up a group of 112 patients with a clear initial diagnosis of anxiety neurosis and found that 44% subsequently suffered from clear-cut depressive episodes.

Treatment studies

An important study by Johnstone et al (1980) was based on a group of 240 neurotic outpatients. They found that depression and anxiety could not be separated either by patients' self-ratings or by ratings derived from psychiatric interviews. They compared treatment with amitriptyline, diazepam, placebo and a combination of amitriptyline and diazepam. All four groups did well, including the placebo-treated group. The added improvement due to an active drug was small and the initial severity of symptoms and the number of life events were better predictors of outcome. The only significant drug effects were for amitriptyline. The authors concluded that:

- Drugs may not be necessary for such conditions at all.
- As far as treatment is concerned a distinction between depression and anxiety is unimportant.
- If a drug is to be given, amitriptyline is preferable to benzodiazepines both in depressions and anxiety states.

Conclusions

There appears to be evidence for both points of view. Much of the confusion may have arisen because research has largely been carried out on patients who present to psychiatrists when the syndromes have reached such a degree of severity that some separation is possible. It may be that anxiety and depressive states early in their respective courses have similar symptom complexes but, as the severity of each condition increases, secondary symptoms appear which allow a distinction between the two to be made. Unfortunately, it may also be that the reverse is the case, and that anxiety and depressive disorders start as relatively discrete syndromes but that gradually chronically anxious patients become depressed and chronically depressed patients become anxious. Perhaps both conditions represent the same sort of reaction to either internal or external stress and the symptom pattern is determined by the personality structure of the individual or by the nature of the external events. Finally, it may be that anxiety and depressive states can be differentiated by age of onset, natural history or treatment outcome but that much of the symptomatology of the two conditions is similar. What is clear is that mixed states are common in general practice and in the community and that no general practitioner or psychiatrist should feel ashamed of making such a diagnosis. ICD-10 has recognised this view with a new category of mixed anxiety/depressive disorder. DSM-IV has not done so. It is also clear that pure anxiety states are uncommon in psychiatric practice compared with depressive or mixed states. See also the NPMS (Jenkins et al 1997), where non-specific disorder is the most common category (Table 21.7). Finally, if anxiety and depression coexist and drug treatment is required, antidepressant treatment is preferable to anxiolytics and the combination of the two has no advantage. A good review is provided by Stavrakaki & Vargo (1986).

Obsessive–compulsive disorder (OCD)

(synonym: obsessional neurosis, compulsive neurosis, obsessional state, psychasthenia)

The last 10 years have seen an enormous increase in the interest in this disorder and major changes have occurred in our understanding of its aetiology and treatment. Of all the disorders in this chapter, it is the one that has been most intensively investigated in the last 5 years.

Epidemiology

Until recently the prevalence of OCD in the general population was generally accepted to be low, at around 0.05%. The incidence in patients presenting to psychiatric outpatient clinics varied from 0.1 to 4% (Black 1974). The disorder was thought to begin in early adulthood (>25 years), with an onset after the age of 35 years being relatively uncommon. Data from the ECA study and other recent studies using the DIS show that OCD is much more prevalent than previously believed. The lifetime prevalence according to the ECA study ranges from 1.9 to 3.1%. This has been confirmed by other DIS studies with the exception of a study from Taiwan which showed lower prevalence rates of 0.3–0.9%. In a study from Edmonton, 6 month prevalence rates for OCD were calculated by age and sex. The authors found that the age prevalence curves were different for the two sexes. Both curves confirmed that OCD is more common in adults, but the peak for women occurs in the 24–35 year age group, whereas that for men occurs later. So far this finding has not been explained or replicated in other studies.

An interesting finding is that the lifetime prevalence of OCD by age does not show a gradual increase. One would expect that, if OCD is such a chronic disorder, cumulative prevalence would slowly increase, whereas this has not been found. One explanation is that OCD is actually getting more common and that patients in older age groups have lived through the risk period before this increase in prevalence began. Another is that patients in the older age cohorts have suffered previous episodes of OCD but have forgotten about them.

The DIS studies all show that the female to male ratio is between 1.2:1 and 2.3:1, with the exception of the Canadian study where the ratio is 1.0:1. It is clear from these studies that many patients who have significant degrees of OCD pathology do not seek treatment. As yet, similar studies using other diagnostic instruments in other cultures have not replicated these findings.

Clinical features

OCD symptoms tend to fall into one of several groups: these may be checking rituals, cleaning rituals, obsessional thoughts alone, obsessional slowness or mixed rituals. Table 17.15 summarises how frequently these patterns occur. Obsessional thoughts may have a number of different presentations. The characteristic features are as follows:

- They come repeatedly into the subject's consciousness against his will.
- They are usually unpleasant and often abhorrent.
- They are always recognised by the patient as his own thoughts, in spite of the first two features, and he often protests that his mind should function in such a silly and senseless fashion.
- They cannot be accepted as harmless and inevitable; the subject feels compelled to try and push them out of his mind and resist them.

The most common obsessions are of contamination and pathological doubting. The majority of patients have multiple thoughts, though one particular pattern may predominate at any given time. The thoughts may have a ruminative quality with a repetitive inconclusive pattern, such as 'What is the meaning of life?' or 'What is God really like?'. Other patients have fears of being unable to resist certain aggressive or sexual impulses so that they fear harming a family member, committing suicide or murdering a child. Sometimes instead of thoughts the patient is preoccupied with vivid images. These can be clearly distinguished from visual hallucinations. The patient sees clear pictures inside his head which he knows are a product of his own mind. These are often violent or sexual in nature. It is important when taking a history to ask about intrusive pictures or images as well as intrusive thoughts.

Obsessional acts or rituals (compulsions) These are repetitive actions based on obsessional thoughts. Their performance is never directly pleasurable. At most they relieve some tension and anxiety. They often have an important symbolic quality, like Lady Macbeth's hand washing.

Obsessional ritual is a better term than compulsive behaviour because the latter is a feature of all obses-

Table 17.15 Frequency of obsessive phenomena
1. Obsessive–compulsive symptoms on admission (n = 250)

Obsessions	Rate (%)	Compulsions	Rate (%)
Contamination	45	Checking	63
Pathologic doubt	42	Washing	50
Somatic	36	Counting	36
Need for symmetry	31	Need to ask or confess	31
Aggressive impulse	28	Symmetry and precision	28
Sexual Impulse	26	Hoarding	18
Other	13	Multiple compulsions	48
Multiple obsessions	60		

2. Course of illness (n = 250)

	Age of onset (years)	Type	Rate (%)	Precipitant	Rate (%)
Male	17.5±6.8	Continuous	85.0	Not present	71
Female	20.8±8.5	Deteriorative	10.0	Present	29
Total	19.8±9.6	Episodic	2.0		

sional phenomena, be they thoughts or actions. It is important to include in the definition of rituals the stipulation that they should not be inherently enjoyable. Without this it would be possible to classify some people who have urges to drink, gamble, masturbate or take drugs as obsessional, though clinically this makes little sense.

Obsessional rituals may consist of repeating, checking, cleaning, avoiding, slowness, striving for completeness, being meticulous or a mixture of these. Rituals of checking, cleaning and avoiding are the most common, each occurring in over 50% of those diagnosed. Frequently missed OCDs are a need for symmetry, exactness, hoarding, sexual imagery and obsessional praying.

Typical examples are counting up to certain predetermined numbers in order to ward off feared consequences, counting all the cracks on the pavement or all the shoes in a shop window. Such rituals may have to be performed many times until the subject is certain he has carried them out correctly. Ritual hand washing is the most common form of cleaning behaviour and is usually a response to fear of contamination. Rituals concerning personal hygiene may result in an individual taking several hours to get ready for work each morning.

It is probably a mistake to attribute a fundamental role to the concept of *resistance* so firmly stated by Aubrey Lewis in the 1930s and repeated in most textbook definitions ever since. Stern & Cobb (1978) found that 46% of their subjects showed little or no resistance to carrying out their rituals and only 30% made a great effort to resist. These authors suggest that Schneider's criterion of *recognition of senselessness* is more important than Lewis' criterion of resistance. Another important finding was that 31% of their patients performed their rituals either exclusively or predominantly in one place, and that the majority of such patients confined their rituals to home. This challenges the widely assumed view that obsessional rituals continue regardless of the environment.

Obsessional slowness Patients who exhibit this pattern are not common, representing only 3 or 4% of referred cases. These patients have to do everything in an exactly correct manner. Their whole behaviour appears to be one slow ritual. They do not repeat behaviour unless their behaviour is interrupted, in which case they may start the whole 'ritual' again. The majority of cases probably do have marked obsessional thought patterns and may be engaging in silent checking. The uniqueness of primary obsessional slowness has recently been questioned by Ratnasuriya et al (1991), who found that such patients could not readily be distinguished from other cases of OCD. Patients who did exhibit slowness nearly always did so in response to mental or overt rituals. It was of interest that 90% of such cases were male and similar high male predominance has been found for OCD cases concerned with symmetry and exactness.

Natural history

The syndrome can begin in childhood but this is unusual. It was infrequent in Rutter's series of 10- and 11-year-old children (Rutter et al 1970). Larger collections of childhood OCD cases are now being published showing an excess of boys, with long histories of symptoms before presentation often going unrecognised as disorder by either parents or child. More commonly it begins in adolescence or early adulthood and may be tolerated for many years before the sufferer seeks treatment.

The largest collection of cases so far published is from Rasmussen & Tsuang (1986). The mean age of onset was 20 years and the mean age of first seeking treatment 27.5 years. The distribution of age of onset appeared to be bimodal, with peaks at 12–14 and 20–22 years of age. Men had an earlier onset than women and only 75 of this cohort of 250 experienced an onset of symptoms after the age of 35 years.

Goodwin et al (1969) reviewed 13 studies, the results of which are summarised in Table 17.16. They show that outcome is more favourable than was thought from earlier work based on inpatient samples. The most common course for patients with symptoms so severe that hospital inpatient treatment was required was a steady one, with occasional exacerbations often related to physical illness or fatigue and with a tendency for the symptoms to gradually wane in severity over many years. Approximately 40% of outpatient samples were symptom-free at follow-up. Only 5–10% were worse and their course seemed to show a progressive decline.

The mode of onset may be acute or insidious and most studies show no clear precipitants in about 30% of cases. Depression is the most common complication but suicide is rare.

Even in outpatients the most common course is a continuous one and episodic obsessive–compulsive neurosis in the absence of an underlying affective disorder is unusual. About 10% of patients have a chronic deteriorating course. Such patients have often completely given up resisting their obsessions. Those patients with a continuous course do experience exacerbations of their symptoms at times of stressful life events. There is a tendency for patients whose illness runs a deteriorating course to be more likely to be male and to have an early age of onset. A need for symmetry or exactness also appears to predict a poor prognosis.

In a follow-up study of children and adolescents 2–7 years after diagnosis and the initiation of treatment (Leonard et al 1993) only 6% were considered to be in remission; 43% still met diagnostic criteria for OCD; 70% were still taking medication. Poor prognosis was associated with three factors:

- More severe OCD symptoms after 5 weeks of clomipramine treatment
- A lifetime history of the disorder
- Parental Axis I diagnosis.

Family history

Studies of family history are sparse. There appears to be a slight excess of first-degree relatives with depressive disorders, but no excess of relatives with anxiety or obsessive–compulsive states. Brown (1942) found a rate of OCD of 6.9% in first-degree relatives. Although a number of concordant monozygotic twin pairs have been reported, there are no systematic twin studies large enough to justify any clear conclusions.

Biological basis

There are three main areas that have contributed to our understanding of the biological basis of OCD: neuroimaging, psychometric testing and neuropharmacological studies.

PET has shown abnormalities of glucose metabolism in the orbital frontal cortex and left caudate nucleus when compared with controls. More recent evidence

Table 17.16 Outcome in obsessional neurosis			
	Condition at follow-up (%)		
Sample	No symptoms	Improved	No improvement
Inpatients only 6 studies (n = 285)	19	41	39
Mixed in- and outpatients 5 studies (n = 385)	19	34	34
Outpatients only 2 studies (n = 146)	40	26	35

Modified from Goodwin et al (1969).

shows that these abnormalities resolve with successful drug treatment. Computerised tomography (CT) has demonstrated decreased caudate nucleus size. Other studies using CT or magnetic resonance imaging (MRI) have shown more diverse abnormalities. Those regions implicated in PET studies are also areas of high serotinergic innervation. Other lines of investigation have implicated serotonin as an important factor in OCD. Low levels of platelet serotonin and cerebrospinal fluid 5-hydroxyindoleacetic acid (5-HIAA) have been found and these appear to reverse with treatment response. MCPP (a serotinergic agonist) may produce an exacerbation of symptoms, whereas metergoline (a serotinergic antagonist) produces a corresponding decrease. Treatment with a wide range of serotonin reuptake blockers has definite antiobsessional effects. All these findings point to hypersensitivity of postsynaptic serotonin receptors. Whether this is in response to low synaptic serotonin concentrations has yet to be determined but it may be that serotonin reuptake blockers exert their action by downregulating postsynaptic receptors.

Neuropsychological studies of OCD have not identified specific deficits but several studies have shown abnormalities suggestive of organic damage when compared with controls. Veale et al (1996) showed that the important cognitive deficits were those associated with frontal lobe dysfunction, such as:

- Being easily distracted by other competing stimuli.
- Excessive monitoring and checking of the response to ensure a mistake does not occur.
- When a mistake does occur, being more rigid at setting aside the main goal and planning necessary subgoals.

They concluded that there was evidence of frontostriatal dysfunction and postulated that OCD patients are less efficient at including relevant feedback, and by checking excessively are collecting too much irrelevant data in their working memory, and that increased distractability and perseveration occur as a result of diminished supervisory frontal lobe activity.

Differential diagnosis

Obsessional behaviour may occur as a normal phenomenon in all age groups. Rituals and superstitions may be less conspicuous in Western society than they used to be but in many cultures they still form a major part of life. Avoiding walking on pavement cracks, laying out toys in certain ways and rituals at bedtime are all normal behaviour in children. Though such behaviour may resemble obsessional rituals, it is different, in that children find it natural and it produces little or no distress.

Many adult obsessionals give a history of obsessional behaviour in childhood. This may be due to the universality of such phenomena, retrospective distortion, or a real relationship between the two; it is not known which. However, a history of tantrums, stealing or truancy in childhood is unusual, indicating that obsessionals may have been unusually good or quiet as children.

Relationship to depression

Obsessional phenomena and depression commonly occur together. Such depressions may be secondary to prolonged obsessional illness, coincidental with it or the primary aetiological factor. In one large series, 31% of severe depressives developed obsessional symptoms. Such patients tend to have normal premorbid personalities and when their depression is treated the obsessional symptoms subside. Their rate of attempted suicide is less than one-sixth that of depressives without obsessions. Depressive illness occurring in a person of obsessional personality may exacerbate obsessional traits to the level of symptoms. It is clear, however, that OCD is not simply a complication of depressive illness. Marks (1969) has reported depressive mood swings occurring frequently in obsessional patients before, during and after treatment and that such depressive episodes continue after successful behavioural treatment for obsessional symptoms. Millar (1980) showed that obsessionals could be differentiated from other neurotics and normals by their markedly negative, isolated and very low opinion of themselves, similar to that found in depressive states. He suggested that obsessional symptoms may represent a neurotic coping device defending against depression.

Perhaps the most powerful evidence is that in all the large recent controlled drug studies the antiobsessional effects of drugs such as fluvoxamine and fluoxetine have not been dependent on an initial level of depression, and the time course of response appears to be a steady but gradual one over 12–16 weeks. Some drugs which are effective antidepressants, such as desimipramine, appear to be ineffective antiobsessional drugs.

Relationship between obsessional fears and phobias

Phobics have fears which are irrational but which are only evoked by the phobic situation. For example, a patient with a fear of hospitals will feel relaxed and not anxious away from hospitals, though he may get anticipatory anxiety prior to a hospital visit. His behaviour would be characterised by avoidance of hospitals and he certainly would not continuously search for them. In contrast, an obsessional who says that he is phobic of dirt and disease will in fact spend much of his time scanning his environment, seeking the very features which alarm him. He will continually look for dirt even in the cleanest of environments. A further distinguising feature has been described by Marks (1969), who states that an obsessional fear is not a direct fear of an object or situation but rather of the imagined consequences thereof. Thus a person with a phobia of dogs will experience extreme anxiety at the sight of a dog, whereas an obsessional will engage in prolonged anxious concern about contamination from the dog. He is also more likely to worry about the dogs he does not see than those he does.

Organic brain disease

Obsessional symptoms can be signs of intracerebral pathology but classical obsessional symptoms are rare in organic states. The obsessional-like manifestations associated with organic brain disease are usually motor, and usually simple stereotyped movements; and often the movement precedes the compulsive thought, if any. A typical example are the OCD symptoms that occur in Sydenham's chorea, again pointing to caudate nucleus involvement.

There is an association between OCD and Gilles de la Tourette's syndrome. Between 11 and 80% of Tourette's patients have obsessional symptoms. Pedigree studies show an unusually high number of cases of Tourette's and OCD in affected families. Conversely, 20% of OCD patients suffer from tics. These findings would fit with the common involvement of the frontal lobes, corpus striatum and caudate nucleus, as suggested from the neuroimaging studies.

Treatment

Simple reassurance may be needed and may have to be given in abundance. It is important not to endorse the patient's unrealistic ideas and behaviour in any way. The chronic nature and fluctuating course of many obsessional illnesses means that long-term supportive psychotherapy is often indicated. Explorative and interpretative psychotherapy seldom help and may make ruminations worse. Offering continuing support and hope, supporting the family, and particularly the spouse, and monitoring the patient's mood for signs of depressive illness are all important aspects of management.

Special behavioural treatments

Vicarious learning or modelling   In this technique the therapist demonstrates 'fearless' behaviour by, for instance, handling 'contaminated' objects. In subsequent sessions the patient is asked to do likewise. It would appear that, in the majority of patients, modelling has little advantage over exposure alone but it may help in some cases.

Response prevention   (synonym: in vivo exposure, real-life exposure)   Observation shows that for many people the frequent performing of rituals does not relieve anxiety but rather increases it. This suggests the possibility that interrupting compulsive behaviour might be therapeutic. Control may be achieved in a variety of ways – by verbal persuasion, continuous monitoring, or engaging in alternative behaviour. Force is counterproductive: it only produces an angry uncooperative patient. Spouses and other family members may be enlisted as cotherapists. Such treatment can be relatively short (3–8 weeks) and seems to have enduring effects.

Relaxation   This does not in itself produce improvement and does not seem to be necessary for improvement during in vivo exposure. Research reports indicate that cognitive-behaviour therapy may be an effective treatment for some patients.

Other psychotherapies   There is general agreement that dynamically oriented psychotherapies are ineffective for OCD.

Antidepressants   Claims have been made for the efficacy of clomipramine in obsessional disorders over the past 10 years. Initially it was not clear whether clomipramine had a specific antiobsessional effect or whether any antidepressant would work as well. Nor was it resolved whether clomipramine primarily relieved depressive rather than obsessional symptoms. Work from Sweden by Thoren et al (1980) has clarified the problem. He and his colleagues found that clomipramine, but not nortriptyline, was significantly superior to placebo in relieving obsessional symptoms. The effect took 5 weeks to develop and could not be predicted from the severity of duration of the illness, from the sex or age of the patient, or from the presence or absence of primary or secondary depressive symptoms. They also found that obsessional symptoms returned when clomipramine was stopped. Clomipramine is a potent (serotonin) reuptake inhibitor, though its most potent active metabolite, n-desmethylclomipramine, is a noradrenaline reuptake inhibitor. Amelioration of obsessional symptoms was positively correlated with reduction of 5-HIAA cerebrospinal fluid concentrations, perhaps reflecting potent 5-HT uptake blockade. Some support for this possibility comes from Stern et al (1980), who found that outcome for obsessional behaviour was related to plasma clomipramine levels, whereas outcome for depressive symptoms was related to plasma n-desmethylclomipramine levels.

It is clear that a robust antiobsessional effect may

require more than 4 weeks to develop. Mavissakalian et al (1985) found symptomatic improvement continued throughout the 12 week trial period. It is also clear that in the absence of significant depressive symptomatology antidepressant drugs are not curative. They ameliorate symptoms and studies report 30–60% pretreatment to post-treatment reduction in symptomatology.

The newer more specific serotonin reuptake blockers, such as fluvoxamine, fluoxetine, paroxetine and sertraline, all appear to be clearly antiobsessional drugs. At present it is not possible to recommend one drug over others in the group, though the balance of evidence is that clomipramine remains the most powerful anti-OCD drug – but often it is not well tolerated because of sedation and weight gain.

Longer-term and follow-up studies following drug treatment are still needed. At present the evidence is that when drugs are discontinued the obsessional symptoms return and that this may occur even after several years of continuous treatment. It may well be that patients with severe OCD need very long-term drug treatment. A sensible clinical alternative is to gain some control over the behaviour using drugs and then to add in specific behavioural and cognitive techniques to help the patient control his behaviour.

Physical treatment Electroconvulsive treatment (ECT) is only indicated for the treatment of depression within this syndrome; there is no evidence that ECT has a specific antiobsessional effect. Severe and crippling obsessional neurosis is always quoted as one of the indications for psychosurgery, and techniques such as bimedial leucotomy, restricted orbital undercutting and stereotactic limbic leucotomy have been advocated. Reported studies are either retrospective, uncontrolled or both. They were also carried out before the advent of modern behavioural therapies. Neurosurgery should only be considered in patients with a history of several years of continuous, crippling symptoms and in whom all other treatments have failed. Postoperatively, an intensive therapy programme should be planned.

Aetiology

Neither learning theory nor psychoanalytic theory provides comprehensive explanations for obsessional phenomena.

Psychoanalytic views Freud believed that obsessional neurosis was more common in men. In his early writings he saw it as the result of early aggressive sexual trauma, obsessional symptoms being conceptualised as disguised self-reproach for some sexual act performed in childhood. Later came the idea that obsessional neurosis represented a regression to the pregenital and sadistic stage of development, obsessional neurotics being seen as individuals concerned with conflicts between aggressiveness and submissiveness, cruelty and gentleness, dirt and cleanliness, order and disorder.

Learning theory views It is clear that obsessional rituals are not simply an avoidance response to some supposed noxious stimulus, as they frequently result in increased rather than decreased anxiety. Teasdale (1974) has suggested that conflict arises because performance and non-performance of rituals have equally aversive consequences for the individual. In other words, the obsessional is constantly having to make a choice between two responses, both of which are negatively reinforced. Whichever choice the individual makes he feels anxious, and this anxiety may in a circular fashion lead to further repetitive behaviour. This may explain in part the intractable nature of obsessional rituals but it does not explain their original appearance.

Personality and OCD It has traditionally been thought that the link between obsessional personality and frank OCD is a strong one and that most patients will show previous obsessional personality traits. Recent studies have challenged this view. Although high levels of previous personality disorder have been found, only a minority have been of a DSM-IIIR compulsive type. In terms of more general personality characteristics, individuals with OCD are said to be characterised by feeling that they constantly fail to live up to perfectionistic ideals, that magic rituals can prevent catastrophies, and by having abnormally high expectations of unpleasant outcomes of events. They tend to give single events undue credence and may have deficiencies in the ability to link concepts and integrate them. The problem with these ideas is that they may be beliefs that are a result of having OCD, rather than in any way being causative.

Somatoform disorders

This section deals with a wide range of syndromes that have one central feature in common: the association of physical symptoms, which mimic physical illness, with psychological stress. For clarity each syndrome is briefly described but the separation into so many different subtypes does not necessarily imply separate or differing aetiologies. Many of these syndromes are closely related and it seems likely that common aetiological processes are involved and that symptom choice may be determined by fairly mundane factors.

Somatoform and dissociative disorders

This group of disorders includes hysterical and hypochondriacal syndromes as well as a group of other related disorders where symptoms are produced without adequate physical cause. Both DSM-III and ICD-10 have abandoned the term hysteria because of its confused and vague meanings. The term functional somatic symptoms (FSS) has also been suggested to cover this group of disorders. ICD-10 has made a clear distinction between dissociative and somatisation disorders and includes all conversion symptoms under the former.

The concept of hysteria Perhaps one of the few things that is certain in psychiatry is that no two psychiatrists can agree on what the terms hysteria and hysterical convey. As individuals we may all think we know what we mean and can recognise a hysteric when we see one. Such confidence is ill-founded.

The term hysteria is currently used in a number of different senses:

- A pattern of behaviour habitually exhibited by certain individuals who are said to be hysterical personalities or hysterical characters.
- To indicate the presence of a physical symptom (usually neurological) produced by the mental mechanism of conversion, viz. conversion hysteria or conversion reaction.
- To indicate that a similar mechanism occurs in dissociative states such as amnesias and fugues.
- As in Briquet's syndrome or 'St Louis hysteria', to describe a syndrome occurring mainly in women with multiple somatic complaints in the absence of bodily disease and running a chronic course (somatisation disorder).
- As a psychoanalytic term, 'anxiety hysteria' used to describe phobic states.
- As in 'epidemic hysteria', a term used to describe the apparently infectious spread of somatic symptoms or odd or disturbed behaviour from individual to individual.
- As a term used by doctors, both physicians and psychiatrists, to indicate that a patient, usually female, is exaggerating or simulating symptoms, or when a doctor feels manipulated by such a patient.
- As a diagnosis in general medicine when all laboratory tests and examinations have proved negative and the symptom cannot be explained.
- As a lay term to indicate the sudden onset of severe distress or tantrums in an individual.
- The term 'hysterical psychosis' is used by some authors to describe syndromes such as latah or amok which occur in specific cultures; and by others to refer to an acute psychotic syndrome, occurring mainly in women in Western cultures, starting and ending abruptly and lasting only a few days.

While the links between some of these uses are obvious, the only thing that others appear to have in common is the term hysteria or hysterical itself.

The concept of somatisation The central feature of somatisation is that symptoms are produced for which there is insufficient or no underlying physical cause. The symptoms are then used for psychological purposes or for personal gain. The broad definition includes both normal and abnormal behaviour and stresses that somatisation is a universal phenomenon.

The gains from somatisation are not mutually exclusive: one or more may operate. None of the mechanisms is exclusive to non-organic illness – all may apply to genuine illness and all of us somatise at times. The gains include:

- The displacement of unpleasant emotions into physical symptoms.
- The use of a symptom to communicate an idea or emotion symbolically, e.g. hysterical paraplegia symbolising helplessness.
- The alleviation of guilt through suffering, e.g. physical pain experienced after the death of an ambivalently regarded individual.
- To manipulate personal relationships, e.g. the spouse who says 'Not tonight dear, I've got a headache' when refusing sexual advances.
- To obtain release from duties and responsibilities, e.g. absence from work or a parental role.
- For financial gain, e.g. compensation after an accident or premature retirement on medical grounds.
- To obtain attention or sympathy.

What follows is an account of the main syndromes that have been described. Essentially, the diagnosis of all these disorders involves a value judgement made by the doctor in deciding that the individual is behaving abnormally; or that the patient is complaining too much, or too long, or complaining of pain or other symptoms without adequate justification.

Somatisation disorder

Multiple somatisation disorder (synonym: Briquet's syndrome or St Louis hysteria) In a series of papers over the past 20 years the St Louis group of Guze, Perley, Woodruff and Clayton has tried to refine and clarify one particular syndrome to which they have given the eponym 'Briquet's syndrome' after the French physician who wrote a monograph on the subject in 1859. This syndrome was included in DSM-III and is now in ICD-10 under the rather ugly title of somatisation disorder. This is a significant advance and the term somatisation disorder should be retained, partly because it separates the syndrome from hysteria and partly because the syndrome originally described by Briquet is characterised principally by multiple physical complaints in various different parts of the body and by appearing to affect different organ systems. The multiple somatic complaints are often dramatically described and almost any symptom can occur, but the most common are chest and cardiac complaints such as dyspnoea, palpitations and chest pain, followed by back and joint pains and by menstrual symptoms such as dysmenorrhoea, irregular periods, excessive bleeding and dyspareunia. Conversion symptoms can occur but they are not essential to the diagnosis. Whether the syndrome is really confined to the female sex, as the St Louis group suggest, is not yet clear.

Such patients usually present first to their general practitioner or to a physician with multiple vague complaints. It is often difficult to get a clear history of onset, or of why the patient has come for help now. These patients tend to be extensively investigated medically and surgically and there is evidence that they eventually undergo three times as many surgical operations as either sick or healthy controls. As well as their physical complaints they have psychiatric symptoms, such as nervousness, anxiety, episodes of depression, moodiness or irritability. Menstrual symptoms, sexual indifference and frigidity are said to be so characteristic that the diagnosis should be made with caution if menstrual and sexual histories are normal. Histories given to different doctors tend to show inconsistencies. It is often a pointless task to try and decide if such patients are deliberately malingering or whether their behaviour is under unconscious control. Marked depression and anxiety are frequently present and may need to be specifically treated.

Symptoms usually begin in adolescence and probably run a lifelong but fluctuating course. The picture is thus very different to conversion disorders with their sudden onset and often quite brief course. The same authors (Woerner & Guze 1968) have found that the syndrome runs in families. The prevalence in the general population of the USA was once thought to be about 1% of females but the ECA study has found a much lower figure. It occurs in about 20% of the first-degree female relatives of index cases. There is also an excess of psychopathic personality and alcoholism in first-degree male relatives. As yet there is no evidence of a true genetic transmission of this disorder, only that it runs in families. It may well be that having a mother who herself continually complained of, and sought treatment for, physical symptoms may be a potent determinant of similar behaviour in the daughter.

Multiple somatisation disorder and undifferentiated somatoform disaster The ICD-10 concept of multiple somatisation disorder is looser than the DSM-

IV category: the patient does not have to have a specific number of symptoms, nor is there a need to have the onset below a certain age. Symptoms do have to be present in the absence of an organic explanation and the essential criteria are 'at least 2 years of multiple and various physical symptoms for which no adequate physical explanation has been found'. Thus, the ICD-10 concept is likely to include a large number of cases who in DSM-IV would fall into the category of 'undifferentiated somatoform disorder'. ICD-10 has a further category of undifferentiated somatoform disorder where cases have 'less striking symptom patterns and the duration of symptoms of less than 2 years'. The validity and reliability of these concepts have yet to be tested but they probably represent a much larger group of patients than the narrower definition, particularly that of DSM-IIIR.

Differential diagnosis The duration of multiple and varying physical symptoms should be at least 2 years. There should have been many contacts with doctors and negative results from numerous investigations, often including invasive procedures and surgery.

It is important to remember that individuals with somatisation disorder have the same chance of developing genuine physical disorders as any other person of that age and they may also suffer from iatrogenic disease. Vigilance is required to ensure that such developments are not overlooked.

Depression and anxiety are common. These are usually secondary to the underlying disorder but may be severe enough to warrant separate treatment. The onset of the syndrome after the age of 40 years is unusual and particular care should be taken not to miss underlying primary affective disorders.

The disorder is differentiated from hypochondriasis because the emphasis is on the symptoms themselves and not on the underlying disease or fear of disease.

Hypochondriasis

Just as the term hysteria has multiple meanings so does the term hypochondriasis. Again the word is used both by clinicians and by the lay public and there is overlap of the meanings:

- It can mean a morbid concern with health and with protecting one's healthy status. Such people may be preoccupied with health foods, patent medicines and remedies to delay ageing and prolong life. Many such people do not complain at all of ill health. In fact they protest their healthiness, linking it to the measures they have taken to protect it.
- It can be used to describe a group of individuals who seem to pursue ill health as a way of life. They

appear to enjoy bad health, collecting new symptoms and shedding others as they progress through life.

- It can describe a conviction of the actual presence of disease or fear of developing a serious disease. It is the latter sense which forms the core of the psychiatric syndrome of hypochondriasis.

Clinical picture The essential feature is a persistent preoccupation with the possibility of having one or more serious and progressive physical disorders. This abnormal attitude to health may take the form of a phobia, an obsession, an overvalued idea (morbid preoccupation) or a delusion.

The unrealistic fear, or belief, of having a disease persists despite medical reassurance and causes impairment in social and occupational functioning. The patient interprets minor symptoms as evidence of major disease. In Kenyon's (1964) series of 512 patients seen over a 10 year period at the Maudsley Hospital with a diagnosis of hypochondriasis, the most common regions of the body involved were the head and neck, abdomen and chest, in that order. The bodily symptoms most affected were musculoskeletal, gastrointestinal and the central nervous system. Where symptoms were unilateral they were predominantly left-sided.

The hypochondriacal reaction may present as a phobia. The patient fears that at some time they may develop breast cancer, have a heart attack or a stroke. Such individuals make repeated requests for examination and reassurance. In ICD-10 these are classified as illness phobias, though few patients indulge in any avoidance behaviour. In fact there is often an obsessional quality to the presentation – for example, the patient suffering with a fear of developing acquired immune deficiency syndrome (AIDS) watching and reading more and more on the subject. Unlike the true obsessional, however, the thoughts are not usually recognised as ego alien and there is little attempt to resist them.

When hypochondriasis presents as a morbid preoccupation it must be distinguished from delusional states. The delusional forms which are usually part of a depressive or schizophrenic disorder are discussed in Chapters 13 and 14 and other delusional states described in Chapter 15.

Differential diagnosis The reader may rightly question the difference between somatisation disorder and hypochondriasis. In somatisation disorder there tends to be a preoccupation with the symptoms rather than fear of having a specific disease or diseases. The patient with hypochondriacal concern will want constant reassurance that he does not have cancer or heart disease. In contrast, the patient with somatisation disorder may never enquire at all about the pathology behind the symptoms and be concerned only with symptom relief. Clearly the overlap between hypochondriacal and hysterical syndromes is great, but is simplistic merely to regard hypochondriasis as hysteria in the male.

Kenyon (1976) in a persuasive review article recommended that the terms of hypochondria and hypochondriasis should be dropped altogether and that hypochondriacal should be retained only as a descriptive term. The great majority of hypochondriacal symptoms appear to be secondary to other disorders, particularly depressive illness, paranoid psychosis, schizophrenia and anxiety states. Neither Kenyon (1964) nor Lader & Sartorius (1968) in two large comprehensive enquiries could isolate a clear-cut primary state of hypochondriasis. In both studies the heterogeneous group of hypochondriacal states could, on close inspection, be allocated to other psychiatric syndromes, of which hypochondriasis was simply a symptom.

In Kenyon's study, primary hypochondriasis, where the admission diagnosis was one of hypochondriasis only, represented 1% of all admissions. The sex ratio was equal and the peak age range was 30–39 years. Even in this group, depression, anxiety and paranoid symptoms were common. In contrast, Pilowsky (1967) described 66 patients with primary and 88 with secondary hypochondriasis. The distinction was an important one, for at follow-up 50% of the primary group described their symptoms as unremitting or continuous, compared with only 17% of the secondary group. The latter were nearly always secondary to an affective disorder.

Unlike multiple somatisation disorder, the sex ratio in hypochondriasis is equal and there is no evidence of a familial tendency.

Psychogenic pain disorder

The complaint of severe prolonged pain which is inconsistent with anatomical patterns of innervation and for which no organic pathology or pathophysiological mechanisms can be detected is the central feature of this syndrome. Patients usually reach psychiatrists after much fruitless investigation. The onset of pain may have some temporal relationship to an emotionally stressful event, may enable the patient to avoid certain activities, and may enable them to get considerable sympathy, at least initially, from friends and relatives.

We must remember that individual pain thresholds vary greatly and that what may not seem painful to one may be very painful to another. Hence the exaggerated or dramatic complaints of pain that come from some patients with minimal organic disease. If we exclude patients in whom there could be some organic aetiology (e.g. some cases of backache), these patients seem to fall into two groups: those in whom the onset of pain precedes depressive symptoms, often by many years, and those in whom pain and depression start together (Bradley 1963). In the latter group, successful treatment with antidepressants or ECT removes both pain and depression. In the former, depression may be relieved but the pain remains, though it is often reported to be more bearable. The same study showed that the previous personality and background of such patients were notable for orderliness, obsessionality, overconscientiousness and anxiety and rigidity, but with no past history of hysterical conversion symptoms, hysterical personality traits or any evidence of gain. The course is very variable, but in some cases the complaints may persist for many years if suitably reinforced by relatives and medical attention.

Dissociative disorders

In ICD-10 this diagnosis has been much expanded to include not just amnesia and fugues but all conversion disorders in which definite physical and not just psychological symptoms are produced. The onset of these disorders is characteristically sudden, but rarely observed and associated with a traumatic life event or chronic, apparently insoluble life stresses.

Conversion and dissociative disorders are often considered together, presumably because the underlying psychogenic mechanisms are thought to be similar, in that 'conversion' occurs in both, the emotional conflict being converted into a physical symptom in one disorder and into an amnesia personality change in the other. In our present state of knowledge, it is rash to invoke such an aetiological mechanism and use it to define the syndrome. However, the term conversion disorder has been retained here because it is so commonly used.

Conversion disorders (synonym: conversion hysteria) The central feature of this syndrome is a loss or impairment of function which appears to be due to a physical cause but is in fact a manifestation of some underlying psychological conflict or need. Almost any physical symptom can be produced but the most common are those that suggest neurological disease, e.g. paralyses, aphonias, seizures, anaesthesias and paraesthesias. Other senses are often impaired, leading to apparent blindness, tunnel vision, loss of smell or deafness. The syndrome is not very common and such patients often present to neurologists rather than psychiatrists. The more dramatic forms described a century ago by Charcot are now unusual.

The syndrome should not be diagnosed just because no organic cause for the physical symptoms can be found, or because all medical investigations have been negative. Follow-up studies by Slater & Glithero (1965) and Merskey & Buhrish (1973) have both shown high rates of overt organic disease in those previously diagnosed as having conversion symptoms. Slater & Glithero studied 85 patients given a diagnosis of hysteria at the National Hospital, Queen Square. At follow-up 9 years later only 39% had no significant organic disease and some of these had received other psychiatric diagnoses such as schizophrenic and endogenous depression. Hysterical pain had been rediagnosed as trigeminal neuralgia, hysterical fits as epilepsy and bizarre paraesthesiae and weakness as Takayasu's disease. Similarly, Merskey & Buhrish examined 89 patients attending a neurology clinic and found that 67% had some organic diagnosis, and in 48% the organic pathology affected the brain. Lewis (1975) found a very different picture when psychiatric patients diagnosed as having hysteria were followed up. Out of 98 subjects 57% were well and working and in those with residual symptoms the pattern of symptomatology was similar to that when the patient was first diagnosed. Relatively few had had a change in diagnosis. Thus, it would seem that a diagnosis of hysteria, when made in a psychiatric hospital, does have some validity and that the clinical picture remains fairly uniform over time.

Conversion hysteria is characterised by the sudden onset of symptoms in clear relation to stress. *La belle indifference* is not often present and is of little diagnostic value. Lader & Sartorious (1968) found that most such patients were highly aroused and anxious. Conversion hysterics were found to be more anxious than either normal controls or patients with phobic and anxiety states. They concluded that conversion was not occurring in the classic psychoanalytic sense, or if it was it was a very imperfect mechanism. There is no definite information available on the sex ratio, but conversion symptoms clearly do occur in men. One particular symptom, globus hystericus, is apparently more common in women.

The course is most often of short duration with sudden onset and complete resolution. The syndrome while it lasts is usually incapacitating. It has recently been suggested that conversion symptoms are now beginning to be less common in non-Western countries, mirroring the gradual decline that has occurred in the West (Nandi et al 1992).

Psychogenic amnesia This uncommon syndrome consists of the sudden onset of memory impairment, usually the forgetting of important personal information. It should only be diagnosed where there is no organic cause for the symptom. The most common type is a failure to recall all events during a circumscribed period. An example might be an individual who walks away unscathed from a major road traffic accident but appears to have no memory for the events surrounding the incident. Less common is a generalised amnesia in which the individual cannot recall anything about his past life. A picture of total personal amnesia, but with preservation of cognitive skills such as reading, writing, and knowing what a telephone is and how to use it is practically diagnostic of psychogenic amnesia. Such complete memory impairment without any other cognitive deficits is very rarely caused by intracranial pathology.

Psychogenic amnesias usually begin and end suddenly. They tend to follow markedly stressful episodes, recovery is usually complete and with no residual memory impairment. Recurrence is unusual. The syndrome is probably commoner in the young. The differential diagnosis is from organic causes, alcoholic amnesia, epilepsy and postconcussional syndromes.

Psychogenic fugue   A fugue involves a travelling away from home or work during an amnesic episode. Unlike the vague wandering that may occur during a period of psychogenic amnesia, an individual's behaviour during a fugue is often purposeful. A new identity may be briefly assumed during the fugue. Such states usually last for just a few hours or at most a few days and involve limited travelling. Occasionally more dramatic pictures are seen with a fugue lasting many weeks. In an extreme case an individual may move away from home, adopt a new identity and live as such for several weeks. Again, fugues are usually precipitated by severe personal stress such as quarrels at home, or the breakup of a relationship. They may be symptomatic of alcohol misuse or depressive illness. The wandering that occurs in temporal lobe epilepsy is usually less complex and there is no tendency to assume a new identity. Recovery from fugue states is usually abrupt and complete. It is probably impossible to distinguish amnesias from conscious malingering unless the patient confesses.

Psychogenic stupor   The patient appears to be stuporose in that they lie or sit motionless for long periods but muscle tone, posture and eye movements indicate that the patient is not asleep or unconscious. The onset is sudden and stress related, unlike manic and depressive stupor which develop more slowly. There should be no evidence of trauma, alcohol or drug abuse.

Multiple personality   This syndrome is extremely rare and some doubt its existence outside literature and psychoanalysis. Essential features are the assumption of one or more new and different personalities which the individual switches into at various times. Each personality is separate from the others and appears to have no knowledge of its rivals. The assumed personality is characteristically widely different from the subject's own. Whereas fugues and amnesias are limited to a single, brief episode, multiple personality may run a prolonged course. The most dramatic cases have been described during the course of the psychoanalytic treatment. The well-published case of Kenneth Blanch, the Californian 'Hillside Strangler', who faked multiple personality and hypnosis to avoid the death penalty and completely fooled many 'expert' psychiatrists and psychologists, was a salutory lesson to supporters of this concept.

Syndromes related to somatoform and dissociative disorders

Compensation neurosis (accident neurosis)   The central feature is the seeking of financial compensation after sustaining a relatively trivial injury. The term compensation neurosis implies that the patient is not faking disability but is suffering from a mental disorder. In an influential paper Miller (1961) showed that men seeking compensation following head injury had more prolonged complaints than those with more serious injuries who were not involved in compensation and that 90% improved after the claim was settled. Claimants were characterised by being unskilled or semiskilled, employed by large impersonal corporations and usually middle aged. Miller's view has held great sway in the courts despite the fact that nearly every subsequent study has obtained contradictory findings.

In fact, return to work is unusual and complete recovery rare. Improvement tends not to occur after the financial settlement. Tarsh & Royston (1985) found that family influences were important in that the more firmly the relatives believed the claimant to be physically ill, the more they relapsed into chronic illness. All authorities agree that the lengthy legal process with its long delays and multiple medical examinations and reports exacerbates the situation and that legal liability should be decided early, or a 'no fault' system of compensation introduced.

Ganser syndrome   This disorder, named after the German psychiatrist who first described it in 1897, is rare and probably not a dissociative or hysterical disorder. Ganser described a small group of prisoners who developed short-lived, florid, psychotic episodes with subsequent retrograde amnesia. The term Ganser syndrome has subsequently been used to apply to any behaviour where dementia or psychosis is simulated or to a similar presentation but restricted to a forensic setting. It has also been used in a more restricted sense to refer to cases of simulated madness or dementia characterised by approximate and absurd answers to questions (*Vorbeireden*). Subject may say, for example, that a horse has five legs or a camel three humps, making it clear that they understand the question they were being asked. Vorbeireden can occur, however, in association with organic brain disease and is not always psychogenic.

Epidemic hysteria (synonym: mass hysteria, communicable hysteria) There are dramatic accounts from history of dancing manias, nuns mewing like cats and biting each other, behaviour spreading from convent to convent, and each year several minor outbreaks occur in the UK and are reported by the media. They have a number of common features: they tend to occur in women, often schoolgirls; they usually arise in an atmosphere of stress or constraint such as a boarding school or other institution; they frequently begin in an individual of high status, with a peer group then developing the same symptoms, which thereafter spread down the status hierarchy, and from older to younger. New cases appear at times of social contact rather than during classes and those who initially deal with the outbreak are often indecisive and anxious.

A typical example occurred at the National Young Brass Band Championships held in the open air near Northampton. The conductor and leader of the favourite all-girls band had left hospital after giving birth to her first child, especially to conduct her band in this prestigious event. During the preperformance rehearsal she felt faint and ill and these symptoms were transmitted to a few players in the band. Several announcements were made over the loudspeakers about not sitting on damp grass, and rumours spread about the toilets being contaminated and, as a result of crop spraying in the adjacent fields the previous day, the grass being poisoned. More and more girls became ill with nausea, diarrhoea, fainting and skin rashes until eventually the competition had to be abandoned. There was no evidence of any viral, bacterial or toxic aetiology and all affected individuals recovered.

There are some reports of the same individual initiating more than one outbreak when moved from school to school.

Combat hysteria (synonym: shell-shock, war neurosis) Overt 'hysterical' symptoms occurred on an unparalleled scale during the trench warfare in the First World War and have probably occurred to some extent in every theatre of war before and since. Although the civilian psychiatrist may have little contact with this syndrome, it is important for a number of reasons. The cases of mutism, paraplegia and blindness that occurred in the trenches spread infectiously from soldier to soldier. They affected men from very different backgrounds with differing levels of intelligence and men who had already shown great bravery. This suggests that, given sufficient stress and sufficient secondary gain, all of us may be liable to such conversion disorders. The life expectancy of a soldier in trench warfare

was only a few weeks, but popular opinion fiercely condemned those who would not fight, while the wounded were praised and esteemed.

Aetiology of somatoform and dissociative disorders

Freud introduced the term *conversion*, by which he meant the rendering innocuous of a dangerous or threatening idea by its conversion into a physical symptom. The conflict itself was said to be unconscious and the resultant physical symptom to have symbolic meaning (e.g. a wife who has murderous impulses towards her husband finds her right arm paralysed so that she cannot attack him). The relief of emotional conflict achieved thereby is called primary gain. Secondary gain refers to the more direct advantages that being ill bring to the patient, such as sympathy, attention and the avoidance of everyday obligations. While such mechanisms may make certain hysterical behaviours in some patients understandable it is doubtful if they have general applicability.

Two sociological concepts provide us with a better understanding of these syndromes. Talcott Parsons in 1951 described the *sick role* and pointed out that in our society it carried with it may privileges. The person who is sick is exempt from normal social obligations. They no longer have to work, or to go school, they are treated with sympathy and understanding by those around them, they are allowed to show weakness and distress. The only obligation on such a sick person is to seek appropriate help and accept the treatment that is offered. Children are particularly adept at prolonging the sick role after minor childhood illnesses and this behaviour is often tolerated for a few days by mothers. Most of us can probably remember the pleasures of being treated as sick, while feeling quite well, after the toxic phase of a childhood illness had passed.

The second concept is that of *illness behaviour* (Mechanic 1962). This term refers to the ways in which given symptoms may be differentially perceived, evaluated and acted (or not acted) upon by different kinds of persons. Illness behaviour therefore describes the actions of the patient. This includes his behaviour when ill. He may be stoical and restrained or histrionic and dramatising. His communication may be entirely verbal or may take the form of physical dysfunction which is displayed for the doctor to see with a minimum of verbal description. It also includes his attitude to those involved in his diagnosis and treatment. He may be hostile, suspicious, fearful, flirtatious, pleading, aloof, or excessively cooperative and agreeable. There are marked cultural and ethnic differences in illness behaviour. Most workers have compared Mediterranean and

Anglo-Saxon cultural groups and found that the former are more likely to show hypochondriacal concern, manifest more conviction as to the presence of serious physical illness and take a more somatic view of illness. Pain thresholds are reported as 'painful' by subjects of Italian or Jewish backgrounds but described as 'warm' by subjects of north European origin.

Illness behaviour may be a learned phenomenon. People's behaviour when ill may depend as much on their previous experience of illness, illness behaviour they have observed in others, and the rewards their previous behaviour has received as on the severity of the illness itself.

If we combine these two concepts we can see much hysterical and hypochondriacal behaviour as a resort to the 'sick role' at times of stress. To a few people the normal demands of life are so onerous that the sick role is preferable most of the time. Such people, because of lack of ability, feelings of vulnerability, insecurity or low self-esteem, may feel that only when ill do they receive sufficient love, sympathy or attention from other people. To others the sick role only becomes attractive at times of particular stress. Stresses may include the impending breakup of relationships, or fear of debt or imprisonment. A good example is what used to be called 'shell shock' or 'combat neurosis' and was reported from many theatres of war. Presumably the advantages of the sick role are greatly increased if you are in active combat where either fighting or deserting may mean that you get shot.

Neither of these concepts involves any judgement by the doctor as to whether the processes involved are conscious or unconscious. Nor is such a decision particularly helpful in the management of patients with these syndromes.

Management of somatoform and dissociative disorders

Doctors, like other people, do not like to feel they are being manipulated or 'conned' by patients and have a tendency when they feel this is happening to confront patients with their views about the basis of their symptoms. Patients are usually very sensitive to any insinuation that their symptoms are not genuine, so such confrontations often end in disaster, with the patient angry and resentful and often discharging himself from treatment. The doctor usually sees such behaviour as a vindication of his point of view and feels content that he has made the right diagnosis. The patient, though, is left with his symptoms and by the very nature of the disorders under discussion will continue to complain and suffer and probably seek help from other specialists. One of the great weaknesses of the psychoanalytic view

of such disorders is that a distinction has to be made between conscious and unconscious motivation. The former is malingering and is therefore strongly disapproved of; the latter is illness, viz. hysteria, which is worthy of concern and treatment. In clinical practice it is usually impossible to make any such clear distinction. It is likely in the majority of cases that the patient's awareness and insight into his behaviour varies with time and with the degree of stress or threat he feels subject to.

The best approach is not confrontation but to emphasise that the symptoms are familiar, that serious physical illness has been excluded and that full recovery can be expected. It is usually unwise to get into arguments about the cause of the symptoms or underlying disorder. Physical, radiological and laboratory examinations should be completed as quickly as possible with the minimum of drama and attention and the symptoms should then be ignored. A team approach to such problems is vitally important: all members of staff and family members who have contact with the patient should adopt the same approach. It is common for such patients to seek out the most junior nurse or medical student who will innocently take great interest in their fascinating symptoms. The main aim is to minimise the advantages of the sick role and to try and ensure that the patient receives no attention or rewards for sick behaviour. Conversely, he should receive praise and interest from staff and family for healthy behaviour. It is important that the patient be allowed to discard his symptoms without losing self-esteem, so gradual recovery should be the aim. With such an approach the relief of conversion symptoms can be confidently expected.

An added advantage of this approach is that it is unlikely to prolong symptoms or create secondary handicaps. Even in more intractable disorders where recovery seems less likely it will often allow a partial recovery of function and will help relatives to deal more firmly and appropriately with the 'sick' member in the family. For example, a bed-ridden patient with weak or paralysed legs would be given a gradual programme of tasks to achieve. Starting with passive leg exercises in bed, gradually moving to active ones 'to build up the muscles', then sitting on the bed with his feet on the floor, standing by the bed with support, standing with a Zimmer frame, walking a few steps with the frame, etc. All complaints of muscle aches and pains should be ignored or answered only briefly and much praise and attention should be given for each task the patient achieves. This may not sound very 'psychological' treatment, but it is likely to be much more effective than attempting to explore the unconscious meaning of the patient's bed-ridden state. This approach, then, concentrates on the patient's adoption of the sick role rather than on the actual symptoms or their psychodynamic significance.

Pilowsky (1983) has suggested that in the management of these disorders it is important to distinguish between illness experience, illness statements and illness behaviours. A patient who makes multiple illness statements may manifest few illness behaviours and be leading a reasonably active and productive life. Hypochondriasis, for example, may be a coping, defensive style and sympathetic listening and reassurance may be what is required. In contrast, a patient with much illness behaviour as well may require different management.

Abnormal stress reactions and adjustment disorders

The ICD-10 classification has three categories: acute stress reaction, post-traumatic stress disorder and adjustment disorder. DSM-IV has only post-traumatic stress disorder, acute and delayed.

Acute stress reaction

After a major stressful event, some individuals develop a characteristic pattern of symptoms. These include a dazed state, with some degree of disorientation and perhaps an impaired ability to comprehend and answer questions. Automatic signs of severe anxiety, such as tachycardia, sweating or flushing occur. There may be apparently purposeless overactivity or agitation or the subject may lapse into stupor, or wander away from the stressful situation in a fugue-like state. Characteristically these symptoms start within a few minutes or at most hours of the stress. There is usually complete resolution within 2–3 days of termination of the stress, or removal from the threatening situation. To make the diagnoses there must be no evidence of a psychiatric disorder immediately prior to the stressful event. Characteristically these reactions follow events, such as natural catastrophes, major accidents, assaults or rape. As yet they have been the subject of little systematic enquiry.

Post-traumatic stress disorder (PTSD)

This is a new category of ICD-10, but was included in DSM-IIIR. It has received much interest because of studies of American Vietnam War veterans and because of a series of major civilian disasters occurring in the mid and late 1980s. It differs from acute stress reactions in that the onset is usually delayed. In other words, there is a latency period which may range from a few weeks to several months following the stress. Both

ICD-10 and DSM-IV suggest that the stressful event must be exceptionally threatening or catastrophic in nature, and likely to cause pervasive distress in almost anyone – for example, a natural disaster, combat, serious accident, witnessing the violent death of someone or being the victim of torture or rape. However, in a study by Horowitz et al (1980) the same distinctive syndrome of re-experiencing the trauma is often present even when the traumatic event is not outside the normal range of experience. The typical features of the syndrome include repeated reliving of the trauma, intrusive memories or flashbacks, and vivid nightmares. These occur against the background of a persisting sense of numbness and emotional blunting. There is usually a marked avoidance of any situation which might resemble that in which the original trauma occurred. Hyperarousal, hypervigilance, insomnia, anxiety and depression are associated features.

Stimuli that resemble or symbolise the original traumatic event may cause exacerbations of the symptoms. Cases have been described where even fairly nonspecific changes may cause this, such as hot, humid, thundery weather in Pacific War veterans.

There is a debate as to whether the clinical features of PTSD sufficiently separate it from generalised anxiety disorder. Clearly the disorders overlap considerably but at the severe end of PTSD the constant intrusive thoughts, the flashbacks, hypervigilance and marked social withdrawal produce a quite different clinical picture to that usually seen in generalised anxiety disorder. PTSD may coexist with major depressive disorder, may present as a combination of the above symptoms and typical grief and often leads to drug and alcohol overuse.

Epidemiology Relatively few studies have looked at the prevalence in the general population but a description of those exposed to the Mount St Helen's explosion in Washington State in the early 1980s showed a level of 1% in men and 3% in women in those who had not been exposed to any danger from the volcano at all. Presumably this background rate is a combination of individuals exposed to previous mass trauma such as the Vietnam War and to individual tragedies. Rates following major disasters vary depending on the nature of the disaster, the degree of exposure to it and whether it is natural or man-made. In circumstances such as the Piper Alpha oilrig explosion in 1988, where only a quarter of the men survived and all survivors had horrific and life-threatening experiences, virtually every survivor had severe PTSD. In most of the major disasters in the UK over the past 10 years the incidents have been sudden, but short-lived. This was not true of the Lockerbie air disaster where a Pan American 747 jet fell on a small Scottish town. There were no survivors from the plane. The local community had to live with the acute effects of the disaster for many weeks as wreckage was sifted through and bodies and bits of bodies removed from the area. In this situation the threat of danger lasts only a few seconds but the continued exposure to the disaster scene and its consequences also produced a high rate of PTSD. In general, man-made disasters appear to produce higher rates than natural ones. It has been suggested that PTSD is a particularly Western disorder and that the high rates following civilian disasters are in part a consequence of the increasing lack of exposure to death and disaster in Western society. Disasters in less developed countries have been much less studied but recent reports from studies in Nicaragua and Sri Lanka do not support this view and show equally high rates and very similar symptom patterns.

The duration of the disorder may be very long. European psychiatrists frequently see patients with 40–50 years of continuous symptoms following concentration camp experiences. In McFarlane's study of firefighters dealing with Australian bush fires, 50% of fire-fighters had some sort of PTSD reaction, a surprisingly high rate in a group of trained men used to dealing with disaster. McFarlane followed this cohort at 4, 11 and 23 months, showing that the most common type of reaction was a delayed onset, with symptoms not being present at 4 months but occurring subsequently. It is difficult to know to what extent such later-onset cases represent the first emergence of PTSD symptoms at this time or whether sufferers tolerate symptoms for several months because they appear understandable and only when they do not begin to wane do they see themselves as having a disorder. The different patterns of traumatisation and the response that occur are important to recognise. Type I trauma describes a one-off, sudden, time-limited event. Type II trauma is prolonged, repeated and, once established, may be helplessly anticipated rather than unexpected. Details of the two types are given in Table 17.17.

Memory and dissociation Under normal or moderately stressful conditions sensory input is synthesised in relation to pre-existing memories and, if personally significant, transcribed into a narrative or personal story. In highly traumatic situations experiences are imprinted as sensations or feelings and not memorised as narratives. This means that traumatic memories are recalled as sensations or emotions and there is often difficulty in giving a verbal account. Because of the way they are stored, such memories may be inaccessible to semantic processing. The processing of a memory in symbolic (language) form may be a prerequisite for integration with other experiences.

These somatic and emotional memories may lead to

Table 17.17   Type I and type II trauma

Type I
Short term, unexplained traumatic event
- Single blow, dangerous and overwhelming events
- Isolated traumatic experiences, often rare
- Sudden, surprising, devastating events
- Limited duration
- For example, rape, natural disasters, car accidents, sniper shooting
- Events become indelibly etched on an individual's mind (recalled in detail) and create more vivid and complete memories than does Type II trauma
- More likely to lead to typical PTSD symptoms of intrusive ideation, avoidance, and hyperarousal reactions
- More likely to lead to classic re-experiencing experience
- Quicker recovery more likely
– Note, however, that Type 1 stressors can trigger or recapitulate an earlier history of victimisation, fears of abandonment, and the like

Type II
Sustained and repeated ordeal stressors
Series of traumatic events or exposure to a prolonged traumatic event
- Variable multiple, chronic, long-standing, repeated and anticipated traumas
- More likely to be of intentional human design
- For example, ongoing physical and sexual abuse, combat
- Initially experience as type I stressors, but as trauma reoccurs, victim expects and fears its reoccurrence
- Feels helpless to prevent it
- Memories are typically 'fuzzy' and 'spotty' because of dissociation; over time dissociation can become a way of coping
- May lead to altered view of self and of the world and accompanying feelings of guilt, shame and worthlessness
- More likely to lead to longstanding characterological and interpersonal problems, as evident in increased detachment from others, restricted range of affect, and emotional liability
- Result in attempts to protect self that may involve the use of dissociative responses, denial and numbing, withdrawal, use of addictive substances
- More likely to lead to 'complex PTSD reaction' and what Van der Kolk (1996) characterise as disorders of extreme stress (DES). Individuals with these reactions have poorer recovery

---

episodes of dissociation and depersonalisation and may also explain why traumatic memories remain unaltered and unprocessed over very long periods (Van der Kolk 1997).

Biological factors Bremner et al (1995) showed decreased right-sided hippocampal volume in Vietnam veterans with PTSD, and that short-term verbal memory impairment was associated with decreased hippocampal volume using structural MRI. Rauch et al (1996), using PET, showed increased activation of the amygdala in response to reading traumatic scripts. The amygdala is central in transforming sensory input into emotional and hormonal responses. Several studies have investigated event-related potentials and have found diminished P300 amplitudes, longer M2 latencies and decreased reaction time.

As yet it is not clear whether these abnormalities have been caused by trauma or represent pre-existing abnormalities which might score as risk factors for the development of PTSD.

These findings are summarised in Table 17.18.

Treatment Most recent disasters have been followed by hurriedly set up postdisaster counselling services and there is now an expectation that such services should be available following a major disaster. Treatment of this type is difficult to evaluate and, although it seems both humane and sensible to provide it, there is no evidence that it protects against the longer-term consequences of the disaster. Several studies are currently under way comparing different types of treatment for well-established PTSD with structured psychotherapies such as cognitive-behaviour therapy being the current psychological treatment of choice. Antidepressant drugs may be of help in chronic, well-established PTSD. They seem particularly useful in coping with the persistent overarousal that may make the disorder self-sustaining.

Finally, it is important that our preoccupation with major disasters does not deflect attention from those individuals who have clear symptoms from an individual catastrophe. It is much more likely that a typical psychiatrist will have to deal with such individuals, who may have been raped, assaulted or involved in car crashes.

Table 17.18   Structural and functional changes in post-traumatic stress disorder

Right-sided activities of amygdala and related structures
Recurrence in left inferior prefrontal activity when traumatic memories activated
Decreased hippocampal volume in chronic PTSD
Decreased P300 amplitude in response to non-trauma-related stimuli
Differential activation of the anterior amygdala in response to potentially threatening stimuli

---

Adjustment disorder

This category is used in the ICD, though not in DSM-IV, to describe the mild and transient states of distress that arise following life changes or stressful life events. These events are such situations as changing school, emigrating, retirement, becoming a parent, etc. The symptoms – which usually consist of depressed mood, anxiety, worry and irritability – are mild and usually develop within 3 months of the event in question. Other symptoms of more serious depression, such as anhedonia, loss of appetite and weight, and loss of drive or interest, are not present.

Miscellaneous syndromes

Dysmorphophobia

This rather clumsy term describes a condition in which an individual insistently complains about some presumed defect in physical appearance which he is convinced is noticeable to others, although in reality his appearance is quite normal. For example, the patient who complains that his nose is too big, too small, hooked or turned up at the end when in fact it looks quite normal is said to be suffering from dysmorphophobia. Plastic surgeons deal with large numbers of patients who wish to have their appearance altered and it is becoming increasingly possible to have such treatment on the National Health Service, especially if the patient is genuinely distressed by his appearance. A psychiatrist will sometimes be asked by the plastic surgeon to help in the selection of patients for surgery. From the few, rather poorly designed follow-up studies published, it would appear that such psychiatric screening is worthwhile. In some individuals, particularly if their appearance is essentially normal, the complaint of bizarre dysmorphophobia is an ominous symptom, for dislike of a bodily part may be the first symptom of a developing psychotic illness.

In others, intractable emotional and interpersonal difficulties have become focused on one particular physical attribute and the patient has entirely unrealistic expectations of how surgery will change his life. A psychiatrist's role in such a consultation is, firstly, to screen for overt psychiatric illness, and, secondly, to make some assessment of how realistic the patient's expectations of operation are. Where a deformity is obvious, surgery is often indicated even though the patient may have unrealistic ideas about the changes to his life that surgery will produce.

Depersonalisation syndromes

Depersonalisation is a quite common experience which

occurs in both healthy and ill individuals. A lengthy but clear definition is as follows (Leading article 1972):

Depersonalisation is a strange, complex and essentially private experience, one characteristic of which is the individual's difficulty in communicating a comprehensible account of it. A prominent feature of the experience is a feeling of change involving either or both the inner and the outer worlds and carrying with it a vague but uncomfortable sense of unfamiliarity. The description 'unreal' or 'detached' is usually accepted, but the experience varies greatly between individuals and between attacks. These phenomena, which occur intermittently, always have the quality of unfamiliarity and discomfort, and are recognised as changes in experience rather than in reality itself. The patient always uses an 'as if' qualification in his often bizarre descriptions of the experience, and one of the serious risks of the condition is it may be misunderstood and a more malign significance attributed to it.

The term derealisation is employed to describe the feeling that changes appear to have occurred in the environment. The patient may say that things appear smaller, larger, closer or further away, or that the room around him appears to have gone flat or two-dimensional. Depersonalisation is sometimes restricted to changes in the individual's perception of himself such as feeling dead, hollow, detached from his surroundings or puppet-like.

When it occurs in normal individuals, depersonalisation may be associated with recent emotional disturbance, fatigue or anxiety. It can occur as a symptom in anxiety states, depressive illness and schizophrenia and may be induced by drugs such as LSD. It may also be a symptom of organic brain disease. Mild depersonalisation without significant impairment of function is estimated to occur at some time in 30–70% of young adults. Depersonalisation and derealisation are usually normal phenomena, or symptoms of some other psychiatric or physical illness. Occasionally, though, attacks of depersonalisation lasting from a few seconds to a few hours form the central feature of a troublesome disorder. In such cases a primary diagnosis of depersonalisation disorder may be justified and DSM-IV contains such a category.

In eliciting the symptom it is probably not sufficient to ask only about feelings of unreality, as this may often produce a positive response. Closer questioning is needed to establish the exact nature of the experience. Depersonalisation can be frightening and distressing but reassurance that the experience is a common one and not a sign of impending madness may be all the treatment that is required. There is no specific treatment for the symptoms, but they generally subside when levels of anxiety are reduced.

REFERENCES

Agras W S, Sylvester D, Oliveau D 1969 The epidemiology of common fears and phobias. Comprehensive Psychiatry 10: 151–156

Agras W S, Chapin H N, Oliveau D 1972 The natural history of phobia. Archives of General Psychiatry 26: 315

Allgulander C, Lavori P W 1991 Excess mortality among 3302 patients with 'pure' anxiety neurosis. Archives of General Psychiatry 48: 599–602

Angst J, Dobler-Mikola A, Schneidegger P 1982 A panel study of anxiety states, panic attacks and phobias among young adults. Paper at research conference on anxiety disorders, panic attacks and phobias. Key Biscayne, Florida, 9 December

APA 1980 Diagnostic and statistical manual, 3rd edn. American Psychiatric Association, Washington, DC

APA 1994 Diagnostic and statiscal manual of mental disorders, DSM-IV. American Psychiatric Association, Washington, DC

Barlow D H, Blanchard E B, Vermilyea J A, Vermilyea B B, Dinardo I A 1986 Generalised anxiety and generalised anxiety disorder: description and reconceptualization. American Journal of Psychiatry 143: 40–44

Bebbington P, Hurry J, Tennant C, Stuart E, Wing J K 1981 Epidemiology of mental disorders in Camberwell. Psychological Medicine 11: 561–579

Black A 1974 The natural history of obsessional neurosis. In: Beech H R (ed) Obsessional states. Methuen, London

Blackman P, Evason E, Melaugh M, Woods R 1989 Housing and health: a case study of two areas in West Belfast. Journal of Social Policy 18: 1–26

Bluglass D, Clarke J, Henderson A S, Kreitman N, Presley A S 1977 A study of agoraphobic housewives. Psychological Medicine 7: 73–86

Bradley J J 1963 Severe localized pain associated with the depressive syndrome. British Journal of Psychiatry 109: 741–745

Bremner J D, Randall P, Scott T M et al 1995 MRI-based measures of hippocampal volume in patients with PTSD. American Journal of Psychiatry 152: 973–981

Brown F 1942 Heredity in the psychoneuroses. Proceedings of the Royal Society of Medicine 35: 785–790

Brown G M, Harris T O 1978 Social origins of depression: a study of psychiatric disorders in women. Tavistock, London

Brown G W, Davidson S, Harris T, Maclean U, Pollock S, Prudo R 1977 Psychiatric disorder in London and North Uist. Social Science and Medicine 11: 367–377

Brown G W, Harris T O, Eales M J 1993 Aetiology of anxiety and depressive disorders in an inner-city population. Psychological Medicine 23: 155–165

Brown T A, Barlow D H, Liebowitz M R 1994 The empirical basis of generalized anxiety disorder. American Journal of Psychiatry 151: 1272–1280

Byrne D S, Harrison S P, Keithley J, McCarthy P 1986 Housing and health. The relationship between housing conditions and the health of council tenants. Gower, Aldershot

Clancy J, Noyes R, Hoenk P R, Slymen D J 1978 Secondary depression in anxiety neurosis. Journal of Nervous and Mental Disease 166: 846–850

Cooper B 1972 Clinical and social aspects of chronic neurosis. Proceedings of the Royal Society of Medicine 65: 509–512

Cooper B, Sylph J 1973 Life events and the onset of neurotic illness: an investigation in general practice. Psychological Medicine 3: 421–435

Crowe R R, Noyes R, Paul D L, Slymen D 1983 A family study of panic disorders. Archives of General Psychiatry 40: 1065–1069

Endicott J, Spitzer R L 1978 A diagnostic interview – the schedule for affective disorders and schizophrenia. Archives of General Psychiatry 35: 837–844

Finlay-Jones R A, Burvill P W 1977 The prevalence of minor psychiatric morbidity in the community. Psychological Medicine 7: 475–489

Fremming K H 1951 The expectation of mental infirmity in a sample of the Danish population. Occasional Papers on Eugenics 7

Freud S 1894a The justification for detaching from neurasthenia a particular syndrome, the anxiety neurosis. In: Early papers Freud S. Hogarth Press 1924, London, vol 1, pp 76–106

Freud S 1894 The aetiology of hysteria. In: Strachey J (ed) Collected papers. Hogarth Press 1946, London, vol I p 183

Garssen B, Rijken H 1986 Clinical aspects and treatment of the hyperventilation syndrome. Behavioural Psychotherapy 14: 46

Garssen B, de Beurs E, Buikhuisen M et al 1996 On distinguishing types of panic. Journal of Anxiety Disorders 10: 173–184

Gelder M G 1986 Neurosis: another tough old word. British Medical Journal 292: 972–973

Gelernter C S, Uhde T W, Cimbulic P et al 1991 Cognitive, behavioural and pharmacological treatments of social phobia. Archives of General Psychiatry 48: 938–945

Goisman R M, Warshaw M G, Steketee G S et al 1995 DSM-IV and the disappearance of agoraphobia without a history of panic disorder: new data on a controversial diagnosis. American Journal of Psychiatry 152: 1438–1443

Goldstein R B, Wickramaratne P J, Horwath E, Weissman M M 1997 Familial aggregation and phenomenology of 'early'-onset (at or before age 20 years) panic disorder. Archives of General Psychiatry 54: 271–278

Goodwin D W, Guze S B, Robbins E 1969 Follow-up studies in obsessional neurosis. Archives of General Psychiatry 20: 182–187

Hagnell O 1966 Incidence and duration of episodes of mental illness in a total population. In: Hare E M, Wing J K (eds) Psychiatric epidemiology. Oxford Press, Oxford

Helgason T 1964 Epidemiology of mental disorders in Iceland. Acta Psychiatrica Scandinavica Supplementum 173

Henderson A S, Duncan Jones P, Byrne D G, Scott R, Adcock S 1979 Psychiatric disorders in Canberra. Acta Psychiatrica Scandinavica 60: 355–374

Hodiamont P, Peer N, Sybe N 1987 Epidemiological aspects of psychiatric disorders in a Dutch health area. Psychological Medicine 17: 495–505

Horowitz M J, Wilner N, Kaltreider N, Alvarez W 1980 Signs and symptoms of post-traumatic stress disorder. Archives of General Psychiatry 37: 85–92

Huxley P J, Goldberg D P, Maguire P, Kincey V 1979 The prediction of the course of minor psychiatric disorders. British Journal of Psychiatry 135: 535–543

International Multicenter Clinical Trial Group on Moclobemide in Social Phobia 1997 Moclobemide in social phobia: a double-blind, placebo-controlled clinical study European Archives of Psychiatry and Clinical Neuroscience 247: 71–80

Jenkins R, Lewis G, Bebbington P, et al 1997 The national psychiatric morbidity surveys of Great Britain – initial findings from the household survey. Psychological Medicine 27: 775–789

Johnstone E C, Cunningham D, Owens D G et al 1980 Neurotic illness and its response to amitriptyline and antidepressant treatment. Psychological Medicine 10: 321–328

Kendler K S, Neale M C, Kessler R C, Heath A C, Eaves L J 1992 Generalized anxiety disorder in women: a population-based twin study. Archives of General Psychiatry 49: 267–272

Kenyon F E 1964 Hypochondriasis: a clinical study. British Journal of Psychiatry 110: 478–488

Kenyon F E 1976 Hypochondriasis: a clinical study. British Journal of Psychiatry 129: 1–14

Kessler R C, McGonagle K A, Zhao S et al 1994 Lifetime and 12-month prevalence of DSM-IIIR psychiatric disorders in the United States. Archives of General Psychiatry 51: 8–19

Klein D F 1993 False suffocation alarms, spontaneous panics, and related conditions: an integrative hypothesis. Archives of General Psychiatry 50: 306–317

Klein D F, Gittelman R, Quitkin F H, Rifkin A 1980 Diagnosis and drug treatment of psychiatric disorders: adults and children. Williams & Wilkins, Baltimore

Lader M, Sartorius N 1968 Anxiety in patients with hysterical conversion symptoms. Journal of Neurology, Neurosurgery and Psychiatry 31: 490–495

Leading article 1972 Depersonalisation syndromes. British Medical Journal 4: 378

Leonard H L, Swedo S E, Lenane M C et al 1993 A 2- to 7-year follow-up study of 54 obsessive compulsive children and adolescents. Archives of General Psychiatry 50: 429–439

Lewis A 1975 The survival of hysteria. Psychological Medicine 5: 9–12

Lewis G, Pelosi A J, Araya R, Dunn G 1992 Measuring psychiatric disorder in the community: a standardized assessment for use by lay interviewers. Psychological Medicine 22: 465–486

Liebowitz M R, Gorman J M, Fyer A J, Klein D F 1985 Social phobia. Archives of General Psychiatry 42: 729–736

Liebowitz M R, Gorman J M, Fyer A et al 1988 Pharmacotherapy of social phobia; an interim report of a placebo-control comparison of phenelzine and atenolol. Journal of Clinical Psychiatry 49: 252–257

McFarlane A 1989 The aetiology of post-traumatic morbidity: predisposing, precipitating and perpetuating factors. British Journal of Psychiatry 154: 221–228

Mann A H, Jenkins R, Belsey E 1981 The twelve-month outcome of patients with neurotic illness in general practice. Psychological Medicine 11: 535–550

Marks I M 1969 Fears and phobias. Heinemann Medical, London

Mavissakalian M, Turner S M, Michelson L, Jacob R 1985 Tricyclic antidepressants in obsessive compulsive disorder: antiobsessional or antidepressant agents. American Journal of Psychiatry 142: 572–576

Mavreas V, Bebbington P E 1987 Psychiatric morbidity in London's Greek Cypriot community. I. Association with socio-demographic variables. Social Psychiatry 22: 150–159

Mazza D L, Martin D, Spacevento L, Jacobsen J, Gibb J H 1986 Prevalence of anxiety disorders in patients with mitral valve prolapse. American Journal of Psychiatry 143: 349–352

Mechanic D 1962 The concept of illness behaviour. Journal of Chronic Disease 15: 189–194

Mellsop G W 1972 Psychiatric patients seen as children and adults: childhood predictors of adult illness. Journal of Child Psychology and Psychiatry 13: 91–101

Merskey H, Buhrish N A 1973 Hysteria: organic brain disease. British Journal of Medical Psychology 48: 359–366

Millar D G 1980 A repertory grid study of obsessionality: distinctive cognitive structure or distinctive cognitive element? British Journal of Medical Psychology 53: 59–66

Miller H 1961 Accident neurosis. British Medical Journal 1: 919–925

Myers J K, Weissman M M, Tischler G L et al 1984 Six month prevalence of psychiatric disorders in three communities. Archives of General Psychiatry 41: 959–967

Nandi D N, Banerjee G, Nandi S, Nandi P 1992 Is hysteria on the wane: a community survey in West Bengal, India. British Journal of Psychiatry 160: 87–91

Noyes R, Clancy J, Hoenk P R, Slymen D J 1980 The prognosis of anxiety neurosis. Archives of General Psychiatry 37: 173–178

Noyes R, Crowe R R, Harris E L, Hamra B J, McChesney C H, Chavomry D R 1986 Relationship between panic disorder and agoraphobia. Archives of General Psychiatry 43: 227–232

Orley J, Wing J K 1979 Psychiatric disorders in two African villages. Archives of General Psychiatry 36: 513–520

Ormel J, Oldehinkel T, Brilman E, van den Brink W 1993 Outcome of depression and anxiety in primary care. Archives of General Psychiatry 50: 759–766

Parsons T 1951 The social system. Free Press, New York

Paykel E S 1978 Contribution of life events to causation of psychiatric illness. Psychiatric Medicine 8: 245–253

Pilowsky I 1967 Dimensions of hypochondriasis. British Journal of Psychiatry 113: 89–93

Pilowsky I 1983 Hypochondriasis. In: Russell G F M, Hersov L A (eds) Handbook of psychiatry Vol 4: The neuroses and personality disorders. Cambridge University Press, Cambridge

Platt S, Martin G, Hunt S 1991 The mental health of women with children living in deprived areas of Great Britain. The role of living conditions, poverty and unemployment. In: Goldberg D, Tantam D (eds) The public health impact of mental disorders. Hogrefe & Huber, Toronto, ch 12

Prusoff B, Klerman G L 1974 Differentiating depressed from anxious neurotic patients. Archives of General Psychiatry 30: 302–309

Rasmussen R A, Tsuang M T 1986 Clinical characteristics and family history in DSM-III obsessive–compulsive disorder. American Journal of Psychiatry 143: 317–322

Ratnasuriya R H, Marks I M, Forshaw D M, Hymas M F S 1991 Obsessive slowness revisited. British Journal of Psychiatry 159: 273–274

Rauch S, Van der Kolk B A, Fisher R et al 1996 A symptom provocation study using positron emission tomography and script driven imagery. Archives of General Psychiatry 53: 380–387

Reiman E M, Raichle M E, Robin S E et al 1986 The application of positron emission tomography to the study of panic disorder. American Journal of Psychiatry 143: 469–477

Robins L N 1966 Deviant children grown up. Williams & Wilkins, Baltimore

Robins L N, Helzer J E, Weissman M M et al 1984 Lifetime prevalence of specific psychiatric disorders in three sites. Archives of General Psychiatry 41: 949–958

Ronalds C, Creed F, Stone K, Webb S, Tomenson B 1997 Outcome of anxiety and depressive disorders in primary care. British Journal of Psychiatry 171: 427–433

Roth M, Gurney C, Garside R F, Kerr T A 1972 Studies in the classification of affective disorders. British Journal of Psychiatry 121: 147–161

Rush B 1812 Medical enquiries and observations upon the diseases of the mind. Kimber & Richardson, Philadelphia

Rutter M L 1972 Relationships between child and adult psychiatric disorders. Acta Psychiatrica Scandinavica 48: 3–21

Rutter M, Tizard J, Whitmore K (eds) 1970 Education, health and behaviour. Longman, London

Shepherd M, Cooper B, Kelton G W, Brown A C 1966 Psychiatric illness in general practice. Oxford University Press, London

Sims A 1978 Hypotheses linking neuroses with premature mortality. Psychological Medicine 8: 255–263

Sims A C P 1985 Neurotic illness: conserving a threatened concept. British Journal of Clinical Pharmacology 19: 95–155

Slater E T O, Glithero E 1965 A follow-up of patients diagnosed as suffering from 'hysteria'. Journal of Psychosomatic Research 9: 9–13

Srole L, Langner T, Michael S, Opler M, Rennie T 1962 Mental health in the metropolis. McGraw-Hill, New York

Stavrakaki C, Vargo B 1986 The relationship of anxiety and depression: a review of the literature. British Journal of Psychiatry 149: 7–16

Stein M B, Walker J R, Forde D R 1994 Setting diagnostic thresholds for social phobia: considerations from a community survey of social anxiety. American Journal of Psychiatry 151: 408–412

Stern R S, Cobb J P 1978 Phenomenology of obsessive–compulsive neurosis. British Journal of Psychiatry 132: 233–239

Stern R S, Marks I M, Mawson D, Luscombe D K 1980 Clomipramine and exposure for obsessive compulsive rituals II: plasma levels, side effects and outcome. British Journal of Psychiatry 136: 161–166

Surtees P G, Deen C, Ingham J G, Kreitman N B, Miller P, Sashidharan S P 1983 Psychiatric disorders in women from an Edinburgh community. British Journal of Psychiatry 142: 238–246

Tarsh M J, Royston C 1985 A follow up study of accident neurosis. British Journal of Psychiatry 146: 18–25

Teasdale J D 1974 Learning models of obsessional–compulsive disorder. In: Beech H K (ed) Obsessional states. Methuen, London

Thoren P, Asberg M, Cronholm B, Jornestedt L, Traskman L 1980 Clomipramine treatment of obsessive–compulsive disorder: a clinical controlled trial. Archives of General Psychiatry 37: 1281–1285

Tyrer P 1984 Classification of anxiety. British Journal of Psychiatry 144: 78–83

Uhlenhuth E H, Balter M B, Millinger G D, Cisin I H, Clinthorne J 1983 Symptom checklist syndromes in the general population: correlations with psychotherapeutic drug use. Archives of General Psychiatry 40: 1167–1173

Van der Kolk B A 1996 Dissociation and information processing in posttramuatic stress disorder. In: Van der Kolk B A, McFarlane A C, Weisaeth L (eds) Traumatic stress: effects of overwhelming stress on mind, body, and society. Guilford Press, New York, pp 303–330

Van der Kolk B A 1997 Psychobiology of posttraumatic stress disorder. Annals of the New York Academy of Sciences 821: 99–113

Vasquez-Barquero J L, Monoz P E, Madoz Javrequi V 1981 The interaction between physical and neurotic morbidity in the community. British Journal of Psychiatry 139: 328–335

Vasquez-Barquero J L, Diez Manrique J F, Pena C et al 1987 A community mental health survey in Cantabria. A general description of morbidity. Psychological Medicine 17: 227–241

Veale D M, Sahakian B J, Owen A M, Marks I M 1996 Specific cognitive deficits in tests sensitive to frontal lobe dysfunction in obsessive–compulsive disorder. Psychological Medicine 26: 1261–1269

Weich S, Churchill R, Lewis G, Mann A 1997 Do socio-economic risk factors predict the incidence and maintenance of psychiatric disorder in primary care? Psychological Medicine 27: 73–80

Weissman M M, Myers J K, Harding P S 1978 Psychiatric disorders in a US urban community. American Journal of Psychiatry 135: 459–462

Weissman M M, Bland R C, Canino G J et al 1997 The cross-national epidemiology of panic disorder. Archives of General Psychiatry 54: 305–309

Wells J E, Bushnell J A, Hornblow A R, Joyce P R, Oakley-Browne M A 1989 Christchurch psychiatric epidemiology study part I: methodology and lifetime prevalence for specific psychiatric disorders. Australian and New Zealand Journal of Psychiatry 23: 315–326

Wheeler E O, White P D, Reid E W, Cohen M E 1950 Neurocirculatory asthenia. Journal of the American Medical Association 142: 878–889

WHO 1974 Glossary of mental disorders and guide to their classification, 8th revision. World Health Organization, Geneva

WHO 1992 Classification of mental and behavioural disorders, 10th revision. World Health Organization, Geneva

Wing J K, Baber T, Brugha T, Burke J, Cooper J E, Giel R, Jablenski A, Regier D, Sartorius N 1990 SCAN: Schedules for Clinical Assessment in Neuropsychiatry. Archives of General Psychiatry 47: 589–593

Wing J K, Cooper J E, Sartorius N 1974 The measurement and classification of psychiatric symptoms. Cambridge University Press, London

Wing J K, Mann S A, Leff J P, Nixon J M 1978 The concept of a 'case' in psychiatric population surveys. Psychological Medicine 8: 203–217

Wittchen H-U, Esau C A, von Zerssen D, Kreig J C, Zaudig M 1992 Lifetime and six-month prevalence of mental disorders: the Munich follow-up study. European Archives of Psychiatry and Clinical Neuroscience 241: 247–258

Wittchen H-U, Zhao S, Kessler R C, Eaton W W 1994 DSM-IIIR generalized anxiety disorder in the national comorbidity survey. Archives of General Psychiatry 51: 355–366

Woerner P I, Guze S B 1968 A family and marital study of hysteria. British Journal of Psychiatry 114: 161–168

Wolff S, Chick J 1980 Schizoid personality in childhood: a controlled follow-up study. Psychological Medicine 10: 85–100

Woodruff R A, Guze S B, Clayton P J 1972 Anxiety neurosis among psychiatric outpatients. Comprehensive Psychiatry 13: 165–170

18

Eating disorders

C. P. L. Freeman

INTRODUCTION

This chapter describes the characteristic psychopathology, clinical course and treatment of the two eating disorders that present most commonly to psychiatrists and psychologists: anorexia nervosa and bulimia nervosa. It also reviews the newly identified binge eating disorder (BED). It does not cover obesity despite the many common areas of interest and overlap, the research and clinical fields of obesity and eating disorders have developed quite separately.

Obesity research has largely had its roots in physiology and the health risks of obesity, whereas eating disorders have been based in the disciplines of psychiatry and psychology. This split is unfortunate and I apologise for repeating it here, but space precludes any meaningful consideration of the diagnosis and management of obesity. The usual justification for separating obesity from the eating disorders is that the majority of the obese population do not have significant psychiatric or psychological disturbance and that any disturbance they do develop is a consequence rather than a cause of the obesity. Nevertheless, much of the work on the regulation and physiology of eating carried out in the obese population has relevance to those with eating disorders. Disturbances of body image have been extensively investigated in anorexia and bulimia but less so in obesity; binge eating is a common behaviour in both groups; and the disorders are also linked because of the strong family history of obesity in both obese and bulimia nervosa subjects. They are divided by the fact that dieting is frequently seen as both the trigger and a maintaining factor in anorexia and bulimia nervosa, whereas it is one of the main methods of treatment for obesity.

Historical perspective

Eating disorders are widely thought to be 20th century Western phenomena. Several detailed reviews have shown this not to be the case (Parry-Jones & Parry-Jones 1995, Silverman 1995, Russell 1997).

In his book *Treatise on Consumption* (1689) Richard Morton describes two cases of anorexia nervosa in an 18-year-old young woman and a 16-year-old young man. The young woman died, though we don't know if this was because of the treatment or the disorder. The outcome of the young man is unknown. He was advised to abandon his studies, move to the country, take up riding and drink an ass's milk diet. In 1767 Robert Whytt, Professor of Medicine at Edinburgh University, described a case in a young woman which appears to have started with a medically prescribed diet. This patient survived and made a complete recovery. There is a description of slow and gradual refeeding to avoid undue gastric dilatation.

The French physician Louis-Victor Marcé, most renowned for his descriptions of postpartum disorders, clearly described the syndrome of anorexia nervosa, though not naming it (Marcé 1860). He recommended that such patients could not be treated without removing them from the family and entrusting their care to strangers, to circumvent the habitual circle of obstinate resistance that such patients and their families present. He recommended that if food refusal continued, intimidation and force should be employed, and, if necessary, the use of an oesophageal sound.

The two physicians whose names are most associated with the description of anorexia nervosa are Charles Lasegue and William Gull. Lasegue, from La Pitié in Paris, described 'de l'anorexie hystèrique'. He warned against giving friendly advice, medicines and most importantly intimidation 'with hysterical subjects a first medical fault is never repairable'. He advised watchful waiting and described in detail the physical symptoms that would develop and the gradual increase in distress in the family and relatives. A point would be reached where the patient herself would receive a shock to her self-satisfied indifference and at this point the physician should carefully move in and resume authority. William Gull's papers appeared a year later (Gull 1874). He described three starving teenage patients, Misses A, B and C. Gull also described gradual refeeding and thought that the main psychopathology in anorexia nervosa was 'perversions of the ego'.

Pierre Janet divided anorexia nervosa into an obsessional and hysterical type. He clearly described the loathing that such women felt for their bodies and their refusal to eat in spite of ravenous hunger. This clearly raises the issue that anorexia is not the correct description for all such disorders.

Hilda Bruch was the first modern author to describe anorexia nervosa and her views still have clear validity and appropriate influence today (Bruch 1962). She described the three core psychological features of the disorder as being:

- Body image disturbance
- Interoceptive disturbance
- Pervasive feelings of ineffectiveness.

Interoceptive disturbance refers to the inability of such individuals accurately to identify and respond to internal sensations, e.g. hunger, fullness, mood states and sexual arousal. Another important modern influence has been Gerald Russell; his work will be referred to later in the chapter.

Earlier descriptions of anorexia nervosa subjects do exist, mainly in early religious literature. Such individuals were often starving to purify themselves or to attain closeness to God and the descriptions lack the characteristic psychopathology described above.

Turning to bulimia nervosa, there is a clear historical starting point when Russell described his 'ominous' variant of anorexia nervosa (Russell 1979). Over the 20 years since that date, bulimia nervosa has emerged as a common disorder affecting nearly 2% of the female population. In a scholarly text, Parry-Jones & Parry-Jones (1991) reviewed the history prior to 1979. Literally translated, bulimia means ox-hunger. They found historical reference to a number of cases occurring in the Middle Ages and up to the beginning of the 19th century where there were clear descriptions of rapid ingestion of food, secret eating, night bingeing, self-induced vomiting and all accompanied by normal weight. St Catherine of Sienna (died 1380) may have been the first case description of bulimia nervosa. She certainly self-induced vomiting by passing straws into her throat. William Cullen (1780) described three types of bulimia, one of which, bulimia emetica, is very similar to the modern concept of bulimia nervosa. Other types of bulimia may have been related to head injury and infestation with worms.

Russell (1997) gives three detailed case descriptions of these early cases. The case of Nadia (Janet 1903); the case of patient D (Wulff 1932); and the case of Ellen West (Binswanger), all of whom may have met modern diagnostic criteria for bulimia nervosa. These cases clearly describe the bodily loathing, the cravings for food, a history of sexual abuse, a family history of depression and the use of other methods of purging such as laxatives to purge.

Diagnostic issues

I will describe the clinical syndromes of anorexia nervosa and bulimia nervosa separately, but it is important to realise that there is much overlap and that individuals during their eating disorders career may move from one disorder to the other, not just on one, but on several occasions (Figs 18.1 and 18.2).

Current diagnostic criteria dictate that anorexia nervosa 'trumps' bulimia nervosa (Table 18.1). In other words, if an individual meets the diagnostic criteria for anorexia nervosa, then this is the primary diagnosis, whether or not they binge or purge. The most common

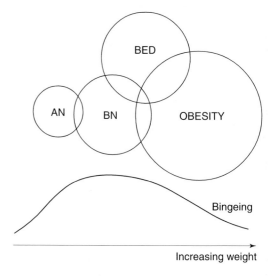

	AN	BN	BED
	1% or less	2–4% depending on population	4–5% depending on definition
Dietary restraint (all 3 groups dieting)	↓↓↓	↓↓	↓
Bingeing	+	+++	++
Purging	++	+++	–

Fig. 18.1 Relationship of eating disorders to each other. AN, anorexia nervosa; BED, binge eating disorder; BN, bulimia nervosa.

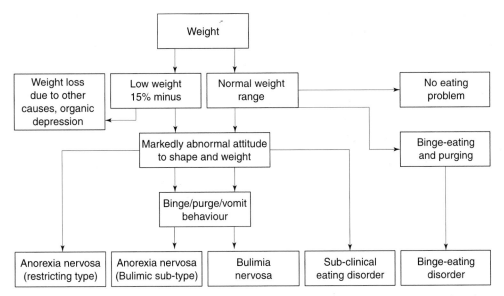

Fig. 18.2 Diagnostic flow chart for anorexia nervosa, bulimia nervosa and binge eating disorder.

Table 18.1 Diagnostic criteria for anorexia nervosa, bulimia nervosa and binge eating disorder. The ruling that anorexia nervosa 'trumps' bulimia nervosa is adopted

	Anorexia nervosa (restricting subtype)	Anorexia nervosa (bulimic subtype)	Bulimia nervosa	Binge eating disorder
Characteristic extreme concerns about shape and weight	Yes	Yes	Yes	Maybe
Behaviour designed to control shape and weight	Yes	Yes	Yes	No
Bulimic episodes	No	Yes	Yes	Yes
Low weight according to population norms	Yes	Yes	No	No
Amenorrhoea	Yes	Yes	Maybe	No

direction of movement is from anorexia to bulimia, with some 50% of those who initially meet the diagnostic criteria for anorexia nervosa graduating to bulimia. Movement in the opposite direction (that is, an individual starting with normal weight bulimia and then developing anorexia nervosa) does occur but is less common.

Tables 18.2 and 18.3 give the diagnostic criteria for the two main disorders according to ICD-10 (WHO 1992). The criteria according to DSM-IV (APA 1994) are similar but less detailed for anorexia nervosa. ICD-10 requires a body mass index of 17.5 or less, whereas DSM-IV only requires a body weight of 85% or less than that which would be expected. ICD-10 gives more detailed criteria for the symptoms to be expected in pre-pubertal anorexia nervosa. DSM-IV subdivides anorexia nervosa into restricting and binge eating/purging type.

For bulimia nervosa, DSM-IV has stricter criteria for a binge in that it has to occur in a discrete period of time (within 2 hours). ICD-10 describes more fully the common earlier history of anorexia nervosa which may have been fully expressed or cryptic. DSM-IV divides bulimia nervosa into a purging type where there is self-induced vomiting or the misuse of laxatives, diuretics or enemas, and a non-purging type where binge eating alternates with other compensatory behaviours such as fasting or excessive exercise.

Binge eating disorder does not yet have separate diagnostic criteria in either DSM-IV or ICD-10, though papers are now regularly beginning to appear on the aetiology, epidemiology and treatment of this disorder. There are research criteria for binge eating disorder in DSM-IV and these are given in Table 18.4. It can be

---

Table 18.2   ICD-10 diagnostic criteria for anorexia nervosa

For a definite diagnosis all of the following are required:

- Body weight is maintained at least 15% below that expected (either lost or never achieved), or Quetelet's body mass index is 17.5 or less. Prepubertal patients may show failure to make the expected weight gain during the period of growth
- The weight loss is self-induced by avoidance of 'fattening foods'. One or more of the following may also be present: self-induced vomiting; self-induced purging: excessive exercise: use of appetite suppressants and/or diuretics
- There is body image distortion in the form of a specific psychopathology whereby a dread of fatness persists as an intrusive, overvalued idea and the patient imposes a low weight threshold on himself or herself
- A widespread endocrine disorder involving the hypothalamic–pituitary–gonadal axis is manifest in women as amenorrhoea and in men as a loss of sexual interest and potency. (An apparent exception is the persistence of vaginal bleeds in anorexic women who are receiving replacement hormonal therapy, most commonly taken as a contraceptive pill.) There may also be elevated levels of growth hormone, raised levels of cortisol, changes in the peripheral metabolism of the thyroid hormone, and abnormalities of insulin secretion
- If onset is prepubertal, the sequence of pubertal events is delayed or even arrested (growth ceases; in girls the breasts do not develop and there is a primary amenorrhoea; and in boys the genitals remain juvenile). With recovery, puberty is often completed normally, but the menarche is late

Atypical anorexia nervosa This term should be used for those individuals in whom one or more of the key features of anorexia nervosa, such as amenorrhoea or significant weight loss, is absent, but who otherwise present a fairly typical clinical picture. Such people are usually encountered in psychiatric liaison services in general hospitals or in primary care. Patients who have all the key symptoms but to only a mild degree may also be best described by this term. This term should not be used for eating disorders that resemble anorexia nervosa but that are due to known physical illness

---

Table 18.3   ICD-10 diagnostic criteria for bulimia nervosa

For a definite diagnosis, all of the following are required:

- There is a persistent preoccupation with eating, and an irresistible craving for food: the patient succumbs to episodes of overeating in which large amounts of food are consumed in short periods of time
- The patient attempts to counteract the 'fattening' effects of food by one or more of the following: self-induced vomiting: purgative abuse: alternating periods of starvation: use of drugs such as appetite suppressants, thyroid preparations, or diuretics. When bulimia occurs in diabetic patients they may choose to neglect their insulin treatment
- The psychopathology consists of a morbid dread of fatness, and the patient sets herself or himself a sharply defined weight threshold, well below the premorbid weight that constitutes the optimum or healthy weight in the opinion of the physician. There is often, but not always, a history of an earlier episode of anorexia nervosa, the interval between the two disorders ranging from a few months to several years. This earlier episode may have been fully expressed, or may have assumed a minor cryptic form with a moderate loss of weight and/or a transient phase of amenorrhoea

Atypical bulimia nervosa This term should be used for those individuals in whom one or more of the key features listed for bulimia nervosa is absent but who otherwise present a fairly typical clinical picture. Most commonly this applies to people with normal or even excessive weight but with typical periods of overeating followed by vomiting or purging. Partial syndromes together with depressive symptoms are also not uncommon, but if the depressive symptoms justify a separate diagnosis of a depressive disorder, two diagnoses should be made

---

As far as other atypical eating disorders are concerned, DSM-IV has only one category, eating disorder not otherwise specified (EDNOS), whereas ICD-10 has five: atypical anorexia nervosa; atypical bulimia nervosa; overeating associated without psychological disturbances; vomiting associated with other psychological disturbances; and other eating disorders. There is very little research on this group and the term 'atypical' includes a number of cases who have partial syndromes of either anorexia nervosa or bulimia nervosa, sometimes referred to as subthreshold disorders. Other disorders classified here would be overeating that leads to obesity, vomiting that may occur in hypochondriacal or

seen that the main differences are concerned with the lack of inappropriate compensatory behaviours such as purging, fasting and excessive exercise.

Table 18.4   DSM-IV research criteria for binge eating disorder

A. Recurrent episodes of binge eating. An episode of binge eating is characterised by both of the following:
   (1) eating, in a discrete period of time (e.g. within any 2 hour period), an amount of food that is definitely larger than most people would eat in a similar period of time under similar circumstances; and
   (2) a sense of lack of control over eating during the episode (e.g. a feeling that one cannot stop eating or control what or how much one is eating)

B. The binge-eating episodes are associated with three (or more) of the following:
   (1) eating much more rapidly than normal
   (2) eating until feeling uncomfortably full
   (3) eating large amounts of food when not feeling physically hungry
   (4) eating alone because of being embarrassed by how much one is eating
   (5) feeling disgusted with oneself, depressed or very guilty after overeating

C. Marked distress regarding binge eating is present

D. The binge eating occurs, on average, at least 2 days a week for 6 months.
   Note: The method of determining frequency differs from that used for bulimia nervosa: future research should address whether the preferred method of setting a frequency threshold is counting the number of days on which binges occur or counting the number of episodes of binge eating

E. The binge eating is not associated with the regular use of inappropriate compensatory behaviours (e.g. purging, fasting, excessive exercise) and does not occur exclusively during the course of anorexia nervosa or bulimia nervosa

dissociative disorders and other types of psychogenic vomiting. Pica of non-organic origin occurring in adults and psychogenic loss of appetite which is not caused by major depression would also be classified here.

The diagnostic criteria for all these disorders are continually under review and it will be interesting to see what emerges in DSM-IVR or DSM-V. Simple changes can make major differences to the size of different diagnostic groups. It was only a few years ago that the diagnostic criteria for anorexia nervosa were altered. The threshold for the amount of weight loss required used to be 25% or greater and is now 15%. This is clearly one way to make a disorder much more common

overnight. Conversely, there are moves to tighten the criteria for bulimia nervosa and only to include the group that are currently described under DSM-IV's binge/purge type. If this happened, the non-purging type of bulimia nervosa would probably be included with binge eating disorder.

ANOREXIA NERVOSA

Epidemiology

Table 18.5 gives the findings of studies that have investigated the incidence of anorexia nervosa.

Clinical features

The core feature of anorexia nervosa is a profound psychological disturbance which centres on an overwhelming concern about body size, shape and weight. Sufferers feel fat even when emaciated, are terrified of any weight gain and preoccupied with elaborate plans to reduce weight further. Such psychopathology has variously been described as hysterical, a phobia of weight gain, an obsessional symptom and clearly delusional. To some extent it simply represents a marked exaggeration of ideas that are widespread in our society and it is perhaps best conceptualised as a set of overvalued ideas. Multiple theories exist as to why these beliefs should be so firmly held. They include fear of maturation, fear of secondary sexual characteristics, fear of separation, usually from a maternal figure, fear of oral impregnation through to addictive and biological models (see Aetiology below). What patients themselves nearly always say is that the central feature for them is that they fear loss of control and that this is countered by the increased sense of self-control from strict dieting and from being able to determine one's size and shape. This of course is one of the many paradoxes of anorexia nervosa: while trying to achieve that sense of autonomy and self-control, sufferers end up trapped in a disorder which profoundly controls them. Patients rarely say that their starvation was designed to make them more attractive to others, though they do feel that gaining even a small amount of weight would make them even less attractive. Weight gain and 'fat' in particular come to symbolise laziness, self-indulgence, lack of control and self-loathing.

As well as self-induced starvation there are a whole range of other behaviours designed to reduce weight. These are summarised in Table 18.6. Many of these behaviours develop into very obsessional or ritualistic patterns so that exercise has to be for a prescribed number of minutes every day and can never be less than that carried out the day before.

Table 18.5	Incidence of anorexia nervosa		
Area	Authors	Period	Annual incidence per 100 000 population
Southern Sweden	Theander (1970)	1931–1940	0.08
		1941–1950	0.19
		1951–1960	0.45
North-east Scotland	Kendell et al (1973)	1966–1969	1.60
	Szmukler et al (1986)	1978–1982	4.06
Zurich canton	Willi & Grossman (1983)	1963–1965	0.55
		1973–1975	1.12
	Willi et al (1990)	1983–1985	1.43
Monroe County,	Kendell et al (1973)	1960–1969	0.37
New York State, USA	Jones et al (1980)	1970–1976	0.64
Rochester, Minnesota, USA	Lucas et al[a] (1991)	1950–1954	4.63[b]
		1980–1984	14.20[b]

[a]Increase in incidence occurred principally in females 10–19 years old.
[b]Figures kindly provided by Dr A. Lucas.

The intense dietary restraint is characterised by a narrowing of the range of foods eaten, a complete avoidance of certain foods which are seen as 'fattening', and usually some method of calorie counting with a predetermined daily calorie limit of well under 1000 calories.

The body image disturbance is an unusual and not very well understood symptom. There are at least two components; the first is a perceptual distortion of body size and shape so that either the whole body or specific parts of the body appear larger or fatter to the sufferer. Anorexia nervosa sufferers can accurately gauge the size of other people's bodies and of inanimate objects but not of their own. There is some evidence that they dis-tort meal size as well. They will often report that when caught unaware by a mirror image they didn't recognise themselves and truly saw a thin emaciated figure. The second component is of body disparagement. This can be generalised or again focused on specific parts. There is an intense dislike amounting to hatred of their own body (for a detailed review see Smeets 1997).

Case history 1: Mr A.B. had been a junior cross-country champion. Even at 14 years he had prided himself on keeping his body fat below 10%. This was measured regularly by his coach using skin callipers. He didn't have to restrict his intake as he ran a half marathon 5 days per week and swam for 2 hours on the other 2 days. At 15 years, while studying for his 'O' grade exams, he had to exercise less and compensated by reducing his intake. By 16.5 years he had the full-blown syndrome of anorexia nervosa with a BMI of 13 and a weight of 35 kgs. He achieved straight As in 'O' and 'A' levels and entrance to medical school.

He presented for treatment towards the end of his first year at medical school, not having been picked up at university entrance and with the headmaster's reference from his school mentioning nothing of his problems. His presenting complaint was pain in his ankles. Examination showed that he had bilateral stress fractures of both ankles, moderately severe osteoporosis and marked lack of secondary sexual characteristics. By this time he was existing on a diet of vitamin pills and white boiled fish. His parents would deliver a crate of fish weekly to his hall of residence. He would eat only one meal per day and

Table 18.6 Behaviour designed to reduce weight in anorexia nervosa

- Marked dietary restraint
- Total fasting
- Increased exercise
- Chewing and spitting of food
- Regurgitation of food
- Vomiting of food after meals
- Excessive use of laxatives
- Use of ipecac to induce vomiting (rare in UK)
- Use of diuretics (mainly over the counter preparations)
- Use of appetite suppressant drugs
- Fluid restriction
- Gastric lavage
- Colonic lavage

would boil the fish for 2 hours, standing with a whole roll of paper towel dabbing the globules of oil and fat that rose to the surface as the fish was being boiled. He could no longer run but he walked at least 5 miles a day in extreme pain. He had kept up his pattern of severely restricted eating for over 4 years, never losing control.

Repeated inpatient treatment programmes in various specialists units around the country produced only modest and short-term improvement, with weight gains of 6–7 kg being lost within 6 months of discharge.

Fifteen years later, Mr A.B., now aged 32 years, has chronic but stable anorexia nervosa with a weight which fluctuates between 37 and 40 kg, a very restricted and stereotyped eating pattern, a rigid plan of exercise and severe osteoporosis, despite several years of testosterone replacement. He did complete a degree, though not in medicine, and leads a lonely isolated life dominated by routine and ritual. He would clearly meet the diagnostic criteria for obsessive compulsive disorder.

Case history 2: Ms C.D. presented at the age of 16 years with severe anorexia nervosa but with only a 9 month history. She had gone on a diet when her first relationship had ended just after her 15th birthday. Other triggering factors appeared to be the loss (at her female boarding school) of a close girlfriend who had become jealous of her relationship with her boyfriend, and the fact that her parents had decided to move to Spain, leaving her and her youngest sister at boarding school in the UK. She had lost just under 17 kg in 9 months and had had amenorrhoea for 6 months.

Physical examination showed she was emaciated, covered in fine downy hair (lanugo) and had bright orange palms and soles (hypercarotenaemia). Her blood pressure was low, with a bradycardia of under 50, and she was markedly depressed. She had not been compulsively exercising or using any other weight control measures.

For the past 3 months she had been existing on cups of tea and coffee with skimmed milk, oxo cubes and plates of boiled vegetables. She would chew the vegetables for long periods but not swallow them, spitting each mouthful out after approximately 10 minutes of mastication.

Her Dexa bone density scan showed no osteoporosis. She had been a very fit and active adolescent with an early puberty and menarche and had fully mineralised her bones by the age of 16 years. Her initial weight loss had been profoundly rewarding. Two other boys in the local village had shown interest in her and she had been able to brush them aside. Her status with her peers at school increased and she moved from just being able to get into size 12 clothes to easily being able to fit into a size 10. She could even wear her younger sisters' clothes. Her more severe weight loss caused her mother to return from Spain and to rent a house close to the school.

Treatment consisted of 10 weekly outpatient sessions followed by monthly follow-ups for the next 9 months. Elements of treatment were the institution of a regular meal plan, self-monitoring with diaries, and two extended family interviews, for one of which her father came back from Spain. She also had repeated medical investigations, the results of which were fed back to her in detail. The individual sessions used both cognitive, behavioural and interpersonal techniques, examining each significant relationship in detail and using cognitive therapy to help her identify her dysfunctional attitudes and beliefs and to challenge them.

Weight gain occurred slowly over the next year and levelled out at about 4 kg less than her predisorder weight, giving her a BMI of just under 20.

Follow-up over the next 9 years has shown no recurrence of her eating disorder, apart from a brief 3 month period of binge eating towards the end of first year at university, again associated with the breakup of a relationship. Menstruation returned within 9 months and fertility has not been impaired. Ms C.D., now aged 24 years, has been in a stable and sexually active relationship for the past 2 years. Interestingly, the first annual bone scan showed a marked drop in bone density into the osteoporotic range, even though weight had been largely restored by this time. Follow-up showed that it was 7 years before she regained the bone density she had had at age 16 years. This occurred without specific treatment.

General psychopathology

Depressed mood and lability of mood are common features, and in more chronic cases hopelessness and thoughts of suicide may be present. Anxiety symptoms, usually related to situations which involve eating, are also encountered and many sufferers develop marked socially phobic symptoms, not being able to eat in public at all. Outside interests are often reduced and there is usually marked social withdrawal. Obsessional features may be present and frequently mean that the food preparation and eating become slow and ritualistic. Work or school performances are often maintained despite increasing impairments of concentration and marked emaciation.

Table 18.7 Physical consequences of anorexia nervosa and bulimia

System	Starvation	Bingeing/purging/vomiting
Cardiovascular	Bradycardia	Arrhythmias
	Hypotension	Cardiac failure
	Sudden death	Sudden death
	Mitral valve dysfunction	
Renal	Mild pitting oedema	Severe oedema
	Electrolyte abnormalities:	Electrolyte abnormalities:
	hypophosphataemia,	hypokalaemia, hyponatraemia,
	hypomagnesaemia,	hypochloraemia, metabolic alkalosis
	hypocalcaemia	(vomitors), metabolic acidosis (with
		laxative abuse),hypomagnesaemia,
		hypophosphataemia,
		hypocalcaemia
	Renal calculi	Renal calculi
	Hypokalaemic nephropathy	Hypokalaemic nephropathy
	Proteinuria	
	Reduced glomerular filtration	
Gastrointestinal	Parotid swelling	Parotid swelling
		Oesophageal erosion
		Oesophageal/gastric perforation
	Delayed gastric emptying	Gastric/duodenal ulcers
	Refeeding pancreatitis	Pancreatitis
	Nutritional hepatitis	
	Constipation	Constipation, steatorrhoea
Skeletal	Osteoporosis	Osteoporosis
	Pathological fractures	Pathological fracture
	Short stature	
Endocrine	Amenorrhoea	
	Low LHRH, LH and FSH	
	Low oestrogen and progesterone	
	Low tri iodothyronine (T_3)	
	High cortisol	
	High fasting growth hormone	
	Erratic vasopressin release	
Haematological	Anaemia	
	Leukopenia	Leukopenia, lymphocytosis
	Thrombocytopenia	
	Bone marrow hypoplasia	
	Reduced serum complement levels	
	Low ESR	
Neurological	Generalized seizures	Generalized seizures
	Confusional states	Confusional states
	EEG abnormalities	EEG abnormalities
	Peripheral neuropathies	Peripheral neuropathies
	Ventricular enlargement	
Metabolic	Impaired temperature regulation	Impaired temperature regulation
	Hypercholesterolaemia	Hypercholesterolaemia
	Hypercarotenaemia	Hypercarotenaemia
	Hypoproteinaemia	Hypoproteinaemia
	Impaired glucose tolerance	Fasting hypoglycaemia
	High β-hydroxybutyrate	High β-hydroxybutyrate
	High free fatty acids	High free fatty acids
	Impaired calcium metabolism	
Dermatological	Lanugo, brittle hair and nails	Calluses on dorsum of hands

Contribution of starvation: the Minnesota experiments

All therapists working with eating disorders should be familiar with a key set of studies carried out towards the end of the Second World War and published nearly 50 years ago by Ancel Keys (Keys et al 1950). Thirty-six men who were the youngest, healthiest and most psychologically normal of 100 volunteers were selected to take part in this study of starvation. By volunteering, the men avoided military service. During the first 3 months they ate normally while their behaviour, personality and eating patterns were monitored. During the next 6 months, the men were restricted to approximately half their former food intake and lost on average a quarter of their former weight. They were thus starved down into the anorexia nervosa range. After 6 months of weight loss, there was a further 3 months of rehabilitation/refeeding with a 9 month poststarvation monitoring occurring, in some subjects.

The importance of this study is that many of the symptoms thought to be characteristic of anorexia nervosa occurred in these men. When treating sufferers it is important to appreciate just how much of the psychological and behavioural symptoms are a result of the starvation state and not a cause of it.

The men became increasingly preoccupied by food: they found it difficult to carry out their usual daily activities because they were plagued by incessant thoughts of food and eating. Food became the principal topic of conversation or reading and of daydreams. The men began to smuggle bits of food out of the dining room, hid food and ate food in secret in long rituals. Men who had no previous interest in food or cooking became intensely interested in menus, cookbooks, dietetics and even food production. The men reported getting vicarious pleasure from watching other subjects eat. Hoarding was not just confined to food but included cooking utensils, recipes and even non-food related items. The men spent much of the day planning how they would eat their daily allotment of food. They made unusual concoctions of food, often ate in silence and ate in a quite ritualistic way, dawdling over food so that even small meals would take several hours.

Other behaviours such as rummaging through garbage cans, binge eating and marked increase in coffee intake were reported in some subjects. Mood swings were common and about a quarter of the men had significant depression. Irritability and frequent outbursts of anger were common. Two subjects developed more serious psychiatric symptoms requiring hospital admission.

During the refeeding phase the behavioural changes did not immediately reverse. In some men they persisted throughout the follow-up period. Some men became more depressed when refeeding. One man chopped three fingers off his hand in a fit of severe depression.

Marked social and sexual changes also occurred so that the men became progressively more withdrawn and isolated with little sense of humour or comradeship. Most men responded to increasing starvation with a decrease in physical activity but a few exercised deliberately, feeling that they would be able to eat a little more if they did so.

Physical complications

Details of these are given in Table 18.7; for a comprehensive review see Sharp & Freeman (1993). The main laboratory abnormalities are also listed.

Most of the many complications associated with anorexia nervosa are found in uncomplicated starvation, and are reversed by return to a normal healthy diet, but there are important differences between anorexia and starvation. In anorexia protein intake is usually adequate but carbohydrates, fats and therefore calories are lacking. Vitamin deficiencies are uncommon.

Cardiac abnormalities may occur at some stage in over 80% of anorexic patients. These include bradycardia, tachycardia, hypotension, ventricular arrythmias, cardiac failure and a variety of ECG changes. Congestive cardiac failure may occur as a terminal event in the disorder but is also a well-recognised complication of refeeding, first described in survivors of the concentration and prisoner of war camps in the Second World War.

Most of the gastrointestinal complications, such as oesophagitis, erosions and ulcers, are a result of frequent exposure to gastric acid. In clinical practice delayed gastric emptying is responsible for the feelings of fullness and bloating reported by patients after eating, which are often wrongly interpreted as the deposition of fat.

Pancreatic disease is uncommon but occasional cases of acute pancreatitis have been reported in the refeeding phase. Liver changes are common in protein-calorie malnutrition. Nutritional hepatitis, manifested by low serum protein and raised serum levels along with raised lactate dehydrogenase and alkaline phosphatase, occur in about a third of subjects.

Pancytopenia is common in severe anorexia, with mild anaemia and thrombocytopenia reported in about-one-third of patients and leucopenia in up to two-thirds.

Patients with early onset anorexia nervosa tend to be shorter than their peers and bone mineralisation can be markedly impaired during adolescence. Osteoporosis and pathological fractures are common and demonstrable osteoporosis can occur within 2 years of the onset of anorexia nervosa.

Anorexia nervosa is one of the most lethal of all psychiatric disorders. Long-term follow-up data indicate that the mortality rate is over 20% at 30 year follow-up (Theander 1985). More recent follow-up studies show mortality rates of between 5 and 10% at 10 years. Two-thirds of patients die of the direct effects of the disorder, one-third from suicide.

Aetiology

Most women who suffer from this disorder will talk about control as being the central issue. They will describe the sense of power and achievement they get from self-induced starvation and denial, particularly when they feel that the rest of their life is out of control. Nevertheless it is clear that anorexia nervosa does not develop from a single cause. When thinking about the aetiology a number of factors have to be considered (Fig. 18.3). The disorder is overwhelmingly one of women; the majority of cases start in adolescence, with the average of onset being 16 years, but it can start at any time from childhood to late middle age. Strict self-starvation is a key feature, but most women do not have a history of obesity. No biological or organic cause has been found and at present we have to conclude that the disorder is mainly psychological in origin.

Genetic factors in both anorexia nervosa and bulimia nervosa run in families. The evidence from twin studies suggests that specific genetic factors are more important in anorexia nervosa and particularly in restricting anorexia nervosa. Concordance rates from monozygotic twins are approximately 65% and for dizygotic is 32%. The vulnerability to anorexia nervosa appears to be a specific one and not a general predisposition to 'neuroticism' or psychiatric disorder. The non-affected twins of monozygotic pairs appear remarkably normal in contrast with bulimia nervosa, there seems to be an inheritance of a more general predisposition with links with substance abuse, affective disorder and obesity. The finding of

high rates of perfectionism in the dizygotic has led to the view that this could be the vulnerability trait.

Sociodemographic factors, social class, parental age, family composition and family size have all been suggested as contributing factors to the development of this disorder; however, none of these have been found consistently across studies. Careful examination of social class distribution (Gard & Freeman 1996) shows that it is only in clinic samples that there is an excess of social classes I–III and that in community samples eating disorders are spread evenly across the social classes. Of the other factors mentioned above, only an association with parental age has some support, with several studies consistently finding that anorexia nervosa sufferers have older parents.

Adverse events

There does not seem to be an excess of childhood sexual or physical abuse compared with other psychiatric disorders, nor is there an excess of parental loss due to death or breakup of a family.

Individual and family pathology

One pragmatic way of viewing the psychology of anorexia nervosa is to see it as an adaptive process. Self-induced starvation serves many positive roles for young women, giving an increased sense of control and autonomy relating to their own body, while at the same time developing increased dependence on their nuclear family. Basic beliefs relating to perfectionism, high achievement and aestheticism are all enhanced, while maturational tasks such as individuation and separation are avoided. Secondary sexual characteristics do not develop and a peripubertal state of development is ensured. It may well be that these psychological factors initiate the disorder and then biological and addictive processes take over, ensuring the chronicity and resistance to treatment.

Family studies, particularly those by Minuchin and Selvini-Palazoli, were very influential in the 1970s and 1980s. Certain characteristic family styles and patterns of interaction were said to increase the likelihood of producing an anorexic daughter. The concept of the anorexogenic mother probably has as much validity as the schizophrenogenic mother and has probably done as much harm. Mothers of anorexic girls already feel profoundly guilty and responsible and theories that blame them are hardly useful therapeutically. Our own studies (Blair et al 1995) comparing normal control families, families with a cystic fibrosis child and families with an anorexic daughter showed little difference between the three groups and the most important

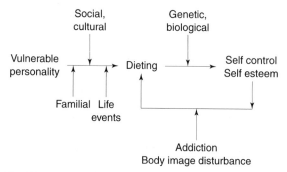

Fig. 18.3 Anorexia nervosa: its multiple aetiology.

finding was that family disturbance increased with the chronicity of the disorder, suggesting it was the disorder which largely caused the family disturbance rather than vice versa. We did not find that classical concepts, such as rigidity, enmeshment, weak generational boundaries, differentiated between the groups. It seems much more likely that these were features of upper middle-class Edinburgh families whether or not they have an ill child.

Biological factors

The hypothalamus has been most frequently cited as the likely organic factor contributing to aetiology but the hypothalamic dysfunction found is similar to that found in starvation due to other causes and tends to return to normal when the patient regains weight. Several studies have found neuropsychological deficits such as reduced vigilance and attention span, impairment of visuospatial processing and impaired associate learning. Again most of these seem to return to normal limits with weight gain. Computerised tomography has shown significant sulcal widening and/or ventricular enlargement, which again appear reversible with renutrition. In a minority of cases these abnormalities do not reverse, even though the degree of abnormality was related to the rapidity of the original weight loss. The most interesting findings are those recently reported by Gordon et al (1997). In a small sample of children and adolescents with anorexia nervosa, 13 of 15 patients had unilateral temporal lobe hypoperfusion as demonstrated by regional cerebral blood flow radioisotope scans. These findings are of particular interest because the abnormalities are unilateral and therefore unlikely to be due directly to starvation. Attempts to link these abnormalities with specific psychopathology, such as impairment of visuospatial processing leading to vulnerability to body image distortion, are at present complete speculation but nevertheless interesting.

Treatment

There is remarkably little research evidence to guide us in this area. There have been very few controlled trials and most of the published work consists of lengthy descriptions of treatment programmes with a striking lack of detail about their effectiveness. One exception to this is the series of trials from the Maudsley Hospital comparing family with individual therapy and different types of family intervention. We therefore have to be guided by what is seen as current best clinical practice. There is general agreement that no one treatment modality is sufficient and that for most moderately severe and severe cases combined treatment approaches are required and that one of the skills is introducing

these claimed elements in sequence so as to provide a coherent treatment programme.

Perhaps the single most skilled task is to engage the patient in treatment in the first place. Many anorexic sufferers feel very strongly that they don't want or need treatment. The following general principles are a consensus of what most specialists would agree.

- The initial interview/assessment and subsequent engagement and treatment is of vital importance and needs time and considerable skill.
- Psychological treatment/psychotherapy is the treatment of choice. Experience in treating such patients is probably much more important than the type of psychotherapy used.
- Inpatient treatment may be required for some patients and a small number will require compulsory treatment to stop them dying.
- Psychological treatment is of little benefit and difficult to administer in severely starving patients who need a degree of weight restoration first.
- The treatment needs to involve significant others (family of origin and/or partner), though this does not need to be in the form of systematised family therapy.
- Treatment needs to be flexible and adapted to suit the patient's needs. Treatment approaches in the past have been too rigid.
- Treatment will not be brief and treatment services need to be organised so as to provide continuity of care through the various phases of treatment.

Inpatient treatment

There is no doubt that weight restoration is the primary goal for emaciated and medically compromised anorexic patients; however, Hsu (1988) has demonstrated that weight restoration to normal or near normal weight is a weak predictor of long term outcome.

It is difficult to tease out what the necessary components are from comprehensive treatment regimens, which often include supervised eating, medication, nutritional education, individual and/or family psychotherapy, operant conditioning methods and coercion. Agras & Kraemer (1983) described 21 published treatment studies which they classified into drug therapy, behaviour therapy and medical therapy. They found that medication did not add benefit to hospitalisation and that behavioural therapy produced more rapid weight gain. Touyz et al (1984) compared the effects of strict versus lenient operant conditioning programmes on weight gain in a sample of 65 anorexic inpatients. The lenient programme produced just as much weight gain and was far more acceptable than the strict programme. It was also associated with higher motivation to participate in other aspects of treatment and required less nursing time.

Indications for inpatient treatment include serious physical complications or suicidal risk. When weight loss is extreme – body mass index (BMI) below 13 – or has been rapid then admission should be considered. Patients can survive at extremely low weights providing the weight is stable and providing there is careful monitoring of white cell count, haemoglobin, electrolytes and creatinine kinase. Other patients whose weight loss has been rapid, particularly after previous refeeding, can be medically compromised at much higher weights. Sometimes hospitalisation is needed because of the need for separation from the family or partner where there is a high degree of negative expressed emotion towards the patient, or where the family feels overwhelmed or helpless. Coercive procedures should be reserved for the very small group of non-compliant patients whose situation is truly life-threatening; if possible they should be avoided altogether.

Involuntary treatment

The legal system in most countries allows the committal of severely emaciated anorexic patients to hospital against their will and patients should not be allowed to die. There is currently an active debate as to whether there could be occasions when, with a severely ill patient with chronic disorder, who has had repeated episodes of refeeding and weight loss over many years, it might be appropriate to let such a patient die with dignity rather than subject her to yet another episode of what would almost be coercive refeeding.

Drug treatment

Nearly all studies in which the efficacy of different types of psychotropic medication have been assessed have shown very disappointing results. Antipsychotics, antidepressants, lithium and minor tranquillisers have all been shown to have little or no value. There has been some recent work showing that fluoxetine may aid refeeding in hospitalised anorexics. This may appear a paradoxical result, given that fluoxetine tends to cause weight loss and increase satiety. If it is effective it may work because it decreases obsessional preoccupation with food and therefore anxiety around eating.

Individual and family therapy

There have been no satisfactory studies comparing different models of individual psychotherapy, either for weight-restored anorexics or for those treated from the start with psychotherapy. Psychotherapy should not be used as a sole treatment. The medical aspects of the disorder need to be closely addressed while psychotherapy is taking place.

Russell et al (1987) showed that one group of patients, those with early-onset anorexia (before the age of 19 years) and with a short history (less than 3 years) fed very much better 1 year after discharge from hospital if they had received family therapy, as opposed to individual supportive psychotherapy, during that year. Another group in this study, those with late-onset anorexia, did slightly better with individual supportive therapy rather than family therapy. The most important finding of this study is that at 5 year follow-up those young patients who had received family therapy were still doing better. Further studies from the same group have confirmed these findings, and a recent study (Dare 1995) showed that those patients who were offered family counselling (a problem-solving approach) did better than those who were offered family therapy using the family systems approach where all the family was involved. More importantly, those families that had a higher degree of disturbance with a high level of criticism of their ill daughter benefited more from family counselling than from conjoint family therapy.

Although cognitive therapy has been widely proposed as part of a multidimensional treatment approach to anorexia, there has only been one controlled trial (Channon et al 1989). This showed no difference between behaviour therapy and cognitive therapy. A large multicentre study is under way in the USA. Currently there is a move towards day-patient or partial hospitalisation rather than inpatient treatment. This is led partly by cost considerations and partly because of the disappointing results of inpatient treatment, the high relapse rate and the repeated need for readmission. There is no doubt that some patients respond to inpatient refeeding by 'eating their way out of hospital'. Although treatment may seem to be partially successful because weight has been restored, the patient feels even more guilt and self-loathing and feels a failure, not just as an individual but as an anorexic, often resolving to starve even more vehemently as soon as discharge is achieved.

BULIMIA NERVOSA

As previously mentioned, Russell (1979) proposed the term bulimia nervosa to describe a disorder which began to appear during the mid-1970s and was characterised by young women presenting with bouts of uncontrolled overeating. Many other names were at first used, including bulimarexia, dietary chaos syndrome, bulimia and binge eating syndrome. The term bulimia nervosa is now the accepted and preferred one. It emphasises the close links between this disorder and anorexia nervosa and it specifies the 'nervosa' part of the syndrome characterised by drive for thinness, distorted body image and body disparagement. The ICD-10 diagnostic criteria are given in Table 18.2.

Clinical features

Like anorexia nervosa this is predominantly a female disorder, and in most clinics male cases of bulimia nervosa are rarer than those of anorexia nervosa. It is a disorder of young people that tends to start most commonly in midadolescence. Cases present for treatment somewhat later, typically in their early 20s. Between a third and a half of cases have previously been through a clear-cut episode of anorexia nervosa or a subclinical episode. The term cryptic anorexia nervosa has been used to describe these latter cases. These are women who would have been at the upper end of the normal weight range for height or mildly obese, who diet so that when they present they are in the middle of the normal weight range. They are classified as normal weight bulimia nervosa but in fact have engaged in marked dietary restraint which has triggered off their binge episodes.

Specific psychopathology

Much of the symptomatology is identical to that found in anorexia nervosa: overvalued ideas concerning shape and weight, and numerous methods of weight control including intense dieting, self-induced vomiting and laxative and diuretic use. There are the same preoccupations with food, eating, shape and weight. There is often less of a preoccupation with intensive exercising compared with anorexia nervosa.

The two main distinguishing features from anorexia nervosa are normal weight and the bulimic episodes themselves. These binges can be massive, involving many thousands of calories, and in severe cases will occur 10–15 times per day.

Bulimic episodes are often planned, the food being bought specifically to binge on. Binges are arranged at a time when they will not be interrupted. Binge foods are usually high-energy, high-fat, sweet foods and may be selected because they are 'easy' to binge on. Binge eating is usually rapid with food being vomited very shortly after it has been consumed. In more severe cases, binge–vomit cycles will go on for many hours. In large case series, the average number of binge episodes is 5–6 per week. Self-induced vomiting is usually induced by activating the gag reflex by inserting fingers into the throat. Many women soon learn to vomit simply by contracting thoracic and abdominal muscles and can then vomit at will and with ease. Some patients find great difficulty in triggering vomiting. Calluses may develop on the knuckles of the index and middle fingers where they are abraded by the palate during repeated efforts to trigger vomiting (Russell's sign). I have had patients who had to use balls of cling film inserted into the throat (a highly dangerous practice) or rolled-up copies of the *Radio Times* because of its rough texture. Gastric lavage is sometimes used instead of vomiting – a patient of mine graduating from aquarium hose to a garden hose and finally to her washing machine waste hose with a diameter of some 3.5 cm. This finally resulted in the rupture of the thoracic oesophagus. The use of ipecacuanha to induce vomiting is not common in the UK; it is used more frequently in the USA.

Figure 18.4 lists the items in a typical binge of over 20 000 calories and shows a number of features. A patient was out with her husband for a social meal. At the point at which she ate the potato salad she crossed her own threshold for her calorie intake for the day of 1000 calories. She deliberately ate the beetroot, thinking this might mark the onset of her bingeing. Everything she ate from this point on was labelled by her as a binge and therefore if she could vomit the beetroot back she would have got rid of all the binge food. She managed to stay in the restaurant for a further half hour, getting increasingly distressed, and then ran out, leaving her husband. The baked potatoes bought on the way home and much of the rest of the food was consumed over the 45 minutes she had at home before her husband arrived. Much of it was straight from the freez-

A BINGE	
1 gin and bitter lemon	2 profiteroles & cream
prawn cocktail	& choc. sauce
roll and butter	1 can diet Coke
2 glasses wine	1 can 7-up
1 slice roast beef	large gin and bitter lemon
1 slice roast pork	5 sandwiches & meat filling
1 slice ham	6 pancakes & butter
portion potato salad	7 scones & butter & jam
portion red cabbage	bowl ice cream (1 litre)
portion sweetcorn	2 slices date & walnut cake
portion coleslaw	1 litre fresh orange
lettuce, cucumber & tomato	3 glasses lemonade
portion curried rice	packet crisps
large baked potato & dressing	cup of tea
1/2 large bakewell tart	2 slices fruit cake
4 oz. Black Magic	4 biscuits
1 lb tablet	packet Polos

Fig. 18.4 A typical binge.

Monday June 11th	Vom	Lax	Other
Breakfast A 2 slices brown toast Primula cheese and marmite 1 medium apple			
A ½lb Muesli/bran type biscuits 1 tin Vienna biscuits (17½oz) 2 slices bread + slices cold butter + 2 tsps. apricot jam 2 mugs milky tea + cup fresh orange juice	1 vomit + 26 Vomit Rinsing Cycles		
Lunch A Scrambled eggs (2 large) on 1 slice (brown) toast + outline marg. 1 tomato. 1 lg. orange ¼lb seedless grapes. Mug milky tea			
A 1 loaf large, brown bread ¼lb butter, 6 heaped tsps golden syrup, 3 oz pate, 8 oz pork pie, tin Heinz coleslaw ½ tube Smarties, mug milky Ovaltine, 2 Farley's rusks 1 large glass orange juice, fresh	1 vomit + 30 cycles		
1 cold large potato, 4 cold sausages, 1 glass diluted Ribena, 4 Opal Fruit sweets, 2 slices cold ham	Rinsing + Vomiting		
A 14 oatcakes + 3 oz chedder cheese 4 boiled potatoes in melted butter, 1 apple, 2 pkts crisps, 2 mugs milky coffee, 4 choc ices, 1 small Aero, mug milky coffee, 1 medium apple	1+ 5 cycles		
A Totals			

Monday June 11th Continued
1 bowl veg soup (Heinz)
3 slices toast and butter
6 pkts crisps, 1 tablet jelly
1 large pkt chocolate digestives
12oz uncooked biscuit mixture:
(Comprising – 12oz margarine
        – 12oz flour
        – 6oz icing sugar
        – 6oz custard powder)
2 cans Fresca drink

}A 1 Vomit + 30 Rinsing and Vomiting cycles

Evening meal
Lettuce, cucumber, tomato
2oz chicken, 2 boiled pots (med)
1oz veg salad (Heinz), 1 beetroot,
2 spring onions, 1 orange (large)
2 slices toast + outline + Marmite
1 5oz flavoured yoghurt.
2 cups tea with milk
mug Ovaltine ½ milk ½ water

1 Vomit

1.30 A.M.
1 loaf bread (toasted) + 6oz butter
½ pot jam + ¼ pot marmalade
6 mugs milk + Ovaltine
1 mug milky tea

}A 2 Vomits

TOTAL CALORIES: 26,000

TOTAL 7 VOMITS + 91 RINSING AND VOMITING CYCLES

Fig. 18.5   Diary pages: bulimia nervosa. **A** binge / purge day; **B** restricting day.

er and semifrozen. She managed to make herself sick just before her husband returned.

Figure 18.5 shows typical diary pages from a patient with severe bulimia nervosa.

Patients are very secretive about their behaviour and may go on for several years before they seek help. Although initially the binges may be exciting, or at least provide some relief from anxiety or depression, as the bingeing progresses there is profound dysphoria, depression, guilt and self-loathing, only partially relieved by self-induced vomiting.

Once established, bulimia nervosa becomes self-sustaining with a number of feedback loops maintaining the disorder (Figure 18.6).

A minority of patients start with self-induced vomiting, progressing subsequently to bingeing. For the majority the vomiting occurs immediately after the first binge or is discovered 'after some months of bingeing'.

Initially vomiting produces a great sense of relief, in that control over bingeing is now less required, but progressively the binges get more and more out of control.

General psychopathology

The most common comorbid symptoms are those of anxiety and mood disorders Laessle (1987) found that 46% of bulimia nervosa subjects had a history of major depression. At presentation, depressive symptoms are certainly common but these are often secondary to the eating disorder and disappear when the eating disorder is treated without the use of antidepressant medication. Clinically the presence of major depressive disorder in patients with bulimia nervosa does not generally imply poor prognosis. Clinical trials of both psychological and drug treatments have found that current or past depressive disorder is not related to outcome. There is an

Day

Wednesday 6th June		Vom	Lax	Other	Comments:
Breakfast 1 cup white coffee (skim milk)				12.5mg Amphet. 1 Sanatogen Multi-Vit	
A *Lunch* 1 cup tea (skim milk) 1 tsp Bio-strath yeast food supplement 1 cup tea (skim milk)					The desire to starve myself today has been:
A					
Evening meal 1 cup tea (skim milk) 1 Oxo cube drink					Today urge to overeat has been:
A 1 Oxo cube drink 1 can diet Coke 1 white coffee (skim milk) TOTAL CALORIES: 88			15 Senakot	Sleeping Pill	Today in general I have felt:
B	Totals				

The desire to starve myself today has been:

not at all — as strong as it possibly could be

Today urge to overeat has been:

not there at all — as strong as it possibly could be

Today in general I have felt:

extremely emotionally upset — not emotionally upset at all

Fig. 18.5 *Cont'd*

excess family history of both major depression and obesity in the families of bulimia nervosa subjects, but no corresponding excess of eating disorders in the families of those with major depression. This indicates that there is not a common pathogenesis in bulimia nervosa and major depression.

A minority of bulimia nervosa sufferers have multiple dyscontrol behaviours indicative of marked personality disturbance. These include cutting, burning, multiple taking of overdoses, alcohol and drug misuse, promiscuity, shop-lifting and other self-damaging behaviours. This subgroup have been given the term multi-impulsive bulimia nervosa by Lacey (1993). Lacey's criteria require at least three of the following behaviours:

- drinking at least 36 units of alcohol per week
- taking heroin, LSD or amphetamines or purchasing street tranquillisers on at least four occasions in the previous year

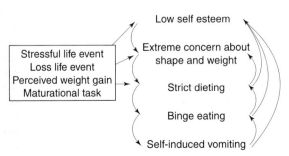

Fig. 18.6 Triggering and maintenance of bulimia nervosa.

- stealing at least 10 times in the previous year
- taking at least one overdose in the previous year; and severe regular self-cutting or self-burning.

These patients also show marked affective dysregulation, with mood swings of depression, anger and elation. They are older when they first seek help and are more likely to have been sexually abused.

Physical complications

Many patients have no physical complaints at all, though bulimia nervosa can be associated with significant adverse medical sequelae. Compared with anorexia nervosa, medical complications are relatively benign, and the mortality seen appears to be very low. Enlarged submandibular and parotid salivary glands resulting in a puffy face occur commonly after bingeing. In the majority of patients these swellings go down after a day or two but in a small number there appears to be permanent hypertrophy. Dental enamel erosion of the palatal surface of the upper teeth can be severe and dentists can easily identify cases of bulimia nervosa by mouth inspection. Dental amalgam is more resistant to gastric acid than the surrounding tooth enamel so fillings tend to protrude above the teeth. The majority of patients who have been vomiting for several years will have obvious evidence of dental enamel erosion. Vigorous toothbrushing is understandable following self-induced vomiting, and may increase dental enamel wear. An alkaline mouthwash should be used.

The other major complication is hypokalaemia. About 50% of bulimia patients have electrolyte abnormalities, which can be detected on routine screening. Frank metabolic acidosis is less common but can occur because of the dehydration and the loss of large amounts of potassium in the urine and chloride in the emesis leading to a picture of raised serum bicarbonate, hypochloraemia and/or hypokalaemia. Metabolic acidosis can also occur in patients abusing large amounts of laxatives. This is caused by the loss of carbonate-rich fluid in the faeces. The hypokalaemia can lead to chest pain and cardiac arrhythmias; we have had one case of cardiac arrest.

Less frequent complications include oesophagitis, oesophageal perforation and Mallory–Weiss tears, in association with vomiting, gastric dilatation and gastric rupture. ECG changes are usually secondary to low potassium.

Menstruation is absent or irregular in about half of severe cases and many demonstrate low oestradiol and progesterone levels. McCluskey (1992) has reported an association with polycystic ovarian disease. See Table 18.7, page 516 for a comprehensive list.

Epidemiology

The point prevalence of bulimia nervosa among young females, using strict diagnostic criteria, is approximately 1000 per 100 000 (1%). A further 1% have significant eating disorder pathology and fewer than half of these are known to their general practitioners. (Fairburn & Beglin 1990). Hoek (1991) found the incidence in primary care in the Netherlands to be 11.4 per 100 000 of the population per year during the period 1985–1989. In the same population he found the 1 year prevalence rate to be 1500 per 100 000 of the population in the community (1.5%). Only 11% of these community cases were detected by general practitioners and half of those were referred on to mental health facilities. It seems that for bulimia nervosa the filter between community and primary care is a very impermeable barrier. Fairburn's studies indicate community cases are no less severe than those detected by general practitioners. This low detection rate appears to be a combination of the secretive and private behaviour of those who suffer from the disorder and low awareness by general practitioners.

The apparent sudden appearance of patients with bulimia nervosa in the late 1970s may be due to the fact that the diagnosis was missed by clinicians before then, or that there has been a large increase in frequency over the past 20 years. Kendler et al (1991) interviewed over 2000 female subjects from a twin register in Virginia, USA. He looked at the lifetime cumulative risk for definite and probable bulimia nervosa in three cohorts: patients born before 1950; those born between 1950 and 1959; and those born after 1959 (Fig. 18.7). The three curves are quite different and show that the lifetime prevalence increases progressively according to recency of birth. Kendler calculated that for those born before 1950 the prevalence of the disorder by the time they were 25 was 0.8%, for those born between 1950 and

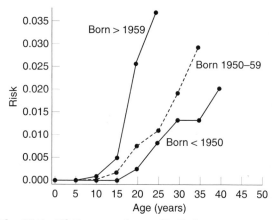

Fig. 18.7 Lifetime prevalence of bulimia nervosa.

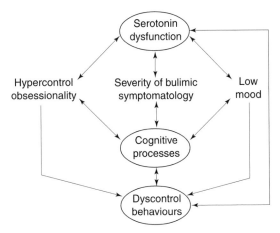

Fig. 18.8 Proposed relationship between bulimia symptoms and dyscontrol behaviours.

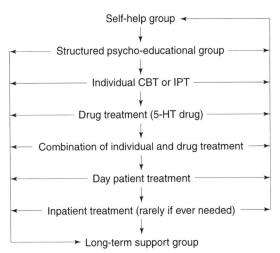

Fig. 18.9 Tiered approach to the treatment of bulimia nervosa.

1959 the prevalence by age 25 was 1.1%, and for the most recent cohort (those born after 1959) it was 3.7%.

These studies and others are reviewed by Fombonne (1996) who comes to the opposite conclusion – that rates have not gone up since 1980.

Aetiology

Given that 50% of patients with bulimia nervosa have a past history of anorexia nervosa, it is clear that the aetiology of the two conditions must have a great deal in common. Nevertheless, there are some factors which may apply preferentially to bulimia nervosa; these include a personal and family history of obesity, a family history of affective disorders and a family history of substance misuse.

If we accept that the prevalence of anorexia nervosa has stayed relatively constant but that of bulimia nervosa has risen, then it may be that cultural and social factors play a more important role in the aetiology of bulimia nervosa and that the increased preoccupation with dieting and slimness is one reason this disorder has become more common. Cowan et al (1996) studied the effect of moderate dieting in healthy women on the prolactin response to the serotonin receptor agonist M-chlorophenylpiperazine (MCCP). This is a measure of the sensitivity of post-5-HT$_{2C}$ receptors. They proposed that dieting in women is associated with the development of a functional supersensitivity of 5-HT$_{2C}$ receptors, probably in response to lower levels of 5-HT (serotonin), and that this might be a vulnerability factor aiding the dysregulation of eating that occurs in some women following dieting. Figure 18.8 shows a suggested method of how serotonin dysregulation and cognitive factors can combine to produce both overcontrol and dyscontrol.

Although frequently cited, there is little evidence that childhood sexual abuse is a specific risk factor for bulimia nervosa. A number of studies and reviews have come to this conclusion. Pope et al (1994) compared young American, Austrian and Brazilian women who suffered from DSM-IIIR bulimia. Childhood sexual abuse was reported by between 24 and 36% of the women in the three countries, though only 15–32% reported abuse before the onset of their bulimia. These rates are no higher than those that occur in general psychiatric populations. It may well be that sexual abuse is a risk factor for psychiatric disorders in general but not specifically for bulimia nervosa. Their study did not find that bulimic women had endured more severe sexual abuse or that sexual abuse was associated with the severity of bulimic symptoms.

Treatment

Despite its relatively recent appearance there are now over 50 good randomised control trials in the literature assessing treatment techniques for this disorder. Four main areas have been investigated: self-help (usually guided self-help); cognitive behavioural therapy (CBT); interpersonal psychotherapy (IPT); and drug treatment using selective serotonin reuptake inhibitors. Nearly all bulimia nervosa patients can be managed on an outpatient basis. Inpatient treatment is only indicated if the patient is suicidal or there is concern about her physical health because of very high frequency vomiting. Very occasionally, patients who have proved refractory to all other methods of treatment may require admission, but this is often extremely difficult to manage on general psychiatric wards because of the type and structure of treatment that is required. The only other indication for inpatient treatment are patients who are early in their pregnancy, as high rates of spontaneous abortions have been reported. Figure 18.9 gives a sequential tiered model for treatment, modifications of which are now in place in most specialist eating disorders treatment centres.

Pharmacological treatment studies

Earlier drug studies evaluated tricyclic antidepressants or phenelzine. Modest efficacy has been demonstrated in the short term for imipramine (Pope et al 1983, Mitchell et al 1990), desipramine (Hughes et al 1986) and phenelzine (Walsh et al 1988). These were all short-term studies with the drug being given usually for 8–12 weeks. Follow-up periods were minimal and there seemed little evidence of any continued gain once the drug was discontinued. Where attempts have been made to assess efficacy (Walsh et al 1991), drop-out and relapse rates have been so high that no conclusions could be drawn. Several of these authors have commented that there are major problems with compliance if antidepressants are the main mode of treatment. Many bulimic patients are reluctant to take medication and side-effects produce a high discontinuation rate.

The largest antidepressant study has been with fluoxetine (Fluoxetine Bulimia Nervosa Collaborative Study Group 1992). Three hundred and eighty-seven women received either 20 or 60 mg of fluoxetine daily or a placebo. Fluoxetine at 60 mg a day was found to be significantly superior to placebo. After 8 weeks of treatment, result with the standard antidepressant dose of fluoxetine 20 mg did not differ from placebo. On the 60 mg dose 63% of women had a reduction of 50% or greater in their binge frequency.

Clinical experience shows that, if drugs are used, they have to be used for periods of up to a year, and that unless other treatments are used in sequence relapse is very high when the drug is discontinued. Even the large fluoxetine study in the USA did not demonstrate any predictors of drug response. It was clear that fluoxetine was working as an antibulimic and not just as an antidepressant agent. Severity of baseline depression was not associated with response.

Psychotherapeutic treatments

Cognitive behavioural psychotherapy (CBT) has been the best evaluated treatment: Several groups in different centres found similar results, with an average reduction in binge and purge frequency of approximately 70% and between one-third and one-half of patients stopping bingeing altogether at the end of 10–16 week outpatient individual therapy (Fairburn et al 1993, Garner et al 1993, Freeman et al 1988). Unlike drug treatments, several studies have had follow-up periods of 1 year. In one study patients were followed up for an average of 6 years. Follow-up shows that treatment gains are maintained; patients with markedly low self-esteem and with severe personality disorder do less well and are more likely to drop out.

Interpersonal psychotherapy (IPT) was developed as a treatment for depression and used in the National Institute of Mental Health study on the treatment of depressive illness. It has been less evaluated than CBT but in one group of studies (Fairburn et al 1993) it has been shown to be as effective as CBT. CBT acted more quickly, with symptom improvement in IPT occurring for up to a year after the end of treatment.

Guided self help

In this treatment approach, patients are given a comprehensive self-help treatment manual and have a limited number of brief sessions with a therapist, who introduces them to the manual and who is available to check on progress and encourage compliance over subsequent weeks. Several studies have shown modest benefits for this approach and it may form a useful first step.

Drug treatment versus psychotherapy

There are no studies that have compared fluoxetine and psychotherapy directly. Mitchell et al (1990) randomised 254 patients to imipramine 300 mg per day maximum; placebo treatment; imipramine plus intensive group CBT; and placebo pills plus intensive group CBT. The main treatment effect was for group CBT; the addition of imipramine did not give additional benefit when compared with group therapy alone, though it did help relieve depressive symptoms. Forty per cent of the patients on imipramine dropped out, mainly because of side-effects.

Agras et al (1992) compared desipramine with cognitve behavioural psychotherapy. Again, psychotherapy alone or psychotherapy in combination with drugs were superior to drugs alone.

REFERENCES

Agras W S, Kraemer H C 1983 The treatment of anorexia nervosa: do different treatments have different outcomes? Psychiatric Annals 13: 928–935

Agras W S, Rossiter E M, Arnow B et al 1992 Pharmacologic and cognitive-behavioural treatment for bulimia nervosa: a controlled comparison. American Journal of Psychiatry 149: 82–87

APA 1994 Diagnostic and statistical manual of mental disorders, 4th edn. American Psychiatric Association, Washington, DC, p 731

Blair C, Freeman C P L, Cull A 1995 The families of anorexia nervosa and cystic fibrosis families. Psychological Medicine 25: 985–993

Bruch H 1965 Anorexia nervosa and its differential diagnosis. Journal of Nervous and Mental Disease 141: 556–566

Channon S, DeSilva P, Hemsley D, Perkins R 1989 A controlled trial of cognitive-behavioural and behavioural treatment of anorexia nervosa. Behaviour Research and Therapy 27: 529–535

Cowen P J, Clifford E M, Walsh A E S, Williams C, Fairburn C G 1996 Moderate dieting causes 5-HT$_{2C}$ receptor supersensitivity. Psychological Medicine 26: 1155–1159

Cullen W 1780 Synopsis methodicae exhibens . . . systema nosologica. Creech, Edinburgh

Fairburn C G, Beglin S J 1990 Studies of the epidemiology of bulimia nervosa. American Journal of Psychiatry 147: 401–408

Fairburn C G, Jones R, Peveler R C, Hope R A, O'Connor M 1993 Psychotherapy and bulimia nervosa: longer-term effects of interpersonal psychotherapy, behavior therapy and cognitive behavior therapy. Archives of General Psychiatry 50: 419–428

Fluoxetine Bulimia Nervosa Collaborative Study Group 1992 Fluoxetine in the treatment of bulimia nervosa: a multicentre, placebo-controlled, double-blind trial. Archives of General Psychiatry 49: 139–147

Fombonne E 1996 Is bulimia nervosa increasing in frequency? International Journal of Eating Disorders 19: 287–296

Freeman C P L, Barry F, Dunkeld-Turnbull J, Henderson A 1988 A controlled trial of psychotherapy for bulimia nervosa. British Medical Journal 296: 521–525

Gard M C E, Freeman C P 1996 The dismantling of a myth: a review of eating disorders and socio-economic status. International Journal of Eating Disorders 20: 1–12

Garner D M, Rockert W, Garner M V, Davis R, Olmsted M O, Eagle M 1993 Comparison of cognitive-behavioural and supportive-expressive therapy for bulimia nervosa. American Journal of Psychiatry 150: 37–46

Gordon I, Lask B, Bryant-Waugh R, Deborah C, Timimi S 1997 Childhood-onset anorexia nervosa: towards identifying a biological substrate. International Journal of Eating Disorders 22: 159–165

Gull W W 1874 Anorexia nervosa (apepsia hysterica, anorexia hysterica). Transactions of the Clinical Society of London 7: 22–28

Hoek H W 1991 The incidence and prevalence of anorexia nervosa and bulimia nervosa in primary care. Psychological Medicine 21: 455–460

Hsu L K G 1988 The outcome of anorexia nervosa: a reappraisal. Psychological Medicine 18: 797–812

Hughes P L, Wells L A, Cunningham C J, Ilstrup D M 1986 Treating bulimia with desipramine: a double-blind placebo controlled study. Archives of General Psychiatry 3: 182–186

Janet P 1903 Les obsessions et la psychasthénic. Vol 1, sect 5: L'obsession de la honte du corps. Germer Baillière, Paris

Kendler K S, Maclean C, Neale M, Kessler R, Heath A, Eaves L 1991 The genetic epidemiology of bulimia nervosa. American Journal of Psychiatry 148: 1627–1637

Keys A, Brozek J, Henschel A, Mickelson O, Taylor H L 1950 The biology of human starvation (2 vols) University of Minnesota Press, Minneapolis

Lacey J H 1993 Self-damaging and addictive behaviour in bulimia nervosa: a catchment area study. British Journal of Psychiatry 163: 190–194

Leassle R G, Kittl S, Fichter M M, Wittchen H, Pirke K M 1987 Major affective disorder in anorexia nervosa and bulimia: a descriptive study. British Journal of Psychiatry 151: 785–789

McCluskey S, Evans C, Lacey J H, Pearce M H, Jacobs H 1991 Polycystic ovary syndrome and bulimia. Fertility and Sterility 55: 287–291

Marcé L V 1860 Note sur une forme de délire hypochondriaque consécutive aux dyspepsies et caractérisé principalement par le refus d'aliments. Annales Medico-Psychologiques 6: 15–28

Mitchell J E, Pyle R L, Eckert E D, Hatzukami D, Pomeroy C, Zimmerman R 1990 A comparison study of antidepressants and structured intensive group psychotherapy in the treatment of bulimia nervosa. Archives of General Psychiatry 47: 149–157

Morton R 1689 Phthisiologia, seu exercitationes de phthisi. Smith, London

Parry-Jones B, Parry-Jones W L 1991 Bulimia: an archival review of its history in psychosomatic medicine. International Journal of Eating Disorders 10: 129–143

Parry-Jones B, Parry-Jones W 1995 The history of bulimia and bulimia nervosa. In: Brownell K D, Fairburn C G (eds) Eating disorders and obesity. Guilford Press, New York, ch 26

Pope H G, Hudson J I, Jonas J M, Yurgelun-Todd D 1983 Treatment of bulimia with imipramine: a double-blind placebo controlled study. American Journal of Psychiatry 14: 554–558

Pope Jr H G, Mangweth B, Brooking N A, Hudson J, Anthanásios C T 1994 American Journal of Psychiatry 151: 732–737

Russell G F M 1979 Bulimia nervosa: an ominous variant of anorexia nervosa. Psychological Medicine 9: 429

Russell G F M 1997 The history of bulimia nervosa. In: Garner D M, Garfinkel P E (eds) Handbook of treatment for eating disorders, 2nd edn. Guilford Press, New York, pp 11–12

Russell G F M, Szmukler G I, Dare C, Eisler I 1987 An evaluation of family therapy in anorexia nervosa and bulimia. Archives of General Psychiatry 44: 1047

Sharp C W, Freeman C P L 1993 The medical complications of anorexia nervosa. British Journal of Psychiatry 162: 452–462

Silverman J A 1995 The history of anorexia nervosa. In: Brownell K D, Fairburn C G (eds) Eating disorders and obesity. Guilford Press, New York, pp 141–144

Smeets M A 1997 The rise and fall of body size estimation research. In: Anorexia nervosa: a review and reconceptualization. Eating Disorders Review 5(2): 75–79

Theander S 1985 Outcome and prognosis in anorexia nervosa and bulimia. Some results of previous investigations compared with those of a Swedish long-term study. Journal of Psychiatric Research 19: 493–508

Touyz S W, Beaumont P J V, Glaun D, Phillips T, Cowie I 1984 A comparison of lenient and strict operant conditioning programmes in refeeding patients with anorexia nervosa. British Journal of Psychiatry 144: 517–520

Walsh B T, Gladis M, Roose S P, Stewart J W, Stetner F, Glassman A H 1988 Phenelzine versus placebo in 50 patients with bulimia. Archives of General Psychiatry 45: 471–475

Walsh B T, Hadigan C M, Devlin M J, Gladis M, Roose S P 1991 Long-term outcome of antidepressant treatment for bulimia nervosa. American Journal of Psychiatry 148: 1206–1212

WHO 1992 The ICD-10 classification of mental and behavioural disorders: clinical descriptions and diagnostic guidelines. World Health Organization, Geneva, pp 176–181

Wulff M 1932 Ueber einen interessanten oralen Symptomen-komplex und seine Beziehung zur Sucht. Internationale Zeitschrift für Psychoanalyse 18: 281–302

19

Sexual disorders

John Bancroft

INTRODUCTION

For the majority of people, the most important relationship in their adult lives is sexual. Many experience problems within such relationships. The general quality or enjoyment of the sexual relationship may be impaired or, more specifically, the physiological responses necessary for satisfactory sex, such as erection or orgasm, may fail. These responses are not only susceptible to psychological influences but can also be affected by a host of physical and pathological processes as well as drugs and alcohol. Sex is, *par excellence*, a psychosomatic process and the understanding of the possible interactions between psychological and physical mechanisms is of fundamental importance. The majority of sexual problems that present for help arise within heterosexual relationships, but other types of sexual difficulty also need to be considered. Homosexuals not only have their share of sexual difficulties but also suffer the consequences of being stigmatised. Other people have sexual preferences which may be incompatible with stable relationships of either a hetero- or a homosexual kind, sadomasochism and fetishism being examples. Occasionally people with such preferences seek professional help. Issues of gender identity are also important with transsexualism or transgender, the most extreme form, presenting particular challenges. Some forms of sexual activity (e.g. sexual assault, sexual abuse of children, or exhibitionism) are illegal and help may be sought to avoid prosecution or, in those who have already been convicted, to prevent further conflict with the law. Those who have been subjected to coercive sex, either as children or as adults, are increasingly likely to seek help for what they believe to be the consequences.

HETEROSEXUAL RELATIONSHIPS

Incidence of problems

It is virtually impossible to establish the true prevalence of sexual difficulties in the general population. There are many ways in which a sexual relationship can be problematic; many such problems reflect transient difficulties in the general relationship. Many couples are relatively disinterested in the sexual dimension of their relationship. Apart from the problems of obtaining representative samples for enquiry, answers to sensitive questions concerning sex will vary considerably in their validity (Bancroft 1989, Clement 1990).

In a substantial and representative early Dutch study, 26% of men and 43% of women reported some problems with sexual enjoyment and arousal, with a further 9% of women expressing actual sexual aversion. A total of 12% of men and 33% of women had difficulty or dissatisfaction with orgasm, with a further 5% of women being anorgasmic (Frenken 1976). In a recent representative American survey, questions were asked about a number of sexual difficulties (Laumann et al 1994). The percentages of men and women reporting each difficulty are given in Table 19.1. For most of these reported sexual difficulties, there was a relationship to general health status. The only problem which showed a clear relation to age was erectile difficulty in men, which was more than twice as prevalent in the over 50s as in the under 50s. The relationship of erectile dysfunction to age was also clearly demonstrated in a study of 40–70-year-old men (Feldman et al 1994). Whereas only 48% denied any problems with erections, complete erectile dysfunctions were reported by 9.6%, with the prevalence from 5% to 15% between the ages of 40 and 70 (Feldman et al 1994).

Obviously the severity and importance of sexual problems vary. Garde & Lunde (1980) interviewed a representative sample of 40-year-old Danish women: 35% reported having sexual problems of some kind, with 15% describing too little motivation, 7% 'derived nothing from intercourse' whilst 6% 'felt it to be an obligation'. Of these women, 11% would have welcomed advice, whilst 5% said they wanted 'sexological treatment'. The proportion who would actually seek such help would no doubt be smaller.

Table 19.1 Percentage of subjects answering 'yes' to whether 'during the last 12 months there has ever been a period of several months or more when you…'

	Men (*n* = 1346)	Women (*n* = 1622)
Lacked interest in sex	15.8	33.4
Had anxiety about performance	17.0	11.5
Climaxed too early	28.5	10.3
Were unable to keep erection	10.4	—
Had trouble lubricating	—	18.8
Were unable to orgasm	8.3	24.1
Had pain during sex	3.0	14.4

Table 19.2 Principal problems of men (*n* = 553) and women (*n* = 577) presenting at a sexual problem service in Edinburgh. (Problems of those presenting as couples, both with problems of equal importance, are not included)

Male problems	Percentage presenting	Female problems	Percentage presenting
Low sexual interest	7	Low sexual interest	35
Lack of enjoyment	1	Lack of enjoyment	12
Other orgasmic problems	5	Orgasmic dysfunction	7
Dyspareunia	1	Dyspareunia	11
Erectile failure	50	Vaginismus	13
Premature ejaculation	13	Sexual aversion	3
Problems relating to homosexuality	3	Problems relating to homosexuality	0.2
Transsexualism	4	Transsexualism	2
Sexual deviance	2		
Sexual offences	3		
Miscellaneous	12	Miscellaneous	15

When we turn to the people who do seek professional help for sexual difficulties, of what do they complain? A consecutive series of 1110 patients presenting at sexual problem clinics in Edinburgh was described by Warner et al (1987). The presenting problems for the men and for the women are shown in Table 19.2. This shows a striking sex difference: a substantial majority of the men present with complaints about their physiological function – erectile or ejaculatory problems; a comparable majority of the women complain about lack of desire or enjoyment, with much less attention to physiological factors. Tiefer (1991) has criticised the diagnostic schema in DSM-IV for sexual dysfunctions, pointing out that diagnosis is based on a very genitally oriented, physiological response concept of sexual interaction. This tallies with how men conceptualise their difficulties, but, according to Tiefer, works to the disadvantage of women. It is certainly true that, whereas diagnostic categories are defined in terms of the 'sexual response cycle' (i.e. desire, arousal, orgasm, according to the ideas of Masters & Johnson 1970 and Kaplan 1974), much of sex therapy is concerned with poor communi-

cation, feelings of emotional insecurity or problems in coping with sexual intimacy. In general, such problems are articulated much more clearly by women than by men and the conventional ways of categorising sexual difficulties in women do not reflect their predominant concerns. (ICD-10 differs from DSM-IV in paying more attention to 'satisfaction and enjoyment' in the sexual relationship.)

There are some obvious reasons for this sex difference: absence of erection or inability to control ejaculation has a much more limiting effect on sexual activity than impaired vaginal response or orgasmic difficulty in the woman. But this nevertheless underlines an important difference in the attitudes of men and women to their sexual relationships. As yet, no method of classifying sexual problems in either sex satisfactorily takes into account the complex interplay of subjective experience and physiological response.

Sexual problems present in a variety of clinical settings. In an Edinburgh study of a family planning clinic population, 75% of 1000 consecutive women attenders completed a questionnaire. Of these women 12% said that they had a sexual problem (Dickerson et al, unpublished data). Studies of gynaecological (Levine & Yost 1976, Frenken & Van Tol 1987), psychiatric (Swan & Wilson 1979), sexually transmitted disease clinics (Catalan et al 1981) and general practice (Golombok et al 1984) reveal a substantial proportion with some sexual problem. It is not always clear whether this is linked to the clinical problem, though in some cases the association is very striking. Thus, up to 50% of male diabetics have problems with erections (McCulloch et al 1980), though diabetic women appear to be relatively immune (Tyrer et al 1983). However, in a study of 1180 males attending a general medical outpatient clinic no less than 34% were found to have some form of sexual dysfunction (Slag et al 1983). Patients with spinal injuries, multiple sclerosis, hypertension, epilepsy, colostomies or ileostomies, mastectomies and those on renal dialysis all appear to have more than their fair share of sexual difficulties. It is nevertheless often difficult to distinguish between direct effects of the disease process on sexual physiology, psychological reactions to the disability, and the sexual side-effects of drug treatment, reminding us once again of the complex psychosomatic nature of sexuality (Bancroft 1989).

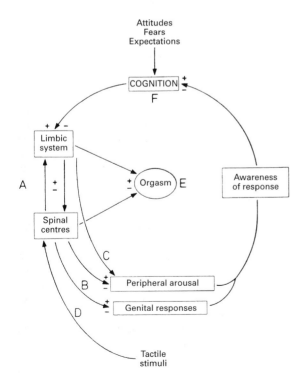

Fig. 19.1 The psychosomatic cycle of sex.

The psychosomatic circle

The psychosomatic nature of human sexuality is represented schematically in Fig. 19.1. Cognitive factors and the sensory input from touch influence the neurophysiological substrate in the limbic system and the spinal centres of the cord. This in turn is responsible for the general bodily changes that follow. Awareness of these bodily changes completes the circle and can be exciting, anxiety-provoking, or in some sense inhibitory. At each point of the system, both excitatory and inhibitory mechanisms are operating. The system can 'reverberate' either positively, with mounting excitement and eventual orgasm, or negatively with inhibition of genital response.

It is possible to identify factors that can interfere at particular points of the circle, e.g. with peripheral control of genital response, or the integrity of spinal centres. But, to understand the effects of such a factor on the sexuality of the individual, one has to consider its impact on the whole system rather than just at the point of action. Thus slight physiological impairment of erectile capacity in one man may cause little psychological reaction in either him or his partner, and hence remain of negligible significance. In another case, when the man or his partner attaches particular importance to erectile performance, similar impairment may lead to a markedly adverse reaction and escalating difficulty to the point of complete erectile failure. Similarly, due to such psychological reverberation in the system, the problem may continue long after the precipitating factor has ceased to operate, e.g. a transient drug effect may lead to persisting problems after the drug is withdrawn. Let us, in summarising the principal aetiological factors, consider each point of this circle in turn.

Central mechanisms

The limbic system and the spinal centres represent the 'black box' of our sexuality; we know very little about their workings. Hormones may play an important part at this level. The role of reproductive hormones in the sexuality of men is becoming increasingly clear. Androgens are necessary for normal levels of sexual interest and for ejaculation. Their effects on erectile function are more complex. Erections occurring during sleep (nocturnal penile tumescence or NPT) are markedly androgen-sensitive, whereas those in response to erotic stimuli in the waking state are much less so (Carani et al 1995). This raises the possibility that the part of the limbic system responsible for sleep erections is linked in some way to the neurophysiological substrate for sexual interest or appetite, and that both are activated by androgens (Bancroft 1988). Drugs may exert sexual side-effects by affecting this part of the system, as may generalised metabolic disturbances and some cases of depressive illness. The role of hormones in female sexuality is much less clear; women appear to vary considerably in their behavioural sensitivity to hormones (Bancroft 1989).

Functional disturbance of the limbic system or spinal cord may affect sexual function, though it is difficult to predict what effect will be produced by a particular lesion. There is a common association between temporal lobe and other types of epilepsy and low sexual interest, at least in men. In some such cases this may result from a lowering of plasma free testosterone induced by anticonvulsant medication (Toone et al 1983).

Genital responses

In both men and women these rely predominantly on vasocongestion. The peripheral blood vessels and the nerves controlling them may be directly affected by disease. Factors affecting the function of the pelvic floor muscles may also be relevant, particularly in women.

One of the consequences of the 'medicalisation' of male sexual dysfunction, and the involvement of surgeons, mentioned earlier, has been an intensive period of investigation of the pathophysiology of erection at the level of the penis. The current view is that penile erection depends on the relaxation of the smooth muscle which is present in abundance in the specialised tissues of the corpora cavernosa, forming the walls of the sponge-like sinusoidal spaces. This relaxation allows the filling and distension of these spaces and the passive compression of the venous drainage between them. This reduction of venous outflow, combined with an associated increase in arterial inflow, results in the buildup of pressure within the corpora close to systolic pressure. Providing the 'hydraulic' integrity of this system is intact, this high pressure, augmented by periodic contractions of the striped muscles enveloping the corpora, produces the rigidity of erection required for effective vaginal entry (Bancroft 1989). Physical causes of erectile failure include insufficient arterial supply due to narrowing or obstruction of the penile or pelvic arteries, damage to the nerve supply that controls these various vascular and smooth muscle responses, and failure of the erectile tissue, for reasons which are not yet well understood, to occlude venous drainage during the development of erection, leading to so-called 'venous incompetence'.

The precise neurotransmitter mechanisms involved in this highly sophisticated example of biological engineering are not yet fully understood. Whereas choliner-

gic and noradrenergic transmission are involved, the former to counteract the inhibitory contractile tone induced by the latter, other neurotransmitters and neuromodulators are probably also involved, including nitric oxide (NO) and vasoactive intestinal polypeptide (VIP). In addition, a variety of drugs, which share in common the capacity to relax smooth muscle, have been found effective in producing erection when injected into the corpora cavernosa. Examples of such drugs are papaverine, phentolamine and prostaglandin E_1. These are now widely used, in diagnostic tests of various kinds, to induce increased blood flow during procedures such as duplex ultrasonography or cavernosography (see Buvat et al 1990 for an authoritative review of these diagnostic methods). Such drugs, given by injection, or, in the case of Prostaglandin E_1, also by the intraurethral route, are also being used as a method of treatment, and will be considered below. The latest potentially important therapeutic development is the drug sildenafil. This inhibits the enzyme phosphodiesterase V, which breaks down the cyclic GMP which serves as the second messenger between NO release and smooth muscle relaxation. This is a novel approach as the drug is only likely to act if natural sexual stimulation occurs (Boolell et al 1996). It is too early to assess its therapeutic value.

The role of drugs in the iatrogenic causation of erectile failure remains uncertain. Whereas direct pharmacological interference with ejaculation is well-established with drugs such as adrenergic blockers, direct interference with the vascular mechanisms leading to erection is less certain. Indirect effects also have to be considered, e.g. via action on the central nervous system or, in the case of hypotensive agents and diuretics, by lowering blood pressure and hence blood flow in restricted vessels (for a comprehensive review of drug effects on sexuality, see Rosen 1991).

In women, pain during intercourse is particularly important. It is commonly caused by vaginal infections or deep pelvic pathology, but may also result from an inadequately lubricated vagina. As this lubrication is normally a response to sexual stimulation, a vicious circle readily becomes established, when anticipation of pain further inhibits lubrication. Many cases of painful intercourse, or dyspareunia, remain ill understood, with a tendency to attribute causation to psychological mechanisms for no adequate reason. This common clinical problem needs more careful study. Oestrogen deficiency in the postmenopausal or lactating woman may certainly cause vaginal dryness and soreness, though the majority of postmenopausal women appear to have enough oestrogen to avoid this problem.

Some women have a particular tendency to react to local pain, or its anticipation from impending vaginal entry, with marked spasm of the pelvic floor muscles. This, if persistent, results in vaginismus, making sexual intercourse painful or impossible. The reason for this tendency to spasm, and the heightened experience of pain associated with it, is usually not clear.

Orgasm is a neurophysiological mystery. Though the physiological basis is probably similar in males and females, an important difference in the male is the association with seminal emission. The combination of emission and the rhythmic muscle contraction that accompanies orgasm results in ejaculation. If for any reason emission occurs without orgasm, then there is no pumping, ejaculatory effect. This may occur with high levels of anxiety and is common among men with severe premature ejaculation. Interference with the nerve supply or pharmacological block may result in orgasm without emission, the so-called 'dry run orgasm'. Occasionally neural disturbance, as in diabetes, may lead to other alterations of ejaculatory function, sometimes resulting in retrograde ejaculation into the bladder (Fairburn et al 1982). Premature ejaculation is very common in young men, but most acquire control as they gain experience. The reasons why some fail to do so are not clear, but any factor that causes the man to be anxious during sexual activity – and anticipation of inadequate ejaculatory control can have that effect – will make the acquisition of control more difficult. In women, the effect of anxiety on orgasm is strikingly different to that in men, usually resulting in a delay. Thus women typically have to learn to let go of control in order to experience satisfactory orgasm while men have to acquire it.

Psychological factors and associated emotional states

It is widely believed that anxiety has a disruptive effect on sexual response. Anger or resentment is also commonly implicated as a cause of sexual difficulty. 'Performance anxiety' or the spectator role, becoming too concerned about how one is responding and not enough about what one is feeling, has also been emphasised as an important factor leading to sexual dysfunction (Masters & Johnson 1970).

Recently, a series of well-controlled laboratory-based studies have investigated the relevance of such emotional states to sexual response in the male (see review by Cranston-Cuebas & Barlow 1990). These have demonstrated that:

- Experimental induction of anxiety often facilitates sexual response, though this is more likely to occur in men who are not already experiencing sexual difficulties.

- Performance demand, induced in the experimental situation again distinguishes 'functional' from 'dysfunctional' men, apparently facilitating response in the former and hindering it in the latter.
- Heightened arousal, induced by whatever means, appears to accentuate the typical pattern. Thus in 'functional' men, who tend to focus on erotic cues in the experimental setting, this focus is enhanced and the sexual response facilitated. 'Dysfunctional' men, who characteristically focus on non-erotic cues in sexual situations, are even more likely to do so. In other words, the arousal increases the response – erotic in the functional group, non-erotic in the dysfunctional.
- Distraction (i.e. being asked to listen to a non-erotic cue while attending to an erotic stimulus) substantially reduces the erotic response in functional men. In dysfunctional men, it makes either little difference or even increases the response. The assumed explanation for this difference is that the dysfunctional men are already attending to non-erotic cues, which may be even more countererotic than the distracting cue.
- When asked to report on their level of genital response to erotic stimuli, 'functionals' tend to report accurately or to overreport their response. 'Dysfunctionals' tend to underreport.

Thus we find 'functional' and 'dysfunctional' men reacting to these emotional states and cognitive processes differently. But we do not know whether that difference is a cause of the dysfunction, representing some characteristic that *precedes* the dysfunction, or is a consequence of dysfunction, so that once men regard themselves as dysfunctional, for whatever reason, they react differently, possibly accentuating the problem in the process. It is becoming increasingly likely, however, that while cognitive mechanisms of the kind studied by Barlow and his colleagues play a part in sexual dysfunction, they are insufficient as an explanation. Other mechanisms, of a more neurophysiological kind, involving direct inhibition of sexual responses are probably involved, and there is now direct evidence to support this conclusion (Bancroft 1997).

Apart from this experimental approach to studying the cognitive and affective mechanisms involved, we can also consider, in a more descriptive way, the types of psychological problem that are commonly associated with sexual difficulties. It is important to remember, however, that demonstrating an association is not the same thing as showing causation. Many individuals have these problems without the sexual difficulties. The mediating mechanisms between psychological process and impairment of sexual response remain obscure.

Nevertheless, these common psychological issues form much of the subject matter of psychological methods of treatment. The therapist aims to identify these issues in each case, to 'work through' them in some sense, and hopes to see behavioural change without necessarily understanding how the change comes about (see Bancroft 1997 for further discussion). We will consider the principles the therapist follows later; let us first consider briefly the common problems.

There are many reasons for feeling anxious, insecure or angry in a sexual context. Some of them are best understood in developmental terms – results of earlier experiences which precede the current sexual relationship. Others reflect the ongoing difficulties in the current sexual relationship. They can be considered under the following headings.

Misunderstandings and ignorance The most frequent are misleading expectations of 'normality' which generate anxiety and guilt if they are not attained. 'Normal' frequency of intercourse, the 'normality' of simultaneous orgasm and female orgasm from vaginal stimulation alone are common examples.

Negative feelings about sex As a result of earlier learning, sex may be viewed as wrong or sexual pleasure as immoral in some way. Sexual pleasure is sometimes confined to 'bad' or at least illicit relationships, making it difficult to enjoy sex in a good, loving relationship. Sexual arousal may threaten the person's need for self-control. This may reflect a general tendency to keep control, as in many obsessional personalities, or more specifically a fear of what will happen during sexual abandonment. Sex may be feared as painful or dangerous. For women in particular, this can become a self-fulfilling prophecy because the resulting muscle spasm can cause pain when intercourse is attempted. The fear of pregnancy is the most rational fear associated with sex and has probably succeeded in spoiling more sexual relationships than any other single factor. But in spite of widespread acceptance of modern methods of fertility control, there are still some women (and occasionally men) who feel that sex unassociated with the possibility of pregnancy is wrong. Fear of venereal disease is adaptive in many situations, but occasionally, in the form of a phobia, it becomes an obstacle to any satisfactory sexual relationship.

With many of these fears and misunderstandings, we have to ask why they persist in spite of experience or information to the contrary. As with most neurotic (i.e. maladaptive) fears, two explanations have to be considered. First, there may be a 'neurotic disposition' which is associated in an ill-understood way with inappropriate learning of anxiety or avoidance (inhibitory) responses. Secondly, the fear may continue because of 'secondary gain'. Thus the avoidance of intercourse because of 'irrational fears' may serve the purpose of avoiding the mature adult sexual role that intercourse symbolises. In such cases, the sexual problem is a manifestation of a more general personality problem.

Low self-esteem This may be specifically related to body image or be more general, as with a person who is depressed. In either case, sexual enjoyment is likely to be impaired. A man who is experiencing failure in his job feels less effective, less 'potent' as a man, and this can adversely affect him sexually. When women feel unattractive or 'unfeminine', for whatever reason, they often find they are less able to enjoy sex. Although low self-esteem, when a manifestation of depression, can have these direct psychological effects, there are probably other ways, as yet not understood, in which depressive illness affects sexual interest and response.

Relationship problems Resentment and insecurity in the sexual relationship are two emotions which cause particular havoc. There are many causes for such emotions but some are sufficiently common to deserve special mention, for example different expectations of marriage. Attitudes to the woman's role in marriage are undoubtedly changing. There are increasing numbers of women who now resent what is traditionally expected of them, often with good reason. It is not unusual to find couples who enjoyed sex before marriage but experienced a decline in the 1 or 2 years after marriage. Beforehand, sex was not taken for granted and could be used by the woman to 'express her love'. After marriage, she is 'contracted to provide it'. In a similar way, many men after marriage feel under pressure to perform sexually.

Many young wives now feel considerable conflict between their role as housewife and mother and their role as an independent career woman. Caring for preschool children is especially stressful and may be compounded by the woman's loss of her previous work role and the social isolation that often ensues. Two people entering marriage usually have a lot of 'personal growth' still to work through. At different times, each person will go through an individual crisis, putting strains on the marital relationship. How a couple deals with these various problems depends not only on the circumstances of the 'here and now' but also earlier experiences, in particular what they have learnt from their parents about close intimate relationships and communicating strong feelings.

Unsuitable circumstances It is easy to overlook the importance of unsuitable circumstances, such as lack of privacy or warmth. Also affecting those who are overworked is lack of appropriate time. Trying to squeeze one's sex life into a few minutes between an exhausting day and badly needed sleep is not the way to maintain a good sexual relationship. The often dramatic improvement in sexual interest and enjoyment that is experienced on holiday is testament to the negative effects of day-to-day pressures.

The effects of earlier sexual abuse or assault

In recent years there has been an extraordinary increase in the number of women (and to a lesser extent men) reporting sexual abuse during their childhood, often within an incestuous relationship. There is little evidence that such abuse has increased, and one must assume that it has become more acceptable and credible to reveal such earlier experiences. While there is general agreement that sexual exploitation of children by adults is unacceptable in any circumstances, it should not be assumed that such experiences will always have long-term adverse consequences. In the American National Health and Social Life Survey (Laumann et al 1994), subjects were asked if they had been 'sexually touched' by an adult when they were a child. Of women who reported such experience, the proportion who also reported recent problems, compared with the women who did not report such childhood experience, are shown in Table 19.3.

This shows, firstly, that the problems were more common in those who had been abused sexually, but also that they were not uncommon in the unabused women and, furthermore, that a substantial proportion of the abused women were not reporting such problems. This study also found that the abused subjects reported a greater variety of sexual experiences during adolescence and adulthood, including a greater likelihood of experiencing coercive sex.

The adverse consequences of such childhood experience have been explained in a number of ways. The trauma of this original experience, and the family reactions to it, can result in a sense of betrayal, guilt or anger that can cause later sexual difficulties. An alternative causal sequence, which has been emphasised by Browning & Laumann (1997), is that this childhood experience has a sexualising effect resulting in earlier onset of adolescent sexual activity, exposure to sexually

transmitted disease, and the negative sexual sequelae of repeated casual sexual encounters in adolescence. The relative importance of these two explanatory models, and the extent to which they overlap, remain to be established. At the same time, there is a possibility, in the present climate, of attributing too many current problems to such early experiences. We have yet to establish the right balance.

Following sexual assault during adulthood, the consequences are less complex and more readily understood. Reactions can often be considered as examples of post-traumatic stress syndrome. Also, there is often a sense of loss that needs to be resolved; for example, loss of one's identity as a sexual person, loss of trust and loss of feelings of emotional safety. Depression is a common sequel (for review, see Becker & Kaplan 1991). One of the main challenges facing the sex therapist is whether to deal with these unresolved issues in individual or couple therapy.

Clinical management

When a sexual problem presents at the clinic, decisions need to be made: first, whether any physical assessment and investigation is required; and, second, whether simple advice or counselling is appropriate, whether more systematic sex therapy is indicated, or whether physical methods of treatment should be considered. The criteria for seeking physical investigations cannot be briefly stated and are outside the scope of this chapter (see Bancroft 1989, Buvat et al 1990) but the occurrence of pain clearly requires assessment. Recent loss of sexual interest in the absence of obvious psychological explanation is also an indication. With erectile dysfunction, the continuation of relatively frequent full erections on waking is a useful clinical indicator of psychogenic causation.

In most cases, the objective of counselling or psychological treatment is the establishment of optimal psychological conditions for the couple to respond sexually. The reduction of performance anxiety or 'fear of failure', increase in feelings of emotional security,

Table 19.3 Recent problems in women who had or had not reported being 'sexually touched' by an adult during childhood (all differences significant at 0.05 level)		
	Not touched sexually ($n = 1361$)	Touched sexually ($n = 247$)
Lacked interest in sex last year	32.1	40.1
Unable to experience orgasm last year	22.2	34.4
Sex was not pleasurable last year	19.1	32.3
Emotional problems interfered with sex last year	40.2	59.2

and the resolution of chronic resentment in the sexual relationship are of paramount importance. The therapist helps to achieve these objectives principally by setting limits (for example, a temporary ban on intercourse), by facilitating communication and by helping in the expression and consequent resolution of resentment. Such an approach, combined with education about sexual function, constitutes the essence of modern sex therapy for couples (see Bancroft 1996, 1997). In some cases, when the basic problems are more intractably rooted in the individual's personality, long-term individual psychotherapy may be indicated.

The physical aspects, however, must not be neglected. Unfortunately there are few physical causes of sexual difficulty which are both common and treatable. Vaginal infections and the sexual side-effects of drugs are probably the most important examples. But it is nevertheless necessary to ensure that physical factors are dealt with properly when they occur. Even in cases where irreversible physical pathology is involved, counselling has an important role to play, with two principal objectives: to establish the optimum psychological conditions to permit the couple to make the best of their sexual relationship within the limits imposed by the physical impairment; and, in the light of any such change, to help the couple decide whether other non-psychological forms of treatment, such as the use of intracavernosal injections or vacuum devices for erectile failure, are appropriate for them. In most respects, these methods do not achieve 'cure' of the problem but rather 'a way round it'.

Whereas full sex therapy is sometimes required in cases where physical factors are important, often more limited counselling is sufficient. The principles of such simple counselling are as follows:

- To provide limited information about sexual response and, when appropriate, the impact of physical disease, in particular to counteract false or misleading expectations.
- To make specific suggestions about approaches to lovemaking that might be useful (e.g. direct clitoral stimulation, agreeing on limits, trying different positions, etc.).
- To give permission and reassurance. Permission is usually implicit in the suggestions made, but is often of crucial importance. Suggestions to use masturbation techniques, for example, may effectively counter the patient's previous belief that masturbation is wrong.
- To facilitate communication. Talking with a couple about sex often provides a model of communication and a vocabulary which makes it easier for them to discuss the issues between themselves.

The main requirement of the counsellor in these circumstances is therefore comfort in talking about sexual matters combined with a reasonable knowledge and understanding of the varieties of human sexual response. Such counselling is largely based on common sense and need only occupy one or two half-hour sessions. It can therefore be provided by a wide range of health professionals who do not have to regard themselves as experts in sex therapy. It is particularly useful at those points in the health care service where ordinary sexual problems are likely to be identified, e.g. family planning clinics, postnatal clinics, vasectomy counselling, sexually transmitted disease clinics, and medical clinics dealing with patients after coronaries or other acute medical episodes. If simple counselling is ineffective, or the problem is obviously complex enough to require more specialist management, sex therapy may be indicated (see Bancroft 1995a for fuller discussion).

Principles of sex therapy

The principles of sex therapy are basically those of behavioural psychotherapy in general, i.e. a combination of 'doing' and 'understanding', getting patients to try things and helping them to understand the difficulties that they have in carrying them out. There are three main components of such treatment: behavioural, educational and psychotherapeutic. They are combined in the following framework which also provides the structure of each treatment session (see Bancroft 1996 for more details).

1. Set appropriate behavioural assignments ('homework'; the behavioural component).
2. Examine the patient's attempts to carry out these assignments.
3. As a result, identify those obstacles (attitudes, fears or other feelings) that underlie the difficulties encountered.
4. Help the patient to modify or reduce those obstacles so that the behaviour can be carried out successfully (the educational and psychotherapeutic components).
5. Set the next behavioural assignments.

The particular strength of this combination is that the setting of relevant target behaviours is a rapidly effective way of uncovering the crucial inter- or intrapersonal problems that underlie the sexual difficulty. Such an approach is a combination of behavioural change and discovery. The therapist can reasonably assume that relevant material will emerge during the course of treatment. It is therefore not necessary to elicit all the information during the initial assessment. This means that there need be no delay in getting the couple or individual patient actively involved and started on a behavioural programme, provided that appropriate assignments suggest themselves. Let us consider the three components of treatment in more detail.

The behavioural component

This is best described for the treatment of couples, when very similar assignments can be given initially whatever the nature of the couple's problem. These early assignments concern the couple's method of communication during lovemaking, both verbally and physically, and their ability to protect and assert themselves to make each other feel secure. The 'sensate focus' stages of Masters & Johnson (1970) are particularly effective for this purpose. The couple are asked to accept limits to their lovemaking, i.e. no direct genital or breast contact or any attempts at intercourse. They are encouraged to take time to touch one another anywhere except the genital areas. Initially the objective of the 'toucher' is to find ways of enjoying touching; the person being touched simply has to protect him- or herself against anything that is unpleasant. At a later stage, the 'toucher' aims to give pleasure as well, and relies on communication from the partner about what or where is enjoyable to the touch. Eventually genital touching is incorporated, following the same principles. These assignments rapidly reveal problems of resentment, feelings of insecurity or lack of trust in the couple (e.g. can the partner be trusted to keep to the limits?), as well as negative feelings about taking the initiative or experiencing pleasure without first giving pleasure.

Once the couple can manage a particular behavioural assignment without difficulty and with emotional comfort, they move on to the next stage. Behavioural progress is often halted for some time whilst crucial inter- or intrapersonal conflicts are resolved. As treatment proceeds, behavioural tasks become more tailor-made for the couple, and specific techniques dealing with premature ejaculation, vaginismus or other special dysfunctions may be incorporated into the programme. Often the most important issues are dealt with before genital touching is attempted. In other cases, the main problems are revealed at the genital stage, when fears of sexual arousal or loss of control and 'performance anxiety' are commonly encountered.

Educational component

Overcoming ignorance and countering false expectations about what is 'normal' or socially acceptable is as important in this context as in the simple counselling approach. A didactic teaching session about normal male and female anatomy and sexual physiology is usually included before the behavioural programme reaches the stage of genital touching. The couple's attention is focused on those aspects of anatomy and physiology which are especially relevant to their problems – for example, the pelvic floor muscles for the woman with vaginismus, or normal ejaculatory physiology for the premature ejaculator. Physical examination, when it is carried out, provides a further opportunity for education.

Psychotherapeutic component

The setting of appropriate behavioural tasks may be all that is required of the therapist for improvement to occur. But in the majority of cases, difficulties in carrying out the behavioural assignments will occur sooner or later and the psychotherapeutic skills of the therapist then become important. This is the aspect of therapy which is most difficult and which has been least well-defined in the literature. This aspect can only be dealt with briefly in this chapter but a much more thorough description of this and other aspects of sex therapy can be found in Bancroft (1989, 1996). The principal psychotherapeutic objectives of the therapist are:

- To facilitate understanding of why the couple or individual has difficulty with specific behaviours
- To make explicit the couple's commitment to specific changes
- To use 'reality confrontation' in which the patient's inconsistencies between attitudes and behaviour or between beliefs and factual evidence are brought out into the open
- To facilitate the expression of affect
- To use an understanding of the relevant background problems to plan further behavioural assignments appropriately.

Efficacy of sex therapy

Assessing the value of a psychological treatment for sexual problems in a relationship is far from straightforward. Attempts to do so have been confounded by a tendency to categorise cases according to the specific type of physiological dysfunction (e.g. erectile dysfunction, orgasmic dysfunction), whereas the goals of sex therapy involve much broader dimensions of the relationship than physiological response. Thus we are faced with a fundamental problem: how does one define success with such treatment? There is also the problem of long-term effects. Relationships are dynamic things which continue to be influenced by a variety of factors over time. Thus, major improvement in a sexual relationship following sex therapy may be obscured by newly developed pressures which create tensions between the couple. Nevertheless, the objectives of sex therapy, in a long-term sense, are to help the couple to learn new and better ways of dealing with their relationship issues when they arise, not simply to reverse current symptoms.

Long-term follow-up has proved difficult. Perhaps couples who have been successfully helped by sex therapy prefer to forget that stage of their lives some years later. Because of these various qualifications, it is only possible, in a short space, to give a crude guide to the efficacy of sex therapy. More detailed analyses of outcome can be found in Arentewicz & Schmidt (1983) and other studies are reviewed in Bancroft (1989) and Hawton (1992). Approximately 50–70% of couples who undergo a reasonable course of sex therapy report substantial benefits. The most consistently good results are for vaginismus, and the worst for low sexual desire. For other types of dysfunction outcome is very variable, reflecting the varied relationship problems that accompany the dysfunction, as well as the often imponderable contribution of physical factors. Also, as discussed elsewhere (Bancroft 1997), sex therapy is well designed to deal with certain aspects of sexual dysfunction and less able to deal with others. Most follow-up studies have been limited by high attrition rates. Hawton et al (1986) were more successful than most in this respect. Of 140 couples treated 1–6 years previously, 75% were contacted (at least one partner). Of these, 75% had experienced a continuation or recurrence of the original problem, though in a third this did not cause concern. Almost a half of them were able to deal effectively with the recurrences, often by adopting strategies learnt during therapy. Of the original group, 13% had separated.

Hawton & Catalan (1986) reported a prospective study of prognostic factors in sex therapy. They found that the quality of the non-sexual relationship, motivation for treatment, particularly in the male partner, and progress by the third treatment session all had prognostic significance. More studies of this kind are required.

Individual therapy

The treatment described above is designed primarily for couples, though the basic principles are equally well applied to individuals. A proportion of patients presenting with heterosexual problems have no current sexual partner, or have partners who won't participate or whom the patient does not want to involve. Individual therapy is appropriate providing that goals of therapy can be chosen which are relevant to that individual alone and not dependent on another particular person. If these individual goals are achieved, and as a consequence the patient becomes more confident and comfortable with his or her sexuality, then positive consequences in sexual relationships may well follow. Quite often the individual problem fits well into the approach outlined above for the couple. If the patient is inhibited about sex, uncomfortable about his or her body and genitals, uneasy about sexual arousal or orgasm, or generally unable to enjoy sexual feelings in a relaxed fashion, then similar behavioural assignments can be followed as for the couple. Individual sensate focus can be used with initial limits on genital touching. In the course of this, relevant attitudes are likely to be revealed. Eventual ability to masturbate to orgasm and feel comfortable and enjoy the experience may be an important step forward for that person. For individuals who have been victims of sexual assault or abuse, either as a child or adult, helping them 'work through' their anger and deal appropriately with their guilt is often necessary before behavioural progress can be made. Various specific techniques can be added to the individual's sensate focus programme, just as they are in couple therapy. Thus the 'stop–start' or 'squeeze' techniques for premature ejaculation can be used if the man tends to ejaculate quickly during masturbation as well as with a partner. Women with vaginismus can use graded vaginal dilation, first with fingers and subsequently with glass or plastic dilators. Men with erectile impotence can sometimes be helped individually if their performance anxiety has affected their ability to obtain erections during masturbation as well as with their partner (see Bancroft 1989 for further details).

Group therapy

The use of group therapy for sexual dysfunction increased appreciably during the early 1980s, but there has been a noticeable decline in this respect over the last few years (Leiblum & Rosen 1989). Usually the group approach involved the same basic principles as described for couple and individual therapy, but applied in a group setting. The advantages of the group are several. The relationship between patient and therapist is less crucial. The group tends to be cohesive, reducing the likelihood of drop-outs from treatment; there is a loyalty to the group or, alternatively, a fear of loss of face that keeps them going. The group may well have shared objectives. Explanations, interpretations and 'permission giving' that come from the group may have more impact than those coming from a therapist. Progress of individual members acts as encouragement for others, whereas individuals experiencing setbacks may get support from the group. There are practical advantages in the economic use of the therapist's time and in provision of educational material (e.g. films).

However, there are also disadvantages. Many people are reluctant to join a group, fearing exposure and loss of confidentiality. Many issues of sex therapy are simply too complex to be dealt with in this format. At the present time, the main interest in groups is for helping the victims and perpetrators of sexual abuse or assault, and for individuals who are troubled by sexual 'compulsions'.

Drug treatment

The last few years have seen a dramatic increase in interest in pharmacological methods of treatment, and there is much ongoing research. The main impact has been the use of drugs injected into the corpora cavernosa of the penis to produce an erection lasting usually for 1–2 hours. Papaverine and prostaglandin E_1, both smooth-muscle relaxants, are the two most widely used for this purpose. Although initially used for diagnosis, repeated self-injections are now mainly being used as a form of treatment (Brindley 1986, Virag et al 1991, Linet et al 1996), and are sometimes irresponsibly marketed by private clinics as 'a cure for impotence'. Obviously this route of administration is not generally acceptable, the reliance on such injections is regarded by many as an 'artificial' form of sexual response, and repeated use may lead to fibrosis within the penis. Recently, transurethral administration of alprostadil has provided a less invasive but possibly less effective method of administration (Padman-Nathan et al 1997). Those direct local methods are welcomed by a proportion of couples, however, particularly those with intractable physical causation such as diabetes or multiple sclerosis. The most interesting, and potentially the most important, development in the pharmacotherapy of erectile dysfunction is the previously mentioned new drug, sildenafil, which is still undergoing clinical trials (Boolell et al 1996). It is claimed that the particular phosphodiesterase inhibited by sildenafil is mainly found in the erectile tissues, so that other effects of this drug are unlikely to be important. In addition, by virtue of its action this drug will only act when sexual excitation has taken place. Thus it promises to be a more physiological way of amplifying and prolonging erectile response. It is, however, too early to know whether its exciting potential will be realised.

The search for a centrally acting drug that will enhance both sexual desire and genital response is continuing. Recent attempts to introduce a new dopamine agonist for this purpose have foundered because of the substantial D_2 side-effects. Several studies have evaluated yohimbine, an α_2-adrenoceptor antagonist, as a treatment for erectile dysfunction, usually with results which are inconclusive but suggestive of modest benefits (e.g. Reid et al 1987, Riley et al 1989). New, more specific α_2-antagonists have undergone a number of experimental studies (see Bancroft 1995b, Riley 1995) which indicate that such drugs do have a complex mixture of effects on erectile response in both functional and dysfunctional men. The parent companies' experience with multicentered clinical trials was, however, not positive enough for them to market the drugs. These mixed effects may reflect the fact that such drugs have both excitatory and inhibitory actions (Bancroft 1995b).

Anxiety-reducing drugs have not been shown to be effective in dealing with the various forms of sexual anxiety, though it should be stressed that they have not as yet been adequately tested. The use of hormones such as testosterone is clearly indicated in male hypogonadism. It may also be beneficial in some eugonadal men complaining of loss of sexual interest, though in such cases counselling is probably also required (O'Carroll & Bancroft 1984).

The role of hormones in the treatment of female sexual dysfunction is much less clear, apart from the use of oestrogens to counter vaginal dryness in postmenopausal women. Some women may benefit from androgens but such effects are very unpredictable and more evidence will be required before clear clinical guidelines emerge (Bancroft 1989).

Other forms of treatment

Surgical implantation of prostheses into the penis as a treatment for erectile dysfunction was widely used for many years. Its use is now declining. The use of external vacuum devices for erectile dysfunction, on the other hand, has increased substantially in the past few years. A study showed these to be more acceptable than self-injection (Turner et al 1991).

HOMOSEXUAL RELATIONSHIPS

It is not known how many people in our society are predominantly homosexual. Figures given by Kinsey and his colleagues (1948) are overestimates because of the inclusion of subgroups (e.g. criminals) with unusually high prevalence. Gagnon & Simon (1973) reanalysed the Kinsey data, concentrating on a more representative group of 2900 young men, of whom 30% had been involved in a homosexual experience in which one or other person had attained orgasm. The large majority of these experiences had occurred in adolescence and more than half before the age of 15. This left about 3% with extensive homosexual as well as heterosexual histories beyond adolescence and 3% with exclusively homosexual histories. A similar reanalysis of the women showed that only 6% (as compared with 30% of the men) had undergone at least one homosexual experience; only 2% had any significant amount of homosexual experience and less than 1% were exclusively homosexual. In the recent British survey (Johnson et al 1994), 1.1% of men and 0.4% of women reported homosexual experiences during the previous year; 6.1% and 3.4%, respectively, reported ever having homosexual experiences. In the US survey (Laumann et al 1994), the figures for the past year were 2.7% of men and 1.3% of women, and for 'ever' were 9.1% and 4.3%. Of the men, 2.8% described themselves as having a homosexual or bisexual identity, with 1.4% of the women doing so. In both studies, these figures are probably underestimates.

A proportion of homosexuals seek professional help for problems in their sexual lives. In the majority of cases, the problems are no different to those experienced by heterosexuals. Masters & Johnson (1979) reported good results in treating sexual dysfunction in gay and lesbian couples, using their usual couple therapy approach. Are homosexual relationships more vulnerable than those of the heterosexual world or are their problems any different? The almost universal nature of the stigma attached to homosexuality is not easy to explain. Legal proscription of homosexuality exists in most Western societies, though the situation is changing in many countries. The law was changed in England in 1967. In Scotland, all forms of male homosexuality remain illegal, although prosecution is unlikely unless privacy is not maintained or the age of consent is breached. In most countries the law does not specifically concern itself with female homosexuality. Even in those countries where the law has changed, legal discrimination persists in various forms. The age of consent tends to be higher (i.e. 21 years) for homosexual than for heterosexual relationships (i.e. 16 years). Men may solicit women but they may not solicit other men. 'Privacy' is defined in a much more restrictive sense for homosexual than for heterosexual acts. The penalties are more severe than for equivalent heterosexual offences. Any form of homosexuality is illegal for members of the armed forces or merchant navy. Admitting to being homosexual in orientation is grounds for dismissal from the services.

Are homosexuals more susceptible to psychological problems? The best evidence comes from large-scale studies by Weinberg & Williams (1974) and Bell & Weinberg (1978) from the Kinsey Institute. They found a higher incidence of loneliness, lower self-acceptance, and more depression and suicidal ideas in their male and female homosexuals than in heterosexual controls.

This was reflected not only in a higher incidence of seeking professional help but also of previous suicidal attempts. It is nevertheless important to stress that these problems were confined to a minority of the homosexuals and most were well adapted and happy. Also, these studies were carried out a long time ago. The situation for gay men and lesbian women has changed in various ways, some for the better, some for the worse. Homosexual men now have to contend with the very substantial threat of human immunodeficiency virus (HIV) infection and acquired immune deficiency syndrome (AIDS). Apart from the fact that, in urban centres where AIDS is common, few homosexual men have escaped the bereavement of a close friend or lover, many gay men are faced with the very uncertain prospect of developing the disease from contacts that occurred some time ago. The stress of such a situation cannot be overestimated. But, apart from the effects of AIDS, if we accept that a homosexual man or woman has a greater likelihood of developing psychological problems than members of the heterosexual community, it is probably in large part a result of the social stigma that they experience.

McWhirter & Mattison (1984), following an in-depth study of 156 long-term male relationships, suggested five developmental stages for male homosexual relationships:

1. blending (year 1)
2. nesting (years 2–3)
3. maintaining (years 4–5)
4. building, (years 6–10)
5. releasing (years 11–20).

Bell & Weinberg (1978) used factor analysis to arrive at a typology of homosexual relationships. They described the 'close-coupled' pair, similar to the happily married and faithful heterosexual couple; the 'open couple' in which a reasonably stable relationship is maintained with a fair amount of 'extramarital' sexuality; 'functionals' were not in stable relationships but enjoyed a wide variety of partners; 'dysfunctionals', conforming to the stereotype of the 'unhappy homosexual', had recurring problems in their sexual relationships, often involving sexual dysfunction or discomfort with their homosexual identity; and 'asexuals' with low sexual interest were inclined to lead a solitary existence. The proportions of males and females in each category in their study is shown in Table 19.4. Apart from the greater number of lesbians in the close-coupled category, there is also evidence that the male homosexuals found the 'open couple' and 'functional' lifestyles easier to cope with than did the lesbians. This study was carried out prior to the 1970s, and it is not clear how relevant their findings are to the situation today. More

Table 19.4 Typology of homosexuality (Bell & Weinberg 1978)		
	Percentage males (*n* = 686)	Percentage females (*n* = 293)
Close-coupled	10	28
Open-coupled	18	17
Functional	15	10
Dysfunctional	12	5
Asexual	16	11
Unclassifiable	29	28

recent studies of gay and lesbian couples have not indicated any obvious change (Kurdek 1995).

Origins of sexual preferences

During normal sexual development, the three main components of our sexuality – sexual responsiveness, the formation and maintenance of emotional dyadic relationships, and 'gender identity' – become integrated into mature adult sexual relationships. Through childhood, these three components remain relatively detached from one another. Around puberty, we normally start to incorporate our sexual responsiveness into our relationships with other people as our sexual preferences become organised. There are a wide variety of factors which may push us away from, or pull us towards, a particular type of relationship; and it is difficult to escape the conclusion that social learning plays an important part in determining our sexual preference. But is there a 'preparedness to learn' either homosexual or heterosexual preferences and, if so, does this result from earlier learning, for example during infancy, or is it determined by innate characteristics? It is a striking fact that, whereas homosexual behaviour is commonplace amongst non-human primates and other mammals, exclusive homosexual preference appears to be a uniquely human phenomenon, and one which probably varies in incidence from one type of society to another. This would suggest that, whereas biological factors may influence whether homosexual activity occurs, the establishment of an exclusive homosexual orientation is probably a result of social learning (Bancroft 1989). Nevertheless, the last few years have seen a new wave of interest in identifying biological determinants of homosexual orientation, particularly reflecting the new technologies that have become available (Bancroft 1994). Whereas studies of twin pairs and family pedigree studies strongly suggest a genetic factor (Bailey & Pillard 1995), modern techniques for identi-

fying DNA markers have produced evidence suggesting a link between a marker on the X chromosome and homosexual orientation in men (Hamer et al 1993). If replicated, this finding will still leave fundamental questions about the nature of the genotype unanswered. Neuroanatomical studies have been focusing on structural differences between male and female brains, and on comparable differences between the brains of homosexual and heterosexual individuals (see Hines & Collaer 1993 for review).

The possibility that hormonal factors are involved in the development of sexual orientation is receding, at least in the male. Pre- and early post-natal exposure to androgenic effects may influence gender role behaviour (Money & Ehrhardt 1972), which may have other consequences for sexual development. Different developmental mechanisms in females, with a greater possibility of a more direct link between hormones and sexual orientation, remain an intriguing possibility (Bancroft 1990).

It is therefore possible that biological factors may *indirectly* affect later sexual preferences by their direct effects on gender role and identity development. There is a consistent body of evidence, both from prospective studies of children with gender non-conformity and retrospective studies of adults, that a substantial proportion of adult homosexuals have shown gender non-conformity during childhood (see Bancroft 1989 for review). This may be an important influence leading to later development of homosexual preferences, though, once again, it is clearly not a *necessary* factor.

Let us consider the ways in which gender identity might affect development of sexual preferences, at least in a proportion of cases, interacting in complex and varied ways with other social factors. In this respect we need to consider not only gender identity of the cross-gender type (e.g. a boy feeling or behaving in a feminine way) but also the lack of confidence in one's assigned gender that may stem from an absent or emasculating father, an overprotective mother, a physical disability, or genital abnormalities during development. Any of these features in a boy could have the following effects:

- Make him unattractive to the opposite sex or undermine his self-confidence in relating to girls, so that attempts at heterosexual contact are likely to be unrewarding or even punishing
- Make him attractive to other males who seek 'unmasculine' partners
- Lead him to escape from the competitiveness of the male world to the homosexual world where there are different criteria for gender success (Hooker 1967).

In a comparable way, we can consider the consequences of sexual anxiety or guilt, particularly in relation to the opposite sex. Such negative feelings may be learnt during childhood, a result of incestuous feelings or experiences, or the consequences of a sexually repressive environment in the home. Such anxiety may act as a 'push' factor away from heterosexual relationships. For those who have had problems in their dyadic relationships, particularly lacking a secure relationship with one or other parent, sexual relations with others may offer them an alternative. Thus, if a boy has never had a good relationship with his father, a close relationship with another male may hold special appeal.

Such explanations, involving relatively 'negative' developmental mechanisms, are unlikely to account for more than a proportion of adults with homosexual orientation. The histories of many individuals simply suggest the relatively early onset of sexual attraction to the same sex. But probably the most crucial additional influence, in determining whether an individual ends up with a homosexual or heterosexual identity, is the socially derived meaning given to homosexuality in any particular culture. If, as in some primitive societies, homosexual interaction is accepted as a normal aspect of sexual behaviour and development (Herdt 1981), then such behaviour is perfectly compatible with the establishment of heterosexual relationships, permitting the expression of a 'bisexual potential'. But in other societies, such as our own, adolescents are strongly encouraged to see themselves as *either* heterosexual *or* homosexual, so that evidence of a capacity for homosexual attraction and enjoyment precludes the possibility of a heterosexual identity. This is the 'social polarisation' effect. One implication of such a view is that sexual orientation, once established, is immutable. There is, however, increasing evidence that many women and, to a lesser extent, men change or modify their sexual preferences at different stages of their lives (Blumstein & Schwartz 1976). There is an increasing tendency to view homosexuality less in terms of 'identity' of the individual, and more in terms of 'relationships' between people (Peplau & Cochran 1990). With the inevitable impact of HIV on sexuality in general, it is difficult to predict how our concepts of sexual orientation will change and evolve over the next decade.

OTHER SEXUAL PREFERENCES

Fetishism and sadomasochism are two types of sexual preference which, while relatively common in some degree, are only seldom presented as problems. They carry less obvious social stigma because they can often be concealed behind an apparently normal heterosexual or homosexual front; but they often conflict with stable sexual relationships, and most often help is requested because of the strain that is imposed on such relationships.

Fetishism

The word fetish, which from its Portuguese origins implies an artistically created artefact, also conveys a special symbolism or 'magical' meaning – the love token or erotic icon. Sexual fetishes, however, vary from a particular physical attribute or body part to a truly inanimate sexual symbol. As the fetishist becomes more preoccupied with his fetish, so his sexual partner becomes less relevant and, in extreme cases, redundant. Hence the fetish serves to weaken the sexual relationship. There are three principal types of sexual fetish to consider:

- a part of the body
- an inanimate extension of the body (e.g. an article of clothing)
- a source of specific tactile stimulation (e.g. a specific texture).

The use of women's clothes as a fetish overlaps with transvestism and will be further considered below. Fetish objects often reflect current fashions. Rubber, leather and shiny black plastic are common fetish textures nowadays. In Kraft-Ebbing's time in the late 19th century, furs, velvets and silks were the popular textures.

It seems likely that fetishism results from a specific conditioning of sexual response to particular stimuli. Penile erection is a peculiarly conditionable response (Rachman & Hodgson 1968, Bancroft 1974) and the lack of any comparable conditionable sexual response in women may account for the apparent rarity of fetishism amongst females. A simple conditioning model is not sufficient, however. Other factors must operate to maintain the response and it remains a mystery why such specific learning occurs in these cases. Does it reflect a peculiarity of learning in certain individuals or does it indicate problems in those people when trying to incorporate sexual responses into their dyadic relationships, resulting in isolation of their sexuality? If conditioning occurs at an early age, before any mature concept of sexuality has developed, are bizarre associations more likely to develop? It is certainly tempting to assume that the fetish object has some significance beyond that of a randomly conditioned stimulus. Occasionally bizarre fetishes are found in association with a neurological abnormality such as temporal lobe epilepsy. In such cases, the stimulus could well be more randomly conditioned as a result of a neurophysiological disturbance of learning.

Sadomasochism

Although the terms sadism and masochism are often used loosely to cover any situation in which an individual gains a reward from either hurting or dominating another person, or being hurt or dominated, the terms are properly used when the rewards involved are clearly sexual. The sadist plays the active role in the infliction of pain, psychological humiliation or ritualised dominance; the masochist, the passive role. Submission is commonly manifested in 'bondage', i.e. being tied up or constrained so that you are unable to protect yourself and are at the mercy of your assailant. Whereas fetishism is distinctly rare amongst women, sadomasochism is by no means unusual, although the more serious use of sadomasochistic sexual activity is rarely found amongst women (Spengler 1977). It is, however, much more common for both men and women to be aroused by the fantasy of such activities than the reality. Moderate pain inflicted as an expression of sexual excitement in the form of the 'love bite' is by no means unusual; this phenomenon is widespread amongst mammals. But for the most part, sadomasochism remains difficult to understand. It is perhaps best seen as a ritualised form of sexual stimulation in which the need for dominance, the psychological significance of passivity, the sexualisation of anger and the arousing effect of pain interact, while the ritual aspects set limits which ensure safety. (For a recent review see Weinberg 1994.)

SEXUAL OFFENDERS

The most important categories of sexual offence are sexual assault and rape, and the sexual abuse of children and minors. Rape offenders seldom present for professional help, even though in some instances a definite sexual preference for assaulting the victim develops (Abel et al 1980). Furthermore, the courts are relatively unlikely to ask for a psychiatric report on a rapist. With sexual abuse of children, however, psychiatric help is frequently sought, either as part of the legal process or in order to avoid it. This reflects an interesting aspect of social attitudes that see sexual abuse of children as more 'pathological' than the sexual assault and rape of adults. The significance of this, and in particular the extent to which social attitudes and expectations about male sexual behavior may foster rape in our society, has been discussed more fully elsewhere (Bancroft 1991a).

Sexual abuse of children

With the recent dramatic increase in the extent to which adults reveal their childhood experiences of being sexually abused, the prevalence of this form of child abuse becomes an issue of some importance. There is no good reason to believe that there has been a substantial increase in such abuse, but certainly we are hearing more about it.

The various prevalence studies leave us with a bewildering range of reported prevalence rates, ranging from 6 to 62% of females and 3 to 31% of males with such experiences (Peters et al 1986). In the recent US survey (Laumann et al 1994), subjects were asked if they had been 'sexually touched' by an adult when they were children: 12% of the men and 17% of the women had, and this proportion did not differ across age groups, suggesting that there had been no increase in such experiences in recent years. In the case of the male, the older person was most likely to be an adolescent; for the female, mostly adult men.

It is difficult to make sense of such disparate rates, although methods of sampling and survey techniques obviously account for a fair amount of the variance. Also, there is likely to be considerable variation in what is regarded as sexual abuse, both by the subject being assessed and by the assessor. Earlier researchers, such as Kinsey, did not assume that a sexual experience involving a child and an adult was *necessarily* harmful to the child. Hence neutral terms were used, and Kinsey et al (1953) reported that 24% of women had described a 'prepubertal sexual experience with a postpubertal male'. Workers in the child sexual abuse field eschew such neutral terminology. Harmful consequences, even if not obvious or immediate, are assumed, and hence all such behaviour, including genital exhibition or verbal communications about sex, is regarded as 'abuse', or in some cases as 'assault' (for example, Katz & Mazur 1979). Children with such experiences are labelled as 'victims'. There can be absolutely no doubt that many if not most cases of sexual exploitation of children by adults are harmful to the child, often to a devastating extent. However, to assume that harm invariably follows any such childhood experience, regardless of its nature, its participants or its immediate consequences, is not only likely to confound 'prevalence rates' of 'abuse' and contribute to the variance in reported figures but, more importantly, may also contribute to a potentially pathogenic situation. This has become a highly contentious area. Wyatt (1991), one of the principal workers in the field, has described the 'schism' between the 'sexual abuse' workers who are struggling to tackle what they see as a frightening and widespread problem, and the more traditional 'sex researchers' who are sceptical about some of the assumptions and assertions.

The problems of evaluating prevalence rates from

surveys of adults pale into insignificance beside the difficulties of evaluating the evidence from young children where sexual abuse is suspected. This problem is not only of crucial importance to any such child, but has an important bearing on social reactions to child sexual abuse. In general, sexual contact between adults and children is an exceedingly emotive topic. Any adult involved in such behaviour is committing an offence and no category of offence is so strongly reviled by the general public. The strength of this social reaction, and the consequences to the alleged perpetrator, are not always just; civil liberties may be endangered. Yet there also seems to be a reluctance to accept that such abuse, particularly when occurring within the family, is anything other than a rare aberration by evil or sick individuals. Evidence that such behaviour might be widespread is probably unacceptable to our society; it threatens too strongly our notion of the sanctity of the family. Masson (1984) presented his controversial historical analysis of the evolution of Freud's ideas about sexual abuse, and in particular Freud's conversion from believing such abuse to be a common cause of neurosis, to regarding accounts of such abuse as 'wish-fulfilling fantasies'. In his book Masson describes the frequency with which physical and sexual abuse of children was reported in the French medical literature of the mid- to late 19th century. He also describes a further literature developing the idea that 'children lie' about such incidents. The implication is that for a while evidence of common and often horrific sexual abuse of children by their parents was publicised, at least in the medical literature. Then came a phase of 'denial', since when, until recently, we have heard relatively little about sexual abuse within the family. Well-publicised episodes, such as the Cleveland affair and the Orkney ritual sexual abuse case in the UK, have shown how quickly public opinion can turn against those who report child sexual abuse as common within the family. At the same time, it is difficult to avoid questioning the approach taken by the professional agencies in some of these cases. Is there any middle ground between believing that children 'never lie' about such matters and regarding their reports as examples of fantasy?

In the meantime, health professionals continue to struggle to help appropriately in such cases, both with the children and the families, and with the adults who are revealing their childhood experiences. Sexual offences considered by the courts are twice as likely to involve girls as boys, possibly because boys are less likely to report the incidents. The major change has been in awareness of intrafamilial child sexual abuse. The taboo against incest appears to be weaker than we had preferred to believe. The explanations for such abuse are not yet well formulated. The concept of the paedophile,

the adult, usually male, who has a sexual preference for a prepubertal or peripubertal child, either female, male or either, is most often useful in explaining cases of extrafamilial sexual abuse. Paedophiles are mainly attracted to girls in the 8–11 years age group, or boys of 11–15 years, the ages when childhood sexuality is probably most noticeable. Many paedophiles have problems establishing satisfactory adult relationships (Mohr et al 1964) and may be attracted to children because they are less threatening. In some cases, there is evidence of a fixation of sexual development at a stage of childhood sexual experimentation; the individual who enjoyed such encounters as a child, and who is unable to progress for one reason or another into a more mature sexual relationship, continues to harbour fantasies of those early positive experiences which form the basis of his adult sexual thoughts and interest. However, there is now increasing evidence that many paedophiles may have been sexually abused by adults themselves when children, which raises the fundamental question of whether such behaviour reflects needs for control over others rather than sexual pleasure per se. A reasonable conclusion from the available evidence is that the origins of paedophilia are not understood.

In the intrafamilial cases involving children close to puberty, the adult's sexual interest in the young person may not be difficult to understand. The 'pathology' lies mainly in the irresponsibility and preparedness to exploit the adult–child relationship. With sexual abuse of very young children, the motivation is usually more difficult, and one wonders to what extent this is a variant of physical abuse, motivated by hostility, need to control, or pleasure in inflicting pain or humiliation.

The effects on the children do depend on the nature of the relationship with the perpetrator. When this occurs within the family, the threat to the family and the enormous responsibility that this places on the child is probably as harmful as the specifically sexual consequences. Summit (1983) has described the 'child sexual abuse accommodation syndrome' which 'allows for the immediate survival of the child within the family but which tends to isolate the child from eventual acceptance, credibility or empathy within the larger society'. There are five components to this syndrome:

- *Secrecy* – the need to keep quiet about the abuse for fear of the consequences of revealing it
- *Helplessness* – the difficulty, in view of the need for secrecy, for the child to avoid further abuse
- *Entrapment and accommodation* – the development of various maladaptive behavior patterns which have a destructive effect on personality development
- *Delayed and unconvincing disclosure* – usually at times of conflict with the family, resulting in rejection of

the child's story and a further damaging sense of being 'unbelieved'

- *Retraction* – the threat of disintegration of the family, following disclosure, leading to retraction of the child's story, resulting in further 'invalidation' of the child.

The effects of such abuse on the sexuality of the child have been described by Friedrich (1988). They depend on the age of the child, the frequency of the abuse, as well as the relationship with the abuser. Abused children may masturbate excessively, show inappropriate sexual knowledge, become preoccupied with sexual thoughts and pursue sexual games with other children. The effects on the sexuality of adulthood were considered earlier in this chapter.

Indecent exposure and exhibitionism

Exhibitionism or 'indecent exposure' is one of the more common forms of sexual offence, and offenders are quite often referred for psychiatric help. It is also a very difficult behaviour to understand. As with many other forms of sexual offence, it is difficult to distinguish between sexual and non-sexual determinants. In certain circumstances, genital display does have a simple sexual significance. It is the most common form of sexual interaction amongst children and may precede sexuality between adults. But, with the exception of exposure by the mentally handicapped, most of these offences are not apparently aimed at establishing further sexual contact with the 'victim'. The theme of mastery and insult is much more noticeable, suggesting that genital display is being used as an expression of hostility. Such display is common amongst many species of primates, especially the males. But, as with sexual assault, the picture is complicated by the 'sexualisation' of the behaviour that is evident in a proportion of cases. Some exhibitionists are sexually aroused at the thought of exposing and use fantasies of exposing while masturbating. It is in these cases that the exhibitionist behaviour is most likely to be persistent. In other cases, the impulse to expose is a more occasional event, occurring against a background of otherwise fairly normal sexual preferences. Other consequences of indecent exposure have to be taken into consideration in understanding its possible determinants. Not only is the offender likely to be punished, but his wife and family will feel humiliated. In many cases one is struck by the apparent need of the exhibitionist to provoke these reactions and one wonders then whether the behaviour would be as likely to occur if it were not regarded as an offence. Certainly, for the vast majority of exhibitionists, their behaviour should be seen as harmless, although unseemly and often tran-

siently unpleasant or frightening for the 'victim'. A large number of women must have witnessed such acts. Gittleson et al (1978) found that 44% of a group of nurses had had this experience, usually in their early teens. Exhibitionism varies in a number of aspects.

The age of the victim A minority of exhibitionists expose persistently to prepubertal girls and in some of them this may lead on eventually to more direct sexual contact with children (Rooth 1973). The most common age of victim is at or around puberty.

The nature of the act Sometimes the exposure is clearly sexual, associated with an erect penis and sexual excitement. Masturbation usually occurs either during the exposure or shortly after. In other cases, the penis is flaccid and there is no obvious sexual arousal. The reaction of the female is important and an exhibitionist may go on exposing until he produces a desired response. Rooth (1971) describes a typical ideal exposure as:

one of dominance and mastery. The exhibitionist, usually timid and unassertive with women, suddenly challenges one with his penis, briefly occupies her full attention and conjures up in her some powerful emotions such as fear and disgust, or sexual curiosity and arousal . . . he experiences a moment of intense involvement in a situation in which he is in control. The reaction that he most dislikes is indifference.

The frequency of exposing behaviour An important distinction, as already mentioned, is between the person who only has occasional urges to expose, often at times of crisis or emotional distress, and those for whom the idea of exposing is always sexually stimulating.

Risk taking Some exhibitionists are careful to avoid being caught or recognised. Others seem to behave in a way that ensures that they are caught, e.g. exposing from their car so that their registration number leads to their arrest. Exhibitionists are unremarkable in their intelligence or social class, though there is some evidence that they are 'underachievers'. Rooth (1971) describes them as 'immature' and suggests that they commonly have dominant, overprotective mothers and passive and ineffectual fathers; they marry women who take over this maternal role, and they have relatively stable marriages of the mother–son type. These must be regarded as clinical impressions but marital sexual problems are undoubtedly common amongst them.

Management of sexual offenders

In the current climate of concern about child sexual abuse and sexual assault, much attention is being given to methods of intervention with the victim. Much less attention has been given to helping the offender, both to avoid further offences and to establish a more accept-able sexual lifestyle. This in part reflects the difficulty of the task. In particular, it reflects our uncertainty and ignorance about why people behave in this way. Unfortunately, it is a minority of such individuals whose behaviour can be understood simply in sexual terms, and more often other factors about need for con-trol, emotional insecurity or feelings of inadequacy are pre-eminent. In the last few years there has been an increase in attempts to help such individuals, mainly in the USA. Abel et al (1992) concluded that for the first-time offenders the most effective methods were those based on cognitive–behavioural principles. It is too early to judge the success of this approach. Appropriate group or special institutional methods may offer the best prospects in certain cases, but this again waits to be demonstrated.

In general the legal process is effective: the large majority of sexual offenders are deterred by their first conviction and are not seen again. But those who reoffend usually present formidable problems. Drugs are sometimes useful for reducing sexual interest and hence lessening the likelihood of sexual offence behav-iour. Although oestrogens were used in the past for this purpose, they have now largely given way to cyproterone acetate, an antiandrogen; benperidol, a butyrophenone; or medroxyprogesterone acetate, a progestagen that has some antiandrogenic effects. None of these drugs is free from side-effects and they should be used with proper supervision, as their effects are difficult to predict in a particular case (Bancroft 1989). They also raise some crucial ethical issues. Although they can be used in the context of a normal doctor–patient relationship and with fully informed consent on the part of the patient, they have frequently been used as a condition of treat-ment imposed by a court, or as part of a process of early release or parole from prison. In such cases it is difficult, if not impossible, to ensure adequate or proper consent and the use of the drug should then be seen as a form of 'social control' rather than medical treatment. This then requires suitable legal scrutiny to ensure that such treatment is not abused (Bancroft 1991b).

TRANSVESTISM AND TRANSSEXUALISM (OR TRANSGENDER)

Gender identity problems, particularly those involving transvestism and transsexualism, deserve separate con-sideration, not only because of their complexity and interest, but also because of the specialised and demanding clinical intervention involved.

Cross-dressing (i.e. dressing in the clothes of the opposite sex) is one factor that these various forms of behaviour have in common. Four categories of cross-dresser can be described, each emphasising one partic-ular aspect of the phenomenon.

The fetishistic transvestite This is a man (proba-bly never a woman) who wears female clothes as fetish objects. The clothes are sexually arousing and, usually, wearing them leads to masturbation. Cross-dressing in this case is a sexual act.

The transsexual A male (or female) who believes himself (herself) to be a woman (or man) or has a strong desire to be accepted as such in spite of his or her anatomy. In this case, cross-dressing is part of the process of expressing one's preferred gender. Both the male and female transsexual are likely to seek medical help to alter their bodies to be consistent with their psy-chological gender (sex reassignment). The term 'trans-gender' is preferred by many individuals because the term emphasises that it is gender and not sexuality or sexual orientation that is at issue.

The 'double-role transvestite' Usually a male who spends part of his life as a normal heterosexual male and part of his life dressing and 'passing' as a woman. Cross-dressing is usually similar to that of the transsexual but there is no desire to change sex permanently.

The homosexual transvestite A man or woman who is sexually attracted to members of the same sex and who cross-dresses, but with less intention of being considered of the opposite sex. This cross-dressing is not necessarily sexual and often takes the form of cari-cature rather than serious impersonation.

These four examples demonstrate the three principal dimensions of the cross-dressing experience: the fetish component; the cross-gender identity and role, and sex-ual orientation. Most of the variety of cross-dressing behaviour can be accounted for by interaction of these three dimensions. There is very little that can be said about the determinants of these behaviours, which remain in most respects ill understood (Green 1974). The most important condition is transsexualism, because of the major and often devastating impact that this has on the individual's life. In males, childhood transsexualism is rare and the majority of such boys fol-lowed into early adulthood have so far shown homosex-ual rather than transsexual identities (Zuger 1978, Green 1985). It remains possible that some of them will eventually adopt the 'transsexual position' and this is one possible route to adult transsexualism. Many others start off with a fetishistic transvestite pattern which, over a period of time, becomes more transsexual, the cross-dressing losing its sexual effects. It is as though the repeated fetishistic cross-dressing undermines or produces conflict with the masculine gender identity, leading in some cases to adoption of a female identity as a solution (Bancroft 1972). In other cases, this process appears to stop, at least for a relatively long time, at the 'double-role transvestite' stage.

In some cases where homosexual attraction is present, but a homosexual identity unacceptable, the transsexual role allows the same attraction to continue while maintaining a heterosexual identity. In many cases, the strength of the transvestite or the transsexual urge varies with the success or failure of the individual's ordinary sexual relationships. Thus a resurgence of these feelings often follows a breakdown in a sexual relationship or marriage rather than precedes it.

In females, transsexualism is less common. The fetishistic dimension is not relevant to the female. In the author's experience, the avoidance of homosexuality is more striking as a causative factor in female transsexuals. They are also more likely than the male transsexual to be involved in a relatively stable sexual relationship. The role of the partner is therefore more relevant. Often the partner's own sexual or gender identity needs are best met by having a transsexual partner, and sometimes the partner may put pressure on the transsexual to seek sex reassignment because of her own need to avoid a homosexual identity.

The gender of the preferred sexual partner is not clearly predicted from the subject's gender identity. Thus, whereas the majority of male-to-female transsexuals, when established in their female role, are sexually attracted to males and regard themselves therefore as heterosexual, some retain the attraction to women that they experienced before gender reassignment. They then regard themselves as lesbian women. The situation is broadly similar for female-to-male individuals. This further emphasises that it is gender rather than sexual orientation that is at issue.

Management

Management of transsexualism presents one of the most demanding challenges in clinical sexology, requiring the collaboration of behavioural, endocrinological and surgical specialists working as a team. Though surgical aspects are complex, it is the psychological management that is most time consuming. It is unlikely that a transsexual will seek help to reduce or eliminate his transsexual feelings. As indicated above, the transsexual urge does wax and wane and there may be relatively prolonged periods when it is unimportant or absent. This in itself makes evaluation of any intervention difficult. Occasionally people have claimed 'cures' of transsexualism but they are usually based on short periods of follow-up and may be no more than a period of remission expedited by treatment. Usually the transsexual wants help with sex reassignment, most tangibly in

the forms of hormone therapy, facial hair electrolysis and surgery to reassign genitalia or remove or augment breasts. The use of such measures remains controversial, but a number of responsible clinicians have worked long enough and cautiously enough in this field to conclude that, with careful selection, at least a proportion of transsexuals will benefit from such reassignment.

In a review of the follow-up literature of sex reassignment surgery, Green & Fleming (1990) concluded that the preoperative factors indicating a favourable outcome include:

- A reasonable degree of psychological stability, with no history of psychosis
- Successful adaptation in the desired role for at least 1 year, with physical appearance and behaviour convincing
- Sufficient understanding of the limitations and consequences of surgery
- Pre-operative psychotherapy in the context of a gender identity programme.

Hormone therapy and facial electrolysis may be introduced at an earlier stage than surgery, but the decision to use surgery should only be made once it has become evident that the individual has the psychological and physical attributes, i.e. outward appearance, to adapt successfully. Hormone therapy involves oestrogens (possibly combined with progestogens) for the male to female, and androgens for the female to male. Oestrogens will probably induce breast growth, redistribution of body fat along more feminine lines, some change in skin texture and some slowing of facial and body hair growth. The extent of these effects is difficult to predict. Oestrogens may also suppress sexual interest and response, which may or may not be acceptable to the patient. The long-term risk should be emphasised. Androgens will increase muscle bulk, deepen the voice and increase body and facial hair growth. Clitoral enlargement is to be expected, often accompanied by an increase in sexual interest and response. Acne may be a problem. Surgical reassignment for the male transsexual involves removal of testes and the corpus spongiosum of the penis, preserving scrotal and penile skin to shape the labia and vaginal barrel, and, with some methods, deploying the corpora cavernosa on either side to provide an erectile base for the labia. Usually some additional skin graft is required to obtain a satisfactory vaginal barrel; some surgeons prefer to use a section of colon for this purpose. Surgical breast augmentation is often required.

The female has fewer options with surgical treatment. Hysterectomy and oophorectomy are usually involved. Mastectomy is often important, as concealment of breasts can be difficult or uncomfortable as well as limiting. Surgical creation of a penis remains surgically difficult, though some progress is being made. The principal problem is in ensuring satisfactory passage of urine through the surgically created urethra without urinary fistulae developing. Once these technical problems are solved, there may be possibilities for erection, at least of an artificial kind.

REFERENCES

Abel G G, Becker J V, Skinner L J 1980 Aggressive behaviour and sex. Psychiatric Clinics of North America 3: 133

Abel G G, Osborn C, Anthony D, Gardos P 1992 Current treatments of paraphiliacs. Annual Review of Sex Research 3: 255–290

Arentewicz G, Schmidt G 1983 The treatment of sexual disorders. Basic Books, New York

Bailey J M, Pillard R C 1995 Genetics of human sexual orientation. Annual Review of Sex Research 6: 126–150

Bancroft J 1972 The relationship between gender identity and sexual behaviour: some clinical aspects. In: Ounsted C, Taylor D C (eds) Gender differences: their origins and significance. Churchill Livingstone, Edinburgh, pp 57–71

Bancroft H 1974 Deviant sexual behaviour: modification and assessment. Clarendon Press, Oxford

Bancroft J 1988 Reproductive hormones and male sexual function. In: Sitsen J M A (ed) Handbook of sexology. Vol 6. Pharmacology of sexual function. Elsevier, Amsterdam, 297–315

Bancroft J 1989 Human sexuality and its problems, 2nd edn. Churchill Livingstone, Edinburgh

Bancroft J 1990 Biological contributions to sexual orientation. In: McWhirter D P, Sanders S A, Reinisch J M (eds) Homosexuality/Heterosexuality. Oxford University Press, New York, pp 101–111

Bancroft J 1991a The sexuality of sexual offending: the social dimension. Criminal Behaviour and Mental Health 1: 181–192

Bancroft J 1991b Ethical aspects of sexuality and sex therapy. In: Bloch S, Chodoff P (eds) Psychiatric ethics, 2nd edn. Oxford University Press, Oxford, pp 215–242

Bancroft J 1994 Homosexual orientation – the search for a biological basis. The neurobiology of sexual orientation. British Journal of Psychiatry 164: 437–440

Bancroft J 1995a Sexuality and family planning. In: Loudon N B, Glasier A F, Gebbie A (eds) Handbook of family planning and reproductive health care 3rd edn. Churchill Livingstone, Edinburgh, pp 339–362

Bancroft J (ed) 1995b Effects of α_2-antagonists on male erectile response. In: The pharmacology of sexual function and dysfunction. Excerpta Medica, Amsterdam, pp 215–224

Bancroft J 1996 Sex therapy. In: Bloch S (ed) An introduction to the psychotherapies. Oxford University Press, London, pp 213–237

Bancroft J 1997 Sexual problems. In: Clark D, Fairburn C (eds) Science and practice of cognitive behaviour therapy. Oxford University Press, London, pp 243–257

Becker J, Kaplan M S 1991 Rape victims: issues, theories, and treatment. Annual Review of Sex Research II: 267–292

Bell A P, Weinberg M S 1978 Homosexualities. A study of diversity among men and women. Mitchell Beazley, London

Blumstein P W, Schwartz P 1976 Bisexuality in women. Archives of Sexual Behavior 5: 171

Boolell M, Gepi-Attee S, Gingell J C, Allen M J 1996 Sildenafil, a novel effective oral therapy for male erectile dysfunction. British Journal Urology 78: 257–261

Brindley G S 1986 Maintenance treatment of erectile impotence by cavernosal unstriated muscle relaxant injections. British Journal of Psychiatry 14: 210

Browning C R, Laumann E O 1997 Sexual contact between children and adults: a life course perspective. American Sociological Review 62(4): 540–560

Buvat J, Buvat-Herbaut M, Lemaire A, Marcolin G, Quittelier E 1990 Recent developments in the clinical assessment and diagnosis of erectile dysfunction. Annual Review of Sex Research 1: 265–308

Carani C, Granata A R M, Bancroft J, Marrama P 1995 The effects of testosterone replacement on nocturnal penile tumescence and rigidity and erectile response to visual erotic stimuli in hypogonadal men. Psychoneuroendocrinology 20: 743–753

Catalan J, Bradley M, Gallway J, Hawton K 1981 Sexual dysfunction and psychiatric morbidity in patients attending a clinic for sexually transmitted diseases. British Journal of Psychiatry 138: 292

Clement U 1990 Surveys of heterosexual behavior. Annual Review of Sex Research 1: 75–92

Cranston-Cuebas M A, Barlow D H 1990 Cognitive and affective contributions to sexual functioning. Annual Review of Sex Research 1: 119–162

Fairburn C G, Wu F C W, McCulloch D K et al 1982 The clinical features of diabetic impotence: a preliminary study. British Journal of Psychiatry 140: 447

Feldman H A, Goldstein I, Hatzichristou D G, Krane R J, McKinlay J B 1994 Impotence and its medical and psychosocial correlates: results of the Massachusetts male aging study. Journal of Urology 151: 54–61

Frenken J 1976 Afkeer van seksualiteit. Van Loghum Slaterus, Deventer (English summary p. 219)

Frenken J, Van Tol P 1987 Sexual problems in gynecological practice. Journal of Psychosomatic Obstetrics and Gynaecology 6: 143–155

Friedrich W N 1988 Behavior problems in sexually abused children. In: Wyatt G E, Powell G J (eds) The lasting effects of child sexual abuse. Sage, Newbury Park, CA, pp 171–191

Gagnon J, Simon W 1973 Sexual conduct: the social sources of human sexuality. Aldine, Chicago

Garde K, Lunde L 1980 Female sexual behavior. A study in a random sample of 40 year old women. Maturitas 2: 255

Gittleson N L, Eacott S E, Mehta B M 1978 Victims of indecent exposure. British Journal of Psychiatry 132: 61

Golombok S, Rust J, Pickard C 1984 Sexual problems encountered in general practice. British Journal of Sexual Medicine 11: 210–212

Green R 1974 Sexual identity conflict in children and adults. Duckworth, London

Green R 1985 Gender identity in childhood and later sexual orientation: follow up of 78 males. American Journal of Psychiatry 142: 339–341

Green R, Fleming D T (1990) Transsexual surgery follow-up: status in the 1990s. Annual Review of Sex Research 1: 163–174

Hamer D H, Hu S, Magnuson V L et al 1993 A linkage between DNA markers on the X chromosome and male sexual orientation. Science 261: 321–327

Hawton K 1992 Sex therapy research: has it withered on the vine? Annual Review of Sex Research 3: 49–72

Hawton K, Catalan J 1986 Prognostic factors in sex therapy. Behaviour Research and Therapy 24: 377

Hawton K, Catalan J, Martin P, Fagg J 1986 Long term outcome of sex therapy. Behaviour Research and Therapy 24: 665–675

Herdt G H 1981 Guardians of the flutes: idioms of masculinity. McGraw-Hill, New York

Hines M, Collaer M L 1993 Gonadal hormones and sexual differentiation in human behavior: new developments from research on endocrine syndrome and studies of brain structure. Annual Review of Sex Research 4: 1–48

Hooker E 1967 The homosexual community. In: Gagnon J H, Simon W (eds) Sexual deviance. Harper & Row, New York

Johnson A M, Wadsworth J, Wellings K, Field J 1994 Sexual attitudes and lifestyles. Blackwell Scientific Press, London

Kaplan H S 1974 The new sex therapy. Brunner Mazel, New York

Katz S, Mazur M A 1979 Understanding rape victims; a synthesis of research findings. Wiley, New York

Kinsey A S, Pomeroy W B, Martin C R 1948 Sexual behaviour in the human male. W B Saunders, Philadelphia

Kinsey A S, Pomeroy W B, Martin C R, Gebhard P H 1953 Sexual behaviour in the human female. W B Saunders, Philadelphia

Kurdek L A 1995 Lesbian and gay couples. In: D'Augelli A R, Patterson C J (eds) Lesbian, gay, and bisexual identities over the lifespan. Oxford University Press, New York, pp 243–261

Laumann E O, Gagnon J H, Michael R T, Michaels S 1994 The social organization of sexuality: sexual practices in the United States. University of Chicago Press, Chicago

Leiblum S R, Rosen R C 1989 Principles and practice of sex therapy, 2nd edn. Guilford, New York

Levine S B, Yost M A 1976 Frequency of sexual dysfunction in a general gynaecological clinic: an epidemiological approach. Archives of Sexual Behavior 5: 229

Linet O I, Ogrinc F G and the Alprostadil Study Group 1996 Efficacy and safety of intracavernosal alprostadil in men with erectile dysfunction. New England Journal of Medicine 334: 873–877

McCulloch D K, Campbell I W, Wu F C, Prescott R J, Clarke B F 1980 The prevalence of diabetic impotence. Diabetologia 18: 279

McWhirter D P, Mattison A M 1984 The male couple. How relationships develop. Prentice-Hall, Englewood Cliffs

Masson J M 1984 The assault on truth. Freud's suppression of the seduction theory. Farrar, Strauss & Giroux, New York

Masters W H, Johnson V E 1970 Human sexual inadequacy. Churchill, London

Masters W H, Johnson V E 1979 Homosexuality in perspective. Little Brown, Company, Boston

Mohr J W, Turner R E, Jerry M B 1964 Paedophilia and exhibitionism. University of Toronto Press, Toronto

Money J, Ehrhardt A A 1972 Man and woman, boy and girl: differentiation and dimorphism of gender identity from conception to maturity. Johns Hopkins University Press, Baltimore

O'Carroll R, Bancroft J 1984 Testosterone therapy for low sexual interest and erectile dysfunction in men: a controlled study. British Journal of Psychiatry 145: 146

Padman-Nathan H, Hellstrom V J A, Kaiser F E et al 1997 Treatment of erectile dysfunction by transurethral alprostadil. New England Journal of Medicine 336: 1–7

Peplau L A, Cochran S D 1990 A relationship perspective on homosexuality. In: McWhirter D P, Sanders S A,

Reinisch J M (eds) Homosexuality/heterosexuality: concepts of sexual orientation. 2nd Kinsey symposium. Oxford University Press, New York

Peters S, Wyatt G, Finkelhor D 1986 Prevalence. In: Finkelhor D et al (eds) Sourcebook on child sexual abuse. Sage, Beverly Hills, pp 15–59

Rachman S, Hodgson R 1968 Experimentally induced 'sexual fetishism': replication and development. Psychological Record 18: 25

Reid K, Surridge D H C, Morales A et al 1987 Double-blind trial of yohimbine in the treatment of psychogenic impotence. Lancet ii: 421–423

Riley A J 1995 Alpha adrenoceptors and human sexual function. In: Bancroft J (ed) The pharmacology of sexual function and dysfunction. Excerpta Medica, Amsterdam, pp 307–322

Riley A J, Goodman R E, Kellett J M, Orr R 1989 Double blind trial of yohimbine hydrochloride in the treatment of erection inadequacy. Sexual and Marital Therapy 4: 17–26

Rooth F G 1971 Indecent exposure and exhibitionism. British Journal of Hospital Medicine April: 521

Rooth F G 1973 Exhibitionism, sexual violence and paedophilia. British Journal of Psychiatry 122: 705

Rosen R C 1991 Alcohol and drug effects on sexual response: experimental and clinical studies. Annual Review of Sex Research II: 119–180

Slag M F, Morley J E, Elson M K et al 1983 Impotence in medical clinic outpatients. Journal of the American Medical Association 249: 1736

Spengler A 1977 Manifest sado-masochism of males: results of an empirical study. Archives of Sexual Behavior 6: 441

Summit R C 1983 The child sexual abuse accommodation syndrome. Child Abuse and Neglect 7: 177–193

Swan M, Wilson L J 1979 Sexual and marital problems in a psychiatric outpatient population. British Journal of Psychiatry 135: 310

Tiefer L 1991 Historical, scientific, clinical and feminist criticisms of 'the sexual response cycle' model. Annual Review of Sex Research II: 1–24

Toone B K, Wheeler M, Nanjee N, Fenwick P, Grant R 1983 Sex hormones, sexual activity and plasma anticonvulsant levels in male epileptics. Journal of Neurology, Neurosurgery and Psychiatry 46: 824

Turner L A, Althof S E, Levine S B, Bodner D R, Kursh E D, Resnick M I 1991 A comparison of the effectiveness of two treatments for erectile dysfunction: self-injection therapy versus external vacuum devices. Paper at annual meeting, International Academy of Sex Research, Barrie, Ontario

Tyrer G, Steele J M, Ewing D J, Bancroft J, Warner P, Clarke B F 1983 Sexual response in diabetic women. Diabetologia 24: 166

Virag R, Shoukry K, Floresco J, Nollet F, Greco E 1991 Intracavernous self-injection of vasoactive drugs in the treatment of impotence: 8-year experience with 615 cases. Journal of Urology 145: 287–293

Warner P, Bancroft J and members of the Edinburgh Human Sexuality Group 1987 A regional service for sexual problems: a 3-year study. Sexual and Marital Therapy 2: 115–126

Weinberg M S, Williams C J 1974 Male homosexuals: their problems and adaptation. Oxford University Press, New York

Weinberg T S 1994 Research in sadomasochism: a review of sociological and social psychological literature. Annual Review of Sex Research 5: 257–279

Wyatt G E 1991 Child sexual abuse and its effects on sexual functioning. Annual Review of Sex Research 2: 249–266

Zuger B 1978 Effeminate behavior present in boys from childhood: 10 additional years of follow up. Comprehensive Psychiatry 19: 363–369

20
Psychiatric disorders specific to women

Jan Scott   Rachel Jenkins

INTRODUCTION

While many mental disorders occur more frequently in women than in men, there is a small group of mental disorders that are specific to women. In each case the onset or exacerbation of psychological symptoms is related to the reproductive cycle. Early classification systems viewed these disorders as discrete categories, but recently (with the exception of the DSM-IV category 'premenstrual dysphoric disorder'), this trend has been reversed. For example, it is increasingly recognised that the symptomatology of postnatal depressive disorders varies little from the symptomatology of depressive disorders presenting at other times. It is the temporal relationship of the onset of the symptoms to clearly defined events that set these disorders apart. The mental disorders associated with childbirth also represent a unique challenge as clinicians try to balance the treatment needs of the parent and the developmental needs of the child.

This chapter explores the clinical features, epidemiology, aetiology and management of mental disorders related to menstruation, pregnancy and childbirth. Additional space is given to the section on premenstrual disorders as relatively few comprehensive reviews exist on this topic, in comparison to the widely available literature on mental disorders associated with childbirth.

PERIMENSTRUAL DISORDERS

Premenstrual syndrome

Menstruation-related changes in mood and behaviour were described by Hippocrates and recognised in the Bible. Unfortunately, progress toward a greater understanding of premenstrual disorders, as opposed to premenstrual symptoms, has been slow. Contemporary research has been hampered by the lack of a consistent definition of the premenstrual syndrome (PMS), and by very different approaches to classification in Europe

and the USA. In ICD-10, 'premenstrual tension syndrome' is classified with 'pain and other conditions' in the section on female genitourinary disorders. In DSM-IV 'premenstrual dysphoric disorder' is described as a mood disorder but is only included in the appendix as a research diagnostic category requiring further study. Thus, the two most widely accepted diagnostic systems offer quite narrow definitions but separate classifications of variants of the premenstrual syndrome (Halbreich 1996). ICD-10 focuses on somatic manifestations and essentially regards premenstrual tension syndrome as a gynaecological disorder; in contrast, DSM-IV primarily requires the presence of at least one premenstrual affective symptom (irritability, depression, anxiety or mood lability) and impairment of day-to-day functioning. As such, the DSM-IV diagnosis can be made in the absence of somatic symptoms.

Both approaches to the classification of PMS have disadvantages. The ICD-10 approach may deter clinicians and researchers from examining the psychological and affective symptoms associated with premenstrual tension or they may fail to adequately differentiate premenstrual tension from other conditions such as painful dysmenorrhoea. Although DSM-IV takes a cautious approach and emphasises the need for further data on premenstrual dysphoric disorder (PMDD), there are still difficulties with the proposed diagnostic category. For example, it is time consuming and tedious to establish that a patient meets the criteria for PMDD, as the diagnostic process requires at least 2 months of prospective daily monitoring of symptoms (Halbreich 1996). Also, the arbitrary number of symptoms (five from a preselected list of 10 features) and severity criteria selected for the diagnosis of PMDD may inappropriately categorise some women with premenstrual symptoms as mentally disordered (Parry & Rausch 1996) or may exclude important subgroups of patients (e.g. those with a different symptom profile) from treatment or research protocols.

Given the uncertainties outlined above and the difficulties of applying these new criteria to the published literature, this chapter will use the acronym PMS and will employ previously published criteria to define the disorder and review its epidemiology, aetiology and treatment (Rubinow & Schmidt 1989, Halbreich 1996, Parry & Rausch 1996).

Definition and epidemiology

Premenstrual syndrome (PMS) is a cyclical disorder of women of reproductive age that recurs at some point between ovulation and menstruation. It is characterised by a combination of affective (e.g. irritability, depression), somatic (e.g. fluid retention, breast tenderness, headache), behavioural (e.g. poor coordination, relationship difficulties) and cognitive (e.g. poor concentration) symptoms. Katherine Dalton (1964) suggested that PMS may also be associated with increased rates of accidents, suicide and criminal activity, but the use of more sophisticated research methods has put these findings into doubt. However, there is a consensus about the key features (Table 20.1) that need to be present to make a diagnosis of PMS (Rubinow & Schmidt

Table 20.1	Key aspects in the diagnosis of premenstrual syndrome
Symptoms	A combination of affective, behavioural, cognitive and/or somatic symptoms should occur in a consistent pattern at some point during most months of the previous year
Timing and cyclicity	Symptoms should occur between ovulation and the onset of menstruation, typically commencing during the last week of the luteal phase and remitting a few days after the start of menses
Severity	Symptoms should be severe enough to disrupt social and/or work roles
Consistency	Prospective monitoring should demonstrate that: • Most of the specified symptoms recur during the designated period of the menstrual cycle • This constellation of symptoms does not occur during other phases of the menstrual cycle • The symptoms do not represent a premenstrual exacerbation of any underlying physical or mental disorder

1989, Halbreich 1996, Parry & Rausch 1996). As shown in Table 20.1, no specific symptoms are pathognomonic of PMS and the diagnosis depends more on the temporal occurrence than on the phenomenology of the disorder (Rubinow & Schmidt 1989).

Rubinow & Schmidt (1989) comment that over 200 potential symptoms of PMS have been identified in different studies. Community surveys suggested that premenstrual complaints were reported by 20–90% of women in their reproductive years (American College of Obstetricians & Gynecologists 1989). However, these studies failed to clearly differentiate premenstrual symptoms from premenstrual disorder, included significant sampling biases and often relied on retrospective ratings of the pattern and timing of occurrence of symptoms. In a study of 240 women identified as suffering from PMS, the five most prevalent symptoms were depression (56%), irritability (48%), anxiety (36%), mood lability (26%) and headaches (23%) (Freeman et al 1985). This study highlights the significant role of affective symptoms in PMS, but can be criticised for failing to employ any measure of symptom severity. Evidence from prospective studies in psychiatric and gynaecological settings demonstrates that the symptom profile and severity of PMS varies considerably between subjects and samples, but about 40% of women meet recognised criteria for PMS (Andersch et al 1986), and 3–8% meet stricter diagnostic criteria that include evidence of impairment of social or occupational functioning (Rivera-Tovar & Frank 1990).

Aetiology

The cause of PMS is uncertain. The linkage of PMS symptoms to biological events (ovulation and menstruation) not surprisingly led to the development of biomedical theories of aetiology that particularly focused on endocrine abnormalities. However, as noted by Rubinow & Schmidt (1989), early studies demonstrating differences between women with PMS and asymptomatic control subjects often selected PMS subjects retrospectively and measured hormone levels using inadequate or non-uniform blood sampling times and intervals.

Endocrine models One of the most frequently quoted early theories of PMS postulated a deficiency of luteal phase progesterone and led to the widespread use of progesterone treatment for PMS sufferers (Dalton 1984). This theory and all others postulating abnormalities in baseline levels of progesterone, oestrogen, gonadotrophins or oestrogen:progesterone ratios have not been substantiated by recent research (Halbreich 1995). However, as women with PMS are reported to be asymptomatic during anovulatory cycles (Backstrom et al 1989), it would be premature to rule out a putative role for gonadal steroids and gonadotrophins (Parry & Rausch 1996). Researchers are currently exploring whether women who develop PMS are biologically susceptible to an exaggerated response to normal levels of gonadal hormones, demonstrate abnormal cyclicity of gonadal hormones, or accumulate higher than expected levels of abnormal progesterone metabolites (Halbreich 1995).

There is no consistent pattern of abnormalities in non-reproductive neuroendocrine markers such as cortisol, thyroid hormones or prolactin. However, one study has demonstrated that women with PMS show similar circadian melatonin secretion patterns to individuals with major depressive disorders (Parry et al 1990).

Neurotransmitter models The accumulated evidence suggests that there are changes in monoamine functioning during the menstrual cycle (Parry & Rausch 1996). Research focused on 5-hydroxytryptamine (5-HT) has demonstrated decreased late-luteal phase uptake of 5-HT in platelets of PMS subjects as opposed to asymptomatic controls (Ashby et al 1988), lower levels of whole blood 5-HT premenstrually in PMS subjects (Rapkin et al 1988) and lowered imipramine receptor binding in platelets of women with PMS when compared with control subjects (Rojansky et al 1991). It is not clear whether these abnormalities identify women specifically at risk of PMS or women at risk of mood disorders in general.

Psychosocial models Although it has been suggested that PMS is associated with high levels of neuroticism, there is no consistent evidence of any association between specific personality traits and PMS (Parry & Rausch 1996). Also there is no empirical evidence to support the influence on the presentation of PMS of cultural factors or public attitudes. Women do show increased reactivity to stress and higher levels of arousal during the late luteal phase (Rubinow & Schmidt 1989) and there is evidence that high levels of stress may exacerbate the symptoms of PMS, while positive environmental changes may reduce the distress associated with PMS (Severino & Moline 1989, Halbreich 1996).

PMS as a variant of affective disorder Most of the hypothesised vulnerability factors found in women with PMS are also found in many patients with other affective disorders (Halbreich 1996). A number of researchers (e.g. Halbreich et al 1982) have also noted the close clinical resemblance of the symptom profile of PMS to atypical depression. These observations have led many to consider that PMS is simply a variant of other recognised mood disorders. Studies of the longitudinal course of PMS (e.g. DeJong et al 1985, MacKenzie et al 1986, Graze et al 1990) confirm a greater than expected lifetime prevalence of depressive disorders (30–60%), and Harrison et al (1985) also identified that there is an increased prevalence of major depressive disorders in first-degree relatives of women with PMS. Unfortunately, most of these studies can be criticised for the methodology employed and further research is required to clarify the relationship between PMS and affective disorders.

PMS as an autonomous mood disorder Schmidt and colleagues (1991) gave a progesterone agonist (mifepristone) to women with prospectively diagnosed PMS. The mifepristone truncated the luteal phase of the menstrual cycle and led to the onset of menses within 72 hours. Although the women now had a peripheral endocrine profile consistent with the early follicular phase of their menstrual cycle, the majority still experienced their characteristic premenstrual symptoms. These results may suggest that PMS symptoms are mediated by hormonal changes that precede the late luteal phase (thus the mifepristone did not influence the development of symptoms). However, an alternative explanation considered by the researchers views PMS as an autonomous cyclical disorder with mood and behavioural changes that are facilitated (entrained) but not caused by the menstrual cycle.

In summary, the aetiology of PMS is under investigation. It is likely that biological and psychosocial factors play a role in the development of PMS, but the relative importance of these different variables has not been established.

Management

Differential diagnosis Before arriving at a diagnosis of PMS, it must be clearly established (preferably prospectively) that the patient is ovulating and experiencing symptoms in the late luteal phase. It is also important to undertake a thorough psychiatric assessment and physical examination to determine whether the individual is suffering from either an underlying medical or mental disorder. Physical problems that may demonstrate cyclicity and can be mistaken for PMS include endocrine disorders (e.g. polycystic ovaries), epilepsy, migraine, endometriosis and various infections (e.g. herpes). The prevalence of comorbid mental disorders with PMS is high, with 70–80% of patients meeting criteria for Axis I disorders (over 50% being affective disorders) and about 10% meeting criteria for Axis II disorders (Parry & Rausch 1996). Often, it is only possible to distinguish premenstrual exacerbation of dysthymic or anxiety disorders by monitoring symptom profile and menstrual cyclicity on a daily basis over 2–3 months. There are no specific laboratory tests to help clinicians diagnose PMS.

Treatment There are more than 50 methods of treatment of PMS described in the literature. For many years, the luteal phase administration of progesterone was advocated as the treatment of choice for PMS. However, double-blind placebo-controlled intervention studies have not shown any additional benefit from this approach as compared with placebo (Halbreich 1996). Few other treatments have been the subject of rigorous research and none is effective or appropriate for all individuals. As shown in Figure 20.1, as the cause of PMS is unknown, the treatment strategy will be determined by the nature and severity of the symptoms and a clinical imperative to select the least invasive intervention.

Mild symptoms If the patient suffers from mild or brief symptoms of PMS, a number of conservative treatment options are available. Psychoeducation sessions focused on education, diet and stress management have been advocated, but the response rate may be no higher than that reported with placebo treatments (Severino & Moline 1989). Increased aerobic exercise (particularly during the luteal phase) has been shown to reduce breast pain and fluid retention and to improve mood-related symptoms, probably as a consequence of increased endorphin levels. The treatment of the physical symptoms of PMS may include bromocriptine (for breast tenderness) and diuretics (for bloating, fluid retention). However, given the potential side-effects of these medications, there is debate about whether such interventions are more beneficial than the use of a support bra and changes in diet and exercise (Halbreich 1996).

The role of dietary and vitamin supplements is uncertain. The results of trials on the benefits of pyroxidine (vitamin B_6) are equivocal and some of the vitamin supplements may be neurotoxic if given in high doses over an extended period of time (Halbreich 1996, Parry & Rausch 1996). However, two well-designed clinical trials have demonstrated additional health gains for women with mild to moderate levels of PMS from the use of magnesium (360 mg q.d.s.) and calcium (1000 mg q.d.s.) supplements respectively.

Moderate to severe symptoms As mood changes are a frequent component of PMS, many researchers have advocated the use of psychotropic agents such as benzodiazepines and antidepressants to treat anxiety and depressive symptoms, respectively. However, most studies supporting the use of these medications were undermined by the inclusion of women with PMS and a comorbid mood disorder and/or women with premenstrual exacerbation of underlying mood disorders. In double-blind placebo-controlled treatment studies of women with pure PMS, only alprazolam (0.25–1.0 mg q.d.s. during the luteal phase) and fluoxetine (20 mg

daily throughout the menstrual cycle) have been demonstrated to be effective (Harrison et al 1990, Steiner et al 1995). The disadvantage of alprazolam is that 10–20% of subjects may experience withdrawal anxiety. If side-effects from selective serotonin reuptake inhibitors (SSRIs) are not tolerable, it may be appropriate to use clomipramine, which has been demonstrated to be effective in smaller scale studies.

Suppression of ovulation may be the most effective intervention for severe PMS that fails to respond to the above treatments (Muse et al 1984). This can be achieved through the long-term administration of oestradiol (either by patches or subcutaneous injection), with progesterone supplements in the last week of the menstrual cycle to prevent endometrial hyperplasia. Danazol, a synthetic androgen, has been shown to be effective in doses of 200–400 mg per day. However, Halbreich (1996) and others recommend caution in its use in women of childbearing age because of androgenic and other side-effects. Gonadotrophin-releasing hormone agonists such as buserilin acetate appear to reduce somatic symptoms in PMS, but are less effective in improving mood-related symptoms. However, Mortola (1991) recommend that this treatment should be combined with oestrogen and progestin supplements (in postmenopausal doses) to reduce the likelihood of menopausal symptoms and bone loss. It may also be necessary to add calcium supplements and increase exercise, or limit the treatment to 6 months. Lastly, for patients with severe, treatment refractory PMS, it is occasionally appropriate to consider surgical hysterectomy and bilateral oophorectomy followed by oestrogen treatment (Casper & Hearn 1990). However, the availability of a number of medical treatments to induce anovulation should mean that clinicians rarely need to resort to irreversible surgery unless PMS is complicated by a comorbid gynaecological disorder (Halbreich 1996).

Summary

The introduction of PMDD into DSM-IV will focus research into the aetiology and treatment of premenstrual symptoms on a more homogeneous population of women. In the interim, clinicians should note that the diagnosis of PMS depends primarily on *when* symptoms occur rather than *what* symptoms are experienced. Diagnosis is best made by careful history taking, physical examination and prospective monitoring of symptom fluctuation during the menstrual cycle. Treatment options for PMS range from lifestyle management (diet and exercise) to antidepressants and ovulation suppressors. Given that treatment is largely determined by symptom profile, it may be necessary to try a number of

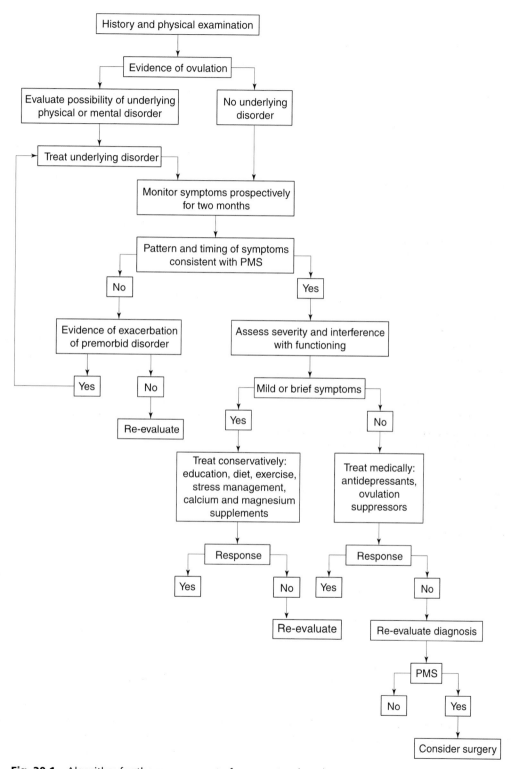

Fig. 20.1 Algorithm for the management of premenstrual syndrome.

options sequentially to find the most beneficial approach for a given individual.

Postmenopausal disorders

It has frequently been suggested that symptoms of depression and anxiety are more common in menopausal women. While there is evidence that women are overrepresented amongst middle-aged individuals attending their general practitioner with psychological symptoms, epidemiological studies do not support the hypothesis that perimenopausal or postmenopausal women are at greater risk of depressive disorder (Kessler et al 1993, Schmidt et al 1996).

Various reasons have been put forward to explain the increased reporting of psychological symptoms. Psychosocial stressors, such as changes in family role and social support, loss events, physical illness and ageing, are associated with the presentation of affective and menopausal symptoms (Cooke & Greene 1981). However, the adverse events reported may be coincidental rather than causal factors. Alternative theories focus on the neuromodulatory effects of gonadal steroids. Changes in levels of gonadal hormones, particularly prolonged perimenopausal exposure to oestrogen or postmenopausal oestrogen deprivation, can exacerbate pre-existing mental disorders and may be associated with the development of mood and behaviour disturbances (Schmidt et al 1996).

The management of perimenopausal depressive disorders requires careful assessment of physical symptoms and present and past psychological problems. Some researchers advocate the use of hormone replacement therapy, but results of depression treatment studies using oestrogen are not conclusive (Pearce et al 1995). Oestrogen replacement may directly improve mood in some women, but in others its beneficial effects are probably due to its impact on physical symptoms (Schmidt et al 1996). For most women with perimenopausal major depressive disorders, effective treatment is usually achieved with the standard antidepressant interventions that are used to treat depressions occurring at other stages of the life cycle.

MENTAL DISORDERS ASSOCIATED WITH PREGNANCY

Normal pregnancy

Although pregnancy has dramatic emotional and psychological consequences for the individual, it is not associated with a significant increase in rates of mental disorders unless there is a pre-existing disorder or the pregnant woman is a teenager (Klein & Essex 1995, Berga & Parry 1996). There is evidence of non-significant increases in the incidence of anxiety and depressive syndromes in the first and third trimester (Gotlib et al 1989, Klein & Essex 1995). Symptoms in the first trimester are usually minor and more typical of an adjustment disorder. In the third trimester anxieties may be expressed about the process of delivery and the safety and development of the fetus. These fears do not necessarily constitute an abnormal reaction.

Research suggests that mental disorders are more common in pregnant women who have a personal or family history of depressive disorders, who are ambivalent about being pregnant, who demonstrate high levels of neuroticism or dysfunctional attributional style, and those who lack marital, family or social support (Kumar 1982, Kitamura et al 1993). Treatment usually focuses on psychosocial interventions that enhance psychological adjustment or improve social support. If antidepressants are required, secondary amine tricyclic antidepressants such as nortryptiline are considered to be relatively safe, but it is recommended that the dose is tapered and withdrawn before delivery to prevent adverse effects on the baby (Berga & Parry 1996). In the rare event of a pregnant women developing severe life-threatening depressive disorder, a course of eletroconvulsive therapy (ECT) may be the most appropriate and rapid method of achieving symptom control and clinical improvement.

Other disorders

Miscarriage and abortion

Spontaneous and therapeutic abortions may be associated with increased rates of psychiatric morbidity, particularly in the first month after the event. Over 50% of women demonstrate features of a grief reaction or a depressive disorder. Symptoms are often typical of adjustment disorders and follow-up studies demonstrate that chronic morbidity is rare. Women at greater risk of disorder are those with a previous history of miscarriage and those who experience conflict related to their religious or cultural beliefs (Clare & Tyrrell 1994).

Hyperemesis gravidum

Katon and colleagues (1980) have reviewed hyperemesis gravidum and concluded that it is a psychosomatic disorder with organic and psychological factors both playing an aetiological role. About 50% of pregnant women report nausea and vomiting in the early stages of pregnancy, but only about 1% experience severe bouts of vomiting and dehydration. Hyperemesis gravidum has a peak incidence between 8 and 12 weeks of pregnancy and is more common in women with a past history of gastrointestinal disorders and also in women who receive less support from their partner or parents. Treatment is supportive and symptomatic and usually focuses on education, restoration of electrolyte and fluid balance (with intravenous fluids where necessary) and reducing nausea and vomiting through the limited and careful prescribing of antiemetics.

Pseudocyesis

This is a rare condition, where the woman erroneously believes she is pregnant and develops associated features such as amenorrhoea and abdominal distension. Pseudocyesis is more common in younger as compared with older females. Once the woman is counselled that she is not pregnant her physical symptoms usually resolve quickly. However, it may take much longer for the patient's underlying belief to shift and there is a greater than expected tendency to recurrence (Small 1986).

MENTAL DISORDERS ASSOCIATED WITH THE PUERPERIUM

Current classification systems vary in the status accorded to mental disorders in the puerperium. In ICD-10, clinicians are discouraged from categorising such disorders as separate from other affective disorders, while DSM-IV includes a course specifier to denote postpartum onset. However, the uncertainty about whether puerperal syndromes represent distinct mental disorders has not impeded clinical and research activity into the special needs of affected women and their children. Disorders of the puerperium are traditionally subdivided into three categories: maternity blues, postnatal depression and postpartum (puerperal) psychosis.

Maternity blues

Maternity blues is the term used to describe a mild, self-limiting episode of psychological disturbance beginning 3–10 days after parturition (peak onset day 5) and remitting by 12–14 days after parturition (Table 20.2). The reported prevalence varies from 30 to 80%. Studies reporting a high prevalence tend to employ very loose diagnostic criteria for maternity blues such as 'crying for five minutes during the first 10 days after delivery of a child' (Yalom et al 1965). Studies reporting lower rates define a syndrome comprising about seven symptoms of at least mild severity (O'Hara et al 1990). The most frequently reported symptoms include depression, mood lability, insomnia, anorexia, fatigue, irritability, anxiety and subjective confusion. The syndrome is so common that many researchers and clinicians regard it as a normal part of childbirth. However, recognition of the syndrome is important as there is evidence that women with more severe symptoms may be at increased risk of developing more serious psychiatric conditions (O'Hara et al 1991).

The aetiology of maternity blues has not been established conclusively. It appears to occur across all races and cultures and is a specific response to childbirth, as opposed to a non-specific response to a comparable stress such as elective surgery (Isles et al 1989). There is no relationship between complications at delivery, but high levels of anxiety and depression in the pregnant woman during the third trimester do appear to reliably predict the occurrence of maternity blues (Kennerly & Gath 1989, O'Hara et al 1991). The most widely held causal theory postulates that the precipitous postpartum fall in oestrogen, progesterone and prolactin (which reach prepregnancy levels within 3 days) leads to destabilisation of neurotransmitter mechanisms involved in mood regulation (Steiner 1996). However, scientific support for this hypothesis is disappointing, with some studies establishing only a weak association between changes in hormonal levels and symptom onset, and others failing to establish any relationship (Heidrich et al 1994).

Table 20.2 Puerperal mood disorders			
	Maternity blues	Postnatal depression	Postpartum psychosis
Incidence	30–80%	10–15%	0.2%
Onset after childbirth	About 3–10 days	About 3 weeks	About 2 weeks
Management	Support and education	Brief cognitive therapy, counselling and/or antidepressants	Admission, education antidepressants, mood stabilisers, antipsychotics, ECT

Given the transient nature of maternity blues, no active treatments are usually recommended. Management comprises education about the nature of the condition, combined with support. Close monitoring is recommended for the small minority of women with severe and persistent symptoms, as about 30% may develop a more serious postpartum depression (Kendell et al 1981).

Postnatal depression

A diagnosis of postnatal depression is restricted to a non-psychotic depressive disorder that usually develops insidiously about 3–4 weeks after childbirth (Table 20.2). The prevalence of depressive disorders is about 10–15% in the 6 months postpartum (O'Hara & Zekowski 1988). Although prospective studies indicate that these rates of depression represent a non-significant increase in puerperal women as compared with non-puerperal controls (Cooper & Murray 1995), the proportion of new onset cases in puerperal women within 1 month of childbirth is significantly increased (Cox et al 1993). Earlier studies suggesting an increased risk of chronicity in postnatal depression (for example, Kumar & Robson 1984) are not supported by recent research which reports that postnatal disorders do not differ diagnostically or in duration from disorders occurring at other times (Cooper & Murray 1995).

The symptoms of postnatal depression are similar to depressive disorders arising at other stages in the life cycle, although the presentation may be coloured by the mother–child interaction (Cox 1992). Weepiness, irritability and anxiety may be more prominent than depressed affect (Pitt 1968). Anxiety may focus on the well-being of the baby, with negative thinking dominated by themes of personal inadequacy or failure to function as a 'good' mother. Suicidal ideation and vegetative symptoms of depression, including loss of libido, are frequent. Sleep disturbance is common, but may be masked by the disruption to normal routines associated with baby care. Physical features resembling those seen in hypothyroidism have also been reported, such as cold intolerance, fatigue and slowed mentation (Harris 1993).

Aetiology

Difficulties in determining the aetiology of postnatal depression may relate to the heterogeneity of the population being studied. Cooper & Murray (1995) suggested that there are at least two distinct subgroups of women who develop nonpsychotic depression after childbirth: those for whom the experience of having a child constitutes a significant causative event; and

those for whom the birth is a non-specific stressor. In their 5 year study of 55 primaparous women and 40 psychiatrically-well control subjects, women whose postnatal presentation was their first ever episode of depression (n = 34) were compared with women for whom the postnatal episode was a recurrence of psychiatric disturbance (n = 21). It was shown that the former group had depressive episodes of short duration and was at increased risk for further postpartum depressions (41%). In contrast, the second group was at increased risk for further non-postpartum episodes (62%) but not for postpartum episodes of depression (18%).

Cooper & Murray (1995) postulated that the short episode duration and specific vulnerability to postnatal depression are consistent with, but not conclusive evidence of, a biological cause. There are empirical studies that support a putative role for sex hormones in the onset of postnatal depression, but there are reports that pituitary dysfunction and suppressed thyroid hormone activity may be associated with its development in a significant minority of patients (Harris 1993, Pedersen et al 1993). Steiner (1996) comments that it is likely that women at risk of postnatal depression show an idiosyncratic individual reaction to postpartum hormonal changes rather than an abnormal pattern of changes per se. However, reviews of biological factors acknowledge the inadequacies of current models and highlight the potential role of psychosocial factors.

Ethnographic studies indicate that postnatal depression is rare in non-Western societies, where social and cultural rituals clearly define the role and expected behaviour of a new mother as well as providing structured social support (Harkness 1987, Oates 1990). European and American studies have shown that psychosocial factors associated with the onset of postnatal depression overlap with those associated with the onset of depression at other times. Women at increased risk for postnatal depression often demonstrate a premorbid personality characterised by high interpersonal sensitivity, a family history or personal history of affective disorders, poor marital relationships, inadequate social support, and report the occurrence of additional stressful life events during pregnancy (O'Hara et al 1990, Paykel et al 1980, Boyce et al 1991). There is no evidence that obstetric complications are associated with postnatal depression, but severe maternity blues may identify women at increased risk of postnatal depression (Cox 1992).

Management

Identification Many of the psychosocial risk factors reported above can be detected at antenatal or early postnatal assessments. In addition, reliable and valid screening questionnaires can be employed to detect postnatal depression, such as the 10 item self-report Edinburgh Postnatal Depression Scale (Cox et al 1987). Most women at risk of non-psychotic postnatal depression will be living in the community at the peak time of onset of the disorder. Therefore, education about vulnerability factors, diagnosis and treatment needs to be targeted at midwives, health visitors and members of the primary care team. It is important that these professionals are able to distinguish postnatal depression from maternity blues or from changes in lifestyle and routine associated with childbearing. Non-mental health professionals also need to be able to sensitively elicit a psychiatric history from women or their significant others who may be reluctant to acknowledge problems because of the perceived stigma associated with unhappiness occurring in the postnatal period.

Prevention Several psychosocial programmes have been developed to help women at risk of postnatal depression. For example, Elliot (1989) recruited women with a previous history of postnatal problems, and offered a psychoeducation and support programme extending from the second trimester to 6 months after the birth of their child. The prevalence of depression in the high-risk group offered the programme (19%) was about half that experienced by vulnerable women who were not offered the intervention (40%). In New South Wales, Barnett & Parker (1985) undertook a project with primaparous women who had been identified to be at greater risk of neurotic and depressive disorders. The women were assigned prenatally to either professional support, lay support or a control condition with no additional help. Both interventions lasted for 12 months postnatally, with gradual reduction in contact over the last 6 months. Overall, those who received professional help showed a significant reduction in postnatal anxiety levels as compared with the other groups; those receiving lay support showed a non-significant reduction in anxiety levels.

As many women at risk of postnatal depression have a past history of affective disorder, Wisner & Wheeler (1994) have also suggested guidelines for pharmacological prevention.

Treatment Psychosocial and medical treatments may be effective in treating postnatal depression. Holden et al (1987) describe the benefits of eight weekly sessions (of 30 minutes) of non-directive counselling by a health visitor. Sixty women with postnatal depression were randomly allocated to counselling or to a control condition. At 3 month follow-up, 69% of women offered counselling met recovery criteria, as compared with 38% of untreated women. However, Cox (1992) comments that only 35% of the treated women responded to counselling alone, and there is a need to

use additional resources such as specialist community mental health team input or day hospital treatment.

Decisions about prescribing antidepressant medication will be influenced by the patient's desire to breast-feed as virtually all these medications are excreted in the breast milk (Steiner 1996). However, this should not be regarded as an absolute contraindication as many studies have established that the amount of tricyclic or related antidepressant medications delivered in breast milk is small, producing negligible plasma levels in the infant with minimal risk of adverse effects (Ito et al 1993). There are fewer data available on SSRIs, but preliminary studies suggest the medication is effective and does not adversely affect the infant (Roy et al 1993). Failure to respond to standard antidepressant regimens usually leads to consideration of the use of ECT or, less often, antidepressant augmentation treatments with lithium, carbamazepine, benzodiazepines and phenothiazines or treatment with thyroid hormones. The medications used to augment antidepressant treatment should not generally be used if a mother is breast-feeding as exposure to these drugs may adversely affect the infant. The use of thyroid hormones may be indicated in women who show abnormal thyroid function tests or who develop a treatment refractory postnatal depression. A typical starting dose would be 0.05 mg of thyroxine per day with weekly monitoring of thyroid functioning (Harris 1993).

Appleby and colleagues (1996) reported a randomized controlled trial of fluoxetine and brief cognitive behavioural counselling in the treatment of postnatal depression. Eighty-seven women satisfying criteria for non-psychotic major depressive disorder 6–8 weeks after childbirth were allocated to one of four treatment cells: fluoxetine or placebo plus one or six sessions of counselling. Highly significant improvements were noted on the Edinburgh Postnatal Depression Scale and the Hamilton Rating Scale for Depression at 1 week, 4 week and 12 week assessments. The outcome data demonstrated that fluoxetine was significantly more effective than placebo and that six sessions of counselling was significantly more effective than one session of counselling. The researchers concluded that brief cognitive behavioural counselling or antidepressants were effective treatments for postnatal depression, producing marked improvement within 4 weeks, but there was no obvious advantage to offering combined treatment.

Family issues There are a number of other individuals and relationships that may be at risk unless a woman with postnatal depression is offered early and aggressive treatment. Murray (1992) reported that babies of women with postnatal depression are significantly more likely than babies of non-depressed mothers to perform poorly on cognitive tests at 9 months.

Field (1992) reported that infants of women with postnatal depression may develop a depressed mood style within 1–2 months of birth and that by the age of 12 months there may be evidence of adverse effects on physical growth and psychological development. Attachment difficulties may also be apparent (Cox 1992). Specialist mother and baby units may be the most effective method of ensuring adequate treatment of postnatal depression while simultaneously monitoring early bonding between a new mother and her baby (Appleby et al 1989). These units may also offer support and education to new fathers, who may be confused, distressed or angered by their partner's reactions (Ballard et al 1994). There is evidence that educating new fathers about postnatal disorders and helping them to adjust may be associated with better prognosis for postnatal depression in their partners (Kumar et al 1995).

Postpartum psychosis

Postpartum psychosis is a rare but severe disorder. As shown in Table 20.2, it is usually distinguished from other postpartum disorders by the incidence, onset, nature and severity of the symptoms. The estimated incidence, calculated from admission rates for psychosis in women within 90 days of parturition, is about one in 500 livebirths (Kendell et al 1987). It is noteworthy that the observed admission rate in women in their first month postpartum represents a sevenfold increase over the admission rate in age-matched non-puerperal women. Postpartum psychosis usually has a rapid onset in the first 1–2 weeks after childbirth but is virtually never reported within the first few days postpartum (Brockington et al 1982). There is a second incidence peak 1–3 months after delivery but the overall risk of hospitalisation for psychosis remains high for up to 2 years postpartum.

Several studies (e.g. Kendell 1985, Marks et al 1992) have explored risk factors for postpartum psychosis. Personal or family history of major mental disorder appear to be the most robust predictors, although lack of social support and single parenthood have also been identified in some studies. Risk is higher in women with a history of bipolar disorder as compared with unipolar disorder. Women with a previous history of postpartum psychosis are at significantly greater risk (1 in 3) of a psychotic episode following a subsequent pregnancy (Cox 1992). These women also carry a 38% risk of experiencing a non-psychotic postnatal depression. The only obstetric risk factor associated with the development of postpartum psychosis is being primaparous. There is no clear evidence that obstetric complications during either pregnancy or the delivery is associated with later development of psychosis.

Platz & Kendell (1988) compared the psychiatric histories of women who had experienced postpartum psychosis with a control group of women who had experienced psychosis unrelated to childbirth. As compared with women with non-puerperal psychosis, the women with postpartum psychosis were less likely to have a family history of mental disorder, and, over 9 years of follow-up, had fewer relapses and were less likely to commit suicide. The latter finding is supported by Appleby (1991).

Three clinical presentations of postpartum psychosis are described in the literature: affective, schizophreniform and acute organic psychosis. Affective syndromes constitute about 80% of postpartum psychoses. As many as half the affective cases present with features of mania and many researchers consider postpartum psychosis as a variant of bipolar disorder. Although schizophreniform syndromes show the typical symptoms of schizophrenia, comorbid affective symptoms are very common and the disorder does not always persist for 6 months (hence not meeting current diagnostic criteria for schizophrenia). Transient organic disorders are reported infrequently in the Western world, although symptoms such as confusion and memory impairment are common in the functional syndromes.

Worsening insomnia is a common prodromal symptom of postpartum psychosis. Psychomotor agitation may also be an early manifestation. However, the most notable feature of postpartum psychosis is the lability of mood, behaviour and psychotic symptoms. Affective states may shift dramatically from elation to depression over a period of hours, while psychotic symptoms may reappear suddenly after a week or more of apparent remission. Paranoid delusions about family, friends or professionals and abnormal ideas about the baby, which appear to be very intense, may change markedly in their content over hours or days. Perplexity, bewilderment and disorientation are common across all three clinical presentations, while other symptoms usually resemble those of the corresponding non-puerperal psychoses. Although suicide and infanticide are rare, suicidal and infanticidal ideation may be a significant problem (Bluglass 1978).

Aetiology

Biological rather than psychosocial factors appear to play a key role in the development of postpartum psychosis (Dowlatashi & Paykel 1990). Current models focus on the impact of falling levels of oestrogen on neuroendocrine and neurotransmitter functioning. Reduction in serum oestrogen (a hormone with anti-dopaminergic effects) is associated with the development of postsynaptic dopamine receptor supersensitivity which may precipitate the onset of psychosis in vulnerable individuals (Deakin 1988, Wieck et al 1991). Other researchers highlight possible associations between the onset of postpartum psychosis and rapid changes in cortisol levels, although the reduction in the serum binding protein transcortin may again be a consequence of the reduction in oestrogen. Stewart & Addison (1988) also note that women with postpartum psychosis have significantly lower levels of tri-iodothyronine in comparison to control subjects.

Management

Prevention Given the 30–40% risk that women with a history of postpartum psychosis will experience an episode of postpartum psychosis or of postnatal depression in a subsequent pregnancy, there is a clear need to identify and monitor this population in the antenatal period. While education and support may help the woman and her significant others, careful assessment is required of the potential risks and benefits of prophylactic medication (Guscott & Steiner 1991). Steiner (1996) identifies that severity and treatment response of previous episodes, stage of gestation and teratogenicity should be reviewed. Anticonvulsant mood stabilisers have a significant teratogenic effect, particularly in the first trimester. Recent evidence suggests the risks of lithium to the fetus are less than previously reported; nevertheless, if lithium is prescribed, very careful monitoring is required (Cohen et al 1994).

Assessment The move to early hospital discharge after childbirth means that postpartum psychosis will usually present to the primary care team. It is important to educate this group of professionals about the presentation, diagnosis, differentiation from postnatal depression and prognosis of postpartum psychosis. Referral and treatment by secondary psychiatric services is advisable given the severity and potential risks to the patient and her new baby. Postpartum psychosis severely impairs day-to-day functioning and admission is required unless highly specialised community services are available (Oates 1988). Hospitalisation should also be considered for cases where assessment is required to establish the diagnosis or to explore further the patient's ideas about and attitudes toward their offspring.

The evaluation of postpartum psychosis should include an assessment of whether the mother and baby will be admitted together or the mother will be admitted alone. The former course of action allows the patient to develop or maintain confidence in her parenting skills, to continue to bond with the infant and to carry on breast-feeding. Admission should be to a specialist mother and baby unit or to a ward where the baby would not be at risk from other patients and where

staff have some experience of caring for small infants. Women with postpartum psychosis are usually admitted alone if they are too disturbed or unpredictable to care for the baby or they represent a significant risk to the child. However, the mother's ability to care for her baby will need to be assessed over an extended period before discharge from hospital.

Treatment Education of the patient and the family is a vital part of the treatment package. Although no randomised controlled trials exist, ECT may be a particularly effective treatment for postpartum psychosis and may benefit women with or without an affective syndrome. Pharmacological interventions are similar to those used for non-puerperal psychoses, although the doses of antipsychotic medication required are often lower. Mood stabilising medications can be restarted immediately postpartum. However, carbamazepine may be preferable in women who are breast-feeding as lithium and valproate are each secreted in sufficient quantities in breast-milk to put the baby at risk of neurotoxicity and hepatotoxicity, respectively (Mortola 1991). As described in the section on postnatal depression, similar consideration needs to be given to the choice of other antidepressant medications.

Family issues Education will help reduce stress in adult relationships, but further input is required to reduce the risks to the new baby. The patient and her significant others must be encouraged to ensure the patient's adherence to prescribed treatments and to participate in postdischarge follow-up to ensure that true remission has been achieved. Although infanticide is rare, difficulties in feeding, bonding and failure to thrive have been demonstrated in women with moderately severe postpartum disorders. As infant morbidity is significantly associated with severity of symptoms, early and active treatment of postpartum psychosis will benefit both mother and baby (Steiner 1996).

CONCLUSIONS

The disorders discussed in this chapter share two important characteristics. First, they are defined by when symptoms occur rather than what symptoms are experienced. Second, the development of symptoms may be associated with changes in levels of gonadal hormones. However, this temporal relationship does not establish a causal link and it seems that the relative contribution of psychological, social and biological factors to the aetiology of the disorders described varies considerably.

Robert Frank (1931) is generally acknowledged as the first psychiatrist of the modern era to define a premenstrual syndrome and to identify the possible aetiological role of hormonal imbalance. Our understanding of PMS has been undermined by the poor research methodologies of early studies. In the future, the more systematic definition of PMS will hopefully lead to more effective treatment strategies. In addition, the current DSM-IV category of premenstrual dysphoric disorder offers a stricter definition of PMS and increases our chances of undertaking research on a homogeneous population of women. The study of a cyclical mood disorder provides considerable opportunities for developing both biological and integrated causal models of affective disorders.

In the 1850s, Marcé suggested that the mental disorders associated with childbirth were quite different syndromes from those that occurred at other times. Later observations recorded by Kraepelin, Bleuler and others, did not share this view and emphasised the similarities rather than the differences between postpartum and non-puerperal mental disorders. About a century later, it is still not clear whether postpartum syndromes are discrete mental disorders or part of a continuum. Despite this uncertainty, Steiner (1996) points out that postpartum disorders do seem to have a definite time course, present unique problems and require special management. Treatment interventions require multidisciplinary input and comprise psychosocial and biological approaches (Guscott & Steiner 1991). Education forms an important plank of the management strategy. Pharmacotherapy for prevention or treatment of acute disorders must only be offered after careful consideration of the risks and benefits to mother and baby. However, this should not lead to a premature shift to short-term psychotherapies. Evidence for their effectiveness is limited and further intervention studies are required before psychological treatments can be advocated as an alternative to pharmacotherapy in any but mild disorders. The treatment of postpartum disorders also poses important questions about how mental health services should be configured. Although mother and baby units have obvious environmental advantages, we do not have evidence that these units are more cost-effective than standard treatment settings (Kumar et al 1995).

Lastly, clinicians and researchers need to understand more about the impact of postpartum disorders on mother–child interactions. This area of research has already demonstrated that significant developmental problems can occur in the offspring of women with postnatal depression and postpartum psychosis. Although these findings need to be confirmed by large-scale longitudinal studies, this research emphasises the need for early treatment of identified cases of postpartum mental disorders and the need to improve our ability to identify prospectively women at high risk of developing such disorders.

REFERENCES

American College of Obstetricians & Gynecologists 1989 Premenstrual syndrome: Committee opinion no 66. ACOG, Washington, DC

Andersch B, Wendestam C, Hahn L, Ohman R 1986 Premenstrual complaints. I. Prevalence of premenstrual symptoms in a Swedish urban population. Journal of Psychosomatic Obstetrics and Gynaecology 5: 39–49

Appleby L 1991 Suicide during pregnancy and in the first postnatal year. British Medical Journal 302: 137–140

Appleby L, Fox H, Shaw M, Kumar R 1989 The psychiatrists in the obstetric unit establishing a liaison service. British Journal of Psychiatry 154: 510–515

Appleby L, Warner R, Whitton A, Faragher B 1996 A controlled study of fluoxetine and cognitive behavioural counselling in the treatment of post-natal depression. British Medical Journal 314: 932–936

Ashby Jr C, Carr L A, Cook C L et al 1988 Alteration of platelet serotonergic mechanism and monoamine oxidase activity in premenstrual syndrome. Biological Psychiatry 24: 225–233

Backstrom T, Hammerback S, Johansson U-B 1989 Etiological aspects of menstrual cycle linked mood changes. In: van Hall E V, Everland W (eds) The free woman. Parthenon, Park Ridge & Carnforth, pp 625–632

Ballard C G, Davis C, Cullen P C, Mohan R N, Dean C 1994 Prevalence of postnatal psychiatric morbidity in mothers and fathers. British Journal of Psychiatry 164: 782–788

Barnett B, Parker G 1985 Professional and non-professional intervention for highly anxious primaparous mothers. British Journal of Psychiatry 146: 287–293

Berga S, Parry B 1996 Psychiatry and reproductive medicine. In: Kaplan, Saddock (eds) Textbook of medicine. Williams & Wilkins, Baltimore, pp 1693–1713

Bluglass R 1978 Infanticide. Bulletin of the Royal College of Psychiatrists 8: 130–141

Boyce P, Parker G, Barnett B, Cooney M, Smith F 1991 Personality as a vulnerability factor to depression. British Journal of Psychiatry 159: 106–114

Brockington I F, Winokur G, Dean C 1982 Puerperal psychosis. In: Brockington I F, Kumar R (eds) Motherhood and mental illness. Academic Press, London, pp 37–69

Casper R F, Hearn M T 1990 The effect of hysterectomy and bilateral oophorectomy in women with severe premenstrual syndrome. American Journal of Obstetrics and Gynaecology 162: 99–105

Clare A W, Tyrrell J 1994 Psychiatric aspects of abortion. Irish Journal of Psychological Medicine 11(2): 92–98

Cohen L S, Friedman J M, Jefferson J W et al 1994 A re-evaluation of risk of in utero exposure to lithium. Journal of the American Medical Association 271: 146–150

Cooke D J, Greene J C 1981 Types of life events in relation to symptoms at the climacterium. Journal of Psychosomatic Research 25: 5–11

Cooper P J, Murray L 1995 Course and recurrence of postnatal depression. Evidence for the specifity of the diagnostic concept. British Journal of Psychiatry 166: 191–195

Cox J 1992 Depression after childbirth. In: Paykel E S (ed) Handbook of affective disorders. Churchill Livingstone, London, pp 569–583

Cox J L, Holden J M, Sagovsky R 1987 Detection of postnatal depression: development of the 10-item

Edinburgh postnatal depression scale (EPDS). British Journal of Psychiatry 150: 782–786

Cox J L, Murray D, Chapman G 1993 A controlled study of the onset, duration and prevalence of postnatal depression. British Journal of Psychiatry 163: 27–31

Dalton K 1964 The premenstrual syndrome. Thomas, Springfield, IL

Dalton K 1984 The premenstrual syndrome and progesterone therapy. Heinemann, London

Deakin J F W 1988 Relevance of hormone–CNS interactions to psychological changes in the puerperium. In: Kumar R, Brockington I F (eds) Motherhood and mental illness. Wright, London

DeJong R, Rubinow D R, Roy-Byrne P P et al 1985 Premenstrual mood disorder and psychiatric illness. American Journal of Psychiatry 142: 1359

Dowlatashi D, Paykel E S 1990 Life events and social stress in puerperal psychoses; absence of effect. Psychological Medicine 20: 655–662

Elliot S 1989 Psychological strategies in the prevention and treatment of postnatal depression. Clinical Obstetrics and Gyncaecology 3: 879–903

Field T 1992 Interventions in early infancy. Infant Mental Health Journal 13: 329–336

Frank R T 1931 The hormonal causes of premenstrual tension. Archives of Neurology and Psychiatry 26: 1053

Freeman E W, Sondheimer S, Weinbaum P J et al 1985 Evaluating premenstrual symptoms in medical practice. Obstetrics and Gynaecology 65: 500

Gotlib I H, Whiffen V E, Mount J H et al 1989 Prevalence rates and demographic characteristics associated with depression in pregnancy and postpartum. Journal of Consulting and Clinical Psychology 57: 269–274

Graze K K, Nee J, Endicott J 1990 Premenstrual depression predicts future major depressive disorder. American Journal of Psychiatry 81: 201

Guscott R G, Steiner M 1991 A multidisciplinary treatment approach to postpartum psychoses. Canadian Journal of Psychiatry 36: 551–556

Halbreich U 1995 Menstrually related disorders: what we do know, what we only believe we know, and what we know that we do not know. Critical Reviews in Neurobiology 9(2&3): 163–175

Halbreich U 1996 Premenstrual syndromes. Baillère's Clinical Psychiatry 2(4): 667–686

Halbreich U, Endicott J, Schact S, Nee J 1982 The diversity of premenstrual changes as reflected in the premenstrual assessment form. Acta Psychiatrica Scandinavica 65: 45

Harkness S 1987 The cultural mediation of postpartum depression. Medical Anthropology Q1: 194–209

Harris B 1993 A hormonal component to postnatal depression. British Journal of Psychiatry 163: 403–405

Harrison W M, Rabkin J G, Endicott J 1985 Psychiatric evaluation of premenstrual changes. Psychosomatics 26: 789

Harrison W M, Endicott J, Nee J 1990 Treatment of premenstrual dysphoria with alprazolam: a controlled study. Archives of General Psychiatry 47: 270–275

Heidrich A, Schleyer M, Springler H et al 1994 Postpartum blues: relationship between non-protein bound steroid hormones in plasma and postpartum mood changes. Journal of Affective Disorders 30: 93–98

Holden J M, Sagovsky R, Cox J L 1987 Counselling in a general practice setting: a controlled study of health visitor intervention in the treatment of postnatal depression. British Medical Journal 298: 223–226

Isles S, Gath D, Kennerley H 1989 A comparison between postoperative women and postnatal women. British Journal of Psychiatry 155: 363

Ito S, Blajchman A, Stephenson M et al 1993 Prospective follow up of adverse reactions in breast-fed infants exposed to maternal medication. American Journal of Obstetrics and Gynecology 168: 1393–1399

Katon W, Reis R, Bokan J, Kleinman A 1980 Hyperemesis gravidas in a biopsychosocial perspective. International Journal of Psychiatry in Medicine 5: 407–416

Kendell R E 1985 Invited review. Emotional and physical factors in the genesis of puerperal mental disorders. Journal of Psychosomatic Research 29: 3–11

Kendell R E, McGuire R J, Connor Y, Cox J L 1981 Mood changes in the first three weeks after childbirth. Journal of Affective Disorders 3: 317–326

Kendell R E, Chalmers J C, Platz 1987 Epidemiology of puerperal psychoses. British Journal of Psychiatry 150: 662–673

Kennerley H, Gath D 1989 Maternity blues: associations with obstetric, psychological and psychiatric factors. British Journal of Psychiatry 155: 367–373

Kessler R C, McGonagle K A, Swartz M et al 1993 Sex and depression in the National Comorbidity Survey I: lifetime prevalence, chronicity and recurrence. Journal of Affective Disorders 29: 85–96

Kitamura T, Shima S, Sugawara M et al 1993 Psychological and social correlates of the onset of affective disorders among pregnant women. Psychological medicine 23: 967–975

Klein M H, Essex M J 1995 Pregnant or depressed? The effect of overlap between symptoms of depression and somatic complaints of pregnancy on rates of major depression in the second trimester. Depression 2: 308–314

Kumar R 1982 Neurotic disorders in childbearing women. In: Brockington I F, Kumar R (eds) Motherhood and mental illness. Academic Press, London

Kumar R, Robson K M 1984 A prospective study of emotional disorders in childbearing women. British Journal of Psychiatry 144: 35–47

Kumar R, Marks M, Platz C, Yoshida K 1995 Clinical survey of a psychiatric mother and baby unit: characteristics of 100 consecutive admissions. Journal of Affective Disorders 33: 11–22

MacKenzie T B, Wilcox K, Baron H 1986 Lifetime prevalence of psychiatric disorders in women with perimenstrual difficulties. Journal of Affective Disorders 10: 15

Marks M N, Wieck A, Checkley S A, Kumar R 1992 Contribution of psychological and social factors to psychotic and non-psychotic relapse after childbirth in women with previous histories of affective disorder. Journal of Affective Disorders 29: 253–264

Mortola J F 1991 The use of psychotropic agents in pregnancy and lactation. Psychiatric Clinics of North America 12: 69–87

Murray L 1992 The impact of postnatal depression on infant development. Journal of Child Psychology and Psychiatry 33: 543–561

Muse K, Cetel N, Futterman L et al 1984 The premenstrual syndrome: effects of 'medical ovariectomy'. New England Journal of Medicine 311: 1345–1349

Oates M 1988 The development of an integrated community-orientated service for severe postnatal partum. General Hospital Psychiatry 11: 328–338

Oates M 1990 Clinical obstetrics and gynaecology:

psychological aspects of obstetrics and gynaecology. Baillière Tindall, London

O'Hara M W, Zekowski E M 1988 Postpartum depression: a comprehensive review. In: Kumar R, Brockington I F (eds) Motherhood and mental illness II. Butterworth, London

O'Hara M W, Zekoski E M, Phillips L H, Wright E J 1990 Controlled prospective study of postpartum mood disorders: comparison of childbearing and non-childbearing women. Journal of Abnormal Psychology 99: 3–15

O'Hara M W, Schlechte J A, Lewis D A, Wright E J 1991 Prospective study of postpartum blues. Archives of General Psychiatry 48: 801–806

Parry B, Rausch J 1996 Treatment of premenstrual mood symptoms. Psychopharmacology16: 829–830

Parry B L, Berga S L, Kripke D F et al 1990 Altered waveform of plasma nocturnal melatonin secretion in premenstrual depression. British Journal of Psychiatry 167: 163–173

Paykel E S, Emms E M, Fletcher J, Rassaby E S 1980 Life events and social support in puerperal depression. British Journal of Psychiatry 136: 339–346

Pearce J, Hawton K, Blake F 1995 Psychological and sexual symptoms associated with the menopause and the effects of hormone replacement therapy. British Journal of Psychiatry 167: 163–173

Pedersen C A, Stern R A, Pate J et al 1993 Thyroid and adrenal measures during late pregnancy and the puerperium in women who have been major depressed or who become dysphoric postpartum. Journal of Affective Disorders 29: 201–211

Pitt B 1968 Atypical depression following childbirth. British Journal of Psychiatry 114: 1325–1335

Platz C, Kendell R E 1988 Matched control follow-up and family study of puerperal psychoses. British Journal of Psychiatry 153: 90–94

Rapkin A J, Buckman T D, Stuphin M S et al 1988 Platelet monoamine oxidase B activity in women with premenstrual syndrome. American Journal of Obstetrics and Gynecology 159: 1536–1540

Rivera-Tovar A D, Frank E 1990 Late luteal phase dysphoric disorder in young women. American Journal of Psychiatry 147: 1634–1636

Rojansky N, Halbreich U, Zander K et al 1991 Imipramine receptor binding and serotonin uptake in platelets of women with premenstrual changes. Gynecologic and Obstetric Investigation 31: 146–152

Roy A, Cole K, Goldman Z et al 1993 Fluoxetine treatment of postpartum depression. American Journal of Psychiatry 150: 1273

Rubinow D R, Schmidt P J 1989 Models for the development and expression of symptoms in premenstrual syndrome. Psychiatric Clinics of North America 12: 53

Schmidt P J, Nieman L K, Grove G N et al 1991 Lack of effect of induced menses on symptoms in women with premenstrual syndrome. New England Journal of Medicine 324: 1174–1179

Schmidt P J, Roca C A, Rubinow D R 1996 Psychiatric disorders during the peri-menopause. Baillière's Clinical Psychiatry 2(4): 710–712

Severino S K, Moline M L 1989 Premenstrual syndrome: a clinician's guide. Guilford Press, New York

Small G W 1986 Pseudocyesis: an overview. Canadian Journal of Psychiatry 31: 452–457

Steiner M 1996 Treatment of psychiatric disorders during pregnancy and post-partum. Baillière's Clinical Psychiatry 2(4): 687–700

Steiner M, Steinberg S, Stewart D et al 1995 Fluoxetine in the treatment of premenstrual dysphoria. Canadian Fluoxetin/Premenstrual Dysphoria Collaborative Study Group. New England Journal of Medicine 332: 1529–1534

Stewart D E, Addison A M 1988 Thyroid function in psychosis following childbirth. American Journal of Psychiatry 145: 1579–1581

Yalom I D, Lunke D T, Moos R H, Hamburg D A 1965 Postpartum blues syndrome. Archives of General Psychiatry 18: 16–27

Wieck A, Kumar R, Hirst A D et al 1991 Increased sensitivity of dopamine receptors and recurrence of affective psychosis after childbirth. British Medical Journal 303: 613–616

Wisner K L, Wheeler S B 1994 Prevention of recurrent postpartum major depression. Hospital and Community Psychiatry 45: 1191–1196

21
Normal and abnormal personality

Ian J. Deary   Michael J. Power

INTRODUCTION

This is an historically important time for personality and personality disorder. In the last two decades we have seen an emerging consensus about the structure of normal personality and in the last decade there has been increasing cooperation between researchers in normal and abnormal personality to discover how the two areas can best combine their knowledge (Costa & Widiger 1994). This chapter offers a summary of what has been established in the field of normal personality research. The area of abnormal personality is at an earlier stage of scientific development and the account reflects this. A description of the clinical classification of personality disorder types is given. Some of the background clinical and basic science research into the different types of personality disorder is discussed. Problems with current conceptions of personality disorder are reviewed. Finally, attempts to combine schemes of normal and abnormal personality are presented. Thus, the chapter covers both basic and applied research with respect to personality. Suggestions are given for more detailed readings in each of the areas mentioned.

APPROACHES TO NORMAL PERSONALITY

The study of personality is an attempt to describe an individual's 'characteristic patterns of thought, emotion, and behavior, together with the psychological mechanisms – hidden or not – behind those patterns' (Funder 1996). Thus personality psychology attempts to provide a descriptive and explanatory framework of non-ability-related aspects of human behaviour. Introductory textbooks on personality psychology typically portray the study of human personality as a number of 'approaches' or 'models' (for example, Engler 1995, Funder 1996). The commonly-cited models of human personality derive from very different theoretical backgrounds and call upon markedly different types of evidence. One of the first options that presents itself to the student of personality is whether to adopt a 'nomothetic' or 'idiographic' approach to human temperament and character.

Nomothetic approaches

A nomothetic approach describes those theories that portray human personality in terms of shared attributes. As such, it is similar to practices in science and medicine. It assumes that humans may be described by a limited number of qualities on which people differ. The two principal subdivisions of nomothetic approaches are type and trait theories. Type theories of personality are those which conceive humans as fitting into discrete categories. Astrology, for example, is a lay type theory which, despite its lack of scientific evidence, is a clear example of the belief that human personality variation may be construed as a limited number of prototypes. Type theories are also found in clinical science: the so-called type A behaviour pattern or 'coronary-prone' personality is often used as a non-continuous typology, and within psychiatry designations of personality disorder are made using the typologies within the DSM and ICD schemes.

Trait theories are similar to type theories in that they posit that human personality variation may be described using a limited number of qualities. However, in trait theories the qualities are continuous. People are described on a number of scales and the person's personality is their position as described on each of these scales. Typically the scales have a normal distribution in the non-clinical adult population and individuals may take any value on the scale as opposed to the dichotomous classification of the type theory. The best-known and most used trait theories include those of Eysenck, Cattell and Costa and McCrae. Because of the pre-eminence of trait theory in modern personality research (Deary & Matthews 1993) most of the space in this section is devoted to it. However, before this, it is necessary to outline the nature of the other approaches to the psychology of personality.

Idiographic approaches

There is a natural objection to the nomothetic approach to personality in terms of each person's individuality. Type and trait theories can easily appear to deny or miss much human idiosyncrasy and there are strains of personality psychology that prefer, instead, to provide a portrait of each individual. There are three principal idiographic strains of personality psychology: psychoanalytic, humanistic and behavioural–cognitive (learning/social learning) approaches. The former two, though well known and much referred to outside the realms of academic personality psychology, have little established scientific validity and attract little empirical research interest. In addition, the influence of these fields on contemporary psychiatry is diminishing.

Psychoanalytic approaches

Psychoanalytic approaches to personality derive from the work of Freud and later psychoanalytic thinkers and practitioners such as Jung, Adler, Horney and Erikson (Pervin 1993). Freud compartmentalised human personality into the id, ego and superego, and attempted to explain human behaviour – especially neurotic symptoms – in terms of the interactions among these three hypothetical entities. Briefly, the unconscious id – working in part on the 'pleasure principle' – contained the energy for the personality system and had strong desires, principally oriented toward sex but also to aggression (life and death instincts; eros and thanatos). The ego, which was partly conscious, carried out functions such as perception and memory. Working on the 'reality principle', its function was to provide a balance between the id, superego and external reality.

The superego, developing later, was the crystallisation of moral values, especially those of parents and authority figures. It is very like lay ideas of conscience and was invoked to account for the fact that people still act morally when there is no one else around. Much of the explanatory power of the Freudian scheme rested on the desires of the id for sex and aggression, which had to be defended against while the business of living was transacted by the ego. In addition to this structural and dynamic model of the adult personality, Freud also described the development of personality as a series of shifting bodily sites of erotic gratification: oral, anal and genital. From these and other constructs – including the important Oedipus complex – various possibilities for abnormal behaviour opened up. In defending against unacceptable impulses from the id one might use various ego defence mechanisms to disguise true desires. One might become fixated in, or regress to, one of the earlier stages of erotic development.

A Freudian would not refer to personality testing as such. However, Freud did have a number of techniques for exploring the mental dynamics of the individual, given that these were not necessarily available to the person through conscious reflection. Thus Freud used free association, dream analysis, analyses of parapraxes (slips of the tongue, of memory, of writing, and so forth) and analysis of transference reactions in order to discover the personality of an individual. These were typically done in the context of psychoanalytic psychotherapy. Most introductory texts on human personality have adequate accounts of Freud's ideas and several of his successors in the field of depth psychology. However, there is no substitute for reading Freud's own writings which provide the clearest exposition of his ideas, concepts, methods and clinical concerns (Freud 1973, 1986).

The chief criticism of the Freudian scheme is that the constructs have not proved amenable to scientific scrutiny. Freud's own data were gathered from a small number of people, largely middle-class, Viennese women with neurotic symptoms whose recollections were recorded some hours after their psychoanalytic sessions. Freud admitted that much of the validity of his scheme rested on patients' acceptances of psychoanalytic interpretations but, fatally, he also admitted that patients were influenced by the therapist into accepting psychoanalytic interpretations as valid (Grunbaum 1984). Psychoanalytic thinkers themselves often split the freudian corpus into two: the clinical theory and the metapsychology (Holt 1985). It is the latter that contains Freud's ideas on personality, and it is this portion that a number of psychoanalytic thinkers have criticised and reformed. Pervin (1993) summarises the main limitations of Freud's psychoanalytic personality theory as follows: it failed to define its concepts clearly; empirical testing of the theory is difficult or impossible; it subscribed to a view of psychological activity that was based on an energy conservation system that has little validity; and the profession's tolerance of some of its adherents' resistance to empirical research.

Therefore, in a contemporary scientific chapter on personality it is important to be clear that Freudian and postFreudian ideas have little scientific standing as accounts of normal and abnormal personality. As we shall see below, psychoanalytic ideas have contributed to the identification and delineation of some personality disorders, though psychoanalytic constructs and theoretical schemes are largely absent from modern research in this area too.

Humanistic approaches

The humanistic approach to personality is also referred to as existential or phenomenological. Humanistic psychology, when it appeared, was called the 'third force' in psychology (Funder 1996). This meant that it was a reaction to psychoanalysis and behaviourism. The latter was seen to offer too mechanistic an account of human behaviour. The former was seen as too pessimistic, with human personality emerging from basic instincts and intrapsychic conflict. Humanistic psychology is usually much more hopeful about the human condition, focusing on human growth and potential rather than deficiency states: indeed, Funder (1996) describes humanistic personality psychology and psychologists as 'modern and cheerful'. Several of the contributors to this line of thinking are associated with types of therapy. Therefore, as we saw with Freud, personality theories and clinical psychotherapies often arise from the same sources.

Arguably, the best-known theorist within the humanistic area is Maslow (1987). Rather than escaping from deficiency, Maslow viewed people as motivated by positive purposes, so recognising that humans seek positive, enriching experiences: curiosity, the unselfish giving of love, and so forth. As opposed to deficiency or 'D' motives, Maslow called these being or 'B' motives. Such motives were structured in response to a hierarchy of needs, the idea being that humans strive for a higher set of needs once a lower set has been met. In order of needs satisfaction the hierarchy is ordered as follows: physiological needs, safety needs, belongingness needs, esteem needs, and self-actualisation needs. As a theory of personality growth, Maslow's complete account applies to a small elite; it is about 1% of people, he reckoned, who achieved self-actualisation. Those who did so were the likes of Thomas Jefferson, Albert Einstein, Eleanor Roosevelt and William James. Typical of self-actualised people is a long list of characteristics including tolerance of others, spontaneity, a life mission, detachment, avoidance of fashions, freshness of appreciation, 'peak' experiences and so forth. Maslow's theory is similar to others of the humanistic persuasion, being conceptually imprecise, lacking empirical research, and based on a small, unrepresentative sample of humans. Maslow adhered to some of Freud's ideas but rejected Freud's pessimism, and self-actualisation may represent Maslow's own idiosyncratic value system. Although the scheme – especially the hierarchy of needs – is popular with the lay public and with some social scientists, the theory has stimulated little psychological research.

Another prominent, optimistic account of human personality in this vein arose from the clinical work of Carl Rogers (1951). His central idea was that humans were motivated by a single positive force to actualise their inner potential and to expand, extend, become autonomous, develop and mature. Antisocial behaviour was largely attributable to external forces, he suggested. The biggest impediment to actualisation according to Rogers was the withholding of positive regard. Therefore, as with Rogers' client-centred therapy, his person-centred theory of personality development stated that humans need unconditional positive regard from important others. Conditional positive regard was deemed to put a person at odds with their 'true self'. This was supposed to lead to conditions of worth being introjected as a part of the personality makeup, resulting in incongruence and defence. The best result one might expect from personality growth in the Rogers' scheme was to be a 'fully functioning person' with no conditions of worth and unconditional positive self-regard. In this eventuality the self is congruent with the totality of experience and one lives wholly and freely in each moment. Such a developmental stage, it was thought, was achieved by people like El Greco, Hemmingway and Einstein, all of whom were quirky but had strong self-belief. Again, Rogers' theory of personality has proved enduringly popular despite its lack of scientific evidence. His constructs are almost absent from current scientific research on personality.

Unlike psychoanalytic theories of personality, humanistic approaches do not rely on unconscious motivations and conflicts. The conscious experience of the moment is the key aspect of the person. Any insights of humanistic approaches to personality are highly specific to individual moments in individual lives. Rychlak (1988) described the typical contribution to the *Journal of Humanistic Psychology* as follows:

> [they] are usually discursive surveys, case-history reports or personal observations. [They believe] the intuition of the investigator [is] above the validation of an experiment in any rank ordering of steps in the scientific enterprise.

Rychlak (1988), a humanist psychology writer and one of the few who attempts experiments in this field, has criticised humanistic personality psychology for attracting people who do not have the self-discipline and effort that a scientific career demands.

Behavioural–cognitive approaches

At its simplest, behaviourist accounts of personality formation and structure are merely the application of learning theories to human behavioural regularities. Classical conditioning ideas deriving from Pavlov and operant conditioning notions deriving from Watson and

Skinner were thought by some to be the bases of personality development. So-called personality traits were seen as the summation of reinforcement histories. The apparent persistence of behavioural patterns – traits when no reward was forthcoming was explained by the principle of partial reinforcement; that is, strong behavioural tendencies can be elicited when the reward for a given behaviour is only intermittent. The behavioural account of personality is associated with the situationist critique of traits and the work of Mischel (1968), which will be discussed below. In essence, situationism stated that a person's behaviour was principally influenced by the situation they found themselves in rather than any inherent, long-standing personality traits.

As the 20th century has progressed there has been a move away from radical behaviourism – in which the main determinant of behaviour was the situation – toward three things:

- the inclusion of internal mental processes into behavioural theories
- a recognition of the importance of social factors in learning
- a compromise with trait theory.

Originally behaviourism denied a role for internal mental states in the determination of behaviour: stimulus–response contingencies combined with learning history were sufficient. Thereafter, behavioural theories of personality began to incorporate internal mental states. For example, Rotter's (1954) expectancy value theory accounted for behavioural differences by appealing to people's expectancies of success following their behaviour and to the value that people placed upon the reinforcement to be got if successful.

The trend toward an inclusion of mentalistic concepts and to a greater focus on social factors in personality may be seen in Bandura's (1971) social learning theory and in the work of Mischel (1968). Both accounts accept the importance of person and situation factors in influencing behaviour. However, within this behavioural–cognitive realm, person factors tend to be expressed as 'cognitive qualities' rather than traits. Such qualities might include a person's competencies, encoding strategies, expectancies, subjective values, and goals and plans.

One such quality that is much used is a person's attributional style; that is, the degree to which a person thinks that events are under his own control. The Attributional Style Questionnaire (Peterson et al 1982) assesses this quality and asks the person to imagine a number of hypothetical situations (e.g. failing an examination) and to make statements as to their likely causes. Internal attributions are beliefs that something in one's self causes the event ('it's my fault'); global attri-butions are beliefs that the effect could generalise to other situations ('it's always my fault'); and stable attributions are beliefs that such effects are unlikely to change ('it will always be my fault'). Aspects of attributional style have been linked to depression; thus, people whose attributional styles are more internal, global and stable were predicted to be more prone to mood disorder, though more recent research has suggested that, although there may be a role for depressogenic attributional style in the maintenance of depression, the evidence for its role in onset is equivocal (Power & Dalgleish 1997).

Behavioural–cognitive accounts of personality have compromised with traits in that they accept the fact of lasting individual differences in behavioural dispositions. Similarly, trait theorists now accept the power of the situation to influence behaviour. The differences between the trait and behavioural–cognitive approaches tend to be those of emphasis and experimental technique. Behavioural–cognitive personality researchers tend to focus on situations and to conduct experimental manipulations. Trait theorists tend to focus on the enduring aspects of the person and to do correlational research. Perhaps the two schools differ most on the origins of behavioural dispositions: trait theorists might emphasise the moderate heritability of traits, whereas behavioural–cognitive researchers would stress that cognitive dispositions are substantially learned.

Trait approaches

The trait approach has emerged as the dominant scientific approach to human personality (Matthews & Deary 1998). The research activity in journals devoted to personality is largely devoted to the structure, origins and consequences of traits. Pure psychoanalytic and humanistic approaches to human personality are all but scientifically moribund, though ideas from both approaches have been incorporated into trait accounts, as we shall see. Behavioural–cognitive approaches to personality are not necessarily inimical and are often complementary to trait approaches. Therefore, the bulk of the consideration of normal personality must be addressed to the achievements of trait theories of personality.

Lay conceptions of traits – the idea that humans have long-standing behavioural predispositions – may be as old as human language. Aristotle's student Theophrastus wrote his book *Characters* in the 4th century BC. He described 30 human personality variants and recent translators have referred to his account as a trait system of personality (Rusten 1993). In the 2nd century AD Galen of Pergamun developed Hippocrates' notion of the four humours to apply to the bases of temperament. Thus, today's metaphorical personality terms, melancholic, sanguine, choleric and phlegmatic, arose from Greco-Roman theories about the bodily bases of character differences. From these origins we can see three aspects of trait approaches that exist today. First, they signal the fact that languages are replete with trait-like terms, words that describe behavioural regularities in individuals. Allport & Odbert (1936) identified almost 18 000 terms in English to describe human personality. Second, early accounts of personality anticipate the motivation to discover the 'right' number of personality traits and their content and structure. Third, Galen's adoption of Hippocrates' humoral theory antedates scientific investigations into the origins of traits, whether these be biological or otherwise.

The Galenic scheme, stripped of its biological associations, was adopted as a psychological typology of temperaments and emotions by the philosopher Kant and the father of modern experimental psychology, Willhelm Wundt. Transforming prescientific notions of traits into the science of personality required:

- the articulation of the hypothesis that valid personality traits might be found in language (Galton, 1884)
- systematic data collection
- multivariate statistical procedures such as factor analysis (Thurstone 1947).

There is not space to discuss these statistical techniques in this chapter; an accessible account is offered by Child (1990). Allport (1937) provided a detailed theoretical and methodological discussion of traits which set the scene for much of the later research.

Schemes and tests

Before assessing the current state of trait theory it is useful to give examples of some popular personality instruments and to describe their origins and the theories that lie behind them. There are hundreds of personality tests, some of which purport to examine most of the important aspects of human personality, some of which assess narrower aspects. In this section we address the more comprehensive models.

Eysenck's three factor theory The origins of Eysenck's theory of personality traits are both clinical and academic. His original concerns were with people's susceptibilities to different types of neurotic illness. In this he partly followed Jung in suggesting that extraverts differed from introverts in being prone to hysteria rather than dysthymic states. He even adopted Jung's distinction of introversion–extraversion, though he intended to make it a more scientific entity. In addition,

Eysenck's earlier writings gather the historical and contemporary evidence for broad personality traits that:

- predispose to negative mood states
- influence the sociability and impulsivity of an individual.

Through the 1940s to the 1960s Eysenck (Eysenck & Eysenck 1969) worked on the production of a two-dimensional system of personality, with neuroticism (N) and extraversion–introversion (E) as two orthogonal (uncorrelated) dimensions of personality. The Eysenck Personality Inventory measured these traits. From the 1970s onward Eysenck has included another dimension called psychoticism (P), a dimension of personality that predisposes to psychosis, antisocial behaviour and creativity. The Eysenck Personality Questionnaire-Revised (EPQ-R) (Eysenck & Eysenck 1991) measures N, E and P. In addition, the EPQ-R has a Lie (L) scale to detect dissimulation or socially desirable responding. Each item in the EPQ-R is posed as a question to which the respondent answers yes or no.

Eysenck's dimensions are very broad, encompassing many lower-level traits which are correlated. Thus neuroticism comprises the following traits: depressed, guilt feelings, low self-esteem, tense, irrational, shy, moody and emotional. Extraversion is made up of: sociable, lively, active, assertive, sensation-seeking, carefree, dominant, surgent and venturesome. Psychoticism is a compilation of: aggressive, cold, egocentric, impersonal, impulsive, antisocial, unempathetic, creative and tough-minded. The former two traits have a normal distribution of scores in the population, and psychoticism is positively skewed, with most people having low scores. Because neuroticism and psychoticism can appear pejorative terms – and can appear to suggest illness when in fact they describe normal personality variation – Eysenck suggested the alternative names emotionality and tough-mindedness versus superego control, respectively.

In addition to psychometric evidence that established the cohesion of Eysenck's three dimensions and their separateness from each other, the structure of personality using the EPQ-R is similar in many different languages and cultures (Eysenck & Eysenck 1982). From an early stage, Eysenck (1967) hypothesised that his personality dimensions, especially N and E, have biological bases. Thus, E is linked to the construct of arousal and the actions of the ascending reticular activating system, and N is linked to the reactivity of the autonomic nervous system. There is more evidence for the former than the latter, though neither trait has a well-established biological basis other than moderately high heritability (Zuckerman (1991). We shall see from other systems that E and N attract near-universal agreement as basic human temperamental traits, but that there is more disagreement surrounding the trait complex captured by Eysenck's P.

Costa & McCrae's five factor model We shall see below that the field of personality research has begun to converge toward a consensus around approximately five basic human personality traits. One of the best known and most used of the five factor models is that of Costa & McCrae (1992a) and their instrument, the NEO Personality Inventory-Revised (NEO-PI-R) (Costa & McCrae 1992b). This inventory has 240 questions, 48 devoted to each of the five dimensions. Eight questions in each dimension are devoted to the dimensions' six facets. The five factors in this model are neuroticism (N), extraversion (E), openness (O), agreeableness (A) and conscientiousness (C). Each of the items in the NEO-PI-R is posed as a statement to which the respondent may 'disagree strongly' – 'disagree' – 'neutral' – 'agree' – strongly agree'. There is a shorter, 60 item questionnaire called the NEO Five Factor Inventory (NEO-FFI) which gives a score for each of the five factors, but not for the facets of each dimension.

Understanding the five dimensions is probably most easily done by describing their facets. Neuroticism comprises anxiety, angry hostility, depression, self-consciousness, impulsiveness and vulnerability. It is very like that of Eysenck's. Extraversion is made up from warmth, gregariousness, assertiveness, activity, excitement-seeking and positive emotions. This is like Eysenck's identically-named factor with the addition of positive emotions. Openness is a mixture of fantasy, aesthetics, feelings, actions, ideas and values. This factor contrasts a willingness to try new things and to be aesthetically minded versus being traditional. It has a modest positive correlation with measured intelligence. Agreeableness has facets of trust, straightforwardness, altruism, compliance, modesty and tender-mindedness. Those scoring low on this scale are tough-minded, independent and blunt. Conscientiousness gathers together competence, order, dutifulness, achievement striving, self-discipline and deliberation.

Unlike Eysenck's model, the five factor scheme of Costa & McCrae is not based in a biological theory, nor is it based in clinical considerations. Rather, it is an attempt to capture agreement from a number of areas in personality. Block (1995) views N and E as coming from the work of Raymond Cattell, O having been developed from embryonic status, and A and C as grafted on to an earlier three factor model because of results from the lexical approach to personality. As we shall see below, among the most dramatic results to come from the work of Costa & McCrae is the overlap

between their five factor system and the traits measured by a large number of seemingly-different personality questionnaires.

Cloninger's seven factor model Cloninger's (1987) original scheme contained only three factors or traits of personality – novelty seeking, harm avoidance and reward dependence. This was measured using the Tridimensional Personality Questionnaire (TPQ). Novelty seeking comprises four subtraits: exploratory excitability versus stoic rigidity (9 items), impulsiveness versus reflection (8 items), extravagance versus reserve (7 items), and disorderliness versus regimentation (10 items). Harm avoidance is made up from four narrower traits: anticipatory worry versus uninhibited optimism (10 items), fear of uncertainty versus confidence (7 items), shyness with strangers versus gregariousness (7 items), and fatiguability and asthenia versus vigour (10 items). Reward dependence is built from four constituent subfactors: sentimentality versus insensitiveness (5 items), persistence versus irresoluteness (9 items), attachment versus detachment (11 items), and dependence versus independence (5 items).

The TPQ was expanded because the original scheme was thought to contain too few aspects of personality as addressed by humanistic writers (Cloninger et al 1993, Svrakic et al 1993). The three biologically based traits were called temperament factors. To the three original temperament dimensions described above a fourth – persistence – was added. The 226 item Temperament and Character Inventory (TCI) – a true–false, self report questionnaire – measures these and also measures so-called character traits of self-directedness, cooperativeness, and self-transcendence. These three factors are different from the temperament traits in that they mature in adulthood and relate to self concepts. Self-directedness is the degree to which the person sees the self as autonomous; cooperativeness is the degree to which the self is integrated with humanity; and transcendence is the degree to which the self is an integrated part of the universe. The original three temperament dimensions were largely uncorrelated, but the introduction of the character traits has led to considerable correlations among the scales (Cloninger et al 1993). Also, whereas the original three scales were well supported by a biological theory, the more humanistic dimensions appear arbitrary and less well supported with evidence. Akin to Eysenck's influences, Cloninger's roots are in clinical concerns and a wish to establish personality traits in biological systems. Thus, Cloninger is keen to find a personality system that will cover both normal and abnormal personality. Also, his assumption is that personality traits refer to evolutionarily important behaviours, each of which has its own main neurotransmitter, brain system, stimuli and responses (Table 21.1).

Table 21.1   Brain systems associated with Cloninger's three temperaments relevant to normal and abnormal personality

Personality dimension	Main neuro transmitter	Brain system	Relevant stimuli	Behavioural response
Novelty seeking	Dopamine	Behavioural activation	Novelty Potential reward Potential relief of monotony or punishment	Exploratory pursuit Appetitive approach Active avoidance, escape
Harm avoidance	Serotonin	Behavioural inhibition	Conditioned signals for punishment, novelty, or frustrative non-reward	Passive avoidance, extinction
Reward dependence	Noradrenaline	Behavioural maintenance	Conditioned signals for reward or relief of punishment	Resistance to extinction

Cattell's 16 factor theory Cattell's work on human individual differences stretches back over 60 years. It covers much more than personality and includes ability, motivation and mood. His original approach to personality was to use personality-descriptive trait terms in the lexicon, but his empirical work has largely been based on questionnaire items, principally as found in his revisions of the 16 Personality Factor Questionnaire (16PF) (Cattell et al 1970). The most uneconomical of the systems we have considered, Cattell found 23 personality factors, one of which was intelligence. The most robust of these were 16 traits (Table 21.2).

Though the Cattellian dimensions have some predictive validity, various problems exist with the theory and the measurement instrument. It must be noted first that, whereas the schemes discussed above include broad dimensions of personality, Cattell's traits are narrower and have much redundancy. Thus, it is statistically possible to reduce them to a smaller number of broader dimensions. Interestingly, this number might be five, as indicated by the latest revision of the 16PF, now called the 16PF5 (Conn & Rieke 1994). Though this was intended to signal the fifth revision, the scoring for the new 16PF allows the extraction of scores for five higher order factors: extraversion, neuroticism, tough poise, independence and control. Second, 16 dimensions have rarely been retrieved statistically from the 16PF, calling into doubt its psychometric structure. Third, there is no explicit series of constructs underlying the various traits measured by the 16PF.

Narrow trait theories The personality theories and the tests associated with Eysenck, Costa and McCrae, Cloninger and Cattell have in common the fact that they attempt to assess human personality com-

prehensively. That is, with respect to their authors' views, each of the above schemes is a relatively complete account of the most important non-ability-related

Table 21.2   Cattell's 16 traits

A	Outgoing and warm-hearted versus reserved and detached
B	Intelligence
C	Unemotional and calm versus emotional and changeable
E	Assertive and dominant versus humble and cooperative
F	Cheerful and lively versus sober and taciturn
G	Conscientious and persistent versus expedient and undisciplined
H	Venturesome and socially bold versus shy and retiring
I	Tough-minded and self-reliant versus tender-minded and sensitive
L	Suspicious and sceptical versus trusting and accepting
M	Imaginative and bohemian versus practical and conventional
N	Shrewd and discreet versus forthright and straightforward
O	Guilt-prone and worrying versus resilient and self-assured
Q1	Radical and experimental versus conservative and traditional
Q2	Self-sufficient and resourceful versus group-dependent and affiliative
Q3	Controlled and compulsive versus undisciplined and lax
Q4	Tense and driven versus relaxed and tranquil

human dimensions of personality. There are other systems in this vein. However, some personality theories and tests make no attempt at a comprehensive account of human personality. Instead, they focus on the theory and measurement of a narrower range of traits that are important in some aspect of human existence. Some schemes examine single traits in isolation. Although there is no necessary contradiction between these single traits and more comprehensive theories, it is always of interest to enquire whether they can be construed with other, more complete, theories. There are many single trait and narrow trait theories, and only a few of the more prominent ones are described here.

Type A behaviour pattern and hostility   This personality trait complex originated from the clinical observations of two cardiologists (Friedman & Rosenman 1974) that people with coronary heart disease (CHD) tended to be aggressive, dominating, driven to achieve goals, time pressured, and workaholic. Large epidemiological studies, such as the Western Collaborative Group Study (Rosenman et al 1975) – in which thousands of men had their type A personality status assessed by clinical interview and were followed up for several years to discover whether or not they developed CHD – seemed to confirm these impressions. However, since such positive early reports, the importance of the type A personality trait for CHD and other aspects of health has become more equivocal. Meta-analytic descriptions of the many studies of type A personality and health have found that: type A personality accounts for 2% or less of the population variance in heart disease; type A personality is a composite trait, with some aspects related to CHD and some not; and that positive results are more likely to emerge from structured interview assessments of type A personality than from self-reports gathered from such instruments as the Jenkins Activity Survey and the Bortner Rating Scale (Miller et al 1991). Of the various facets of the type A personality conglomerate, the most important with respect to illness proneness would appear to be hostility (Miller et al 1996).

Locus of control   An influential distinction made by Rotter (1966) was that between internal and external locus of control. Individuals who have a character internal locus of control see themselves able to control the occurrence of events, whereas individuals with an external locus of control see events to be controlled by luck, chance and other people. Rotter proposed that locus of control was a relatively enduring and cross-situationally consistent characteristic. He also developed a widely used 29 item locus of control scale that has been adapted for a number of health-related beliefs and conditions. However, there are a number of criticisms of the concept, despite the continuing use of the related scales. In particular, Weiner (1986) and others have agreed that the concept is not unidimensional but confounds, for example, locus (internal–external) and controllability (controllable–uncontrollable). One of the best-known applications of the locus of control and related attribution theories has been in Abramson and colleagues' (1978) reformulated learned helplessness theory, which we mentioned earlier. Abramson et al followed Weiner's suggestion that locus of control should be divided into two dimensions of locus and controllability and in addition added further dimensions of stability and globality. However, although Abramson et al conceptually distinguished locus and control, in the questionnaire designed to assess attributional style (the Attributional Style Questionnaire, Peterson et al 1982), they surprisingly failed to assess perceived controllability.

Consensus?

From the above descriptions of influential personality schemes it might appear that there was little agreement as to the structure of human personality. Cattell's 16 factors are not the worst disagreements with the more economical 3, 5 or 7 factor systems. The 18 factors of the California Personality Inventory (CPI) (Gough 1987) or the 31 traits in the Occupational Personality Questionnaire (OPQ) (Saville et al 1984) signal more uncertainty. However, each of these instruments deals with primary traits, of narrow behavioural content, and each set of traits may be reduced to a smaller number with factor analysis, just as was discussed in relation to Cattell's narrow traits. In addition, neither the CPI nor the OPQ's psychometric structure was verified by factor analysis.

In fact, the last 10 years or so have seen a remarkable consensus on the approximate number and nature of broad personality traits. Two different streams of research have converged on a five factor model of personality, the traits sometimes called the 'big five'. The first stream is the so-called lexical approach in which personality trait adjectives – as found in the lexicons of different languages – are examined for their correlational structure when they have been used to rate a person's personality. Whether people rate their own traits, or whether this is done by others who know them well or little, the correlational structure of the traits appears to show five broad groups or factors of personality terms (Tupes & Christal 1961, Digman & Takemoto-Chock 1981). These are very similar to the five factors seen in the NEO-PI-R (p. 570). Using the terminology of the lexical model, the five factors are as follows (Goldberg 1993):

- Surgency (or extraversion)

- Conscientiousness
- Agreeableness
- Emotional stability (the opposite of neuroticism)
- Culture or intellectence.

Only the last of the five factors has seen any real disagreement as to its exact structure and content. A similar trait structure has been found in other languages and cultures, indicating that human languages tend to contain five broad groups of personality descriptive adjectives. This includes non-Indo-European languages such as Hungarian. The most recent studies in the lexical approach have been done by Goldberg (Goldberg 1993, Goldberg & Saucier 1996) who, apart from confirming the five factor structure of personality descriptive adjectives, has provided useful lists of adjectives that may be used to compile personality trait questionnaires.

The second source of confirmation of a five factor model of human personality is the personality questionnaire research spearheaded by Costa & McCrae (1992a). They have applied their NEO-PI-R and other questionnaires too numerous to list – including the Guildford–Zimmerman Temperament Survey, the Minnesota Multiphasic Personality Inventory and the California Personality Inventory – to samples of subjects and have found very impressive agreements. That is, despite other personality questionnaires appearing to contain different numbers and types of personality traits they all, largely, have much overlap with the five factor model. Overlap with the five factor model has also been found with the inventories of Cattell, Comrey, Eysenck, Murray, Wiggins, the Jungian Myers–Briggs Type Inventory and the Occupational Personality Questionnaire.

In summary, the converging consensus around the five factor model signals the exciting possibilities that disparate human languages might all contain approximately the same personality trait descriptive system and that different personality questionnaires might merely be indexing variants of the five factor model. As might be expected, lexically-derived factors and NEO-PI factors have moderate to high correlations when assessed in the same subjects. Costa & McCrae (1992c) have discussed 'four ways the five factors are basic'. First, that longitudinal and cross-sectional studies find five robust dimensions of behavioural disposition that endure over time. Second, similar five factor schemes are found in different personality theories and languages. Third, the five factor model fits in different ages, sexes, races and language groups. Last, there is evidence for the heritability of all five personality factors.

There are objectors to the five factor consensus.

Eysenck (1992) objected to the five factor theory. He had no disagreement with neuroticism and extraversion and, indeed, these two traits appear so frequently and prominently in most personality systems that it is clear they are important sources of human variation in all cultures. Agreeableness and conscientiousness, Eysenck suggested, are primary traits associated with psychoticism, and openness is too closely linked to intelligence. Moreover, he notes that the five factor model is merely descriptive, having no background in theory, biological or otherwise. Block (1995) suggested that the five factor model might be an artefact of 'prestructuring' of personality data sets; essentially his worry was that researchers might have inadvertently selected only groups of synonyms based around the five broad factors, thus ensuring a five factor model. This may be countered by the finding of a five factor model in entirely unprestructured data sets (Saucier & Goldberg, 1996).

Stability of personality

Traits by definition are long-standing behavioural dispositions. Therefore, to be valid, trait measurements must be stable across time and must be able to predict behaviour. A major critique of traits came from the movement known as situationism, which suggested that people's behaviours were principally a result of the situation rather than personality traits. This idea dates back even before the classic studies of Hartshorne & May (1928), who showed little consistency in moral behaviours across different situations. The high tide of situationism came with Mischel's (1968) book *Personality and Assessment*. In his detailed and thoughtful critique of traits he first acknowledged that people form trait-like descriptions of themselves and others and that these were stable. However, he insisted that, for trait terms to be valid, one must find cross-situational consistency, and one must also find that traits can predict behaviours in situations. It was these two latter desiderata that were not met; he found that individuals showed little consistency in their responses in different situations and that personality traits rarely correlated with behaviours above about $r = 0.3$.

The situationist critique, though, fails to take account of the importance of behavioural aggregation, as emphasised by all trait theorists (Epstein 1977). This principle states that single situations contain too much noise or error variance to act as estimates of traits or for measured traits to predict them with a high correlation. Therefore, it is the aggregated behaviour of an individual over a number of relevant situations that would suggest their dispositions, and it is this same aggregated behaviour that should be used to correlate with trait ratings from questionnaires. Epstein (1977) showed that, when people rated their emotions, impulses and behaviours over 20 days the median reliability for all categories was 0.72. Moskowitz (1988) showed that highly reliable trait and behavioural disposition ratings could be achieved for dimensions of friendliness and dominance after studying subjects in only six situations. Moreover, the correlations between trait ratings and behaviours was over 0.5.

Mischel's research subsequent to his situationist critique used trait terms to predict behaviours with some success (Wright & Mischel, 1987). He has shown, for instance, that trait ratings of children's aggression and withdrawal can correlate highly with their trait-relevant behaviours. Correlations are especially high when the behaviours being counted are central to the trait, and when the situation makes particular demands on the trait. Mischel's more mature research, then, has shown that traits do significantly contribute to the prediction of behaviours and that behaviours are stable across time. In addition, it is clear that the situation is also relevant. Such a compromise, also accepted by trait theorists (Eysenck & Eysenck, 1980), is called interactionism, which recognises the part played by long-standing behavioural dispositions (traits) and situations in determining behaviours. Therefore, personality traits should be seen as a part of a larger person–situation interaction theory of behaviour, one which is accepted by trait theorists and social psychologists alike (Carson 1989). A more radical social psychology critique is that traits are mere solipsistic fictions that we construct for ourselves. This may easily be refuted by the evidence that our self-ratings of traits agree strongly with other people's ratings of our trait levels (Kenrick & Funder 1989).

The stability of personality that has been addressed thus far is relatively short term. However, it is important to know about the longer term stability of personality. If traits are predictive of behaviour, they should show some medium- to long-term stability. Stability has two meanings: it may mean stability of mean levels in a population over time, or it may mean stability of individual differences over time, irrespective of whether the population level is changing. With regard to the former, there is little change in personality trait levels after age 30 years, though there are some small decreases in neuroticism, extraversion and openness between age 20 and 30 (McCrae & Costa, 1994).

Stability of individual differences in extraversion over a 10 year interval ranged from 0.7 to 0.8, and for neuroticism from 0.6 to 0.7 (Costa & McCrae, 1977). The 7 year stability of traits measured in the NEO-PI are as follows: neuroticism = 0.67, extraversion = 0.81, openness = 0.84, agreeableness = 0.63, and conscientiousness = 0.78 (Costa & McCrae, 1992b). Costa & McCrae's (1992b) reports from the Baltimore Longitudinal Study of Aging suggest 24 year stabilities between 0.7 and 0.9 for scales from the Guildford–Zimmerman Temperament Survey. Eysenck's traits show similar levels of stability: over 6 years the stability coefficients were psychoticism = 0.61, extraversion = 0.84, neuroticism = 0.73, and lie scale = 0.75. The high stability of personality scales from many questionnaires is demonstrated in the large review compiled by Schuerger at al (1989). In summary, individual differences in personality traits are stable over many years, with extraversion having especially high stability.

Genes, environment and biology in normal personality

The techniques of behaviour genetics and molecular genetics have been applied to personality traits to discover the relative contributions of heredity and environment to the patterns of human temperament. An accessible summary of the methods and results of behaviour genetic research applied to personality is offered by Loehlin (1992), who used extraversion to exemplify the different research designs in this type of research.

Loehlin (1992) first addressed twin studies. He attempted to fit the same model of genetic and environmental influences to personality trait data from five different twin studies, conducted in the UK, USA, Australia, Sweden and Finland. These included sets of monozygotic and dizygotic twins who had been given different personality inventories, though all had included measures of extraversion. The range of heritability estimates was between 54% and 80%. That is, over half of the variance in extraversion in these groups was due to genetic effects. The proportion of variance not accounted for by genetic effects can be attributed to two sources: environment and error variance. The effects of the environment may be separated into the effects of the family (called the between family effect or shared environment) and the unique effects of the environment on the individual (called the within family effect or individual environment). On fitting the data from the five twin studies of personality, Loehlin (1992) found that there was no contribution from the shared environment. This surprising result indicated that the effect of the environment on personality trait levels is largely due to the unique environmental experience of members within a family.

There is an interesting anomaly in the personality trait results found in twin studies. The correlations of monozygotic twins are typically considerably more than twice as great as those of dizygotic twins, despite their genetic similarity being only twice as great on average. Two factors may be invoked to account for this, though they are not exclusive. The first is non-additive genetic variance, the recognition that phenotypic similarity between two individuals might rise in a non-linear fashion with rises in genetic similarity. This is called epistasis and it recognises that some human traits are the outcome of complexes of many individual genetic effects at distant loci and that it is the total effect of the pattern of genes that produces the personality trait level. The phenomenon has been called emergenesis (Lykken et al 1992). When Loehlin (1992) introduced an epistasis parameter to the analysis of the five large twin studies of personality he found that the additive genetic effect on extraversion reduced to 36% and that the epistasis effect added another 12%, giving a broad heritability of 48%. The second effect that could explain the greater similarity of monozygotic twins' personalities is non-equal environment effects. That is, it might be the case that the environments of monozygotic twins were so similar that this explained their greater-than-twice similarity over dizygotic twins. Such a parameter fits the data, and can replace the epistasis effect, but Loehlin (1992) was unable to adduce evidence to show that greater environmental similarity had any effect on personality traits.

Loehlin (1992) analysed the data from a number of other research designs. He found that three large adoption studies of personality – one in the UK and two in the USA – gave an additive genetic contribution estimate of 36% for extraversion, similar to that obtained from twin studies. Two twin family studies – where twins and their biological relatives are studied – gave heritability estimates of 37% for additive genetic effects and 14% for epistasis effects. Again, family environment made no contribution to extraversion levels. Interestingly, the correlations between one member of a monozygotic pair and his/her own children and the cotwin's children were almost identical. Loehlin's (1992) analyses of twins reared apart reveal substantial genetic effects, but the non-additive genetic effects account for the majority, making them at odds with the above data.

Loehlin (1992) applied similar analyses to all of the five factor model traits and arrived at the heritability estimates shown in Table 21.3. These show that the additive genetic effects are sizeable, but less than 50%. It is not possible at this stage to separate the contribution of non-additive genetic effects and the special environment shared by monozygotic twins, though either or both of these effects make a modest contribution. Finally, the effect of shared environment (family upbringing) is small or negligible. Bouchard's (1994) data from the Minnesota study of twins reared apart

Table 21.3 Genetic and environmental contributions (percentage variance) to personality dimensions in the five factor model of personality (Loehlin 1992)

	h^2	c_{mz}^2	c_s^2
Models assuming unequal MZ/DZ environments			
Extraversion	36	15	0
Neuroticism	31	17	5
Agreeableness	28	19	9
Conscientiousness	28	17	4
Culture	46	5	5
	h^2	i^2	c_s^2
Models assuming non-additive genetic effects			
Extraversion	32	17	2
Neuroticism	27	14	7
Agreeableness	24	11	11
Conscientiousness	22	16	7
Culture	43	2	6

MZ, monozygotic; DZ, dizygotic; h^2, heritability; c_{mz}^2, shared environment of MZ twins; c_s^2, shared environment of any siblings; i^2, epistasis. Remaining variance (100 minus row totals) is due to the individual's unique environment and error.

offer similar conclusions for the heritability of the 'big five' personality traits.

The heritability of personality traits, therefore, is moderately large. However, behaviour genetic studies do not offer evidence about the mechanisms of genetic effects. Such evidence may be obtained from molecular genetic findings. There have been few such studies applied to personality traits to date, and the initial findings have not proved replicable. The finding that novelty-seeking traits and aspects of extraversion were related to variations in the dopamine D_4DR receptor gene (Ebstein et al 1996, Benjamin et al 1996) was in agreement with the biological personality theory of Cloninger, but was not replicated in a subsequent study (Malhotra et al 1996). Similarly, the finding that variations in the 5-hydroxytryptamine (5-HT) transporter gene were linked to neuroticism levels (Lesch et al 1996) was not replicated in a subsequent report (Ball et al 1997).

As molecular genetic studies progress, they promise insights into the biological underpinnings and mechanisms of human personality variations. To date, the principal biological accounts of personality are offered by Eysenck (1967), Cloninger (1987) and Zuckerman (1991). Variously, these accounts link personality traits to evolutionary strategies, neurotransmitter-receptor systems and functional brain systems. None of them has met to date with conspicuous success, though there is some evidence to link differences in extraversion with differences in cortical arousal (Zuckerman 1991).

PERSONALITY DISORDERS

Some individuals present to mental health services despite having no mental illness, that is no Axis I disorder in the DSM system. Such people may have long-standing maladaptive behaviour patterns and suffer distress themselves or cause others distress. This raises the question of whether there are recognisable patterns of such personality disorder and, if so, how many disorders are there? Another interesting question is whether personality disorder patterns show overlap with normal personality dimensions. That is, do we require different systems, as we have now, of personality to describe normal and abnormal personality? These are the questions to which we now turn.

Writers sometimes refer to the satirical descriptions of annoying personality types by Theophrastus (Rusten 1993) as the beginnings of a descriptive system for personality disorders. In fact, present day lists and definitions of personality disorder are the blossoming of clinical observations from about the beginning of the 19th century. A helpful account of the evolution of personality disorder ideas was given by Berrios (1993), who drew on many foreign language texts. Berrios describes how the French psychiatrist Pinel, writing in 1809, articulated the concept 'manie sans délire' to describe outbursts of aggression in the absence of mental illness, though the concept was not well understood by other clinicians. Further, the English physician Pritchard's concept of moral insanity, which is sometimes taken to be the progenitor of antisocial personality disorder, was related to mood disorder (Whitlock 1982). Koch's (1891) diagnosis of psychopathic inferiority contained reference to antisocial behaviour. Among the more developed early accounts of personality types that suffered themselves or made others suffer are those by Schneider (1923) and Henderson (1939). Schneider, in his book *Psychopathic Personalities*, described the following types of psychopathy: hyperthymic, depressive, insecure, fanatical, lacking in self-esteem, labile in affect, explosive, wicked, aboulic and asthenic. In Henderson's book *Psychopathic States* there were three types of psychopathy: aggressive, passive and creative.

Types and classifications

As with mental illnesses, the two principal classificatory schemes for personality disorders are the American Psychiatric Association's (APA 1994) Diagnostic and Statistical Manual, edition IV (DSM-IV) and the World Health Organization's (WHO 1992) International Classification of Diseases, edition 10 (ICD-10). The personality disorder diagnoses of each system are shown in Table 21.4. The 10 diagnoses in the DSM-IV system are gathered into three clusters. The 'odd and eccentric' cluster A contains paranoid, schizoid and schizotypal personality disorders. The 'dramatic and emotional' cluster B contains antisocial, borderline, histrionic and narcissistic types. The 'anxious and fearful' cluster C contains avoidant, dependent and obsessive–compulsive categories. The APA defines personality disorder as:

> an enduring pattern of inner experience and behaviour that deviates markedly from the expectations of the individual's culture, is pervasive and inflexible, has an onset in adolescence or early adulthood, is stable over time, and leads to distress or impairment.

As a part of Axis II in the DSM system, personality disorders may coexist with mental disorders and individuals may qualify for as many personality disorders as they meet the criteria for. Information for the DSM system for personality disorders is gathered by the Personality Disorders Work Group who review literature, reanalyse data and oversee field trails of criteria proposed for the personality disorder categories; for examples of their literature reviews, field trials, deliberations and reports see Livesley (1995a). It is not enough merely to meet the criteria for personality disorder types: in the DSM-IV system the personality disorder must also be stable and of long duration, be broadly expressed, lead to distressed or impaired functioning, and not be due to a mental illness, physical illness or drugs.

The first clear contrast with most theories of normal personality is the fact that personality disorders are diagnosed as types, or categories, with little room for capturing the degree to which a person shows each of the types of disorder. There are clear indications that this will change in future revisions. The APA recently devoted a book to the relations between the five factor model of personality and personality disorders (Costa & Widiger 1994), and the DSM-IV manual explicitly discusses the issue of construing personality disorders as traits. Another notable difference from systems of normal personality is the heterogeneity of the concepts captured within the APA and WHO systems. Whereas it is typical for personality researchers to work with constructs that cover a system that includes most of the important sources of human personality variation, and

Table 21.4   Comparison of DSM-IV and ICD-10 personality disorder classifications

ICD-10 description	DSM-IV description	DSM Cluster
Paranoid Excessive sensitivity, suspiciousness, preoccupation with conspiratorial explanations of events, with a persistent tendency to self-reference	*Paranoid* Interpretation of people's action as deliberately malevolent, leading to distrust and suspiciousness	*Cluster A* Odd/eccentric
Schizoid Emotional coldness, detachment, lack of interest in other people, eccentricity, and excessive introspection and fantasy	*Schizoid* Detachment from social relationships and a restricted range of emotional experience and expression	
No equivalent	*Schizotypal* Acute discomfort in interpersonal relations with peculiarities of ideation, appearance and behaviour	
Histrionic Self-dramatisation, shallow mood, egocentricity and craving for excitement, with persistent manipulative behaviour	*Histrionic* Excessive emotionality and attention seeking	*Cluster B* Dramatic/emotional
Dissocial Callous unconcern for others, with irresponsibility, irritability and aggression, and incapacity to maintain enduring relationships	*Antisocial* Disregard for and violation of the rights of others with evidence of conduct disorder before the age of 15 years	
No equivalent	*Narcissistic* Pervasive grandiosity, lack of empathy and need for admiration	
Emotionally unstable *Impulsive* Inability to control anger or to plan ahead, with unpredictable mood and quarrelsome behaviour *Borderline* Unclear self-image, involvement in intense and unstable relationships, unpredictable mood, threats or acts of self-harm	*Borderline* Pervasive instablity of affect, interpersonal relationships, self-image, and excessive impulsivity	
Anakastic Indecisiveness, doubt, excessive caution, pedantry, rigidity and perfectionism	*Obsessive–compulsive* Preoccupation with perfectionism, orderliness, and control	*Cluster C* Fearful/anxious
Dependent Failure to take responsibility for actions, with subordination of personal needs to those of others, with need for constant reassurance and feelings of helplessness when a close relationship ends	*Dependent* Persistent clinging and submissive behaviour relates to an excessive need for care	
Anxious/avoidant Persistent tension, self-consciousness, exaggeration of risks and dangers, hypersensitivity to rejection, and restricted lifestyle because of insecurity	*Avoidant* Pervasive social discomfort, fear of negative evaluation and timidity	

to conduct psychometric and experimental work to validate the traits in the system, the concepts that are gathered together in the present – day personality disorder schemes have a wide range of origins. Tyrer et al (1991) describe how: antisocial personality arose from developmental research in children with conduct disorders; borderline and narcissistic concepts came from clinical studies by psychodynamic psychiatrists; European clinical phenomenology gave schizoid and obsessive–compulsive concepts; academic psychology contributed avoidant personality disorder; and schizotypal disorder came from genetic research and psychodynamic studies.

Individual personality disorders

Paranoid personality disorder

This is 'a pattern of distrust and suspiciousness such that others' motives are interpreted as malevolent' (APA 1994). The disorder begins by early adulthood and at least four of the following characteristics are displayed:

- Suspicious that others are exploiting, harming or deceiving but without sufficient basis
- Doubts the trust or loyalty of friends or associates
- Fear of confiding
- Reads hidden or threatening meaning into events
- Bears grudges
- Oversensitive to attacks on character
- Recurrent unjustified suspicions about fidelity of partner.

A review of research concerning this personality disorder is provided by Bernstein et al (1995). They note that clinical writings since Kraepelin's have noted a personality type characterised by a 'pervasive and unwarranted mistrust of others'. Key clinical writers such as Kretschmer, Schneider, Sheldon and Millon added features including sensitivity to criticism, antagonism, aggressiveness, hypervigilance and excessive need for autonomy. Unresolved matters include the possibilities that paranoid personality disorder lies on the schizophrenia spectrum, might be a risk factor for more severe delusional and paranoid disorders, and might overlap with schizotypal personality disorder. Among patients, paranoid personality disorder is more common in males (Alnaes & Torgersen 1988). Bernstein et al (1995) note that the 11 clinical studies that used DSM-III criteria found prevalences between 1% and 20% with a median of 5% for paranoid personality disorder. However, using DSM-IIIR criteria the figures from four studies were 15–30% with a median of 18%. Among non-clini-

cal adult samples the prevalence is about 3% or less (Coryell & Zimmerman 1989, Bernstein et al 1993).

Although there are overlaps between several DSM-IV and ICD-10 criteria, there are items in each system that have no equivalent in the other. For example, the expectation of being exploited or harmed has no equivalent in ICD-10, whereas the preoccupation with conspiratorial explanations has no place in DSM-IV. Only about 25% of people with paranoid personality disorder do not receive a further concurrent personality disorder diagnosis, and substantial overlaps are found with schizotypal (17–71%; Widiger et al 1986), narcissistic (2–75%), borderline (0–100%), avoidant (8–86%) and passive–aggressive personality disorders (17–53%). These figures are taken from the review of six clinical studies reviewed by Bernstein et al (1995). The range of the figures is a cause for concern, and it is clear from their data that there are, in fact, substantial overlaps between paranoid and almost all personality disorders. In outpatients, people with paranoid personality disorder are 3.5 times more likely to have agoraphobia without panic (Alnaes & Torgersen 1988), and relatives of people with paranoid personality disorder may have a specific increase in bulimia (Coryell & Zimmerman 1989). There is some evidence for a shared genetic basis for paranoid personality disorder and delusional disorder (Torgersen 1995). Paranoid traits are found to be about 40% heritable (Kendler & Hewitt 1992).

Schizoid personality disorder

This is 'a pattern of detachment from social relationships and a restricted range of emotional expression' (APA 1994). It includes at least four of the following:

- Avoids close relationships
- Chooses solitary activities
- Avoids sexual experiences with others
- Has few pleasurable activities
- Lacks confidants
- Indifferent to praise or criticism
- Is emotionally cold or affectively flat.

Bleuler (1924) first used the term schizoid and suggested a link with schizophrenia. Kretschmer defined two types; those that were insensitive and those that had inner sensitivity. Kalus et al (1995) emphasise a central difficulty of this disorder in that it refers to a subjective lack of concern toward criticism rather than some more objective state. They also point out that the DSM-III system lacked some features that some clinical writers would see as important in this disorder, such as asexuality, autistic thinking, fragmented self-identity and derealisation/depersonalisation (for example, Guntrip 1969). These deficiencies were addressed for the DSM-IIIR and DSM-IV revisions. The same authors review the compatibility between DSM and ICD-10 criteria and find this to be high.

Non-patient samples show prevalence rates of schizoid personality disorder between 0.5% and 7%, and among clinical samples assessed with DSM-IIIR criteria in four studies prevalence rates ranged from 1% to 16% (median 8.5%) (Kalus et al 1995). Torgersen (1995) reports that, whereas the prevalence of DSM-III schizoid personality among psychiatric outpatients was 2%, this has risen to 15% for DSM-IV criteria. Kalus et al (1995) review seven studies examining comorbidity of schizoid personality disorder with other personality disorder and find substantial overlaps with schizotypal (2–80%), avoidant (23–88%), paranoid (0–62%), antisocial (0–40%) and borderline (0–60%). There is little study of Axis I comorbidity with schizoid personality disorder, though a small study of seven relatives of people diagnosed with schizoid personality disorder found two cases of alcohol abuse/dependence, one case of mania and one case of drug abuse/dependence (Coryell & Zimmerman 1989). Kalus et al (1995) review genetic and family studies and suggest that it is unclear whether schizoid personality disorder lies on the schizophrenia spectrum. Moreover Torgersen and colleagues' (1993a) twin family study found no such relationship.

Schizotypal personality disorder

This is 'a pattern of acute discomfort in close relationships, cognitive or perceptual distortions, and eccentricities of behavior' (APA 1994). The disorder begins by early adulthood and includes at least five of the following:

- Ideas of reference
- Odd beliefs or magical thinking
- Unusual perceptual experiences
- Odd thinking and speech
- Suspiciousness
- Restricted or inappropriate affect
- Eccentric appearance or behaviour
- No confidants
- High levels of social anxiety associated with paranoid fears.

Schizotypal personality disorder is related to the Axis I disorder schizophrenia in terms of phenomenological, genetic, outcome and treatment response characteristics (Siever et al 1995). The inclusion of this personality disorder in DSM-III came about because the definition of borderline conditions was too vague, including both affective and schizophrenia-type traits (Spitzer et al 1979). The aim was to capture a type of personality with chronic psychosis-like characteristics,

perhaps biologically related to people with schizophrenia. However, the association between schizotypal personality disorder and schizophrenia lies not so much with the positive (psychotic-type) as with the negative (social withdrawal) characteristics (Siever et al 1995). Torgersen (1995) surveys the evidence suggesting a heritable component to schizotypal personality disorder and finds that the negative features are more heritable than the positive (perceptual/cognitive features).

Various studies reviewed by Siever et al (1995) show that up to about a half of patients with schizotypal personality disorder may also suffer from a major depressive disorder at some point. The overlap with schizophrenia was similar. Some suggest that about 25% of patients with schizotypal personality disorder may go on to develop chronic schizophrenia, though others find much lower rates (Siever et al 1995). The shared genetic diathesis between schizophrenia and schizotypal personality disorder is demonstrated by adoption (Kendler et al 1985) and family studies (Schulz et al 1986). Relatives of people with schizophrenia show more schizotypal personality disorder (Kendler et al 1989). Abnormalities of smooth pursuit eye tracking and performance in perceptual backward masking tasks are found in schizophrenia and schizotypal personality disorder, but not in controls or other personality disorder categories (Braff 1986, Siever et al 1990). Siever et al (1995) review further shared biological features between schizophrenia and schizotypal personality disorder, such as platelet monoamine activity, galvanic skin orienting response and CT-estimated ventricular:brain ratio. They suggest that worse outcomes in schizotypal personality disorder are associated with paranoid symptomatology and social impairment. Siever et al (1995) provide a thoughtful discussion of whether, in future, schizotypal personality disorder might move to Axis I as a part of the schizophrenia spectrum.

Overlaps with other personality disorders are substantial and many. There is much comorbidity with other Cluster A DSM personality disorders, as noted above. However, other personality disorders that involve social isolation also show overlap; that with avoidant ranges from 15% to 88% in seven studies reviewed by Siever et al (1995). The same review shows a very large overlap with borderline personality disorder (33–91%), suggesting that the intention to separate borderline states into affective and schizophrenia-like divisions has not been successful.

Antisocial personality disorder

This is 'a pattern of disregard for, and violation of, the rights of others' (APA 1994). The disorder applies to individuals who are 18 years or older but who have shown evidence of conduct disorder before the age of 15 years. In addition, at least three of the following characteristics are present:

- Non-conformity to social norms with repeated unlawful behaviour
- Deceitfulness
- Impulsivity
- Instability and aggressiveness
- Disregard for safety
- Irresponsibility
- Lack of remorse.

One of the major debates surrounding the antisocial personality disorder is the possible overemphasis of criminal acts as criteria for the disorder and the lack of inclusion of psychopathic personality traits (Blackburn 1988, Widiger & Corbitt 1995). Nevertheless, DSM criteria do agree with clinicians' ratings of antisocial personality disorder (Skodol et al 1991) and correlations between DSM-III and DSM-IIIR ratings and scores on the more psychological trait-based Psychopathy Checklist (PCL) are moderately high, between 0.54 and 0.63 (Hare et al 1991). The prototypical items for this disorder, according to clinicians, are unstable interpersonal relationships, failure to learn from experience, disregard for the consequences of actions, and so forth (Livesley et al 1987).

Widiger & Corbitt (1995) review what they term the 'overdiagnosis' of antisocial personality disorders within prison and forensic settings. Using clinical criteria the rates of diagnosis in prisons are often over 50% and can be as high as 70–80%. Rates tend to be rather lower – about 33% – when prisoners are diagnosed using more psychological criteria such as are found in Hare's PCL (Hare 1985). In the Epidemiological Catchment Area (ECA) Study 47% of people who met the DSM-III criteria for antisocial personality disorder had a significant arrest record (Robins et al 1991). Widiger & Corbitt's (1995) survey of lifetime prevalence among normal population samples shows rates between 2.1% and 3.7%. In five ECA areas the 1 month prevalence ranged from 0.3% to 0.8% (Regier et al 1988).

The two most prominent alternatives to the DSM-IV criteria for personality disorder are those of Hare (Hare et al 1991) in the PCL-Revised (Table 21.5) and those of the dissocial personality disorder in the ICD-10 criteria (Table 21.6). Both of these lay more stress on the psychological traits than on social acts. The PCL-R has good reliability and predictive validity in terms of predicting recidivism and in being associated with laboratory tests thought to relate to psychopathy (Hare et al 1991). Hare & Hart (1995) have suggested that the changes made to DSM-IV leave the gap between the social act-oriented DSM system and the psychologically-oriented ICD-10 and PCL systems as wide as they were previously.

Borderline personality disorder

This is 'a pattern of instability in personal relationships, self-image and affects, and marked impulsivity' (APA 1994). The disorder begins by early adulthood and includes at least five of the following:

- Fear of abandonment
- Unstable interpersonal relationships
- Disturbance of self-identity

Table 21.5   Items from Hare's Psychopathy Checklist-Revised (Hare et al 1991)

Factor 1	Factor 2
Glibness/superficial charm	Need for stimulation/proneness to boredeom
Grandiose sense of self-worth	Parasitic lifestyle
Pathological lying	Poor behavioural controls
Conning/manipulative	Early behaviour problems
Lack of remorse or guilt	Lack of realisitic, long-term goals
Shallow affect	Impulsivity
Callous/lack of empathy	Irresponsibility
Failure to accept responsibility for actions	Juvenile delinquency
In addition	
Revocation of conditional release	
Promiscuous sexual behaviour	
Many short-term marital relationships	
Criminal versatility	

Table 21.6 ICD-10 criteria for dissocial personality disorder: at least three must be present to make the diagnosis

- Callous unconcern for the feelings of others
- Gross and persistent attitude of irresponsibility and disregard for social norms, rules and obligations
- Incapacity to maintain enduring relationships, though with no difficulty in establishing them
- Very low tolerance to frustration and a low threshold for discharge of aggression, including violence
- Incapacity to experience guilt, or to profit from adverse experience, particularly punishment
- Marked proneness to blame others, or to offer plausible rationalisations for behaviour that has brought the individual into conflict with society

- Impulsivity
- Recurrent self-harm
- Labile affect
- Chronic feelings of emptiness
- Uncontrollable anger
- Stress-related paranoia or dissociation.

Original descriptions of so-called borderlines emphasised 'brief psychotic regression experiences' (Kernberg 1967, Masterson 1972). Considerable debate has ranged since about the clusters of symptoms/features that should be included in the disorder. Table 21.7 shows the prevalence of certain features of borderline personality as noted in nine studies summarised by Gunderson et al (1995b). In particular this survey seemed to establish the fact of cognitive/perceptual problems in people with borderline personality disorder. Also, Dahl (1995) comments that the original core

idea of 'identity diffusion' in borderline personality disorder was narrowed to self-image and the sense of self, whereas Kernberg's original concept of identity diffusion included sexual orientation, long-term goals, types of friends and values. Dahl (1990) has argued that the DSM committee has given too little attention to the validity of the borderline concept (essentially copied by the ICD-10 classification) and suggests that a broader borderline concept could be envisaged that included most of the Cluster A and B diagnoses in the DSM scheme. In the ICD-10 system, borderline type is one of two emotionally unstable personality disorders – the other being impulsive – and their criteria are shown in Table 21.8. Gunderson et al (1995b) note the huge amount of work devoted to this relatively new personality disorder and the unusual meeting of an essentially psychodynamic concept with modern empirical psychiatry.

The disorder is more frequently diagnosed in women (75% of diagnoses), and the prevalence ranges from 2% in the general population, 10% in psychiatric outpatient clinics, 20% among psychiatric inpatients to 30–60% among people with personality disorders (APA 1994). This diagnosis demonstrates considerable comorbidity. Prior to the introduction of DSM-IV criteria the overlap with histrionic personality disorder was as great as 50% with DSM-III and 23% with DSM-IIIR (Gunderson et al 1995b). There have also been substantial overlaps with antisocial, self-defeating and avoidant personality disorders. Axis I overlaps include mood disorders (Gunderson & Phillips 1991). Dahl (1995) suggested that the large comorbidity that involves borderline personality disorders brings into question the validity of this construct. He has suggested that a dimensional model might be more appropriate and that borderline personality disorder might be viewed as extreme neuroticism.

Table 21.7 Prevalence of features of borderline personality as noted in nine studies summarised by Gunderson et al (1995b)

Cognitive/perceptual problem	Number of studies involved	Range (%) of presence of feature
Depersonalisation	6	30–85
Derealisation	6	30–92
Paranoid experiences	6	32–100
Hopelessness/worthlessness	3	77–88
Visual illusions	5	24–42
Muddled thinking	1	52
Magical thinking	3	34–68
Ideas of reference	3	49–74
Odd speech	2	30–59
Disturbed thoughts	2	39–68

Table 21.8 ICD-10 criteria for emotionally unstable personality disorder types: in both cases three criteria of the impulsive type must be met before the diagnosis may be made; in addition, for borderline type diagnosis to be made, two of the borderline criteria must be present

Impulsive type
- Marked tendency to act unexpectedly and without consideration of the consequences
- Marked tendency to quarrelsome behaviour and to conflicts with others, especially when impulsive acts are thwarted or criticised
- Liability to outbursts of anger or violence, with inability to control the resulting behavioural explosions
- Difficulty in maintaining any course of action that offers no immediate reward
- Unstable and capricious mood

Borderline type
- Disturbances in and uncertainty about self-image, aims and internal preferences (including sexual)
- Liability to become involved in intense and unstable relationships, often leading to emotional crises
- Excessive efforts to avoid abandonment
- Recurrent threats or acts of self-harm
- Chronic feelings of emptiness

Histrionic personality disorder

This is 'a pattern of excessive emotionality and attention seeking' (APA 1994). The disorder includes at least five of the following characteristics:

- Needs to be the centre of attention
- Seductive interpersonally
- Shallow emotional expression
- Preoccupied with physical appearance
- Impressionistic speech, lacking detail
- Self-dramatisation
- Suggestible
- Misjudges intimacy in relationships.

This personality disorder has its roots in psychoanalytic writings and has been traced back to Freud's notion of hysteria (Pfohl 1995). Among the key contributors to the delineation of the concept and the empirical research into the clusters of traits that go to make up the disorder were Kernberg (1967) and Lazare et al (1966, 1970). Early factor analytic studies of 'hysterical personality' suggested the following traits: aggression, emotionality, oral aggression, exhibitionism, egocentricity and sexual provocativeness. These are similar to the DSM-IIIR histrionic personality disorder. Pfohl (1995) remarks on the lack of predictive validity studies using DSM histrionic personality disorder criteria, though scales to assess related concepts – usually 'hysteria' – such as the Lazare–Klerman Trait Scale and the Hysteroid–Obsessoid Questionnaire, suggest a high rate of low mood, somatisation, and sensitivity to comments about sex role adequacy. Those with the disorder may have a worse outcome of major depression (Pilkonis & Frank 1988) which may be due

to the fact that they are less likely to be taking antidepressants at follow-up (Pfohl et al 1987).

The sex ratio for the disorder appears to be about equal, despite many of the original descriptions referring to women, though sometimes the gender neutral items in structured questionnaires are applied unequally to the sexes (Pfohl 1995). The general population prevalence is about 2–3% and that in outpatient and inpatients clinic settings is 10–15% (APA 1994). There is comorbidity with somatisation disorder (Lilienfeld et al 1986). In the survey of five studies conducted by Pfohl (1995), there are substantial overlaps with antisocial (10–49%), borderline (44–94%) and narcissistic (8–44%) personality disorders. Kernberg (1988) suggested that histrionic and borderline personality disorders were on a continuum rather than separate entities.

Narcissistic personality disorder

This is 'a pattern of grandiosity, need for admiration, and lack of empathy' (APA 1994). At least five of the following characteristics are present:

- Grandiose self-importance
- Fantasies of success, power, brilliance, beauty or ideal love
- Belief that self is 'special'
- Need for excessive admiration
- Sense of entitlement
- Interpersonally exploitative
- Lacks empathy
- Envious
- Arrogant.

This concept was introduced to the DSM system for the first time in edition III. It is another personality disorder concept to arrive from psychoanalytic writings. Horney's (1937) aggressive–expansive type of personality has some of the features of narcissistic personality disorder. Kohut and especially Kernberg (1976) made contributions to the concept that were formalised in the DSM concept of narcissistic personality disorder. The diagnosis does not appear in ICD-10. Paris (1995) suggests that there was insufficient attempt at empirical investigation into this concept prior to DSM-IV, perhaps indicating a too-willing acceptance of some psychoanalytic ideas to a field dominated by descriptive phenomenology.

This is an unusual principal diagnosis in the clinical setting. The general population prevalence is about 1% and that within clinical populations is very dependent on the criteria used, with ranges from 2% to 16% (Gunderson et al 1995a). The overlap with other personality disorders is considerable, up to 50% with other 'dramatic' cluster diagnoses, and high overlap is also found with passive–aggressive, schizotypal and paranoid personality disorders. Gunderson et al (1995a) in their review of the construct note that two key types of studies are lacking from the literature: the degree to which modern, systematic conceptions of the disorder match with the ideas of expert clinicians; and predictive validity studies that might investigate whether the disorder affects the course of and response to Axis I disorders.

Avoidant personality disorder

This is 'a pattern of social inhibition, feelings of inadequacy, and hypersensitivity to negative evaluation' (APA 1994). The disorder is characterised by at least four of the following:

- Avoids occupations requiring interpersonal contact
- Only becomes involved if certain of being liked
- Restrained in intimate relationships
- Fear of criticism or rejection
- Feelings of inadequacy in new interpersonal situations
- Self perceived as inferior and socially inept
- Avoids personal risk because of embarrassment.

This disorder presents in about 0.5%–1% of the general population and in about 10% of mental health outpatients (APA 1994). Though traceable to ideas of Bleuler and Schneider, it was named by Millon (1969) and first introduced to the DSM system in its third edition. Millon & Martinez (1995) liken the concept to the hyperaesthetic schizoid type described by Krteschmer. These authors also list many psychoanalytic writers

who contributed to this concept and who delineated patients for whom 'there is an intolerable strain in associating with people and solitude becomes primarily a means of avoiding it' (Horney 1945). However, they also point to the lack of a large empirical dataset or well-articulated theory to inform the revision of the construct. Whether the key to the disorder is anxiety or narcissistic vulnerability remains a matter of debate (Pilkonis 1995).

The disorder shows significant overlaps with borderline, schizoid, schizotypal, dependent, paranoid and self-defeating personality disorders (Millon & Martinez 1995), though much of this overlap may be due to shared diagnostic features. The overlap with the Axis I disorder social phobia is discussed below.

Dependent personality disorder

This is 'a pattern of submissive and clinging behavior related to an excessive need to be taken care of' (APA 1994). The disorder includes at least five of the following:

- Indecisive
- Hands responsibility to other
- Fear of disagreeing with other
- Lacks initiative
- Excessive need for nurturance
- Fear of being alone
- Shifts quickly to a new relationship when a close relationship ends
- Preoccupation with fears of abandonment.

This personality disorder is among the more common personality disorder diagnoses made in mental health settings, though prevalence estimates are variable, ranging from 5% to 55% (Millon & Martinez 1995). According to Hirschfeld et al (1995) the roots of the disorder lie in psychoanalytic theory, social–psychological theory and ethology. These authors identify conceptual overlaps with borderline (the fear of abandonment) and avoidant and histrionic personality disorders (need for reassurance). Most empirical studies find an overlap of more than 50% with borderline personality disorder, and confirm the suggested overlaps with avoidant and histrionic disorders. Few patients receive a sole diagnosis of dependent personality disorder (Hirschfeld et al 1995). Livesley et al (1990) used factor analytic techniques to identify two key dimensions of the dependent personality disorder – attachment and dependency – and these were correlated at 0.62. Though Hirschfeld et al (1995) view this as evidence for the validity of the DSM personality disorder construct, Livesley (1995b) counters with the view that it, with much other evidence, suggests that personality disorders as a whole would be better described as a series of dimensions.

Obsessive–compulsive personality disorder

This is 'a pattern of preoccupation with orderliness, perfectionism, and control' (APA 1994). The disorder includes at least four of the following characteristics:

- A preoccupation with details or rules
- Perfectionism
- Overemphasis on work and productivity at the expense of leisure
- Overconscientiousness
- Hoarding
- Inability to delegate
- Miserliness
- Rigidity and stubbornness.

This has a prevalence of approximately 1% in general population samples and between 3% and 10% of psychiatric patient samples. Pfohl & Blum (1995) describe the origins of this concept in Freud's writing on the anal character type, and in Abraham's recognition of a type of person who was fastidious, made lists, could not throw away old objects, tended to postpone decisions and actions and is rigid in interpersonal relationships (Oldham & Frosch 1988). Through intermediate attempts to provide scales to measure the disorder (Lazare et al 1966), the original features of the disorder have remained recognisable in the DSM criteria.

As might be expected, some studies report that over 50% of people with obsessive–compulsive Axis I disorder also meet the criteria for obsessive–compulsive personality disorder, though other studies report lower rates (Pfohl & Blum 1995). The review by Baer et al (1990) suggests that these disorders are distinct entities, though most studies of obsessive–compulsive disorder find that such patients have at least one Axis II diagnosis. There are substantial overlaps with paranoid, histrionic, borderline, narcissistic and avoidant personality disorders (Pfohl & Blum 1995).

Personality disorder not otherwise specified

This is a category used in cases where a person has features of several different personality disorders but does not meet the diagnostic criteria for any single disorder, and where a person meets the criteria for a personality disorder not included in the above scheme (e.g. passive–aggressive personality disorder).

Measurement instruments for personality disorder

There is a large and growing number of instruments for the diagnosis and assessment of personality disorders. There are self-rated instruments and structured interviews; there are schemes based on DSM, ICD and other personality disorder nosologies; and there are different amounts of evidence for the validity of each. A useful survey and critical review of many instruments is provided by Zimmerman (1994) and a shorter buyer's guide to some commonly used inventories and interviews is given by Loranger et al (1997). In the rest of this section some frequently used instruments are described.

The structured clinical interview for DSM-IIIR (SCID-II, Spitzer et al 1990) follows a 113 item self-report personality questionnaire that covers the criteria for all of the DSM-IIIR personality disorders. The clinical interview that follows picks up on any questions that the patient has endorsed. Hyler and colleagues have developed a self-report questionnaire modelled on the DSM-IIIR criteria, the Personality Diagnostic Questionnaire 4 (PDQ-4) (Hyler 1994). When compared with the SCID and Personality Disorder Examination (see below) it tended to produce false-positive results, leading the authors to suggest that it might be an effective screening instrument (Hyler et al 1990).

The International Personality Disorder Examination (IPDE) is based upon the ICD-10 personality disorder classification (Loranger et al 1997). The interview is preceded by a screening questionnaire that has 59 items. The interview itself covers the operational criteria for the ICD-10 personality disorders, sometimes with multiple questions to cover those criteria that have multiple-part items. Basic psychometric data have been reported from 716 patients in 11 countries in the four major continents. The reliability and temporal stability is similar to that of the major Axis I categories. There is moderately good agreement with DSM-IIIR categories.

The Personality Assessment Schedule (PAS) is an interview based on 24 aspects of personality and is unique in using primarily the evidence of informants to make ratings (Tyrer 1988). The interview takes about 1 hour and assesses the following traits: pessimism, worthlessness, optimism, lability, anxiousness, suspiciousness, introspection, shyness, aloofness, sensitivity, vulnerability, irritability, impulsiveness, aggression, callousness, irresponsibility, childishness, resourcelessness, dependence, submissiveness, conscientiousness, rigidity, eccentricity and hypochondriasis. With respect to diagnosis the prime concern is the set of dimensions that causes the greatest social impairment. The higher order structure of the PAS finds sociopathic, passive-dependent, anankastic and schizoid types, which is in agreement with others (Mulder & Joyce, 1996). The PAS is not directly linked to DSM or ICD systems, which might account for its limited use.

The Dimensional Assessment of Personality Problems – Basic Questionnaire devised by Livesley and colleagues (1992) represents an attempt to be comprehensive in covering all clinically relevant aspects of personality pathology and to construe these in a psychometrically valid multidimensional format. It comprises 290 items, each based on a five point response scale. It is discussed in more detail below.

A narrower instrument is the Diagnostic Interview for Borderlines which concentrates on this important personality disorder (Zanarini et al 1989). Its 186 questions divide into aspects of affect, cognition, impulse action patterns and interpersonal relationships. The rater uses responses to these to rate 22 statements capturing aspects of borderline personality disorder.

Zimmerman (1994) summarised his findings with various personality disorder instruments as follows. Unstandardised clinical evaluations of personality disorders are unreliable. Joint interview agreement is good, especially where the developers of the interview are involved in the assessment. The longer the period between interviews and the more symptomatic improvement that has occurred, the less reliable the personality disorder ratings, though antisocial personality disorder ratings are less affected than others. There are substantial differences in the coverage of personality disorder facets among widely used instruments. The patient's acute state biases both self-report scales and interviews.

Problems with current categorical schemes

Critiques of personality categories range from moral objections to the pejorative labelling of people, a priori criticisms of the personality disorder classification and individual categories, problems of measurement, and empirical findings that contradict the clinical classification schemes. The proper classification of phenomena is the prerequisite to their scientific study and, in medicine, their specific treatments and estimations of prognoses. However, in the field of personality disorders the classification of the disorders is far from settled.

An example of how powerful a pejorative label a personality disorder diagnosis can be was demonstrated by Lewis & Appleby (1988). Their objections to personality disorder diagnoses were that diagnoses were unreliable, that attributing personality disorder diagnoses led to therapeutic neglect, and that because people with these disorders were deemed to be in control of their actions they received little sympathy for their distress. Their empirical study involved sending psychiatric case vignettes to 240 psychiatrists and asking them about their opinions and management decisions. The vignettes were identical except that some mentioned the presence of an unspecified personality disorder and some did not. Whenever personality disorder was mentioned in a vignette the patient was seen in a much less favourable light: as manipulative, attention-seeking, disliked, a difficult management problem, annoying, unlikely to improve, responsible for their own life problems, not meriting medical staff time, uncompliant with advice and treatment, not a suicide risk and not meriting antidepressant treatment despite having symptoms of low mood. Even when psychiatrists offered a diagnosis of depression for the case vignette, if personality disorder was mentioned then they were assessed less favourably. The authors concluded that the 'clinical diagnosis of personality disorder has no justification and should be abandoned'. The study evoked much comment, including Widiger's (1989) opinion that the psychiatrists' responses validated personality disorder diagnoses, because the manipulativeness, annoyingness and attention-seeking tendencies were traits used in the diagnostic procedure.

There has long been a worry about tautology in personality disorder diagnosis. That is, a person is said to have a given personality disorder because they tend to engage in certain acts, and their engaging in these acts is 'explained' by the person's having the specified personality disorder. Blackburn's (1988) discussion of psychopathy and antisocial personality disorder is instructive. In the many competing diagnostic schemes for antisocial/psychopathic personalities there are two clear origins for the diagnostic items. Some of the items are behavioural traits, and some are social acts. His opinion is that the inclusion of social acts is inappropriate in diagnosing personality: social acts belong to a moral frame of reference and amount to judgements about the appropriateness of behaviour. Instead he suggests, as did Cleckley (1976) and writers cited above in the section on antisocial personality disorders, that the focus on personality disorder diagnosis should be the inferred behavioural tendencies. Thus, in antisocial personality the focus might be on traits such as superficial charm, insincerity, affective poverty, and so forth, rather than criminality, delinquency, hedonism, etc. This separation of personality traits from social acts might allow the personality disorder to be defined in one domain (psychological traits) and used to predict behaviours in another (social acts).

Further a priori criticisms of personality disorder schemes were made by Widiger & Costa (1994). They commented that, unlike normal personality concepts, there was heterogeneity within personality disorders with respect to the numbers of constructs each contained. Thus, borderline personality disorder involved issues of identity, affectivity and impulsivity, whereas avoidant personality disorder was much narrower. It is not clear, therefore, whether personality disorder schemes have properly considered whether each category is at the same level of description; perhaps some are broad dimensions whereas others are narrow or primary traits. They further comment that the three clusters of personality disorder do not cohere conceptually and support this theoretical comment by evidence that the clusters do not emerge in empirical studies of personality disorder ratings; even this most basic aspect of the DSM classification system might be fiction.

Other critiques of personality disorders are that the schemes for diagnosis have changed too quickly, without sufficient reference to empirical data. The process of change within the DSM system of personality disorders is given in detail by Livesley (1995a) and for the ICD system by Loranger et al (1997). At the clinical level it has long been known that personality disorder diagnoses tend to be made idiosyncratically by psychiatrists, with different clinicians having a few favoured diagnoses (Walton & Presly 1973). The increasing clarity of operational criteria in systems such as DSM and ICD can solve this but has led to other problems. Tyrer et al (1991) welcomed the inclusion of clear operational criteria for personality disorders in DSM-III but feared that reliability of diagnosis was being achieved at the cost of decreased validity with respect to key personality disorder traits. Morey (1988) demonstrated the effect of changing criteria from DSM-III to DSM-IIIR (Table 21.9). This shows that there were very large increases in rates among psychiatric patients of diagnosis for narcissistic, avoidant, dependent, paranoid, and schizoid,

some almost eightfold. Such large increases in prevalence are evidence of a system that is far from stable and validated. Other indicators of the instability of personality disorder systems are the removal of passive–aggressive personality disorder from DSM-IIIR and DSM-IV and the removal of sadistic and self-defeating personality disorder which appeared in the appendix to DSM-IIIR. Moreover, narcissistic, borderline, schizotypal and avoidant personality disorders were all new to DSM-IIIR (Widiger & Costa, 1994). In fact, if the rationales provided for the changes from DSM-IIIR to DSM-IV are examined in detail (Livesley 1995a) one sees that there is a heavy focus on descriptive validity, but much less emphasis on the predictive and construct validity of each personality disorder diagnosis.

A problem in personality disorder conceptualisation and clinical practice is the degree to which they overlap with Axis I mental illness categories. Widiger & Shea (1991) emphasise confusion in four categories. There is evidence that schizotypal personality disorder might be a part of the schizophrenia spectrum, making it unclear whether it is a personality or illness concept. This is supported by the genetic link between schizotypal personality disorder and schizophrenia (Nigg & Goldsmith 1994). Borderline personality has a close relationship with mood disorder and it is not clear whether it is a mood disorder variant (since some dysphoric mood states can be very long-lasting) or a personality type akin to the neuroticism trait that leads frequently to low mood states. Further, borderline personality disorder has some criteria that overlap with bulimia. There are overlaps between antisocial personality disorder and substance use disorders and it is not clear whether their frequent co-occurrence is caused by true comorbidity of two different disorders, the giving of two names to a single underlying concept, or the artefactual co-occurrence of two real disorders whose operational criteria have been insufficiently distinguished. Perhaps the largest overlap discussed by Widiger & Shea (1991) was that between avoidant personality disorder and social phobia. In both of these categories social contact is avoided because of fears of embarrassment following the evaluation of others. The course of the disorders does not help to distinguish them – because social phobia, like a personality trait, may be continuous from late adolescence – nor does treatability, because there have been attempts to 'treat' avoidant personality disorder with alprazolam (Reich et al 1989). Widiger & Shea (1991) suggested various answers to these problems of overlap that might help to validate personality disorder criteria. More use of exclusion criteria – for example, not diagnosing schizotypal personality disorder in the presence of schizophrenia or borderline personality disorder in the presence of depression – was considered to

Table 21.9 Effect of changing from DSM-III to DSM-IIIR criteria on the percentage of patients with various personality disorder diagnoses (Morey 1988)		
	Patients with diagnosis (%)	
Personality disorder	DSM-III	DSM-IIIR
Borderline	32.0	33.3
Narcissistic	6.2	22.0
Histrionic	24.6	21.6
Antisocial	5.8	6.2
Avoidant	11.3	27.1
Dependent	14.1	22.3
Compulsive	8.9	7.9
Passive–aggressive	8.2	7.9
Paranoid	7.2	22.0
Schizoid	1.4	11.0
Schizotypal	17.2	9.3
Atypical, mixed	29.2	22.3

be arbitrary, and not conducive to validating categories. Shifting the placement of personality disorders to Axis I – as with the cyclothymic personality of DSM-II that became cyclothymia in DSM-III – is again arbitrary. Deleting overlapping criteria to reduce personality–illness overlaps might add distinctiveness but is indefensible; imagine, for example, removing pyrexia from all but one physical illness category just to achieve sharper illness boundaries. Adding differentiating criteria to personality disorder categories is their strongest suggestion, and in essence reflects the scientific attempt to find core features of the various personality types. An example of this research is that of Hare et al (1991) on the psychology of psychopathy. Widiger & Shea's last suggestion was that the method for conceptualising personality disorders might be shifted from categories (types) to dimensions (traits). This possibility is discussed in the next section.

Apart from Axis I–Axis II comorbidity, the overlap among personality disorders themselves is considerable, as was seen above in the sections devoted to each disorder. This large redundancy problem has been described as a major threat to the validity of the entire personality disorder scheme (Paris 1995).

Dimensionality of personality disorders

Given that the concept of personality traits (or dimensions or factors) has proved valid and useful in describing normal personality variation (Matthews & Deary 1998), it is increasingly being considered whether this might also be the right approach for the scientific study of personality disorders. Torgersen (1995) favours a move toward a factor analytic approach to delineating personality disorder. In DSM-IV it is explicitly recognised that personality disorder categories might be viewed also as 'dimensions representing spectra of personality dysfunction' (APA 1994). In addition, the DSM workgroup acknowledges that two issues require and are receiving active investigation: the degree to which personality disorders are continuous with Axis I mental disorders, and the relationship between normal and abnormal personality dimensions. In considering how to improve the validity of personality disorder concepts, Widiger & Shea (1991) suggested that it might be useful to move from categories to dimensions. Though categories might be good for describing illness states that are qualitatively different from normal states, and which might remit and relapse with normal functioning in-between, they suggest that they offer misleading, too-rigid stereotypes in describing personality. Moving to a dimensional system would allow the retention of cut-off points for making diagnoses, but would be more informative by allowing continuous ratings of people on

a number of valid dimensions. Thus a richer scheme for personality assessment could emerge, with each person having a profile rather than a category. One problem with such a scheme is that clinicians are not used to dimensional approaches – a point also emphasised by Tyrer et al (1991). However, this is not strictly true, since clinicians measure blood pressure along a dimension and then apply cut-offs for treatment, and, in any case, the 'true' structure of personality and personality disorders is a matter for discovery rather than invention or clinical convenience.

In searching for a dimensional solution to personality disorders there are immediate questions that must be addressed: How many dimensions are there? Should they be primary or broad traits? Is the structure of personality disorder traits the same in clinical and healthy populations (and different only in the mean levels of dysfunction found)? Should separate research efforts be aimed at individual areas of personality disorder or should the entire scheme be the subject of comprehensive investigations?

In moving to studies which have examined the dimensional structure of personality disorder it is interesting to see the same issue of the proper number and nature of dimensions being emphasised, much as it has been in studies of normal personality. Among the most economical proposals is that of Blackburn (1988) who suggested that the DSM personality disorder categories refer chiefly to different amounts of hostility and dominance and that each could be construed using a simple two-dimensional model with orthogonal dimensions of hostile–friendly versus dominant–submissive. Some support for this proposal came from a reanalysis of the Personality Deviance Scales (PDS) of Bedford & Foulds (1978). In Foulds' theory, personality deviance, as he called it, was trait-like and could be assessed along the dimensions of intrapunitiveness, extrapunitiveness and dominance. Deary et al (1995) reanalysed data from the PDS in a large sample of normal individuals and found only two clear factors: hostility and submissiveness/low self-confidence. The main objection to such a two factor system is that it omits consideration of the personal distress that is important in various personality disorders.

Factor-analytic studies of personality disorders conducted in clinical and non-clinical settings point quite strongly toward about four or five replicable dimensions of personality disorder. In a now-classic study that presaged most of the developments of the following years to date, Presly & Walton (1973) argued that categories should be replaced with dimensions in personality disorder. They converted personality disorder symptoms to item scales on which each patient might be rated. Thereafter, they subjected ratings to principal components analysis and found four basic factors underlying the item markers of the different categories. Their first factor included items such as egocentricity, lack of regard for the consequences of acts, inability to learn from experience, irresponsibility, impulsiveness and conscience defect, and was called social deviance. Factor two was called submissiveness and included timid, meek, submissive, avoid competition, intropunitive, indecisive, low officiousness, low need for attention and low extrapunitiveness. Factor three was named obsessional–schizoid and contained items such as stubborn, overindependence, meticulous, officious, attachment, suspicious, insensitive and lack of suggestibility. Factor four included ingratiation, need for attention, excess emotional display, unlikeability and insincerity. It was called hysterical, though today would have attracted narcissistic and/or histrionic labels. Presly & Walton (1973) argued that, whereas psychiatrists are good at recognising and rating individual personality disorder traits, they are poor at combining them to form valid syndromes. They argued that a reliable method of assessing traits was required, that traits must be expressed as dimensions, and that patients should be profiled across these dimensions.

One of the largest and most systematic attempts to move from the clinical knowledge contained in present-day personality disorder categories to valid dimensions of abnormal personality is that undertaken by Livesley and his colleagues. An overview of their research is given in Livesley & Jackson (1992). Livesley's programme has three main phases: constructing a theoretical classification of personality disorders and selecting items to represent the constructs on the classification; demonstrating empirically whether the constructs combine to form the expected classificatory scheme; and demonstrating validity of the classificatory scheme and its constructs by clinical prediction, generalisation to other groups, and so forth (Livesley & Schroeder 1990). In more detail, the research programme gathered items to index personality pathology using the following steps:

- Conducting a content analysis of the literature
- Having psychiatrists indicate which features of each personality disorder were most prototypical
- Organising personality disorder features into a theoretical taxonomy of personality pathology
- Writing behavioural questionnaire items to represent features of each disorder
- Conducting psychometric analyses to establish internally consistent and distinctive sets of items for each dimension of personality pathology
- Conducting factor analyses to discover which were the basic dimensions of personality within this

comprehensive set of personality disorder features (Livesley et al 1992).

Schroeder & Livesley (1991) gathered 79 descriptors to cover the 11 DSM-IIIR personality disorder categories. Multiple items were written to assess each descriptor. When 11 factors were specified in clinical and normal population samples the resemblance of the solution to DSM-IIIR personality disorder categories was limited. However, between 15 and 18 primary personality disorder traits have been identified and are measured by the Dimensional Assessment of Personality Problems – Basic Questionnaire (DAPP-BQ, Schroeder et al 1992). These are: affective lability, anxiousness, callousness, cognitive distortion, compulsivity, conduct problems, diffidence, identity problems, insecure attachment, interpersonal disesteem, intimacy problems, narcissism, passive oppositionality, rejection, restricted expression, self-harm, social avoidance and stimulus seeking.

We now meet a similar problem of level of description that was found in normal personality: that is, systems that contain large numbers of quite narrow traits usually have much overlap and can be analysed further to discover broader, independent traits. Thus, Schroeder & Livesley (1991) found that a higher-order solution of their personality disorder traits resulted in four factors, named psychopathic entitlement, dependent emotionality, social avoidance and compulsiveness. It is notable that, despite differences in methodology (e.g. self-report versus interview), subject samples (clinical versus normal population) and starting points (DSM criteria versus other systems) these same four higher order factors of personality tend to appear quite consistently. They are similar to those found by Presly & Walton (1973), Tyrer & Alexander (1979) and Mulder & Joyce (1997; and see Table 21.10). Therefore, as with normal personality, the level of description we choose may vary, but at the most general level there is some consistency. Mulder & Joyce have argued that there might be four As in personality disorder: antisocial, asocial, asthenic and anankastic. Also, with respect to the broad versus narrow traits problem, Torgersen et al (1993b) suggest that a hierarchical structure of personality disorders might be constructed. For example, a broad category or dimension of affect constricted personality disorder might be defined and then divided further to reflect specific variants.

Integrating normal and abnormal personality?

It can be seen that there is some consensus about the major dimensions of normal personality and some early but growing consensus about possible major dimensions of abnormal personality. It may be asked, therefore, if there is some overlap between normal and abnormal personality traits and whether the same systems of assessment might be used in these two domains that have until recently been seen as entirely separate. Support for such an integration comes from the finding that the structure of personality traits is very similar in both clinical (personality disorder) and general population samples (Livesley et al 1992). An American Psychiatric Association book has been devoted to studying the links between the five factor model of normal personality and personality disorders (Costa & Widiger 1994). There seems to be willingness to learn from the successes in normal personality on the part of personality disorder researchers, and it seems possible that both normal and abnormal personality will be construed, in the future, in terms of dimensions and that there will be some overlap between the two schemes (Shea 1995).

There is evidence to show that most of the major models of normal personality can account for much of the variance in personality disorder ratings. Schroeder et al (1992) studied normal personality with the Costa & McCrae (1992a) NEO-Personality Inventory-Revised (NEO-PI-R, a measure of the five factor model) and abnormal traits with the Dimensional Assessment of Personality Problems – Basic Questionnaire (DAPP-BQ) in a large group. A combined analysis of these instruments revealed five factors. Neuroticism from the NEO-PI-R was associated strongly with anxiousness, affective lability, diffidence, insecure attachment, social avoidance, identity problems, narcissism and passive oppositionality

within the DAPP-BQ. This demonstrates the pervasive influence of subjective distress – high neuroticism – among many aspects of personality disorder. Extraversion from the NEO-PI-R was associated with stimulus seeking from the DAPP-BQ. Agreeableness from the NEO-PI-R was associated negatively with interpersonal disesteem, rejection, suspiciousness and conduct problems from the DAPP-BQ. This captures the antisocial elements of personality disorders. Conscientiousness from the NEO-PI-R was associated with compulsivity (positively) and passive-oppositionality (negatively) from the DAPP-BQ, capturing the anankastic aspects of personality disorders. Social avoidance, restricted expression, identity problems and intimacy problems from the DAPP-BQ had modest negative associations with extraversion and openness factors from the NEO-PI-R. This combination of traits appears to capture the asocial (Mulder & Joyce, 1996) aspects of personality disorders. Similarly, there is significant overlap between the personality trait systems of Cloninger (Svrakic et al 1993) and Eysenck (O'Boyle 1995) and DSM-based dimensions of personality disorder.

Treatment

A number of different treatment approaches have been used in the treatment of personality disorders, including psychodynamic, behavioural, cognitive and pharmacological. Millon (1996) describes a large range of treatment strategies at length. In the majority of cases however there have been few if any systematic evaluations of the particular approaches, but, instead, support for the use of the theory is based on individual case

Table 21.10 Comparable, higher order dimensions of personality disorder as found in various psychometric studies

Walton & Presly (1973)	Tyrer & Alexander (1979)	Schroeder & Livesley (1991)	Deary et al (1995)	Mulder & Joyce (1996)	Relationship to normal personality dimensions?	
					Five factor model	Eysenck's factors
Social deviance	Sociopathy	Psychopathic entitlement	Hostility	Antisocial	Agreeableness (–)	Psychoticism
Submissiveness	Passive dependence	Dependent emotionality	Submissiveness	Asthenic	Neuroticism	Neuroticism
Obsessional–schizoid	Anankastic Schizoid	Compulsiveness Social avoidance		Anankastic Asocial	Conscientiousness Extraversion (–)	— Extraversion (–)
Hysterical						

studies. A repeated theme throughout all of the work has been the extraordinary difficulties faced in the treatment of personality disorders; most approaches that have proven successful with Axis I disorder require substantial modification when applied to personality disorders. One exception to the lack of systematic evaluation has been the use of so-called Dialectical Behavior Therapy (DBT), which has been evaluated in the treatment of borderline personality disorder and which is now being increasingly adapted for use in a range of settings. Our review therefore will concentrate first on DBT as a model for the development and evaluation of other therapies. Other therapies will then be reviewed, including cognitive therapy, psychodynamic therapies and pharmacotherapies.

Dialectical behavior therapy

Dialectical Behavior Therapy (DBT) is a complex integrative therapy developed by Marsha Linehan (1993). It draws on behavioural, cognitive and psychodynamic approaches to therapy, but also incorporates elements from Eastern philosophy and meditation techniques. Although DBT to date has been used primarily with borderline personality disorders, the collection of techniques allow it to be adapted both for other personality disorders and for a variety of outpatient and institutional settings (Linehan 1993). Linehan argues that at the core of borderline personality disorder lies a problem with emotional regulation, a problem that in fact lies at the heart of a range of Axis I and Axis II disorders (Power & Dalgleish 1997). This emotional dysregulation consists of hypersensitivity to emotional events, extreme emotional responses, and slow recovery following emotional arousal. The dysregulation is considered to arise from an innate temperamental vulnerability in interaction with 'invalidating environments'. The most extreme invalidating environment is that of sexual and physical abuse, high rates of which are consistently reported in borderline disorder (Herman et al 1989). The net effect of this interaction, according to Linehan, is that the individual's emotional development is dysfunctional, leading to a range of affective, cognitive and interpersonal problems.

The therapy itself consists of a combination of individual and group therapy formats lasting for a minimum of 12 months and with sets of aims at different stages in therapy, as outlined in the following points.

Pretreatment: orientation and commitment Negotiation of and commitment to therapy and psychoeducational input.

Stage 1 The explicit primary aim in DBT is the reduction of suicidal and other self-harming behaviours. Any parasuicidal episode is recorded by the patient and becomes the focus for the following individual therapy sessions. Exploration of the external and internal antecedents to the act occurs, and a variety of techniques is used to consider alternative problem-solving strategies for parasuicide. In addition to individual therapy sessions, there is also a weekly DBT skills group, preferably run by a different therapist. The aim of the group is to teach basic skills rather than to explore other issues, for which the individual sessions are intended. Basic skills focus on developing tolerance for distress, emotion regulation and interpersonal skills. One of the main skills taught is 'mindfulness training' based on Eastern meditation techniques. In cognitive terms, mindfulness training involves the development of a conscious tolerance or acceptance of aversive states (especially overwhelming emotions) that individuals would normally attempt to rid themselves of in dramatic ways.

Stage 2 Whereas stage 1 in DBT is primarily focused on the here-and-now, in stage 2 the patient is helped with the emotional processing of previous traumatic experiences. Only when the patient has developed the stage 1 skills does this uncovering occur, though the exploration of earlier traumatic experiences may often require further practice in the use of those skills.

Stage 3 The main aims for this stage are to help the individual develop self-esteem and to help set and work towards realistic future goals. The borderline patient typically has very poor self-esteem and general identity problems. These problems are often thought to be a consequence of the extreme invalidating traumatic experiences experienced in childhood by these individuals, therefore the final goals in therapy are to help the individual develop a more resilient self concept.

There are many other features of DBT that are described in the overview of DBT and the accompanying skills training manual (Linehan 1993). The most impressive aspect of the approach however has been its systematic evaluation in a randomised control trial of DBT versus treatment as usual (Linehan et al 1991). The study showed that there were very low drop-out rates from DBT (in contrast to findings from most treatment studies of personality disorders). After 1 year's treatment, DBT patients had lower levels of parasuicide and less severe parasuicide attempts if they did occur; they reported less anger, more social adjustment and better work performance. The overall superiority of DBT was maintained at 6 month and 12 month follow-ups (Linehan & Kehrer 1993).

Cognitive therapy

There have been two major adaptations of cognitive therapy for work with personality disorders by Beck et al (1990) and by Young (1990). The two approaches clearly have considerable overlap, though each has added considerably to the therapeutic approach used in traditional cognitive therapy for depression. Both Young (1990) and Padesky (1994) have emphasised the importance of 'early maladaptive schemata' in personality disorders. Young has argued that, whereas schemata in affective disorder are often conditional and of the form 'If X, then Y' (e.g. 'If someone important criticises me, then I am unlovable'), in personality disorders they are typically unconditional and of the form 'I am unlovable'. The fact that these schemata are formed early, often preverbally, makes them more difficult to work with. For this reason in its application to personality disorder cognitive therapy has an increased focus on the therapeutic relationship, it has adapted a number of insights from psychodynamic work with personality disorders, it has a greater emphasis on interpersonal schemata (or 'cognitive-interpersonal cycles'), and it has been extended to be of medium-term rather than short-term duration, typically lasting a year or more (Pretzer 1994). As Pretzer (1994) has summarised, there are as yet no randomised control trials of cognitive therapy for personality disorders, though there have now been a number of promising reports based on single case designs.

People with borderline and antisocial personality disorders are viewed as particularly difficult to manage. For these patients Davidson & Tyrer (1996) developed a relatively brief cognitive therapy based upon the ideas of Beck, Young and Linehan, as described above. Their series of case studies indicates relatively fast improvement in most individuals in aspects such as improving quality of relationships, reducing self-harm, increasing self-esteem and employing more adaptive and constructive behaviours. However, the changes were rarely statistically significant and this type of brief, eclectic therapy requires more study.

Psychodynamic therapies

As in the case of cognitive therapy, the application of psychodynamic therapies to personality disorders has witnessed considerable alteration in classical psychoanalytic views. The traditional 'blank therapist' standpoint is perceived as too depriving for work with personality disorder patients. Therefore, modified psychoanalytic approaches, as in the work of Kernberg and Kohut, see the therapist taking a more active and directive stance, using problem-solving strategies, and using more supportive interventions including a range of other therapies, as appropriate. These developments demonstrate that different schools of therapy are converging in their views on the optimal methods for work-

ing with personality disorders. However, as with the cognitive therapies, there are as yet no controlled trial outcome studies of these modified dynamic psychotherapies, only promising case studies and reports from treatment centres such as the Menninger Clinic (Wallerstein 1986). The use of primarily psychodynamic therapy for borderline and narcissistic personality disorders is reviewed and discussed by Higgitt & Fonagy (1992).

Miscellaneous therapies

There are several other approaches to therapy that are currently being modified or that have been tried in the past with limited success. These therapies include behaviour therapy (e.g. social skills training), interpersonal psychotherapy and pharmacotherapy. In addition, there have been numerous milieu and residential treatment programmes that have ranged from hospital inpatient wards, to therapeutic communities, to day-treatment programmes. The residential and milieu treatment programmes have often adapted ideas from a range of treatment approaches and are difficult to evaluate by strict research outcome criteria. The participants in such programmes have typically presented with a wide range of Axis I and Axis II disorders, so it is normally impossible to draw conclusions specifically about the treatment of personality disorder. See Piper et al (1996) for a recent summary of some of these programmes together with an account of their own day-treatment programme. Also informative and practically useful is the description of the inpatient psychotherapy unit for severe personality disorders given by Norton & Hinshelwood (1996).

Mention will be made therefore of two of the highlighted approaches, interpersonal psychotherapy and pharmacotherapy, given their undoubted usefulness in the treatment of personality disorder. Interpersonal psychotherapy is a treatment method developed by Klerman and his colleagues (Klerman et al 1984) for use in depression. Its rise to international prominence followed its successful use in the National Institute of Mental Health Treatment of Depression study; subsequent analysis of the outcome data showed that the 35% of depressed participants who also had at least one Axis II disorder did almost as well as those without personality disorders (Shea et al 1990). These and other subsequent findings have led to the adaptation of interpersonal psychotherapy for the treatment of personality disorders. However, we again await the outcome of systematic treatment trials before deciding on the usefulness of the approach with specific personality disorders.

Pharmacotherapy is often used in the treatment of personality disorders, though its use may be best indicated where there are accompanying Axis I disorders. For example, antidepressants may be used where there is evidence of mood disorder, whether or not an Axis I diagnosis can be made. Much of the research has focused on the treatment of borderline personality disorder (BPD) with the inevitable problems of the overlap with mood disturbance. Stein (1994) found little evidence for the effectiveness of neuroleptics or tricyclic antidepressants in BPD, though there were few placebo-controlled studies with validly diagnosed patients. There was some evidence for beneficial effects of monoamine oxidase inhibitors (MAOIs), but their effects were not separable from the 'informal psychotherapy' effectively offered by the studies involved. Additionally, there was some evidence for beneficial effects of selective serotonin reuptake inhibitors (SSRIs) on some aspects of BPD patients' behaviours. Like Stein (1994), Soloff (1994) reviewed the use of neuroleptics, antidepressants (tricyclics, MAOIs and SSRIs), lithium carbonate, carbamazepine and benzodiazepines in borderline personality disorder. There was evidence for efficacy in acute crises, though no one drug emerged as the treatment of choice and there was little evidence concerning effective maintenance treatment. He recommended that drug treatment be used as an adjunct to psychotherapy, as did Koenigsberg (1994), and that treatment efficacy be studied with respect to the various traits incorporated in the borderline concept.

Personality disorders can adversely affect treatment of comorbid Axis I disorders. Concurrent personality disorders – especially Cluster C – are associated with poorer outcomes in the drug and electroconvulsive therapy (ECT) treatments of major depression (Ilardi & Craighead 1994/5). Also, antisocial personality disorder is associated with poor outcomes in the treatment of drug abuse (Leal et al 1994). Further, the presence of obsessive–compulsive personality disorder can adversely affect the outcome of pharmacological treatment of obsessive–compulsive disorder (Cavedini et al 1997).

REFERENCES

Abramson L Y, Seligman M E P, Teasdale J D 1978 Learned helplessness in humans: critique and reformulation. Journal of Abnormal Psychology 87: 49–74

Allport G W 1937 Personality: a psychological interpretation. Holt, New York

Allport G W, Odbert H S 1936 Trait names: a psycho-lexical study. Psychological Monographs: General and Applied 47 (1, whole number 211)

Alnaes R, Torgersen S 1988 DSM-III symptom disorders (axis I) and personality disorders (axis II) in an outpatient population. Acta Psychiatrica Scandinavica 78: 348–355

APA 1994 Diagnostic and statistical manual of mental disorders, 4th edn. American Psychiatric Association, Washington, D C

Baer L, Jenike M A, Ricciardi J 1990 Standardized assessment of personality disorders in obsessive compulsive disorder. Archives of General Psychiatry 47: 826–830

Ball D, Hill L, Freeman B et al 1997 The serotonin transporter gene and peer-rated neuroticism NeuroReport 8: 1301–1304

Bandura A 1977 Social learning theory. Prentice-Hall, Englewood Cliffs

Beck A T, Freeman A, Associates 1990 Cognitive therapy of personality disorders. Guilford Press, New York

Bedford A, Foulds G 1978 Manual of the personality deviance scales. NFER-Nelson, Windsor

Benjamin J, Li L, Patterson C, Greenberg B D, Murphy D L, Hamer D H 1996 Population and familial association between the dopamine D4 receptor gene and measures of novelty seeking. Nature Genetics 12: 81–84

Bernstein D P, Cohen P, Velez C N, Schwab-Stine M, Siever L 1993 The prevalence and stability of the DSM-IIIR personality disorders in a community based survey of adolescents. American Journal of Psychiatry 150: 1237–1243

Bernstein D P, Useda D, Siever L J 1995 Paranoid personality disorder. In: Livesley W J (ed.) The DSM-IV personality disorders. Guilford Press, New York

Berrios G E 1993 Personality disorders: a conceptual history. In: Tyrer P, Stein G (eds) Personality disorder reviewed. Gaskell, London

Blackburn R 1988 On moral judgments and personality disorders: the myth of the psychopathic personality revisited. British Journal of Psychiatry 153:505–512

Bleuler E 1924 Textbook of psychiatry. Brill A A (trans). Macmillan, New York

Block J 1995 A contrarian view of the five factor approach to personality description. Psychological Bulletin 117: 187–215

Bouchard T J 1994 Genes, environment and personality. Science 264: 1700–1701

Braff D L 1986 Impaired speed of information processing in nonmedicated schizotypal patients. Schizophrenia Bulletin 7: 499–508

Carson R C 1989 Personality. Annual Review of Psychology 40: 227–248

Cattell R B, Eber H W, Tatsuoka M M 1970 Handbook for the sixteen personality factor questionnaire. Institute for Personality and Ability Testing, Champaign, IL

Cavedini P, Erzegovesi S, Ronchi P, Bellodi L 1997 Predictive value of obsessive–compulsive personality disorder in antiobsessional pharmacological treatment. European Neuropsychopharmacology 7: 45–49

Child D (1990) The essentials of factor analysis. Cassell, London

Cleckley H 1976 The mask of sanity, 6th edn. Mosby, St Louis, MO

Cloninger C R 1987 A systematic method for clinical description and classification of personality. Archives of General Psychiatry 44: 573–588

Cloninger C R, Svrakic D M, Przybeck T R 1993 A psychobiological model of temperament and character. Archives of General Psychiatry 50: 975–990

Conn S R, Rieke M L 1994 The 16P F fifth edition technical manual. Institute for Personality and Ability Testing, Champaign, IL

Coryell W H, Zimmerman M 1989 Personality disorder in the

families of depressed, schizophrenic and never-ill probands. American Journal of Psychiatry 146: 496–502

Costa P T, McCrae R R 1977 Age differences in personality structure revisited: studies in validity, stability and change. Aging and Human Development 8: 261–275

Costa P T, McCrae R R 1992a NEO-PI-R professional manual. Psychological Assessment Resources, Odessa, FL

Costa P T, McCrae R R 1992b Trait psychology comes of age. Nebraska Symposium on Motivation 39: 169–204

Costa P T, McCrae R R 1992c Four ways five factors are basic. Personality and Individual Differences 13: 653–665

Costa P T, Widiger T A 1994 Personality disorders and the five factor model of personality. American Psychiatric Association, Washington, DC

Dahl A A 1990 Empirical evidence for a core borderline syndrome. Journal of Personality Disorders 4: 192–202

Dahl A A 1995 Commentary on borderline personality disorder. In: Livesley W J (ed.) The DSM-IV personality disorders. Guilford Press, New York

Davidson K M, Tyrer P 1996 Cognitive therapy for antisocial and borderline personality disorders: single case study series. British Journal of Clinical Psychology 35: 413–429

Deary I J, Matthews G 1993 Personality traits are alive and well. Psychologist 6: 299–311

Deary I J, Bedford A, Fowkes F G R 1995 The personality deviance scales: their development, associations, factor structure and restructuring. Personality and Individual Differences 19: 275–291

Digman J M, Takemoto-Chock N K 1981 Factors in the natural language of personality: re-analysis, comparison and interpretation of six major studies. Multivariate Behavioral Research 16: 149–170

Ebstein R P, Novick O, Umansky R et al 1996 Dopamine D4 receptor (D4DR) exon III polymorphism associated with the human personality trait of novelty seeking. Nature Genetics 12: 78–80

Engler B 1995 Personality theories: an introduction, 4th edn. Houghton Mifflin, Boston

Epstein S 1977 Traits are alive and well. In: Magnusson D, Endler NS (eds) Personality at the crossroads. Erlbaum, Hillsdale, NJ

Eysenck H J 1967 The biological basis of personality. Thomas, Springfield, IL

Eysenck H J 1992 Four ways the five factors are not basic. Personality and Individual Differences 13: 667–673

Eysenck H J, Eysenck S B G 1969 Personality structure and measurement. Routledge & Kegan Paul, London

Eysenck H J, Eysenck S B G 1982 Recent advances in the cross-cultural study of personality. In: Spielberger C D, Butcher J N (eds) Advances in personality assessment. Erlbaum, Hillsdale, NJ

Eysenck H J, Eysenck S B G 1991 The Eysenck personality questionnaire revised. Hodder & Stoughton, Sevenoaks

Eysenck M W, Eysenck H J 1980 Mischel and the concept of personality. British Journal of Psychology 71: 191–204

Friedman M, Rosenman R H 1974 Type A behavior and your heart. Knopf, New York

Freud S 1973 Introductory lectures on psychoanalysis. Penguin, Harmondsworth

Freud S 1986 Historical and expository works on psychoanalysis. Penguin, Harmondsworth

Funder D C 1996 The personality puzzle. Norton, New York

Galton F 1884 Measurement of character. Fortnightly Review 36: 179–185

Goldberg L R 1993 The structure of phenotypic personality traits. American Psychologist 48: 26–34

Goldberg L R, Saucier G 1996 Evidence for the big five in analyses of familiar personality adjectives. European Journal of Personality 10: 61–77

Gough H G 1987 California personality inventory administrator's guide. Consulting Psychologists, Palo Alto, CA

Grunbaum A 1984 The philosophical foundations of psychoanalysis. University of California Press, Berkeley

Gunderson J G, Phillips K 1991 Borderline personality disorders and depression: a current overview of the interface. American Journal of Psychiatry 148: 967–975

Gunderson J G, Ronningstam E, Smith L E 1995a Narcissistic personality disorder. In: Livesley W J (ed.) The DSM-IV personality disorders. Guilford Press, New York

Gunderson J G, Zanarini M C, Kisiel C L 1995b Borderline personality disorder. In: Livesley W J (ed.) The DSM-IV personality disorders. Guilford Press, New York

Guntrip H 1969 Schizoid phenomena, object relations and the self. International Universities Press, New York

Hare R D 1985 A comparison of procedures for the assessment of psychopathy. Journal of Consulting and Clinical Psychology 53: 7–16

Hare R D, Hart S D 1995 Commentary on antisocial personality disorder: the DSM-IV field trial. In: Livesley W J (ed.) The DSM-IV personality disorders. Guilford Press, New York

Hare R D, Hart S D, Harpur T J 1991 Psychopathy and the proposed DSM-IV criteria for antisocial personality disorder. Journal of Abnormal Psychology 100: 391–398

Hartshorne H, May M A 1928 Studies in deceit. Macmillan, New York

Henderson D K 1939 Psychopathic states. Norton, New York

Herman J L, Perry J C, van der Kilk B A 1989 Childhood trauma in borderline personality disorder. American Journal of Psychiatry 146: 490–495

Higgitt A, Fonagy P 1992 Psychotherapy in borderline and narcissistic personality disorder. British Journal of Psychiatry 161: 23–43

Hirschfeld R M A, Shea M T, Weise R 1995 Dependent personality disorder. In: Livesley W J (ed.) The DSM-IV personality disorders. Guilford Press, New York

Holt R R 1985 The cuurent status of psychoanalytic theory. Psychoanalytic Psychology 2: 289–315

Horney K 1937 The neurotic personality of our time. Norton, New York

Horney K 1945 Our inner conflicts. Norton, New York

Hyler S E 1994 PDQ-4. New York State Psychiatric Institute, New York

Hyler S E, Skodol A E, Kellman H D, Oldham J M, Rosnick L 1990 Validity of the personality diagnostic questionnaire-revised: comparison with two structured interviews. American Journal of Psychiatry 147: 1043–1048

Ilardi S S, Craighead W E 1994/5 Personality pathology and response to somatic treatments for major depression: a critical review. Depression 2: 200–217

Kalus O, Bernstein D P, Siever L J 1995 Schizoid personality disorder. In: Livesley W J (ed.) The DSM-IV personality disorders. Guilford Press, New York

Kendler K S, Hewitt J 1992 The structure of self-report schizotypy in twins. Journal of Personality Disorders 6: 1–17

Kendler K S, Gruenberg A M, Tsuang M T 1985 Psychiatric illness in first degree relatives of schizophrenic and surgical control patients: a family study using DSM-III criteria. Archives of General Psychiatry 42: 770–779

Kendler K S, Walsh D, Su Y et al 1989 The Roscommon

family and linkage study of schizophrenia: preliminary report. Abstracts of the 28th Annual Meeting of the American College of Neuropsychopharmacology, p. 56.

Kenrick D T, Funder D C 1989 Profiting from controversy: lessons from the person–situation debate. American Psychologist 43: 23–34

Kernberg O 1967 Borderline personality organisation. Journal of the American Psychoanalytic Association 15: 641–685

Kernberg O 1976 Borderline conditions and pathological narcissism. Aronson, New York

Kernberg O 1988 Hysterical and histrionic personality disorders. In: Cooper A, Frances A, Sacks M (eds) The personality disorders and neuroses. Lippincott, Philadelphia

Klerman G L, Weissman M M, Rounsavilee B J, Chevron E S 1984 Interpersonal psychotherapy of depression. Aronson, New York.

Koch J A 1891 Die psychopathischen Minderwertigkeiten. Maier, Ravensburg

Koenigsberg H W 1994 The combination of psychotherapy and pharmacotherapy in the treatment of borderline patients. Journal of Psychotherapy Practice and Research 3: 93–107

Lazare A, Klerman G, Armor D 1966 Oral, obsessive and hysterical personality patterns. Archives of General Psychiatry 14: 624–630

Lazare A, Klerman G, Armor D 1970 Oral, obsessive and hysterical personality patterns: replication of factor analysis in an independent sample. Journal of Psychiatric Research 7: 275–279

Leal J, Ziedonis D, Kosten T 1994 Antisocial personality disorder as a prognostic factor for pharmacotherapy of cocaine dependence. Drug and Alcohol Dependence 35: 31–35

Lesch K-P, Bengel D, Heils A et al 1996 Association of anxiety-related traits with a polymorphisn in the serotonin transporter gene regulatory region. Science 274: 1527–1531

Lewis G, Appleby L 1988 Personality disorder: the patients psychiatrists dislike. British Journal of Psychiatry 153: 44–49

Lilienfeld S, Van Valkenburg C, Larntz K, Akiskal H 1986 The relationship of histrionic personality disorder to antisocial personality and somatization disorder. American Journal of Psychiatry 143: 718–722

Linehan M M 1993 Cognitive–behavioral treatment of borderline personality disorder. Guilford Press, New York

Linehan M M, Kehrer C S 1993 Borderline personality disorder. In: Barlow D H B (ed.) Clinical handbook of adult psychological disorders. Guilford Press, New York

Linehan M M, Armstrong H E, Suarez A, Allmon D, Heard H L 1991 Cognitive–behavioral treatment of chronically parasuicidal borderline patients. Archives of General Psychiatry 48: 1060–1064

Livesley W J (ed.) 1995a The DSM-IV personality disorders. Guilford Press, New York

Livesley W J (ed.) 1995b Commentary on dependent personality disorder. In: The DSM-IV personality disorders. Guilford Press, New York

Livesley W J, Jackson D N 1992 Guidelines for developing, evaluating, and revising the classification of personality disorders. Journal of Nervous and Mental Disease 180: 609–618

Livesley W J, Schroeder M L 1990 Dimensions of personality disorder: the DSM-IIIR cluster A diagnoses. Journal of Nervous and Mental Disease 178: 627–635

Livesley W J, Reifer L I, Sheldon A E R, West M 1987 Prototypicality ratings of DSM-III criteria for personality disorders. Journal of Nervous and Mental Disease 175: 395–401

Livesley W J, Schroeder M L, Jackson D N 1990 Dependent personality disorder and attachment problems. Journal of Personality Disorders 4: 232–240

Livesley W J, Jackson D N, Schroeder M L 1992 Factorial structure of traits delineating personality disorders in clinical and general population samples. Journal of Abnormal Psychology 101: 432–440

Loehlin J 1992 Genes and environment in personality development. Sage, Newbury Park, CA

Loranger A W, Janca A, Sartorius N 1997 Assessment and diagnosis of personality disorders: the ICD-10 international personality disorder examination (IPDE). Cambridge University Press, Cambridge

Lykken D T, McGue M, Tellegen A, Bouchard T J 1992 Emergenesis: genetic traits that may not run in families. American Psychologist 47: 1565–1577

McCrae R R, Costa P T 1994 The stability of personality: observations and evaluations. Current Directions in Psychological Science 3: 173–175

Malhotra A K, Virkkunen M, Rooney W, Eggert M, Linnoila M, Goldman D 1996 The association between the Dopamine D_4 receptor (D_4DR) 16 amino acid repeat polymorphism and novelty seeking. Molecular Psychiatry 1: 388–391

Maslow A 1987 Motivation and personality, 3rd edn. Harper & Row, New York

Masterson J 1972 Treatment of the borderline adolescent: a developmental approach. Wiley, New York

Matthews G, Deary I J 1998 Personality traits. Cambridge University Press, Cambridge

Miller T Q, Turner C W, Tindale R S, Posavac E J, Dugoni B L 1991 Reasons for the trend toward null findings in research on type A behavior. Psychological Bulletin 110: 469–485

Miller T Q, Smith T W, Turner C W, Guijarro M L, Haller A J 1996 A meta-analytic review of research on hostility and physical health. Psychological Bulletin 119: 322–348

Millon T 1969 Modern psychopathology. W B Saunders, Philadelphia

Millon T 1996 Disorders of personality: DSM-IV and beyond. Wiley, New York

Millon T, Martinez A 1995 Avoidant personality disorder. In: Livesley W J (ed.) The DSM-IV personality disorders. Guilford Press, New York

Mischel W 1968 Personality and assessment. Wiley, New York

Morey L C 1988 Personality disorders in DSM-III and DSM-IIIR: convergence, coverage and internal consistency. American Journal of Psychiatry 145: 573–577

Moskowitz D S 1988 Cross-situational generality in the laboratory: dominance and friendliness. Journal of Personality and Social Psychology 69: 915–924

Mulder R T, Joyce P R 1997 Temperament and the structure of personality disorder symptoms. Psychological Medicine 27: 99–106

Nigg J T, Goldsmith H H 1994 Genetics of personality disorders: perspectives from personality and psychopathology research. Psychological Bulletin 115: 346–380

Norton K, Hinshelwood R D 1996 Severe personality disorder: treatment issues and selection for in-patient psychotherapy. British Journal of Psychiatry 168: 723–731

O'Boyle M 1995 DSM-IIIR and Eysenck personality measures among patients in a substance abuse programme. Personality and Individual Differences 18: 561–565

Oldham J M, Frosch W A 1988 Compulsive personality disorder. In: Michels R et al (eds) Psychiatry. Lippincott, Philadelphia

Padesky C A 1994 Schema change processes in cognitive therapy. Clinical Psychology and Psychotherapy 1: 267–278

Paris J 1995 Commentary on narcissistic personality disorder. In: Livesley W J (ed.) The DSM-IV personality disorders. Guilford Press, New York

Pervin L A 1993 Personality: theory and research. Wiley, New York

Peterson C, Semmel A, von Baeyer C, Abramson L Y, Metalsky G I, Seligman M E P 1982 The attributional style questionnaire. Cognitive Therapy and Research 6: 287–300

Pfohl B 1995 Histrionic personality disorder. In: Livesley W J (ed.) The DSM-IV personality disorders. Guilford Press, New York

Pfohl B, Blum N 1995 Obsessive–compulsive personality disorder. In: Livesley W J (ed.) The DSM-IV personality disorders. Guilford Press, New York

Pfohl B, Coryell W, Zimmerman M, Stangl D 1987 Prognostic validity of self-report and interview measures of personality in depressed patients. Journal of Clinical Psychiatry 48: 468–472

Pilkonis P A 1995 Commentary on avoidant personality disorder: temperament, shame, or both? In: Livesley W J (ed.) The DSM-IV personality disorders. Guilford Press, New York

Pilkonis P, Frank E 1988 Personality pathology in recurrent depression: nature prevalence, and relationship to treatment response. American Journal of Psychiatry 145: 435–441

Piper W E, Rosie J S, Joyce A S, Azim H F A 1996 Time limited day treatment for personality disorders: integration of research and practice in a group program. American Psychological Association, Washington

Power M J, Dalgleish T 1997 Cognition and emotion: from order to disorder. Psychology Press, Hove

Presly A S, Walton H J 1973 Dimensions of abnormal personality. British Journal of Psychiatry 122: 269–276

Pretzer J 1994 Cognitive therapy of personality disorders: the state of the art. Clinical Psychology and Psychotherapy 1: 257–266

Regier D A, Boyd J H, Burke J D et al 1988 One-month prevalence of mental disorders in the United States. Archives of General Psychiatry 45: 977–986

Reich J, Noyes R, Yates W 1989 Alprazolam treatment of avoidant personality traits in social phobic patients. Journal of Clinical Psychiatry 50: 91–95

Robins L N, Tipp J, Przybeck T 1991 Antisocial personality. In: Robins L N, Regier D A (eds) Psychiatric disorders in America. Free Press, New York, p. 258

Rogers C 1951 Client-centred therapy: its current practice, implications and theory. Houghton Mifflin, Boston

Rosenman R H, Brand R, Jenkins D, Friedman M, Straus R, Wurm M 1975 Coronary heart disease in the Western Collaborative Group Study: final follow up of 8.5 years. Journal of the American Medical Association 233: 872–877.

Rotter J B 1954 Social learning and clinical psychology. Prentice-Hall, Englewood Cliffs

Rotter J B 1966 Generalised expectancies for internal versus external central reinforcement. Psychological Monographs 80, no.1

Rusten J 1993 Theophrastus: Characters. Harvard University Press, Cambridge

Rychlak J F 1988 The psychology of rigorous humanism, 2nd edn. New York University Press, New York

Saucier G, Goldberg L R, 1996 Evidence for the big five in analyses of familiar English personality adjectives. European Journal of Personality 10: 61–77

Saville P, Holdsworth R, Nyfield G, Cramp L, Mabey W 1984 The occupational personality questionnaire (OPQ). Saville & Holdsworth, London

Schneider K 1923 Psychopathic personalities. Cassell, London

Schroeder M L, Livesley W J 1991 An evaluation of DSM-IIIR personality disorders. Acta Psychiatrica Scandinavica 84: 512–519

Schroeder M L, Wormworth J A, Livesley W J 1992 Dimensions of personality disorder and their relationships to the big five dimensions of personality. Psychological Assessment 4: 47–53

Schuerger J M, Zarrella K L, Hotz A S 1989 Factors that influence the temporal stability of personality by questionnaire. Journal of Personality and Social Psychology 56: 777–783

Schulz P M, Schulz S C, Goldberg S C, Ettigi P, Resnick R J, Friedel R O 1986 Diagnoses of the relatives of schizotypal outpatients. Journal of Nervous and Mental Disease 174: 457–463

Shea M T, Pilkonis P A, Beckham E, Collins J F, Elkin I, Sotsky S M, Docherty J P 1990 Personality disorders and treatment outcome in the NIMH Treatment of Depression Collaborative Research Program. American Journal of Psychiatry 147: 711–717

Shea T 1995 Interrelationships among categories of personality disorders. In: Livesley W J (ed.) The DSM-IV personality disorders. Guilford Press, New York

Siever L J, Keffe R, Bernstein D P et al 1990 Eye tracking impairment in clinically identified schizotypal personality disorder patients. American Journal of Psychiatry 147: 740–745

Siever L J, Bernstein D P, Silverman J M 1995 Schizotypal personality disorder. In: Livesley W J (ed.) The DSM-IV personality disorders. Guilford Press, New York

Skodol A E, Oldham J M, Rosnick L, Kellman H D, Hyler S E 1991 Diagnosis of DSM-IIIR personality disorders: a comparison of two structured interviews. Methods in Psychiatric Research 1: 13–26

Soloff P H 1994 Is there any drug treatment of choice for the borderline patient? Acta Psychiatrica Scandinavica 89(suppl): 50–55

Spitzer R L, Endicott J, Gibbon M 1989 Crossing the border into borderline personality and borderline schizophrenia: the development of criteria. Archives of General Psychiatry 36: 17–24

Spitzer R L, Williams J B W, Gibbon M, First M 1990 User's guide for the structured clinical interview for DSM-IIIR. American Psychiatric Association, Washington DC

Stein G 1994 Physical treatments of the personality disorders. Current Opinion in Psychiatry 7: 129–136

Svrakic D M, Whitehead C, Przybeck T R, Cloninger C R 1993 Differential diagnosis of personality disorders by the seven-factor model of temperament and character. Archives of General Psychiatry 50: 991–999

Thurstone L L 1947 Multiple factor analysis. Chicago University Press, Chicago

Torgersen S 1995 Commentary on the cluster A personality

disorders. In: Livesley W J (ed.) The DSM-IV personality disorders. Guilford Press, New York

Torgersen S, Onstad S, Skre I, Evardsen J, Kringlen E 1993a 'True' schizotypal personality disorder: a study of co-twins and relatives of schizophrenic probands. American Journal of Psychiatry 150: 1662–1667

Torgersen S, Skre I, Onstad S, Evardsen J, Kringlen E 1993b The psychometric–genetic structure of DSM-IIIR personality disorder criteria. Journal of Personality Disorders 7: 196–213

Tupes E C, Christal R E 1961 (reprint 1992) Recurrent personality factors based on trait ratings. Journal of Personality 60: 225–251

Tyrer P 1988 Personality disorders: diagnosis, management and course. Wright, Boston

Tyrer P, Alexander I 1979 Classification of personality disorder. British Journal of Psychiatry 135: 163–167

Tyrer P, Casey P, Ferguson B 1991 Personality disorder in perspective. British Journal of Psychiatry 159: 463–471

Wallerstein R S 1986 Forty-two lives in treatment: a study of psychoanalysis and psychotherapy. Guilford Press, New York

Walton H J, Presly A S 1973 Use of a category system in the diagnosis of abnormal personality. British Journal of Psychiatry 122: 259–268

Weiner B 1986 An attributional theory of motivation and emotion. Springer, New York

Whitlock F A 1982 A note on moral insanity and psychopathic disorders. Bulletin of the Royal College of Psychiatrists 6: 57–59

WHO 1992 International statistical classification of diseases and related health problems, 10th revision. World Health Organization, Geneva

Widiger T, Frances A, Warner L, Bluhm C 1986 Diagnostic criteria for the borderline and schizotypal personality disorders. Journal of Abnormal Psychology 95: 43–51

Widiger T A 1989 Psychiatrists' responses to personality disorder. British Journal of Psychiatry 154: 266

Widiger T A, Corbitt E M 1995 Antisocial personality disorder. In: Livesley W J (ed.) The DSM-IV personality disorders. Guilford Press, New York

Widiger T A, Costa P T 1994 Personality and personality disorders. Journal of Abnormal Psychology 103: 78–91

Widiger T A, Shea T 1991 Differentiation of axis I and axis II disorders. Journal of Abnormal Psychology 100: 399–406

Wright J C, Mischel W 1987 A conditional approach to dispositional constructs: the local predictability of social behavior. Journal of Personality and Social Psychology 53: 1159–1177

Young J 1990 Cognitive therapy for personality disorders: a schema-focused approach. Professional Resource Exchange, Saracota

Zanarini M C, Gunderson J G, Frankenburg F R, Chauncey D L 1989 The revised diagnostic interview for borderlines: discriminating BPD from other axis II disorders. Journal of Personality Disorders 3: 10–24

Zimmerman M 1994 Diagnosing personality disorders: a review of issues and research methods. Archives of General Psychiatry 51: 225–245

Zuckerman M 1991 Psychobiology of personality. Cambridge University Press, Cambridge

22
Learning disability

Walter J. Muir

INTRODUCTION

The last decade has witnessed a huge change in the care of people with learning disability. Ideas about the locus of care, and the types of medical and social intervention that are appropriate, are in continuing flux and even the nomenclature used to describe an individual's complex patterns of disabilities has changed. Our large institutions that provided accommodation and the day-to-day needs of so many individuals, for so much of their lives, are rapidly becoming a thing of the past. More than ever it is a time when the psychiatrist involved in the medical care of this large and important group of people must reassess his or her role in providing for their multifaceted needs. The pressures of community care are different from those of the institution, and often more complex and difficult to deal with. Nevertheless there are also aspects which are invariable. The majority of people with learning disability, whether children or adults, live at home with their families. The role of the family in the care and support of the person is thus pivotal, and helping the family is often as integral to the part played by the psychiatrist as helping the person with the disability directly.

It is impossible in this chapter to cover all aspects of learning disability that may be important to the psychiatrist. To understand learning disability it is really necessary to understand the huge variety of conditions with which it is associated. There have been great advances in molecular genetics, leading to significant progress in our understanding of the cause of many of these conditions, especially the two most common genetic conditions in which learning disability is a component – Down's syndrome and fragile X. These conditions are paradigms for other causes of learning disability and will be discussed in some detail.

It is also a time to reassess our concept of disorder and disease with reference to learning disability. In the past it was often, either openly or implicitly, considered a disease. The problem with the person was said to be his or her 'learning disability', and treatments and interventions were based on an assumption that common denominators permeated this group of people and could be acted on in the same sorts of ways. Thus our hospitals which cared for large numbers of people with learning disability were often divided into wards for people with 'special needs' or 'challenging behaviours' with similar uniformity in therapies. Such broad groupings are no more representative of the underlying conditions than the term mental illness is of the multifarious collection of psychiatric disorders. This simple use of the term learning disability cannot do for the future. To understand the role learning disability plays in a person's life, we must consider what it means with respect to that person's adaptation to the internal and external environments present at a given time, and think more broadly than in terms of the patient-focused medicine taught in the traditions of Osler. Barton Childs (1995) has championed this important change in our view of disease, the originator being Garrod, who was the pioneer in the study of inborn errors of metabolism that underlie many of the disorders causing learning disability. The competency of any person's adaptation to the world, at any point in time, is a composite of three main histories or time frames, the proximate cause of disease depends on the immediate molecular (and thus genetic) and sociocultural situation, the second time frame is the developmental history, and the third, the genetic and cultural inheritance patterns. The factors are interlinked – the present biochemical and biophysical constitution is the product of the developmental interactions between inherited genetic factors and the external environment. For a given situation, disease or disorder is seen as an incongruence between these factors and the present environment, and thus it is hard to imagine a condition which does not have a dependence on genetic factors for its appearance. This concept of disorder as incongruence is epitomised by learning disability, and the move away from simple definitions based only on intellectual impairment, to include problems with social adaptation, is congruent with this model. Learning disability is a common denominator in many conditions, and it is with the conditions and their psychiatric and medical associates that the focus should rest. In this chapter important conditions which have learning disability as a component will be examined. In people with severe and profound learning disability, even where an underlying condition cannot apparently be found, an organic cause can nearly always be presumed. Even in mild learning disability, previously thought to be multifactorial (and often, by implication, indefinable in simple molecular terms), there is increasing evidence for the involvement of organic pathologies.

THE DEVELOPMENT OF THE CONCEPT

Learning disability is a concept rather than a condition, and a vast variety of specific and non-specific pathologies include it as part of their clinical state. Definitions have used administrative and social outcomes as their constructs and learning disability, in itself, is not a disease or illness. A confusion between learning disability and mental illness continues, and is still present in our legal definitions, with the terms mental disorder or mental impairment used to encompass both ideas. Alternatively, there was a school of thought, now rapidly disappearing, that regarded mental illness and learning disability as mutually exclusive, and signs and symptoms of mental illness in people with learning disability were interpreted as behavioural or adaptive problems – a source of considerable inappropriate treatment and distress for the individuals concerned.

However, it has long been recognised that there are certain common denominators in the definition of learning disability, the most important being a combination of intellectual impairment, an associated degree of social or adaptive dysfunction, and an onset before adulthood. Many people with intellectual impairment without social or adaptive problems do not become involved with the special services for people with learning disability, and so are never classified as having learning disability. On the other hand, it is recognised that many people who come to use such services may have no measurable reduction in intellectual skills, but by default of their social or adaptive problems, and especially problems in living independently, attract the label of having learning disability, a label that, if incorrectly given, is every bit as hard for that person to shake off as the misdiagnosis of a mental illness. The number of people in learning disability hospitals with IQ measures in the normal range was the most obvious and notorious result of incorrect labelling (Castell & Mittler 1965), and their detention in hospital was legitimised by the concept of moral insanity.

That many children and adults suffered from this triad of core difficulties in varying degrees and combinations had been recognised for centuries. Descriptions of learning disability have been found from ancient Egyptian texts, and concern for the welfare of those with 'weak minds' was an ancient duty, noted especially in writings dating from at least the first millennium BC from the Far East (China, Confucius; Persia, Zoroaster). A distinction between those with mental illness and people with what we would now call learning disability was made early (Clarke 1975) and enshrined in English legislature at the time of Edward II ('King's Prerogative', De prærogativa regis, 1325) for the purposes of managing a person's estate. The 'born fool' was to have his estate managed for him; the person whose mental state fluctuated between periods of lucidity and madness was to have his estate held in trust until he was ready to reassume it. Berrios has pointed out (1994) that attempts at a medical subdescription of disorders associated with learning disability began during the 17th and 18th centuries. Cullen studied the various heterogeneous classifications of learning disability and classified congenital amentia as being present from birth. By the early 19th century the problems of understanding learning disability taxed those same psychiatrists studying mental illness. Pinel advanced the idea of acquired and congenital forms of learning disability. Esquirol proposed a developmental rather than disease-oriented model, and Séguin was the major advocate of an interventionist and educationalist approach to treatment. In Britain, Pritchard did not consider learning disability to be a form of mental illness and stressed that the developmental delay was present from birth. He also graded the extent of the intellectual impairment from the profound through to the normal. However, in Europe the confusion between mental illness and learning disability meant that the then current idea that degeneration was a part of the natural history of psychoses was extended to learning disability, culminating in the eugenic arguments and mass sterilisation programmes which started as early as 1907 in some states of the USA.

NOSOLOGY

Much confusion has occurred over the correct term to describe people who have a combination of intellectual impairment and adaptive dysfunction, which has left a number of terms in concurrent use within any one country, completely different terms used in others, or the same terms used to mean different things. All our major classification systems use the term mental retardation. At present the term learning disability has wide acceptance in Britain, and has largely, although not yet legally, replaced the term mental handicap. It is used throughout this chapter, although it should be remembered that for the person the most important qualifiers are their first and second personal names and not a descriptive label.

Over the last century the terminology used has been interlinked with legislature, and various legal definitions have been introduced as the older terms were (slowly) replaced. For instance the term 'simpleton', which was adopted by Duncan for those whom we would now regard as having mild learning disability, was later replaced with the term 'moron' by Goddard, as it was felt that the former term was too derogatory (Penrose 1954). This in turn was later replaced with 'feeble-minded'. In the UK the Idiots Act, (1886) made for the 'provision of asylums for care, education and training of those classed as idiots and imbeciles from birth or from an early age'. The Lunacy Act, 1890 however continued to confuse the mentally ill with the learning disabled. A lunatic was 'an idiot or person of unsound mind'. Many of the now unacceptable terms used to describe the extent of a person's learning disabilities were enshrined in the Mental Health Act of 1913. The act defined the classes of 'mental defectives', using the terms idiots, imbeciles and feeble-minded persons roughly corresponding to profound/severe, moderate and mild degrees of learning disability. A fourth term, moral defective, was also included. This could be interpreted as a person with learning disability and seriously irresponsible aggressive or criminal behaviour, but the act only implied, and never stated, that the person who was a 'moral defective' should also have learning disability, leading to the admission to hospital of many without learning disability.

The amended act (1927) gave a definition of mental deficiency as 'a condition of arrested or incomplete development of mind' existing before the age of 18 years whether arising from inherent causes or induced by disease or injury. If mind is taken to encompass both social, adaptive and intellectual functioning then the definition is surprisingly close to that used today. A Royal Commission (1954/55), in part set up to account for the number of compulsory admissions with a diagnosis of moral deficiency, recommended revising terminology and abolishing the term moral deficiency. It's key recommendations were to allow voluntary admission to hospital, improved facilities for community care with an emphasis on training rather than occupation, the provision of suitable hostels for adolescents, that early certification of children should be avoided and they should be provided with welfare services as for normal children, the coordination of hospital and local authority services in the care of the learning disabled,

and a system whereby appeals against detention could be heard by independent tribunals. Most of these ideals are still held today. The 1959 and 1960 Mental Health Acts introduced the terms mental subnormality (England and Wales) and mental deficiency (Scotland). More recently, the 1983 and 1984 Acts have introduced the terms of mental impairment and mental handicap, although they are both classified as forms of mental disorder along with mental illness. This is unfortunate, as it tends to maintain the confusion that learning disability is a congener of mental illness.

The transcultural confusion in terminology also began early. Fifty years ago 'feeble-minded' equated to mild learning disability in the UK, but was a blanket term for all types of learning disability in the USA. (Baker & Cantwell 1995). In Germany and Scandinavia the term 'oligophrenia' was widely employed. Oligophrenia was used by Kraepelin to signify all levels of learning disability. Bleuler (1923) recognised the heterogeneity of oligophrenia and that it included both congenital and childhood acquired learning disability.

For research purposes the most widely used term is mental retardation, which has the merit of being understandable irrespective of culture. The terms learning disability or learning difficulties used in the UK mean specific and different Axis I disorders in the USA. Even in the UK learning difficulties have been applied to conditions as disparate as profound degrees of intellectual impairment and specific reading disorder. It would seem wise to restrict the terminology to learning disability for general purposes (and this is generally preferred by people with learning disability), and accept the use of mental retardation in research.

Systems of classification: ICD-10, DSM-IV and the AAMR

The terminology used to describe and categorise people with learning disability has advanced considerably with the multiaxial systems of DSM-IV (APA 1994) and the American Association on Mental Retardation criteria (AAMR 1992). ICD-10 (WHO 1992, 1993) also uses similar criteria, although not a multiaxial approach. All three systems are similar in their requirements for diagnosis and in stressing the duality of problems – intellectual impairment coupled with diminished social adaptive functioning. In DSM-IV the term mental retardation is used for learning disability and is coded on Axis II, as opposed to specific clinical conditions such as learning disorders and pervasive developmental disorders which are coded on Axis I. Thus a person with autistic disorder on Axis I can be qualified as also having mental retardation (Axis II) which may be mild, moderate, severe or profound. The person may also have another medically relevant condition such as epilepsy, which would be coded on Axis III; psychosocial and environmental problems are noted on Axis IV, and Axis V allows an overall assessment of adaptive functioning. DSM-IV defines mental retardation as being characterised by:

- intellectual impairment (IQ of 70 or less)
- impaired adaptive functioning
- onset before 18 years of age.

The AAMR classification uses the same three basic criteria as DSM-IV but is more complex, with extensive definitions of patterns and degrees of support needs. ICD-10 again uses the term mental retardation and lists it amongst the mental and behavioural disorders. Although it states that the impairment occurs during the developmental period, there is no age criterion as in the other two systems. Any other disorders that can be identified as being present can be used to generate an independent additional code. The same IQ bands used in DSM-IV are used to define the degrees of intellectual impairment. The DSM-IV guidelines are perhaps the most useful, certainly for research in learning disability. The definition of mental retardation as an Axis II label, rather than a primary disorder, also fits best with its highly heterogeneous causation (Bregman & Harris 1995).

PREVALENCE AND EPIDEMIOLOGY

Bearing in mind the dual nature of the definitions of learning disability – the intellectual impairment and the problems of adaptive functioning – it is difficult to give an overall picture of how many people have learning disability, and in practice most weight is given to the intellectual deficit, which has the simple merit of being quantifiable. The best measure of intellectual impairment is still IQ testing, and although the pattern of strengths and weaknesses within the overall test result are perhaps more important, the global score is used to define the subgroups of learning disability. It is important to remember that any IQ score will have an error value of plus or minus 5 points, which renders the cut-off levels defining mild, moderate and severe levels arbitrary for any individual. However, for a population an IQ of 70 is around two standard deviations from the mean, and can be considered distinctive. Using this definition, about 3% of the population should have learning disability. In practice differential mortality and diagnostic changes with time mean that this estimate is too high and a widely accepted figure is around 1–2% (Bregman & Harris 1995). Recently introduced short forms of the standard Wechsler Adult Intelligence Scale

are highly correlated with results using the entire test (Nagle & Bell 1995), and their ease of use may result in more accurate estimates.

It has long been known that the distribution of IQ in the population is not gaussian but asymmetric, with more people having low and very low IQ values than expected. The easiest explanation is that the lower tail of the curve comprises two overlapping distributions and this has led to a 'two-group' interpretation. Numerically the greater group is that defined by the gaussian tail (i.e. the expected 2.27% of the population with IQ less than 70), and this has been called 'sociocultural' learning disability or 'physiological' learning disability based on the assumption that it is determined by similar multifactorial influences controlling IQ levels over 70.

Estimates of the prevalence of mild learning disability tend to differ from expectation, sometimes to surprisingly low levels, indicating the difficulty in defining caseness. In studies of children in Gothenburg the very low level of 0.4% was reported, and in northern Finland it was 0.55% (Hagberg et al 1981, Rantakallio & von Wendt 1986). In over 50% of people with mild learning disability no cause can be attributed. Around 15–20% had perinatal hypoxia, and congenital causes are present in 10%. Only 5% have a defined genetic syndrome, including trisomies. In the Scandinavian studies, about the same number had the fetal alcohol syndrome.

The excess at more severe levels of disability is considered to be due to an organic or pathological group with a cluster of disorders of definable aetiology, including genetic causes and environmental agents such as hypoxia, trauma and infections. Some people in this group will have disorders such as autism, cerebral malformation syndromes and cerebral palsy without a yet defined cause, but assumed to have definite biological factors in their genesis. The 'organic' group comprises around 0.3–0.4% of the general population and 10–20% of those with learning disability.

Causes of 'sociocultural' learning disability

IQ is not the sole criterion in determining learning disability, and there must be problems with social adaptation before the label is given; thus many with IQ below the 70 point cut-off will never be involved with the health or social services. The number who will require special education will likewise vary, but obviously to a lesser extent. IQ scores are not stable over time and the intellectual development of the individual is highly complex and plastic. IQ is, however, heritable. Twin studies have shown a high degree of concordance in IQ between twins reared together and apart (Bouchard et al 1990). Adoption studies have suffered from methodological shortcomings but Horn et al (1979) looked at the relation between the IQ of children who were adopted within a few days of birth and the IQ of their biological and adoptive mothers. The heritability was high for young children but became less for older children. The children were also largely adopted into affluent homes, and the adoptive parents had IQs well above average. Mild learning disability is known to be overrepresented in families from social classes IV and V, especially where sibships are large, where the rooms are relatively overcrowded and there is an association with poverty (Birch et al 1970, Blackie et al 1975). Related to such findings are the reports of a higher prevalence of all levels of learning disability amongst black 10-year-old children from Atlanta, Georgia compared with white controls (Murphy et al 1995). For children with mild learning disability around 50% of the variance was related to economic status, the education level of the mother, birth order and maternal age at childbirth (Yeargin-Allsopp et al 1995). The social interpretation is changing, however, and more recent studies suggest up to 45% of people with mild learning disability may have definite organic factors, including subtle chromosome rearrangements and perinatal insults from toxins such as alcohol. Thus estimates of the importance of polygenic factors and social disadvantage may have to be revised downwards, although it is clear that they are crucial factors in increasing the risk of mild learning disability. At present there are a number of ongoing trials which aim to alter the outcomes by removing the sociocultural and educational disadvantages for children with mild learning disability. A comprehensive intervention programme for low birthweight infants during the first 3 years of life seemed to increase the intellectual development measured at 3 years (Blair et al 1995) but longer term outcomes are awaited. A programme for early educational and social intervention for children from disadvantaged families has been followed up to the age of 15 and the results have been compared with those for a control group without such interventions, with encouraging results (Campbell & Ramey 1995). The findings, if confirmed, have profound implications for the support and care of children at risk of mild learning disability.

PREVENTION

An obvious aim is to prevent a child developing learning disability. The control of neonatal infections and improvements in obstetric care in developed countries have limited many associated factors. There has also been a substantial (but not uniform) increase in survival of small-for-date deliveries, without a concomitant increase in the numbers with learning disability. However, other environmental associates, such as poverty and social disadvantage, are not so easily remedied, and more recently recognised prenatal insults, such as the fetal alcohol syndrome and the teratogenic effects of substance abuse and associated infections such as those caused by the human immunodeficiency virus (HIV), may be a major problem for the future. The prenatal diagnosis of disorders associated with learning disability is becoming applicable to many genetic and metabolic conditions, especially with the advent of molecular diagnostics based on the polymerase chain reaction, in association with improved methods of amniocentesis, chorionic villus biopsy and cell sorting methodologies. However, this must be tempered by the knowledge that the only 'treatment' available for many is termination, and therapies based on gene targeting or even product replacement are still to be developed.

Prenatal testing

A wide range of conditions, especially those associated with large scale chromosome abnormalities or anatomical malformations, can be detected in utero. Specific examples are Down's syndrome and the neural tube defects, discussed later in this chapter.

Newborn screening

In 1962 Guthrie developed an assay to measure phenylalanine concentrations in small amounts of blood and paved the way for the widespread neonatal diagnosis of phenylketonuria, an inherited inborn error of metabolism frequently associated with learning disability. The detection, from a small blood sample spotted on to filter paper (the Guthrie test), allowed early treatment of phenylketonuria, with a drop in the incidence of associated learning disability. Soon afterwards, Guthrie developed a series of other tests for maple syrup urine disease, histidinaemia and galactosaemia. Today, screening for metabolic disease has developed into a fine art. The tests are deliberately set to be oversensitive to avoid false negatives and further investigations are needed to confirm the diagnosis in any positive cases. Screening can also be done for congenital hypothyroidism, a previously widespread cause of learning disability (cretinism). Usually the initial screen is for a low thyroxine level and, if positive, this is followed by thyrotrophin estimation. It seems from such programmes that congenital hypothyroidism may occur in 1:3600–1:5000 newborns (Rovet et al 1987).

Carrier or heterozygote screening

Advances in genetics allow the inheritance of many conditions to be studied, and carriers of a condition, who may not display any clinical consequences themselves, can be identified and counselled. This is the province of the clinical geneticist, but the psychiatrist may be called to advise and help on those conditions specifically associated with learning disability. For treatable conditions, studies on the extended family of the proband may help allay anxieties and fears about possible transmission of the condition. However, where adequate treatments are not available, and this applies to most inherited conditions associated with learning disability, the situation is much more difficult, and carriers may be stigmatised. Such diagnosis is available for the fragile X syndrome. Diagnosis of this in a young child has tremendous implications for the rest of the family (see below) and requires careful genetic examination, counselling and possibly long-term follow-up. Mass screening programmes are more problematic. They will have to undergo extensive cost–benefit analysis if the conditions are not directly treatable.

AETIOLOGY

Associated chromosomal abnormalities

Although human chromosomes have been studied for over 100 years it was only in the middle of the 20th century that the correct human somatic and meiotic counts were established (Tijo & Levan 1956). Advances in cell culture techniques and the advent of DNA staining methodologies allowed the delineation of chromosome abnormalities in association with a wide variety of clinical conditions associated with learning disability, and chromosome banding still lies at the heart of the cytogenetic services. In the last decade genetic advances have allowed the development of the discipline of molecular cytogenetics, and a new era of discovery is occurring. An outline of various chromosomal conditions associated with learning disability is given in Table 22.1.

The trisomies

Classical chromosomal abnormalities are found to occur in around 0.6% of newborn infants. Trisomies are the most common single type of human chromosome abnormality, and in addition to occurring in at least 0.36% of all births (autosomal trisomies 0.12%; sex chromosome aneuploidies 0.24% – see Evans 1977), they are found in over 25% of spontaneous abortions, and are thus the leading cause of pregnancy loss. Trisomies of the large chromosomes are rare, usually lethal in utero, but occur more frequently in early spontaneous abortions. Trisomies of the smaller chromosomes, and especially 13, 18, 21 and the sex chromosomes, are compatible with a full-term pregnancy. Patau's syndrome (trisomy 13) and Edward's syndrome (trisomy 18) are associated with severe congenital abnormalities and profound learning disability. Children with trisomy 13 usually die around 4 months of age, with few surviving into the first years of life. Trisomy 18 is also lethal and most die in the first year. Trisomy 16 is of interest in that its occurrence seems almost entirely related to maternal age. Trisomy 8 is being increasingly described, especially with newer methods of fetal investigation and diagnosis, but the fetus rarely survives until birth. There is an excess of male fetuses and mosaicism is usual. In surviving trisomy 8 there is a moderate degree of learning disability. However, in terms of both numbers affected, and the importance to the specialist in the psychiatry of learning disability, trisomy 21 or Down's syndrome holds first place. Numerically the individual trisomies of the sex chromosomes are next in rank.

Partial trisomies, involving duplication of a segment of the chromosome or an entire chromosome arm, are known for many chromosomes; those of 4p, 5p, 6p, 7q, 9p, 10p, 10q, 11q, 12p, 13q, 14q, 15q and 20p, although rare, are the most important (de Grouchy & Turleau 1990). Deletion of a whole autosome is usually lethal. A partial deletion leads to monosomy of that segment of the chromosome, and partial monosomy of 4p, 4q, 5p, 9p, 11q, 12p, 13q, 18p, 18q, 21p and q have been described. The unitary features of all these rare syndromes are learning disability of varying degrees and growth retardation. With the advent of more sensitive fluorescent hybridisation studies of karyotype, new syndromes associatied with more restricted chromosomal rearrangements are being regularly described.

Down's syndrome

Down's syndrome is pictured in 17th century paintings (Zellwiger 1968) but the first detailed description of the condition was given by James Langdon Down (1866), who used the term mongolian idiocy. The epithet, with its incorrect and racial assumptions of origin, has been changed to Down's syndrome (or Down syndrome). Shuttleworth (1909) studied the associates of the condition and found that people with Down's syndrome tended to be the youngest in their sibship, and that there was clear association with advanced maternal age at the time of birth. A variety of causes were later put forward to account for the development of Down's syn-

Table 22.1 Some important chromosomal abnormalities associated with learning disability

Chromosome involved	Type of rearrangement	Common name	Comments
21	Trisomy	Down's syndrome	Rare forms due to robertsonian translocations
13	Trisomy	Patau's syndrome	Robertsonian translocations in around 20%
18	Trisomy	Edward's syndrome	Nearly all due to full trisomy
8	Trisomy		Usually mosaic, variable learning disability, rare
X	Sex chromosome monosomy	Turner's syndrome	Learning disability rare
XXX	Sex chromosome trisomy	Trisomy X	Mild learning disability to normal
XXY	Sex chromosome aneuploidy	Klinefelter's syndrome	Mild learning disability to normal, male phenotype
XYY	Sex chromosome aneuploidy		Mild learning disability to normal, male phenotype
5p	Partial monosomy	Cri du chat syndrome	Profound learning disability, microcephaly
4p	Partial monosomy	Wolf–Hirschhorn syndrome	Severe learning disability, many survive to adult
17p11.2	Small deletion	Smith–Magenis syndrome	Usually seen on general microscopy, self-injurious behaviours
16pter–p13.3	Small deletion	α-Thalassaemia mental retardation	Cryptic terminal deletion
15q11–q13	Microdeletion	Prader–Willi syndrome	Contiguous gene syndrome – paternal origin of deletion; rarely uniparental disomy – maternal
15q11–q13	Microdeletion	Angelman's syndrome	Contiguous gene syndrome – maternal origin of deletion; very rarely uniparental disomy – paternal
17p13.3	Microdeletion	Miller–Dieker syndrome	Profound learning disability, lissencephaly
22q11.2	Microdeletion	DiGeorge's / Velo-cardio facial syndrome	Mild to moderate learning disability / behavioural, psychiatric disorders

drome, ranging from maternal alcoholism to tuberculosis and hypothyroidism (Smith & Berg 1976). The cause is now known to be, in nearly all cases, the presence of an extra full or partial chromosome 21.

Genetics That non-disjunction of genetic factors could be a cause of Down's syndrome was early and presciently suggested by Waardenburg (1932) but full corroboration had to await the advent of karyotyping methodologies. Lejeune (1959) showed that an extra acrocentric chromosome existed in the fibroblasts of people with Down's syndrome, and in parallel studies this was also found to be a feature of bone marrow cells from men and women with Down's syndrome by Jacobs and her coworkers in Edinburgh (1959); all studies from a variety of populations have shown that Down's syndrome is associated with an extra copy of chromosome 21.

Studies on the molecular origins of the extra chromosome show it to be maternal in over 90% of cases (Koehler et al 1996), but there is still uncertainty as to whether the error occurs in the first or second meiosis. Currently it seems that 75% of maternal errors occur during the first meiotic division, whereas most paternal errors (around 60%) occur at the second. Mitotic errors account for around 5% of cases. The mechanism involved in the creation of the trisomy is uncertain. It is clear that in maternal first meiosis-derived trisomies aberrant (reduced rate) recombination occurs between chromosomes that will undergo eventual non-disjunction, and this is especially prominent in exchanges near the centromere, leading to reduced chiasma formation in this zone. One hypothesis is that an aberrant pattern of recombination down the chromosome may lead to a greater susceptibility for bivalents to segregate abnormally. In the ageing ovum there may be an increased dependence on the correct pattern of chiasma formation to ensure normal segregation of chromosomes, with the maternal age effect seen as a double-hit phenomenon with ageing oocyte factors acting on a predisposed chromosomal set-up.

Nearly 95% of people with Down's syndrome have full trisomy 21. Robertsonian translocations involving acrocentric chromosomes account for another 5%. Some of these (around 45%) are due to a robertsonian fusion chromosome (usually between chromosomes 14 and 21) being inherited from a balanced carrier parent, leading to a trisomy of the long arms of chromosome 21, which contains most of the genes for this chromosome (depending on the whether the fusion is mono- or dicentric, some component of the short arms of 21 may also be present). Phenotypically the individual has full Down's syndrome. The small short arms of the acrocentric chromosomes contain many repetitive sequences and show a great deal of sequence homology, which may be related to the tendency to form fusion chromosomes. The fusion and its normal homologue are able to pair during meiosis. Other robertsonian translocations arise de novo and most of these are of maternal origin (Shaffer et al 1992). The formation of these de novo chromosomes does not seem to have a maternal or paternal age association. The situation is even more complex in that proximal 21q loci usually show a great deal of homozygosity, even if the parent chromosomes were heterozygous for alleles in this region. Fusion with chromosomes 21 and 22 can occur but much more rarely. A familial balanced carrier of a robertsonian (21;21) fusion is especially unfortunate as all offspring will have Down's syndrome (monosomy 21 being non-viable).

A further 5% of people with Down's syndrome will have two cell lines in their body, one with full trisomy 21 and one with a normal karyotype. Such mosaicism may arise from loss of a chromosome 21 in a trisomic cell early in embryogenesis or from an early mitotic non-disjunction. Mosaicism is a complex phenomenon with varying percentages in different cell lines (lower in white cells than fibroblasts, for example) and varies with time within the same cell line.

Prenatal screening   The relation of trisomy 21 to maternal age is well established, but it is important to remember that up to 80% of children with Down's syndrome are born to women under 35 years. Maternal age considerations are thus only one factor in preventing Down's syndrome. In the UK, screening of mothers over the age of 35 is routine, but this is not the case for younger mothers. The most commonly used marker for fetal Down's syndrome is a lowered level of α-fetoprotein in the mother's serum (Merkatz et al 1984). More recently a combination of maternal α-fetoprotein, human chorionic gonadotrophin and urinary oestriol has been used to calculate the risk for a younger mother of carrying a fetus with Down's syndrome (Wald et al 1988). A very large prospective study of over 25 000 mothers combined serum screening with ultrasound and was able to detect 58% of fetuses with Down's syndrome (Haddow et al 1992). A more invasive technique is amniocentesis guided by ultrasound scanning, with the culturing and karyotyping of fetal cells obtained from a sample of amniotic fluid. The main indication for this is advanced maternal age. Tests for fragile X and other conditions can also be made using DNA from the sample. The test is carried out between 15 and 22 weeks of pregnancy and carries a risk (0.5%) of losing the pregnancy which adds to the risk of spontaneous second trimester miscarriage. Chorionic villus sampling is a method of obtaining placental tissue through trans-cervical or transabdominal routes; it also carries an increased risk of fetal loss. Its main advantage over amniocentesis is that it is an earlier procedure (10–12 weeks of pregnancy). Very early chorionic villus sampling has been associated in some reports with the prevalence of fetal limb abnormalities (Firth 1991) and it requires a highly experienced operator for its success.

Advances in ultrasound, especially colour Doppler imaging, have led to an increasing detection rate of systemic abnormalities associated with fetal Down's syndrome. Heart defects and gastrointestinal abnormalities (especially duodenal atresia) can be detected. These features in a fetus would indicate screening for trisomy, but may only be detectable later in pregnancy. More subtle variations such as thickening of the nuchal skin fold and cystic hygromas (Nicolaides et al 1992) hold promise of a higher sensitivity in specialist centres.

It is now possible to use the polymerase chain reaction to specifically amplify small amounts of fetal DNA from the maternal circulation. Basically the method involves isolating nucleated red blood cells contributed by the fetus, using a flow sorting method to identify those carrying specific fetal cell surface protein markers. The method needs to be established to ascertain the false-positive and false-negative rates, but holds great promise in allowing the early identification of a number of conditions associated with learning disability, including Down's syndrome (Rose 1996).

In vitro fertilisation allows the possibility of pre-implantation diagnosis of aneuploidies. Attempts have been made to use fluorescent in situ techniques to identify aneuploidy, as yet with mixed results.

Clinical features Down's syndrome can be considered as a paradigm of a multisystem disorder. The clinical variety is associated with a multiplicity of metabolic and developmental disorders resulting from the presence of the extra chromosome and its genes, and almost every organ system in the body can be involved. It is important to have some working knowledge of these, as the interplay between the various systems can be extensive and confusing. The physical features of someone with full trisomy 21 are usually well enough developed at birth to allow immediate diagnosis.

There is a generalised disturbance of growth. The mean height for adult men with Down's syndrome is around 1.5 metres, and for women 1.4 metres. Growth is reduced more in the limbs than the trunk. There is, however, the complication that the rate of growth may differ at different ages, and in spite of the reduced stature the intrinsic bone development seems normal. In fact the height at 10 years, as in normal individuals, predicts the final adult height in children with Down's syndrome (Rarick & Seefeldt 1974) and plasma growth hormone is not reduced. However, serum insulin-like growth factor (IGF-1) remains at a constant level throughout life, rather than showing the normal twofold difference between adult and childhood levels (Sara et al 1983). Over 30% of both sexes tend to be overweight and in one sample nearly 50% were obese (Prasher 1995a). This was related to living at home rather than in supported accommodation.

The outcome of differential growth anomalies in Down's syndrome is especially seen in the shape of the head and the features of the face. The head shows a marked brachycephaly, which develops after birth, with a reduction in anteroposterior diameter. The maxilla is also decreased in size relative to the mandible (Allanson et al 1993). The bridge of the nose may be underdeveloped and the eyes close together, with the characteristic slope and presence of an epicanthic fold. The hypopharynx is narrowed and there is a greater susceptibility to sleep apnoea, especially in young people (Howenstine 1992). Psychological disturbance, such as excessive daytime restlessness and behavioural difficulties, in association with snoring can indicate this diagnosis, for which remedial treatments are available. The joints of the neck should also be a focus of attention in young adults and adolescents. Instability of the atlantoaxial joint is associated with transverse ligament weakness and causes symptoms in around 1.5% (Pueschel & Scola 1987). The X-ray diagnosis can be difficult and require repeated films from different views to establish it. It is often asymptomatic even when seen on X-ray, and intervention is controversial. There is a general consensus that it should not overtly restrict physical activity, save in those sports where there is a high risk of

neck strain. Isolated cases of death in association with medical procedures due to this anomaly continue to be reported, including death during tracheal intubation and in physical restraint. The need for, and the use of, physical restraint procedures in adolescents and adults with Down's syndrome and severe behavioural disturbance needs to be very carefully evaluated.

One of the most striking features of the newborn child with Down's syndrome is the muscular hypotonia, some degree of which is an almost constant finding. Involuntary reflexes that participate in forming the background muscle tone are reduced in intensity, as is voluntary muscle control such as hand grip. The decrease in tone, which is thought to be central in origin, continues in older children (Morris et al 1982). Hypotonus and feeding difficulties during the neonatal period are important correlates of early mortality. In a large Californian follow-up study of the predictors of mortality in people with Down's syndrome (Eyemann et al 1991), individuals with one or more major medical problem (such as heart and gastrointestinal abnormalities) can expect to survive to at least the age of 31. If there is no major medical problem survival to at least 50 years can be expected.

Congenital heart disease occurs in around 50% of children with Down's syndrome and is still a leading cause of infant mortality (Mikkelsen et al 1990) which requires early detection and treatment if pulmonary hypertension is to be avoided. The echocardiogram can reveal most defects (Wells et al 1994). Gastrointestinal anomalies are less prevalent and can be of a variety of types. The incidence of congenital duodenal obstruction is strikingly raised to nearly 300 times that in the general population but the indications for treatment are the same.

The skin shows characteristic developmental anomalies which once played a key part in the diagnostic process. The dermatoglyphs of the palm and sole are arranged in specific ways, with ulnar loops on the second finger and an arched tibial pattern on the hallucis of the foot, and there is often a marked transverse palmar crease. The use of these in diagnosis is now limited but they are of interest in that they represent developmental problems that occur during the third month of fetal life. The skin itself is soft in children with Down's syndrome, and the hair is soft and fine but has a tendency to dryness in adults; this may also occur in association with hypothyroidism. The circulation to the extremities is often poor and acrocyanosis in cold weather is frequent.

It is unfortunate that the peripheral sensory systems are very often affected in Down's syndrome. In the eye, squints are common (up to 20%) and may require surgical correction. Myopia and other refractive errors are also present in over one-third of patients. A large number of other conditions have also been described and may be missed on general screening (Roizen et al 1994). With the importance of visuospatial learning in children with Down's syndrome the correction of such abnormalities is essential. Later in life cataracts become more common. Keratoconus, an acute and painful inflammation of the cornea leading to scarring and the formation of a cone-shaped protrusion, is rarer but sight-threatening. There seem to be two peaks of incidence – one in late teenage years and one after the age of 40.

Hearing difficulties are also marked. Otitis media affects many children, and this may be exacerbated by structural anomalies of the ear. Audiometry and auditory short latency (brainstem) evoked potential studies have shown that the majority of children have a unilateral or bilateral hearing loss to some degree (Squires et al 1986). This hearing loss is added to by the later onset of sensorineural deafness. The more profoundly disabled can find using corrective hearing aids and spectacles difficult, but as they facilitate communication, efforts should be made to encourage their use. The provision of appropriate specialist audiometry services can help greatly (Yeates 1995).

The immune system in Down's syndrome is also commonly affected (Ugazio et al 1990) and deficiencies in immunological competence and surveillance may be a common denominator for several disorders, including infections, tumours and endocrine disturbances. Infection, especially pneumonia, is still the leading cause of death in Down's syndrome and the mortality rate from infections is markedly raised when compared with that of the general population. Although B lymphocytes appear to have normal morphology there is a tendency to raised levels of IgG and IgM antibodies. Cell-mediated immunity is also altered, with a small decrease in T lymphocyte numbers. The thymus is often severely dysmorphic, and there is an associated T cell maturation delay. A high frequency of transient leukaemoid reactions occur in the newborn, and the white cells involved always seem to be fully trisomic for chromosome 21 (Siebel et al 1984). The risk of true leukaemia is raised in both children and adults, and apart from the first year, where acute non-lymphocytic leukaemia predominates, the spectrum of types is similar to that seen in the general population (McCoy & Epstein 1987). The treatment response in people with Down's syndrome may differ and methotrexate may be toxic at even standard doses.

Probably related to the immune disturbance is the increased prevalence of thyroid dysfunction (usually hypothyroidism) at all ages. Some cases are congenital but most are of later onset, and the presence of thyroid antibodies is variable. However, up to 20% of adolescents and adults with Down's syndrome may suffer from it, and it is a crucial differential diagnosis to be eliminated in the presentations of behavioural disturbance, depression and dementia in these age groups. Diabetes mellitus is also more prevalent, and again is postulated to have an autoimmune basis.

The central nervous system   The overall average weight of the brain is decreased by around 10–20%. Other changes are more subtle. There is a decrease in the number of gyri, cortical thinning in some areas and the middle lobe of the cerebellum tends to be underdeveloped. The fine structure is also altered and there is a decrease in neuronal numbers in a rather patchy fashion but including in the cerebellum, locus coeruleus and basal forebrain. In the last area the decrease is thought to be specific to cholinergic systems (Holtzman et al 1996). Individual neurone morphology is also altered, with abnormal dendrite formation. There are also anomalies in neurone-associated cells, including glial cell enlargement.

The development of the brain in Down's syndrome involves abnormal degrees of neuronal differentiation, abnormal cortical lamination (Golden & Hyman 1994) and a decrease in the number of neurones eventually formed (Wisniewski et al 1986). Studies of cultured fetal neurones (Busciglio & Yankner 1995) show normal initial differentiation but subsequent degeneration and programmed cell death (apoptosis). The cell death may involve defects in the mechanisms that scavenge free radicals in the cell. Such defects may underlie not only the developmental anomalies that occur in Down's syndrome but also predispose to the development of dementia. Free radical excess is certainly one key candidate hypothesis for the development of Alzheimer's disease in the normal population, and one of the triplicated genes on chromosome 21 is superoxide dismutase, which performs a scavenging function. The presence of pathological features of Alzheimer's disease including neurofibrillary tangles and amyloid-containing plaques is well documented and these have been found in practically all individuals with Down's syndrome over the age of 35 on whom postmortem studies have been performed (Wisniewski et al 1985). The brain distribution of these lesions is similar to that of Alzheimer's disease of the normal population. The dementia associated with Down's syndrome is further discussed below.

Associated learning disability   Intellectual disability becomes apparent during the first few months of life and increases as the child becomes older, with a progressive increase in the delay in attaining developmental milestones (Share & Veale 1974). Very early milestones, such as smiling at faces, may be delayed for only a few months, but later milestones, especially language related such as the ability to form a sentence of three words, may be delayed for up to 2 years. After the first decade the intellectual disability tends to remain relatively static or only slowly progressive, with some late teenagers showing a second growth phase followed by a period of stability until the decline with advancing years, which, in many cases, is accelerated by dementia (Gibson 1978, Shepperdson 1995). At around 5 years of age most children will have test scores in the high moderate to mild range of learning disability, and early educational and psychological interventions may be a key to maintaining this (see below). The variability in intellectual attainment is well demonstrated by children with Down's syndrome who are not mosaic in karyotype having test scores in the normal (low average) range (Kouseff 1978). There is evidence that the parents' educational levels, which partly reflect their IQs, have an association with the degree of intellectual disability of their Down's syndrome children (Libb et al 1983, Sharav et al 1985).

Early intervention and intellectual and social achievement

Although the earlier studies on the comparative upbringing of children with Down's syndrome suffered from methodological difficulties, the general conclusion is that children brought up in their own homes do better than those in institutions or foster care. One study has shown an increase of over 17 IQ points at about the age of 10 years if the child is brought up at home (Ludlow & Allen 1979). In the comparative longitudinal survey reported by Shepperdson (1995) the attainment levels were linked to the social class of the parents, and were also higher for children of younger mothers who gave greater stimulation.

A single measure such as IQ is, however, grossly inadequate for understanding the profile of disability experienced by the person with Down's syndrome. Some consensus findings are emerging from studies of the neuropsychological strengths and weaknesses associated with Down's syndrome. There seems to be a preservation of visuomotor skills and coordination (Thase et al 1984). Haxby (1989) found that young adults with Down's syndrome, without confounding medical problems, did better on tests of short-term memory based on visual and spatial (Corsi's block tapping tests) rather than verbal tasks. Other adults with learning disabilities but without a specific syndrome showed the opposite effect. Wang & Bellugi (1994) compared groups of adolescents with Down's syndrome and William's syndrome and confirmed that the subjects with Down's syndrome did less well on the digit span test and better on the block tapping test. The young adults with Down's syndrome also performed better on tests of manual dexterity and sequencing of movements. The relative deficit in auditory short-term memory may be important in overall attainment, and is compounded by the hearing problems that children and adults with Down's syndrome are susceptible to (Gravel & Wallace 1995). A detailed speech, language and hearing assessment should thus be part of the background to any educational intervention programme for children with Down's syndrome, and strategies should be adopted that combine written and oral communication methods. Computer-based teaching could be helpful in this context.

Psychiatric disorders

There is an increasing realisation that people with Down's syndrome are affected by the same types and numbers of psychiatric disorders as anyone in the general population. Overall prevalence figures vary. Myers & Pueschel (1991) found psychiatric disorders of some form in nearly 18% of children and 27% of adults with Down's syndrome. In a large study (using World Health Organization criteria) of over 200 adults, psychiatric disorders occurred at a rate approaching 30% (Prasher 1995b). In the study by Myers & Pueschel (1991) around 6% had major depressive disorder. Collacott et al (1992) found a higher incidence (11%) when all types of depression were included, and this was nearly three times greater than in a matched learning disability control group. Previous reports suggesting that adults with Down's syndrome were less prone to mania (Sovner et al 1985) were possibly due to underreporting of bipolar disorder rather than a true decrease in incidence. Clinically the depression tends to present with marked biological features (Pawlarczyk & Beckwith 1987, Myers & Pueschel 1995), with prominent sleep disturbance, psychomotor slowing or agitation. Much less apparent are the cognitive associates such as loss of interest in day-to-day activities, poor concentration, or thoughts of guilt or worthlessness. Suicidal thoughts are uncommon. Hallucinations (auditory and visual), however, may occur in a substantial percentage. The relative lack of cognitive and subjective symptoms of depression means that the differential diagnosis can be difficult. The functioning of those who have depressive illness seems to be poorer than matched groups, with continuing problems in adaptive behaviour even after recovery (Collacott & Cooper 1992). The main alternatives are dementia, physical disorders including hypothyroidism, and bereavement reactions. Dementia and depression may coexist and some have suggested a definite relationship between the two in Down's syndrome (Burt et al 1992). Bereavement is an especially common occurrence for adults with Down's syndrome. There are two contributing factors. Firstly, the maternal ageing effect means many parents are older when their child is born; secondly, and more importantly, the adult with Down's syndrome is usually looked after by his or her parents no matter what age they are. The response to tricyclic antidepressants is usually good, with some claims as to the greater effectiveness of those with predominant actions on the serotonergic system. Sometimes a trial of antidepressants is needed to help establish the diagnosis.

Schizophrenia has been long described as co-occurring with Down's Syndrome (Neville 1959) although it is not commonly diagnosed (Duggirala et al 1995). Small-scale studies suggest that a chronic negative outcome is not common (Cooper et al 1995).

Other disorders reported in adults with Down's syndrome include obsessive–compulsive disorder and Tourette's syndrome but the true incidence of these is uncertain. Children with Down's syndrome also seem at increased risk from autism (Howlin et al 1995) but, again, whether there is a definite causal relationship, whether there is an increased incidence or whether the co-occurrence is truly sporadic, is not certain.

Alzheimer's disease   The development of dementia in adults with Down's syndrome was noted only 10 years after Langdon Down's original report (Fraser & Mitchell 1876), and the pathological features of Alzheimer's disease were described at postmortem examination in an adult with Down's syndrome in 1929 (Struwe 1929). In fact plaques and neurofibrillary tangles occur in the brains of almost 100% of adults with Down's syndrome (Kolata 1985, Wisniewski et al 1985a, 1985b) and the anatomical distribution of these lesions is similar to that seen in Alzheimer's disease in elderly subjects from the general population. These changes, however, can begin as early as the second decade of life in adults with Down's syndrome, and have even been described in a 12 year old (Cork 1990). The main component of the amyloid in Down's syndrome is the amyloid $\beta A4$ protein with 42 amino acid residues ($A\beta_{42}$). This is coded for by the amyloid precursor protein (APP) gene on chromosome 21, mutations in which are the cause of a class of relatively rare, early-onset familial dementia in the general population (Goate et al 1991). APP exists in three isoforms. In the brain of the fetus with Down's syndrome there is an almost fivefold increase in the expression of the APP-95 variant (Neve et al 1988), and a fourfold increase in the APP-751 and APP-770 forms. These latter two isoforms have structures suggesting that they may act as protease inhibitors, and levels are increased in the hippocampus and striatum of adults with Down's syndrome (Neve et al 1990). The role of the APP in the development of pathology is still unclear, and there must be some mechanism to explain why the plaques and tangles do not, on average, appear until the third decade, whereas the APP levels are persistently high throughout life.

Teller et al (1996) showed that the abnormal accumulation of $A\beta_{42}$ occurs from the 21st week in utero, long before the formation of any plaques, right through to the 61st year of life – a feature that is not seen in matched control subjects. Normally the APP is processed into $A\beta_{40}$ with only small amounts of $A\beta_{42}$ produced. However, in Down's Syndrome the $A\beta_{42}$ peptide is present even in the absence of amyloid plaques. They suggested that in Down's syndrome a mechanism must exist to degrade this protein and prevent it aggregating, and that it may be this mechanism that fails with age, rather than the protein deposition into plaques being the proximate cause of the disease. Another candidate is the copper–zinc-requiring superoxide dismutase gene (CuZnSOD) that lies in close proximity to the APP gene on the long arm of chomosome 21. SOD acts as a free radical scavenger of forming hydrogen peroxide, which is the substrate for other enzymes to break down to water. Defective metabolism of reactive oxygen species is certainly a feature of fetal Down's syndrome neurones. Duplication of this gene itself is not a necessary factor involved in producing the learning disability but occurs in nearly all subjects with Down's syndrome. Gliosis is also a prominent feature in Down's syndrome and the gene coding for a key glial calcium binding protein subunit ($S100\beta$) is also found on chromosome 21. Interleukin 1 is a cytokine produced by macrophages and promotes gliosis. It is also involved in the cellular regulation of APP uptake. Interleukin 1-containing cells are markedly increased in people with Down's syndrome and it may be a clue linking a defective immune response to the regulation of already aberrantly expressed proteins. It is also conceivable that all these factors may act together to induce the histological changes and the temporal sequence of the disease.

Clinical dementia in adults   The signs and symptoms of clinical dementia do not occur with the same frequency as the histopathological changes; a broad range of prevalences, from 6% to 75%, has been reported (Rabe et al 1990), probably reflecting differences in diagnostic criteria and tests used, and cohort effects in a period where the longevity of the person with Down's syndrome has markedly changed. At the beginning of the 20th century the average life expectancy for someone with Down's syndrome was around 9 years (Holland et al 1993). Now nearly 15% of men with Down's syndrome and around 20% of women are over the age of 55 (McGrother & Marshall 1990), with most of this change occurring in the last 30 years. There is a need to separate the effects of normal ageing in Down's syndrome not due to Alzheimer's pathology from those of the pathology itself. It is perhaps unfortunate that the concept of premature ageing has been applied widely to all the clinical changes in adults with Down's syndrome, when in fact most of the evidence for this concept is, as Epstein (1995) points out rather circuitously, based on Alzheimer's neuropathology. The problem is further compounded by the difficulty of diagnosis of dementia using standard criteria in adults with Down's syndrome, and the fact that the presentation may show several features that are atypical of dementia in the general population (Dalton et al 1993).

Longitudinal studies have shown that adults over the age of 50 with Down's syndrome showed a greater rate of loss of adaptive behaviours than comparison groups with other causes of learning disability (Zigman et al 1996a), and that the adaptive loss is global rather than specific. Some studies found little evidence for deterioration in cognitive measures, including short-term memory, in Down's syndrome adults (Devenny et al 1992, Burt et al 1995), but in these studies Alzheimer-type dementia was an exclusion criterion, and they focused on an age group largely below 50 years (Zigman et al 1996b). Studies looking at a wider age spread do show definite declines, especially in tasks involving planning and attention (Das et al 1995). Overall there is now considerable evidence from a wide range of cross-sectional and longitudinal studies that dementia develops in a sizeable proportion of adults with Down's syndrome, and is especially likely over the age of 50 (Berg et al 1993).

Prediction of who will and who will not develop dementia amongst adults with Down's syndrome is not possible at present, although some studies have attempted to address this question. Changes in neuropsychological measures and in the timing of late auditory event-related potentials over a 2 year time period have been described, and a marked increase in the latency of the P300 waveform may indicate the onset of dementia before clinical signs are apparent (Blackwood et al 1988, Muir et al 1988). However, the high prevalence of hearing loss in older subjects with Down's syndrome makes such tests difficult. The alleles of genetic polymorphism associated with the apolipoprotein E gene on chromosome 19 may act as weighting factors for the development of senile dementia (reviewed in Pericak-Vance & Haines 1995). The protein produced by this gene binds to amyloid β peptide in the plaques and tangles of Alzheimer's disease. The most common allele in Western populations is termed APOE3. Being homozygous or heterozygous for a less common allele, APOE4, is associated with an increased risk and decreased age of onset of late-onset forms of Alzheimer-type dementia in the general population, but studies on adults with Down's syndrome have yielded conflicting results. The rarest allele, APOE2, is associated with a protective effect against the development of dementia both in the general population and in Down's syndrome. Although it is a promising development the APOE genotype still needs further validating research before it can be considered as a clinical test to add to the dementia screening repertoire in Down's syndrome.

Although there has been recent progress through brain imaging in the identification of structural (Schapiro et al 1992) and functional (Deb et al 1992) correlates of changes that precede its clinical appearance, the diagnosis at present is almost entirely clinically based. Estimates of the incidence of presenile dementia in adults with Down's syndrome obviously rely on valid indicators of the condition. The incidence is age related, with most follow-up studies indicating that around 10% of adults with Down's syndrome above the age of 40 will show clinical evidence of dementia per year. This leads to an overall prevalence of around 40% for clinical dementia in adults over the age of 40, which correlates well with the numbers found in practice. Knowledge of the number of persons in a given region who have Down's syndrome is surprisingly limited, at least in the UK. A survey of adult training and resource centres, voluntary agency-run day centres, clients on the lists of community learning disability nurses, and information on children known to the Scottish Down's Syndrome Association in 1995 (Table 22.2) found 343 persons with Down's syndrome in community settings in the Lothian Region of Scotland, of whom 139 were over 36 years old. These are minimum numbers, and between 30 and 40% of these will be showing some clinical signs of dementia. These figures are broadly comparable with those found in Lanarkshire and Ayrshire by Irving (1992). The increase in the number of adults with Down's syndrome

Table 22.2 Number of people in the community with Down's syndrome by age in Lothian Region, Scotland (minimum figures)	
Age range (years)	Number
Under 10	61
10–15	26
16–25	40
26–35	77
36–49	109
50–59	28
Over 60	2
Total	343
Total over 36 years	139

is projected to continue and peak at least 50% above 1990 levels between the years 2000 and 2020 (Steffelaar & Evanhuis 1989). For a presenile dementia this will represent a considerable number of affected people.

For diagnosis of any form of dementia there must be a demonstrable deterioration in short-term and later long-term memory, along with a worsening ability to focus attention and maintain personal orientation (Geldmacher & Whitehouse 1996). However, it is apparent that the person with Down's syndrome is very different in many ways from people in the general population with presenile dementia or the dementia of old age. Not only does he or she have a different metabolic and genetic background, but usually also differs in upbringing, education, language acquisition, work placements and social support structure. Thus the dementia, whether it is classically Alzheimer's disease or not, will be acting on a different substrate, and thus can be expected to produce different effects in all areas of functioning. Disturbance of memory may not be the initial symptom. Irving (1992) conducted a comprehensive survey of adults with Down's syndrome and dementia in two areas of Scotland, and found difficulties over multiple areas of function, with a deterioration in self-care skills being the most common, followed by loss of social and language skills and then memory loss. Various behavioural difficulties are very common (including wandering), and may arise for the first time or may represent an exacerbation of long-term behavioural disorders. In common with other forms of dementia, psychotic features such as auditory and visual hallucinations are quite frequent, although the degree of learning disability may make their interpretation difficult. Epilepsy may also arise for the first time, and in a few cases may be the initial sign of dementia. Although generalised seizures can occur, it is a clinical impression that myoclonic epilepsy is a feature of the dementia associated with Down's syndrome. There may be a diurnal pattern, with a prominence of the fits on awakening. Although the usual antiepileptic medications are useful, the epilepsy is sometimes difficult to treat (Tangye 1979). Difficulties with speech production and the use of language are often important signs, ranging from a simplification of speech through to mutism. The rate of progression of the dementia is variable, but often rapid. In the later stages the person will sometimes be immobile without help, and doubly incontinent.

In the assessment of adults with Down's syndrome or any other cause of learning disability the establishment of a baseline level of functioning is important, but may be a difficult and, at present, usually a retrospective process. The work-up must be extensive, making full use of information from key informants from the person's place of occupation and home as well as from the clinical, physical and psychological examination of the person himself. Psychological assessment using scales such as the Vineland (Sparrow et al 1984) can be a very useful adjunct to clinical diagnosis (Crayton & Oliver 1993) but as yet there are no specific tests that allow diagnosis. Dementia is a process of change, and the subject must be followed up over what will sometimes be a considerable period of time to allow a diagnosis to be made. Brain imaging studies, including computed tomography and magnetic resonance imaging, need to be repeated and can clearly show changes typical of the progression of Alzheimer's disease. The differential diagnosis includes major depressive disorder and anxiety disorder, both of which are common in adults with Down's syndrome and are the mental health problems that most commonly go unrecognised in people with learning disability (Moss et al 1991), and endocrine disorders – especially hypothyroidism. Both mental health problems and medical disorders may occur in the presence of dementia and require vigorous treatment. Indeed there is some evidence that adults with Down' syndrome and dementia are at greater risk of developing hypothyroidism than those without dementia (Percy et al 1990).

After the diagnosis is confirmed the psychiatrist has a role to play in working with and supporting the family or carers, treating the behavioural or psychiatric components of the condition, and also advising on the suitability of the particular environments that the person encounters. Many of the current care settings do not produce a compatible environment for the person with dementia. For instance, the adult training centre (or resource centre in some parts of the country) can serve large numbers of changing clients. The noise levels are often high, and open plan design can lead to increased confusion and behaviour disturbance. Similarly, hospitals usually have high ambient noise levels, multiple staff changes and, to an already confused person, present an additional source of fear and disorientation. Sadly, eventual hospital placement still too often occurs for the wrong reasons and at the wrong stage of the illness, simply due to the unavailability of an appropriate alternative. Placement on wards for the care of the elderly is certainly neither generic or appropriate and leads to distancing of the person from the social work and health care services for adults with learning disability, and the allied specialist therapies that are appropriate to their needs.

The condition puts a tremendous stress on the family or carers of the person, especially the parents, who themselves may be experiencing problems of ageing – a situation Janicki has described as 'two-generation ageing'. The situation is inverted from normal ageing and dementia, where the sufferer is usually looked after by the children. Every attempt should be made to allow the person to continue to live at home and to support the parents in the immediate practical aspects of health care, and also in making plans for future care. The carers are especially troubled by restlessness, loss of speech, incontinence and wandering (Prasher & Filer 1995) and these behavioural problems need careful management. Parents are also highly concerned as to who will look after their son or daughter when they themselves die, whether or not the person suffers from dementia. After parental loss, it is in fact still the family that usually look after the person with Down's syndrome, and usually the siblings (most often a sister) take over the role of carer. In the final stages of the condition the health needs may become overwhelming and there is a great need for specialist provision of respite and terminal care for the person. Studies on good palliative care for people with learning disability are in their infancy.

Sexual development and its problems Sexuality and sexual expression are part and parcel of the normal development of the adolescent with Down's syndrome, as for anyone else. The sexual development of men with Down's syndrome seems to follow a normal course, with the development of primary and secondary sexual characteristics. Girls with trisomy 21 start menstruating at around the same age as others, and cycles are usually regular and associated with regular ovulation (Scola & Pueschel 1992). However, most men seem to have a problem in spermatogenesis, with varying degrees of impairment from the very mild to complete arrest with reduced sperm counts. The oft quoted statement that men with full trisomy 21 have never been known to father a child is wrong in absolute fact (Sheridan et al 1989) but correct in principle. Men with mosaic Down's syndrome, however, are fertile and have been known to have children. The cause of the defective spermatogenesis is unknown. Women with full trisomy 21 can be fertile (at least two dozen children have been reported). Some, however, have problems with ovulation or slowed follicle growth.

Sex education is as appropriate for young people with Down's syndrome as it is for any other person. It is as important that they should learn and understand about the formation and problems of human relationships, and marriage, heterosexuality and homosexuality, as about the mechanistic aspects of intercourse and body function. Their learning disability in combination with increased independence makes them vulnerable to abuse and exploitation, and the dangers should be included as part of their education, whether mainstream or special.

Sex chromosome aneuploidies

Abnormalities of the number of sex chromosomes are not uncommon, at around 1 in 500 livebirths. The trisomies are more common at birth than monosomy X (Turner's syndrome, XO) but the latter is the most common chromosome abnormality in spontaneous abortions, whereas the former are rarely found (Hassold & Jacobs 1984).

Only one X chromosome is active in any cell. The second chromosome in normal females exists in a largely inactive state, after compaction and the formation of a heterochromatic Barr body in the late blastocyst stage of embryo development. This inactivation is now thought to be mediated, at least in part, by sequences in the so-called X inactivation centre (XIC) situated in the Xq13.3 region of the X chromosome to be inactivated, and including a key gene termed XIST, an acronym of 'inactive X specific transcripts' (Brown et al 1991). The XIST gene may act via binding RNA rather than coding directly for a protein. The key features of the inactivation process are: that the active gene(s) for inactivation are *cis* acting, that is act on the chromosome on which they reside; that activation of the genes causes a spreading inactivation of the chromosome paralleled by a methylation of CpG islands down the chromosome; and that the inactivation 'skips' key regions on the partly inactivated X chromosome, including the pseudoautosomal region, which continue to exhibit gene activity. The homologous active X chromosome does not express XIST activity and is spared. The pattern of X inactivation is normally thought to be random, and females cells are usually a mosaic, from the active X chromosome point of view, of paternal X derived and maternal X derived lines. However, the extremes of the normal distribution may mimic non-random inactivation and explain why some heterozygous carriers of X-linked disorders may be very severely or minimally affected. Rarely there seem to be true non-random inactivation patterns which can run in families. In disorders with relevance to learning disability, some families with the Lesch–Nyhan syndrome have multiply affected females who are thought to arise through this mechanism (Marcus et al 1992). Another, and more common, type of non-random inactivation can occur in identical female twins and can explain some of the clinical discordancy in the phenotype of X-linked disorders that can be found in some pairs.

With the sex chromosome aneuploidies, all the extra X chromosomes, if present, are inactivated, so that the phenotypic consequences must be due to the higher copy number of the genes on those chromosomes that are spared from inactivation. The autosomes in some way contribute to the inactivation process, and the correct count is needed to inactivate any extra X chromosomes. In triploidies (cells with 69 chromosomes) the extra X chromosome is not inactivated (Jacobs et al 1979). Of the anomalies of sex chromosome number, only those leading to an increased number will show an association with learning disability. Females with Turner's syndrome (XO) have a distribution of IQ indistinguishable from the general population; in fact, mosaicism, which occurs in around a quarter of cases, may on average confer a slightly higher than normal IQ. The clinically important aneuploidies have the karyotypes 47, XXY, 47,XXX and 47,XYY. Various mosaic karyotypes (the other cell line usually being normal) are also found. Higher number aneuploidies are rarer.

Klinefelter's syndrome

The Karyotype 47,XXY occurs in around 1:1000 men, and is thus a relatively common and important condition. Around half the non-disjunctions are paternal and half maternal in origin. Three-quarters of the maternally derived cases show a maternal age effect, and most of the paternally derived cases are associated with advancing age of the father. The original clinical description predated cytogenetic analysis (Klinefelter et al 1942) and the original classification was later found to include men who did not have XXY. The key criteria are now held to be an XXY karyotype and male hypogonadism. Diagnosis often occurs at puberty, with a variable degree of development of secondary sexual characteristics, or through referral to an infertility clinic. Nearly 90% may have scant facial hair, and gynaecomastia may occur in around 50% (Frøland 1969). The adult with Klinefelter's syndrome is usually taller than average by around 4 cm (with especially long lower limbs) and an asthenic body build. The average IQ of adults is around 90 and thus slightly below normal, and a relatively large number will fall into the learning disabled range. The disability is usually mild and most have IQ levels above 60. Specific learning disorders are probably more common, and require intervention, although the usual delay in diagnosis predicates against this. The postulated relationship of Klinefelter's syndrome to psychiatric disorders, especially psychoses, was based on the studies of individuals in institutions: the true relationship is uncertain.

Trisomy X

This karyotype (47,XXX) is found in around 1:1000 women. That any syndrome is associated with this karyotype is controversial. Generally there is little clinical evidence to suggest any abnormality (a slight increase in height may occur, but this also correlates with parental height). However, up to 70% may have learning disorders (Ratcliffe & Paul 1986) and learning disability is overrepresented, in association with a slight decrease in average IQ from normal values. Some women have reduced fertility, but most do not, and their children have normal karyotypes. The reports of an increased incidence of schizophrenia are interesting, and not necessarily associated with learning disability.

47 XYY Males

Again this occurs in around 1:1000 men. Men with this karyotype have even less phenotypic correlates than trisomy X, and yet it has engendered a controversial status out of proportion to its clinical importance. Studies on populations of men in maximum security psychiatric hospitals in the 1960s seemed to show an excess of men with this karyotype as well as men with Klinefelter's syndrome (Witkin et al 1976). However, studies lacked adequate comparison groups, and the high prevalence of XYY in the general population meant that doubts were soon cast on causal inferences relating karyotype to criminal behaviour. IQ may be very slightly lower, on average, than in the normal population, which may account in small part for a general increase in behavioural problems in this group.

Sex chromosome polysomies and other abnormalities

Where the number of X chromomes and/or Y chromosomes increases above 2 then definite phenotypic consequences result. X chromosome tetrasomy (48,XXXX) and pentasomy (49,XXXXX) are rare but well described. 48,XXXY and 49,XXXXY are more common. The general finding is of a marked degree of learning disability and a variety of physical abnormalities. The greater the number of X chromosomes, the more profound the learning disability tends to be. The extra X chromosomes all seem to be maternal in origin in these conditions. All the extra X chromosomes are also inactivated, and the phenotype must largely be due to an increased copy number of those genes escaping inactivation.

Ring X and supernumary marker chromosomes derived from the X chromosome are generally also associated with learning disability in the carrier. In some cases they may fail to inactivate, due to lack of XIC. Thus the genotype is producing a disomy of regions of the X chromosome that would not normally be present even with multiple full copies of the X chromosome.

Deletions and duplication of parts of chromosomes

Loss of a whole autosome (monosomy) is usually disastrous for fetal development, and few survive to birth. A great variety of deletions (partial monosomy) and duplications (partial trisomy) of segments of an autosome have been observed. These range from the whole of a chromosomal arm down to very small deletions and duplications that require specialised methods for detection. In the extreme case a deletion may only become apparent on molecular analysis.

Many of the larger deletions and duplications are associated with learning disability, and there are some paradoxical findings, such as that of partial trisomy 8, which is associated with a greater degree of learning disability than full trisomy 8. These conditions are rare and only two at the extremes of the cytogenetically detectable spectrum will be described.

Partial monosomy of the short arm of chromosome 5 (cri du chat syndrome: 5p-) This occurs in around 1:50 000 newborns. The infant has a characteristic cry which is said to be like that of a kitten, hence the epithet. Microcephaly is usually pronounced, and dysmorphisms include hypertelorism and micrognathia, the latter associated with dental malocclusion (Niebuhr 1978). The learning disability is profound in degree, and its depth may increase in some cases with ageing. Many people with cri du chat syndrome live well into adult life and puberty occurs normally. In the vast majority of cases the deletion is a sporadic occurrence, but rarely it can be inherited as the unbalanced form of a parental translocation.

William's syndrome Learning disability is a common associate of this condition, which also includes growth retardation, characteristic facial features ('elfin' facies), a hoarse voice and premature wrinkling and sagging of the skin, and vascular anomalies especially aortic stenosis. More relevant to the future understanding of other conditions associated with learning disability is the highly variable pattern of cognitive impairments that form a specific profile of weaknesses and abilities (Ashkenas 1996). As children, these individuals' ability to recognise faces is good, but they do badly on the ability to assemble a whole object from component parts, given a model to follow. Like many genetic conditions associated with learning disability, the phenotype is inconstant and diverse. This has often led to a tacit assumption that such conditions are necessarily of polygenic effect. In the case of William's syndrome there is usually a deletion of a small region (around 2 cM) of the long arm of chromosome 7 leading to hemizygosity, in that the implicated region is only represented by one chromosome. One of the deleted genes is that for elastin, which may therefore suffer from a reduction in expression and account for vascular changes. Elastin is not found in the brain, however, and specific defects of the elastin gene are not associated with learning disability or even the skin changes of this condition (Morris et al 1993, Olson et al 1995). It is likely that William's syndrome is a contiguous gene deletion disorder and that the other genes deleted determine the phenotype. Parental imprinting may be important in determining some of the outcomes of the deletion in William's syndrome. Those in whom the deletion is maternally derived are smaller in height than if the deletion is paternally derived. Unusual cases of William's syndrome with smaller deletions have been described (Frangiskakis et al 1996) and are not associated with learning disability but there are quite specific and remarkable problems with the visuospatial task described above. The strongest candidate gene is a kinase (LIMK1) which is widely expressed in the nervous system and codes for a highly unusual protein with two zinc-finger domains. There is currently much interest in the function of protein kinases in memory and cognition, and William's syndrome may be a key to our understanding of the link between relatively simple genetic abnormalities and specific alterations in highly complex cognitive functions.

Contiguous gene syndromes Major advances have been made using molecular cytogenetics in the detection of syndromes based on chromosomal microdeletions, microduplication and cryptic translocations. Most of these syndromes are associated with learning disability, and include the Prader–Willi/Angelman syndromes of chromosome 15 and other, as yet seemingly rarer, conditions. They are described in more detail in Chapter 7. It is probable that the number of these conditions will rise dramatically as the methodologies are applied to people with learning disability without known aetiologies, and perhaps especially to those with more severe degrees of handicap.

Associated genetic disorders showing mendelian inheritance patterns

It is impossible to list here the large number of inherited conditions that are associated with learning disability. Very detailed accounts are given in relevant genetic texts (Scriver et al 1995). An outline of some important disorders following autosomal dominant, recessive and sex-linked inheritances is given in Table 22.3.

Autosomal dominant conditions

The phakomatoses These are a cluster of conditions with neurocutaneous signs and a variety of

Table 22.3 Selection of inherited disorders associated with learning disability. (In total, including those not associated with learning disability, there are over 2000 dominant and 600 recessive disorders)

Inheritance pattern	Common name	Comments
Dominant	Tuberous sclerosis	Variable association with learning disability, three different disorders
Dominant	Neurofibromatosis	Variable association with learning disability
Recessive	Hurler's syndrome	Lysosomal storage disease – mucopolysaccharides
Recessive	Sanfillipo disease	Lysosomal storage disease – mucopolysaccharides, four different disorders
Recessive	Sialidosis	Lysosomal storage disease – glycoproteins
Recessive	Niemann–Pick disease	Lysosomal storage disease – sphingomyelins
X-linked dominant	Fragile X syndrome	FRAXA – triplet repeat expansion disorder, shows anticipation
X-linked dominant		FRAXE – triplet repeat expansion disorder, mild learning disability
X-linked recessive	Hunter' disease	Lysosomal storage disease – mucopolysaccharides
X-linked recessive	Fabry' disease	Lysosomal storage disease – trihexosylceramides

causes (Riccardi 1990). The main disorders in this grouping are neurofibromatosis, tuberous sclerosis, Von Hippel–Lindau disease and the Sturge–Weber syndrome. Neurofibromatosis and tuberous sclerosis are genetic and heterogeneous conditions. Neurofibromatosis consists of several genetic conditions and is a relatively common autosomal dominant disorder (around 1:4000). Although learning disability may be a component it is not a major association of the condition, and the condition is very pleiomorphic even within the same family. Von Hippel–Lindau disease is also genetic but rare, and is associated with the development of angiomatous tumours in various areas of the body. The Sturge–Weber syndrome is apparently not inherited, and clinically features port-wine stain of the face, and angiomas of the meninges in the temporal and occipital regions leading to learning disability, epilepsy and sometimes hemiparesis. There have been some suggestions that dysfunctional cells in these disorders arise from the neural crest, but consistent supportive evidence for this is lacking. From its strong association with learning disability, tuberous sclerosis is the most relevant to the present discussion.

Tuberous sclerosis This group of disorders has been known for well over a century. Their prevalence is estimated at around 1:10 000, although this figure is likely to be too low because the conditions are extremely variable in clinical presentation and penetrance within families. Males and females are equally affected. Clinically the key features are learning disability of all degrees, seizures, hamartomas of the central nervous system (including the retina), depigmented skin patch-

es (ash leaf spots) and fibromas of the nails. Sometimes tumours also occur in the heart muscle and kidneys. The most common feature is skin depigmentation (over 96% cases), which is especially noted under ultraviolet light. Seizures are very common (90%) and often the initial presentation in an infant, with 'salaam attacks' (infantile spasms) being characteristic. However, all other types of epilepsy, including partial and general seizures, may occur. The partial and general epilepsy can persist throughout to adulthood. Learning disability is present in up to 50% of people with tuberous sclerosis, and can vary from profound to mild. There are often associated behavioural disorders.

Three forms of tuberous sclerosis exist. Tuberous sclerosis 1 (TSC1) is caused by a gene on chromosome 9 near the ABO blood group locus (Fryer et al 1987). A gene has been cloned for tuberous sclerosis type 2 (TSC2) and occurs on chromosome 16. This form of tuberous sclerosis is said to be more often associated with psychiatric and behavioural disorders than TSC1. A third and rare type of tuberous sclerosis (TSC3) has been described in individuals with a chromosomal translocation involving chromosome 12.

Most studies have focused on TSC1. There seems to be no evidence for imprinting. Sampson et al (1989) found a prevalence rate of around 1:12 000 in the west of Scotland for children under 10 years of age. A high percentage (60%) of cases were said to be new mutations, as neither parents showed any signs of the condition. However, it is now clear that obligate carriers may show no clinical evidence of the condition, and the extended family of any new case, or indeed any case that has not been fully investigated, now needs genetic examination.

Autosomal recessive conditions

A vast number of single gene metabolic disorders associated with learning disability show a recessive inheritance pattern. Individually most are rare or very rare. The most common, at around 1:15 000 newborns (Levy 1991), is phenylketonuria, which holds a special place as the first to have its metabolic consequences described. This is an aminoacidopathy (there are 47 others known) with several genetic causes, and its consequences including learning disability require long exposure. Supervised early dietary phenylalanine restriction helps prevent this. At special risk are children of mothers who are homozygous for the gene and who may have poorly controlled phenylalanine levels. The embryo in such cases is at risk in utero. Once learning disability is established it cannot be reversed.

A large number of lysosomal storage diseases have also been described (Suzuki 1996). Of those involving mucopolysaccharide storage, Hurler's disease is the classic, with severe learning disability and characteristic skeletal abnormalities of short stature, kyphosis, flexion deformities, a long head and characteristic facies. The internal organs, especially the spleen and liver, may be grossly enlarged. The defect is in the enzyme α-iduronidase. The other lysosomal storage diseases include a group involving the storage of sphingolipids (e.g. Tay–Sachs disease) and glycoproteins (e.g. sialidosis). Most but not all of these rare conditions are autosomal recessive, and thus will be expressed more frequently in societies where cousin marriages are more common.

Mendelian and non-mendelian disorders associated with the sex chromosomes

A growing number of conditions causing learning disability have been linked to the X chromosome. In addition to specific mendelian single gene disorders (e.g. Hunter's and Fabry's diseases amongst the storage disorders), many factors pointed to an excess of sex-linked conditions. By far the most important are the fragile X syndromes which do not show true mendelian inheritance. A major advance in our understanding of the causes of conditions associated with learning disability has come through an understanding of the gene disorder that leads to the fragile X syndrome. The work on this condition heralded the identification of an ever growing number of inherited disorders associated with triplet repeat expansion, including Huntington's disease. The inheritance of fragile X, which proved

difficult to understand before the genetic disruption was pinpointed, is now relatively well understood, and recent work on the molecular pathology of the condition has raised important new questions about the stability of genetic mutations.

It has long been known that more men than women suffer from moderate and severe degrees of learning disability. Last century Johnson noted this from the data provided by a census in the USA, and this has been amply confirmed since then. In a large study of X-linked learning disability Lehrke (1972, 1974) showed that the sex ratio in surveys of people with learning disability has always been biased towards men, and that in families with more than one offspring with learning disability the number of male–male sibling pairs was greater than the number of male–female. A variety of factors could explain this gender difference, including the increased rates of premature birth, neonatal morbidity (and mortality) and congenital abnormalities. X-linked genetic conditions that are associated with learning disability will also tend to be expressed to a greater extent in men, due to the lack of a second compensating X chromosome. In females there are two possibilities to balance the effects of a deleterious gene mutation. First, there is a random inactivation pattern of the X chromosomes (Lyon hypothesis) that means only a percentage of subjects will be expressing the chromosome with the mutation. Second, in cases where the aberrant gene lies in a region which is spared inactivation (e.g. the pseudoautosomal region), and as both genes are active, there will be a compensatory normal gene as well as the aberrant gene.

Fragile X syndrome

Familial disorders, with learning disability mainly in men, have been described for some time. Martin & Bell (1943) found a family in which 11 of the men had a common set of clinical features including learning disability, and similar families were subsequently identified (Renpenning et al 1962). In some of these individuals it was later found that a cytogenetic abnormality of the X chromosome could be induced under certain lymphocyte culture conditions, notably folate deprivation or thymidilate stress (Lubs 1969, Sutherland 1977). A very faintly staining and seemingly constricted region near the end of the long arm, and located more precisely on the banding pattern map of the chromosome at Xq27.3, appeared in a percentage of cells. The apparently tenuous nature of the anomaly earned it the tag of 'fragile site' and other such folate-dependent sites are now known, both on the X chromosome and on autosomes. The identification of the abnormality was important as its inheritance within a family could be studied, and its presence linked individuals with quite widely variable clinical features.

Turner and her colleagues (1992) systematically looked for fragile X chromosomes in a large number of learning disabled individuals in New South Wales, yielding rates of around 1:2600 men and 1:4200 women. In Coventry, Webb et al (1986) found a rate of 1:1000 schoolchildren. These rates were approximate, as the expression is so dependent on culture conditions and is especially subject to false positives. A more recent reanalysis of the positives in the Coventry sample (Morton et al 1995) yielded a frequency of around 1:2200, and the most recent molecular-based studies give a lower figure of 1:4000 males. However, this still places the fragile X syndrome as the most common inherited disorder associated with learning disability.

Physical features These are very variable and overlap considerably with the normal population. The most consistent are the large testicles and ears seen in around 80% of adult men with the condition. The increase in testicular volume may be dramatic – up to and over 120 ml. A disorder of connective tissue may account, at least in part, for the large prominent (anteverted) ears, and also for other, less consistent findings, including a very smooth skin, hyperextensible finger joints, flat feet and mitral valve prolapse. The face tends to be long and narrow with a relative underdevelopment of the midface. These features tend to be most prominent after puberty; up to 20% of children with the fragile X karyotype may show no clinical features. Most will show some degree of cupping of the ears, although the macro-orchidism is a postpubertal feature which continues thereafter (Hagerman 1991, Butler et al 1992). Macrocephaly to a slight degree seems to be a very stable finding (Patton reported in Bailey & Nelson 1995). In females with full fragile X syndrome the features tend to be less prominent, but similar in type with large ears and the other facial features. As with males, these features tend to become more prominent after puberty.

Associated learning disability and behavioural features Learning disability is usually the first feature detected in male children with fragile X syndrome but is highly variable, from profound to borderline. Hagerman and his colleagues have reported a decline in the IQ scores with growth (Hagerman et al 1989, Hodapp et al 1990) and have found that, although 44% of preschool boys with fragile X tested in the non-learning disabled range (IQ > 70; Freund et al 1995), this reduced to 13% of all boys with fragile X tested out of a total group of 250 males, and only seven individuals maintained this into adulthood, of whom three had an unusual mutation. In fact most adults with fragile X syndrome will test within the moderate to severe

range of learning disability. Such declines in IQ scores have been noted by others (Lachiewicz et al 1987, Fisch et al 1991) but the reasons for this apparent change in the degree of learning disability are not clear, and such changes are not restricted to the fragile X syndrome (Hodapp & Zigler 1994). Females with full fragile X syndrome attain generally higher IQ scores, in the mild range, or may not suffer from learning disability but instead have specific learning disorders.

A behavioural profile has been described. Hand flapping or waving and repetitive mannerisms are sometimes seen in men with fragile X, and, coupled with shyness, social anxiety, gaze avoidance and poor relations with their peer groups, have suggested an overlap with autism, although the social adaptation does not seem to be so disturbed. Neurological and imaging findings (see below) suggest that there may be a true link between the two conditions rather than each being a phenocopy of the other. Women with fragile X also tend to be shy and anxious and a percentage of females with a diagnosis of autism test positive for fragile X (Bailey et al 1993). Communication difficulties exist, with conversational rigidity and perseveration, and some have noted a cluttered and overdetailed form of speech (Grigsby et al 1990). The incidence of mood and personality disorders is said to be raised, including schizotypal personality disorder, but the numbers studied are small. In contrast, people with fragile X also have areas of great relative strengths. Their domestic and daily living skills are especially well preserved and often improve in adulthood (Dykens 1995).

Genetics Early studies on the inheritance of fragile X syndrome revealed several peculiarities that made its interpretation along classical mendelian lines impossible. The penetrance of the condition seemed very low when compared to other X-linked disorders. Sherman and her colleagues (1985) studied over a hundred families with fragile X syndrome. They found that the daughters of women who must be obligate carriers of the disordered gene had a much greater chance of having learning disability than the daughters of unaffected male carriers (the so-called normal transmitting males). The daughters of normal transmitting males, in fact, were practically never intellectually affected. They could identify fragile X chromosomes, by karyotype directly or inferred from intellectual impairment, in only around half of the female obligate carriers. Further, on examining the structure of the pedigrees the degree of learning disability in fragile X seems to increase in the younger generations – they exhibited the phenomenon of genetic anticipation and in the case of fragile X this was called the Sherman paradox. The gene disrupted in fragile X was finally cloned and sequenced in 1991 (Kremer et al 1991, Oberlé et al

1991, Verkerk et al 1991) and given the designation FMR-1, an acronym for fragile X mental retardation gene type 1. It is now clear that disruption of the function of this gene alone is sufficient to cause fragile X syndrome. Nearly all cases of fragile X are associated with a large sequence of multiply-repeated DNA nucleotide base pair triplets (cytosine – guanine – guanine or guanine – cytosine – cytosine, depending on the strand chosen). The most common nomenclature used to describe this repeated triplet is $(CGG)_n$ where n is the copy number of the triplet of base pairs within the brackets. This non-coding sequence of DNA is found in the 5' untranslated end of the FMR-1 gene. In men with the full fragile X syndrome the copy number of the triplet was found to be very large, from over 230 to well over 1000, which represents 690 to well over 3000 base pairs of DNA. With such large repeats in the gene the cytosine residues of CG base pairs are very highly methylated (by enzyme action), not only in the repeat itself but also in the surrounding areas of DNA in the gene, including the CpG island and promoter region of the gene, which is essential for correct DNA polymerase binding and thus DNA transcription. The consequence of such a degree of methylation is to inactivate or silence the gene, and no transcription occurs, and therefore no gene product (protein) is formed. Rare individuals have been described who have other FMR-1 disruptions, such as deletions of the gene, intragenic mutations, even a single base pair mutation, all silencing the gene, and produce the full clinical phenotype of fragile X syndrome. Thus it is the specific lack of the protein product (called FMRP, fragile X mental retardation protein) that is causal in fragile X syndrome.

When the repeat region DNA from the normal population (that is from other than fragile X subjects and their families) was examined it was found to be much smaller and variable in size from individual to individual – on average from 6 to 50 repeated triplets with a mean value of around 30. Normally this size of the repeat is stable when passed on from one generation to another. These triplets are mostly CGG but around 1 in 10 is AGG. Thus there are two sources of variation in the population: the number of CGG triplets and the number of interspersed AGG (Fu et al 1991, Snow et al 1993). It is now known that lack of AGG sequence (which will increase the number of 'perfect' CGG repeats) or an increase in the number of CGGs towards the 3' end of the sequence tends to make the inheritance less stable, and the repeat sequence can expand in size when passed on in the normal population (Hirst et al 1994). This may be one source of a slow increase in size of small triplet repeats in the general population.

In the families of subjects with fragile X syndrome

the size of the repeated triplet is different. Normal transmitting males and obligate carrier females were found to have between 60 and 200 repeats. Repeats in this size range are termed premutations and are highly unstable when transmitted by a mother to her child. This transmission nearly always causes the premutation to undergo a large expansion, and is the key to understanding the unusual inheritance patterns. Smaller sized premutations may expand (further CGG triplets are added to the 3' side) by maternal transmission to large premutations, and large premutations to the very large mutation seen in individuals with full fragile X syndrome. Passage by paternal transmission shows a limited amount of instability and the premutation may have a small gain or loss in size. Thus the daughters of normal transmitting males will have the premutation of much the same size as their fathers. However, when they pass an X chromosome to their offspring then the triplet repeat premutation will be expanded to a great degree and usually the full very large mutation results with, on average, 50% of their sons having full fragile X syndrome and 50% of their daughters being heterozygous for the mutation. An increased number of interspersed AGG triplets (or rather a decreased length of 'perfect' CGG triplets in the 3' direction) confers stability on the premutation and reduces its likelihood of full expansion (Eichler et al 1994). Thus both sequence and size of the premutation contribute to the likelihood of the development of full fragile X syndrome.

The exact time and locus of the expansion of the premutation during mother-to-child transmission is not clear. Men with full fragile X have a premutation in their X carrying sperm and not the full mutation (Reyniers et al 1993) and they are thus presumably technically able to father a daughter who would not have full fragile X. The implications of this are very important. Either a regression in size of the mutation has occurred, the mechanism of which would be of great interest in gene therapy, or the mutation expansion has occurred postzygotically, sparing the clonal germ cell line. FMRP does not seem necessary for correct spermatogenesis and so a third hypothesis, an active selection against mutation-containing sperm during spermatogenesis, would have to rely on some component other than FMRP as a trophic factor. Whatever the case, some imprinting mechanism is needed, specific to female transmission, to recognise the premutation as compared to a normal sized repeat. Another feature that still needs to be accounted for is the quite sizeable frequency of somatic mosaicism in people with the mutation and premutation. The most recent evidence (Malter et al 1997) has found that intact ovaries from fetuses with full fragile X syndrome carry the full mutation which is unmethylated. This suggests that the germline is not a protected environment for the expansion and that there must be some form of contraction in fetal testes. Further, the expansion must precede the methylation, and must be a germline or a very early event in zygote development.

The cytoplasmic protein normally produced by this gene (FMRP) has structural features suggesting it is able to bind RNA, and its widespread and very general distribution in adult tissues is consistent with a general housekeeping function (Devys et al 1993). Higher levels occur in brain (cortex and especially cerebellum) and testes. The role it plays in development, and the effects of its deficiency, are not yet clear, but studies in mice with knock-out mutations of the gene are underway. Adults with fragile X syndrome were early known to have abnormal brain electrical activity shown by EEG (Wisniewski et al 1991) and event-related potentials (St Clair et al 1987, Muir et al 1988). Brain imaging has subsequently revealed that the posterior cerebellar vermis is smaller in both men and women with fragile X syndrome compared with matched controls. They also seem to have abnormally large hippocampi, as well as larger caudate nuclei and, in males, increased lateral ventricular volume (Reiss et al 1994,1995). The involvement of the cerebellar vermis is of interest as this has also been postulated as a region disturbed in autism. Hippocampal involvement would be consistent with delays in late evoked potentials, but these can be disturbed by many other mechanisms.

Epidemiology of the mutation and its place in diagnosis Another unusual feature, for an X-linked condition, is the apparent low rate of new mutations and evidence for a founder effect (common ancestor), especially in well studied Swedish and Finnish families (Oudet et al 1993, Malmgren et al 1994). It appears that the premutation can be carried silently over many generations, which at first seems at odds with the high frequency of the condition, but there may be a slow overall 'creep' in size of the premutation over generations. The haplotypes of markers close to the mutation can be used, as well as the sequence of the mutation itself, to follow the disorder down families. These markers show linkage disequilibrium in a variety of populations. The French ancestors may have been different from the Finnish and Swedish, who may have shared at least one common ancestor. Studies in the UK, however, have shown a wider diversity of haplotypes, and evidence for a common ancestor is not so strong (Macpherson et al 1994). It may be that a different process can account for the increase here, with occasional stepwise 'jumps' upward in the size of the premutation. These indications of population differences make generalisations about the absolute numbers of people carrying the premutation difficult. However, in a very large study from Quebec (Rousseau et al 1995) the mutation size was examined in over 10 000 females. A premutation size of 66 triplets or over was found in around 1:500 females. A similar frequency was found for repeats from 55 to 63 triplets long, which are at lower risk of mutation in one generation at least. The predicted number of children carrying a full mutation from these figures is around 1:2900, broadly compatible with the figure seen in the general population.

The mutation can now be studied directly from a venous blood sample. The repeat can be detected and sized, either on a gel after restriction enzyme digestion or by direct amplification by the polymerase chain reaction (Oostra et al 1993). Many individuals who may have fragile X have not yet been screened, and it is only in the last few years that the tools for accurate diagnosis have become available. The lack of screening is probably most apparent in adults with learning disability. If there are physical features and/or if there is a family history of learning disability it is important to test for fragile X and obtain genetic counselling for the family. Prenatal screening is possible but controversial if the fetus is female, when prediction of outcome is limited. A recent antibody test for the full mutation would allow a routine screening in the newborn, but like all new procedures will require a cost–benefit analysis. It is often very difficult to detect fragile X syndrome until the child is several years old and shows significant delays in attaining developmental milestones.

Education and support of the family There is at present no cure or therapy for the fragile X syndrome itself, and the diagnosis, like all associated with learning disability, is a major event in the parents' life. The family will need support, and this may also apply to the extended family as the implications of the disorder become clear. If parents have a son with fragile X syndrome then they will have to consider the effects on their other children if they have any, or are planning to have any. The possible delay in the appearance of problems must be addressed both for the son and also for any daughters who may carry an expanded premutation or the full mutation. Obviously early access to clinical genetic counselling is important.

There is much that can be done to alleviate the associated problems and capitalise on adaptive strengths of someone with fragile X syndrome. At present, however, strategies are very general and designed to help people with learning disability in the widest sense. A greater understanding of the profile of learning disability in fragile X will help in maximising the educational potential of those with the condition, and the way ahead seems to lie in identifying the particular constellation of weaknesses, strengths and natural histories of syndromes such as fragile X that have associated learning disability. When such knowledge is gained then appropriate, and disorder-specific, interventions can be designed.

Other disorders associated with fragile sites

Amongst the folate-sensitive fragile sites two on the X chromosome and one on chromosome 16 have been studied in detail. All are associated with a large GCC triplet expansion that is methylated. The original fragile X syndrome is now called FRAXA to distinguish it from FRAXE and FRAXF on the X chromosome. The presence of FRAXE is associated with a mild degree of learning disability, but the causal gene has not yet been isolated. FRAXF and FRA16 have yet to be associated with any clinical disorder.

FRAXE lies some 600 kb further towards the tip of the X chromosome long arm than FRAXA. The GCC repeat that it contains is polymorphic and has a similar pattern to the FRAXA repeat (Knight et al 1994). Maternal line expansion seems to occur and the full mutation contains between 200 and 1000 triplets and is methylated. A candidate gene sequence has recently been identified (Gedeon et al 1995). FRAXE-associated X-linked mental retardation occurs at a rate of around 1:100 000 (Allingham-Hawkins & Ray 1995).

Non-genetic causes

Injury to the central nervous system can be caused by a wide variety of non-genetic mechanisms (Table 22.4). Although the brain is a plastic organ, especially during childhood, severe insults will have profound implications for cognitive development. The toxic damage can be done in utero, in the perinatal period, or in childhood itself.

Intrauterine and neonatal damage

Infections A growing number of infections by viruses or bacteria are known to be associated with the later development of learning disability. Those that can infect the developing embryo itself can cause a considerable range of congenital disabilities. The most commonly known, and feared, are the rubella and cytomegaloviruses. Other agents such as that of toxoplasmosis, and other viruses such as hepatitis B and herpes simplex, may also be implicated. Infection with the syphilis bacterium, formerly an important cause of congenital abnormalities, is now very rare and should be detected early with current screening programmes, and the increase (although still rare) in HIV carrier status in pregnant mothers may supplant it as a cause of

learning disability in their children. The HIV virus and the acquired immune deficiency syndrome (AIDS) may occur in up to 30% of infants of HIV-positive mothers, who also have higher rates of carriage of other infections. There is an overlap in the destructive consequences of such infections. Sequelae such as deafness, blindness, microcephaly or hydrocephalus with associated mild to very profound learning disability and epilepsy are usually associated with obvious infection. Silent infections, of which cytomegalovirus is the most common, are more insidious and chronic forms, as detected by antibody assays, may be associated with progressive developmental delays, without early clinical signs of infection (Peckam et al 1983). The infections which do not seem to cross the placenta, such as measles, mumps, the coxsackie viruses and influenza, seem to able to produce damage, and thus later learning disability, by the secretion of toxins or perhaps by stimulation of an immune response at critical developmental periods. Rarely an encephalitis may result after routine immunisation, with consequent learning disability. Severe encephalitis and meningitis are also important causes of learning disability at any stage of childhood.

Toxins and irradiation Severe damage to the fetus can result from high levels of alcohol ingestion by the mother, associated with the development of the fetal alcohol syndrome. That alcohol can affect the fetus has been known for a considerable time (Lemoine et al 1968), and although the term fetal alcohol syndrome was coined almost quarter of a century ago (Jones & Smith 1973), it is only in recent years that its importance as a leading cause of learning disability has been recognised. A characteristic set of features occurs in the newborn of mothers who have severe dependency on alcohol and who continue to drink heavily through their pregnancy. They have small heads and are small in overall length. The eye fissures are small, as are the maxilla and mandible, and there may be cleft palate and joint deformities. The neonatal mortality of such infants is high, and a degree of learning disability is usually found in those who survive. Alcohol crosses the placenta but its mode of toxicity is unclear. The effects of smaller amounts of alcohol are hard to judge but some have estimated the fetal alcohol syndrome to be an extremely frequent cause of learning disability (Schenker et al 1990).

A variety of other substances can also harm the fetus and lead to learning disability. Cocaine abuse in the mother can be associated with a varied degree of learning disability in the child. Lead and other metal poisoning is now rare. Some prescription drugs, including antiepileptics such as phenytoin, have a well-known potential to damage the fetus. Exposure to high doses

Table 22.4   Selection of non-inherited conditions associated with learning disability

Cause	Specific type	Timing of insult	Comments
Infective agents	Cytomegalovirus	Pre and postnatal	Persistent carriage rate of around 1%
	Rubella virus	Pre natal	Immunisation programme important in decreasing incidence, rare cases postnatal
	Toxoplasma gondii	Pre and postnatal	Postnatal, especially with HIV infection through vertical transmission
	Syphilis	Prenatal	Now rare, vertical transmission
	Herpes simplex	Neonatal and Childhood	
	Listeria monocytogenes		
	Other causes of meningitis and encephalitis		A whole variety of cerebral infections can lead to permanent damage
CNS and skull developmental information	Micro- and macrocephalies	Prenatal	
	Spina bifida	Prenatal	Learning disability often secondary to infections
	Hydrocephalus	Pre and postnatal	With meningomyelocoele and Arnold–Chiari malformation
	Craniostenosis	Pre and postnatal	
	Callosal agenesis	Prenatal	
	Lissencephalies		
	Holoprosencephalies		
Toxins	Maternal alcoholism	Prenatal	Fetal alcohol syndrome
	Lead encephalopathy	Infancy / Childhood	Much rarer than previously
	Bilirubin and haem products	Neonatal	Rhesus incompatibility is now much less common than formerly
Teratogens	Coumarin anticoagulants	Prenatal	
	Phenytoin	Prenatal	
Hypoxic damage	Small-for-date infants		Along with other developmental problems
	Severe prematurity		Along with other developmental problems
	Birth trauma		
Uncertain origin	Cerebral palsies		
	Autism	Infancy	
	Rett's syndrome	Infancy	
	Childhood disintegrative disorder	Infancy	

of ionising radiation during pregnancy is also associated with learning disability in the child.

Injury and hypoxia   Any condition causing severe degrees of hypoxia in the fetus or infant has the potential to induce learning disability. Prolonged and difficult labour, respiratory difficulties and cerebral cyanosis from a wide variety of other conditions can thus lead to brain damage. Some cases of cerebral palsy probably result from such mechanisms. Severe epilepsy, and especially prolonged status epilepticus, can also be associated with severe hypoxia. Any direct injury to the developing brain can also lead to damage. Thus neonates who experience birth trauma, and later those unfortunate children who suffer trauma from accidental or deliberate severe injury to the head, can sometimes develop learning disability.

Developmental and anatomical abnormalities of the central nervous system

Neural tube defects   These are fairly common conditions (around 1–9:1000) in which the developing neural tube fails to close completely, a process usually achieved by the end of the fourth week of fetal development. Learning disability, which can range from mild to profound, is not caused directly by these conditions but is a secondary consequence of an associated hydrocephalus or ascending meningitis. The learning disability itself is often made more complex by the presence of paralyses and sensory impairments.

The most severe form, anencephaly, occurs when the axis fails to close at the head end, and the condition results in stillbirth, or at most a survival measured in hours. At more caudal levels, failure of closure can result in an encephalocele, with protrusion of the meninges covered in a layer of skin. This is relatively uncommon but is usually associated with severe learning disability, and sometimes blindness. Failure to close at a still more caudal level results in spina bifida cystica with a myelocele or open meningomyelocele. Most have an associated Arnold–Chiari malformation at the base of the brain and there is resultant hydrocephalus in 80% (Laurence 1990). This can progress very swiftly and, if untreated, can result in interruption of the spinal cord, with double incontinence, lower limb paralysis, sensory anaesthesia, developmental pelvic and lower limb abnormalities, and a markedly increased risk of meningitis. Where the protruding meninges are covered with skin or a thick membrane however, there may be minimal neurological and cognitive deficits. A single vertebral anomaly may appear lower down the spine as spina bifida occulta, and may not be associated with clinical disorder.

The epidemiology of neural tube defects is complex, with well-defined regions of increased incidence such as the west of Scotland and Ireland, and the south of Wales. In such pockets the heritability of the condition is lower than elsewhere, implying that environmental factors are especially important. Overall the causes are complex and multifactorial. There is an excess of affected females, but twinning is very rare, possibly due to the increased lethality of a double pregnancy. A variety of environmental insults, such as hypoxia, radiation, drugs and even potato blight, have been suspected, all of which interact with the genetic background, which in some cases shows a familial pattern. Recently, folic acid deficiency has been shown to play a role, and maternal supplements may help reduce the recurrence risk if given before the 28th day of pregnancy. The open neural tube causes raised levels of α-fetoprotein which are used, in combination with ultrasound and amniocentesis, to make in utero diagnoses in midtrimester. The uptake of screening is high and in some areas of the UK there has been a dramatic reduction in the rate of neural tube defects.

Congenital hydrocephalus In addition to its association with neural tube defects, hydrocephalus can result from of a variety of other conditions, ranging

from specific anatomical abnormalities (aqueductal stenosis, Dandy–Walker malformation) and congenital infections to idiopathic cases. The incidence is around 1:2000 livebirths, though it is markedly increased in stillbirths. Surgical shunt insertion has revolutionised prognosis but learning disability is still a problem, especially in cases where secondary infection has occurred.

The cerebral palsies and the profound and multiply handicapped This term is used here for want of one more appropriate, and is restricted to people with varying degrees of spastic diplegia or quadriplegia following brain injury from a number of different causes, including hypoxia and birth trauma. Its non-specific phenomenology hides a multitude of causal factors. Where present, the associated learning disability can range from the mild to the profound. The most difficult situation is where profound learning disability coexists with deep degrees of quadriplegia. This is often associated with other motor (including swallowing) and autonomic control problems, and sensory impairments that can range to cortical blindness and deafness. In such cases of profound and multiple handicaps the care needs are intense, and can sometimes only be met in an intensive nursing environment. Management of long-term tube feeding, oral and tracheal suction, physiotherapy to prevent pressure sores and contraction deformities, and the difficulties in communication can be a very harrowing experience for both the family and health care staff involved, and counselling and psychological support is essential. For those people who are cared for at home, regular respite is needed, and community care provision should be adapted to include the medical needs, which often cannot be met in standard nursing home facilities.

DISORDERS OF UNKNOWN, PRESUMED BIOLOGICAL, AETIOLOGY

Autism and pervasive developmental disorder

Pervasive developmental disorder is a fairly recently introduced concept that, in the DSM-IV classification, embraces autistic disorder, childhood disintegrative disorder, Rett's syndrome, Asperger's syndrome, and unspecified forms of autism (Campbell & Shay 1995). Unfortunately there is no clear evidence for causal links between these conditions, and autistic disorder, or autism, is itself heterogeneous in origin. At present they sit in a grey area of psychiatric classification, encompassed by both child psychiatry and learning disability, and with a multitude of aetiogenic theories existing to explain their origin and development from psychodynamic constructs, psychological dysfunctions through to biological and genetic diatheses.

Autism is a disorder of major concern to the adult psychiatrist specialising in learning disability. Kanner's early assumption of a good cognitive prospect for children with autism by treatment of the supposed psychogenic disturbance is not tenable. Between 75 and 80% of children and adults with autism have learning disability, and on average this is moderate in degree.

Autism

Development of the concept

The condition was first described over half a century ago by Leo Kanner (1943), who considered that it exhibited five characteristics – 'a profound lack of affective contact with other people', 'an anxiously obsessive desire for the preservation of sameness', 'a fascination for objects which are handled with skill in fine motor movements', 'mutism or a kind of language that does not seem intended to serve interpersonal communication', and 'the retention of an intelligent physiognomy and good cognitive potential manifested, in those who can speak, by feats of memory, or in the mute children, by their skill on performance tests, especially the Séguin form board' (Kanner & Eisenberg 1956). Kanner, as Wing points out (1991), did not recognise learning disability as a component part of the syndrome, but rather explained failure on tests of IQ on the basis of lack of cooperation. It is unfortunate that many myths about the syndrome that developed during the 1950s still hold sway, even with members of the medical profession. Bertelheim (1956) introduced the idea that the prime cause of autism was an unloving and threatening relationship with the parents in the earliest years – the so-called 'refrigerator mother'. Kanner also felt that he could detect some autistic traits in the child's parents that could contribute to this supposed abnormal bonding. The idea that the mother and her upbringing of the child is the root cause of the autism has probably been as damaging as Bateson's theories of the double-bind as a cause of schizophrenia. There is no evidence that the parents of autistic children are less affectionate or caring than others, and even at its conception the idea could not explain why other children in the family were completely normal. However, even today there are parents who suffer from guilt based on this erroneous idea.

The use of the terms childhood schizophrenia and childhood psychosis to describe autism have also caused problems. The term autistic, in the sense of autistic aloneness or social withdrawal, was first conceived by Bleuler (1950) as one of the four primary diagnostic symptoms of schizophrenia. The psychody-

namic base to the origin of autism was questioned in the early 1960s, and it is now clear that it is a disorder of developmental neurobiology and consequent developmental psychology. Autism is not a variant of schizophrenia (Rutter 1978), this being an outdated concept based on presumed psychodynamic origins of schizophrenia. Schizophrenia beginning in childhood is a very clear disorder, and very rare. The term childhood schizophrenia should be restricted to mean this, and the important restriction was introduced into DSM-III. The terms infantile psychosis and infantile autism should probably be abandoned, as the person grows to become an autistic teenager and then an autistic adult.

Classification

Current definitions all revolve around dysfunction in three main areas – Wing's triad of two-way social interactions, communication, and restricted, repetitive behaviour. (Rutter & Schopler 1987).

The current revision of the international classification of mental and behavioural disorders, ICD-10 (WHO 1992), has created a classification group of pervasive developmental disorders which includes childhood autism (F84.0) and atypical autism (F84.1) within the larger grouping of disorders of psychological development. The disorders also include Rett's syndrome, Asperger's syndrome and overactivity disorder with learning disability and stereotyped movements. The definition of autistic disorder in ICD-10 requires an onset before the age of 3 as well as the triad.

The interaction deficits include an inadequate appreciation of social cues and/or a lack of adjustment of behavioural response in accordance with social context, and especially marked problems in initiating and sustaining two-way relationships. There is also a lack of appropriate social use of whatever language skills have developed, the poor use of conversation and relatively little reciprocal exchange. There is a lack of appropriate response to other peoples verbal and non-verbal cues, and the tonality of speech is restricted or unusual with little use of emphasis, cadence or accompanying gestures. There are also stereotyped and repetitive patterns in behaviours, interests and activities. These are restrictive and tend to impose a rigidity and routine on a wide range of daily activities, and there is a great resistance to change in these functions. In children there may be a specific attachment to unusual objects and at all ages motor stereotypies may occur, such as flapping and rocking movements.

This definition mirrors that found in DSM-IV (APA 1994) for autistic disorder (299.00), which has a well defined set of diagnostic criteria, and it is useful to paraphrase these here. A total of at least six items from three groups is required for diagnosis:

- At least two items from a series of qualitative impairments of social interaction. They show a marked impairment in the use of multiple non-verbal behaviours, such as eye-to-eye contact, facial expressiveness, body posture, and gestures used to regulate social interaction. They fail to develop relationships appropriate to their developmental level with their peer group. There is a limitation in their ability spontaneously to seek out and share enjoyments, interests or achievements with other people. They fail to reciprocate appropriately in social or emotional interactions.

- At least one item from a series of qualitative impairments in communication. They do not develop, or show a delay in developing, spoken language, which is not accompanied by attempts to compensate through other ways of communicating, e.g. by gestures, or signing, or imitation. Where speech has developed adequately they have a marked impairment in the ability to initiate or sustain a conversation. They show a stereotyped and repetitive use of language, or idiosyncratic and peculiar language. They lack varied spontaneous make believe play or social imitative play appropriate to their level of development.

- At least one of the following restricted, repetitive and stereotyped patterns of behaviour, interests and activities. They display an all-encompassing preoccupation with one or more stereotypes and restricted pattern of interest, abnormal in intensity or focus. They have an apparently inflexible adherence to specific and (seemingly) non-functional routines or rituals. There are stereotyped and repetitive motor mannerisms. They have a persistent preoccupation with parts of objects.

With DSM-IV, autistic disorder moved from being an Axis II disorder to an Axis I disorder, in part due to the increasing acceptance of its origin in disturbance of developmental and neurobiological processes. Learning disability is not required for its diagnosis, and when present, is classed as an Axis II associated condition. However, people with autistic disorder who do not have learning disability are very much the minority.

These criteria have been validated in a large multi-centre study by Volkmar et al (1994) of 1000 young people, including 454 with autism and 240 with other pervasive developmental disorders. Another large study of over 700 children with developmental disorders or learning disability (Waterhouse et al 1996) compared a variety of classification systems (DSM-III, DSM-IIIR, DSM-IV and ICD-10) and found that all were able to identify autistic core groups with significantly lower IQ and adaptive functioning levels. Within the autistic diagnoses two separate groups could be identified, one with lower and one with higher degree of functioning. A possible relation between the high functioning group and Asperger's syndrome needs further study. A study from Norway (Sponheim 1996) confirmed the validity of the DSM-IV subgroups of pervasive developmental disorder, and for autism in ICD-10. The former classified slightly more cases as autistic disorder, whereas the latter tended to put these into the other (and for ICD-10 more numerous) groupings included in pervasive developmental disorder. There were some difficulties with the diagnosis of Rett's syndrome by ICD-10 criteria but the agreement about the diagnosis of autistic disorder between the two instruments was high.

Epidemiology

The estimated prevalence of autism very much depends on the diagnostic criteria used. As a label, it has been incorrectly applied to many children and adults with learning disability, and especially those who have been in institutions for extensive periods, who show some of features resembling autism, especially the stereotyped movements and the development of rigid and repetitive behaviours. Studies on hospitalised patients have shown that up to one-third may have autistic spectrum disorders and this group also tends to have severe behavioural difficulties. Studies have also focused on children, when it is clear that autism continues into adulthood. The early studies (Lotter 1966) gave a rate for the full syndrome of 2:10 000 children. More recent studies have shown on average a much higher prevalence, between 10 and 20 per 10 000 children (Wing & Gould 1979, Gillberg et al 1986 – Rutter's criteria; Tanoue et al 1988 – using DSM-III criteria). The latter figures, if replicated, place autism as a rather common disorder with a rate of between 1:1000 and 1:500 children. If adults with autism were also considered the figures would obviously be considerably greater. Consistently more males than females are affected, with the sex ratio reported to be between 2:1 and over 3:1. The predominance of men is even more pronounced in those with the mildest learning disability. A heterogeneous causation could explain this finding, with a subgroup of autism associated with mild degrees of learning disability due to an X-linked disorder. The true cause is however unknown. Kanner's original postulate of a link to higher social class in the parents of these children has received no support from recent studies.

Clinical features

Most of the behavioural changes that we associate with autism require the development of complex abilities in children and thus the diagnosis of autism is rarely made in the youngest years, and usually not until the child is around 4 years old. The implication that autism was present at an earlier age is usually based on a retrospective analysis of the developmental history. Lister (1992 MD thesis reported in Happé 1994) looked at a large cohort of over 1000 children at 12 months, 6 years and 12 years for predictors of autism, but found nothing at 12 months associated with the later development of autism. Johnson et al (1992), in a retrospective analysis, again found very few problems and normal socialisation at 12 months in those who were later diagnosed as having autism, but at 18 months they were beginning to show specific problems in social interactions, and high-risk studies on the siblings of autistic children also indicate that deficits may start to appear at around 18 months (Baron-Cohen et al 1992).

The clinical picture is very variable, and the atypical case seems more common than the full classical picture, especially when associated with more severe degrees of learning disability. It is clear that autism is not restricted to childhood but can continue right through adulthood (Shah et al 1982), and, if associated with learning disability, can cause immense social problems for the person. The social difficulties can be manifest as aloneness and indifference to the social presence of others through to a highly passive stance in social interaction. The gaze avoidance, stressed in the earliest descriptions, is often not a feature: there is, rather, an inappropriateness of eye contact, sometimes with long periods of staring. The structure of the social interaction is disorganised, sometimes in very subtle ways, so that it takes detailed analysis to pinpoint what has happened. The person may use social cues and body language inappropriately; for instance, one person breaks into song or whistling at odd points of a conversation, and is, at first glance, over-friendly, staring directly and openly welcoming, which later is seen as a stereotyped and inappropriate approach to making initial contact with people. In children any play that exists is not influenced by other children, and does not display normal degrees of imaginative development. Speech may never develop, especially in those with more severe learning disability, but sometimes in those whose development in other areas is much greater. The presence of mutism in such a person can be disconcerting, sometimes extending even to the utterances of cries of pleasure or pain, although the facial expression of emotions may be relatively intact. In those who are able to develop speech it can be very repetitive in its content and echolalic. The repertoire of themes for conversation can be very narrow, but within these can be surprisingly developed, to the extent of an obsession with the intrinsic detail and facts of the specific topic. The conversation is held on this topic, usually despite attempts by the correspondent to change the subject. Stereotyped movements are again more prominent in those with severer degrees of learning disability, but mannerisms and tic-like activity (which, to the person is purposeful and aware) can be seen even in those with mild degrees of handicap. Hand flapping, gazing and body rocking are among the most common. Some people may spin around repetitively, sometimes with their hands outstretched. There is often a fascination for objects which may form part of their mannerisms, for instance the twirling of sticks or feathers in the hand. Objects may be collected repeatedly and hoarded – records, cards, envelopes – and may be arranged in special patterns. There may be a preoccupation with a temporal routine. The person must rise at a specific time, must go to certain places at definite times of the day, and will tend to incorporate rituals and mannerisms around a specific timetable. In some people with autism there also an increased need for personal space. In adults, at least, a feature of our hospitals for people with learning disability has often been a great deal of external space, and some people with autism seem driven to use this to the utmost extent, walking in fixed routes over the grounds. Attempts to change such behaviours by psychological interventions, or even physical limitation of activity, have not been entirely successful, and often seem to cause a great deal of anguish and meet with exceptional resistance from the person with autism. There is an important view that we should accept that the person with autism has specific environmental and temporal needs, and although these may differ from the general norms, they should be met and accepted, rather than frustrating attempts made to change them.

Biology

Autistic disorder, like schizophrenia, probably comprises a group of conditions that share the same clinical picture. At present most of our understanding is based on the natural history of the condition in children, and continuing studies through adulthood are needed. Autism is more frequent in males, suggesting a sex linkage of the condition in a percentage of cases. Autism also shows a tendency to run in some families. Overall the rate of autism in the siblings of a proband is around 3% – a marked increase over the rate in the general population – and other cognitive impairments including language disorder are also raised in sibs (Bolton & Rutter 1990). If atypical autism and Asperger's syndrome are included the rate is around 6%; if other forms of pervasive developmental disorders are also included then nearly 7% of sibs will be affected (Waterhouse et al 1996). Twin studies also indicate a genetic component. The concordance rate for monozygotic twins is much higher than for dyzygotic twins (Folstein & Rutter 1988), but is not full, and other factors must play a role. In studies of families multiply affected with autism (Ritvo et al 1985, Spence et al 1985) an autosomal recessive inheritance has been suggested, however the heterogeneity of the condition must make such interpretations difficult. Medical illnesses that involve the central nervous system have been found in up to one-half of cases of autism, especially those with the more profound degrees of disability (Reiss et al 1986, Wing 1994). They include tuberous sclerosis, untreated phenylketonuria, neurofibromatosis and neuronal damage caused directly by infections such as congenital rubella and herpes simplex, or perhaps indirectly via immune mechanisms with cytomegalovirus (Stubbs 1988). It is unclear whether these associations are real or coincidental but it is reasonable to assume that some will be true phenocopies. Of relevance to the excess of males with autism is a suggested association with the fragile X syndrome (Le Couter 1988), though recent studies have not revealed any triplet expansions in autism. Holden et al (1996) looked at 19 families with at least two boys with autism or pervasive developmental disorders and found no evidence for expansion of triplet repeats at three fragile sites on the X chromosome.

Brain imaging in autism has revealed a number of non-specific abnormalities. Some studies have implicated the cerebellar vermis (Courchesne et al 1988), which also has been reported abnormal in fragile X syndrome. Postmortem studies have shown Purkinje and granule cell loss in the cerebellar vermis and cerebellar hemispheres. There are also cytoarchitectural abnormalities in the hippocampus and amygdala which have led to comparisons of autism with features of the Klüver–Bucy syndrome. In the hippocampus the cellular abnormality suggests immature brain development, perhaps during the first 6 months of pregnancy. The occurrence of autism after herpes simplex encephalitis, which has specificity for hippocampal structures, may also be related to damage in this area.

Such abnormalities in brain development might be expected to influence neurotransmitter systems. Serotonin has been found to be increased in autism (Young et al 1982), but such a change is not specific to this condition and is found in many other people with learning disability. Trials of serotonin-lowering agents such as fenfluramine have not produced evidence for consistent effect in double-blind cross-over trials (Ho et al 1986, Kohler et al 1987). Endorphins have also been reported as increased in the cerebrospinal fluid (Gillberg 1988). The prevalence of stereotypies and mannerisms has also suggested hyperactivity in dopaminergic systems, based on comparison with motor dysfunctions in animal studies. Most studies have not found consistent differences in the levels of dopamine metabolites in autism, but neuroleptics are sometimes useful in control of mannerisms in people with learning disability in general.

Abnormalities of psychological development

A number of psychological theories have been developed or adapted to try and explain the psychological deficits in autism, but our limited knowledge about the neural processes involved in communication and social interactions has limited the testability of these models; the idea that a single common process underlies the genesis of the three areas of difficulty in autism may be over-simplistic. Currently the theory with the greatest explanatory power as to the development of the symptoms and signs is the 'theory of mind' where people with autism are said to have difficulties in attributing mental states as part of the self or independently as belonging to others – in other words, difficulties in developing cognitive representations of such abstract concepts as self and non-self, essential to the understanding of social interactions and their cognitive repercussions. The ability to recognise that mental sets can exist in other people independent of the self is said to be critical to socialisation, communication and imagination (Frith 1992). Autistic children fail on tests such as the Sally-Ann task designed to test their ability to generate secondary abstractions about mind-sets, tests that children of comparable mental age with Down's syndrome and control children seem able to cope with. This important finding is made even more interesting by the fact that some children with autism seem to do better than controls on tests that set out to investigate beliefs about objects rather than other peoples mind-sets (Leslie & Thaiss 1992), suggesting the problem may be specific to the ability to correctly attribute belief systems to other people. Most of the subjects tested were at the mild end of the learning disability spectrum, and some studies have really been on very able children, who perhaps would fall into the Asperger's syndrome category. With the probable differences in the aetiology of autism, and the sex differences related to the ability level, the generality of the results awaits further study.

Associated behavioural and psychiatric problems

Most of the behavioural difficulties that are associated with autism seem to result when changes are made in the predictable routines of day-to-day life. Aggression to others or self-injurious acts are usually a response to fear, either fear of change or as a reaction to change underway. Problems with communication, especially lack of speech, often mean that the person with autism has to use other ways of imparting his or her concerns, such as screaming. The understanding of the meaning of such outbursts, which may otherwise be interpreted as temper tantrums, is important in helping the person. The introduction of new environments and routines is best done over a long timescale, with gradual changes in day-to-day living building up to the eventual goal. The needs of someone with autism are very different from the needs of others, and the concept of normalisation for them does not usually mean that they should be forced to adopt the norms of general society. They have a right to have their own specific needs met, and this means the design of an appropriate environment and routine.

There is some indication that psychiatric problems increase in people with autism as they grow into their teens and adulthood. Bipolar disorder and major depressive disorder have been reported as starting in adolescence, as well as an increase in the severity of some behavioural symptoms such as obsessions, and an apparent lack of motivation. There are no reports of any increase in schizophrenia.

Therapies

The main aim with children is to allow as full an education as possible. Help with language acquisition is especially important, and requires a highly individualised educational programme. Intervention may be required to reduce any behavioural disorders that may interfere with learning, and the full cooperation of the family is needed to make a success of these. Behavioural therapies may need to be carried out on a one-to-one basis, and although the person can fully exist in a group, and often in group living, there is often little constructive or understanding interaction with others. The general treatment focus at present is on helping the person to generalise social skills, to target the development of expressive language, and to use task analysis to aid day-to-day living (Matson et al 1996). The importance of involving parents, siblings and peers is recognised, as well as situating the intervention in the person's natural environment, and the concept of identifying and tackling the pivotal behaviours around which others evolve is helpful.

At all ages the management of change is a difficult issue. Change can be of three basic sorts – change in living environment, change in the temporal structure of the daily routine, and change in social contacts and carers. The effects of the last are often forgotten when the person is living in supported accommodation away from home. The effects of a high staff turnover may be noticeable in increased behavioural difficulties. Even though there may be difficulty in forming relationships, the person with autism has a need, like all other people with learning disability, for consistency.

Drug therapies have a limited role in autism. Antipsychotics, especially haloperidol, have been said to have a beneficial effect in reducing anger and irritability in children, with facilitation of language development. Long-term movement disorders, including tardive dyskinesia, are a significant problem with such medication in this group. In adults antipsychotics are used widely and in wide-ranging doses, often as a last resort to try and reduce behaviour disturbance or severe stereotypic movements and mannerisms. There is a well-known tendency to continue such medication on a long-term basis once started. Antipsychotics are probably helpful in a subgroup of people with autism, especially to reduce agitation when enforced change occurs, but the need should be regularly reviewed, and it is usually better to try and examine the environmental needs of the person to see if these can be met and a routine maintained. Trials of serotonin blockers have shown equivocal beneficial effects but may help in individual cases.

Rett's syndrome and childhood disintegrative disorder

Rett's syndrome and childhood disintegrative disorder are progressive conditions, the latter being exceedingly rare. Most children with these syndromes eventually develop severe to profound degrees of learning disability. Rett's syndrome nearly always affects girls, and there is a disastrous loss of previously acquired skills after the age of 5 months. Movement disorders develop and are helped by haloperidol. In the late stages the severe handicap may be accompanied by epilepsy, decreased mobility and growth retardation. The cause is as yet unknown.

OTHER ASSOCIATED CONDITIONS

Epilepsy

Epilepsy is common in people with learning disability – it may be found in over 40% of hospitalised patients –

and reflects the degree of developmental damage to the brain. It is impossible to cover the field here, but several points are important to the psychiatrist. Epilepsy may begin at any age, and its presentation may change with time, and be of multiple forms in the same person. In tuberous sclerosis, for example, early infantile spasms may later be replaced with grand mal seizures and simple or complex partial seizures. The epilepsy in some cases may become progressively worse with time, in association with progress of hamartomas in the brain. Temporal lobe seizures can produce a variety of behavioural manifestations from limited tics and stereotypies through to complete motor automatisms and psychosis-like behaviour. The peri-ictal period is often difficult for the person whatever the seizure type. Confusion and discomfort may lead to apparent aggression and outbursts. The person with a prolonged recovery period is best nursed in a quiet and familiar environment. Attention should be paid to soiling and wetting associated with a seizure: many people with learning disability are very conscious of their appearance and can be very distressed at the loss of dignity.

Treatment of the multiple forms of epilepsy may be difficult. Newer antiepileptic drugs, such as lamotrigine, vigabactrin and gabapentin, are sometimes very helpful in adjunctive control of refractory epilepsy and have been used with marked success in many people with learning disability. However, drugs such as vigabactrin can be psychotropic and precipitate behavioural and mood disturbances in predisposed people. Carbamazepine can be used if mood control is needed, and is a useful alternative to lithium in some cases. Status epilepticus, or serial repeated seizures, is a medical emergency. Rectal diazepam may abort the condition, but some need intravenous benzodiazepines for control. If there is any difficulty in obtaining speedy resolution the person is best transferred to the appropriate medical unit. That repeated status attacks can lead to further brain damage is a controversial issue, but a clinical impression is that it can occur if associated with repeated episodes of severe cyanosis. The management of complex and severe epilepsy in those with learning disability is best done by a specialist, in some areas a neurologist; in other areas specialist epilepsy services for people with learning disability have been successfully established with clinics based in health centres or general practices.

Dual diagnosis: the occurrence of psychiatric illness

Psychiatric disorders, and especially the most severe disorders such as schizophrenia and bipolar illness, can not only be diagnosed in people with learning disability, but occur at a much more frequent rate than in the general population. In the past the two conditions were thought to be mutually exclusive (Shapiro 1979), as the necessary communication skills to allow full presentation of a psychosis were not present in someone with learning disability. The definition of psychiatric disorders in the learning disabled has also suffered from diagnostic overshadowing (Reiss & Syszko 1983, Sovner 1986), leading to a substantial level of underdiagnosis (Reiss 1990), further confused by the historical distinction between primary and secondary handicaps.

Currently there is a tendency to use the term dual diagnosis to embrace those with learning disability and a major psychiatric illness. At the most superficial level, a psychosis is a particular combination of behaviour and communication disturbances, and the patterns and intensities of these within such a disturbance, combined with their development over time, lead to the application of a specific diagnosis such as schizophrenia or bipolar disorder. In people with learning disability, efforts have been made to separate similar disturbances into those considered to be behavioural disorders and those which are psychiatric disorders, with the implication that the former are reactive events to external and environmental circumstances. There is little evidence that such a division is useful or has meaning, and if a person's symptoms and signs fall into a classifiable grouping within the terms of DSM-IV or ICD-10 then that particular diagnosis should be used (Szymanski 1994).

The level of psychiatric morbidity in people with learning disability is, in fact, high at all ages. In children and adolescents with learning disability recent studies have confirmed previous reports (Ruedrich & Menolascino 1984) of high rates of psychiatric disorder. In a study in New South Wales, Einfeld & Tonge (1996) found that over 40% of those aged between 4 and 18 had severe emotional or behavioural disorder or psychiatric disorder. Most (90%) of the parents of these children reported great difficulty in obtaining appropriate specialist help. There is a lack of adequate longitudinal studies following children through to adulthood to identify predictors of different psychiatric outcomes.

Schizophrenia

Kraepelin originally introduced the term Propfschizophrenie to describe those cases of dementia praecox arising in people with learning disability, and thought the conditions coexisted in about 7% of people with learning disability. He felt that this psychosis was of especially early onset and itself led to the development of intellectual disability. Bleuler was later to deny that there was a true association, an idea that persisted, and was further confused by the later use of the term childhood schizophrenia in the context of autism.

It is now widely accepted that the incidence of schizophrenia is raised in those who also have learning disability. On average the rate is raised threefold over the general population. Many of the earlier studies were hospital based. Reid (1972b) found a 3% rate of schizophrenia or paranoid psychosis in hospital residents, using a clinical diagnosis. On follow-up, he felt the disorder ran a more benign course than in non-learning disabled individuals. In the Camberwell studies Corbett (1979) found schizophrenia at similar levels in hospital and community settings, at a rather higher level than other reports, of around 6%. Most studies have been hampered by a lack of adequately validated rating scales for psychiatric disorder in those with intellectual disability. There is a great awakening of interest at present in the relationship between schizophrenia and learning disability and the other dual diagnoses, especially in the implications they have for future service provisions in the community. However, the proposition that mental health problems of the learning disabled are greater than in others has not been accepted with open arms by professions other than psychiatry, and there is a continuing need to refine the diagnostic process and clarify the true prevalence of schizophrenia and other psychiatric disorders.

Clinical features   There is little overall difference in the presentation of schizophrenia between those with mild learning disability and those in the general population (Meadows et al 1991), but the age of onset is significantly earlier (on average 23 years). Thought disorder and complex persecutory delusions are probably less evident. In persons with moderate degrees of learning disability hallucinations may occur, and, in combination with persecutory feelings, may lead to fear, social withdrawal and rarely aggressive outbursts.

In people with severe or profound learning disability a lack of communication skills means that diagnosis on conventional lines is often impossible. However, unless one holds the view that a degree of intellectual development is absolutely necessary for the presentation of schizophrenia, there is no reason to suppose that they cannot suffer from the same disorder. Acting on a different neurological substrate, this produces a behavioural disturbance that can be very distressing for the person and the carers. There may be aggressive outbursts or bizarre behaviours in response to apparently fearful stimuli, mood lability, an increase in stereotypies and mannerisms, or an onset of these anew. After extensive investigation there may be no physical or environmental reasons for the change in the person, nor any consistent precipitants. The diagnosis is always difficult, and will remain as unspecified functional psychosis, but the symptoms often show a response to a trial of neuroleptics. A detailed family history can be useful and familial schizophrenia is not uncommonly found.

Aetiology   In common with schizophrenia in the general population the cause is unknown, and is likely to be multiple. The two striking features of schizophrenia in people with learning disability, the increased incidence (which is perhaps an underestimate, as those with severe and profound learning disability are excluded) and the earlier age of onset, could be explained by one (or all) of several mechanisms. There could be the coincidental occurrence of schizophrenia and learning disability. However, this would not explain the increased rate. The schizophrenia could be a result of developmental insult in learning disability encroaching on the anatomical areas that are involved in the genesis of schizophrenic symptoms – thus schizophrenia would be secondary to the cause of learning disability. The learning disability could be a consequence of a very early and severe form of schizophrenia (as originally proposed by Kraepelin), and the age of onset is certainly earlier. Or, finally, the coassociation between schizophrenia and learning disability may be a true one with one a common cause. One such common cause could be a contiguous gene deletion syndrome which resulted in the loss of genes needed to prevent both disorders. These syndromes tend to be non-inherited however, and one feature of people with dual diagnosis is a strong family history, often for both disorders. The familial coassociation can be complex and coexist with other disorders or chromosome rearrangements (Holland & Gosden 1990, Sharp et al 1994, Mors et al 1997), and a final possibility is that the disorders are actually different facets of one underlying inherited genetic condition.

Bipolar disorder

Bipolar disorder disproportionately affects those with learning disability but not, it seems, to the same degree as schizophrenia. Depression as a symptom is extremely common in those with learning disability (Sovner & Hurley 1983). The prevalence rates for bipolar illness and depression are uncertain, and estimates vary widely from 2 to 12% of the learning disabled population (Reid 1972a, Heaton-Ward 1977, Corbett 1979). These figures are in general higher, however, than the general population prevalence of around 0.8%. Reliable diagnosis can be difficult in those with learning disability but in those with mild to moderate degrees of learning disability the standard diagnostic criteria can be valid (Fraser & Nolan 1994). Unlike schizophrenia, even in those with severe degrees of learning disability the diagnosis can be usefully made using the biological features of depression and mania (King et al 1994). As in schizophrenia, the presence of a family history in such cases is also helpful (Sovner 1989) in increasing the likelihood of correct diagnosis. There have been few studies comparing the symptom profile of bipolar disorder in adults with learning disability with illness in the general population and very little is known of the natural history of the disorder. However, it is generally thought that the symptoms of depression are modified by learning disability, and certain behaviours (hyperactivity and wandering, mutism, unexplained temper tantrums, etc.) may be symptomatic of depression in this group – behaviours that are not seen in depression in the general population ('depressive equivalents': Cole & Hardy 1985).

Major depressive disorder

The increased susceptibility of adults with Down's syndrome to depression has already been noted. Depression can occur in any person with learning disability, and is found in children as well as adults. The biological features are sometimes more marked than the subjective feelings of depression, but a low mood is a frequent symptom even in the more severely disabled. Suicidal thoughts and acts can occur in people with mild and borderline learning disability, but are not frequent and indeed seem to be rare in the more severely disabled, and may be difficult to separate from a form of self-injurious or ritualistic behaviour. A time chart of sleep, activity pattern, eating and cyclical changes in mood associates (aggressive, self-injurious behaviour, sexual behaviour, irritability, anhedonia, apathy and withdrawal) as well as observed mood changes can help to establish diurnal or other circadian rhythms and point to the diagnosis. In more severely handicapped adult women the time course associated with the menstrual cycle must be considered, and a painful premenstrual period or menses themselves can be mistaken for mood disorder.

Other disorders

Chronic anxiety disorder can occur but is difficult to distinguish from depression. Low self-esteem may be a confusing feature of both conditions. Personality disorder is difficult to define. Reid & Ballinger (1987) felt that it was present in some form in over 20% of those with mild to moderate handicap in hospital. The relevance of this diagnosis in people with overall developmental delays is uncertain, and it is difficult to say whether features such as passiveness and dependence are the product of an abnormal personality development or part of the cluster of symptoms that characterise specific aspects of the person's learning disability. The approach to help the person, who may be very vulnerable when these features are predominant in their presentation along with learning disability, is supportive and there is the danger that appending the diagnosis of a personality disorder, unless the clinician is on very certain grounds, may lead to an exclusion of the individual from the required services. Attention deficit/hyperactivity disorder is a prominent feature of children (and adults) with learning disability, and the criteria for this condition can be met in up to 20%. The use of stimulant medications may help in the mildly learning disabled who meet the full criteria, but their effectiveness in the many children who have only some symptoms, and in people with severe or profound learning disability, has not been shown.

There have been reports of increased levels of obsessive–compulsive disorder in learning disability (Vitiello et al 1989) and it is said that the phenomenon of hand washing is less common than in the general population. The distinction from the ritualistic behaviours associated with autism requires care however, and the psychological consequences of the obsessions and compulsions need to fit clearly with the diagnostic criteria for obsessive–compulsive disorder.

Treatment issues

Oral and depot neuroleptics are frequently used in treating psychiatric and behavioural disturbance in people with learning disability. Between 5 and 10% of those in hospitals (Wressel et al 1990) and up to 5% of those known to community learning disability health services (Thinn et al 1990) may receive depot neuroleptics, and overall psychotropic drug use may be as high as 30% in the community. The most common indication is schizophrenia or schizophreniform psychosis (Gravestock 1996), which account for around 50% of those on depot, but a significant minority (23%) do not have psychosis. A major worry in those who have epilepsy is a reduction in seizure threshold, but this is by no means a contraindication and the adjustment of the dose of neuroleptic or anticonvulsant can usually allow such cotherapy. Long-term use is associated with the possibility of chronic movement disorders, including tardive dyskinesia, which may superimpose and worsen existing movement abnormalities, or be confused with stereotypies intrinsic to the condition producing the learning disability. Although chlorpromazine, thioridazine and haloperidol remain in extensive use, the newer neuroleptics such as sulpiride and risperidone seem to be well tolerated in people with mild learning disability and psychosis. Clozapine is useful as a therapy in resistant cases, although the intensive initial monitoring of blood parameters is sometimes difficult if the person is unwilling to undergo repetitive venepuncture (a problem which is rather more widespread than admitted in subjects with severe and profound degrees of handicap). Very low doses of medications will obtain an effect in some people with learning disability, presumably as a result of differences in metabolism. Clinical experience has shown that syrup or liquid formulations are helpful, and hospital pharmacies may be able to make up very low dose suspensions of some neuroleptics such as sulpiride.

Mood-stabilising medications are frequently used in treating various behavioural problems in the learning disabled (Crabbe 1994), often empirically or on the basis of cyclical behavioural changes. The use of antidepressants is governed by the same criteria as in the general population, always keeping in mind the increased likelihood of epilepsy in this population and of cardiac or other systemic problems, especially in adults with Down's syndrome. Lithium can be used in bipolar illness but possible interactions with systemic disorders (e.g. hypothyroidism) must be taken into account. Carbamazepine is increasingly used as a mood-stabilising agent, and is useful in those who also have epilepsy. The dose levels needed to control mood may be slightly lower than those for epilepsy in some cases and should be titrated individually.

Behavioural disorders: challenging behaviours

The concept

As with psychiatric disorders, behavioural problems are overrepresented in people with learning disability. The term 'challenging behaviour' is used to describe a vast number of different maladaptive behaviours, ranging from minor antisocial behaviours leading to some disruption of day-to-day living up to serious aggressive outbursts against others or the person themselves. The reported prevalences of such behaviours are high, as is their persistence (Einfeld & Tong 1996). Studies on people with learning disability in seven health districts in north-west England (Qureshi 1994) used a set of criteria to define when a behaviour could be considered challenging – at least one of the following should hold true:

- At some time must have caused more than minor injuries to themselves or others or destroyed their immediate living or working environment.
- At least weekly had a behaviour that required intervention by staff or placed them in physical

danger, or caused damage that could not be rectified immediately or caused at least an hour's disruption.
- Caused over a few minutes' disruption at least daily.

Seven per cent of people with learning disability met the criteria overall, with those in hospital showing a higher prevalence (14%) than those in community placements (5%). People aged between 15 and 34 years were especially prominent, with 15–19-year-olds being the greatest problem in the community, and 25-29-year- olds in hospital. Most of the people were classified as having severe to profound learning disability, and only a small percentage of these were said to have mental illness, but most of those within the small group of mild to borderline learning disability were said also to have mental illness. This may reflect the difficulties of diagnosis of mental illness in the more severely handicapped, but also indicates that a substantial percentage of people who exhibit challenging behaviour may not have a concurrent psychiatric disorder. Reid & Ballinger (1995) have followed up a group of 100 severely handicapped men and women since 1975 and found a worrying persistence of many problems, especially symptoms of the autistic type, such as emotional withdrawal, stereotypies and avoidance of eye contact, in the 67 surviving people. Noisiness, overactivity, irritability and social withdrawal were also persistent.

Types

The numbers and forms of challenging behaviour are truly legion, as are their causes and meaning, so that the usefulness of any descriptive typology is open to debate. It is postulated that many behaviours are related to institutionalisation; however, they are also found in people who have never been in hospital, and a persistent decrease on resettlement from hospital to community has yet to be adequately described.

The minor disorders are often of an antisocial rather than destructive nature but their chronicity and form can be highly degrading to the person and prejudice social acceptance and integration. Shouting and screaming may simply be ways of either attracting attention or, conversely, protecting the personal space of an individual. Repetitive extreme noisiness is wearing for the person, other residents and care staff. Anal poking and faecal smearing are often due to difficulties in toileting or to constipation rather than a behavioural disturbance per se, but are extremely distressing. Similarly, self-induced vomiting and other food-related behaviours such as deliberate choking are unacceptable in a normal living environment. Stealing, often of food or hot drinks, is important in hospital settings, and perhaps often genuinely produced by them. It can be a game which some use to create attention, but has attendant dangers of scalding. True caffeine addiction may result in some cases, and the resultant dysphoria misinterpreted as psychiatric illness.

Aggressive outbursts can be against person or property, and while severe physical violence is fortunately rare, it is a major limiting factor in community provision for people with severe degrees of learning disability, especially if there are no factors that predict outbursts.

Self-injurious behaviour is a worrying problem that can range from simple skin picking through to severe eye gouging, head banging and face beating. Repetitive self-injury and self-mutilation is perhaps the most distressing of all the problems that present to psychiatrists in learning disability. It is much more common in people with severe and profound degrees of learning disability (Reid et al 1978), and in this group it is associated with the presence of other challenging behaviours such as noisiness, overactivity, irritability and stripping. The overall prevalence may be around 10% in all forms, and between 1 and 2% for the most severe (Corbett 1975).

Aetiology

This is complex and all factors tend to interact, so that one particular type of behaviour may relate to different causal mechanisms at different times.

Associated biological disorders

Since challenging behaviours are most prevalent in people with severe learning disability, definite biological disorders might be expected to be associated with them. The discipline of behavioural phenotypes that attempts to relate clusters of behaviours with particular clinical syndromes is an emerging one. However, behavioural associations for the two most important disorders with a defined biological basis, Down's syndrome and the fragile X syndrome, have proven difficult to define and validate. Even in discrete disturbances such as in phenylketonuria, the metabolic changes lead to non-specific and variable behavioural consequences. At present only two conditions stand out as being associated with a definite constellation of behaviours.

The Lesch–Nyhan syndrome (Johnson & Patel 1996) is extremely rare, but has assumed prominence out of proportion to its incidence owing to the striking degree of self-mutilation associated with it. At birth such children appear healthy, but by 3–4 months dystonias become apparent, along with a delay in attaining developmental milestones. The later development of spasticity, choreiform movements and transient hemiparesis

can lead to the diagnosis of cerebral palsy, but the appearance, at around 2 years, of self-destructive biting of the lips, the inside of the mouth and the fingers, points to the correct diagnosis. The degree of learning disability is variable. The condition follows an X-linked recessive inheritance pattern and is due to a mutation in the HPRT (hypoxanthine phosphoribosyltransferase) gene with a near total lack of the enzyme and an associated hyperuricaemia. Dopamine levels are reduced in the basal ganglia and in synaptic terminals, but not in the cell bodies in the substantia nigra. The other monaminergic systems seem intact. Treatment studies using oral 5-hydroxytryptamine (5-HT) have been claimed to reduce the incidence of self-mutilation, but other studies have not been able to reproduce this. Behavioural interventions have produced similarly disappointing results. The peripheral consequences such as hyperuricaemia are treatable but the centrally mediated behaviours persist. The gene can be genetically inactivated ('knocked-out') in mice but these do not display symptoms similar to those seen in man. Thus the link between aberrant dopamine levels and severe self-mutilation is still to be uncovered, and most people who self-mutilate do not have this syndrome.

The Prader–Willi syndrome occurs in around 1:14 000 children and is usually due to deletions or uniparental disomy of an imprinted region of chromosome 15. The inheritance of the condition is described in Chapter 7. The overeating behaviour exists in nearly all cases, but to varying degrees, and studies suggest that abnormal time patterns or control of satiety may play a role. Overeating can lead to enormous degrees of obesity (Holland 1991).

Psychological associates

At the root of many psychological interventions for challenging behaviours is the concept that both the behaviours and ways of modifying them are learned and maintained by positive or negative reinforcers (Bailey & Pyles 1989). Reinforcers are divided into primary ones, such as food, drink and pain, associated with basic biological needs, and secondary ones that result from a pairing with primary reinforcers. Social reinforcers (praise, pleasant environments, aversive stimuli, etc) are generally thought to be secondary in type. The antecedents of a behaviour can be difficult to determine, and the use of a given behaviour may generalise beyond the original inducing stimuli and reinforcers. However, it is important to try and understand both the origin of the behaviour, its original maintaining factors, the present maintaining factors, and the meaning it has for the person. This last has often been neglected, with the focus on changing the behaviour rather than viewing it as a form of communication (Durand 1990) or as an expression of frustration at difficulties in communication. It is important also to consider whether the behaviour is a consequence of physical, emotional or sexual abuse (Turk & Brown 1993), whether by family, carers or other people with learning disability. Other inducing stimuli include undetected or untreated pain (for example, a person may scratch the face in response to earache, or bite others when they have soiled themselves). Epilepsy has been postulated as a cause of challenging behaviour (Gedye 1989), and in clinical practice good epilepsy control can help reduce disturbances arising during periods of peri-ictal confusion. The behavioural automatisms during ictus in temporal lobe epilepsy should be considered as part of the illness rather than a challenging behaviour. Social reinforcers, including positive responses as well as aversive ones when the behaviour occurs, have often been shown to be maintaining factors. The linking of unwanted behaviours to positive reinforcements such as warm social responses, or concern, often leads to the person being labelled as attention seeking, and ignored, rather than a focus being made on the cause of the anomalous responses.

Environmental factors

The living situation can play an important role in maintaining a behaviour or preventing the adoption of alternative wanted behaviours. Much of the concepts of chronic institutionalisation lodged against hospital care can be viewed as the presence of a non-therapeutic physical and personal environment where the person does not have opportunities to develop the skills to alter behaviours. Some behaviours may be an ethological response to surviving in large groups of people where interactions with staff are few. On the other hand, some environmental needs, such as stability and continuity of day-to-day living patterns and adequate personal space based on individual needs, may be lacking in community placements and may also contribute to behavioural problems. To alleviate rather than contain severe behavioural disturbance it is essential to design the living and personal environment to the person. Two of the most prolific precipitants of behavioural disturbance are multiple residential placements in a short period of time (which can occur, for instance, as a person with developing dementia is shuttled from one care placement to another as they are successively unable to cope with a rapid rate of decline) and multiple changes of care staff over short periods of time, as can happen both as hospitals close and in the community where organisations have to employ staff on short-term contracts because of budgetary uncertainties.

Assessment and treatment

Assessment must address the possibility of psychiatric disorder. In people with profound degrees of handicap the presence of a family history of psychosis and a cyclical component in the behaviour pattern may indicate the diagnosis. Medical problems such as incontinence, constipation, infections, epilepsy, endocrine disturbances and sources of pain should be assessed. Sensory impairments and, if present, the way in which they are influenced by the living environment should be considered. A restricted range of communication skills may mean that the behaviour is a way of attracting attention to problems. For people who have no, or limited, verbal skills, the use of Makaton or Sign-along forms of sign language for people with learning disability is very helpful but facility in these modified forms of British sign language for the deaf is not a common skill in psychiatrists. The use of an interpreter, the advocate if the person has one, is essential here. The carer can make detailed behavioural diaries, or use the aberrant behaviour checklist or other psychometric instruments to chart the periodicity and relatedness of the behaviours. It is often helpful for the clinical psychologist and psychiatrist to work together on diagnosis and management.

Treatments should address the possible causes, stimuli and reinforcers of the behaviour, and the environment in which it occurs. In general, outcomes are better for people with milder disabilities where teaching of anger management and self-management skills and the self-monitoring of unwanted behaviours can be combined with operant interventions to replace unwanted with wanted responses. Interventions with people with severe and profound degrees of learning disability have been less successful on the whole, and it can be considerably more difficult to implement a behavioural treatment programme within the necessary restrictions of the person's own home or place of work than in a specialist behavioural unit. Whether the treatment programmes successful in such situations can generalise in place and time to the normal living environment is also largely untested. Physical restraint used to be quite widely used as a treatment rather than an emergency measure in people with learning disability, especially in those with severe self-injurious behaviour. Restraint can mean anything from the wearing of splints and protective headgear controlled by the person themselves, through to gloves for repetitive picking of skin, to full-blown devices to secure limbs in those who beat themselves, and the use of isolation and 'time out' rooms (Harris 1996). Where the device can be applied and taken off by the persons themselves, the result is sometimes surprisingly good. In such situations the extra physical control seems to provide an extra psychological barrier against self-injury. Recently there have been questions as to any superior efficacy of imposed restraint when compared with other methods, as well as moral questions as to acceptability. Emergency restraint for short periods by trained staff may be needed to protect the person from severe injury, but repeated use should be thoroughly reviewed. Positive programming methods (LaVigna et al 1989) are an altenative that use non-aversive programmes based on the teaching of skills functionally equivalent or related to target behaviours to establish a more socially appropriate repertoire.

Pharmacotherapy is still often used, even when psychiatric disorder has been eliminated as a diagnosis. In profoundly handicapped people a trial of neuroleptic is sometimes used with severe disturbance without recognisable precipitants, and is successful in some cases, with the secondary interpretation of an underlying psychiatric disturbance. Unfortunately the use of such medications tends to become long term in some cases in spite of the increased risk of tardive diskinesia. Good practice would advocate periodic attempts at drug dose reduction, and clinical experience would suggest this can be succesful if done very slowly, and by small incremental amounts. Complete drug washout, in hospital if necessary to ensure safety, can help in those maintained on high doses of medication for long periods. There is little indication that people with learning disability as a whole are any more, or any less, susceptible to the extrapyramidal effects of neuroleptic medications, and concurrent rather than emergency prescriptions of anticholinergics are not warranted save in cases of high sensitivity. It should also be remembered that both neuroleptics and anticholinergics will reduce the seizure threshold in a person with epilepsy. There is currently much interest in the use of selection serotonin reuptake inhibitors (SSRIs) in the management of various forms of challenging behaviour but the results so far have been conflicting, and often anecdotal. Clomipramine has been used to decrease self-injurious behaviour in a very small controlled study (Lewis et al 1996), but more selective agents such as fluoxetine have been claimed to increase aggressive behaviours (Troisi et al 1995).

DEVELOPMENT OF SEXUALITY AND RELATIONSHIPS

Sexuality is an inevitable part of development, and no less so in those with learning disability. Sex education and counselling are very important for them, as is the development of stable interpersonal relationships. The taboos of the past were applied in extremis to people with learning disability, and any form of sexual activity was often seen as unacceptable. Families often had (and still have) extreme difficulty in talking about the sexual development of the person with learning disability, and a whole range of genuine and unwarranted fears were repressed. People with learning disability are more prone to sexual exploitation, but this is all the more reason to ensure an understanding of their own sexuality and development, and also the issues of consent. The field is covered in detail by Craft (1994). The law has clear boundaries on various sexual practices, and the person should appreciate these. The law also defines valid sexual relations as based on an ability to consent; this is usually lacking in severe and profoundly disabled people, and any sexual activity with them by others would constitute an offence (Gunn 1994).

Education can be in a group or on individual basis, and finding the best contraception for the person is essential. Family planning clinics can offer advice, and community learning disability nurses serve an important liaison function. There are now numerous instances of people with learning disabilities marrying, and in some cases having children. Where inherited syndromes are a risk factor, then genetic counselling is appropriate.

Some sexual behaviour may be unacceptable due to the locus of behaviour (e.g. open masturbation in public places) or because of its direction (e.g. exhibitionism in public, or in front of children). The meaning of such problems for the person may be completely different to such behaviours in a person of normal intelligence, and in many cases is due to inappropriate education or unawareness of age appropriateness of a behaviour. However, it is also important to define when these are not the root of the problem, and people with mild learning disability can commit offences in public, or with children, for the same reasons as those without learning disability. It is rare that sexual problems are due to psychiatric illness but the psychiatrist in learning disability is often called to assess and treat such difficulties (see below).

THE FAMILY

The person with learning disability is usually cared for by the family, and the needs of the family often go unrecognised in the face of the needs of the child. Tizard & Grad's (1961) findings are still true: most children with learning disability do not impose intolerable management problems on their family; most parents wish to keep the child at home; it is not inevitable that the parents will always wish to care for their children at home. The reason for the last finding has changed however, and has moved from considering the alternative as being institutional provision to that of independent living.

The first crisis is when the family learns the child has learning disability. The way in which they are first told, or more frequently have their suspicions confirmed, can have a lasting influence on the way they perceive the child, but it is still sometimes done abruptly without detailed explanation of the implications or support needed. The phases of adaptation to the diagnosis parallel grief reactions, going through shock, denial, anger and eventual adaptation (Cunningham 1983). Psychiatrists are little involved in helping families at this time, most of the work being the province of the obstetrician or paediatrician. Some families can find support from others who have gone through the same problems, and the voluntary agencies can provide support groups and peer counselling. The community paediatrician plays a vital role in both providing direct help and coordinating services for the child's health needs. The effectiveness of some early intervention programmes has been mentioned above. Even with early intervention the stress to a level of clinical significance can be very high (Beckman 1991). The family's, and especially the mother's, strategies for coping with child's problems and the mother's own levels of social support are important factors in determining the eventual self-sufficiency of the person (Sloper & Turner 1996), but the reciprocal effects of the person on other important areas of family life, including the parents, marriage and perceived satisfaction with life must also be noted (Sloper et al 1991). The other area is the effect of the child on the siblings. There may be role reversal in the family where a younger sibling takes care of an older one with learning disability. However, it does not seem that there is a reduction in the quality of social relationships or time outwith the family for other siblings. Parental and family teaching workshops or teaching of skills in their own homes (Portage schemes) can achieve a high level of success in assisting parents to learn and to teach their children necessary living skills. Portage schemes can start before the child is 1 year old, and be instigated by health visitors or community learning disability nurses.

The next family milestone is schooling. The parents usually wish their child to attend mainstream schools, and can have great difficulty in accepting that he or she may be failing in such circumstances, or may need special educational provision, which to many is an additional stigma to the diagnosis. Although assisted learning at normal schools is an educational goal, the reality is that it is not universally available, and chronic class failure may be detrimental and delaying to the child who needs a specifically adapted educational curriculum.

Adolescence can also be problematic, and behavioural and emotional difficulties are as apparent in the person with learning disability as in any other teenager. Often these are interpreted as challenging behaviours to be treated, rather than as an intrinsic part of the development of emotional maturity. There is little difference in quality from the non-learning disabled adolescent, but the difficulties may be more intense due to problems in communication and understanding, or may occur at different times, with apparently teenage problems lasting into the subsequent decade. The last phase is the transition to adulthood and ageing. The transition is not only personal but also one in terms of service provision. The health services for the child are usually unified under paediatrics, but those for adults are diverse, and access may be difficult. The transition is also a time of 'letting go', with its implied increased risk taking, for the parents, and it is often harder for them to do so with their adult 'child' with learning disability than their other children. The parents (and the siblings after bereavement) remain the main carers for adults with learning disabilities, and with dual ageing, older parents usually become more and more concerned at the future for their child when they are not around, but are faced with conflicting feelings as the relationship is as important a source of support to them as it is to the child. People in their fifties and sixties staying with their octogenarian or even older parents are not unknown, and much tact and understanding has to be used in assessing and developing the person's own self-care skills and in the discussion of future placements. There is a change in attitude with younger parents however, and more are able to come to terms with a future independent life for their child. School programmes are now designed with independence in mind, with self-care and work skill development as well as self-travel and the use of community facilities. To ensure success the parents must play a full role, and it is essential for them to be involved in participating in the assessment and choice of the future home for their child.

Bereavement

It has been mentioned that behavioural problems can be precipitated by the death of a parent. A (false) assumption in the past was that people with learning disability did not understand death and thus did not grieve. There are now several studies which show that this is not the case (McLoughlin, 1986) and it is clear that not only do people with learning disability recognise death but that they also go through a grieving process that may appear aberrant due to the different communication styles used to express their emotions and feelings. The degree of understanding which shapes the concept of death and dying may be related to the level of cognitive development, as proposed by Piaget, rather than the actual age of the person. Group work with others who have been bereaved may be helpful, but often individual support is needed. Cathcart (1995) has reviewed this area and suggests support systems. She also discusses the complementary subject of how to support staff when someone with learning disability, for whom they have cared for over long periods of time, dies.

SERVICES

Residential and respite facilities

It has been known for a considerable time that most people with learning disability live in the community, usually at home with their parents and family no matter how old they may be themselves (Kushlick 1966). This even applies to those referred to specialist psychiatric services, of whom in the region of 50% stay with their families (Bouras et al 1994). Other residential facilities are provided by a variety of organisations, including social work hostels and voluntary agency-run homes through to social work-funded individual placements with other families. Overall care in the community is in general much more costly than care in a hospital setting, with an average of between two and three and a half times as much spent per head, and the desirable staffed smaller settings usually have the highest budgets (Turner et al 1995). Hostels still tend to house similar numbers of people to hospital wards, and the trend is to smaller groups in more domestic-type environments. The provision of respite services is an essential lifeline for many families. In the past these would have been provided in hospitals and by social workers, but increasingly voluntary agencies are providing good respite services. The use of the respite service may be initiated by the family, or by the person themselves, and regular planned periods of stay can be more useful in helping a family to 'recharge their batteries' than emergency use at periods of extreme stress. With the closure programme for most hospitals there is a need to develop alternative resources for people with multiple complex health needs, and cooperation between health and social agencies in joint ventures offers one solution.

Education

The role of the psychiatrist in learning disabilities in the education of children with learning disabilities has decreased as our service has become more adult orien-

tated, and it is rightly the province of the teacher and the educational psychologist. However, it is important to be aware of the changes in education and especially the trend to greater degrees of integration in mainstream settings. There has long been a tradition of special education for people with learning disabilities in the UK, and no one is now considered to be unable to benefit from education of some form. Early preschool intervention and education is probably vital to later development. A variety of preschool factors, including parenting styles, the parents' interpretation of the value of education, and the home learning environment, may have some influence on eventual educational outcome (Bryant & Maxwell, 1996). The goal for many, of attending mainstream schooling, is often attainable, with some able to attend mainstream classes with special tuition, and some helped by individually designed curricula in special needs classes. The Warnock Report (1978) redefined educational problems in terms of special educational needs, instead of starting from the assumption of learning disability, and in some ways helped the recognition that specific educational difficulties, including those defined in DSM-IV as learning disorders, can occur in any child. Independent special school provision still plays a major role in the education of those with more severe degrees of disability and associated problems, but there is an increasing degree of integration of special and mainstream education in the same setting. Education continues long after the person is of school-leaving age. In some cases, especially in special educational settings, the person may continue at secondary school well past leaving age. The transition from secondary schooling to further education (either in college settings or training centres) or to work placements is a critical time, and it is important that the person's future is planned in advance and with their involvement (Kohler & Rusch, 1996). The family's involvement is also important and the family acts as a stable and continuing factor during a period of change (Rusch & Millar 1996). Failure to plan, with prolonged periods without further education, can lead to skill loss, especially in areas such as signing in people without oral vocabularies. Tertiary educational establishments often have learning support departments that can offer further skill training for people with learning disabilities. Locality-based colleges usually offer a variety of special classes, either full time, or part time in association with other placements, in reading and literacy, numeracy and basic computing skills, through arts and drama, to specific work-related training. There are also attempts currently being made to integrate with mainstream classes, and projects such as that at Edinburgh's Telford College have shown that some students, even with profound multiple disabilities, can find useful education in such circumstances and are in general well accepted by other students of the college.

Day services and work experience

Traditionally, day services have been a social work responsibility, and in most areas adult training centres or adult resource centres provide daily work and skill development-related activities for large numbers of people. These are of great benefit to many with learning disability, and often serve as a staging post to more normal employment. They are also therapeutic in themselves, and can help provide a structured activity setting for people whose challenging behaviour or health-related needs make it difficult to integrate into current normal work settings. A usual practice is for a maximun of 4 days a week to be spent at the centre, with the fifth day at home. For some groups of people the adult training centre can be a difficult environment. The noise levels are usually high, and especially so at meal times, and the number of people attending is large. For people with Down's syndrome and dementia, and for some users who are simply getting older and less tolerant, the centre can be a confusing and frightening place. Smaller, quieter areas within the main centre are one way of improving the environment to meet their needs. Voluntary agencies are also now providing day care, and the type of provision depends on the ethos of the organisation. There are some who provide a very structured and sheltered working day, with small numbers of people, and these can be very suited to meeting the needs of those with autism. Many, and perhaps in the future most, people with learning disability do not need to attend such centres but can work alongside others in the general population. Such work placements are often very beneficial to the person's self-esteem, and behavioural problems in other environments may disappear. The type of work needs to be matched to the person's abilities but there is no reason why the role played by the person with learning disability should not be every bit as important as that played by colleagues.

Advocacy

Making themselves and their rights heard has never been easy for people with learning disability, and they have suffered considerably from the assumption that they cannot make choices for themselves. The advocacy movement, where a specified person gets to know and understand a person with learning disability, can communicate with and for them, and can advance the person's rights and feelings when needed, is one step in trying to remedy these problems. In many cases the advocacy movement started with concerns over medical

research on subjects unable to give informed consent, and especially those with mental disorder. In the UK, voluntary organisations involved with learning disability have provided the impetus for the formation of independent advocacy groups, and give a structure that can monitor and assess an individual's ability as an advocate. Difficulties have arisen in some areas, and in the USA conflicts between advocacy groups and the scientific community have been long-standing and have impeded the formation of agreed ethical guidelines in this area, with widely disparate practices existing (Bonnie 1997).

The move from hospital to community

In the UK over the 13 years from 1980 until 1993 the number of people resident in hospitals for learning disability decreased by over 26 000 (Emerson & Hatton 1994), reflecting a change in what is considered as the most appropriate type of residential care and support for the person with learning disability, a change which predated the current and centrally driven process of community care. By the 1970s most hospitals had changed from being institutions with large numbers of children into having a mainly adult population. The initial moves into the community for many residents occurred in that decade, with the discharge of large numbers of people, usually with mild degrees of learning disability and low levels of challenging behaviours or mental illness. Community absorption was largely into existing facilities, or those being developed in parallel for people already based in the community. The second phase began in the 1980s and is continuing; it has the aim of relocating residential care of most of the remaining people with learning disability away from large hospitals. In theory this should be on the basis of developing services according to the needs of the individual, rather than fitting them to available resources. The move away from large wards to small domestic-type environments is likely to be beneficial to all people with learning disability, no matter the severity, and for people with mild disabilities proper social skills training and support systems can allow many to live in unstaffed or minimally staffed domestic accommodation – in other words their own homes (O'Brien 1994).

For those with greater dependency needs, staffed accommodation is the more likely option. Overall the person discharged from a large hospital may expect to have more opportunities to use and develop new living skills, although longer term studies indicate that these may level off or even fall (Cambridge et al 1993). They will also have more contacts with other people, although these still tend to be people with learning disabilities. Many studies in the past indicated that the total time staff spent in direct interaction with residents was low, and this is increased on discharge. This seems to be related to the particular motivation of the staff group involved, and does not relate to the ratio of carers to residents (Felce & Repp 1992). There is more to integration into a community than having a residential placement. The use of community resources is almost invariably increased on discharge, but this may be at a superficial level, and less for those with more severe disabilities.

Care staff have to be selected with caution and receive practical training in the skills needed to support the individuals they will care for, although there are some indications that any improvement in care so produced may be temporary. The involvement of staff with residents well before they are discharged from hospital is important, and the transition phase can often be helped by involvement of hospital staff in the new setting. It is useful to employ staff with a wide experience in detecting mental health problems and challenging behaviour, through to an ability to manage epilepsy with the use of rectal medication if needed. The legal issues of such interventions have to be considered in each case, and the situation is very different from that of parents who have looked after their children since birth and have become experts in particular aspects of health care. Working stress and staff turnover in community settings may actually be higher than in hospitals (Murphy et al 1991), with negative repercussions on many with learning disability who react badly to change. Further investigation into such effects is needed to ensure the success of community care.

Some agencies, especially in the voluntary sector, may feel unhappy at providing levels of care with an extensive health component; others, with support from specialist community learning disability teams, become highly proficient.

The major problems for successful community living away from hospital arise when the person has severe challenging behaviours. The incidence of stereotypic behaviours, such as rocking, do decrease on discharge, but the more severe problems, including aggression, do not, save in very small, intensively staffed community settings (Felce et al 1994). It is a general impression that hospital readmissions for those discharged from long-stay care are usually due to levels of aggressive behaviour unacceptable to the care groups, and it is often difficult to re-establish that person with that particular care group who may perceive themselves to have failed. The problem of chronic severe behavioural disturbance, at present, still merits the provision of small long-stay residential facilities that are managed by health care staff skilled in behavioural methodologies, and able and willing to use them to ensure the safety of the person. In fact it should be accepted that small numbers of people will always need, and have a right, to be cared for in a hospital setting. Those formally detained under sections of the mental health or criminal procedures acts require hospital provision, and there are those with similar degrees of behavioural or psychiatric problems who, due to the severity of their handicap, are cared for as informal patients. The setting does not however need to be institutional, and this term is best applied to the type of care rather than the locus. Institutionalisation can easily become a facet of poor community care and one of the challenges for the future will be to monitor the quality of health and social service provision and delivery to guard against such problems.

Psychiatric and health care provision

Proponents of complete normalisation for people with learning disabilities have argued that psychiatric disorders should be managed by, and within, general psychiatric services (Newman & Emerson 1991). In other areas such as social work, provision is now largely by the non-specialist. However, attempts to introduce such models in practice have not been successful (Day 1994b), and there is little evidence that people with learning disability would receive better psychiatric care in mainstream facilities. In fact the opposite is likely, and it is the right of people with learning disability to have their specialist needs recognised and treated appropriately. The psychiatrist has a major role in the diagnosis and management of psychiatric and behavioural disorders in people with learning disability. In spite of the reduction in long-stay hospital accommodation, there is a continuing need for inpatient and daypatient places for the assessment and treatment of people with severe psychotic illnesses and behavioural disorders. These should be designed to be proactive as well as reactive, and accept both informal and elective admissions in addition to formally detained patients. People who have learning disability and behavioural disorders are also especially likely to need much longer hospital treatment than is the case in general psychiatry, and this should be taken into account when bed numbers are considered; it would be inappropriate to remove entirely the small number of long-stay places.

The main service is, however, and will increasingly be, community based. Specialist community mental health teams for adults with learning disability already exist in most areas, and have long been multidisciplinary. Ideally they comprise a consultant in the psychiatry of learning disability (and the Royal College of Psychiatrists recommends one full-time consultant in the psychiatry of learning disability for every 100 000 population, recognising the considerable extra work-load involved in helping people with learning disability), community nurses (usually registered learning disability nurses), a clinical psychologist, and sessional inputs from specialist occupational therapists, speech and communication therapists, physiotherapists and dieticians. Specialist therapies, such as art and music therapists, are extremely useful and have important roles in facilitating and interpreting communication with people with learning disability, as well as forming part of individual treatment modalities. Strong links with the area social work departments are needed, and joint health and social work meetings on a regular basis help in joint prediction and planning for problems. Most of the work of community teams is done in the person's home or work setting, and the multidisciplinary nature can offer a wide range of treatment types and environmental modifications that may be needed to assist the complex nature of the person's problems.

THE LAW

The Mental Health Acts in the UK allow compulsory admission to a hospital for treatment of mental illness or behaviour disorder in people with learning disability, and are described elsewhere in this volume. In England and Wales, the term used to signify learning disability is mental impairment, which is defined as a state of arrested or incomplete development of mind including a significant impairment of intelligence and social functioning. Severe mental impairment is defined as severe impairment of intelligence and social functioning. The distinction is left to the psychiatrist but in practice is usually used to divide those with mild to upper moderate degrees of learning disability from those with more severe conditions. In Scotland, mental disorder is taken to encompass mental illness and mental handicap. Mental handicap is defined as mental impairment along the lines of the English definition. Under both acts the person with learning disability also needs to have a mental illness or manifest seriously aggressive or irresponsible behaviours.

Many severely and profoundly learning disabled people have an inability to understand or give informed consent to any procedure. Such 'incompetent' patients (common law) also often have no insight into their own personal safety in the domestic environment, or into road safety. The care of such people demands that they be provided with a safe environment, which may involve securing dangerous areas or preventing them from wandering off without supervision, and this can be done in good faith without recourse to formal procedures. However, it is probably good practice, where

treatments are considered for severe escalations of mental illness or behavioural disorder, for application be made for detention under the appropriate section of the act, which would protect the person's rights by proscribing the treatments allowed by a second psychiatrist. Elective (as opposed to emergency medical) physical and psychiatric treatments, including sterilisation, are not permitted without a court order.

Offences committed by people with learning disability

There is little to distinguish in those offences committed by people with very mild learning disability and they shade into those in the general population. People with mild learning disability are, however, more liable to problems associated with lack of understanding and adherence to society's social conventions and norms, and are prone to low self-esteem. The chances of offending are increased if the home circumstances of the person are socially disadvantaged, and the association of poor social conditions and mild learning disability has been noted above. Some of the studies which indicated that repeated criminality was associated with mild learning disability may have reflected a differential arrest and conviction rate compared with the general population, rather than a true effect.

It is rare for a person with severe or profound learning disability to be charged with an offence. It is generally recognised that in such situations, where such people are involved, insight into the nature and consequences of offending is severely limited by intellectual and social impairment. In rare cases where persons with profound learning disability are also severely aggressive to themselves (self-injury) or others, and who would otherwise meet the legal definition of an incompetent patient, there may be a need to use the Mental Health Act to safeguard their rights, especially if neuroleptic medication or physical methods including restraint are thought useful in treatment.

There are two important offence groupings in which people with mild learning disability are overrepresented. The first is in sexual offences, and especially males (Day 1990, 1994a). There may be problems with immaturity and the tendency to offend against persons of an emotional rather than actual age match. The person's understanding of the nature and gravity of the offence is important, and whereas sex education may be appropriate in minor offences such as single episode exhibitionism, the rarer but very serious repeated attacks on women or children may involve prolonged treatment as a formal patient in a secure or special hospital setting. The second serious group is arson and related offences, the most worrying of which is repeated, apparently motiveless, fire setting. This seems to be more common in the late teens or early adulthood and in men with mild learning disability (Higgins 1995). The danger to others in such cases is very high – even a simple fire can endanger the lives of many. Unfortunately long-term treatment on a formal basis may again be required. The long-term needs of these two groups of people with learning disability need to be acknowledged in our plans for community care. Some are cared for in our special hospitals and will continue to be so, but there will also be a continuing need for long-term hospital provision outwith these.

The appropriate adult

Although statutory and common law rights apply to any person, people with learning disability are especially vulnerable when they are accused of, or witness to, or victim of a crime. They may be readily confused, especially with the stress of the situation, and may easily make self-incriminatory, erroneous or conflicting statements. It is important to judge whether the person is able to understand the significance of questions put, whether he knows of his rights to have a lawyer and relative contacted if detained, and whether he understands the concepts of arrest, caution and charging. If the proceedings reach the point where the person has to attend court, the situation is compounded by the adversarial system of interviewing adopted as standard practice in the UK. The 'appropriate adult' scheme was devised to circumvent some of the problems arising from such situations, and it is mandatory for police in England and Wales to have an appropriate adult present if they suspect the person of having a mental disorder (Police and Criminal Evidence Act, 1984). In Scotland, at present, it is a code of good practice rather than mandatory. The appropriate adult should be a trained person (and training must be multidisciplinary, involving police, psychiatric, legal and social work professionals) and is there to facilitate the process of interview for both the individual and the police – acting to interpret and clarify questions and meanings to both parties. The appropriate adult should be present when a person is charged. His attendance is especially important if the person is to be searched or intimately examined, especially if there is any indication that the person has been sexually abused or assaulted. During an interview he is not a substitute for a lawyer, nor is he expected to provide the emotional support of a relative, but he would indicate whether he felt a line of questioning was likely to lead to unreliable answers, read any documents or statements signed by the person, and note on this anything felt to be inaccurate. He would also indicate whether the person needed medical assistance, or a rest period to recover

from stress. There is still much to be done to develop and assess such services on a national basis. It is also important to clarify the difference between the appropriate adult's role and that of an advocate. The former functions in a clearly defined observational and interpretative role and can provide moral support for the person, in contrast to the much wider remit of the advocate to provide emotional support, and interpret and be a voice for, and active participant in safeguarding, a person's rights, interests and feelings.

REFERENCES

AAMR 1992 Mental retardation: definitions, classification, and systems of support, 9th edn. American Association on Mental Retardation, Washington, DC

Allanson J E, O'Hara P, Farkas L G, Nair R C 1993 Anthropometric craniofacial pattern profiles in Down syndrome. American Journal of Medical Genetics, 47: 748–752

Allingham-Hawkins D J, Ray P N 1995 FRAXE expansion is not a common etiological factor among developmentally delayed males. American Journal of Human Genetics 56: 72–76

APA 1994 DSM-IV diagnostic and statistical manual of mental disorders, 4th edn. American Psychiatric Association, Washington, DC

Ashkenas J 1996 Williams syndrome starts making sense. American Journal of Human Genetics 59: 756–761

Bailey A, Bolton P, Butler L et al 1993 Prevalence of the fragile X anomaly amongst autistic twins and singletons. Journal of Child Psychology and Psychiatry 34: 673–678

Bailey D B, Nelson D 1995 The nature and consequences of fragile X syndrome. Mental Retardation and Developmental Disabilities Research Reviews 238–244

Bailey J S, Pyles D A M 1989 Behavioral diagnostics. In: The treatment of severe behavior disorders. Behavior analysis approaches. American Association on Mental Retardation, Washington, DC, pp 85–107

Baird P A, Sadovnick A D 1985 Mental retardation in over half-a-million consecutive live births: an epidemiological study. American Journal on Mental Deficiency 89: 323–330

Baker L, Cantwell D P 1995 Learning disorders, motor skills disorder and communication disorders. In: Kaplan H I, Sadock B J (eds) Comprehensive textbook of psychiatry, 6th edn. Williams & Wilkins, Baltimore, pp 2243–2276

Baron-Cohen S, Allen J, Gillberg C 1992 Can autism be detected at 18 months? The needle, the haystack and the CHAT. British Journal of Psychiatry 161: 839–843

Beckman P J 1991 Comparison of mothers' and fathers' perceptions of the effect of young children with and without learning disabilities. American Journal on Mental Retardation 95: 585–595

Berg J M, Karlinsky H, Holland A J 1993 Alzheimer's disease, Down syndrome, and their relationship. Oxford University Press, Oxford

Berrios G E 1994 Mental illness and mental retardation: history and concepts. In: Bouras N (ed.) Mental health in mental retardation. Recent advances and practice. Cambridge University Press, Cambridge, pp 5–18

Bettelheim B 1956 Childhood schizophrenia as a reaction to extreme situations. Journal of Orthopsychiatry 26: 507–518

Birch H G, Richardson S A, Baird S, Horobin G, Illsley R 1970 Mental subnormality in the community. Williams & Wilkins, Baltimore

Blackie J, Forrest A D, Witcher G 1975 Subcultural mental handicap. British Journal of Psychiatry 127: 535–539

Blackwood D H R, St Clair D M, Muir W J, Oliver C J, Dickens P 1988 The development of Alzheimer's disease in Down's syndrome assessed by auditory event-related potentials. Journal of Mental Deficiency Research 32: 439–453

Blair C, Ramey C T, Hardin J M 1995 Early intervention for low birthweight premature infants: participation and intellectual development. American Journal on Mental Retardation 99: 542–554

Bleuler E 1923 Textbook of psychiatry. Brill A A (trans). Allen & Unwin, London

Bleuler E 1950 Dementia praecox or the group of schizophrenias. Zinkin J (trans). International Universities Press, New York

Bolton P, Rutter M 1990 Genetic influences in autism. International Review of Psychiatry 2: 67–80

Bonnie R J 1997 Research with cognitively impaired subjects. Unfinished business in the regulation of human research. Archives of General Psychiatry 54: 105–111

Bouchard T J, Lykken D T, McGue M, Segal N L, Tellegen A 1990 Sources of human psychological differences in the Minnesota study of twins reared apart. Science 250: 223–228

Bouras N, Brooks D, Drummond K 1994 Community psychiatric services for people with mental retardation. In: Bouras N (ed.) Mental health in mental retardation. Recent advances and practice. Cambridge University Press, Cambridge, pp 293–299

Bregman J S, Harris J C 1995 Mental retardation. In: Kaplan H I, Sadock B J (eds) Comprehensive textbook of psychiatry, 6th edn. Williams & Wilkins, Baltimore, pp 2207–2241

Brown C J, Ballabio A, Rupert J L et al 1991 A gene from the region of the human X inactivation centre is expressed exclusively from the inactive X chromosome. Nature 349: 38–44

Bryant D M, Maxwell K L 1996 Early intervention. Current Opinion in Psychiatry 9: 317–321

Burt D B, Loveland K A, Lewis D R 1992 Depression and the onset of dementia in adults with mental retardation. American Journal on Mental Retardation 96: 502–511

Burt D B, Loveland K A, Chen Y W, Chuang A, Lewis K R, Cherry L 1995 Aging in adults with Down syndrome: report from a longitudinal study. American Journal on Mental Retardation 100: 262–270

Busciglio J, Yankner B A 1995 Apoptosis and increased generation of reactive oxygen species in Down's syndrome neurons in vitro. Nature 378: 776–779

Butler M G, Bruschwig A, Miller L K, Hagerman R J 1992 Standards for selected anthropometric measurements in males with fragile X syndrome. Pediatrics 89: 1059–1062

Cambridge P, Hayes L, Knapp M 1993 Care in the community: Five years on. PSSRU, Kent

Campbell F A, Ramey C T 1995 Cognitive and school outcomes for high-risk African American students at middle adolescence. American Educational Research Journal 32: 743–772

Campbell M, Shay J 1995 Pervasive developmental disorders. In: Kaplan H I, Sadock B J (eds) Comprehensive textbook of psychiatry, 6th edn. Williams & Wilkins, Baltimore, pp 2277–2293

Castell J H F, Mittler P J 1965 Intelligence of patients in subnormality hospitals: a survey of admissions in 1961. British Journal of Psychiatry 111: 219–225

Cathcart F 1995 Death and people with learning disabilities: interventions to support clients and carers. British Journal of Clinical Psychology 34: 165–175

Childs B 1995 A logic of disease. In: Scriver C R, Beaudet A L, Sly W S, Valle D (eds) The metabolic and molecular bases of inherited disease. McGraw-Hill New York,. pp 229–257

Clarke B 1975 Mental disorder in earlier Britain: exploratory studies. University of Wales Press, Cardiff

Cole J O, Hardy P M 1985 Organic states. In: Achatzberg A F (ed.) Common treatment problems in depression. American Psychiatric Association, Washington, DC

Collacott R A, Cooper S A 1992 Adaptive behaviour after depressive illness in Down's syndrome. Journal of Nervous and Mental Disease 180: 468–470

Collacott R, Cooper S A, McGrother C 1992 Differential rates of psychiatric disorders in adults with Down's syndrome compared with other mentally handicapped adults. British Journal of Psychiatry 161: 671–674

Cooper S A, Duggirala C, Collacott R A 1995 Adaptive behaviour after schizophrenia in people with Down's syndrome. Journal of Intellectual Disability Research 39: 201–204

Corbett J A 1975 Aversion for the treatment of self injurious behaviour. Journal of Mental Deficiency Research 19: 79–95

Corbett J A 1979 Psychiatric morbidity and mental retardation. In: James F E, Snaith R P (eds) Psychiatric illness and mental handicap. Royal College of Psychiatrists, London

Cork L C 1990 Neuropathology of Down syndrome and Alzheimer's disease. American Journal of Medical Genetics Supplement 7: 282–286

Courchesne E, Yeung-Courchesne R, Press G A, Hesselink J R, Jernigan T L 1988 Hypoplasia of the cerebellar vermal lobules VI and VII in autism. New England Journal of Medicine 318: 1349–1354

Crabbe H 1994 Pharmacotherapy in mental retardation. In: Bouras N (ed.) Mental health in mental retardation. Cambridge University Press, Cambridge

Craft A 1994 Practice issues in sexuality and learning disabilities. Routledge, London

Crayton L, Oliver C 1993 Assessment of cognitive functioning in persons with Down syndrome who develop Alzheimer's disease. In: Berg J M, Karlinsky H, Holland A J (eds) Alzheimer's disease, Down syndrome, and their relationship. Oxford University Press, Oxford.

Cunningham C C 1983 Early support and interventions: the HARC infant project. In: Miltler P, McConachie (eds) Parents, professionals and mentally handicapped people, approaches to partnership. Croom Helm, London

Dalton A J, Seltzer G B, Adlin M S, Wisniewsky H M 1993 Association between Alzheimer's disease and Down syndrome: clinical observations. In: Berg J M, Karlinsky H, Holland A J (eds) Alzheimer's disease, Down syndrome, and their relationship. Oxford University Press, Oxford.

Das J P, Divis B, Alexander J, Parrila R K, Naglieri J A 1995 Cognitive decline due to aging among persons with Down syndrome. Research in Developmental Disabilities 16: 461–478

Day K 1990 Mental retardation: clinical aspects and management. In: Bluglass R, Bowden P (eds) Principles and practice of forensic psychiatry. Churchill Livingstone, Edinburgh. pp 399–418

Day K 1994a Male mentally handicapped sex offenders. British Journal of Psychiatry 165: 630–639

Day K 1994b Psychiatric services in mental retardation, generic or specialised provision. In: Bouras N (ed) Mental health in mental retardation. Recent advances and practice. Cambridge University Press, Cambridge, pp 275–292

Deb S, de Silva P N, Gemmel H G, Besson J A, Smith F W, Ebmeier K P 1992 Alzheimer's disease in adults with Down's syndrome: the relationship between regional cerebral blood flow equivalents and dementia. Acta Psychiatrica Scandinavica 86: 340–345

de Grouchy J, Turleau C 1990 Autosomal disorders. In: Emery A E H, Rimoin D L (eds) Principles and practice of medical genetics, 2nd edn. Churchill Livingstone, Edinburgh, vol 1, pp 247–271

Devenny D A, Hill A L, Paxot O, Silverman W P, Wisniewski K E 1992 Ageing in higher functioning adults with Down's syndrome: an interim report in a longitudinal study. Journal of Intellectual Disability Research 36: 241–250

Devys D, Lutz Y, Rouyer N 1993 The FMR-1 protein is cytoplasmic, most abundant in neurons, and appears normal in carriers of the fragile X premutation. Nature Genetics 4: 225–240

Down J L H 1866 Observations on an ethnic classification of idiots. Clinical Lectures and Reports, London Hospital 3: 25

Duggirala. C, Cooper S-A, Collacot R A 1995 Schizophrenia and Down's syndrome. Irish Journal of Psychological Medicine 12: 30–33

Durand V M 1990 Severe behavior problems. Guilford Press, New York

Dykens E M 1995 Adaptive behavior in males with fragile X syndrome. Mental Retardation and Developmental Disabilities Research Reviews 1: 281–285

Eichler E E, Holden J J A, Popovich B W et al 1994 Length of uninterrupted CGG repeats determines instability in the FMR-1 gene. Nature Genetics 8: 88–94

Einfeld S L, Tonge B J 1996 Population prevalence of psychopathology in children and adolescents with intellectual disability: II Epidemiological findings. Journal of Intellectual Disability Research 40: 99–109

Emerson E, Hatton C 1994 Moving out. The impact of relocation from hospital to community on the quality of life of persons with learning disabilities. HMSO, London

Epstein C J 1995 Down syndrome (trisomy 21). In: Scriver C R, Beaudet A L, Sly W S, Valle D (eds) The metabolic and molecular bases of inherited disease. McGraw-Hill, New York, pp 749–794

Evans H J 1977 Chromosome anomalies among livebirths. Journal of Medical Genetics 14: 309

Eyemann R K, Call T L, White J F 1991 Life expectancy of persons with Down syndrome. American Journal on Mental Retardation 95: 603–612

Felce D, Repp A 1992 The behavioural and social ecology of community houses. Research in Developmental Disabilities 13: 27–42

Felce D, Lowe K, de Paiva S 1994 Ordinary housing for people with severe learning disabilities and challenging behaviours. In: Emerson E, McGill P, Mansell J (eds) Severe learning disabilities and challenging behaviours: designing high quality services. Chapman & Hall, London

Firth H V 1991 Severe limb abnormalities after chorionic villus sampling at 56–66 days gestation. Lancet 337: 762–763

Fisch G S, Arinami T, Froster-Iskenius U, Fryns J P, Curfs L 1991 Relationship between age and IQ among fragile X males: a multicenter study. American Journal of Medical Genetics 38: 481–487

Folstein S, Rutter M 1988 Autism: familial aggregation and genetic implications. Journal of Autism and Developmental Disorders 18: 8–30

Frangiskakis J M, Ewart A K, Morris C A et al 1996 LIM-kinase 1 hemizygosity implicated in impaired visuospatial constructive cognition. Cell 86: 59–69

Fraser J, Mitchell A 1876 Kalmuc idiocy: report of a case with autopsy and notes on 62 cases by A. Mitchell. Journal of Mental Science 22: 161–162

Fraser W, Nolan M 1994 Psychiatric disorders in mental retardation. In: Bouras N (ed.) Mental health in mental retardation. Cambridge University Press, Cambridge, pp 79–92

Freund L S, Peebles C D, Aylward E, Reiss A L 1995 Preliminary report on cognitive and adaptive behaviors of preschool aged males with fragile X. Developmental Brain Dysfunction 8: 242–251

Frith U 1992 Cognitive development and cognitive deficit. The Psychologist 5: 13–19

Frøland A 1969 Klinefelter's Syndrome. Costers Bogtrykkeri, Copenhagen

Fryer A E, Chalmers A, Connor J M et al 1987 Evidence that the gene for tuberous sclerosis is on chromosome 9. Lancet i: 659–661

Fu Y H, Kuhl D P A, Pizzuti A et al 1991 Variation of the CGG repeat at the fragile X site results in genetic instability: resolution of the Sherman paradox. Cell 67: 1047–1058

Gedeon A K, Keinänen M, Adès L C et al 1995 Overlapping submicroscopic deletions in Xq28 in two unrelated boys with developmental disorders: identification of a gene near FRAXE. American Journal of Human Genetics 56: 907–914

Gedye A 1989 Episodic rage and aggression attributed to frontal lobe seizures. Journal of Mental Deficiency Research 33: 369–379

Geldmacher D S, Whitehouse P J 1996 Evaluation of dementia. New England Journal of Medicine 335: 330–336

Gibson D 1978 Down's syndrome. The psychology of mongolism. Cambridge University Press, Cambridge

Gillberg C 1988 The role of the endogenous opioids in autism and possible relationships to clinical features. In: Wing L (ed.) Aspects of autism: biological research. Gaskell/The National Autistic Society, London, pp 31–37

Gillberg C, Persson E, Grufman M, Themner U 1986 Psychiatric disorders in mildly and severely retarded urban children and adolescents: epidemiological aspects. British Journal of Psychiatry 149: 68–74

Goate A, Chartier-Harlin M-C, Mullan M et al 1991 Segregation of a missense mutation in the amyloid precursor protein gene with familial Alzheimer's disease. Nature 349: 704–706

Golden J A, Hyman B T 1994 Development of the superior temporal neocortex is anomalous in trisomy 21. Journal of Neuropathology and Experimental Neurology 53: 513–520

Gravel J, Wallace I 1995 Early otitis media, auditory abilities and educational risk. American Journal of Speech–Language Pathology 4: 89–94

Gravestock S 1996 Depot neuroleptic usage in adults with learning disabilities. Journal of Intellectual Disability Research 40: 17–23

Grigsby J P, Kemper M B, Hagerman R J, Myers C S 1990 Neuropsychological dysfunction amongst affected heterozygous fragile X females. American Journal of Medical Genetics 35: 28–35

Gunn M 1994 Competency and consent. The importance of decision making. In: Craft A (ed) Practice issues in sexuality and learning disabilities. Routledge, London, pp 116–134

Haddow J E, Palomaki G E, Knight G J et al 1992 Prenatal screening for Down's syndrome with use of maternal serum markers. New England Journal of Medicine 329: 821–827

Hagberg B, Hagberg G, Lewerth A, Lindberg U 1981 Mild mental retardation in Swedish school children I: prevalence. Acta Paediatrica Scandinavica 70: 441–444

Hagerman R J 1991 Physical and behavioural phenotype. In: Hagerman R J, Silverman A C (eds) Fragile X syndrome: diagnosis, treatment and research. Johns Hopkins University Press, Baltimore, pp 3–68

Hagerman R, Schreiner R, Kemper M, Wittenberger M, Zahn B, Habicht K 1989 Longitudinal IQ changes in fragile X males. American Journal of Medical Genetics 30: 377–392

Happé F 1994 Autism, an introduction to psychological theory. UCL Press, London

Harris J 1996 Physical restraint procedures for managing challenging behaviours presented by mentally retarded adults and children. Research in Developmental Disabilities 17: 99–134

Hassold T J, Jacobs P A 1984 Trisomy in man. Annual Review of Genetics 18: 69–98

Haxby J V 1989 Neuropsychological evaluation of adults with Down's syndrome. Patterns of selective impairment in non-demented old adults. Journal of Mental Deficiency Research 33: 193–210

Heaton-Ward W A 1977 Psychosis in mental handicap. British Journal of Psychiatry 130: 525–533

Higgins J 1995 Crime and mental disorder II. In: Chiswick D, Cope R (eds) Seminars in practical forensic psychiatry. Gaskell/Royal College of Psychiatrists, London

Hirst M C, Grewal P K, Davies K E 1994 Precursor arrays for triplet repeat expansion at the fragile X locus. Human Molecular Genetics 3: 1533–1560

Ho H H, Lockitch G, Eaves L, Jacobson B 1986 Blood serotonin concentrations and fenfluramine therapy in autistic children. Journal of Pediatrics 108: 465–469

Hodapp R, Zigler E 1994 Past, present and future issues in the developmental approach to mental retardation and developmental disabilities. In: Chirchetti D, Cohen D I (eds) Developmental Psychopathology. Vol 2: Risk, disorder and adaptation. Wiley, New York, pp 299–331

Hodapp R M, Dykens E M, Hagerman R J, Schreiner R, Lachiewicz A, Leckman J F 1990 Developmental implications of changing trajectories of IQ in males with fragile X syndrome. Journal of the American Academy of Child and Adolescent Psychiatry 24: 214–219

Holden J J A, Wing M, Chalifoux M et al 1996 Lack of expansion of triplet repeats in the FMR1, FRAXE and FRAXF loci in male multiplex families with autism and pervasive developmental disorders. American Journal of Medical Genetics 64: 399–403

Holland A J 1991 Learning disability and psychiatric/behavioural disorders: a genetic perspective. In: McGuffin P, Murray R (eds) The new genetics of mental illness. Butterworth-Heinemann, Oxford, pp 245–258

Holland A, Gosden C (1990) A balanced chromosomal

translocation partially co-segregating with psychotic illness in a family. Psychiatry Research 32: 1–8

Holland A J, Karlinsky H, Berg J M 1993 Alzheimer disease in persons with Down syndrome: diagnostic and management considerations. In: Berg J M, Karlinsky H, Holland A J (eds) Alzheimer disease, Down syndrome, and their relationship. Oxford University Press, Oxford

Holtzman D M, Epstein C J, Mobley W C 1996 The human trisomy 21 brain: insights from mouse models of Down syndrome. Mental Retardation and Developmental Disabilities Research Reviews 2: 66–72

Horn J M, Loehlin J C, Willeman L 1979 Intellectual resemblance among adoptive and biological relatives: the Texas adoption project. Behavioural Genetics 9: 177–201

Howenstine M S 1992 Pulmonary concerns. In: Pueschel S M, Pueschel J K (eds) Biomedical concerns in persons with Down syndrome. Brookes, Baltimore, pp 197–104

Howlin P, Wing L, Gould J 1995 The recognition of autism in children with Down syndrome: implications for intervention and some speculations about pathology. Developmental Medicine Child Neurology 37: 406–413

Irving M 1992 The effects of ageing upon individuals with Down's syndrome. Scottish Down's Syndrome Association, Edinburgh

Jacobs P A, Baikie A G, Court Brown W M, Strong J A 1959 The somatic chromosomes in mongolism. Lancet i: 710

Jacobs P A, Matsuyama A M, Buchanan I M, Wilson C 1979 Late replicating chromosomes in human triploidy. American Journal of Human Genetics 31: 446

Johnson L T, Patel P I 1996 Lesch–Nyhan syndrome: an overview of pharmacologic and molecular genetic aspects. Mental Retardation and Developmental Disabilities Research Reviews 2: 147–154

Johnson M H, Siddons F, Frith U, Morton J 1992 Can autism be predicted on the basis of infant screening tests? Developmental Medicine and Child Neurology 34: 316–320

Jones K L, Smith D W 1973 Recognition of the fetal alcohol syndrome in early infancy. Lancet ii: 999

Kanner L 1943 Autistic disturbance of affective contact. Nervous Child 2: 217–250

Kanner L, Eisenberg L 1956 Early infantile autism 1943–1955. American Journal of Orthopsychiatry 26: 55–65

King B H, DeAntonio C, McCracken J T, Forness S R, Ackerland V 1994 Psychiatric consultation in severe and profound mental retardation. American Journal of Psychiatry 151: 1802–1808

Klinefelter Jr H F, Reifenstein Jr E C, Albright F 1942 Syndrome characterized by gynecomastia, aspermatogenesis without a-Leydigism and increased excretion of follicle-stimulating hormone. Journal of Clinical Endocrinology and Metabolism 2: 615–627

Knight S L, Voelckel M A, Hirst M C, Flannery A V, Monda A, Davies K E 1994 Triplet repeat expansion at the FRAXE locus and X-linked mild mental handicap. American Journal of Human Genetics 55: 81–86

Koehler K E, Hawley R S, Sherman S, Hassold T 1996 Recombination and nondisjunction in humans and flies. Human Molecular Genetics 5: 1495–1504

Kohler J A, Shortland G, Rolles C J 1987 The effect of fenfluramine on autistic symptoms. British Medical Journal 295: 885

Kohler P D, Rusch F R 1996 Secondary educational programs and transition perspectives. In: Wang M C,

Reynolds M C, Walberg H J (eds) Handbook of special education: research and practice, 2nd edn. Elsevier, Oxford, pp 108–130

Kolata G 1985 Down syndrome – Alzheimer's linked. Science 230: 1152–1153

Kouseff B G 1978 Trisomy 21 with average intelligence? Birth Defects, Original Article Series 14:323

Kremer E J, Pritchard M, Lynch M, Holman K, Baker E, Warren S T 1991 Mapping of DNA instability at the fragile X to a trinucleotide repeat sequence (pCCG)n. Science 252: 1711–1714

Kushlik A 1966 Social problems of the mentally subnormal. Social Psychiatry 1: 73–82

Lachiewicz A M, Gullion C M, Spiridgliozzi G A, Aylsworth A S 1987 Declining IQs of young males with the fragile X syndrome. American Journal on Mental Retardation 92: 272–278

Laurence K M 1990 The genetics and prevention of neural tube defects and 'uncomplicated' hydrocephalus. In: Emery A E H, Rimoin D L (eds) Principles and practice of medical genetics, 2nd edn. Churchill Livingstone, Edinburgh, vol 1

LaVigna G W, Willis T J, Donnellan A M 1989 The role of positive programming in behavioral treatment. In: The treatment of severe behavior disorders. Behavior analysis approaches. AAMR, Washington, DC, pp 59–83

Le Couter A 1988 The role of genetics in the aetiology of autism, including the findings of the links with the fragile X syndrome. In: Wing L (ed.) Aspects of autism: biological research. Gaskell / The National Autistic Society, London, pp 38–52

Lehrke R G 1972 A theory of X-linkage of major intellectual traits. American Journal of Mental Deficiency 76: 611–619

Lehrke R G 1974 X-linked mental retardation and verbal ability. Birth Defects: Original Article Series 10: 1–100

Lejeune J 1959 Le mongolisme: premier example d'abberation autosomique humaine. Annals Génétique Seminars Hôpital 1: 41–49

Lemoine P, Harousseau H, Borteyru J P, Menuet J C 1968 Les enfants de parents alcooliques: anomalies observées à propos de 127 cas. Ouest-Medicine 25: 477

Leslie A M, Thaiss L 1992 Domain specificity in conceptual development: evidence from autism. Cognition 43: 225–251

Levy H L 1991 Screening of the newborn. In: Tausch H W, Ballard R A, Avery M E (eds) Diseases of the Newborn. W B Saunders, Philadelphia, pp 111–119

Lewis M H, Bodfish J W, Powell S B, Golden R N 1996 Clomipramine treatment for self-injurious behaviour of individuals with mental retardation. A double-blind comparison with placebo. American Journal on Mental Retardation 100: 654–665

Libb J W, Myers G J, Graham E, Bell B 1983 Correlates of intelligence and adaptive behavior in Down's syndrome. Journal of Mental Deficiency Research 27: 205

Lotter V 1966 Epidemiology of autistic conditions in young children. I Prevalence. Social Psychiatry 1: 124–137

Lubs H A 1969 A marker X chromosome. American Journal of Human Genetics 21: 231–244

Ludlow J R, Allen L M 1979 The effect of early intervention and preschool stimulus on the development of the Down's syndrome child. Journal of Mental Deficiency Research 23: 29

McCoy E E, Epstein C J 1987 The oncology and immunology of Down syndrome. Liss, New York

McGrother C W, Marshall B 1990 Recent trends in incidence, morbidity and survival in Down's syndrome. Journal of Mental Deficiency Research 34: 49–57

McLoughlin I J 1986 Bereavement in the mentally handicapped. British Journal of Hospital Medicine October 36: 256–260

Macpherson J N, Bullman H, Youings S A, Jacobs P A 1994 Insert size and flanking haplotype in fragile X and normal populations: possible multiple origins for the fragile X mutation. Human Molecular Genetics 3: 399–405

Malmgren H, Steen-Bondeson M L, Gustavson K H et al 1994 Strong founder effect for the fragile X syndrome in Sweden. European Journal of Human Genetics 2: 103–109

Malter H E, Iber J C, Willemsen R et al 1997 Characterization of the full fragile X syndrome mutation in fetal gametes. Nature Genetics 15: 165–169

Marcus S, Steen A M, Andersson B, Lambert B, Kristofersson U, Francke U 1992 Mutation analysis and prenatal diagnosis in a Lesch–Nyhan family showing non-random X inactivation interfering with carrier detection tests. Human Genetics 89: 395

Martin J P, Bell J 1943 A pedigree of mental defect showing sex linkage. Journal of Neurology 6: 154–157

Matson J L, Banairdez D A, Stabinsky-Compton L, Paclawskyj T, Baglio C 1996 Behavioral treatment of autistic persons: a review of research from 1980 to the present. Research in Developmental Disabilities 17: 433–465

Meadows G, Turner T, Campbell L, Lewis S W, Reveley M A, Murray R M 1991 Assessing schizophrenia in adults with mental retardation: a comparative study. British Journal of Psychiatry 158: 103–105

Merkatz I R, Nitowsky H M, Macri J N, Johnson W E 1984 An association between low maternal serum alpha-fetoprotein and fetal chromosome abnormalities. American Journal of Obstetrics and Gynecology 148: 886

Mikkelsen M, Poulsen H, Nielsen K G 1990 Incidence, survival and mortality in Down syndrome in Denmark. American Journal of Medical Genetics Supplement 7: 75–78

Morris A F, Vaughan S E, Vaccaro P 1982 Measurement of neuromuscular tone and strength in Down's syndrome children. Journal of Mental Deficiency Research 26: 41

Morris C A, Loker J, Ensing G, Stock A D 1993 Supravalvular aortic stenosis cosegregates with a familial 6;7 translocation which disrupts the elastin gene. American Journal of Medical Genetics 46: 737–744

Mors O, Ewald H, Blackwood D, Muir W 1997 Cytogenetic abnormalities on chromosome 18 associated with bipolar affective disorder or schizophrenia. British Journal of Psychiatry 170: 278–280

Morton N E, Rindl P M, Bullock S et al 1995 Fragile X syndrome is less common than previously estimated. Journal of Medical Genetics 32: 144–145

Moss S, Goldberg D, Simpson N, Patel P 1991 Psychiatric and physical morbidity in older people with severe mental handicap. Hester Adrian Research Centre, University of Manchester, Department of Psychiatry, Manchester

Muir W J, Squire I, Blackwood D H R et al 1988 Auditory P300 response in the assessment of Alzheimer's disease in Down's syndrome: a two year follow-up study. Journal of Mental Deficiency Research 32: 455–463

Murphy C C, Yeargin-Allsop M, Decouflé P, Drews C D 1995 The administrative prevalence of mental retardation in 10-year old children in metropolitan Atlanta. American Journal of Public Health 85: 319–323

Murphy G, Holland A, Fowler P, Reep J 1991 MIETS: a

service option for people with mild mental handicaps and challenging behaviour or psychiatric problems. Mental Handicap Research 4: 41–66

Myers B A, Pueschel S M 1991 Psychiatric disorders in a population with Down syndrome. Journal of Nervous and Mental Diseases 179: 609–613

Myers B A, Pueschel S M 1995 Major depression in a small group of adults with Down syndrome. Research in Developmental Disabilities 16: 285–299

Nagle R J, Bell N L 1995 Clinical utility of Kaufman's 'amazingly' short forms of WAIS-R. Jounal of Clinical Psychology 51: 396–400

Neve R L, Finch E A, Dawes L R 1988 Expression of the Alzheimer amyloid precursor gene transcript in the human brain. Neuron 1: 699

Neve R L, Dawes L R, Yankner B A, Benowitz L I, Rodriguez W, Higgins G A 1990 Genetics and biology of the Alzheimer amyloid precursor. In: Coleman P, Higgins G, Phelps C (eds) Progress in brain research. Elsevier, New York, vol 86, pp 257–267

Neville J 1959 Paranoid schizophrenia in a mongoloid defective: some theoretical considerations derived from an unusual case. Journal of Mental Science 105: 444

Newman I, Emerson E 1991 Specialist treatment units for people with challenging behaviours. Mental Handicap 19: 113–119

Nicolaides K H, Azar G, Snijders R J M, Gosden C M 1992 Fetal nuchal oedema: associated malformations and chromosomal defects. Fetal Diagnosis and Therapy 7: 123–131

Niebuhr E 1978 The cri du chat syndrome. Epidemiology, cytogenetics and clinical features. Human Genetics 44: 227

Oberlé I, Rousseau F, Heitz D et al 1991 Instability of a 550-base pair DNA segment and abnormal methylation in fragile X syndrome. Science 252: 1097–1102

O'Brien J 1994 Down stairs that are never your own: supporting people with developmental disabilities in their own homes. Mental Retardation 32: 1–6

Olson T M, Michels V V, Urban Z et al 1995 A 30 kb deletion within the elastin gene results in familial supravalvular aortic stenosis. Human Molecular Genetics 4: 1677–1679

Oostra B A, Jacky P B, Brown W T, Rousseau F 1993 Guidelines for the diagnosis of fragile X syndrome. National Fragile X Foundation. Journal of Medical Genetics 30: 410–413

Oudet C, Von Koskull H, Nordstrom A M, Peippo M, Mandel J L 1993 Striking founder effect for the fragile X syndrome in Finland. European Journal of Human Genetics 1: 182–189

Pawlarczyk D, Beckwith B E 1987 Depressive symptoms displayed by persons with mental retardation: a review. Mental Retardation 25: 325–330

Peckham C, Coleman J C, Hyurley R, Chin K S, Henderson K, Preece P M 1983 Cytomegalovirus infection in pregnancy: preliminary findings from a prospective study. Lancet i: 1352–1355

Penrose L 1954 The biology of mental defect, 2nd edn. Sidgwick & Jackson, London

Percy M, Dalton A, Markovic V et al 1990 Auto-immune thyroiditis associated with mild 'subclinical' hypothyroidism in adults with Down's syndrome: a comparison of patients with and without manifestations of Alzheimer's disease. American Journal of Medical Genetics 36: 148–154

Pericak-Vance M A, Haines J L 1995 Genetic susceptibility to Alzheimer disease. Trends in Genetics 11: 504–508

Prasher V P 1995a Overweight and obesity amongst Down's syndrome adults. Journal of Intellectual Disability Research 39: 437–411

Prasher V P 1995b Prevalence of psychiatric disorders in adults with Down's syndrome. European Journal of Psychiatry 9: 77–82

Prasher V P, Filer A 1995 Behavioural disturbance in people with Down's syndrome and dementia. Journal of Intellectual Disability Research 39: 432–436

Pueschel S M, Scola F H 1987 Atlantoaxial instability in individuals with Down's syndrome: epidemiologic, radiographic and clinical studies. Pediatrics 80: 555–560

Qureshi H 1994 The size of the problem. In: Emerson E, McGill P, Mansell J (eds) Severe learning disabilities and challenging behaviours. Designing high quality Services. Chapman & Hall, London, pp 17–36

Rabe A, Wisniewski K E, Schupf N et al 1990 Relationship of Down's syndrome to Alzheimer's disease. In: Application of basic neuroscience to child psychiatry. Plenum Press, New York, pp 325–340

Rantakallio P, von Wendt L 1986 Mental retardation and subnormality in a birth cohort of 12 000 children in northern Finland. American Journal of Mental Deficiency 90: 380–387

Rarick G L, Seefeldt V 1974 Observations from longitudinal data on growth on stature and sitting height of children with Down's syndrome. Journal of Mental Deficiency Research 18: 63

Ratcliffe S G, Paul N 1986 Prospective studies on children with sex chromosome aneuploidy. Birth Defects, Original Article Series 22: no. 3

Reid A H 1972a Psychoses in adult mental defectives. I: Manic depressive psychosis. British Journal of Psychiatry 120: 205–212

Reid A H 1972b Psychoses in adult mental defectives. II: Schizophrenia and paranoid psychoses. British Journal of Psychiatry 120: 213–218

Reid A H, Ballinger B R 1987 Personality disorder in mental handicap. Psychological Medicine 17: 983–989

Reid A H, Ballinger B R 1995 Behaviour symptoms among severely and profoundly mentally retarded patients: a 16–18 year follow-up study. British Journal of Psychiatry 167: 452–455

Reid A H, Ballinger B R, Heather B B 1978 Behavioural syndromes identified by cluster analysis in a sample of 100 severely and profoundly retarded adults. Psychological Medicine 8: 399–412

Reiss S 1990 Prevalence of dual diagnosis in community-based day programs in the Chicago metropolitan area. American Journal on Mental Deficiency 94: 578–585

Reiss S, Szysko J 1983 Diagnostic overshadowing and professional experience with mentally retarded persons. American Journal on Mental Deficiency 87: 396–402

Reiss A L, Feinstein C, Rosenbaum I C 1986 Autism and genetic disorders. Schizophrenia Bulletin 12: 724–738

Reiss A L, Lee J, Freund L 1994 Neuroanatomy of the fragile X syndrome: the temporal lobe. Neurology 44: 1317–1324

Reiss A L, Abrams M T, Greenlaw R, Freund L, Denckla M B 1995 Neurodevelopmental effects of the FMR-1 full mutation in humans. Nature Medicine 3: 393–398

Renpenning H, Gerrard J W, Zalenski W A, Tabata T 1962 Familial sex-linked mental retardation. Canadian Medical Association Journal 87: 954–956

Reyniers E, Vits L, De Boulle K et al 1993 The full

mutation in the FMR-1 gene of male fragile X patients is absent in their sperm. Nature Genetics 4: 257–260

Riccardi V M 1990 The phakomatoses. In: Emery A E H, Rimoin D L (eds) Principles and practice of medical genetics, 2nd edn. Churchill Livingstone, Edinburgh, vol 1

Ritvo E R, Spence M A, Freeman B J, Mason-Brothers A, Mo A, Marazita M L 1985 Evidence for autosomal recessive inheritance in 46 families with multiple incidences of autism. American Journal of Psychiatry 142: 187–192

Roizen N J, Mets M B, Blondis T A 1994 Ophthalmic disorders in children with Down's syndrome. Developmental Medicine and Child Neurology 36: 594–600

Rose N C 1996 Pregnancy screening and prenatal diagnosis of fetal Down syndrome. Mental Retardation and Developmental Disabilities Research Reviews 2: 80–84

Rousseau F, Rouillard P, Morel N-L 1995 Prevalence of carriers of premutation-size alleles of the FMR-1 gene and implications for the population genetics of the fragile X syndrome. American Journal of Human Genetics 57: 1006–1018

Rovet J, Glorieux J, Heyerdahl S 1987 Summary of presentations and discussion on the psychological follow-up of CH children identified by newborn screening. In: Therell B L (ed.) Advances in neonatal screening. Excerpta Medica, Amsterdam

Ruedrich S, Menolascino F J 1984 Dual diagnosis of mental retardation and mental illness: an overview. In: Menolascino F, Stark J (eds) Handbook of mental illness in the mentally retarded. Plenum Press, New York, pp 45–81

Rusch F R, Millar D M 1996 The transition to adulthood and the world of work by youth with mental retardation. Current Opinion in Psychiatry 9: 328–331

Rutter M 1978 Diagnosis and definition of childhood autism. Journal of Autism and Childhood Schizophrenia 8: 139–161

Rutter M, Schopler E 1987 Autism and pervasive developmental disorders: conceptual and diagnostic issues. Journal of Autism and Developmental Disorders 17: 159–186

St Clair D, Blackwood D H, Oliver C J, Dickens P 1987 P3 abnormality in fragile X syndrome. Biological Psychiatry 22: 303–312

Sampson J R, Scahill S J, Stephenson J B P, Mann L, Connor J M 1989 Genetic aspects of tuberous sclerosis in the west of Scotland. Journal of Medical Genetics 26: 511–516

Sara V R, Gustavson K-H, Annerén G, Hall K, Wetterberg L 1983 Somatomedins in Down's syndrome. Biological Psychiatry 18: 803–811

Schapiro M B, Haxby J V, Grady C L 1992 Nature of mental retardation and dementia in Down syndrome: study with PET, CT and neuropsychology. Neurobiology of Aging 13: 723–734

Schenker S, Becker H C, Randall C L et al 1990 Fetal alcohol syndrome: current status of pathogenesis. Alcohol Clinical and Experimental Research 14: 635

Scola P S, Pueschel S M 1992 Menstrual cycles and basal body temperature curves in women with Down syndrome. Obstetrics and Gynaecology 79: 91–94

Scriver C R, Beaudet A L, Sly W S, Valle D 1995 The metabolic and molecular bases of inherited disease, 7th edn. McGraw-Hill, New York

Shaffer L G, Jackson-Cook C J, Stasioniski B A, Spence J E, Brown J A 1992 Parental origin determination in thirty de novo robertsonian translocations. American Journal of Medical Genetics 43: 957–963

Shah A, Holmes N, Wing L 1982 Prevalence of autism and related conditions in adults in a mental handicap hospital. Applied Research in Mental Retardation 3: 303–317

Shapiro A 1979 Psychiatric illness in the mentally handicapped: a historical study. In: James F E, Snaith R P (eds) Psychiatric illness and mental handicap. Royal College of Psychiatrists, London

Sharav T, Collins R, Schlomo L 1985 Effect of maternal education on prognosis of development in children with Down's syndrome. Pediatrics 76: 387

Share J B, Veale A B 1974 Developmental landmarks for children with Down's syndrome. University of Otago Press, Dunedin

Sharp C W, Muir W J, Blackwood D H R, Walker M, Gosden C, St Clair D M 1994 Schizophrenia and mental retardation in a pedigree with retinitis pigmentosa and sensorineural deafness. American Journal of Medical Genetics 54: 354–360

Shepperdson B 1995 Two longitudinal studies of the abilities of people with Down's syndrome. Journal of Intellectual Disability Research 39: 419–431

Sheridan R, Llerena J R, Matkins S, Debenham P Cawood A, Bobrow M 1989 Fertility in a male with trisomy 21. Journal of Medical Genetics 26: 294–298

Sherman S L, Jacobs P A, Morton N E et al 1985 Further analysis of the fragile X syndrome with special reference to transmitting males. Human Genetics 69: 289–299

Shuttleworth G E 1909 Mongolian imbecility. British Medical Journal 2: 661

Siebel N L, Sommer A, Miser J 1984 Transient leukemoid reactions in mosaic trisomy 21. Journal of Pediatrics 104: 251

Sloper P, Turner S 1996 Progress in social-independent functioning of young people with Down's syndrome. Journal of Intellectual Disability Research 40: 39–48

Sloper P, Knussen C, Turner S, Cunningham C 1991 Factors related to stress and satisfaction with life in families of children with Down's syndrome. Journal of Child Psychology and Psychiatry 32: 655–676

Smith G F, Berg J M 1976 Down's anomaly. 2nd edn. Churchill Livingstone, Edinburgh

Snow K, Doud L K, Hagerman R, Pergolizzi R G, Erster S H, Thibodeau S N 1993 Analysis of a CGG sequence at the FMR-1 locus in fragile X families and in the general population. American Journal of Human Genetics 53: 1217–1228

Sovner R 1986 Limiting factors in the use of DSM-III criteria with mentally ill / mentally retarded persons. Psychopharmacology Bulletin 24: 1055–1059

Sovner R 1989 The use of valproate in the treatment of mentally retarded persons with typical and atypical bipolar disorders. Journal of Clinical Psychiatry 50: 40–43

Sovner R, Hurley A D 1983 Do the mentally retarded suffer from affective illness? Archives of General Psychiatry 40: 61–67

Sovner R, Hurley A N, Labrie R 1985 Is mania incompatible with Down's syndrome? British Journal of Psychiatry 146: 319–320

Sparrow S, Balla D, Cicchetti D 1984 Vineland adaptive behavior scales (survey form). American Guidance Service, Circle Pines, MN

Spence M A, Ritvo E R, Marazita M L, Funderburk Sj, Sparkes R S, Freeman B J 1985 Gene mapping studies with the syndrome of autism. Behavioural Genetics 9: 527–542

Sponheim E 1996 Changing criteria of autistic disorders: a comparison of ICD-10 research criteria and DSM-IV with DSM-IIIR, CARS and ABC. Journal of Autism and Developmental Disorders 26: 513–525

Squires N, Ollo C, Jordan P 1986 Auditory brain stem responses in the mentally retarded. Audiometric correlates. Ear and Hearing 7: 83–92

Steffelaar J, Evanhuis H 1989 Epidemiological study of estimated numbers of older patients with Down's syndrome in 1990–2025. Nederlandse Psyschrift voor Geneeskunde 133: 1121–1125

Struwe F 1929 Histopathologisch untersuchungen uber Entstehung und Wesen der senilen plaques. Zeitschrift Gesamte Neurologie Psychiatrie 122: 291–244

Stubbs E G 1988 Does intrauterine cytomegalovirus plus autoantibodies contribute to autism? In: Wing L (ed.) Aspects of autism: biological research. Gaskell / The National Autistic Society, London, pp 91–101

Sutherland G R 1977 Fragile sites on human chromosomes, demonstration of their dependence on the type of tissue culture medium. Science 197: 265–266

Suzuki K 1996 The genetic lysosomal diseases: Tay–Sachs disease as the prototype. Mental Retardation and Developmental Disabilities Research Reviews 2: 167–176

Symanski L 1994 Mental retardation and mental health: concepts, aetiology and incidence. In: Bouras N (ed.) Mental health in mental retardation. Recent advances and practice. Cambridge University Press, Cambridge, pp 19–33

Tangye S R 1979 The e.e.g. and incidence of epilepsy in Down's syndrome. Journal of Mental Deficiency Research 23: 17–24

Tanoue Y, Oda S, Asano F, Kawashima K 1988 Epidemiology of infantile autism in southern Ibaraki, Japan: difference in prevalence rates in birth cohorts. Journal of Autism and Developmental Disorders 18: 155–166

Teller J K, Russo C, DeBusk L M et al 1996 Presence of amyloid β-soluble peptide precedes the amyloid plaque formation in Down's syndrome. Nature Medicine 2: 93–95

Thase M E, Tigner R, Smeltzer D J, Liss L 1984 Age-related neuropsychological deficits in Down's syndrome. Biological Psychiatry 19: 571–585

Thinn K, Clarke D J, Corbett J A 1990 Psychotropic drugs and mental retardation: 2. A comparison of psychoactive drug use before and after discharge from hospital to community. Journal of Mental Deficiency Research 34: 397–407

Tijo J H, Levan A 1956 The chromosome number of man. Hereditas 42: 1–6

Tizard J, Grad J C 1961 The mentally handicapped and their families. A social survey. Institute of Psychiatry, Maudsley Monographs no 7. Oxford University Press, London

Troisi A, Vicario E, Nuccetelli F, Ciani N 1995 Effects of fluoxetine on aggressive behavior of adult inpatients with mental retardation and epilepsy. Pharmacopsychiatry 28: 73–76

Turk V, Brown H 1993 The sexual abuse of adults with learning disabilities: results of a two year incidence survey. Mental Handicap Research 6: 193–216

Turner G, Robinson H, Laing S et al 1992 Population screening for fragile X. Lancet 339: 1210–1213

Turner S, Sweeney D, Hayes L 1995 Developments in community care for adults with learning disabilities: a

review of 1993/1994 community care plans. HMSO, London

Ugazio A G, Maccario R, Norarangelo L D, Burgio G R 1990 Immunology of Down syndrome: a review. American Journal of Medical Genetics Supplement 7: 214–212

Verkerk A J M H, Piretti M, Sutcliffe J S et al 1991 Identification of a gene (FMR-1) containing a CGG repeat coincident with a breakpoint cluster region exhibiting length variation in fragile X syndrome. Cell 65: 905–914

Vitiello B, Spreat S, Behar D 1989 Obsessive–compulsive disorder in mentally retarded patients. Journal of Nervous and Mental Desease 17: 232–236

Volkmar F R, Klin A, Siegel B et al 1994 Field trial for autistic disorder in DSM-IV. American Journal of Psychiatry 151: 1361–1367

Waardenburg P J 1932 Das menschliche Auge und seine Erbanlagen. Martinus Nijhoff, The Hague

Wald N J, Cuckle H S, Densem J W et al 1988 Maternal serum screening for Down's syndrome in early pregnancy. British Medical Journal 297: 883–887

Wang P P, Bellugi U 1994 Evidence from two genetic syndromes for a dissociation between verbal and visual-spatial short term memory. Journal of Clinical and Experimental Neuropsychology 16: 317–322

Warnock Report 1978 Special educational needs. Report of the committee of enquiry into the education of handicapped children and young people. HMSO, London

Waterhouse L, Morris R, Allen D et al 1996 Diagnosis and classification in autism. Journal of Autism and Developmental Disorders 26: 59–88

Webb T, Bundey S, Thake A et al 1986 The frequency of fragile X chromosome among schoolchildren in Coventry. Journal of Medical Genetics 23: 396–399

Wells G L, Barker S E, Finley S C, Colvin E V, Finley W H 1994 Congenital heart disease in infants with Down's syndrome. Southern Medical Journal 87: 724–727

WHO 1992 The ICD-10 classification of mental and behavioural disorders. Clinical descriptions and diagnostic guidelines. World Health Organization, Geneva

WHO 1993 The ICD-10 classification mental and behaviour disorders. Diagnotic criteria for research. World Health Organization, Geneva

Wing L 1991 The relationship between Asperger's syndrome and Kanner's autism. In: Frith U (ed.) Autism and Asperger's syndrome. Cambridge University Press, Cambridge, pp 93–121

Wing L 1994 The autistic continuum. In: Bouras N (ed.) Mental health in mental retardation. Recent advances and practice. Cambridge University Press, Cambridge, pp 108–125

Wing L, Gould J 1979 Severe impairments of social interaction and associated abnormalities in children: epidemiology and classification. Journal of Autism and Developmental Disorders 9: 11–29

Wisniewski K E, Wisniewski H M, Wen G Y 1985a Occurrence of neuropathological changes and dementia of Alzheimer's disease in Down's syndrome. Annals of Neurology 17: 278–282

Wisniewski K E, Dalton A J, Crapper McLachlan D R, Wen G Y, Wisniewski H M 1985b Alzheimer's disease in Down syndrome: clinicopathological studies. Neurology 35: 957–961

Wisniewski K E, Laure-Kamionowska M, Connell F, Wen G Y 1986 Neuronal density and synaptogenesis in the postnatal stage of brain maturation in Down syndrome. In:

Epstein C J (ed.) The neurobiology of Down syndrome. Raven Press, New York, pp 29–44

Wisniewski K E, Segan S M, Miezejeski C M, Sersen E A, Rudelli R D 1991 The fra(X) syndrome: neurological, electrophysicological and neuropathological abnormalities. American Journal of Medical Genetics 38: 476–480

Witkin H A, Mednick S A, Schulsinger F et al 1976 Criminality in XYY and XXY men. Science 193: 547–555

Wressell S E, Tyrer S P, Berney T P 1990 Reduction in antipsychotic drug dosage in mentally handicapped patients: a hospital study. British Journal of Psychiatry 157: 101–106

Yeargin-Allsop M, Drews C D, Decouflé P, Murphy C C 1995 Mild mental retardation in black and white children in metropolitan Atlanta: a case–control study. American Journal of Public Health 85: 324–328

Yeates S 1995 The incidence and importance of hearing loss in people with severe learning disability: the evolution of a service. Mental Handicap 23: 79–84

Young J G, Kavanagh M E, Anderson G M, Schaywitz B A, Cohen D J 1982 Clinical neurochemistry of autism and associated disorders. Journal of Autism and Developmental Disorders 12: 147–165

Zellwiger H 1968 Is Down's syndrome a modern disease? Lancet ii: 458

Zigman W B, Schupf N, Sersen E, Silverman W 1996a Prevalence of dementia in adults with and without Down syndrome. American Journal on Mental Retardation 100: 403–412

Zigman W, Silverman W, Wisniewski H M 1996b Aging and Alzheimer's disease in Down syndrome: clinical and pathological changes. Mental Retardation and Developmental Disabilities Research Reviews 2: 73–77

23

Psychiatric disorders in childhood

Peter Hoare

INTRODUCTION

Child psychiatry is concerned with the assessment and treatment of children's emotional and behavioural problems. These problems are very common, with prevalence rates of 10–20% in several community studies (Rutter et al 1970a, Richman et al 1982). This means that the majority of disturbed children are not seen by specialist psychiatric services, but by general practitioners, community health doctors and paediatricians along with other professionals such as teachers and residential care staff. Consequently, knowledge about the range and variety of emotional and behavioural problems shown by children is important for all doctors involved in the care of children. Again, the everyday work of the paediatrician provides clear evidence of the stressful effects of illness on the child's and family's psychological well-being and adjustment. The paediatrician should therefore be alert to such problems and also be sufficiently competent to help the child and his family adapt to the impact of illness. Knowledge about the psychology of childhood is essential to accomplish this task successfully.

For the psychiatrist in training, knowledge of child development and experience in child psychiatry are important for several reasons: first, in demonstrating that childhood experiences are influential in the development of the adult personality; second, in providing an explanation for the continuity or discontinuity of psychopathology between childhood and adult life; third, in showing the ways in which parental psychiatric illness can adversely affect the child's development. This last can happen either directly through the effects on the parent–child relationship or indirectly through the child's exposure to deviant parental role models. For both these reasons, the child is at greater risk of becoming disturbed. Fourth, they provide the basis for evaluating the significance or otherwise of childhood experience in the development of adult psychopathology. Finally, they give the trainee the competence to assess families and their functioning.

Psychiatric disturbance in childhood is most usefully defined as an abnormality in at least one of three areas: emotions, behaviour or relationships. However, unlike in most other branches of medicine, it is *not* helpful to regard these abnormalities as strictly defined disease entities with a precise aetiology, treatment and prognosis. Rather, it is preferable to regard them as deviations or departures from the norm which are distressing either to the child or to those involved with his welfare. Although child psychiatric disorders do not conform to a strict medical model of illness, it does not mean that these disorders are trivial or unimportant. Some disorders such as autism or conduct disorder have major implications for the child's development and adaptation in adult life.

In childhood, the distinction between disturbance and normality is sometimes imprecise or arbitrary. Isolated symptoms are common and not pathological. For example, many children will occasionally feel sad, unhappy or have temper tantrums. This does not mean that they are disturbed, as disturbance is characterised by the number, frequency, severity and duration of symptoms rather than by the form of symptomatology. In addition, disturbed children rarely have unequivocally pathological symptoms such as hallucinations or delusions. In clinical practice, it is often more important to establish why the child is the focus for concern than it is to adopt the more narrow perspective of whether the child is disturbed or not.

Another important feature of psychiatric disturbance in childhood is that several factors rather than one factor contribute to the development of disturbance. This makes assessment and treatment more difficult so that an essential prerequisite for successful treatment is the correct evaluation of the relative contribution of the different aetiological factors. Aetiological factors are usually categorised into two groups: constitutional and environmental. The former include heredity factors, intelligence and temperament. The three major environmental influences are the family, schooling and the community. Another factor, physical illness or handicap, if present, can have a profound effect on the child's development and on his vulnerability to disturbance.

Three other considerations are of general importance in understanding children's behaviour: the situation-specific nature of behaviour; the impact of current stressful circumstances; and the role of the family. Several studies have shown that children's behaviour varies markedly in different situations, that is, it is situation specific. For instance, a child may be a major problem at school but not at home, or vice versa. Consequently, there may well be an apparent discrepancy between accounts of the child's behaviour from the parents and from the teachers. The most likely explanation for this discrepancy is that the demands and expectations upon the child in the two situations are different. It is therefore essential to obtain several independent accounts about the child's behaviour wherever possible in order to derive a more accurate and realistic assessment of the problem. This situation-specific nature of the behaviour has implications for treatment, as it is important to explain to parents and to teachers the reasons for the discrepancy, thereby lessening the likelihood of misunderstanding.

Children are immature and developing individuals whose capacities and coping skills change markedly during childhood. Childhood is also a period of life characterised by change, challenge and the necessity for adaptation. Consequently it is not surprising that symptoms of disturbance may arise at times of stress when the demands on the child are excessive. Research in the past 15 years (Goodyer 1990) has shown that life events are associated with an increased psychiatric morbidity among children, a finding similar to that reported for adults. Some stresses, such as the birth of a sibling or starting school, are of course normal and inevitable, whereas others, such as marital break-up or life-threatening illness, are serious, with long-term implications for the child's well-being.

The child may, however, cope successfully with the stress, thereby enhancing his self-esteem and confidence. Alternatively, the child may be over-whelmed, responding with the development of symptomatic behaviour. The latter may involve regressive behaviour, i.e. behaving in a more immature, dependent fashion, or more specifically maladaptive, e.g. aggression, excessive anxiety or withdrawal. A crucial feature of assessment is the identification of stressful factors that may be contributing to the problem, as this will influence treatment strategies and also the prognosis.

The family is the most potent force for the promotion of health as well as for the development of disturbance in the child's life. Assessment of parenting qualities, the marital relationship and the quality of family interaction are essential components of child psychiatric practice. It is a frequent observation that it is the parents who are disturbed and not the child. One consequence of this observation is that in many cases the focus of treatment is likely to be the parents, or the whole family, rather than the child. Indeed in many instances the main emphasis of treatment is the promotion of normal healthy family interaction as much as the specific treatment of the child's disturbed behaviour.

Finally, many disturbed children do not complain about their distress nor admit to problems, but rather it is their parents or other adults involved with their care who bring the child to the attention of professionals. Disturbed children more commonly manifest their distress or unhappiness indirectly through symptoms such as abdominal pain, aggression or withdrawal. Direct questioning of the child on first acquaintance is also unlikely to reveal the true extent of the child's feelings and his degree of distress. Sensitive observation during the interview and the use of indirect techniques, such as play, are necessary to elicit a more accurate view of the child's feelings. This is only likely to be successful once a relationship of trust has been established between the child and the doctor.

NORMAL AND ABNORMAL PSYCHOLOGICAL DEVELOPMENT

Children are developing individuals. They are not small adults. A child of 2 is very different from a child of 12, whereas an adult of 25 may not differ that much from one of 35. During childhood, the child undergoes a remarkable transformation from a helpless, dependent infant to an independent self-sufficient individual with his own views and outlook, capable of embarking on a career and living separate from his family. Knowledge about the *mechanisms*, *processes* and the *sequences* underlying these events is necessary in order to understand the nature of psychological disturbance in childhood. This knowledge also helps to define more clearly what is age-appropriate behaviour and to distinguish the pathological from the normal.

Developmental theories

It is useful to define some terms at the outset as they are often used interchangeably. *Growth* refers to the incremental increase of a character, feature or attribute; *maturation* is that aspect(s) of development that is mainly due to innate or endogenous factors; *development* describes those changes in an organism's structure and behaviour that are systematically related to age. Many behaviours, for example walking and talking, have a substantial maturational component, whereas others, for instance emotional and social development, are strongly influenced by environmental factors. The continuous interaction between maturational and environmental factors throughout childhood helps to mould the personality development of the child.

Developmental theories tend to focus on at least one of the following areas: cognitive, emotional and social. They differ widely in theoretical orientation, supporting empirical evidence and in the relative importance attributed to experience in influencing development. No single theory is satisfactory, so that most clinicians use some parts of the various theories to explain different aspects of development. The theories are usually described as stage theories, implying that they regard development as a series of recognisable phases of increasing complexity through which the child progresses. Table 23.1 summarises the important stages of the various theories.

Cognitive development

Piaget, a Swiss psychologist, has elaborated the most comprehensive theory about cognitive development. Many of his conclusions were based on experiments conducted on his own children over a number of years. He has had a tremendous impact on educational concepts and teaching, particularly in primary schools, over the last 30 years. More recently, the theoretical basis and validity of Piaget's conclusions have been questioned by further empirical studies (Bee 1996). Despite these criticisms, Piaget's views remain the most useful account of cognitive development.

Piaget's theory is based within a biological framework. In order to survive, the individual must have the capacity to adapt to the demands of the environment. Cognitive development is the result of interaction between the individual and the environment. Four factors influence cognitive development: increased neurological maturation, enabling the child to appreciate new aspects of experience and to apply more complex reasoning as he gets older; the opportunity to practise newly acquired skills; the opportunity for social interaction and to benefit from schooling; and the emergence of internal psychological mechanisms or *structures* that allow the child to construct successively more complex cognitive models based on maturation and experience.

Piaget describes two types of intellectual structure: schemas and operations. The former are present at birth, and the latter arise during childhood. *Schemas* are internal representations of some specific action, for instance sucking or grasping, whereas *operations* are internal rules of a higher order which have the distinctive feature that they are *reversible*, for instance multipli-

cation is reversible by division. There are two ways whereby the child adapts his cognitive structure to the demands of the environment, *assimilation* and *accommodation*. The former refers to the incorporation of new objects, thoughts and behaviour into existing structures, whereas the latter describes the change of existing structures in response to novel experiences. The child attends and learns most when his environment has a degree of novelty that challenges his curiosity but is not so strange that it becomes too confusing.

Piaget describes four main phases: sensorimotor, preoperational, concrete operational and formal operational. The age range given for each stage is the average, though this can vary considerably depending upon intelligence, cultural background and social factors. However, the order is assumed to be the same for all children. Schemas predominate in the sensorimotor and preoperational stages, whereas operations predominate in the concrete operational and formal operational stages.

Sensorimotor (birth–2 years) Initially, behaviour is dominated by innate reflexes such as feeding, sucking and following, hence the name for this period. Gradually, the infant realises the distinction between *self* and *non-self*, namely where his body ends and the world outside begins. The infant also realises that his behaviour can influence the environment, so that intentional and purposeful behaviour begins. Finally, the infant achieves *object permanence*, whereby he recognises that an object still exists even although it is no longer visible.

Preoperational period (2–7 years) Language development greatly facilitates cognition so that the individual begins to represent objects by symbols and words. Thinking is, however, *egocentric* and *animistic*. The former refers to the child's tendency to regard the world solely from his own position, along with the inability to see a situation from another viewpoint. Animistic thinking describes the child's tendency to regard everything in the world as endowed with feelings, thoughts and wishes. For instance, the moon is watching over you when you sleep, the child says 'naughty door' when he bangs into the door.

The child has problems with the principles of conservation for number, volume and mass. The essential principle underlying conservation is that the number, volume or mass of an object are not changed by any visual alteration in their display or appearance. For instance, the child readily believes that the more widely spaced of two rows of counters has more counters than the denser packed row, or that there is more water in a tall beaker when it has been poured there from a shorter, more squat beaker.

The child also believes that every event has a preced-

Table 23.1 Summary of cognitive, emotional and social development

	Age (years)				
	0	2	6	9	12 + upwards
Cognitive (Piaget)	*Sensorimotor* Differentiates self from objects Begins to act intentionally Achieves object permanence	*Preoperational* Learns to use language and to represent objects by image and words Thinking is egocentric (unable to see other viewpoint) and animistic (everything has feelings including inanimate objects)	*Concrete operational* Thinking is more logical and less egocentric Achieves conservation of number (age 6), volume (age 7) mass (age 8) Able to arrange objects in rank order		*Formal operational* Able to think in abstract manner about propositions and hypotheses
Emotional (Freud)	*Oral* Main concern is initially with satisfaction of basic needs such as hunger Later on, attachment to caregiver	*Anal* Cooperative activity with caregiver Satisfaction with increased self-control and achievement	*Phallic* Learns to interact with peers, often leads to rivalry Aware of own sexuality causing Oedipal conflict, resolved by identification with the same-sex parent Conscience begins to form	*Latency* Reduced sexual interest with main concerns about peer relationships and position within peer group	*Genital* Revival of earlier conflict, especially sexual conflict Four main tasks: separation from parents, sexual role, career choice, identity
Social and personality development	Social smiling (8 weeks) Attachment (6 months) Stranger anxiety (10 months) Erikson's stage of trust versus mistrust	Cooperative play (3 years) Erikson's stage of autonomy versus shame and doubt	Strong preference for same sex friends with stereotyped expectations (6–7 yrs) Erikson's stage of initiative versus guilt	Erikson's stage of industry versus inferiority	Enduring relationships (8 years onwards) Erikson's stage of identity versus role diffusion

ing cause, rejecting the concept of chance or coincidence. Again, the child's moral sense is rigid and inflexible, so that punishment is invariable, irrespective of the circumstances. The child's concept of illness is radically different from that of the adult, with illness being a consequence for misdeeds, a punishment for a misdemeanour.

Concrete operational (7–12 years) Thinking becomes more logical and less dominated by immediate perceptual experience or by changes in appearance. Conservation of number, weight and mass is successively achieved during this period. The child becomes less egocentric, capable of seeing events from another person's standpoint. The child is able to appreciate and utilise reversibility, for example if 2 and 2 equals 4, then 4 minus 2 must equal 2.

Formal operational (12 years and upwards) This stage represents the most complex mode of thinking. Its main characteristics are the ability to think in an abstract fashion, to formulate general rules and principles and to devise and test hypotheses, an approach similar to that used in mathematics or in scientific investigation. An example of such reasoning is the following: Joan is fairer than Susan; Joan is darker than Anne. Who is the darkest? (Answer: Susan). Prior to the formal operational stage, the child would require the aid of dolls to solve this problem. It should be pointed out that not everyone achieves this stage of thinking, even as an adult! The content of thinking also alters markedly with an emphasis on the hypothetical, the future and ideological issues.

Critical comment on Piaget Recently, Piagetian model has been criticised extensively for the lack of evidence to support the existence of the internal structures necessary for the concrete and formal operational stages as well as the elaboration of alternative explanations for the child's inability to carry out conservation tasks successfully before a certain age (Matthews 1994). These criticisms are substantial, but they do not detract from the major conceptual contribution that Piaget has made to knowledge about cognitive development in children.

Recent developments in cognitive theory Psychologists and psychiatrists have become increasingly interested in the development and application of cognitive theory to the understanding and treatment of psychiatric disorders (Hawton et al 1995 and Ch. 2). The main principles underlying this theory are that an individual's beliefs about himself, the future and the world influence his mood and behaviour, an idea similar in some ways to the Piagetian concept of schemas. When a person is depressed, his thoughts are self-defeating and he commits certain cognitive errors. Two common types of cognitive error are *personalisation* and *dichotomous thinking*. The following two statements are

examples of these two errors respectively: 'The reason my parents separated is all because of me' and 'I'm no good at tennis, so I'm bound to be useless at any other sport.'

A major extension of these ideas in childhood is the notion of the *self-concept*. By the age of 6 or 7 years, most children have very definite and clear ideas about themselves and their qualities. For example, they are able to compare themselves with other children with respect to popularity, attractiveness, scholastic ability, and so on. Self-concept is a construct similar to that of a schema in Piaget's theory. Another important facet of self-concept is the favourable or unfavourable evaluation that the child makes of himself, an aspect called *self-esteem*. Children with high self-esteem appear to do better in school, regard themselves as in control of their own destiny, have more friends and get along better with their families (Bee 1996).

Emotional and social development

Sigmund Freud elaborated the most comprehensive theory about emotional development, while Erikson, also a psychoanalyst, applied psychoanalytic concepts within a social and cultural framework. Freudian theory emphasises the biological and maturational components of development with an invariable sequence to development for everyone. Like Piaget, it is a stage or phase theory with the individual progressing successively through each phase. A major criticism of Freudian theory is that its concepts do not lend themselves readily to scientific investigation, so that it is difficult to prove or disprove the validity of the theory.

Freud proposed that the individual goes through five stages prior to adulthood: oral, anal, phallic, latency and genital. These terms refer to the major developmental task or potential conflict that the individual has to achieve or resolve during this period. Table 23.1 describes the important features of the different stages, e.g. during the phallic stage, the oedipal crisis arises. At this time, around 3–4 years, the child becomes aware of his own sexual feelings and also that he is attracted in a sexual manner to the parent of the opposite sex. Moreover, the child is simultaneously aware that the parent of the same sex is a rival for the attention of the other parent. The conflict arises because the child is caught between the desire for one parent and the wrath of the other. The conflict is successfully resolved by the child identifying with the parent of the same sex, thereby eliminating the rivalrous feelings.

Erikson's major contribution has been to place psychoanalytic concepts in a social and cultural dimension (Table 23.1). For Erikson, the most important task for the individual is to achieve a coherent sense of identity, a balanced and mature appraisal of one's abilities and limitations, with a recognition of the importance of previous experience and with realistic expectations for the future. Such a task occupies the individual throughout his lifetime. The individual passes through a series of developmental stages, all of which are polarised into two extremes, one successful and adaptive and the other unsuccessful and maladaptive. The two poles of the first stage are *trust* and *mistrust*. The former refers to the child's belief that the world is safe, predictable, and that he can influence events towards a favourable outcome, whereas a sense of mistrust implies a world that is cruel, erratic and unable to meet his needs. The role of the caregiver, usually the mother, is crucial to the achievement of a successful outcome. Erikson also believed that the individual carries forward the residues of earlier stages into the present, thereby giving the past an influence on contemporary behaviour. Erikson's writings are a compelling and coherent account of development. A major weakness is, however, the lack of empirical evidence to support the conclusions.

Development of social relationships (Bee 1996)

A characteristic of human beings is their predisposition to establish and maintain social relationships. Although Freud and Erikson refer to social relationships, it is only with the recent elaboration of *attachment theory* by Bowlby (1969) and by Ainsworth (1982) that a plausible theory for this phenomenon has been described. Attachment theory proposes that social relationships develop in response to the mutual biological and psychological needs of the mother and the infant. Mother–infant interaction promotes social relationships. Each member of the dyad has a repertoire of behaviour that facilitates interaction: the infant by crying, smiling and vocalisation; the mother by facial expression, vocalisation and gaze. A mother can regulate the infant's state of alertness, for instance rocking and stroking to soothe the child, talking and facial expression to stimulate the child.

The term *attachment* describes the infant's predisposition to seek proximity to certain people and to be more secure in their presence. Bowlby maintains that there is a biological basis for this behaviour, as it has been found extensively in other primates as well as in most human societies. It has considerable survival and adaptive value for the species, as it enables the dependent infant to explore from a secure base and also to use the base as a place of safety at times of distress. From 6 months onwards infants develop selective attachment to people, usually the mother initially, but not exclusively to her. This first relationship is regarded as the prototype of subsequent relationships, so that its success or failure may have long-term consequences. Clinicians distinguish between *secure attachment* and *anxious attachment*, with the former referring to healthy and the latter to potentially unsatisfactory relationships.

Bonding refers to the persistence of relationships over time, namely the child's capacity to retain the relationship despite the absence of the other individual. Much of the infant's behaviour promotes the development of attachments by ensuring close proximity and interaction with the mother. These ideas have many implications for obstetric and paediatric practice, for the reduction of stress associated with hospitalisation and for possibly explaining the origins of non-accidental injury to children.

Other aspects of development

Gender and sex role concepts Gender identity is a part of self-concept, but the development of the child's understanding about 'boyness' or 'girlness', the sex role concept, is a more elaborate process. Children usually acquire *gender identity* (correctly labelling themselves and others) by about age 2 or 3, followed by *gender stability* (permanence of gender identity) by about 4. *Gender constancy* (gender identity unalterable by change in appearance) appears around 6 years, similar to other conservation-like concepts. Children show clear evidence of sex role stereotyping from an early age, with an excessively rigid concept for a brief period around 6 or 7 years. Freudian theory explains these findings on the basis of identification whereby the child imitates the same-sex parent, thus acquiring appropriate sex-typed behaviour. Alternative explanations emphasise the importance of social reinforcement or of cognition whereby the child acquires a schema about the respective roles and behaviour of boys and girls.

Moral development The acquisition of moral or ethical values is an important aspect of the socialisation of children. Freud and Piaget both described how this process happens. Freudian theory maintains that the superego or conscience develops during the phallic stage around 4–5 years. At this time, the child is identifying strongly with the same-sex parent in order to resolve the oedipal conflict and in consequence acquires parental values and prohibitions. In contrast, Piaget hypothesises a much more gradual or stage-like sequence to the acquisition of moral values. The child around 3 years old bases his judgement on the outcome rather than the intention of an act, with an emphasis on punishment following on from a misdemeanour. Subsequently, the child adopts a more conventional morality based upon conformity with family values. Finally, the adolescent derives a personal value system that combines his own idiosyncratic values with those of his family and of society with the intention of achieving the 'greatest good for the greatest number'.

Developmental psychopathology

This long-winded phrase refers to two important dimensions necessary to evaluate children's behaviour: first, whether the behaviour is age appropriate, namely the developmental aspect; and second, whether the behaviour is abnormal, the psychopathological. For example, separation anxiety is a normal phenomenon among children between 9 months and 4 years approximately, whereas it would be abnormal in a child aged 6 years.

The tripartite division of disturbance into abnormalities of behaviour, emotions or relationships provides a useful way of analysing disturbance. Many behavioural problems can be conceptualised in terms of deficits or excesses. For instance, children with encopresis or enuresis can be regarded as having failed to acquire the skills necessary to use the toilet appropriately. Similarly, the aggressive child is showing excessive belligerent or assertive behaviour at an inappropriate time. This approach also has implications for treatment, as the latter is often based on behavioural techniques designed to promote certain behaviours or alternatively eliminate others.

Anxiety is central to the understanding of emotional disturbance. It has physical manifestations, such as palpitations and dry mouth, as well as psychological, such as fear and apprehension. Anxiety is a normal, indeed essential, part of growing up. It may occur in many situations: in response to external threat; new or strange situations; or in response to the operation of conscience. Anna Freud (1936) developed the concept of *defence mechanisms* to explain how the individual deals with excessive anxiety. This response is entirely healthy and appropriate in many situations, only becoming maladaptive when it is used exclusively or excessively, thereby preventing the individual from learning how to cope with a normal amount of anxiety. Common defence mechanisms include *denial, rationalisation, regression* and *displacement*. Denial is the child's reluctance or inability to accept the psychological impact of a particular event or situation. For instance, a child refuses to admit to stealing even though it is obvious that he is responsible, as the resultant loss of self-esteem and overwhelming guilt makes this impossible. Rationalisation is the attempt to justify or minimise the psychological consequences of an event. 'I don't really like football, so that I am not bothered about playing for the team' is an example of the way the child may deal with a failure to gain selection for the school team.

Regression occurs when a child behaves in a more developmentally immature manner, often at times of stress, for example becoming enuretic at the start of primary school. Displacement is the transfer of hostile or aggressive feelings from their original source on to another person, for instance getting angry with a sibling rather than with an adult.

Social relationships are often impaired among disturbed children. This may be a primary failure in some instances, such as autism, or more commonly a secondary phenomenon. Children with neurotic or conduct disorders are usually isolated and unpopular with their peer group as they either exclude themselves or are themselves excluded as a result of their deviant behaviour. In addition, the behaviour usually brings them into conflict with parents or other adults such as teachers.

GENERAL FEATURES OF PSYCHIATRIC DISTURBANCE

Diagnostic classification

A single cause is rarely responsible for the development of disturbance. The usual pattern is for several factors to be involved, with a broad distinction into constitutional and environmental factors. The important constitutional factors are intelligence and temperament, while current life circumstances, the family, schooling and the community are the major environmental influences. One consequence of this multiple causation is that it is inappropriate to devise a diagnostic classification on the basis of aetiology, as the relative contribution of each factor is often unclear.

Diagnostic practice is therefore descriptive or phenomenological, with three main categories of abnormality: *emotions, behaviour* and *relationships*. In addition, these abnormalities should be of sufficient severity that they impair the individual in his daily activities and/or cause stress to the individual or to those responsible for his well-being. A commonly used definition of disturbance is as follows: an abnormality of emotions, behaviour or relationships which is sufficiently severe and persistent to handicap the child in his social or personal functioning and/or to cause distress to the child, his parents or to people in the community.

Another feature of contemporary diagnostic practice in child psychiatry is the adoption of a multiaxial framework to describe the various abnormalities or handicaps that are frequently present together in one child. This is also a further recognition of the multifactorial nature of disturbance in childhood. The two most common systems are the ICD-10 (WHO 1992) and DSM-IV (APA

Axis	DSM–IV	ICD–10
I	Clinical syndrome	Clinical syndrome
II	Mental retardation Personality disorders	Disorders of psychological development
III	Physical disorders / illnesses	Mental retardation
IV	Psychosocial and environmental problems	Medical illness
V	Global assessment of functioning	Abnormal psychosocial conditions
VI		Psychosocial disability

Table 23.2   DSM-IV and ICD–10 classification systems (modified for child psychiatry)

1994) (Table 23.2). DSM-IV is used extensively in North America, whereas ICD-10 is popular in the UK. The two systems have similar underlying principles with an emphasis on a clinical–descriptive approach to diagnosis and the categorisation of children along several dimensions, with every child having a position on each dimension, even when there is no abnormality. ICD-10 uses a glossary and DSM-IV uses operationally defined criteria to provide the basis for diagnosis. An important difference between ICD-10 and DSM-IV is that the latter allows for more than one diagnosis on the clinical syndrome axis, whereas ICD-10 prefers a single diagnosis, an approach more widely used.

DSM-IV places pervasive developmental disorders, including autism and developmental disorders such as specific reading disorder, on Axis I, whereas ICD-10 groups these conditions on a separate Axis II, disorders of psychological development. The following list shows a convenient way to classify the important psychiatric syndromes in childhood:

- Conduct disorders
- Emotional disorders
- Mixed disorders of conduct and emotions
- Hyperkinetic disorders
- Disorders of social functioning
- Tic disorders
- Pervasive developmental disorders
- Miscellaneous disorders.

Conduct disorder is characterised by severe, persistent, socially disapproved of behaviour, such as aggression or stealing, that often involves damage to or destruction of property and is unresponsive to normal sanctions. The main feature of emotional disorder is a subjective sense of distress, often arising in response to stress. This group is further divided into phobic, anxiety, obsessional, conversion states and severe reactions to stress. Many disturbed children show a mixture of emotional and behavioural symptoms, so that a mixed category is clinically useful. Hyperkinetic disorders cover a range of disorders characterised by overactivity, distractibility,

impulsivity, aggression and short attention span. Large differences in the prevalence of this syndrome have been reported between the USA and the UK (see section on overactivity and hyperactivity). Disorders of social functioning comprise conditions such as elective mutism and attachment disorders. Pervasive developmental disorders includes childhood autism, Rett's syndrome, childhood disintegrative disorder and Asperger's syndrome. The miscellaneous group contains a diverse group of problems such as encopresis, enuresis and developmental disorders. Other important but uncommon conditions such as schizophrenia and mood disorders are categorised in a similar fashion as that for adults, providing that the diagnostic criteria are fulfilled.

Epidemiology

Epidemiological research has been an important research interest in the UK for the past 30 years. It has provided accurate information about the frequency and distribution of disturbance throughout childhood and adolescence (Rutter et al 1970a), the differences between urban and rural areas (Rutter et al 1975) and the effects of illness and handicap on vulnerability to disturbance (Rutter et al 1970b), as well as providing clues about the relative importance of various aetiological factors (Rutter et al 1975).

Most studies have shown prevalence rates of between 10 and 20% depending on the criteria for deviance. The first and most influential study was the Isle of Wight (IOW) study carried out by Rutter and his colleagues (1970a). Using strict definitions of disorder, they found rates of approximately 7% among 10–11-year-old children. Follow-up of these children into adolescence indicated a prevalence rate of around 7%, with more than 40% of the children with conduct disorder continuing with major problems. Disorders arising for the first time during adolescence were more adult-like in presentation, with a preponderance of females. Over 80% of the disorders were in the emotional, conduct or mixed categories. Emotional disorders were more common among girls, with anxiety as the most common type. By contrast conduct disorders, and to an important extent mixed disorder, were more common among boys, with an association with specific reading retardation. A comparative study of 10-year-olds living in London (Rutter et al 1975) showed a rate of disturbance over twice that on the IOW. This study also showed that the difference in prevalence rate was entirely accounted for by the increased frequency of predisposing factors among children and their families in London compared with those on the IOW. These factors were family discord, parental psychiatric disorder, social disadvantage and inferior quality of schooling.

The IOW study (Rutter et al 1970b) also showed that children with chronic illness or handicap had much higher rates of disturbance than healthy children. For instance, children with central nervous disease such as epilepsy or cerebral palsy had a rate over five times that of the general population, while children with other illnesses such as asthma or diabetes were twice as likely to be disturbed as healthy children.

Studies of preschool children, most notably by Richman et al (1982), have found that about 20% of children have significant behaviour problems, with 7% classified as severe. Follow-up studies of these children indicated that about 60% persisted, most commonly among overactive boys of low ability. An important association was found between language delay and disturbed behaviour. Finally, problems were more likely to persist when there was marital discord, maternal psychiatric ill-health and psychosocial disadvantage such as poor housing and large family size.

ASSESSMENT PROCEDURES

Assessment is more time consuming in child psychiatry than in other branches of psychiatry. It has three components: history taking and examination; psychological assessment; and information about the child and family from other professionals.

History taking and examination

This has many similarities to traditional methods, though with important modifications. Interview skills are essential to the elucidation, understanding and treatment of emotional and behavioural problems in children. Training in interview skills should be an important part of medical undergraduate and postgraduate training. Points of general importance include: clarification about the nature of the problem and the

reason for referral; obtaining adequate factual information; eliciting emotional responses and attitudes about past and current events; observing behaviour during the interview; establishing trust and confidence of the child and family; providing the parents with a summary of problems and a provisional treatment plan at the end of the initial interview.

There are no absolute rules about interviewing, indeed flexibility is essential. However, the following guidelines are useful:

- The interview room should be large enough to seat the family comfortably and also to allow the children to use the play material in a relaxed manner.
- Avoid having a desk between the interviewer and the family, i.e. put the desk against the wall of the interview room.
- Do not spend the interview writing down notes but rather encourage eye-to-eye contact, taking the minimal notes necessary.
- The play material must be suitable for a wide age range and include crayons and paper, jigsaws, simple games, books (provides rough estimate of reading ability), doll's house, play telephones and miniature domestic and zoo animals.
- The play material should be gradually introduced as appropriate and not left around in a haphazard manner.
- Interview parents and young children together.
- Older children and adolescents like to be seen separately from parents at some point during interview.
- Older children and adolescents are able to talk about problems openly once trust in the interviewer has been established.
- Too direct questions usually elicit denial from the child, so open-ended questions are much preferable.

The interview should provide information about the following (italic type indicates essential facts):

1. *Presenting problem(s): frequency, severity, onset, course, exacerbating/ameliorating factors, effect on family, help given so far*
2. Other problems or complaints
   a. General health: eating, sleeping, elimination, physical complaints, fits or faints
   b. Interests, activities and hobbies
   c. *Relationship with parents and sibs*
   d. Relationship with other children, special friends
   e. Mood – happy, sad, anxious
   f. Level of activity, attention span, concentration
   g. Antisocial behaviour
   h. *Schooling: attainments, attendance, friendships, relationship with teachers*

i. Sexual knowledge, interests and behaviour (when relevant).
3. *Any other problems not previously mentioned*
4. Family structure
   a. *Parents: ages*, occupations, *current physical and psychiatric state*, previous physical and psychiatric history
   b. Sibs: ages, problems
   c. Home circumstances
5. Family function
   a. *Quality of parenting; mutual support and help; level of communication and ability to resolve problems*
   b. *Parent–child relationship: warmth, affection and acceptance; level of criticism, hostility and rejection*
   c. Sibs' relationship
   d. Pattern of family relationships
6. Personal history
   a. Pregnancy and delivery
   b. Early mother–child relationship; postpartum depression; early feeding patterns
   c. Temperamental characteristics: easy or difficult; irregular, restless baby and toddler
   d. Developmental milestones
   e. *Past illnesses and injuries, hospitalisation*
   f. Separations greater than 1 week
   g. Previous schooling
7. *Observation of child's behaviour and emotional state*
   a. *Appearance: nutritional state, signs of neglect or injury*
   b. Activity level; involuntary movements; concentration
   c. Mood: expressions or signs of sadness, misery, anxiety
   d. Reaction to and relationship with the doctor: eye contact, spontaneous talk, inhibition and disinhibition
   e. Relationship with parents: affection/resentment, ease of separation
   f. Habits and mannerisms
   g. Presence of delusions, hallucinations, thought disorder
8. Observation of family relationships
   a. Patterns of interaction
   b. Clarity of boundaries between parents and child
   c. Communication
   d. Emotional atmosphere of family: mutual warmth/tension, criticisms
9. Physical examination
   a. Screening neurological examination
      (i)   Note any facial asymmetry
      (ii) Eye movements: ask child to follow a moving finger and observe eye movement for jerkiness, incoordination
      (iii) Finger–thumb apposition: ask child to press the tip of each finger against the thumb in rapid succession; observe clumsiness, weakness
      (iv) Copying pattern: drawing a man
      (v)   Observe grip and dexterity in drawing
      (vi) Observe visual competence when drawing
      (vii) Jumping up and down on the spot
      (viii) Hopping
      (ix) Hearing: capacity of child to repeat numbers whispered 2 metres behind him
   b. Further medical examination (if relevant).

Formulation

At completion of the assessment, the clinician should be able to make a formulation. This is a succinct summary of the important features of the individual case. The formulation consists of the following: a statement of main problems; the diagnosis and differential diagnosis; the relative contribution of constitutional and environmental factors to the aetiology; the probable short-term and long-term outcome; further information required (including special investigations); the initial treatment plan. The formulation should be included in the casenotes, thereby providing the clinician with a record of his views at referral.

Psychological assessment

Psychological assessment, carried out by child psychologists, is an invaluable and integral part of the overall assessment of a child's problems in many situations. It can provide information about three aspects of development: general intelligence, educational attainments and special skills. Assessment is usually based upon the administration of standardised assessment tests. These are either norm referenced or criterion referenced. The former compares the child's ability with other children of the same age, whereas the latter is on a pass/fail basis, for instance whether he can tie his shoelaces. Ideally, the test items should have good discriminatory value (distinguish between children of different ability), be reliable (give similar results when repeated) and valid (in agreement with other independent evidence). An important aspect of the assessment is that the tasks are carried out in a standardised fashion, thereby increasing reliability and validity.

Intellectual ability

Developmental assessment in infancy and early childhood The commonly used tests are the Bayley scales of infant development (Bayley 1969), Griffiths mental development scale (Griffiths 1954) and the

Denver developmental screening test (Frankenberg et al 1975).

Assessment of general intelligence in school-age children The most popular test is the Wechsler intelligence scale for children – revised form (WISC-R) (Wechsler 1992). This covers an age range from 6 to 16 years. Ten subtests are usually used, measuring different aspects of the child's ability. Commonly, the tests are divided into 'verbal' and 'performance' categories yielding a 'verbal IQ' and a 'performance IQ'. The 'verbal' subtests commonly used are *information, comprehension, arithmetic, similarities* and *vocabulary*, while the 'performance' are *picture completion, picture arrangement, block design, object assembly* and *coding*. Each subtest has a mean score of 10 so that combining the 10 tests gives a 'full scale' IQ of 100 with a standard deviation of 15. The 'normal' distribution of the test scores means that it is possible to state that 66% of children will be within the IQ range 85–115, 95% within IQ range 70–130, 99% within IQ range 55–145. Other tests used include the Stanford–Binet (Form L-M) (Thorndike 1973) and the British ability scales (BAS) (Elliott et al 1983).

Educational attainment

There are two commonly used reading tests: the Schonell graded word reading test (Schonell & Schonell 1950) and the Neale analysis of reading ability (Neale 1958). The latter is more comprehensive, though taking longer to administer. It provides information about speed, accuracy and comprehension of reading. The scores are transformed into reading ages of so many years and months, for instance 6 years 11 months. Other attainment tests include the Schonell graded spelling test (Schonell & Schonell 1950). There is no satisfactory standardised test of mathematical skills, although appropriate subtest scores of the WISC-R or the BAS can be used as a guide to mathematical ability.

Specific skills

Reynell development language scale (Reynell 1969), Bender motor gestalt test and the Vineland social maturity scales are examples of tests to assess the child's acquisition of certain abilities and skills. These are often helpful with some specific problems.

Limitations of assessment

Caution should always be exercised in the interpretation of test results. It is wrong to attribute undue significance to a single result, most often done with the IQ score. Many factors influence test results, including fatigue, poor testing conditions and the use of inappropriate tests. The results should be evaluated in the context of the overall assessment and the report from the child psychologist. A great deal of harm, upset and distress can arise for a child when he is incorrectly classified or labelled as either too able or too dull on the basis of an unreliable psychological assessment.

Additional information

A distinctive feature of child psychiatry practice is the importance attached to obtaining independent evidence about the child's behaviour. This is for two reasons: first, a child's behaviour varies from one situation to another, so that it is helpful to have information about the child's behaviour in several contexts; second, parental accounts of the child's behaviour are likely to be distorted in many cases, as it is the parents who are disturbed rather than the child. Consequently, an important part of assessment is to obtain reports from other professionals involved with the family, such as school teachers, health visitors or general practitioners. Another common practice is the use of questionnaires to supplement information provided by referrers and other more formal reports. Several questionnaires (Rutter et al 1970a, Richman et al 1982, Achenbach & Edelbrock 1983) have been devised to assess different age ranges and have satisfactory psychometric properties. The most commonly used questionnaires for school-age children in the UK are the Rutter parents' and teachers' scales, also known as Rutter A and Rutter B, respectively. These scales have established reliability and validity as well as classifying children into neurotic or emotional conduct or antisocial and mixed categories.

DISORDERS IN PRESCHOOL CHILDREN

Except for rare but severe disorders such as childhood autism, psychiatric disorders in this age group are mostly deviations or delays from normality rather than psychiatric illness as such. Moreover, the child's behaviour and development are so influenced by the immediate surroundings that it is often the environment which is responsible for the problems rather than the child.

Aetiology

Four types of factor contribute to problems in varying degrees in the individual child: temperamental factors; physical illness or handicap; family psychopathology; and social disadvantage. The New York Longitudinal Study (Chess & Thomas 1990) showed clearly that children with certain types of temperamental characteristics, the so-called 'difficult child' and the 'slow to warm up child' profile, were more likely to develop problems. Again, physical illness or handicap can reduce activity, directly or indirectly affect developmental progress and increase parental anxiety, all of which potentiate the likelihood of behavioural disturbance. Parental psychiatric illness, marital disharmony and poor parenting skills are instances where disturbances in the parents adversely affect the child's behaviour. Richman et al (1982) showed high rates of depression among mothers of preschool children. Social disadvantage such as poor housing or inadequate recreational facilities increases the risk of disturbance among preschool children.

Frequency of problems

Table 23.3 shows the prevalence of common problems among 3- and 4-year-olds in the general population (Richman & Lansdown 1988). Problems are mainly about eating, sleeping and elimination, with a marked decrease in wetting and soiling over the 1 year period. Affective symptoms such as unhappiness and relationship problems are much less common, but probably more significant. Community studies (Richman et al 1982) indicate that 20% of children are regarded by their mothers as having problems, with 7% rated as severe.

Table 23.3 Problem behaviours in 3- and 4-year-olds (Richman & Lansdown 1988)		
Behaviour	3-year-olds (%)	4-year-olds (%)
Poor appetite	19	20
Faddy eater	15	24
Difficulty settling at night	16	15
Waking at night	14	12
Overactive and restless	17	13
Poor concentration	9	6
Difficult to control	11	10
Temper	5	6
Unhappy mood	4	7
Worries	4	1
Fears	10	12
Poor relationships with siblings	10	15
Poor relationships with peers	4	6
Regular day wetting	26	8
Regular night wetting	33	19
Regular soiling	16	3

Common problems

This section discusses those problems that are particularly frequent among the preschool child, while others such as soiling, which occur in older children as well, are discussed in a later part of this section of the chapter.

Temper tantrums

These usually arise when the child is thwarted, angry or has hurt himself. They can occur in isolation or as part of a wider problem. They comprise a variety of behaviours, including screaming, crying, often with collapse on to the floor and banging of the feet. A child can be aggressive towards other people around him, but the child only rarely injures himself. Most tantrums 'burn themselves out', so that specific intervention is not necessary. If it is, then the following points are useful: if necessary, restrain from behind by folding arms around child's body; minimise any additional attention to the child; only respond and praise when behaviour is back to normal.

Feeding problems

These range in severity from a minor problem such as the finicky child to the severe disabling problem of non-organic failure to thrive. Minor problems will usually respond to patient and attentive listening to the parents' concerns, counselling and specific advice. Severe non-organic failure to thrive (prevalence 2%) is a complex problem requiring comprehensive assessment and a large amount of time and resources to remedy (Skuse et al 1992). Several factors are responsible in most cases, including poor mother–child relationship, often in the context of more widespread emotional and social deprivation, and factors in the child, including temperamental factors and aversion to feeding. *Pica*, the ingestion of inedible material such as dirt or rubbish, is a normal transitory phenomenon during the toddler period. Persistent ingestion is found amongst mentally retarded, psychotic and socially deprived children. Lead poisoning, though always mentioned, is a possible but uncommon danger from pica.

Sleep problems

These are common, with up to 20% of 2-year-olds waking at least five times per week (Eaton-Evans & Dugdale 1988). The two most frequent problems are reluctance to settle at night and persistent waking up during the night. Several factors contribute to the problem, including adverse temperamental characteristics in the child, perinatal problems and maternal anxiety. It is also important to distinguish between those factors responsible for the onset of the problem and those for maintaining the problem. Medication such as trimeprazine and promethazine are frequently prescribed but are usually ineffective. Their only genuine indication is to provide a brief respite for the parents as well as ensuring that the child has an uninterrupted night's sleep. The most successful management is a behavioural strategy (see treatment section).

Psychiatric aspects of child abuse

Originally this was restricted to the 'battered baby syndrome' but it has now been extended to include physical abuse, emotional abuse, sexual abuse and neglect. Several enquiries and controversies during the 1980s, particularly the Cleveland affair (Butler-Sloss 1988), have highlighted the importance of this topic for all doctors involved in the care of children (general practitioners, paediatricians, school doctors and child psychiatrists). The main professional responsibility for child protection is social work, though other professionals are frequently involved at various stages in an individual case.

It is important to remember that the different aspects of child abuse are frequently present in the same child and family and that many comments about the detection, management and treatment apply equally well to all aspects of child abuse. Several recently published books (Bentovim et al 1988, Cicchetti & Carlson 1989, Jones 1992, Monck et al 1995) provide very useful accounts of current practice about various aspects of child abuse, particularly in relation to sexual abuse.

Physical abuse

Diagnostic awareness and suspicion are the key elements in the detection and recognition of physical abuse. The following list summarises the common characteristics of abused children and their families, although the most important factor to recognise is that child abuse occurs in any family irrespective of class, colour or creed.

Risk characteristics in the abused child:

- Product of unwanted pregnancy
- Unwanted child in family
- Low birth-weight
- Separation from mother in neonatal period
- Mental or physical handicap
- Habitually restless, sleepless or incessantly crying
- Physically unattractive.

Risk characteristics in the parent(s):

- Single parent
- Young
- Abused themselves as children
- Low self-esteem
- Unrealistic expectations of child and his development
- Inconsistent or punishment-orientated discipline.

Risk characteristics in social circumstances:

- Low income or unemployment
- Social isolation
- Current stress such as housing crisis, domestic friction, exhaustion or ill-health
- Large family.

Management

Most cases of child abuse do not require the involvement of a child psychiatrist, as the principal concerns are the protection of the child, practical support for the family and help with parenting skills. The child psychiatrist can make a useful contribution in two ways: first, in acting as an outside consultant to other professionals and agencies working with the family on various aspects of detection, management and treatment; second, in providing individual and family therapy for the child, the parents or the family in particular instances, depending upon the assessment.

In addition to its immediate effects, child abuse may have medium-term and long-term sequelae. Many abused children continue to be exposed to emotional abuse and neglect throughout their childhood, so that they often show symptoms of disturbance such as unhappiness, wariness, untrusting, low self-esteem and poor peer relationships. This childhood experience in turn predisposes abused children to become abusing parents when adults.

Emotional abuse

This term has been introduced to describe the severe impairment of social and emotional development resulting from repeated and persistent criticism, lack of affection, rejection, verbal abuse and other similar behaviour by the parent(s) to the child. Affected children display a variety of symptoms: low self-esteem, limited capacity for enjoyment, severe aggression, impulsive behaviour.

Sexual abuse

This became a topic of major public and paediatric concern in the late 1980s (Butler-Sloss 1988). A commonly used definition is as follows: 'the involvement of dependent children and adolescents in sexual activities they truly do not comprehend, to which they are unable to give informed consent, and which violate social taboos of family roles'.

Fundamental to child sex abuse is the misuse of adult power. The range of activities includes fondling, masturbation, rape and buggery. The term also covers some activities not involving physical contact such as posing for pornographic photographs or films. The abuser is frequently known to the child and is often a member of the family (incest).

The presentation of sexual abuse varies widely depending on the nature of the abuse and on the relationship between the abused child and the perpetrator. Open disclosure is more likely when the offender is outside the family, whereas physical symptoms involving the anogenital region and or emotional or behavioural disturbance are more common when a family member is responsible. As with physical abuse, diagnostic awareness and suspicion are the key elements in the detection and recognition of the abuse.

Investigation (see Bentovim et al 1988) Sensitivity and tact are clearly essential when conducting the examination and interview of the child during the initial investigation. Separate detailed questioning and interviewing of the parents is also necessary.

Management (see Bentovim et al 1988) The same principles apply in sexual abuse as for physical abuse. The role of the child psychiatry team is more important here, as interviewing skills, psychotherapeutic expertise and the use of specialised equipment (anatomically accurate dolls) are often necessary at the detection and the treatment stages of management. Detailed accounts of this work, including the use of the anatomical dolls, are described in the books by the Great Ormond Street child sex abuse team (Bentovim et al 1988, Monck et al 1995). The establishment of specialised assessment teams in every locality was another important recommendation of the Cleveland enquiry (Butler-Sloss 1988).

Neglect

This varies markedly, ranging from relative inadequacy and incompetence in providing basic care, love and security for the child to severe failure in the provision of basic essentials, often combined with emotional and social deprivation. Though more difficult to quantify than physical or sexual abuse, the condition is certainly more common, at least in its milder forms, than these other two forms of abuse. Additionally, it may be more long-lasting with potentially more serious consequences for the child's development. It is often noticed or reported by relatives, neighbours, health visitors or teachers. Adverse social circumstances and poor parenting are usually found, with the necessity for alternative family placement for the child in the long term in many cases.

Munchausen's syndrome by proxy (Meadow 1995)

This remarkable variant of physical abuse often occurs against the same background of parental psychopathology and social disadvantage as other forms of abuse. The essential feature of this syndrome is the fabrication of physical illness in the child by the parent(s), usually the mother. Common examples include factitious recurrent bleeding or unstable control of diabetes or epilepsy. Extensive investigation and admission to hospital are carried out, with fruitless results. It is only when the possibility of parental abuse is recognised that the explanation becomes apparent.

Management As soon as the diagnosis is established, the parents should be confronted with the situation. The main priority is the protection of the child, including where necessary the removal of the child from the family home. The immediate and longer-term aims of treatment are similar to that for child abuse as the underlying psychopathology and social circumstances are similar. The role of the child psychiatrist is usually confined in most cases to offering counselling for the parents and/or family therapy when indicated.

PERVASIVE DEVELOPMENTAL DISORDERS, SCHIZOPHRENIA AND OTHER PSYCHOSES (LORD & RUTTER 1994, GILLBERG 1995)

These conditions have been previously combined under the general term 'childhood psychosis', as they are severe and disabling, with clear-cut abnormalities. However, autistic children do not experience hallucinations nor delusions, the characteristics of psychosis, and moreover have had the abnormalities from early infancy. For these reasons, ICD-10 and DSM-IV have separated out childhood autism from other psychotic conditions in childhood into a new diagnostic category called pervasive developmental disorders. This also includes Rett's syndrome, disintegrative disorder and Asperger's syndrome.

Childhood autism

Kanner's (1943) original description of 11 children with 'an extreme autistic aloneness' has not been improved upon, with its astute observation of 'inability to relate in an ordinary way to people and to situations' and 'an anxiously obsessive desire for the maintenance of sameness'. Subsequently, opinions have fluctuated about the diagnosis, aetiology and treatment. Most authorities now agree that three features are essential to the diagnosis: general and profound failure to develop social relationships; language retardation; ritualistic and compulsive behaviour. Additionally, these abnormalities should be manifest before 30 months of age.

Prevalence

Epidemiological studies in childhood have found prevalence rates of 2/10 000 increasing to 20/10 000 when individuals with severe mental retardation and some autistic features are included. Boys are three times more affected than girls.

Clinical features

Impaired social relationships Parental recollections of infancy often reveal that, as an infant, the child was slow to smile, unresponsive and passive, with a dislike of physical contact and affection. Contemporary social deficits include the failure to use eye-to-eye gaze and facial expression for social interaction, rarely seeking others for comfort or affection, rarely initiating interaction with others, a lack of empathy (the ability to understand how others feel and think) and of cooperative play. The children are aloof and indifferent to people.

Language abnormalities Language acquisition is delayed and deviant, with many autistic children never developing language (approximately 50%). When present, language abnormalities are many and varied, including immediate and delayed echolalia (repetition of spoken word(s) or phrase(s)), poor comprehension and use of gesture, pronominal reversal (the use of the third person when 'I' is meant) and abnormalities in intonation, rhythm and pitch.

Ritualistic and compulsive behaviour Common abnormalities are rigid and restricted patterns of play, intense attachments to unusual objects such as stones, unusual preoccupations and interests (timetables, bus routes) to the exclusion of other pursuits and marked resistance to any change in the environment or daily routine. Tantrums and explosive outbursts often occur when any change is attempted.

Other features Autistic children often exhibit a variety of stereotypies including rocking, finger twirling, spinning and tiptoe walking. They are often overactive with a short attention span. Seventy per cent of autistic children are in the retarded range of intelligence, with only 5% having an IQ above 100. Occasionally, some have remarkable abilities in isolated areas, for instance computation, music or rote memory. About 20% will develop epilepsy during adolescence, though not usually severe.

Association with other conditions Autistic behaviour occurs in some patients with a diverse group of conditions including fragile X syndrome, rubella, phenylketonuria, tuberous sclerosis, neurolipoidoses and infantile spasms (Lord & Rutter 1994). Rett's syndrome, with its marked autistic features, has been described (Hagberg et al 1983, Kerr & Stephenson 1985).

Aetiology

Most people favour an organic basis for the following reasons: neurological abnormalities are common; the association with epilepsy and various neurological syndromes; the increased rate of perinatal complications; and the higher concordance among monozygotic compared with dizygotic twins (Rutter & Schopler 1988, Lord & Rutter 1994). Application of new investigative techniques such as computerised tomography, magnetic resonance imaging and positron emission tomography are beginning to reveal abnormalities in the frontal lobe region, with distinctive deficits on tests of executive function (Pennington & Ozonoff 1996). The relationship between autism and the fragile X syndrome is also unclear, as the different rates in the various studies may be a reflection of the degree of mental handicap rather than of any aetiological significance. A most interesting psychological perspective on the autistic deficit is provided by the work of Baron-Cohen (1995) and Hobson (1993). They maintain from the results of experiments with autistic children that the primary deficit in autism is a lack of empathy, namely the inability to perceive and interpret emotional cues in social situations.

Treatment

The explanation of the diagnosis is a vital first step in helping parents to accept the presence of handicap, with the consequent lessening of the parental guilt about aetiology. Counselling and advice are likely to be necessary throughout childhood. Lord & Rutter (1994) suggested that treatment aims should have four components: the promotion of normal development; the reduction of rigidity and stereotypies; the removal of maladaptive behaviour; and the alleviation of family stress. Behavioural methods, including operant conditioning and shaping (see behavioural treatment section), are the most likely ways to achieve some success with the first three aims while counselling is important for the fourth. Special schooling, where the child's special social and educational needs are recognised, is very beneficial, sometimes on a residential basis. Drugs do not have an important part in management.

Outcome

Many autistic individuals are unable to live independently, with only 15% looking after and supporting themselves as adults. Many are placed in institutions for the mentally handicapped, though government policy now favours community care. Autistic children with an IQ of at least 70, receiving proper education and coming from middle-class families do better than other groups. In most individuals there is some improvement in social relationships, though many are still handicapped. Parents often find it helpful to join the National Society for Autistic Children.

Other pervasive developmental disorders

Asperger's syndrome / schizoid personality

This condition, originally described by Asperger (1944), shows some similarities to childhood autism in that there is an impairment of social relationships, with a lack of reciprocal social interaction and a restricted, stereotyped repetitive repertoire of interests and activities. However, the children differ diagnostically from those with childhood autism in two important respects: there is no general intellectual retardation; and the language development is normal. Other characteristics include male preponderance and poor motor coordination with marked clumsiness. The condition is now regarded as one of the autistic spectrum disorders (Gillberg 1995), with the impairment in social relationships persisting into adult life.

The term 'schizoid' personality of childhood was coined by Wolff & Chick (1980) to describe a small number of children with unusual but distinctive personality characteristics, similar in some ways to children with Asperger's syndrome. These 'schizoid' children are described as aloof, distant and lacking in empathy. Other features include: obstinate and aggressive outbursts when under pressure to conform, often at school; undue rigidity; sensitivity to criticism; and unusual interests to the exclusion of everything else. More recently, Wolff (1991) has argued from follow-up studies of these children that they form a separate diagnostic category, the schizoid personality of childhood, similar to but distinct from childhood autism and Asperger's syndrome. As adults, Wolff (1991) found that they showed features of the schizotypal disorder.

Rett's syndrome

Rett (1966) described 22 mentally handicapped children, all girls who had a history of regression in development and displayed strikingly repetitive movements of the hands. He thought that the children were autistic with progressive spasticity, and proposed that diffuse cerebral atrophy was the underlying cause. More recent reports (Hagberg et al 1983, Kerr & Stephenson 1985) have indicated this syndrome is more common than previously believed, with a prevalence rate of 1/30 000 (1/15 000 girls).

Clinical features The condition, which has only been described in girls, shows a characteristic clinical picture: a period of normal development up to around 18 months followed by a rapid decline in developmental progress and the rapid deterioration of higher brain functions. Within the following 18 months there is evidence of severe dementia, loss of purposeful use of the hands, jerky ataxia and acquired microcephaly. After this rapid decline, the condition may stabilise, with no further progression for some time. Subsequently, more neurological abnormalities appear, including spastic paraplegia and epilepsy.

Aetiology Rett originally believed that high levels of ammonia were responsible for the condition, though subsequent studies have not confirmed this observation. The most commonly proposed explanation is that it is due to a dominant mutation on one X chromosome, and that the condition is non-viable in the male.

Prognosis The majority of children are left profoundly retarded with severe neurological impairments. Many succumb to intermittent infections or to the underlying neuropathological disorder.

Disintegrative disorder

Clinical features (Corbett et al 1977, Lord & Rutter 1994) This term refers to a group of conditions characterised by normal development until around 4 years of age, followed by profound regression and behavioural disintegration, loss of language and other skills, impairment of social relationships and the development of stereotypies. It can follow on from a minor illness or from more definite neurological disease such as measles encephalitis. The prognosis is poor owing to the underlying degenerative pathology in many cases. Most individuals are left with severe mental retardation.

OTHER RELATED CONDITIONS

Many children with mental retardation show some

autistic features. In clinical practice it is often difficult to know whether they fulfil the criteria for pervasive developmental disorder in addition to that for intellectual retardation. It is clear that there is a wide diversity in the severity of these 'autistic features', so that it is often arbitrary whether the label childhood autism is applied to these children. Many of them also show features of hyperactivity and aggression. For these reasons, ICD-10 has made two additional categories: overactive disorder associated with mental retardation and stereotyped movements; and pervasive developmental disorder unspecified.

Schizophrenia (see Chs 13 and 24)

This is a rare disease during childhood. Even during adolescence, it has a frequency of less than 3/10 000. Symptomatology consists of delusions (fixed, false beliefs), hallucinations (perceptual experience in the absence of relevant sensory stimulus), distortions of thinking (thought insertion and withdrawal) and of movement, most commonly catatonia. It can present with acutely disturbed behaviour or insidiously with gradual withdrawal and failing schoolwork. There is good evidence of a genetic component, with approximately 10% of relatives having the disease. Diagnostically it can often be difficult to distinguish from a major mood disturbance such as manic–depressive psychosis or a drug-induced episode.

Treatment

Treatment must be comprehensive, including drug treatment with major tranquillisers, such as chlorpromazine or haloperidol and antiparkinsonian drugs, and individual and family therapy, as well as help with education. Favourable prognostic factors include high intelligence, acute onset, precipitating factors and normal premorbid personality.

Delirium-like conditions

Delirium-like conditions, with impairment of consciousness, hallucinations and illusions, are common among children with acute infections. Rarely, a non-infective agent, for instance acute intermittent porphyria, is responsible.

EMOTIONAL DISORDERS

The primary abnormality is a subjective sense of distress due to anxiety, which can be expressed overtly as in anxiety disorders or covertly as in somatisation or conversion disorders. This group of disorders is similar in many respects to neurotic disorders in adults. They are further divided into the following categories: anxiety and phobic states; obsessional disorders; conversion disorders, dissociative states and somatisation disorders; and reaction to severe stress and adjustment disorders. Many children often show a mixed pattern of symptoms, so that a clear-cut distinction into a single category is not possible. The IOW study (Rutter et al 1970a) found a prevalence rate of 2.5% with a female preponderance. Prognosis is generally favourable as many problems arise from an acute stress, so that the problems should resolve once the stressful effects lessen.

Anxiety states

Clinical features

This is the most common type of emotional disorder. Anxiety has physical and psychological components, with the former referring to palpitations and dry mouth and the latter to the subjective sense of fear and apprehension. Somatic symptoms, particularly abdominal pain, are common. Again, many symptoms may represent the persistence and exaggeration of normal developmental fears, ranging in severity from an acute panic attack to a chronic anxiety state over several months. Predisposing factors include temperamental characteristics, overinvolved and overconcerned parents and the 'special child syndrome'. This last refers to children who are treated differently by their parents. This may arise in several circumstances, for instance if the child is much wanted, or there has been previous ill-health during pregnancy or infancy, resulting in 'anxious' attachment between the child and parents. In turn, 'anxious' attachment may lead to the parents inadvertently reinforcing normal fears and anxieties.

Treatment

Several approaches, including individual, behavioural and family therapy, are used, often in combination, depending upon the assessment and formulation. Anxiolytic drugs such as diazepam do not have a major role except in certain situations and for a specified period.

Phobic states

Clinical features

Phobias are common and normal among children. For instance, toddlers are fearful of strangers, whereas adolescents are anxious about their appearance or weight. Pathological fears often arise from ordinary fears that are exacerbated by parental and/or social reinforcement. A phobia is defined as a special form of fear for specific objects or situations, for instance dogs or heights. Its characteristics are that it is out of proportion to the situation, is irrational, is beyond voluntary control and leads to avoidance of the feared situation. This avoidance behaviour is the main reason the fear is maladaptive as it leads to increasing restriction and limitation of the child's activities.

Treatment

A behavioural approach using graded exposure to the feared situation is the most commonly used treatment. The rationale of this approach is that continued exposure to the feared stimulus reduces the anxiety associated with the stimulus, thereby decreasing avoidance behaviour. The success of this method often depends on the ability of the therapist to devise a treatment programme that combines gradual exposure without inducing too much anxiety. Occasionally, anxiolytic drugs are used in conjunction with this behavioural approach.

School refusal

This term, also known as school phobia, refers to the child's irrational fear about school attendance. It is also known as the masquerade syndrome as it can present in a variety of disguises, including abdominal pain, headaches and viral infection. The child is reluctant to leave home in the morning to attend school, in contrast to the truant who leaves home but does not arrive at school. It occurs most commonly at the commencement of schooling, change of school, or the beginning of secondary school.

Most cases can be understood in terms of the following three mechanisms, often in combination: first, separation anxiety, whereby the child and/or the parent are fearful of separation, of which school is an example; second, specific phobia about some aspect associated with school attendance, such as travelling to school, mixing with other children, or some part of the school routine, for instance certain subjects, gym, or assembly; third, an indication of a more general psychiatric disturbance such as depression or low self-esteem. The latter is more frequent among adolescents. Typically, most school refusers have good academic attainments, are conformist at school, but oppositional at home. School refusal can present acutely or insidiously, often becoming a chronic problem in adolescence.

Treatment

The initial essential step is to recognise the condition itself, namely to avoid unnecessary and extensive investigations for minor somatic symptoms or to advise prolonged convalescence following minor illness. For the acute case, early return to school with firm support for the parents and liaison with the school is the most successful approach. For the more intractable cases, extensive work with the child and parents, along with a graded return to school, is advisable. A specific behavioural programme for the phobic elements may be necessary, as well as the use of anxiolytic drugs in some instances. The chronic problem often requires a concerted approach, sometimes involving a period of assessment and treatment at a child psychiatric inpatient unit. Many clinicians also use family therapy to tackle the major relationship problems that exist in many cases.

Outcome

Two-thirds usually return to school regularly, while the remainder, usually adolescents from disturbed families, only achieve erratic attendance at school at best. Follow-up studies into adult life have found that approximately one-third continue with neurotic symptoms and social impairment.

Obsessive–compulsive disorders (Fig. 23.1)

Definition

An obsession is a recurrent, intrusive thought that the individual recognises is irrational but cannot ignore. A compulsion or ritual is the behaviour(s) accompanying these ideas, the aim of which is to reduce the associated anxiety.

Clinical features

Most children display obsessional symptoms to a minor degree at some time, for instance avoiding cracks on paving stones or walking under ladders. They have no significance. It is when the behaviour interferes with ordinary activities that it amounts to an illness. Common obsessional rituals are hand washing and dressing. Obsessional thoughts often have a foreboding quality, for instance that 'something could happen' to a parent or sibling, that he might die, or get run over. The rituals are maintained, though maladaptive, because they produce temporary reduction in anxiety. Commonly, the child involves other members of the family in the performance of rituals, so that the child assumes a controlling role within the family. The illness

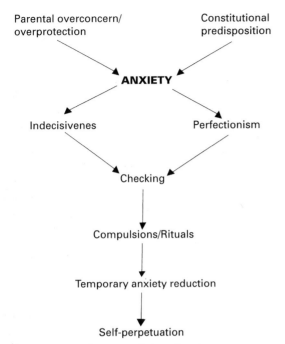

Fig. 23. 1 Development of obsessional symptoms.

is rare (community prevalence 0.3%) but more common among older children and adolescents, with an acute or gradual onset. In addition to anxiety symptoms, many children exhibit depressive features.

Treatment

Behavioural methods, particularly response prevention, are successful in eliminating the obsessive–compulsive behaviour. Response prevention consists of training the child to become aware of the cues that trigger the symptom and then using distraction techniques to make the performance of the ritual impossible. Medication, usually clomipramine, is helpful sometimes for anxiety and depressive symptoms. Involvement of other members of the family, whether specifically in family therapy or to assist the child in the elimination of rituals, is necessary. Some cases require inpatient admission.

Outcome

Two-thirds do well, with the remainder continuing to have problems, usually in a fluctuating fashion.

Conversion disorders and dissociative states

Clinical features

These are rare in childhood. Conversion disorder refers to the development of physical symptoms, usually of the special senses or limbs, without any pathological basis in the presence of identifiable stress and/or affective disturbance. The emotional conflict is said to be 'converted' into physical symptoms which are less threatening to the individual than the underlying psychological conflict. A dissociative state is the restriction or limitation of consciousness due to psychological causes; examples include amnesia and fugue. It is, however, extremely dangerous to diagnose the condition solely by the exclusion of organic disease as follow-up studies have found that a minority subsequently develop definite organic illness. There should always be positive psychological reasons to explain the development of the symptoms. Common reasons include major life events or stresses for the child, a similar illness among other family members/peers, or an underlying depressive disorder.

Minor degrees of these disorders are extremely common and frequently occur as a transitory phenomenon during the course of many illnesses. A more general term, 'abnormal illness behaviour', has been coined to describe the situation when the individual persists with and exaggerates symptoms following on from an illness, akin to the physician's phrase 'functional overlay'.

Treatment

Successful treatment depends upon the recognition that the symptoms are 'real' for the child: psychic pain is as distressing as physical pain. Anger and confrontation are unhelpful. A firm sympathetic approach with little attention to the symptom per se, as well as avoiding rewarding the symptom, is probably best. Allow the child to give up his symptoms with good grace, often providing the child with some face-saving reason for improvement. Identify and treat any affective disturbance. The outcome is good for the individual episode, though other psychological problems may persist.

Somatoform disorders (Lask & Fosson 1989)

Clinical features and management

Many children complain of somatic symptoms which do not have a pathological basis. Common symptoms are abdominal pain, headaches and limb pains, with community prevalence rates of approximately 10% (Faull & Nicol 1986). This condition is usually managed by general practitioners, though it sometimes results in a referral for a specialist opinion. Management involves the minimum necessary investigation to exclude any pathology, the identification of any stressful circumstances and a sensitive explanation of the basis for the symptoms. The prevention of restrictions and the active encouragement of normal activities are essential.

When somatic symptoms are persistent, chronic and involve several systems of the body, ICD and DSM use the term somatisation disorder. While it is doubtful whether this disorder occurs in childhood, there is no doubt that persistent unexplained physical complaints are a common reason for children being taken to see the doctor. In many cases, there is clear evidence of underlying anxiety or recent stressful events.

Reaction to severe stress and adjustment disorders

This group of disorders arises in response to an exceptionally stressful event or a significantly adverse life change. The clinical features of the different syndromes vary considerably, with a preponderance of affective symptoms in most cases.

Adjustment disorder

Definition   This is a maladaptive response occurring within 3 months of an identifiable psychosocial stressor. The maladaptive response must be of sufficient severity to impair daily activities such as schooling, hamper social relationships and be greater than expected given the nature of the stressor. Finally, the reaction must not last longer than 6 months.

Clinical features   By definition, the symptoms vary, with ICD and DSM recognising more than six categories. Clinical practice shows that anxiety and depressive symptoms, often combined, are the most frequent categories. Common stressors include parental divorce, unemployment, family illness or family move.

Predisposing factors   Age has different effects depending on the type of stressor. For instance, separation is more upsetting for the younger child than for the adolescent, whereas a loss or change of heterosexual relationship is far more important for an adolescent than for the younger child. Boys are also more vulnerable to the adverse effects of stress than girls. Temperamental characteristics, such as 'difficult' or 'slow to warm up' style, probably influence susceptibility as well. Again, the child's previous experience and repertoire of coping skills affect the response to the current stressor. For instance, if the child has successfully coped with adversity in the past, his resilience and ability to withstand the present situation are enhanced. Finally, the family, particularly the parents, can magnify or minimise the impact of a stressor, depending on their resourcefulness and coping style.

Outcome   By definition, the disorder can only last for 6 months, after which time the diagnostic category must change. The more important clinical consideration is not the change in diagnostic category, but the adverse effect that chronic or repeated stresses can have on the child's long-term adjustment.

Post-traumatic stress disorder (PTSD) (Yule 1991)

The 'epidemic' of disasters which have involved British children over the past 10 years (the capsize of the *Herald of Free Enterprise*, the sinking of the cruise ship *Jupiter*, the Pan-Am Lockerbie air crash and the crushing disaster at the Hillsborough football stadium) have made clinicians acutely aware of this syndrome. Clinicians are now familiar with the wide symptomatology often found and have also become involved in treatment programmes to reduce the distress in the immediate aftermath and also in the longer term.

Definition   This disorder arises following exposure to a stressful event of an exceptionally threatening or catastrophic nature that would cause pervasive distress in almost anyone. The events include accidents or disasters, as well as more personal trauma such as witnessing murder, rape or torture. In clinical practice, children who have been sexually abused commonly present with symptoms falling within the diagnostic category of PTSD.

Clinical features   These include 'flash backs' (the repeated re-enactment of the event with intrusive memories, dreams or nightmares); a sense of detachment, 'numbness' and emotional blunting; irritability, poor concentration and memory problems. Following disasters, many survivors often experience an increased awareness of danger, a foreshortened view of the future ('only plan for today'), a feeling of 'survivor' guilt (self-reproach about own survival, while companions died) and acute panic reactions.

Yule (1991) indicates that between 30 and 50% of children show significant psychological morbidity after disasters, with symptoms persisting for several months (Yule et al 1990).

Individual vulnerability factors   Important modifying factors are probably age, previous experiences, current life situation and availability of help. Though cognitive immaturity may protect the child from appreciating the implications of the disaster, it may also be disadvantageous as the child may not be given the opportunity to talk about the event. The child's previous experience of stressful events and their outcome, successful or otherwise, are likely to influence the response to the disaster. Similarly, coexisting adverse circumstances such as family disharmony or school problems reduce the child's capacity to cope with the new situation.

Management Though most research is anecdotal rather than systematic, the available evidence (Yule 1991) suggests that postdisaster 'debriefing' sessions on an individual or group basis are helpful. Specific counselling sessions to help the child deal with phobic, anxiety or depressive symptoms are frequently necessary as well. Cognitive/behavioural approaches are particularly suitable for this pattern of symptoms.

MOOD DISORDERS

Depression (Goodyer 1995) (see Chs. 14 and 24)

There is an important distinction between sadness and unhappiness on the one hand and a depressive disorder on the other. Transitory mood swings are a normal phenomenon affecting many children, particularly adolescents. Moreover, sadness and unhappiness are features found in several other psychiatric disorders including chronic anxiety and conduct disorder. By contrast, depressive disorder is characterised by a sustained lowered mood, anhedonia (inability to derive pleasure from life), low self-esteem, suicidal ideas and disturbances of eating and sleeping.

Until recently, it was thought that this syndrome did not occur in prepubertal children, except perhaps following certain illnesses such as infectious mononucleosis. However, the development of reliable interview schedules and questionnaires (Rutter 1988) has changed this view, so that it is recognised that depressive illness does occur, though uncommonly (less than 1%). Bipolar or manic depressive illness is even more infrequent.

Assessment

A comprehensive assessment involving individual and family interview(s) is essential, along with information from the school. The interview(s) with the child has particular importance as it can involve the disclosure of suicidal ideas and also provide the opportunity for the child to unburden himself, as well as establishing a trusting relationship with the therapist. The assessment of suicidal risk is important (see Ch. 26). Detailed enquiry should be made about current stresses, particularly life events involving threat and loss of self-esteem, and also about recent illnesses, particularly viral infections.

Treatment

Tricyclic antidepressants (imipramine or amitriptyline) are successful for some children with definite depressive disorder, though the problems with side-effects are common and occasionally disabling. The newer classes of antidepressants such as fluoxetine and paroxetine are now being used with some success, but controlled trials have not been carried out so far. Individual and family therapy are also used in most cases. Attempts should be made wherever possible to ameliorate any contributory stressful factors. Recently, some clinicians have also attempted to use cognitive behavioural approaches in older children and adolescents.

Outcome

Approximately two-thirds will respond to treatment, with the remainder continuing either to show symptoms or to be vulnerable to further episodes.

CONDUCT DISORDER

Clinical features

This is usually defined as persistent antisocial or socially disapproved of behaviour that often involves damage to property and is unresponsive to normal sanctions. The IOW study (Rutter et al 1970a) found a prevalence rate of 4% when the mixed disorder category was included as well, with a marked male predominance (at least 3:1). There is no absolute criterion for deviance as societal and cultural values determine the seriousness or importance that is attached to antisocial behaviour. Common symptoms include temper tantrums, oppositional behaviour, overactivity, irritability, aggression, stealing, lying, truancy, bullying and wandering away from home/school. Delinquency (a legal term referring to a child or young person committing an offence against the law) is a frequent feature among older children and adolescents. Stealing, vandalism, arson and firesetting are common forms of delinquency (male:female 10:1).

Traditionally, a distinction has been made between socialised and unsocialised behaviour. The former describes behaviour that is in accord with peer group values but contrary to those of society, for instance antisocial gang behaviour such as stealing and vandalism. Unsocialised antisocial behaviour implies more disturbed behaviour as it is often carried out by the individual against a background of parental rejection or neglect and poor peer relationships. Learning difficulties, especially specific reading retardation, occur more commonly among children with conduct disorders. This is a further reason why school is unpopular and a source of discouragement for these children. Additionally, many children with conduct disorder have affective symptoms such as anxiety or unhappiness, as well as low self-esteem and poor peer relationships. When these symptoms are prominent, it is often appropriate to classify the disorder as mixed, implying both emotional and behavioural symptomatology.

Aetiology

Four factors, the family, the peer group, the neighbourhood and constitutional, make some contribution in most cases, but the family is usually the most important. Families of children with conduct disorder are characterised by a lack of affection and rejection, marital disharmony, inconsistent and ineffective discipline, and parental violence and aggression. The families are often of large size, which aggravates the problems of supervision and care. Constitutional factors present in some cases include low intelligence and learning difficulties, along with adverse temperamental features such as overactivity and impulsiveness. Oppositional peer group values are an important feature in older children and adolescents. Many children with conduct disorder live in areas of urban deprivation with poor schooling. The intractable and chronic nature of these problems is a major reason for the continuation of conduct disorder into adolescence and adult life.

Treatment

Help for the family, by counselling for the parents or by family therapy, is often used. Again, a behavioural approach for some symptoms, such as aggression, is often successful. Educational support through remedial teaching or the provision of special education can be important in some cases. For many families however, the role of psychiatric services is limited to practical support for rehousing in order to alleviate the social disadvantage which is often an important contributory factor.

Prognosis

Two-thirds continue to show problems into adult life. Bad prognostic features are many and varied symptoms, problems at home and in the community and antiauthority and aggressive attitudes.

DISORDERS OF ELIMINATION

Enuresis

This term refers to the involuntary passage of urine in the absence of physical abnormality after the age of 5 years. It may be nocturnal and/or diurnal. Bed wetting continuously, though not usually every night, since birth is termed primary enuresis, whereas when there has been a 6 month period of dry beds at some stage, the recurrence of the bed wetting is termed secondary or onset enuresis. Diurnal enuresis is much less common than nocturnal, but more common among girls and among children who are psychiatrically disturbed. Depending upon definition, approximately 10% of 5-year-olds, 5% of 10-year-olds and 1% of 15-year-olds will have nocturnal enuresis. The majority of children with nocturnal enuresis are not psychiatrically ill, though a substantial minority, approximately 25%, have signs of psychiatric disturbance.

Aetiology

A combination of individual factors such as positive family history (approximately 70%), developmental delay, psychiatric disturbance and small bladder capacity, along with environmental factors such as recent stressful life events, large family size and social disadvantage, are present in most cases.

Treatment

It is important to exclude any physical basis for the enuresis by history, examination and, if necessary, investigation of the renal tract. Assuming no physical pathology, the most important initial step is to minimise the handicap, namely to point out to the parents the very favourable natural outcome of the condition, and to relabel the child's enuresis as immaturity rather than laziness or wilfulness. A star chart, which ensures the accurate recording of the enuresis as well as giving positive reinforcement for dry nights, provides an accurate baseline, and is also a successful treatment in its own right. An enuretic alarm is successful with older cooperative children. The success of this approach is probably because the child becomes more aware of the sensation of a full bladder, along with the encouragement from parents for dry nights. The newer models of the buzzer are extremely compact and do not require a pad placed between the sheets, thereby increasing patient compliance considerably. It is useful to combine a buzzer with a star chart. Tricyclic antidepressants such as imipramine, 25–50 mg nocte, are very effective at stopping enuresis, though their major limitation is that the enuresis returns when they are stopped. Many paediatricians, however, believe it is wrong to prescribe such drugs, as they may be lethal when taken in an overdose, either accidentally or intentionally.

Soiling and encopresis

Most children are clean and continent of faeces by their fourth birthday. Encopresis is the inappropriate passage of formed faeces, usually on to underwear, in the absence of physical pathology after 4 years of age. Soiling, the passage of semisolid faeces, is often used synonymously with encopresis. Symptoms vary widely in severity, ranging from slight staining of underwear to encopresis together with the smearing of faeces, usually on to walls. It is uncommon, with a community prevalence among 8-year-olds of 1.8% for boys and of 0.7% for girls. Psychiatric disturbance is common among children with encopresis. Enuresis may also be present.

Clinical features

Figure 23.2 shows a convenient way to classify encopresis, with a broad distinction into children who retain faeces with eventual overflow incontinence and those who deposit faeces inappropriately on a regular basis. Some children have never achieved continence, a situation called continuous or primary encopresis, while others have had periods of cleanliness followed by relapse, the so-called discontinuous or secondary encopresis. Figure 23.2 also lists the common different patterns of interaction found among encopretic children and their parents. For instance, children with retentive encopresis have often been subjected to coercive and obsession-

al toilet training practices, so that the encopresis is seen as a reaction, often of anger and aggression, towards this practice. Similarly, many children with continuous non-retentive encopresis come from disorganised chaotic families where regular training and toileting are not the norm. Again, encopresis can arise in some children as a response to a stressful situation. Finally, encopresis can reflect a poor parent–child relationship, often of long standing and usually associated with other aspects of psychiatric disturbance. The clinical picture is often, however, not as clear-cut, with the different elements each making some contribution. There may be a previous history of constipation and occasionally anal fissure.

Treatment

A physical aetiology such as Hirschsprung's disease must be excluded before commencement of psychological treatment. The assessment must include an account of previous treatments and, most importantly, the current attitude of the parents and the child to the problem. Treatment has two aims: the promotion of a normal bowel habit; and the improvement of the parent–child relationship. Initially, bowel washout and/or microenemas may be necessary to clear out the bowel. Judicious use of bowel smooth muscle stimulants (Senokot), stool softeners (Dioctyl) and bulk agents (lactulose) is helpful for the child with retention. Again, suppositories are often useful from time to time. This medical approach should also be combined with an educational package for the parents and child, emphasising the importance of dietary fibre. The psychological component includes behavioural (star chart), individual psychotherapy to gain the trust and cooperation of the child and parental counselling or family therapy to modify critical attitudes and hostile interactions between the child and his parents.

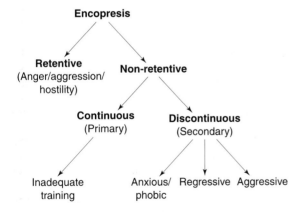

Three patterns are common:
- Child with primary encopresis
- Child with retentive encopresis
- Child with secondary encopresis

Fig. 23. 2 Types of encopresis and their psychopathology. Three patterns are common: the child with primary encopresis; the child with retentive encopresis; and the child with secondary encopresis.

Prognosis

It usually resolves by adolescence, though other problems may persist. Occasional case reports of persistence into adult life have been published (Fraser & Taylor 1986).

OVERACTIVITY AND HYPERACTIVITY
(Taylor 1994, Gillberg 1995)

Clinical features

Terms such as overactivity or hyperactivity, hyperkinetic disorder and attention deficit disorder are used interchangeably, so that it is important to define the usage in each instance.

In the UK, hyperkinetic disorder is restricted to the small number of children (less than 1%) who show severe, pervasive (present in all situations) hyperactivity, and are impulsive and distractible with a short attention span. They are often aggressive, with marked mood swings. Other associated features are male predominance (at least 3:1), developmental delay with learning difficulties and evidence on examination or investigation of neurological impairment. The hyperactivity is at its peak between the ages of 3 and 8 years.

Attention deficit disorder is a term mainly used in North America where it refers to a large group of children (approximately 5–10% of the population) whose principal abnormalities are a short attention span and distractibility. They are frequently hyperactive, though only in some situations, aggressive and have learning difficulties.

Extensive studies (reviewed by Taylor 1994) indicate that it is a difference in terminology rather than a true difference in prevalence that explains the difference between the UK and the USA. Again, many disturbed children have overactive or hyperactive behaviour as part of the clinical picture, but only in certain situations. British psychiatrists would probably classify these children within the conduct disorder category, whereas North American clinicians would include them as attention deficit disorder.

Overactivity or hyperactivity can therefore be most usefully conceptualised in several different ways: a symptom in the uncommon pervasive hyperkinetic syndrome; a feature of many children with conduct disorder; a reflection of developmental delay or immaturity on its own or in association with general intellectual retardation; one extreme of the normal temperamental variation; an uncommon response to high anxiety or tension; a symptom in childhood autism; and rarely as a reaction to some drugs, for example barbiturates or benzodiazepines.

Treatment

Medication, usually with stimulant drugs such as methylphenidate (up to 0.3 mg/kg/day) can be very valuable for children with the hyperkinetic syndrome, but it should be restricted to this group of children and not prescribed for every child with overactivity. Most importantly, treatment should be combined with behavioural approaches. Side-effects of methylphenidate include loss of appetite, insomnia, reduced growth rate and labile moods. Drug 'holidays', whereby the drug is stopped for periods of time, are very useful, not only to minimise side-effects but also to show whether medica-

tion is still necessary. Other drugs such as dexamphetamine, pemoline and imipramine are useful alternatives when methylphenidate is not effective or side-effects are too severe.

Behavioural techniques, parental counselling and the alteration and manipulation of the child's environment, particularly at school, to reduce and minimise distraction are the main components of treatment programmes in most cases. An alternative approach adopted by some clinicians has been the use of exclusion diets, on the basis that the child is allergic to certain substances, commonly tartrazine. Evidence for the efficacy of these exclusion diets other than as a placebo response is unconvincing, though Egger et al (1992), using a sophisticated methodological design, showed that children with severe hyperactivity and mental retardation did respond. It is, however, unclear whether these results would apply to children of normal intelligence with less severe problems who make up the majority of overactive children.

Outcome

Hyperactivity and attention deficits lessen considerably by adolescence, though other major problems such as learning difficulties and behaviour problems persist. A substantial minority continue to have problems in adult life, mainly of an antisocial nature. There is also increasing evidence for the efficacy of methylphenidate in adults in whom the diagnosis of attention deficit disorder was missed in childhood or who have continued on treatment from childhood (Biederman et al 1993, Spencer et al 1995).

MISCELLANEOUS DISORDERS

Developmental disorders

Language disorders (Campbell & McIntosh 1997)

Children with language disorders are more vulnerable to disturbance, mainly because of the associated anxiety and embarrassment caused by the disorder. Specific language delay (5–6/1000) is twice as common in boys than girls, with a strong association with large family size and lower social class. Richman et al (1982) found that approximately 25% of 3-year-olds with specific language delay had behavioural problems.

Stuttering, an abnormality of speech rhythm consisting of hesitations and repetitions at the beginning of syllables and words, is a normal, though transitory phenomenon occurring at around 3–4 years of age. When it persists (approximately 3% of the general population), often due to inadvertent parental attention, it leads to anxiety and low self-esteem.

Elective mutism   This is not strictly a language disorder, as the main problem is the child's refusal to talk in certain situations, most commonly at school, rather than an inability to speak. Mild forms of the disorder are common but transitory, usually at the commencement of schooling, while the severe form occurs in about 1 in 1000. Other features include previous history of speech delay, excessively shy but stubborn temperament and parental overprotectiveness.

A combination of behavioural and family therapy techniques to promote communication and the use of speech is most commonly used, though some cases require inpatient assessment. Prognosis is good for approximately 50%, with failure to improve by the age of 10 years a poor prognostic sign.

Reading difficulties

Though mainly of educational concern, the child psychiatrist may get involved because of the associated behavioural or emotional problems. The two main categories are found: general reading backwardness, when the retardation is a reflection of general intellectual delay; and specific reading retardation, when the attainment in reading is significantly behind that expected on the basis of age and intelligence. The problem is usually 'significant' when the delay is at least 2 years. Dyslexia is a concept similar to that of specific reading retardation, implying a neuropsychological substrate for the specific reading difficulties. The use of this term is contentious, so that the more bland expression, specific reading retardation, is preferred by many clinical psychologists.

The aetiology is multifactorial, involving genetic, social, perceptual and language deficits. A noteworthy feature is the strong association between specific reading retardation and conduct disorder. The behaviour problem most likely arises secondarily to the frustration and disillusionment associated with the reading difficulty. Treatment involves the detailed assessment of the precise nature of the problem by a psychologist, followed by an individualised remedial programme carried out by a specialised teacher in collaboration with the psychologist. Help with the behavioural problem is also necessary in order to prevent more serious problems arising during adolescence.

Tic disorders

Tics are rapid, involuntary, repetitive muscular movements, usually involving the face and neck, for instance blinks, grimaces or throat clearing. Simple tics occur as a transitory phenomenon in about 10% of the popula-

tion, with boys outnumbering girls by 3:1 and with a mean age of onset around 7 years. They range in severity from simple tics involving head and neck through to complex tics extending to the limbs and trunk, and finally to the Gilles de la Tourette syndrome. The latter comprises complex tics accompanied by coprolalia (uttering obscene words and phrases) and echolalia (the repetition(s) of sounds or words). Like stammering, tics are made worse at times of stress and may be exacerbated by undue parental concern. The differential diagnosis of tics in childhood is principally from chorea, where the movements are less coordinated and predictable, are not stereotypic in form and cannot be suppressed. Other features of tics are positive family history and a previous history of neurodevelopmental delay. Many tics resolve spontaneously, but those that persist can be extremely disabling and difficult to treat.

Treatment   Several approaches are used alone or in combination, depending on the assessment. Medication is effective but should be reserved for severe cases. Haloperidol (0.5–1.5 mg b.d.) is the drug of choice for the Tourette syndrome. If unsuccessful, alternative drugs are pimozide and clonidine. Many children with simple tics respond to explanation and reassurance along with advice for the parents. Individual and/or family therapy may be indicated when anxiety and tension are clearly making important contributions to the problem. Behaviour therapy in the form of relaxation and or massed practice can also be helpful.

Prognosis   Simple tics have a good outcome with complete remission, whereas in the Tourette syndrome the condition fluctuates in a chronic manner, with 50% continuing with symptoms into adult life.

Habit disorders

Finger or thumb sucking and nail biting

These are extremely common and usually of no pathological significance. Excessive finger/thumb sucking can lead to deformity of teeth and fingers. Occasionally, they are signs of a more serious disturbance which itself requires treatment.

Rocking and head banging

Many normal otherwise healthy toddlers indulge in these habits when they are in their cot, causing much anxiety and distress to their parents who are also embarrassed by neighbours' complaints about the noise. Most children spontaneously cease these habits by around the fourth birthday so that reassurance and support for the parents are usually effective.

More serious self-injurious behaviour occurs among

some severely retarded children, some blind children and children with the Lesch–Nyhan syndrome.

Masturbation

This usually attracts attention and concern when it happens excessively. Most infants and toddlers engage in and enjoy touching their genitalia. During middle childhood, this appears less common and/or the child is more discrete. At adolescence, masturbation is probably universal among boys, though less common among girls. Excessive masturbation requires investigation and help. Causes include: local skin irritation, particularly among infants; sexual abuse among older children; and emotional deprivation, when the masturbation represents an attempt by the child to obtain some pleasure from an otherwise unloving environment. Some mentally retarded adolescents cause much embarrassment to their parents by masturbation in public. Clear guidance for the parents about what is acceptable, and what is not (for instance, masturbation in private is allowable), is the best way to help, along with encouragement to parents to enforce these rules.

Sleep disorders (see section on preschool children as well)

Night terrors

The usual pattern is for the child to wake up in a frightened, even terrified state, not to respond when spoken to, nor appear to see objects or people. Instead, he appears to be hallucinating, talking to and looking at people/things not actually present. The child may be difficult to comfort, with the period of disturbed behaviour and altered consciousness lasting up to 15 minutes, occasionally longer. Eventually the behaviour settles, with or without comfort, and the child goes back to sleep, awakening in the morning with no recollection of the episode. The latter point is invaluable in helping to allay parental anxiety about the episodes. Night terrors arise from stage 4 or deep sleep. The peak incidence is between 4 and 7 years, with a continuation of 1–3% in older children. It is also helpful to identify and ameliorate any identifiable stresses that may occasionally contribute to the problem. Lask (1988) described an apparently novel successful behavioural approach relying on waking the child 15 minutes before the expected time of the night terror.

Nightmares

These are frightening or unpleasant dreams, occurring during REM (rapid eye movement) sleep. The child

may or may not wake up but there will be a clear recollection of the dream if he does wake up, and in the morning. There is no period of altered consciousness or inaccessibility as there is with night terrors. Again, daytime anxieties and/or frightening television programmes in the evening may be contributory factors.

Sleep walking (somnambulism)

The child, usually aged between 8 and 14 years, calmly arises from his bed with a blank facial expression, does not respond to attempts at communication and can only be awakened with difficulty. The child is in a state of altered consciousness at the deep level of sleep (stages 3 or 4). Any contributory anxiety should be treated, as well as giving the parents some advice about the safety and protection of the child during these episodes.

Eating disorders (see also preschool section and Ch. 18)

Obesity

This is a common problem affecting around 10% of children, depending upon definition. Psychological problems may be responsible for the onset of the obesity and/or may arise secondarily to the obesity. The role of the psychiatrist or psychologist is to identify and treat these problems and, more importantly, to enlist the cooperation of the child and family in adherence to a dietary regimen. Other treatment components include a behavioural programme to modify eating patterns, for instance making the child more aware of the cues associated with excessive eating. A major problem with treatment programmes is that they may not modify the eating habits sufficiently to ensure that the weight loss is maintained when the programme is finished.

Anorexia nervosa

This condition, defined as a morbid fear of being fat accompanied by behaviour designed to produce weight loss, does occur in prepubertal children, girls and boys, though much less frequently than among adolescents. Again bulimia, defined as periodic bouts of 'binge eating' or the consumption of high calorific food over a brief period, often followed by self-induced vomiting, rarely occurs in children. The main features of these conditions are discussed in Chapter 18.

PSYCHOLOGICAL EFFECTS OF ILLNESS AND HANDICAP

Approximately 15% of children have some form of

chronic illness or handicap. The IOW study (Rutter et al 1970b) showed clearly that this group of children were much more at risk for disturbance, namely a rate of 33% among children with chronic illness affecting the central nervous system and of 12% among children with chronic illness not affecting the central nervous system, compared with 7% among the general population. The IOW study also showed that children with chronic illness or handicap had the same range of disorders as other disturbed children, thereby implying that the mechanisms involved with this increased morbidity are probably indirect and non-specific rather than direct and specific to each illness or handicap.

Illness or handicap imposes psychological stress on the child and family not only at the time of diagnosis (see later) but also in the long term. These effects are discussed with regard to the child himself and to other family members, though the two effects interact with each other.

Effects on the child

Three aspects are important: the acquisition of skills and outside interests; the development of self-concept; and the development of adaptive coping behaviour. Many illnesses or handicaps inevitably limit and restrict the child's ability or opportunity to acquire everyday skills and to develop interests and hobbies. For example, the child with cerebral palsy by definition is motor handicapped. Other examples are the dietary restrictions of diabetes, the exercise limitations of asthma and the avoidance by children with epilepsy of some activities such as cycling or swimming. Additionally, educational problems are common among this group of children for a variety of reasons, including increased absence from school, specific learning difficulties, especially among children with epilepsy, and low expectations of parents and teachers.

Illness and handicap can adversely affect the child's self-concept in several ways through the effects on the child's body image, his self-esteem and his ideas about the causation of the disability. Many children have a distorted view of their body believing the handicap to be very prominent or disfiguring. These ideas can often be reinforced by comments from parents and peers. Self-esteem can also be impaired due to a faulty cognitive assessment of the situation and to a pessimistic and despondent response to that evaluation. This leads the child to have low self-esteem with a gloomy view about his illness and about his prospects for the future. This is particularly likely and also potentially very disabling among older children and adolescents. The other factor influencing the child's self-concept is his explanation for the cause of his disability. Young children below the

age of 6 years often regard their disability as a punishment for some misdemeanour, while during middle childhood the child commonly thinks he has 'caught' the illness from someone or something. It is only from around 10 years onward that adult-like ideas of causation begin to appear.

Successful adaptation to a disability depends upon the acquisition of a range of coping behaviours and defence mechanisms in order to reduce the anxiety to an acceptable level. Effective coping strategies include rationing the amount of stress into manageable amounts, obtaining information from several sources, rehearsing the possible outcomes of treatment and assessing the situation from several viewpoints. Parents, nursing staff and paediatricians have an important role in promoting this repertoire of skills among children with disability. Additionally, defence mechanisms such as denial, rationalisation and displacement can be helpful for the child during the initial stages of adjustment to the illness or disability.

Effects on the parents

The parents can respond in various ways in the short term (see later) and also in the long term. Most parents eventually achieve some degree of adaptation, though for a minority maladaptive behaviour patterns emerge and are prominent. The common reaction is overprotection, whereby the parent(s) is unable to allow the child to experience the normal disappointments and upsets inevitable during childhood, so that the child leads a 'cotton wool' existence. Less frequently, the parent(s) may be rejecting and indifferent to the child because the child's disability is so damaging to the parent's self-esteem or because the disability has exacerbated an already precarious parent–child relationship. Overprotection and rejection are sometimes combined together in the parental reaction to the child's disability.

The parents may also find it difficult to provide appropriate discipline and control as they fear, irrationally, that such control may aggravate the child's illness. For example, parents of children with epilepsy may think that not giving in to the child's demands, thereby increasing the child's frustration, may induce an epileptic fit.

Finally, the stress of coping with the child's illness may exacerbate parental marital disharmony, though in a minority it may paradoxically unite them as they face the adversity together.

Effect on siblings

This can manifest itself in several ways: the oldest sibling may be given excessive responsibility, such as looking after the handicapped sib; the siblings may lose friendships because they are reluctant to bring their friends home in case their handicapped sib is an embarrassment; finally, the sibling's own developmental needs may be neglected, with consequent resentment and frustration.

Breaking bad news to parents

This distressing but inevitable aspect of paediatrics comes in various guises, such as the birth of a child with Down's syndrome or the diagnosis of cystic fibrosis. Unfortunately, most undergraduate and postgraduate training includes little teaching about this important subject. Though the details vary with each case, the following general principles are important:

- Information should be given by the most senior and experienced doctor involved with the child's care.
- Both parents must be seen together if at all possible, as this reduces misinformation and allows the parents to be mutually supportive from the outset.
- Allow adequate time for interview (*not* 10 minutes at the end of a ward round).
- Privacy is essential, not only as a matter of courtesy and dignity but also because it allows parents to express their emotions more easily.
- Begin the interview by asking the parents to tell you what they know about the problems.
- Tell parents frankly and honestly in simple and non-technical language the nature of the problem, explaining the reasons for the investigations and the basis for the diagnosis.
- Encourage the parents to ask questions (by asking them some open-ended questions).
- Emphasise the positive as well as the negative aspects of the diagnosis, for instance the child will have access to physiotherapy and special equipment, will be able to go to school and to have effective control for any pain.
- Facilitate the expression of emotions by the parents, namely respond sympathetically and sensitively to the parents' distress and crying.
- Make a definite offer of a further appointment to talk things over again.
- Many parents find it helpful to continue the discussion with a nurse or social worker after the interview.

Reactions to hospitalisation

Admission to hospital is a common experience during childhood, with approximately 25% admitted by the age of 4 years. For most children this is a short admission for a brief treatable illness, while a minority (approximately 4%) remain in hospital for at least a month. While most parents and their children cope successfully with the admission, some, particularly those with repeated admissions for minor illnesses, show evidence of disturbance, which may in turn have been the reason why the child was admitted in the first place.

Admission to hospital can have adverse effects in the short term as well as in the long term. The contributory factors can be grouped under three headings: the child and family; the nature of the illness; the attitudes and practices of the hospital and its staff. Important child and family factors include age, temperament of the child, previous experience of hospital, previous parent–child relationship and current family circumstances. Children between the ages of 1 and 4 years are particularly stressed by separation from familiar figures. Similarly, children with adverse temperamental characteristics, such as poor adaptability and irregularity of habits, are more vulnerable. If the child had a favourable experience when in hospital previously, this will ease the burden for any subsequent admission. If the parent–child relationship was poor before admission, hospitalisation is likely to exacerbate this problem because of the additional stress. Adverse family circumstances, for instance financial, may also be aggravated by admission.

The nature of the illness, particularly the associated pain and the necessity for painful procedures, influences the child's response. Again, an acute admission is likely to be more stressful than an elective procedure.

The attitudes of the staff and hospital practices can minimise considerably the distress for the child. Helpful and favourable aspects include: good rooming-in facilities; adequate preparation for painful or unpleasant procedures; nursing and medical staff trained to minimise distress and to be available to offer comfort when required. The ward should be organised so that parents and sibs are encouraged to visit, and there should be play leaders and teachers available on the ward. Medical and nursing staff should also have access to social work resources as well as to psychological and psychiatric services. Finally, joint liaison between the medical and psychiatric team and the establishment of a staff support group to enable staff to discuss their own anxieties about working in a stressful environment are likely to be beneficial.

MISCELLANEOUS TOPICS

Stillbirth and neonatal death

Parental responses vary considerably, though most couples are profoundly shocked initially, followed by a bereavement response for the loss of the child. Hospital staff should be sensitive and responsive to the parents' feelings and wishes. The issue of a certificate of still-birth or a death certificate and the funeral arrangements are extremely distressful for the parents. Mourning is facilitated by the parents seeing and holding their dead child, as well as having a photograph to remember the child. The results of investigations, including the post-mortem examination, should be communicated to the parents to allay their anxiety and to advise about future pregnancies.

Sudden infant death syndrome (SIDS)

This is the most common cause of death for infants between 1 month and 1 year. The sudden and unexpected nature of the event produces profound shock, disbelief and numbness, followed by a bereavement response. The mourning may continue for several months. The family doctor and health visitor usually have important roles for the family over the ensuing months. Skilled counselling is essential, as most parents inevitably feel responsible for the child's death and are overcritical of themselves in consequence. The provision of home monitoring facilities requires careful consideration and discussion because false alarms are frequent, thereby increasing parental tension and anxiety.

Care of the dying child

Parents usually undergo two periods of grief response: first at the time of diagnosis (initial phase) and then at the approach of death (terminal phase). These phases have the features of a grief response, namely shock and numbness, denial, development of somatic symptoms and/or affective features such as anger, anxiety or depression, followed by some degree of acceptance. Most concern is often expressed about what to tell the child. This is obviously influenced by the child's age and intelligence. Generally speaking, current hospital practice is to facilitate discussion with the child about his illness and its implications. Parental wishes should, however, be respected, while indicating to the parents the advantages of a more open attitude. Consequently, there are no absolute rules but rather that a sensitive and flexible approach is most likely to be best.

TREATMENT METHODS

Several factors are usually responsible for the development of disturbance, so that it is unlikely that one treatment method will resolve the problem completely. All treatment approaches also rely upon common elements that are not only necessary but also essential for a successful outcome. These elements include active cooperation between the therapist, child and family, agreement with them on the goals of treatment, and a mutual trust to enable these goals to be achieved. Again, the relative efficacy of different treatments is not clearly established, so that the choice of treatment is often a reflection of the therapists' training and experience rather than an absolute indication in any particular instance. Careful analysis of the following elements is therefore necessary in order to devise an effective treatment programme:

- Individual
  - Physical illness or handicap
  - Intellectual ability
  - Type of symptomatology
- Family
  - Developmental stage (for instance a family with preschool children or one with adolescents)
  - Psychiatric health of parents
  - Marital relationship
  - Parenting qualities
  - Communication pattern within the family
  - Ability to resolve conflict
  - Support network, for instance availability of extended family
- School
  - Scholastic attainments
  - Child and parents' attitude to the authority of the school
  - Peer relationships
- Community
  - Quality of peer relationships and of role models
  - Neighbourhood and community resources.

The formulation of the problem along these four dimensions determines the suitability and likely success of treatment.

The three main types of treatment approach available are *drug treatment*, the *psychotherapies* and *liaison* or *consultation work*. The last refers to the common practice whereby the child psychiatrist or a member of the psychiatric team does not have direct contact with the referred child, but rather helps those involved with the child to understand and modify the child's behaviour. Psychotherapies are treatments that use a variety of psychological techniques to ameliorate disturbance. They include individual therapy, behaviour therapy, family therapy and group therapy as well as counselling and advice for parents.

Drug treatment

This does not have a major treatment role in child psychiatry. Moreover, drugs should only be used to treat specific symptoms and for a defined period of time only. They are most likely to produce symptomatic relief rather than have a curative effect. Table 23.4 summarises the important indications and side-effects of various drugs used in child psychiatry.

Psychotherapies

These are the most common treatment approach in contemporary child psychiatric practice.

Individual psychotherapy (Wolff 1996)

Though there are several theoretical orientations, including psychoanalytic (Freud 1946) and Rogerian (Reisman 1973), the therapist still has the same therapeutic tasks. These are: to develop a trusting, non-judgemental relationship with the child; to enable the child to express his feelings and thoughts; to understand the meaning of the child's symptoms, including his behaviour during the therapeutic session; and finally to provide the child with some understanding and explanation for his behaviour. The indications for individual psychotherapy are not clearly established, though most usually it is for children with a neurotic or reactive disorder rather than for those with a constitutionally based disorder. For younger children the medium for communication is play, such as sand play, or through drawing, while for older children verbal exchange and discussion are possible.

Behavioural psychotherapy

This approach is based upon the application of the findings from experimental psychology, particularly learning theory, to a wide range of problems such as

Table 23.4 Drug treatment in child psychiatry

Drug	Usage	Comment
Anxiolytics	Anxiety/phobic conditions	Short-term adjunct to behaviour treatment
Neuroleptics Phenothiazines (e.g. chlorpromazine)	Schizophrenia/hyperkinetic syndrome	Extrapyramidal side-effects common
Butyrophenones (e.g. haloperidol)	Complex tics/Tourette's syndrome	Extrapyramidal side-effects common
Tricyclics Imipramine/amitriptyline	Enuresis	Effective, but high relapse rate
Clomipramine	Major affective disorder	Most useful with persistent and sustained mood disturbance
Stimulants Methylphenidate	Hyperkinetic syndrome	Effective short-term. Long-term side-effects on growth, sleep and appetite
Fenfluramine	Pervasive developmental disorder	Effectiveness not established. Side-effects include irritability, anorexia and weight loss
Hypnotics (e.g. trimeprazine/promethazine)	Persistent sleep disorder in preschool children	Only short-term
Lithium	Recurrent bipolar affective disorder	Close supervision of blood level and for signs of toxicity
Laxatives (e.g. bulk-forming, Methylcellulose; stimulants, Senna; softener, Dioctyl)	Encopresis with constipation	Facilitates formation and passage of faeces
Central α-agonist (e.g. clonidine)	Unresponsive Tourette's syndrome	Sedation and rebound hypertension

enuresis, encopresis, tantrums and aggression. Its characteristics are as follows:

- Define problem(s) objectively with reference to the antecedents, the behaviour itself and the consequences (the ABC approach)
- Emphasis on current behaviour rather than on past events
- Set up hypotheses to account for the behaviour
- Pretreatment baseline to determine the frequency and severity of the problem
- Devise behavioural programmes on an individual basis to test the hypothesis
- Evaluate outcome of treatment programmes
- Tackle one problem at a time.

As with other psychotherapies, success depends upon the establishment of a trusting relationship with the patient and the close supervision of the treatment programme, together with the involvement of teachers and parents in many cases.

Family therapy (Barker 1992 and Ch. 24)

This is an extremely popular treatment approach now. The rationale underlying family therapy is that the child's disturbed behaviour is symptomatic of the disturbance within the family as a group. There are many different theoretical approaches and techniques (see Barker 1992) but all usually involve interviewing the whole family on each occasion for about 1 hour. Most family work is short term, lasting about 6 months, with approximately monthly sessions. The emphasis is on current behaviour, verbal and non-verbal, observed during the session rather than on past events. The main aim is to improve communication within the family so that dysfunctional patterns of behaviour are replaced by more healthy and adaptive behaviour.

Group therapy (see Ch. 24)

Older children and adolescents often benefit from group therapy when the aim is to improve interpersonal relationships, particularly with the peer group, using a variety of theoretical models, for instance psychodynamic and social skills.

Supportive psychotherapy and counselling

The former is frequently used for children with chronic illness or handicap: the focus may be the child or the parents. It is especially beneficial at the time of diagnosis but also in the longer term when the implications of the disability become more evident. Parental counselling is also used to help the parents understand their child's behaviour problems, the factors that may have led to them and that are responsible for their continuation, along with an emphasis on the parent–child relationship and the improvement of parenting skills. Counselling may therefore help parents to devise and implement a behavioural programme to modify the child's behaviour as well as to promote normal development.

Liaison and consultation psychiatry (Lask 1994)

This is a collaborative approach between the child psychiatry team and the professionals directly involved with the child, for instance hospital staff, teachers and residential care staff, in order to help these professionals to understand the child's disturbed behaviour and their own possible contribution to the problem and to suggest ways to improve the situation. Although the child psychiatrist may see the referred child in the first instance, subsequent contact is usually with the staff rather than with the child. This approach can also include the establishment and supervision of a staff support group whose aim is to look at the attitudes and emotional responses of the staff towards the behaviour shown by the children under their care.

REFERENCES

Achenbach T M, Edelbrock C S 1983 Manual for child behaviour checklist and revised behaviour profile. Achenbach, Burlington, VT

Ainsworth M D S 1982 Attachment: retrospect and prospect. In: Parkes C M, Stevenson-Hinde J (eds) The place of attachment in human behaviour. Basic Books, New York

APA 1994 Diagnostic and statistical manual of mental disorders, 4th edn. American Psychiatric Association, Washington, DC

Asperger H 1944 Die 'autistischen Psychopathien' im kindesalter. Archive für Psychiatrie und Nervenkrankheiten 117: 76–136

Barker P 1992 Basic family therapy, 3rd edn. Collins, London

Baron-Cohen S 1995 Mindblindness. MIT Press, London

Bayley N 1969 Bayley scales of infant development: birth to two years. Psychological Corporation, New York

Bee H 1996 The developing child, 8th edn. Harper, New York

Bentovim A, Elton A, Hildebrand J, Tranter M, Vizard E 1988 Child sexual abuse within the family: assessment and treatment. Wright, Bristol

Bierderman J, Faraone S, Spencer T et al 1993 Patterns of comorbidity, cognition, and psychosocial functioning in adults with attention deficit hyperactivity disorder. American Journal of Psychiatry 150: 1792–1798

Bowlby J 1969 Attachment and loss. Vol 1: Attachment. Hogarth Press, London

Butler-Sloss E 1988 Report of the inquiry into child abuse in Cleveland (1988). HMSO, London

Campbell A, McIntosh N (eds) 1997 Forfar & Arneil's

textbook of paediatrics, 5th edn. Churchill Livingstone, Edinburgh

Chess S, Thomas A 1990 The New York longitudinal study: the young adult periods. Canadian Journal of Psychiatry 35: 557–561

Cicchetti D, Carlson V 1989 Child maltreatment. Theory and research on the causes and consequences of child abuse and neglect. Cambridge University Press, New York

Corbett J, Harris R, Taylor E, Trimble M 1977 Progressive disintegrative psychosis of childhood. Journal of Child Psychology and Psychiatry 18: 211–219

Eaton-Evans J, Dugdale A E 1988 Sleep patterns of infants in the first year of life. Archives of Disease in Childhood 63: 647–649

Egger J, Stolla A, McEwan L 1992 Controlled trial of hyposensitisation in children with food-induced hyperkinetic syndrome. Lancet 339: 1150–1153

Elliott C, Murray D J, Pearson L 1983 The British abilities scales (new edition). NFER-Nelson, Windsor

Faull C, Nicol R 1986 Abdominal pain in six year olds: an epidemiological study in a new town. Journal of Child Psychology and Psychiatry 27: 251–261

Frankenberg W K, Dodds J B, Fandal A W, Kazuk E, Cohrs M 1975 Denver screening test. Ladoca Project & Publishing Foundation, Denver

Fraser A M, Taylor D C 1986 Childhood encopresis extended into adult life. British Journal of Psychiatry 149: 370–371

Freud A 1936 The ego and the mechanisms of defence. Hogarth Press, London

Freud A 1946 The psychological treatment of children. Imago, London

Gillberg C 1995 Clinical child neuropsychiatry. Cambridge University Press, Cambridge

Goodyer I 1990 Life experiences, development and childhood psychopathology. Wiley, Chichester

Goodyer I 1995 The depressed child and adolescent: developmental and clinical perspectives. Cambridge University Press, Cambridge

Griffiths R 1954 The abilities of babies. McGraw-Hill, New York

Hagberg B, Aicardi J, Dias K, Ramos O 1983 A progressive syndrome of autism, dementia, ataxia and loss of purposeful hand use in girls: Rett's syndrome. Archives of Neurology 14: 471–479

Hawton K, Salkovskis P, Kirk J, Clark D 1995 Cognitive behaviour therapy for psychiatric problems: a practical guide, 2nd edn. Oxford University Press, Oxford

Hobson P 1993 Autism and the development of mind. Erlbaum, Hove

Jones D 1992 Interviewing children who have been sexually abused, 4th edn. Royal College of Psychiatrists/Gaskell Press, London

Kanner L 1943 Autistic disturbances of affective contact. The Nervous Child 2: 217–250

Kerr A M, Stephenson J 1985 Rett's syndrome in the West of Scotland. British Medical Journal 291: 579–582

Lask B 1988 Novel and non-toxic treatment for night terrors. British Medical Journal 297: 592

Lask B 1994 Paediatric liaison work In: Rutter M, Taylor E, Hersov L (eds) Child and adolescent psychiatry: modern approaches, 3rd edn. Blackwell, Oxford

Lask B, Fosson A 1989 Childhood illness: the psychosomatic approach. Wiley, Chichester

Lord C, Rutter M 1994 Autism and other pervasive developmental disorders. In: Rutter M, Taylor E, Hersov L (eds) Child and adolescent psychiatry: modern approaches, 3rd edn. Blackwell, Oxford

Matthews S 1994 Cognitive development In: Bryant P, Colman A (eds) Developmental psychology. Longman, London

Meadow R 1995 What is, and what is not, 'Munchausen syndrome by proxy'? Archives of Disease in Childhood 72: 534–538

Monck E, Bentovim A, Goodall G, Hyde C, Lwin R, Sharland E 1995 Child sexual abuse: a descriptive and treatment study. HMSO, London

Neale M D 1958 Neale analysis of reading ability manual. Macmillan, London

Pennington B, Ozonoff 1996 Executive functions and developmental psychopathology. Journal of Child Psychology and Psychiatry 37: 51–88

Rett A 1966 Uber ein eigenartiges hiratrophisches Syndrom bei Hyperammonarnie ein Kinderalten. Weiner Mediginiske Wockenschrift 116: 723–726

Reisman J M 1973 Principles of psychotherapy with children, 2nd edn. Wiley, New York

Reynell J 1969 Reynell developmental language scales. NFER, Windsor

Richman N, Lansdown R 1988 Problems of pre-school children. Wiley, Chichester

Richman N, Stevenson E J, Graham P 1982 Pre-school to school: a behavioural study. Academic Press, London

Rutter M 1988 Depressive disorders. In: Rutter M, Tuma A M, Lann I S (eds) Assessment and diagnosis in child psychopathology. Fulton, London

Rutter M, Schopler E (eds) 1988 Autism: a reappraisal of concepts and treatment. Plenum Press, New York

Rutter M, Tizard J, Whitmore K 1970a Education, health and behaviour. Longmans, London

Rutter M, Graham P, Yule W 1970b A neuropsychiatric study of childhood. Clinics in developmental medicine 35/36, SIMP/Heinemann, London

Rutter M, Yule B, Quinton D, Rowlands O, Yule W, Berger M 1975 Attainment and adjustment in two geographical areas: III. Some factors accounting for area differences. British Journal of Psychiatry 126: 520–533

Schonell F J, Schonell F F 1950 Diagnostic and attainment testing. Oliver & Boyd, Edinburgh

Skuse D, Wolke D, Reilly S 1992 Failure to thrive. Clinical and developmental aspects In: Remschmidt H, Schmidt M (eds) Child and youth psychiatry, European perspectives. Vol II: Developmental psychopathology. Huber, Stuttgart

Spencer T, Wilens T, Biederman J, Faraone S, Ablon S, Lapey K 1995 A double-blind crossover comparison of methylphenidate in adults with childhood-onset attention deficit hyperactivity disorder. Archives of General Psychiatry 52: 434–443

Taylor E 1994 Syndromes of attention deficit and overactivity. In: Rutter M, Taylor E, Hersov L (eds) Child and adolescent psychiatry: modern approaches, 3rd edn. Blackwell, Oxford

Thorndike R L 1973 Stanford Binet intelligence scale, form L-M, 1972 norms tables. Houghton Mifflin, Boston

Wechsler D 1992 Manual for the Wechsler intelligence scale for children, 3rd UK edn (WISC-III UK). Psychological Corporation, Kent

WHO 1992 The ICD-10 classification of mental and behaviour disorders: clinical descriptions and diagnostic guidelines. World Health Organization, Geneva

Wolff S 1991 Schizoid personality in childhood and adult life.

III: The childhood picture. British Journal of Psychiatry 159: 629–635

Wolff S 1996 Child psychotherapy. In: Bloch S (ed) Introduction to the psychotherapies, 3rd edn. Oxford University Press, Oxford

Wolff S, Chick J 1980 Schizoid personality in childhood: a controlled follow-up study. Psychological Medicine 10: 85–100

Yule W 1991 Work with children following disasters. In: Herbert M (ed.) Clinical child psychology. Wiley, Chichester

Yule W, Udwin O, Murdoch K 1990 The 'Jupiter' sinking: effects on children's fears, depression and anxiety. Journal of Child Psychology and Psychiatry 71: 1051–1062

24
Psychiatric disorders of adolescence

W. Parry-Jones

INTRODUCTION

Adolescent psychiatry is closely allied with both child and adult psychiatry, having overlap in aetiology, assessment and treatment. However, clinical work is uniquely different, due to the effects of the maturational stage of adolescence, which is commonly regarded as a time of turmoil, unhappiness, rebellion and antisocial behaviour. While many adolescents experience personal suffering and misery, emotional and behavioural disturbance is not a prerequisite. However, misbehaviour, alienation and apparent unhappiness is a focus source of concern. Inevitably, the adolescent psychiatrist deals with a wide range of young people whose mental state and behaviour are considered abnormal or unacceptable. The term 'adolescent disturbance' is used to cover this spectrum of conditions. Involvement with family members is almost invariable and skills in interviewing parents and conducting family interventions are intrinsic. There is a need to collaborate closely with other services and agencies, and clear definition of the adolescent psychiatrist's central role and responsibilities is required. If interdisciplinary work is to be effective, psychiatrists have to be confident about the nature of their contribution and able to convey this to colleagues. Only a small proportion of adolescent disturbance calls for active psychiatric intervention, especially if this is viewed in orthodox clinical terms. However, distinctive psychiatric skills are called for in consultation with other disciplines.

Specialisation in adolescent psychiatry has a brief history (Parry-Jones 1994). During the second half of the 19th century, childhood mental disorders began to be described, distinguishing psychological and organic factors. Puberty became regarded increasingly as a physiological cause of mental disturbance, and pubescent or adolescent insanity was referred to frequently. Adolescents were admitted routinely to asylums, receiving no special age-related care until the late 1940s, when the first adolescent units opened. Exclusively adolescent inpatient services developed rapidly in the

UK, on a regional basis, in the late 1960s, in response to concern about the welfare of adolescents in adult mental hospital wards. Subsequently, there has been remarkable growth of adolescent services, and hospital treatment of serious adolescent mental disorder is usually in age-appropriate surroundings. The future of the specialty is assured (Parry-Jones 1995), although significant deficiencies remain, reflecting the tendency for health services to be slower in providing for adolescents than for children or adults. Psychiatric services are variable and incomplete, especially for acute disturbance, emergencies, rehabilitation and long-term care. Particular shortcomings include limited provisions for older adolescents, those with learning disability, aggressive, conduct-disordered and highly dangerous teenagers and drug abusers. Accessibility of services, especially inpatient units, is often unsatisfactory and overlap with adult services tends to be inadequate and unplanned. Joint planning and coordination of services delivered by mental health, education and social services and voluntary organisations can be limited (NHS Health Advisory Service 1986). Outside psychiatry, a voluminous literature relates to adolescent health care and welfare (Parry-Jones 1997).

As adolescent psychiatry is relatively new, there is considerable variation in thinking about optimal ways of understanding and managing disturbance, and selecting the most effective approach for personal practice and wider service organisation is difficult. As a medical specialty, its proper boundaries and functions fall conventionally within a medical remit. The clinical psychiatric model, emphasising individual disorder and treatment, has advantages. Traditional reliance on detailed diagnostic assessment enables both psychiatric and non-psychiatric problems to be identified, intervention planned systematically, with clarification of the contributions of psychiatrists and associated professionals. Although popular in many services, the adoption of a single theoretical and treatment model restricts the range of disorders treated. In view of the variable, incomplete nature of current adolescent services and the diversity of presenting problems, an eclectic approach is advocated. Continuities between adolescent psychiatry and the child and adult fields mean that the adolescent psychiatrist should be a generalist theoretically and practically.

SCOPE OF ADOLESCENT PSYCHIATRY

Concept and definition of adolescence

Although the physical and psychological characteristics of adolescence have been described for centuries, its current format emerged in the late 19th century, influenced by social, cultural and economic factors (Parry-Jones 1994). It carried new age-related expectations and problems, generated by lengthening compulsory education, delayed assumption of adult responsibilities and associated dependence on parents. By the end of the 19th century, adolescence was a popular focus of study, and phase-specific forms of psychiatric disorder became well established.

In Western society, there is no satisfactory definition of adolescence, which is regarded usually as extending from the onset of puberty to attainment of physical maturity and adult status. Broadly, it covers the age range of 12–20 years, incorporating early (12–15 years), mid (14–16 years) and late adolescence (17–20+ years). There is growing recognition of the value of the concept of youth psychiatry, covering the 16–25 year age range. In many parts of the world, however, adolescence is not clearly designated, with children introduced early to adult social and economic responsibilities, and little transition between childhood and adulthood.

Adolescent development

Adolescent disturbance comprises specific psychiatric disorders and reactions to developmental and situational stresses. It is necessary to consider the interrelationship between these components and to take the broadest view of causation. Effective understanding of adolescent disturbance, identification of psychopathology and its management require thorough familiarity with phenomena of normal adolescence, information about the lives of adolescents and their families, and appreciation of internal and external stressors. A fundamental clinical task is disentangling essentially normal, age-appropriate behaviour from psychopathology.

Adolescence is characterised by rapid biological and psychological changes, intensive readjustment to family, school, work and social life, coupled with unrelenting progression to adulthood. Clinically, the concept of adolescence as a period demanding completion of a sequence of phase-specific tasks is valuable, creating a frame of reference for assessment and treatment. Particularly significant for psychiatric treatment are cognitive changes, with acquisition of the capacity for abstract thought. The theme of normal development pervades adolescent psychiatry, but it is not discussed separately in this chapter, since it is covered comprehensively elsewhere (Bancroft & Reinisch 1990, Coleman & Hendry 1990, Lewis & Volkmar 1990). Instead, emphasis is placed on clinical aspects of adolescent and family development when relevant to causation, diagnosis, treatment and prognosis. Particular attention is given to the clinical significance of maturational stress.

Psychiatric disorder in adolescence

No psychiatric disorders are unique to adolescence. Disorders include conditions commencing in infancy and childhood and those arising in adolescence, with symptoms resembling those in adulthood. In this chapter, emphasis is placed on distinctive features of adolescent presentations and the disorders prominent at this time. During early adolescence, therefore, the main manifestations are of childhood disorders, in conjunction with those beginning to appear, e.g. anorexia nervosa, substance abuse and stress-related disorders accompanying biological and social change. By late adolescence, conditions such as schizophrenia emerge. Common manifestations of adolescent disturbance take the form of emotional upset, delinquent or antisocial behaviour, conflict with parents, change in friendship patterns, alienation, school difficulties, eating problems, substance abuse and sexual problems. No single theory provides a sound rationale for assessment, classification and intervention. The most satisfactory model is all encompassing, involving interaction of biological, psychological and social factors in causing and maintaining problems.

Difficulties related to the process of adolescent development may arise variously. For example, on entering puberty, children with pre-existing medical, psychiatric, developmental or temperamental difficulties may experience particular problems. There may be issues relating to the timing of puberty, or problems generated by physical, cognitive, emotional, social, psychosexual and moral maturation. Developmental changes have the capacity of being either stressful or supportive. Wide variation in age of onset and rate of growth spurt, for example, and impact of both early and late development, may have positive or negative effects. In boys, delayed maturation can generate inferiority feelings and, in girls, early menarche may be experienced negatively, or positively – signifying maturity.

At all stages, adolescence is influenced by facilitating or obstructive family influences and, in assessment and treatment, this interactionary process needs consideration. For example, concurrence of adolescence with parental midlife changes frequently impairs parental function. Conflict between adolescents and parents is rarely long-standing and, generally, parental influence remains significant throughout adolescence. Nevertheless, adolescent challenge to parental standards and attainments can pose a major threat, destabilising family homeostasis. Similar processes occur in recombined, reconstituted and nuclear families.

Estimation of prevalence and incidence of adolescent psychiatric disorder is still limited, especially in specific populations, such as those with learning disability or developmental problems. Variation in prevalence rates relates to differences in sampling methods, case definition criteria and assessment procedures (Costello 1989, Brandenburg et al 1990). Nevertheless, findings suggest that up to 25% of children and adolescents have clinically identifiable psychiatric disorders.

CLINICAL ASSESSMENT

Adolescents are unlikely to acknowledge problems, finding it difficult to request help. Self-referral is infrequent and, generally, referral is initiated by others, presenting problems often reflecting contravention of parental expectations or social rules and requirements. Preparation for the initial interview, by the general practitioner or other referrer, is especially important in clarifying the patient's reasons for requiring help. However, the psychiatrist is wise to assume limited preliminary preparation, until the position is clarified at first interview. The obtrusiveness of adolescent disturbance, its arousal of anxiety in others, and the adolescent's sense of urgency about resolving difficulties, generate the need for rapid clinical response. Prompt consultation and planned emergency provisions are essential.

Assessment should be broad based and the following sequence provides a framework for the initial meeting:

1. Joint interview with the adolescent and parents, clarifying reasons for referral, the psychiatrist's role and plans for the session, establishing the history of presenting problems, the adolescent's personal history, including developmental and medical aspects, and the family history
2. Interview with the adolescent
3. Physical examination
4. Interview with parent(s) either singly or together
5. Assembly of additional information from school or other sources, with appropriate consent.

Initial professional contact, including correspondence and telephone calls, is particularly important. Attention needs to be given to the reception of the young person and parents and to stage management of the first interview. Joint meetings assist alliance building, by clarifying the purpose and structure of the interviews, while facilitating preliminary observations about the adolescent's mental state, parental attitudes and interactive features. Predictable feelings and attitudes of the parents need consideration, with a sensitive response to their predicament. Disappointment about the adolescent's progress, and anger, recrimination and guilt about past events may be expressed. There may be ambivalence about consultation and its connotations of parenting failure, with annoyance and relief at the prospect of intervention. Clinic refusers are frequent and steps need to be taken to minimise non-attendance. Success is likely to be related to adequate preparation of adolescents and parents by the referrer. If serious opposition to attendance is anticipated, a home visit may be indicated.

Particular attention has to centre on establishing trust and confidence, especially with youngsters who are withdrawn, uncommunicative, angry, sulky or fearful of being thought 'mad'. Adolescents quickly detect phoniness and resist an 'open up, trust me, all will be well' approach. Content of early interviews should be as unambiguous as possible, with clear evidence that the consulting room is neutral and the intention is to be unbiased, without attributing blame or undermining adolescent values and convictions. The most constructive approach is to regard assessment and treatment as a collaborative process, each step being explained and discussed, in intelligible terms, with verbal consent being sufficient in most situations. Face-to-face interviews can be daunting and imaginative use has to be made of strategies for reducing tension and confrontation.

Legal and ethical issues need to be given thorough consideration, especially where there are no clear guidelines. Confidentiality is of central importance, with clarification of the extent to which revelations will remain private. Boundaries of personal and public thoughts and feelings in families need to be reflected explicitly in the stage management of interviews. Reassurance about confidentiality has to be tempered by reality, indicating that, under some circumstances, information may have to be conveyed to others. In contacts with schools or employers, written consent is preferable. Adolescents under 16 years of age, with sufficient understanding of the proposals, may consent to examination, with or without parental agreement (Gillick competence: *Gillick* v. *West Norfolk & Wisbech AHA* [1985]). Consent of a young person over 16 years is sufficient in itself and separate permission from parent or guardian is unnecessary (England & Wales: Family Law Reform Act, 1969; Scotland: Act of Legal Capacity (Scotland) Act, 1991). Imposition of intervention without consent occurs only when emergency action is needed because of threatened or actual life endangering behaviour caused by major disturbance of thinking or perception. It is conventional under such circumstances, with young people under 16 years, to accept authority of parents or guardians. In the absence of such consent, or with young people over 16 years, appropriate compulsory powers provided by mental health legislation should be utilised.

Mental state examination

Despite the greater degree of informality and flexibility necessary with adolescents, mental state examination needs to be conducted systematically, using the framework employed with other age groups. Recording of the examination should include reference to physical appearance, behaviour and manner of relating, speech, mood, thinking, perception, orientation, attention and concentration, memory and insight.

Physical examination

The physical health of adolescent patients must not be overlooked. Physical examination represents an important medical contribution in multidisciplinary work. While it is undertaken routinely on adolescent inpatients, it is not always deemed necessary for outpatients. Fears about complicating the therapist's role are misplaced and examination can establish credible evidence of interest in the patient. Even if the yield of abnormalities is small, examination provides opportunity to discuss physical changes of adolescence, facilitating revelation of personal health worries. Specific indications for examination include known or suspected physical illness or anomalies, self-concern about illness and evidence of precocious, or delayed, puberty. If the family believes the adolescent's illness is due to physical causes, it is wise to undertake detailed examination. Routine use of growth charts is recommended, with rating of pubertal stages.

Special investigations

Differential diagnosis may necessitate special medical and psychological investigations, which need to be selected carefully and completed swiftly, with appropriate explanation to the adolescent and parents, for example, if there was disturbance of growth, weight loss or the possibility of seizure disorder. It is becoming increasingly possible to make selective use of neuroimaging (Peterson 1995) and new techniques for visualising chromosomes have increased interest in molecular genetic screening for inherited disorders. Referral questions to child psychologists must be explicit, in relation, for example, to the requirement for testing intellectual capacity and educational attainment, or neuropsychological screening.

Interviewing parents and siblings

Information from parents about the adolescent, their personal histories, their marriage, the nuclear and extended family, home background and friends is essential in assessment. Problems of parents, especially single or adoptive, quality of parenting and the nature of adolescent–parent interaction require exploration. Attention needs to be paid to the family's developmental stage and capacity to cope with the adolescent's challenge. Reasons for interviewing or involving siblings should be clear. Such action requires the consent of the adolescent, parents and the siblings themselves, and the usual rules of confidentiality apply. This lays the foundation for extending assessment to include joint meetings with part, or whole, family groups. Throughout, the psychiatrist has responsibility to provide feedback to parents about the adolescent's progress.

Assembling additional information

Diagnosis and treatment planning is improved by sampling behaviour and mental state in settings outside the consulting room. Information from teachers and, sometimes, school visits can be helpful in evaluating day-to-day social and academic functioning, providing an effective index of degree of disturbance and enhancing understanding of relationships with peers and adults. Elective home visits extend the scope of assessment and treatment, e.g. assessing housebound adolescents or undertaking specific therapeutic tasks, such as setting up response prevention programmes or modelling management of anorectic patients in family meals, as part of treatment relocation from clinic to home. Home visiting is intrusive and expensive in time, requiring well thought out reasons and objectives for cost effectiveness.

Standardised interviews and rating scales

Clinicians and researchers have access to an increasing range of diagnostic tools (Orvaschel 1985, Gutterman et al 1987), usually comprising separate parent and adolescent versions. Highly structured patient interviews include the Diagnostic Interview for Children and Adolescents (DICA) (Boyle et al 1993). Semi-structured interviews include the Kiddie Schedule for Affective Disorders and Schizophrenia (K-SADS) (Endicott & Spitzer 1978) and the Child and Adolescent Psychiatric Assessment (CAPA) (Angold 1989). Rating scales which cover a range of psychopathology are the Behavior Problem Checklist for Children and Teachers (Quay 1983), the Conners Parent and Teachers Questionnaires (Conners & Barkley 1985), the Child Behavior Checklist (Achenbach 1991) and the Revised Children's Manifest Anxiety Scale (Reynolds & Richmond 1978). There are several self-report inventories and scales for use with adolescents.

DIAGNOSIS AND CLASSIFICATION

The diagnostic process does not differ from that employed in other age groups. There may be reluctance to diagnose psychiatric disorder in adolescents from fears of the adverse effects of medical labelling, reflecting misapprehension of the meaning and application of the diagnostic process. Diagnosis is sometimes viewed as especially difficult and unreliable, as adolescent disorders are regarded as atypical versions of more clearly defined adult forms. This is not necessarily the case, although adolescent presentations are often complex and not immediately part of recognisable nosological entities. It is essential to accept that typical adolescent presentations occur, with characteristics shaped by pathoplastic effects of maturation. In view of possible clinical ambiguity in adolescent disturbance, diagnostic precision is vital in improving communication, understanding causation, treatment planning and prognostic evaluation. The non-hierarchical diagnostic approach implicit in DSM-IV and ICD-10 has revealed that many adolescents display psychopathology fulfilling criteria for several disorders, e.g. depression associated with conduct disorder, eating disorders, substance abuse and anxiety.

A formulation is useful in all cases and the following framework is commended:

1. essential features
2. differential diagnosis
3. causation, identifying predisposing, precipitating, perpetuating and protective factors
4. management and treatment plan, including investigations needed
5. prognosis.

Although the last is influenced by maturational processes and associated disturbances, it relates principally to the nature and course of the disorder and its suscepti-

bility to existing treatments. Prognostic pointers need serious consideration, and overoptimism about outcome, because adolescence is transient, is misplaced. Without attention to prognosis, decisions about intervention either risk over-reacting too urgently, or underestimating the seriousness of the problem, because the adolescent will 'grow out of it'.

CLINICAL SYNDROMES

Follow-up studies of preschool and older children indicate that a significant proportion of early-onset disorders persist into adolescence and beyond. These include disorders of empathy, such as autism and autistic-like conditions, conduct disorder, psychoses and some developmental disorders. In autistic children, for example, there may be maturational gain in adolescence but, generally, there is behavioural deterioration with social and cognitive deficits and a risk of seizures. Similarly, a high proportion of children with attention deficit and hyperactivity disorder remain disabled in adolescence and adulthood (Barkley et al 1990).

Neurotic, stress-related and somatoform disorders

Concepts of emotional disorder and neurosis

Although all adult neurotic disorders occur in adolescence, generalised anxiety, with regressive symptoms, is the common presentation. Phobic, hysterical or obsessive–compulsive features may present transiently, preceding clinical pictures with more enduring features. More clearly defined disorders of late adolescence merge with those typical of adulthood. It is important, however, to recognise poorly differentiated, early adolescent emotional disorder, although outcome is generally good. In ICD-10, the concept of 'developmental appropriateness' is used to distinguish between such emotional disorders, with childhood or early adolescent onset, from neurotic disorders.

Anxiety disorders

The commonest presentation is that of the overanxious teenager, showing excessive, non-specific worrying and fearful behaviour, concern about the future, excessive demands for reassurance, inability to relax, preoccupation with past behaviour, and somatic complaints. Separation anxiety can arise suddenly, with unrealistic worries about harm occurring to an attached person or fears of their non-return. Commonly, such anxieties are associated with reluctance or refusal to go to school.

Some anxious youngsters display persistent and excessive shrinking from contact with strangers, interfering with social functioning and peer relationships. Phobic anxiety, particularly social phobias and agoraphobia, may originate in adolescence. Although true school phobia may be manifested, it is not necessarily a feature of school refusal (Berg 1991). Specific fears can present acutely as panic disorder.

Crucial to management is clarification of the pattern and causation of symptoms. It may be sufficient to identify the problem and support existing coping methods. With serious symptoms, a more systematic approach relieving distress and disability involves behavioural techniques, e.g. relaxation training and desensitisation. Anxiety management training is useful in treating panic attacks. Although brief use of benzodiazepines may be beneficial, caution is needed because of dependency risk.

Obsessive–compulsive disorder (OCD)

OCD generally begins in adolescence or young adulthood, sometimes in mid-childhood. Onset is usually gradual, with no special premorbid personality. The clinical picture is essentially the same as in adults (Rapoport 1989). Odd behaviours are usually the first features, with obsessional ideas becoming evident on enquiry. Ruminations and rituals are likely to be recognised by the adolescent as alien and senseless. Obsessional slowness may be present and, commonly, a phobic component. The disorder can be seriously handicapping, interfering with social activities, relationships, education and work. Involvement of family members in rituals can cause distress and, sometimes, dominate the household. OCD can be associated with anxiety and depression, and adolescents with anorexia nervosa and Tourette's syndrome have high rates of obsessional symptoms.

The prevalence of OCD in adolescents is approximately 2% (Flament et al 1988). Diagnosis is missed easily and frequency of the disorder, especially milder forms, may be much higher. The connection between OCD and compulsive behaviour in normal children and adolescents is unclear and learning theories provide inadequate theoretical explanation. Genetic and family factors have been implicated and the strongest case for a physical basis concerns altered serotonin function.

Diagnostically, the absence of another psychiatric disorder is critical, because obsessional symptoms occur more widely than the disorder and can be associated with other clinical features. Internal resistance is not a diagnostic requirement (Allsopp & Verduyn 1989). The Leyton Obsessional Inventory is suitable for adolescents. Where there are bizarre ideas and behaviours, schizophrenia may be suggested and morbid rumination may indicate depression. Separation from Tourette's syndrome and primary phobic disorders can be difficult.

Treatment needs to consider the relative severity of obsessional thoughts, compulsions and family disruption. Psychotherapeutic techniques are a common component in establishing relationships and in family work (Bolton et al 1983). Treatment relies primarily on cognitive–behavioural therapy (March1995). Responses of family members can perpetuate disorder, and counselling and support of parents and siblings, with frequent feedback, are required in addition to treatment strategies involving the parents. The most important drug is clomipramine (Leonard et al 1988), but increasing experience is being obtained with fluoxetine, fluvoxamine and other selective serotonin reuptake inhibitors (SSRIs) (Riddle et al 1992).

Follow-up suggests poor outcome, with a chronic but variable course, associated with episodic remissions. There is strong continuity from childhood to adulthood, that for obsessive–compulsive symptoms being stronger than for the disorder itself (Zeitlin 1986).

Reaction to severe stress and adjustment disorders

Stresses accompanying maturational changes of adolescence can provoke healthy, transient, adjustment reactions, associated with prominent emotional and behavioural manifestations, such as irritability, depression and temper outbursts. Provided symptoms are not persistent and there is no significant disturbance of daily functioning, it is unnecessary to categorise such states as psychiatric disorders.

Acute stress reaction

Exceptional physical or mental stress, such as produced by natural catastrophe, assault or multiple bereavement, can lead to transient disorders, usually subsiding within hours or days.

Post-traumatic stress disorder (PTSD)

The essential feature is the development of characteristic symptoms in response to a distressing event, outside the range of usual human experience and 'likely to cause pervasive distress in almost anyone' (ICD-10). The DSM-IV definition of the stressor criteria is more precise, requiring 'exposure to an extreme traumatic stressor involving direct personal experience of an event that involves actual or threatened death or serious injury, or other threat to one's physical integrity; or witnessing an event that involves death, injury, or a threat to the physical integrity of another person; or learning about unexpected or violent death, serious harm, or threat of death or injury experienced by a family member or other close associate. The person's response to the event must involve intense fear, helplessness, or horror (or in children, the response must involve disorganized or agitated behavior)'. Increased reporting of traumatic experiences provides greater opportunity for the study, in juveniles, of the effects of personal injury and abuse and consequences of witnessing fearful scenes. Characteristic symptoms of PTSD comprise: persistent re-experiencing of the traumatic event; persistent avoidance of stimuli associated with the event, or numbing of general responsiveness; and manifestations of increased arousal, sleep difficulties, impaired concentration, exaggerated startle response, irritability and anger outbursts. Anxiety and depressive symptoms are common and may warrant separate diagnosis. Diagnosis is not made if the disturbance lasts less than 1 month (Eth & Pynoos 1985, Lyons 1987, Yule & Williams 1990, Terr 1991).

Adult diagnostic criteria have been applied, but influence of developmental stage generates differences. Adolescents often present in a depressed, moody state. Manifestations of guilt are more salient than in younger children, together with a tendency to alternate between compliant withdrawal and aggressiveness.

Not all adverse reactions to major traumatic events meet PTSD criteria and other diagnoses need to be considered, including adjustment disorder, anxiety and depression, phobic states; exacerbation of pre-existing conditions and comorbidity occurs commonly (Di Gallo et al 1997). PTSD is increasingly important in compensation litigation. There are no entirely satisfactory screening and diagnostic instruments and it is best to use a variety of measures of anxiety, fears and depression, additional to specific measures of PTSD, including the Impact of Event Scale (Horowitz et al 1979) and the Child Post-traumatic Stress Reaction Index (Pynoos & Eth 1986) .

Adjustment disorders

These are mild, transient conditions, without antecedent psychiatric disorder, related closely in time and content to recognisable stresses, within the range of common experience. They are generally reversible, lasting only a few months. Death of a close friend or relative is an important precipitant and is likely to be a potential risk factor for subsequent psychopathology. Individual adolescent vulnerability plays a major part in shaping manifestations. This diagnosis has been overused frequently as a non-stigmatising label for responses to a wide range of normal and abnormal stressors.

Treatment

Objectives involve reduction of the stressor, provision of physical safety and care, early psychosocial intervention and family contact. Individual treatment should be directed primarily towards supporting the adolescent's coping strengths. There is growing evidence of the benefits of crisis intervention and counselling to ameliorate acute trauma and minimise risks of subsequent disorder. Intervention is required within 24 hours, if possible, before maladaptive responses become established (Parry-Jones 1996a).

In the management of potentially traumatised adolescents, a spectrum of interventions is required, ranging from psychological first-aid in the immediate aftermath of the event, to long-term psychotherapy. In treating established PTSD, the essential component is re-exposure to traumatic cues, in a structured, supportive fashion, with attempts to enhance coping strategies for dealing with intrusive phenomena. Generally, there is scope to work with parents and possibly whole families. Long-term treatment may involve group work, intensive individual psychotherapy and psychotropic medication. Despite the potential for chronic disabling symptoms, difficulty in establishing therapeutic alliance with PTSD sufferers is common.

Dissociative (conversion) disorders

The disorder may be construed variously, by reference to conversion and dissociation, individual response to intolerable predicaments and abnormal illness behaviour. The latter seems most pertinent in the management of young people, providing a more credible and pragmatic explanation for adolescents than reliance on the concept of unconscious motivation. Clinical features of adolescent hysterical states include abnormalities of gait and posture, aphonia and fits resembling epileptic seizures. Such presentations need to be taken seriously and responded to promptly, with thorough physical examination and investigation. Careful differential diagnosis is crucial to eliminate the possibility of physical disorder.

Effective treatment is likely to involve combined use of dynamic and behavioural psychotherapy (Brooksbank 1984). Exploratory psychotherapy may progress to an examination of the psychological meaning of the illness, but is unlikely to be helpful in adolescents who are poorly motivated or low intelligence. If successful, firm prediction of recovery and continuing support may be sufficient. Various retraining techniques may be employed, often calling for considerable ingenuity, e.g. biofeedback confirming return of motor function in limb paralysis.

Hypochondriacal disorder

Although some adolescents are health conscious, preoccupation with fear of disease, despite medical reassurance, in the absence of physical disorder, is an uncommon feature of adolescent emotional disorders, but may occur in anxiety or depression. In young people preoccupied with health worries, there should be appropriate physical examination and investigation. Underlying emotional difficulties need to be understood and it is often useful to interpret symptoms in terms of the avoidance of difficulties. Nevertheless, in such cases, there is a risk of chronic disability associated with somatisation (Eminson et al 1996). The onset of *body dysmorphic disorder*, in which there is preoccupation with an imagined, or slight defect, in appearance, is often during adolescence, when body changes are marked.

Chronic fatigue syndrome

Occasionally, adolescents present with complaints of mental or physical fatigue and weakness, in the absence of anxiety or depression, commonly following physical illnesses such as influenza or glandular fever. Causation, diagnosis and treatment of chronic fatigue syndrome presents problems in view of the viral, toxic, environmental or psychological factors implicated. Whatever the aetiology, prolonged fatigue symptoms can generate psychological problems for the adolescent and the family. These provide a legitimate focus for a range of behavioural and cognitive treatment techniques, without disputing the origins of the disorder. Conflicting advice about the need for rest results in uncertainty in coping with fatigue symptoms.

Depersonalisation and derealisation

Both occur within the range of normal adolescent experience, under conditions of fatigue, excitement or stress and may feature in acute anxiety, panic disorder, phobic and depressive states. Very rarely, depersonalisation occurs as an enduring syndrome, beginning in adolescence. Anxiety management techniques or psychotropic drugs are likely to be most effective, especially when symptoms are secondary to other disorders.

Conduct disorder

Conduct disorder is characterised by persistent dyssocial, aggressive or defiant behaviour, representing serious violation of age-appropriate social expectations. It may arise initially in adolescence or continue from childhood and needs to be viewed in the context of the adolescent's life history, as well as current factors. Its significance is often difficult to assess, since unreasonable behaviour and poor impulse control is likely during adolescence, and complaints may reflect a low tolerance threshold by the adults. Transient manifestations and occasional minor forms of public disorder must be distinguished from persistent, pervasive symptoms constituting conduct disorder. Problems are more serious than in mischievous, rebellious behaviour, in which basic rights of others are not violated. Conduct disorder is not the equivalent of juvenile delinquency and cannot be equated with antisocial behaviour as part of adjustment reactions or personality disorder. Types of behaviour forming the basis of the diagnosis include repeated lying, stealing, severe destructiveness, fire-setting, excessive fighting and bullying, cruelty to persons or animals, truancy, running away, severe temper tantrums, defiant provocative behaviour and persistent disobedience. In classification, the socialised–unsocialised distinction is retained because of the prognostic importance of problems in peer relations and integration. The condition can overlap with emotional disorders and mixed categories are listed in ICD-10.

There is limited evidence about prevalence because of difficulties in case definition and the changing nature of conduct disturbance during development. Conduct disorder in adolescents needs to be taken seriously, in terms of the wide range of emotional, social and relationship problems that can ensue, although not all youngsters displaying antisocial behaviour continue to do so in adult life (Robins 1978, 1991). Influential causative theories focus on the sociological bases of antisocial behaviour, a view supported by high rates of such behaviour in inner-city areas, characterised by social disorganisation and family instability. Parental psychopathology has been implicated, but precise causal connections are difficult to establish. Other factors include neurological impairment and underlying psychotic features. Since multiple influences contribute to the presentation of conduct disturbance, diagnostic assessment needs to be comprehensive, incorporating a detailed medical history and neurological examination.

Types of conduct disorder

Deliberate fire-setting is particularly dramatic and dangerous. Most perpetrators are boys who have experienced abnormal family life, and it is usually symptomatic of wider conduct disturbance (Jacobson 1985a, 1985b). It is crucial to assess the degree of dangerousness and differentiate between high- and low-risk fire-setters. Recidivists are likely to have high levels of curiosity about fire, involvement in fire-related activities, greater antisocial behaviour and may reveal overt revenge fantasies and sexual excitement. Residential assessment and treatment requires constant vigilance to minimise risks. *Runaways* present complex management problems, especially when leading alienated urban lifestyles. Generally, they have a background of social alienation and parental estrangement, and share common motivations in their flight from situational stresses. Repetitive running away, associated with serious personal risk, may be a suicidal equivalent. Runaways are likely to express loneliness, fear and resentment, but are difficult to engage in consistent treatment (Tomb 1991). Victims of *bullying* are more likely to be encountered by the psychiatrist than the perpetrators, but it is important to consider characteristics of both groups (Besag 1989). Distinction has to be made between bullying by a small number of individuals, and mobbing, involving a large group of the victim's peers. *Stealing* may occur, with or without confrontation of the victim, the latter being characteristic of mugging, purse snatching and armed robbery. Persistent *truancy* is usually associated with educational backwardness, family disadvantage and delinquency. There is little evidence about effectiveness of clinical treatment (Berg 1985). Law-breaking behaviour is widespread among young people but, when it leads to conviction, the term *juvenile delinquency* is applicable (Rutter & Giller 1983).

In *family-based conduct disorder* (ICD-10) there should be no significant disturbance or abnormalities of social relationships outside the family. Types of behaviours involved include persistent negativistic, hostile, defiant, provocative, destructive behaviour, violence against family members and fire-setting within the home. It is unclear whether situation-specific emphasis facilitates prognosis. Adolescent disturbance is often characterised by conflict with parents or substitute caregivers, with complaints about the adolescent's anger, defiance or unmanageability. Family disputes may be attributed to adolescent demands for independence, parental disapproval and disappointment with the adolescent's behaviour, and developing personality and overreaction to the teenage lifestyle. Angry outbursts and temper tantrums, however, occur frequently in adolescents coping with biological changes and mounting academic and family responsibilities, and may be age-appropriate, despite parental complaints of its obtrusiveness. Parent–adolescent alienation does not necessarily lead to psychiatric disorder, although there may be complete breakdown of communication and trust. 'Dropping out' from activities desired by parents, truancy, recurrent staying out late or absconding may

occur. Complete parental estrangement, withdrawal from the peer group and loss of career orientation generally appear in late adolescence, following depression, severely disturbed family relationships and wider social, economic and cultural influences. Unemployment prospects heighten alienation from work, with reluctance to strive for employment, poor punctuality and unwillingness to conform to employers' requirements. Prolonged unemployment can lead to depression and the stigma of not belonging to any workforce.

Treatment

Management and treatment need to match specific medical, family, psychodynamic or environmental vulnerabilities. Evidence concerning precursors of antisocial behaviour (Farrington 1995) indicate the value of early intervention and attempts have been made to encourage prosocial behaviour, using the peer group, parents and residential communities. No specific medication is indicated, although short-term empirical use of neuroleptics is justifiable in aggressive or hyperactive youngsters. With multiple intervention strategies, and the complexity of measuring effectiveness, it is difficult to comment usefully on outcome (Kazdin 1995).

Personality disorders

From infancy, temperamental and personality qualities become increasingly identifiable, e.g. degree of dependence, sociability and frustration tolerance. Personality is formed by genetic factors and the influence of physical and psychological experience. Reciprocal responses between child, parents and others, and the effects of life events are crucial. The question of personality dysfunction hardly arises in infancy and childhood, but by adulthood, abnormal personalities are identifiable and distinguishable from mental disorders. During adolescence, the scope for diagnostic uncertainty is considerable. By the age of 20 years, emotionally healthy people have completed the bulk of their maturation, but this may be delayed or impeded by disrupted childhood and poor parenting. Not all juveniles with problems in personality development exhibit personality disorders as adults, but some abnormalities are overtly persistent, even by early adolescence (Bernstein et al 1993). There is a popular view that it is improper to diagnose personality disorder while the young personality is being formed. Without recognition of early prognostic indicators to long-term personality difficulties, however, the pace and form of therapeutic intervention may be inappropriate. Nevertheless, it is difficult to define and categorise personality disorders unequivocally in this age group, and measurement is problematic. The nature of the deficit needs to be focused on, and distinction made between personality variation and personality disorder. The relationship between temperament, normal personality variation, personality accentuation and personality disorder is unclear and is probably not a simple continuum (Rutter 1987).

Types of personality disorder

Current classification of personality disorder is inadequate for adolescence since, at this stage, forms of disorder have not crystallised. Although features suggesting paranoid, obsessive–compulsive, cyclothymic, histrionic or antisocial personality disorder occur, manifestations most commonly encountered include poor socialisation and communication, low self-esteem, frustration tolerance and impulse control, and tension discharge outbursts. Coping capacity with negative life events is often critical. Origins of difficulties are obscure, little being known, for example, about the development of negative self-concepts. Children with abnormal social development and 'schizoid' features, which may be reflected in their antisocial behaviour, are identified inadequately (Wolff & Cull 1986).

Borderline personality disorder (Ludolph et al 1990) is a controversial concept in British psychiatry, whose trend goes against diagnostic ambiguity. The DSM-IV definition refers to 'instability of interpersonal relationships, self-image, and affects, and marked impulsivity' and the criteria include transient psychotic symptoms. For those aged under 18 years, the imprecise term 'identity disorder' has often been employed. Features include poor anxiety tolerance, fears of being alone or close to others, educational deterioration, substance abuse, chaotic interpersonal relationships, disorders of eating and sexual behaviour and defiant oppositional acts. Causation is speculative, involving possible genetic, constitutional and developmental factors. Compared with antisocial personality disorder and dysthymic disorder, borderline personality is more likely to be associated with exposure to chronically disturbed caretakers, prolonged separation, abuse and neglect (Zanarini 1989).

Assessment and diagnosis

Diagnostically, evidence is required, from adolescence or earlier, of enduring, maladaptive behaviour patterns covering a wide range of activities, causing subjective discomfort, abnormal responses and recognisable difficulties in relationships and coping with age-appropriate expectations. Assessment requires detailed history taking, with corroboration from schools and other sources.

A range of interview schedules, involving subjects and informants, is available (Tyrer 1988), but minimal use has been undertaken with adolescents. Significant comorbidity can exist, e.g. with depressive disorder, although caution has to be exercised because clinical depression can influence personality assessment during acute episodes.

Treatment

Intervention tends to be discouraged by diagnostic ambivalence, connotations of poor prognosis, few guidelines concerning techniques, doubts about treatment effectiveness and lack of outcome research. Treatment is rendered difficult by problems in relating, and gaining access, to young people. Realistic therapeutic objectives require recognition of the potentially lifelong nature of problems, their complex aetiology and the unlikelihood of complete resolution. Strategies are essentially psychotherapeutic, involving subjects individually or in groups, the family and other contextual factors, such as the school peer group. Sometimes, it may be feasible to consider ways of reversing processes that perpetuate and consolidate disorders. Individual psychotherapy in borderline disorders requires considerable experience and the capacity to set clear objectives and firm limits (Egan 1986). Social skills and cognitive behavioural techniques may facilitate development of self-control and ability to 'stop and think before one acts' (Kendall & Braswell 1985).

Pathological gambling

In the UK, there are no legal restrictions on young people gambling on fruit machines. This may develop into a major problem for some adolescents and, in a small number, lead on to stealing and other criminal behaviour to support the habit (Griffiths 1990).

Psychoactive substance abuse

In most adolescent populations, drug and alcohol use is a serious social concern and a major public health problem. Alcohol and drugs are overused with no evidence of abating and, in many parts of the world, adolescents grow up in an environment where substance abuse is commonplace. Abuse is increasing in all age groups and contributes significantly to adolescent morbidity and mortality. Precise prevalence rates are difficult to achieve, particularly since drug use patterns change rapidly. First drug and alcohol experiences occur earlier, and are perceived, like tobacco smoking, as 'grown-up' habits, providing a vehicle for challenge. Peer group pressures, family influences, easy access, media glamorisation, and natural curiosity make refusal difficult, and adolescents are expected to experiment. The decision whether or not to do so can now be regarded as a developmental test.

Drugs and alcohol provide psychological relief from newly experienced emotional turmoil, yet experimentation is dangerous and dependency unpredictable. Addictive behaviours are maintained by powerful motivation, and interventions need to be highly effective. Concern about drugs like marijuana is justified clinically, but alcohol abuse is more prevalent, its effects are cumulative, possibly more chronic. Principal medical complications of drug misuse involve physical trauma, intentional and accidental overdosage, withdrawal effects and the hazards of parenteral use, including human immunodeficiency virus (HIV) infection. The main psychiatric consequences are depression, suicidal ideation, attempted suicide and drug-induced psychosis. Accidents, homicides and suicides have strong correlation with drug and alcohol abuse.

Alcohol

Young people are drinking earlier, more often, and have established a greater than average increase in such indicators of alcohol-related harm as drunkenness offences and road accident deaths. In one study, 20% of 11–15-year-old girls and 22% of boys had had a drink in the previous week and the proportions rise rapidly with age (Marsh et al 1986). Fifty-three per cent of 16–19-year-olds consider themselves to be regular drinkers (Rudat et al 1993).

There is no single theory why alcohol misuse begins. Pressures to conform with peer group habits are high and alcohol features prominently in entertainments and recreation, with rapid growth in retail outlets, including the sale of 'alcopop' drinks. At least one-half of young drinkers are likely to have had their first drink at home and parental models are, therefore, crucial. Young people whose parents make significant use of alcohol, drugs and tobacco are more likely to use these themselves and to have psychiatric and social difficulties. Equally, there is evidence that children from households where alcohol is forbidden can be at risk. Many who start drinking outside the home, in school, parks, clubs and in the company of peers, emerge, ultimately, as the heaviest drinkers and have problems in parental relationships and hostility towards authority.

Coexisting conduct and personality problems and emotional disturbance are major contributory factors. Many young people regard alcohol as an escape from loneliness and stress, and shy youngsters find it assists social mixing. There may be feelings of parental rejection or indifference, lack of peer acceptance, emotional isolation and low self-esteem. Increasing alcohol intake

may be a clue to suicide risk. Substance abuse to ward off reality during this stage may compromise seriously further ability to make adequate adjustment to an increasingly complex society and to deal with daily problems and frustrations.

Hawker (1978) showed that, in most young people, alcohol caused no problems for themselves or others, although some displayed socially disruptive behaviour under its influence. Four per cent of boys and 3% of girls drank because they liked getting drunk, and 10% reported episodic amnesia. Frequent drinkers got drunk relatively more often than infrequent drinkers and experienced greater hangover symptoms. In the long-term, critical milestones are age at first drinking, daily regular drinking and age of experiencing amnesia.

Management follows that used with adults. Cognitive strategies are useful in strengthening abstinence, e.g. by self-definition as a non-drinker and viewing other drinkers negatively. Avoidance of high-risk situations and engagement in alternative activities is important. Effective prevention requires changes in the law relating to drinking and driving offences, drunkenness and licensing, and increased tax on alcohol. Scope for health education is considerable, despite the dilemma concerning total abstention or safe limits, the objectives should include moderation, drinking only in appropriate circumstances, social disapproval of drunkenness and greater acceptance of abstention.

Cannabis

Cannabis is widely used among older adolescents. Only a minority develop dependence and intermittent use does not appear to be adverse, although acute psychoses can be precipitated.

Stimulants

Frequently abused stimulant drugs include cocaine, amphetamines, methylphenidate, phenmetrazine, diethylpropion and ephedrine. Acute paranoid psychotic states, resembling schizophrenia, can occur following chronic use. Rapid rise in cocaine use is of special concern. It is a short-acting stimulant, generating powerful dependence, which can be swallowed, injected or inhaled, especially as crack. The latter can produce acute respiratory failure and bronchial spasm.

Hallucinogens

This group includes lysergic acid diethylamide (LSD), psilocybin ('magic mushrooms'), mescaline, phencyclidine (PCP or 'angel dust') and methylenedioxymethamphetamine (MDMA or 'ecstasy'). Enduring affective and psychotic disorders can occur, sometimes with flashbacks. In small dosage, PCP induces drunkenness; higher levels produce excitement, aggressiveness and hallucinations. The widespread use of ecstasy is a cause for serious concern because, in addition to inducing a general sense of well-being, it can result in depression, anxiety and paranoid psychosis, and a number of deaths have been reported.

Opiates

This group includes heroin, morphine, codeine and synthetic opiates, which can be swallowed, smoked, inhaled or injected. Tolerance develops rapidly, resulting in increasing dosage. Serious adverse effects include constipation, nausea, vomiting, respiratory depression and coma.

Depressants

Commonly abused drugs include benzodiazepines, notably temazepam, barbiturates and other hypnotics and sedative psychotropic drugs. Use reduces anxiety, inducing a feeling of freedom from tension and aggression.

Caffeine

There is widespread consumption of caffeine in soft drinks, coffee, tea, cocoa and 'over-the-counter' medications. Effects of caffeinism include restlessness, insomnia, flushing, diuresis, muscle twitching, gastrointestinal disturbance, rambling speech, tachycardia or cardiac arrhythmia. Reduced intake can produce withdrawal symptoms, e.g. irritability, lethargy and headaches, but rapid discontinuation is usually achievable.

Inhalants

Despite considerable preventive efforts, there is little evidence of reduction in the use of, or mortality from, the deliberate inhaling of solvents, gases and other volatile substances (Watson 1986, Ashton 1990). Solvents implicated have been toluene and acetone, included in glues, typewriting correction fluids and aerosols. Use has also been made of petrol, paint stripper and butane gas. It is estimated that 3.5–10% of adolescents have experimented with solvents and 0.5–1.0% of secondary school pupils are abusers (Ramsey et al 1989).

Occasional abusers form the largest group and experimental misuse is usually transient in youngsters with various personality problems. Habitual abusers are chiefly boys aged 13–15 years, with high rates associated with single parent families, paternal alcoholism, unemployment, large families and low socioeconomic status. Masterton (1979) differentiated between socially determined abuse, the product of the subculture and social disorganisation, and psychologically determined abuse, responding to individual underlying disorder.

Inhalation produces excitement, disinhibition, delusions and perceptual disturbance and aggressive, risk-taking behaviour. Large dosage causes increasing drowsiness, convulsions and coma. Death results from accidents, suicide, or respiratory depression, due to inhalation of vomit, vagal inhibition and cardiac arrhythmia. Despite concern about brain damage, misuse of volatile solvents, as commonly practised by secondary school pupils, is unlikely to result in neurological or neuropsychological impairment (Chadwick et al 1989). Nevertheless, annual deaths in Britain from volatile substance abuse are increasing.

Assessment and diagnosis of drug abuse

Accurate identification of drug-related problems is critical in the differential diagnosis and management of adolescent disturbance. The presence and extent of abuse is difficult to establish, as such problems are likely to be denied strongly, necessitating highly specific questioning. There is a danger of misinterpreting events as essentially 'normal' adolescent disturbance. Parents and professionals may overlook substance abuse or deny its connection with emotional, social and behavioural problems. Ultimately, crises such as law breaking, running away or school expulsion may precipitate treatment (Williams et al 1989). Warning signs include unusual mood lability and reported 'personality changes'. Impaired school performance occurs commonly, with absenteeism and truancy. There may be evidence of uncharacteristic delinquency, alienation from 'straight' friends, and deteriorating family relationships. Physical changes, e.g. in eating and sleeping routines, may be noticeable. Full physical examination is required, confirming or excluding the presence of intoxication or withdrawal, clarifying routes of drug administration and identifying medical consequences. Urinary drug screening should be undertaken with, if appropriate, more extensive testing, e.g. for HIV and hepatitis B antigen.

Treatment of drug abuse

Treatment should commence in the least restrictive programme. Initially, short-term abstinence needs to be assured and, for individuals who evade confrontation and need a restricted environment, hospitalisation is required, although suitable facilities are scarce. During this period, adolescents can begin to examine the impact of abuse and acknowledge need for treatment. The next step is assessment of problems involved in the maintenance of abstinence. Outpatient treatment is the preferred option, despite compliance problems. It calls for experienced staff, a range of individual, group and family treatments, school liaison and a climate of free expression and spontaneous action (Friedman & Glickman 1986). Reduction of high-risk behaviour among intravenous drug users is crucial. Long-term aftercare is essential to maintain behaviours learned in treatment, and recovery requires consistent family involvement. Major efforts have been made at preventive education starting in the preadolescent period. Effectiveness is reduced by the high-dependency effects and cash returns to dealers, which are powerful reinforcers.

Sexual disorders, offences and abuse

Disorders of gender identity and sexual preference

Gender identity refers to the sense of belonging to one sex and awareness of being male or female. It is learned at an early stage and needs to be distinguished from sex role identity, concerning the consistency with male or female behaviour of a particular culture, which develops later in childhood or early adolescence. There is no reliable information about the prevalence or incidence of adolescent gender identity disorders. Problems include: transsexualism; cross-gender identification, without acknowledged homosexual orientation or a desire to change sex; and established homosexual behaviour or orientation (Zucker & Green 1992).

Various treatments have been employed, including behaviour therapy, individual psychotherapy, family therapy and parent counselling (Zucker 1990), but prospects of successful outcome are limited and difficulties arise in setting therapeutic objectives. While it may be possible to achieve agreement about short-term goals, e.g. reducing social difficulties, the long-term goals, e.g. changing sexual orientation, are problematic. Parents, concerned whether effeminate behaviour in boys might forecast homosexuality, generally will be reluctant to accept plans for adaptation to homosexual orientation (Green 1987).

Sexual offences

Indecent exposure, like other adolescent sexual problems, may reflect clumsy, immature attempts to achieve sexual gratification and recognition. Cases of voyeurism

and the touching or fondling of strangers may be similarly explicable. Prevalence of sexual abuse and assault of, or by, adolescents remains unclear because of underreporting. Offences include rape, incest, paedophilia, sexual homicide and involvement in pornography and prostitution.

In assessment and management of sexually abused adolescents, including the male victims of female perpetrators, the principles outlined earlier in this chapter apply, and need to include particular attention to comorbid depression and PTSD. Rigorous care has to be taken, in cases of alleged abuse, before accepting unsubstantiated accounts. Despite the requirement to report juveniles suspected of being at risk, and the overriding necessity for protection, difficult decisions, and the potential loss of the therapeutic alliance, may arise with older adolescents having a history of sexual abuse by a family member, but who are no longer at risk.

Teenage parenthood

Sexual maturity is occurring earlier and births and abortions in teenage girls are increasing. After the teenage birth rate fell until the mid-1980s, it rose to 33.2 in 1991 in England and Wales and to 31.9 per 1000 in 1990 in Scotland. In 1991, 24 per 1000 women aged 16–19 in England and Wales, and 6 per 1000 aged 14–15 had an abortion (Woodroffe et al 1993). There is no evidence of specific psychopathology leading to schoolgirl pregnancy or substantial evidence of positive intent (Shaffer et al 1978). However, neonatal mortality is higher, and there is evidence that children of teenage parents have higher rates of cognitive deficits and psychosocial problems. Runaway girls are particularly vulnerable to the risks of prostitution and pregnancy. Few physical disadvantages accompany teenage childbearing, provided antenatal care is adequate. Educationally, however, girls may be seriously disadvantaged, employment difficulties are likely and teenage marriage lacks stability. There are fewer teenage fathers, because many teenage pregnancies are fathered by men aged over 20 years, some of whom fail to acknowledge paternity. Generally, teenage fathers are affected less adversely than mothers.

Eating disorders

Problems with eating, body weight and shape are referred frequently to adolescent psychiatrists. Anorexia nervosa may arise in prepubertal children (Fosson et al 1987), but occurs typically in mid- or late adolescence. Bulimia nervosa is increasingly common among late adolescents. Obesity is rarely the main referral reason, despite its high prevalence and damaging effects on self-esteem and peer relationships. Rumination disorder and pica occur rarely in isolation, other than in mentally retarded adolescents, but may feature with anorexia nervosa or bulimia nervosa.

Anorexia nervosa

Girls predominate, especially during late adolescence, accounting for 90–95% of cases. Prevalence rates of 0.5–1.0% have been recorded, but evidence concerning increasing incidence is controversial. Diagnosis and management resembles that in adults. Outcome is poor in a large proportion of patients (Steinhausen 1997).

Complex sociocultural causative factors need to be related to underlying psychobiological and maturational processes. Adolescence in girls is accompanied by increased deposition of adipose tissue, and consequent feelings of fatness may predispose to dieting. Abstinence has a powerful manipulative effect in family relationships and, at a time of age-appropriate turmoil, the sense of personal control from relentless dieting appeals to some adolescents. Persistent self-induced weight loss may become a maladaptive way of coping with maturational changes, associated with fears about adult sexuality and autonomy. Since teenage slimming is widespread, it is difficult initially to distinguish psychopathology from transient age-appropriate behaviour. The extent to which an overwhelming fear of fatness exists is the most useful index of serious disorder. If dieting fails to maintain the desired weight, there may be complete breakdown of control, with bingeing, and self-induced vomiting or purging.

Family interaction and issues concerning autonomy, emancipation and maturity fears usually feature prominently in treatment. Family-based treatment is most effective in young patients with disorders of short duration, but less beneficial with older adolescents (Russell et al 1987). Depending upon the severity of weight loss and its medical consequences, treatment may need to begin in hospital and progress to outpatient care. Some programmes avoid explicit emphasis on weight restoration, focusing on personal and interpersonal issues and normalisation of eating and related behaviours. While these may be appropriate with adults, structured weight-oriented programmes are often required with younger patients and weight restoration alone may succeed.

Weight gain is a complex, prolonged process, complicated by ambivalence towards treatment and change. Programmes require dietary counselling and psychoeducational, behavioural, cognitive and psychotherapeutic strategies, e.g. concerned with problems of meal completion, manipulative conduct, and conformity to social functions of eating. Parental or family involvement is often crucial. There should be planned progression from minimal responsibility to full control of food intake and weight management. There is no consensus about frequency of weighing or whether patients should be informed about exact weight. Target weight needs to be seen as appropriate, reflecting the uniqueness of individual physique and weight, so that power struggles between therapist and patient diminish and treatment goals are understandable. Consideration needs to be given to the most effective method of calculating target weight, matching it to the patient's age, sex, height, maturational stage, eating attitudes, shape, weight gain and physical and nutritional knowledge. Using several methods, including Quetelet's body-mass index, to corroborate the chosen target is most helpful. In postmenarchic girls, non-negotiable, long-term target weights, concerned largely with menstrual onset, are likely to achieve the greatest compliance (Parry-Jones 1991).

Bulimia nervosa

This disorder has a prevalence of approximately 1.0% in adolescents (Fairburn & Beglin 1990). Anorexia nervosa may have occurred previously, but body weight, although a focus of concern, is usually normal. It is a chronic, often secretive, disorder, requiring prolonged treatment, especially in patients with concomitant psychopathology, and long-term outcome is unclear. Its management resembles that for anorexia nervosa. Hospitalisation is required only when bingeing, vomiting and purging are out of control, if there is a major weight loss or if there are serious medical complications.

Obesity

Obesity, usually defined as the body weight being 20% above normal, affects 20–30% of young people (Parry-Jones 1988). Causation is multifactorial, including physiological predisposition, family eating patterns and overeating in response to anxiety, depression, disturbed relationships and maturational stress. In addition to medical complications and increased vulnerability to other eating pathology, obesity generates personal and family problems. Teasing and bullying by peers can lead to self-consciousness and isolation. Family tensions may be generated by maintaining reducing diets. Treatment outcome is discouraging, lost weight being regained rapidly unless there is consistent family support and strong motivation. Cognitive and behavioural methods, involving the family, and if possible, the school peer group, are the most successful.

Mood disorders

Depression

Presentation of adolescent depression is often complex and, initially, not clearly part of the 'adult' entity. Several characteristic patterns are distinguishable, e.g. lowering of mood is more influenced by environment and is less fixed, reflecting typical adolescent mood fluctuation. Continuities with childhood and adult disorder, however, should not be overlooked. Although depressive behaviour may be displayed from early childhood, capacity to articulate feelings of lowered mood emerge increasingly with adolescent cognitive maturity. Nevertheless, adolescents are often unwilling to talk spontaneously about deeper feelings and, rather than lowered mood, may refer ambiguously to a sense of emptiness or absence of feelings. Research on depression in young people has expanded (Goodyer 1995). Systematic interview schedules have been developed and the similarity between adolescent and adult depression has been confirmed, although puberty has modifying effects on psychological markers of depression (Puig-Antich 1986) .

Prevalence Data on prevalence of adolescent depressive disorders in non-clinic populations are inadequate, although there is more information about the frequency of depressive symptoms. Kashani et al (1987) reported a prevalence of 4.7% for major depression and 3.3% for dysthymic disorder, significantly higher than rates for preadolescents. Rutter et al (1976) revealed a 1 year prevalence of affective disorder of 1.4 per 1000 in 10–11-year-olds, and a threefold increase in the rate from preadolescence to adolescence. A sharp rise in depressive feelings during pubescence was also demonstrated. During adolescence, the sex ratio changes progressively, girls outnumbering boys by up to 4:1. Some studies suggest that about 25% of adolescent psychiatric patients suffer clinical depression.

Mild depressive episode Coping with pubertal changes, separating from the family, developing intimate relationships and preparing for work may produce an unhappy, demoralised state. Relinquishment of childhood gratifications has to be mourned, the ending of school years can be unsettling, and a new awareness of the problems facing humanity increases the emotional burden. Usually, such maturational tasks are achieved comfortably, with only transient mood lowering and little interference with everyday functioning. Some adolescents experience persistent sadness, hopelessness and apathy, which interferes with performance and leads to personal suffering. Although usually mild, there may be expressions of self-denigration, and feelings of loneliness and hopelessness may precipitate suicidal ideas. Fears of failure may be prominent, such as not becoming an effective adult, or making a successful sexual relationship. In the background, there are likely to be behavioural problems, and difficulties with school, family and peers.

Depressive episodes may follow bereavement or personal setbacks and disappointments, such as breaking up a close relationship or academic failure, with loss of an important hope or ambition. Problems in the adolescent's social life at home, school or in the peer group may be precipitants, the intensity of depression depending on the degree of loss and susceptibility to the implications of reversal. Personality features predisposing to depression may be recognised during adolescence and depressive cognitions can commence in late childhood. Adolescents who habitually adopt these ways of thinking and lack self-esteem are more likely to become depressed when faced with reversals. Processes interacting with cognitive development to produce low self-esteem and negative self-evaluation are ill-understood and the significance of these apparent vulnerability factors is uncertain.

Lowered mood may not always be conspicuous or described spontaneously, although characteristic depressive symptoms are confirmed on detailed inquiry. For such presentations, the unsatisfactory term 'masked depression' has been used (Carlson & Cantwell 1980). While this is not a separate diagnostic entity, retaining the term in adolescent practice emphasises that depression can go unrecognised. Presentations concealing depression can take the form of restless boredom, persistent search for new activities, fatigue, bodily preoccupations and physical symptoms. Alternatively, there may be uncharacteristic antisocial and risk-taking behaviour, promiscuity or drug abuse. There may be association between depression and both substance abuse and conduct disorder (Kovacs et al 1988).

Moderate and severe depressive episode Serious depressive episodes are rare before puberty, increasing in mid- and late adolescence to adult levels. Developmental processes accounting for this change are ill-understood. Clinical features are essentially the same as in adulthood, comprising single or recurrent episodes of depression, with or without psychotic symptoms, and depression alternating with mania or hypomania. As in adults, moderate–severe depression has prominent somatic symptoms, but retardation may not be as salient. Compared with depression, largely understandable in reactive terms, there is likely to be less mood changeability. A family history of affective disorder is often present.

Recognition of the first episodes of bipolar disorder is

often difficult, especially in younger adolescents, until a cyclical pattern emerges. Instead, attempts may be made to construe symptoms in terms of personal and interpersonal difficulties. In differential diagnosis, affective disturbance in early schizophrenia has to be considered. Although little is known about the course of adolescent depressive disorders and prediction of relapse is difficult, adolescent depression can be a chronic, recurring and debilitating condition, persisting into adulthood.

Diagnostic assessment Depressive disorder requires disentangling from age-appropriate reactions. Consideration needs to be given to evidence of change in behaviour and mental state, the extent to which these are in keeping with age and development, and the frequency, persistence and pervasiveness of abnormalities. Physical examination is essential because depressive symptoms can follow physical diseases. Measures suitable for use with adolescents include the Hamilton Rating Scale for Depression, the Children's Depression Inventory (CDI) and the Depression Self-rating Scale.

Treatment   Most depressed teenagers are manageable at home, only a small proportion requiring hospitalisation for intensive assessment and treatment. It is important not to overreact to minor, age-related mood swings, when what is required is reassurance of parents or other significant adults. Intervention in 'understandable' depression ranges from direct practical help in resolving personal, situational and relationship problems, to individual psychotherapy, systematically planned to develop a more assertive and confident outlook and to enhance self-esteem. When there is a chronically negative self-view it may be difficult to shift the focus to assets and achievements, away from losses, regrets and inadequacies. Cognitive-behaviour therapy can be effective because it is problem-oriented, concerned with current experiences and discourages dependency and regression, but the effects may be short-term (Wood et al 1996). The burden borne by parents and siblings can be considerable. Parents may feel responsible for the adolescent's state and unsure how to deal with mood disturbance in a young person who is cut off and unaffected by reassurance. However, elaborate family involvement is not appropriate in all cases, especially with older adolescents.

The role of pharmacotherapy remains controversial and there have been few well-controlled studies of antidepressants in adolescents and no evidence of significant differences between placebos and tricyclic antidepressants (Remschmidt & Schulz 1995). The present consensus is that treatment should be started with an SSRI, e.g. fluoxetine, because of fewer side-effects, increased safety in overdose, and reported efficacy. Clinical experience, however, suggests that medication may be beneficial for a small number of patients with biological or psychotic symptoms. If a tricyclic antidepressant is used, because of failure to respond, it should be administered in maximum dosage for 6–10 weeks, with ECG monitoring, before concluding it is ineffective. Caution is needed not to undermine attempts to cope constructively with painful feelings by resorting to medication. Lithium is as effective in adolescents as it is in adult manic–depressive disorder (Youngerman & Canino 1978) and, following several major affective episodes, it is appropriate for long-term prophylactic treatment, although compliance may be poor. Minor tranquillisers and hypnotics are best avoided. Electroconvulsive therapy (ECT) may be effective in severe, protracted depression, resistant to other treatments.

Manic episodes

Despite doubts about the occurrence of mania in children, its adolescent presentation, as manic episodes or part of bipolar disorder, is well established, with prevalence of 0.6–1.0% in mid- and late adolescence (Carlson & Kashani 1988). Hypomania and mania in adolescents is similar to that in adults, although difficulties may arise in identifying the first episode (Carlson 1990). Differential diagnosis includes substance abuse and schizophrenia. Hospitalisation is usually necessary in severe mania to ensure patient safety. Treatment of the acute condition is by neuroleptics or lithium, although the latter is best used prophylactically.

Suicide and suicidal behaviour

Suicide is very rare before puberty, but the incidence rises rapidly and it becomes the third leading cause of death for adolescents, following accidents and homicides (Hawton 1986). Male suicides outnumber females at all ages and in all cultures, and rates have been increasing in males. This pattern is reversed in attempted suicide, although female rates appear to be declining. Methods vary widely, according to country and culture, with drug overdose, hanging, jumping from heights, car exhaust fumes and shooting being most frequent. Self-poisoning is the commonest form of parasuicide, the usual agents being analgesics and psychotropic drugs. There is likely to be a background of broken homes, disturbed relationships with parents and family history of suicidal behaviour. Precipitants include multiple losses or changes, such as fears of failure, recent quarrels, break-up with a boy- or girlfriend, trouble with teachers or school work, or social embarrassment. Few adolescents who make suicide attempts actually have psychiatric disorder and serious suicidal intent is often low. Instead, there may be a range of motives, such as relief from intolerable stress, retaliation or manipulation. Suicide of a friend or relative, or media coverage of the death of a cult figure, may be influential. Suicide pacts are infrequent.

Assessment

Serious attention should be given to subtle or blatant verbal warnings referring to dying or suicide, and behavioural warnings, such as suicide notes or isolating behaviour. Key risk factors are male sex, previous self-destructive behaviour, psychiatric disorder, especially mood disorder, conduct disorder, substance and alcohol abuse, suicide plans, family history of depression or suicide, isolation and alienation from family, friends or other social support systems, school problems and selection of a violent method, carried out in isolation with little likelihood of interruption. When depression is associated with conduct disorder, impulsivity, and drug and alcohol abuse the risk may be higher.

Management

Not all young persons are assessed psychiatrically, although this is recommended practice. Examination in hospital, at the crisis point, is most effective, and delayed appointments are often unsuccessful. Difficulty in engagement is common, often due to negative family attitudes. Some psychiatrists hospitalise all suicidal adolescents, irrespective of risk, but a discriminating approach is preferable, provided immediate outpatient treatment is available. In addition to treating depression, attention needs to be given to self-esteem deficits, to developing more effective coping and problem-solving behaviour and to intervention with dysfunctional families (Brent 1997). Ten per cent of adolescents who attempt suicide repeat within a year (Hawton et al 1982). Repeaters have higher rates of drug and alcohol abuse, associated psychiatric disturbance, long-term problems, poor peer relationships, early parental loss and are likely to live away from home.

Self-mutilation

Self-injuring activities include cutting, scratching, cigarette burns, tattooing, bruising, biting and inserting needles. Additional to its occurrence in schizophrenia and learning disability, it arises typically in teenage girls displaying personality problems with impulsive-aggressive behaviour, poor relationships and low self-esteem, often in association with eating disorders, appearing to relieve intolerable tension or relationship impasse (Solomon & Farrand 1996). A sequence can be identified, involving buildup of tension, anticipatory excitement at the prospect of injury, feelings of detachment on self-injury, discharge of tension and calmness, even sleep, before experiencing shame and guilt.

Self-mutilation is notoriously difficult to treat. The least possible response should be made that is compatible with essential first aid. Psychiatric treatment addresses the underlying emotional and personality problems, although this may be complicated by poor verbal communication. Intervention should involve a search for more adaptive strategies for alleviating tension and achieving gratification, e.g. relaxation techniques.

Schizophrenia and schizotypal disorders

There is no unique adolescent psychosis and the view that adolescent 'turmoil' represents a 'normal psychosis' is outdated (Rutter et al 1976). Adolescent disorders need to be seen in the context of all psychoses occurring in children and adults, and adult diagnostic criteria are applicable. Adolescence has a pathoplastic influence, giving disorders staged characteristics and colouring the content of symptoms. Schizophrenia is rare in childhood, but there is a remarkable increase after puberty, and the usual age of onset is 15–45 years (Remschmidt et al 1994). In the initial clinical picture, first-rank symptoms may be fleeting, difficult to elicit or absent (Garralda 1985). The common presentation is the acute syndrome, with falling off in social and academic performance, mood disturbance, incoherent speech, bizarre actions, hallucinations, delusions and preoccupation with inner thoughts.

Differential diagnosis

Careful syndromal diagnosis is essential, but it is characteristic of adolescent psychoses that precise diagnosis may be difficult, and lengthy observation and assessment necessary. Adolescents with severely disturbed emotional and personality development are hard to understand and may appear incoherent, but few develop psychotic disorders. Diagnostic problems arise if there are affective features, insidious personality deterioration or clouding of consciousness. Distinguishing between first episodes of schizophrenia and mania is particularly difficult, but this should encourage rigorous diagnostic endeavours. Not uncommonly, apparently affective disorders emerge as schizophrenia. Paranoid states, without typical schizophrenic features, are unusual. Acute and transient psychotic disorders attributable to stressful experiences occur, but distinction from schizophrenia is uncertain. Possible organic causes of psychosis, e.g. toxic confusional and drug-induced states and rare neurodegenerative conditions, need investigation. Early signs of subacute sclerosing panencephalitis may resemble schizophrenia, until progressive dementia with myoclonus and epilepsy supervenes. Seizure disorder, especially with temporal lobe involvement, can be associated with schizophrenia-like disorder, and some anticonvulsants can produce psychotic states.

Treatment

Treatment is concerned with a wider range of problems and handicaps than the schizophrenic process and intervention has to be tailored pragmatically to symptoms and needs. The overall aim is outpatient or day hospital care, but hospitalisation is commonly necessary. Management of a few schizophrenic adolescents in a general-purpose, multidisciplinary unit may generate problems (Parry-Jones 1992), due to differing staff attitudes towards the concept of psychosis, fears about diagnostic 'labelling', disagreement about the patient's capacity to control psychotic behaviour and ambivalence about antipsychotic drugs.

Individual intervention centres on straightforward communication about the disorder, as well as maturational, social and educational problems. It should be supportive and non-confrontational, and stressful group therapy is inappropriate. Family-based treatment should provide information and support, reducing high expressed emotion, encouraging realistic expectations, acceptance of relapses and long-term disabilities.

Treatment with typical neuroleptics is the mainstay in acute and chronic schizophrenia and allied disorders, with depot preparations for maintenance when there is unreliability with oral medication. Although clozapine has superiority in the treatment of both positive and negative symptoms, especially in treatment-refractory states, its toxic effects require close monitoring (Kumra et al 1996). There is scope for behaviour modification, particularly reducing withdrawn, socially unacceptable behaviour. Appropriate educational provisions, especially residential, are hard to find, and there are difficulties in obtaining employment. Facilities for rehabilitation and long-term care of teenagers with chronic schizophrenia are unsatisfactory, and overlap with adult services is often unplanned. Even after vigorous treatment, adolescents with schizophrenia are likely to display a fluctuating course, with progression to a chronic stage, characterised by negative symptoms. Favourable prognostic pointers include acute onset associated with stress, affective features, higher intelligence and good premorbid personality. Generally, the younger the onset, the worse the prognosis (Kydd & Werry 1982).

Sleep disorders

In addition to sleep disturbance associated with psychiatric disorder, such as anxiety, depression and PTSD, adolescents may suffer from other conditions which have received little attention (Anders & Eiben 1996). Many adolescents have difficulty sleeping regularly through the night and have an increased need for daytime sleep (Carskadon & Dement 1987). Normal daytime somnolence has to be distinguished from narcolepsy and hypersomnolence occurring in the Kleine–Levin syndrome. Sleepwalking and night terrors may start in early adolescence, but are usually outgrown. Terrifying dreams or nightmares may be precipitated by frightening experiences occurring during acute stress and anxiety.

Tic disorders

Tics beginning in adolescents are usually short lived and recovery takes place without treatment. Sometimes symptoms persist for a longer period, although recovery usually occurs within a few years. Tourette's disorder has usually appeared by early adolescence, characterised by motor and vocal tics, coprolalia, palilalia, sleep disturbance, learning difficulties and behaviour disorder. Association with OCD has been established (Leckman et al 1997). Tics need to be distinguished from other movement disturbances and neurological disorders, such as Huntington's chorea.

In the treatment of Tourette's disorder, emphasis needs to be given to supporting the adolescent and family and enabling normal daily life and schooling to proceed. Haloperidol is an established treatment, but other drugs have been used, including pimozide, clonidine, risperidone and fluoxetine (Cohen et al 1988).

Organic disorders

Assessment and differential diagnosis of suspected organic psychiatric disorder in adolescents, e.g. disorders associated with head injury, intracranial infections, cerebral tumours, endocrine and metabolic disorders, does not differ from that for adults. Detailed physical examination and neuropsychiatric assessment is essential, with selective use of special investigations.

Dementing disorders occur rarely in childhood and adolescence. Huntington's chorea can arise, although generally commencing after the age of 25 years. Neurological signs, especially choreiform movements, usually precede psychiatric symptoms, including depressive and schizophrenia-like features, culminating in progressive intellectual impairment. Other causes of dementia include the lipoidoses, leucodystrophies, hepatolenticular degeneration and subacute sclerosing panencephalitis. Although the pace of deterioration varies, the outcome is fatal or results in profound intellectual impairment. Occurrence after a period of normal function heightens the distress of parents and siblings, emphasising the need for family support during relentless deterioration. The opportunity for individual work is variable, but there may be scope for medication, e.g. neuroleptics in Huntington's chorea.

Psychiatric disorders associated with chronic physical illness

Adjustment problems can arise in long-term illnesses such as epilepsy, diabetes mellitus, asthma, ulcerative colitis, rheumatoid arthritis, cystic fibrosis, muscular disorders and physical deformities. Depression may be associated with multiple sclerosis, and organic causes of secondary mania have been described. While chronic illness is not necessarily associated with overt psychological disturbance (Kellerman et al 1980, Zeltzer et al 1980), there may be many concealed psychosocial problems, e.g. following head injury (Bogan et al 1997). Responses may be more critical in life-threatening diseases, such as leukaemia, which can interrupt normal maturation, prolong dependence and interfere with peer group activities. Treatment refusal may occur as part of an autonomy struggle with parents and staff. The psychiatrist's role involves individual work and provision of explanation and support to parents and staff. Participation in groups of adolescents with similar disorders provides peer support, facilitating adaptation to disability and treatment compliance.

Epilepsy

Accurate diagnosis is essential before any form of psychiatric treatment is undertaken. Social management is particularly important in adolescent onset. Adolescents resent being stigmatised and overprotected and their need for control may lead to refusal of medication. Consideration needs to be given to the effects of anticonvulsants, injuries sustained during seizures and attitudes of family, peers, school staff and employers. Parents require help in reducing anxiety and overprotection, while adolescents need support and guidance in anticipating, reasonably confidently, a fairly normal life. Special psychiatric aspects concern emotional disturbance in temporal lobe disorders and schizophrenia-like psychoses.

Acne

Acne can be associated with intense anxiety, shame, depression and despair, aggravated by inappropriate self-treatment. Sufferers may fail to receive adequate care if the condition is dismissed as a passing teenage problem. Topical treatment, usually with benzoyl peroxide, is generally employed before using antibiotics or retinoids.

Cancer

Increased chances of long-term survival have rapidly changed the pattern of presenting psychological problems in adolescents (Koocher et al 1980). These vary with the type of cancer, sites affected, course and forms of treatment. Feelings of inferiority and difference from peers occur. Painful diagnostic and therapeutic procedures, like biopsies and bone marrow aspirations, and concern about disfigurement and residual cosmetic defects following surgery, cause anxiety. Problematic side-effects of treatment commonly arise from cytotoxic chemotherapy and radiotherapy. Consequences of repeated hospitalisation and treatment include interruption of ordinary peer relations, school absences and boredom and stress in hospital. Worry about uncertain outcome is less problematic than for the parents.

Psychiatric input involves mental state assessment and identification of adjustment difficulties, with treatment emphasis on normalisation and psychosocial rehabilitation. Most worries and conflicts are resolvable by ventilation of feelings and brief, focused help, fostering the adolescent's coping skills and self-help capacity. Specific treatment techniques, e.g. relaxation training and systematic desensitisation, are indicated with depression, procedure-related pain and anxiety and school difficulties. Reaction to adverse cosmetic effects of treatment and persistent maladaptive thinking may necessitate prolonged psychotherapy. The psychiatrist is well placed to work with parents and siblings, and in supporting and training specialist staff, especially those involved in terminal care.

Surgical treatment

Teenagers should receive personal preparation for surgery to reduce preoperative anxiety and distress and aid postoperative adjustment and recovery. Management of postoperative pain is an appropriate area for psychiatric input.

Sensory handicaps

Early-onset deafness interferes with language and speech development, and deaf children and adolescents have increased rates of emotional and behavioural disorders. Undetected partial deafness should be considered in academic underachievement. In assessment and management, principal issues are overcoming communication difficulties and understanding the practical, day-to-day problems of young people and their families (Gregory et al 1995). Rates of psychological problems in visually impaired children and adolescents are also higher than in the general population (Freeman 1977), with 45% showing disorder.

HIV infection and acquired immune deficiency syndrome (AIDS)

There is limited information about HIV seroprevalence rates among adolescents, but approximately 1% of all AIDS cases are adolescent (Hein 1989). Adults suffering from AIDS were often exposed to the virus as teenagers, and many adolescents, particularly runaways and gay males, are exposed to HIV infection by risky sexual behaviour and drug abuse. Young male prostitutes are particularly vulnerable. Although, with improved health education, most teenagers are likely to know that the disease is transmitted by sexual intercourse and reused needles, there may be misconceptions and ignorance. Knowledge about safer sex practices, e.g. abstinence, reduced number of sexual partners and encounters and condom use, is likely to be limited. HIV-infected haemophiliac adolescents, and their distressed parents, present particularly difficult management problems.

Neuropsychiatric features include possible early subacute encephalitis and the AIDS dementia complex (ADC). In adolescents, this may present with impaired attention, concentration and memory, and frontal lobe dysfunction. The infected teenager is susceptible to a wide range of intercurrent infections. The psychiatrist's role in HIV spectrum disease, becoming clarified with increasing clinical experience (Krener & Miller 1989), requires full integration into the multidisciplinary team, with specialised knowledge of the chronic illness (Krener 1991).

EFFECTS OF GENERAL HOSPITALISATION

Despite recommendations for specialised medical adolescent inpatient services, there has been limited development of such resources in Britain. Generally, adolescents requiring hospital treatment are managed in paediatric or adult wards. While technical care may be of a high order, adolescents may encounter problems in both settings in relation to privacy, age-appropriate freedom, involvement in decision making and consent, and understanding and communication by staff lacking specific familiarity with maturational needs (Gillies & Parry-Jones 1992).

LEARNING DISABILITY

Incidence of psychiatric disorders and disturbed behaviour in adolescents with learning disability is higher than in the general population. Diagnostic interviewing needs to be flexible, taking into account effects of limited cognitive capacity on communication and understanding, and direct observation of behaviour is required. Difficulties in assimilating information, experimenting socially and conforming to peer group behaviour, with lack of expressive ability, can leave mentally retarded teenagers isolated and socially rejected. Although disorders resemble those in non-retarded adolescents, there may be diagnostic difficulties, e.g. identifying schizophrenia in the presence of severe disability. A wide range of disturbed behaviour occurs. Violent, aggressive, self-stimulating and self-injurious behaviour is a major concern and constitutes the most frequent reason for pharmacological control. The overriding treatment emphasis is on acceptance and integration in the community and improvement in living skills.

TREATMENT

General principles

Treatment is usually multimodal and flexibility and versatility are crucial. An eclectic approach permits a range of techniques, adapting intervention to individual needs. Psychiatric intervention is necessary only within a small section of the spectrum of adolescent mental health problems and disorders, and input at the point of service delivery frequently requires joint work with other services and agencies. Collaboration is enhanced by familiarity with their functions, resources and practice, and reduction of interprofessional tensions is facilitated by acknowledging the distinctive competences and central role responsibilities of each discipline (Parry-Jones 1986).

Referral reasons are often more concerned with not knowing what to do than with intrinsic disorders. However, clear courses of therapeutic action are rarely available and the risk:benefit ratio of intervention should be considered against likely outcome without treatment. The necessity and timing of psychiatric treatment is controversial, because of difficulties distinguishing healthy behaviour from disorder, but residual ambiguity does not negate intervention. Decisions are essential concerning design and implementation of interventions, treatment adherence, progress monitoring, and termination. Non-adherence to treatment can be a major challenge, and engaging commitment is facilitated by focusing on clearly relevant issues and actions to produce change. Unnecessary prolongation of outpatient contact risks increased dependency and, generally, it is best to withdraw with further progress still to be made.

Therapeutic relationship

Development of trust depends on the therapist's honesty, even-handedness and respect for confidentiality. Being 'tough', expressing negative views or criticism will not necessarily jeopardise good relationships. Difficult decisions, threats of absconding, dropping out of treatment or acting out are best countered by openness and directness. Future appointments need to be clear, with full expectation that they will be kept. Drop-out rates and prematurely terminated treatment is not necessarily higher than with adults. Alleged proclivity to drop out of psychotherapy can often be explained in terms of the therapist's emotional response to unilateral termination and failure to acknowledge adolescent attempts at independence. Follow-up of some non-attenders, especially suicide attempters, is essential.

Location of treatment

Most adolescents are manageable as outpatients, but some treatments need to be home based, e.g. response prevention programmes for OCD. Despite careful definition of selection criteria, inpatient admission has to fulfil diverse purposes (Steinberg 1982). Twenty-four hour observation and assessment is crucial, especially if there is a safety requirement. Residential treatment facilitates initiation and monitoring of intensive techniques which would be impracticable on an outpatient basis. Limited development of day care has been achieved.

Main therapeutic approaches

A wide therapeutic perspective avoids factionalism, resolving the dichotomy between physical and psychodynamic approaches. Rigorous attention should be paid to evidence of evaluative research. Although psychological methods predominate, combined or sequential psychotherapy and pharmacotherapy has to be considered.

Managing emergencies

Prompt response is necessary because disturbed behaviour can be obtrusive and deemed uncontainable in the home, school or neighbourhood. Certain circumstances necessitate urgent intervention, including risk of serious self-harm, acute alcohol or drug intoxication, aggressive and violent behaviour, absconding and homelessness (Steinberg 1989). Clinical emergencies may be precipitated by acute psychotic episodes, severe mood disturbances and acute stress reactions.

The priority is ensuring the safety of the adolescent and others. General or psychiatric hospitalisation, or an alternative place of safety, may be indicated and time-limited crisis intervention should be provided utilising rapid assessment and focused, flexible, short-term strategies. Adolescents and families are more amenable to therapeutic intervention following unexpected hospitalisation, violence, attempted suicide or family breakdown.

Ethical and legal issues

Rigorous confidentiality needs to be maintained. Clarification of authority for intervention is important, since few adolescents seek help themselves. Whenever possible, the adolescent's full agreement should be obtained (see above). Parental agreement is desirable with young people of any age, but alternative authority may be derived from a Care Order, whereby the local authority has parental responsibility, the Mental Health Act, 1983 or the Mental Health (Scotland) Act, 1984. Consent has to be based on detailed explanation of what treatment entails. Special issues arise in family therapy: for example, involvement of family members, not registered as patients, in a way amounting to personal treatment; the use of personally disturbing procedures; and failure to provide adequate explanation of strategies and a range of treatment options. Meticulous clarification of the reasons for intervention and definition of the participative basis of family members is essential.

Transfer to adult services

This should be planned carefully, with attention to the timing, allowing opportunity for the patient, relatives and staff to adjust to the transition. Limited resources in some adolescent units necessitate temporary admission of violent or self-destructive patients to adult wards. Such transfers are usually urgent and well-established links with adult services forestall difficulties.

Psychological and social treatments

Professional relationships with patients and families

Intervention involves staff of different disciplines and experience and psychotherapies need to be eclectic and flexible. Staff may experience anxiety, ambivalence, irritation and anger in handling disturbed adolescents, and establishing emotional empathy may be difficult. Constructive use of dependency problems is often avoided by staff, who are trained to steer clear of becoming 'overinvolved'. Particular problems may arise between parents and staff, who may appear to blame or depreciate the parents, and flaunt easy relationships with previously uncommunicative or oppositional teenagers. Staff need opportunities to acknowledge difficulties, with skilled support and supervision.

Individual work

The best received approach is likely to be brief, focused intervention, with short-term goals concerned with problem solving and developing and maintaining a sense of control. This recognises that, for many adolescents, talking about intimate feelings is an unaccustomed task, whereas 'action-oriented' techniques are more acceptable. Treatment of silent, non-productive adolescents poses a serious challenge.

Insight-oriented psychotherapy requires consideration of the teenager's capacity to verbalise thoughts and feelings and think conceptually. Some psychotherapists doubt the treatability of certain adolescent disorders from a psychoanalytic viewpoint, favouring other supportive and educational techniques to avoid unforeseen failures or aggravation. Transference issues can present problems, especially in multidisciplinary residential settings. Integrating different forms of psychotherapy makes treatment more specific to problems and development, e.g. individual psychodynamic and behavioural methods in eating disorders or behavioural and family techniques in OCD. Current adolescent psychotherapy lacks empirical demonstration of efficacy, tending to display an expectation that benefits can be taken on trust.

Limit setting and control

Limit setting is important in staff adolescent relationships and the need for clear boundaries requires therapeutic use of authority in management. Deficient authority, evident in the lives of many adolescents, occurs symptomatically, for example in school non-attendance and limit-testing antisocial behaviour. As part of a phase of treatment, assertion of authority can enable the re-establishment of a school routine or regaining healthy weight.

Younger staff may experience difficulties in being authoritative, fearful of jeopardising good relationships built on an 'equal footing' basis. In residential units, adolescents are likely to regard the staff as more restrictive and less tolerant than the staff views itself. Parents need to see staff use of authority as complementing, not usurping, their control.

Small group work

Group work is used frequently, especially as an adjunct to therapeutic community participation. It poses special problems for the therapist and there is little information about outcome, indications and contraindications, or selection criteria. Emphasis on action, rather than introspection, encourages structured activities, such as role play. Once alliance is established, attachments and differences can emerge and individuals share common experiences and practice interaction in a supportive environment. Indiscriminate inclusion of patients in open groups has limited clinical justification. Group therapy may benefit youngsters who are difficult to engage individually, with interpersonal problems or showing withdrawal and isolation, and the chronically physically ill.

Therapeutic communities

It is questionable how far the ethos of the adult therapeutic community is transferable to adolescent work, requiring control and leadership, but the principles have found application in many residential training and therapeutic institutions (Parry-Jones 1998). Evaluation is difficult, but the method appears most beneficial for long-stay, homogeneous populations. However, this would restrict the diversity of patient intake and pace of treatment necessary for effective general-purpose units.

Behavioural and cognitive therapies

There is considerable scope for behavioural therapy in disorders, such as obsessional states and single phobias, either alone or with other treatments (Werry & Wollersheim 1989). Reported use of cognitive therapy with adolescents is growing and experience suggests its usefulness in depression, anxiety and panic disorder. Use of self-monitoring and behavioural assignments appeals to young patients. Self-instructional training can be used with adolescents with deficits in self-control, who are impulsive, attention disordered, disobedient and aggressive (Kendall & Braswell 1985).

Anxiety management training

Anxiety management combines relaxation training, symptom explanation and techniques for controlling intrusive anxious thoughts. The latter is achieved by distraction or by repeating reassurance to neutralise their content.

Social skills training

Approaches involving instruction, role play, modelling and feedback are particularly appropriate and successful with adolescents. Despite considerable face value appeal, evidence about long-term effectiveness remains limited, with few evaluative studies (Hansen et al 1989).

Self-management

Many adolescent treatment procedures are adaptable for self-management, making them more acceptable and enjoyable, enhancing a sense of personal responsibility. It applies particularly to behavioural approaches, such as self-directed response prevention in OCD (Brigham 1989).

Creative and experiential therapies

Therapeutic use of art ranges from opportunities for recreation and disinhibition, to psychotherapy (Merry 1986). Using role play to clarify feelings and behaviour, or rehearse new responses, is constructive. Psychodrama is generally a group activity and, like sculpting and role play, requires experienced leadership (Wynn 1986). Various exercises and activities are used for enhancing the sense of belonging within groups, promotion of responsibility, trust and self-esteem. Long-term benefits, however, are unproven.

Parental and family work

Intervention with parents or families needs planning in the light of the overall diagnostic formulation, since elaborate family involvement is not always appropriate. Time allocated to the adolescent, the parents, or the whole, or part, family group requires careful balancing. Most adolescents accept family interviews as an appropriate medium for issues impinging on all family members. This permits separate sessions with the adolescent and parents, preserving privacy of personal disclosures. The form of conjoint intervention should match the stage reached in the adolescent–parent relationship, acknowledging the changing balance of responsibility and independence. With all adolescents, it is appropriate to emphasise responsibility for their own thoughts,

feelings and actions. Despite expectation of increasing acceptance of adult responsibilities, the inevitable ambiguity of this transitional stage generates adjustment difficulties for both parties.

Intervention with parents

Parents play a key part in supporting treatment and as agents of change. Intervention with parents has to be differentiated from family therapy, parent education and marital therapy. This approach emphasises the appropriate and adaptive development of parenting and the modification of attitudes and responses to the adolescent's behaviour, especially where they perpetuate dysfunction.

Parental willingness and capacity to form a treatment alliance needs evaluation. Knowledge of individual and marital histories clarifies the relationship between parenting styles and the parents' personal and developmental difficulties. Intervention objectives need to be agreed, with an explicit focus on parenting, not individual psychopathology. Parental attitudes towards adolescence require exploration. It may be viewed negatively, as a period to be endured until the young person is old enough to pursue adult life. At a personal level, earlier painful feelings and unresolved conflicts may be aroused. At the interpersonal level, implications of adolescent detachment for the marital relationship may be problematic and counselling may be indicated. Regarding the adolescent's capacity for emancipation, there may be separation-inducing perceptions and expectations, conveying confidence in the ability to grow and become independent, or separation-inhibiting perceptions, conveying lack of confidence.

Exercise of parental authority and control may be the principal therapeutic focus in parent–adolescent conflict and estrangement. Some degree of challenge and confrontation is appropriate to adolescent maturation and need not be seen as a personal assault by parents, especially at a time of reappraisal in their own lives. A positive view of adolescence, as a creative force in the family, is encouraging, and parental morale and successful coping has to be fostered. Individual or couple therapy should be arranged formally, or referral made to other services.

Family-based treatments

The most commonly used forms are psychodynamic methods, structural or strategic family therapy, behavioural methods and various eclectic approaches which represent typical practice in adolescent psychiatry (Will & Wrate 1985, Barker 1986). A problem-oriented method, with pragmatic objectives, benefits from greater flexibility and is particularly suitable in issues regularly precipitating family conflict. Identifying reciprocal changes and planning their implementation provides a model for family negotiation and communication. There are insufficient scientific grounds for an exclusively family-oriented approach. Evidence is weak for causal links between observable family interaction and presenting adolescent psychopathology, and there has been limited evaluation of family-based treatments (Diamond et al 1996). Adolescent disorder is infrequently best understood in terms of family psychopathology, although family factors can precipitate, exacerbate or maintain problems in predisposed individuals. Particular indications include issues specific to adoption and divorce. In the selection of family-based treatments there has to be full awareness of positive and negative aspects.

Physical treatments

Psychopharmacology in adolescence

There is limited information about the use and response to psychotropic drugs (Campbell et al 1985). Licensing restrictions, applying to marketing of psychotropic drugs for children, are unclear regarding adolescents, but use has been limited on ideological grounds and from fear of side-effects. There is scope for the judicious use of some drugs, avoiding polypharmacy (Rosenberg et al 1994).

Consent and compliance

Oral or written consent should be obtained, based on information about the respective risks and benefits with, and without, medication. To promote compliance, adolescents need active engagement and information about expected changes and monitoring.

Psychotropic medication

Anxiolytics, sedatives and hypnotics Although safe and effective for brief administration, prolonged use of benzodiazepines produces adverse effects. There is no place for the use of barbiturates and it is rarely necessary to prescribe hypnotics. Beta blockers are indicated in the short-term treatment of anxiety with prominent autonomic symptoms.

Anticholinergics and antihistamines There is no evidence that these drugs warrant a place in adolescent treatment, apart from the use of anticholinergic drugs in treating acute dystonic and parkinsonian effects of antipsychotic drugs.

Antidepressants The current view, based largely on uncontrolled studies, is that antidepressants are less effective in adolescent than in adult depression (Ryan 1990). There is evidence, for example, that despite a wide range of plasma levels, imipramine is not an effective antidepressant in adolescent major depression (Ryan et al 1986). With careful identification of target symptoms, however, medication may prove useful. Relatively little is known about adolescent response to antidepressants and suggested usage relies on adult data. Imipramine and amitriptyline have ceased to be standard antidepressants for this age group, especially since the SSRIs, such as fluoxetine and fluvoxamine, have fewer side-effects and a better safety profile. The latter are reported to be effective in OCD. Dietary precautions with monoamine oxidase inhibitors make them unsuitable for adolescents. Baseline measurements of blood pressure and pulse rate should be recorded before administration, with an electrocardiogram and continued ECG monitoring, especially using tricyclics, because of the known cardiotoxicity of tricyclic antidepressants. Monitoring of antidepressant plasma levels is unlikely to be useful clinically.

Psychostimulants Dextroamphetamine and methylphenidate hydrochloride are used in the treatment of hyperactivity in children, but there have been fewer studies of their effects in adolescents. In the latter, there is risk of abuse and dependence, and the possibility of reduction in growth velocity (Biederman 1988).

Neuroleptics There is no contraindication to the use of the phenothiazines and butyrophenones in psychotic states, the guidelines being those applicable to adults. Side-effects, particularly acute dystonic reactions, tardive and withdrawal dyskinesia and neuroleptic malignant syndrome are the main concern. Use of neuroleptics for behaviour problems and aggressiveness remains controversial and is to be discouraged or applied selectively.

Lithium It is appropriate to consider the use of lithium treatment for bipolar disorder (Kafantaris 1995), with close cooperation between doctor, patient and family ensuring compliance. Treatment may produce hypothyroidism, but current lower lithium doses and serum levels generate fewer side-effects (Ch. 4).

Anticonvulsants Additional to seizure control, anticonvulsants have been employed in treatment of behaviour disorders. Carbamazepine is most widely used, but its benefit in hyperactivity, aggression and impulsivity awaits assessment.

Electroconvulsive therapy

There have been few studies of the use of ECT in adolescents and, currently, attitudes towards its use are likely to be unfavourable. It is rarely indicated, except in severe, prolonged major depression or uncontrolled mania (Bertagnoli & Borchardt 1990).

RESIDENTIAL TREATMENT AND CARE

Psychiatric inpatient hospital treatment

The optimal role of inpatient units has remained controversial, because of the potential diversity of admission policies and therapeutic regimens. The NHS Health Advisory Service (1986) clarified the nature of the required residential service, emphasising the benefits of general-purpose units. Clinical practice in such units is demanding and stressful, the organisation of interdisciplinary work is complex, and maintenance of a stable therapeutic ethos requires perceptive management (Steinberg 1986). In the UK, changes in the organisation of the NHS have imposed new pressures on the viability of inpatient units (Parry-Jones 1995). Nevertheless, guidelines for health service commissioning authorities emphasise the fact that young people under 16 years should only exceptionally be accommodated in adult wards (NHS Health Advisory Service 1995). Future planning needs to consider the range of poorly delineated demands relating to the care of disturbed adolescents, and current lack of uniformity in the organisation of residential services, causing gaps and unplanned overlap (Parry-Jones 1996b).

Reasons for referral and selection criteria

Reasons for referral reflect differing views about the function of hospitalisation and admission policies of individual units. The latter may be unclear because units are small, highly selective, operate outside mainstream psychiatry and have infrequent use by general practitioners, adult psychiatrists and paediatricians. The varied needs of hospital referrals include educational appraisal, care, control and provision of a safe place, diagnostic assessment, treatment and further work with involved adults (Steinberg 1982). These relate to identifiable psychiatric disorder and unmanageable behaviour, of which the latter is not necessarily within the scope of the psychiatric service, whose principal resource is 24 hour medical and nursing care.

Operational policies vary widely in relation to treatment and length of stay. Hospitalisation cannot provide the definitive treatment and, wherever possible, intervention should be focused on the changes necessary for short stay. All patients should be assessed prior to admission and intervention decisions related to the definite, or possible, presence of individual psychiatric disorder unequivocally requiring 24 hour nursing and medical care. Highly selective admission policies, in short-stay, general-purpose units, possessing inadequate staffing and secure facilities, have limited provision for severely disturbed adolescents. Local authority resources for 'difficult to place' patients have diminished, and demand for places in youth treatment centres exceeds availability.

Therapeutic objectives and outcome

Hospitalisation should be undertaken with great discrimination so that the therapeutic objectives are clearly defined. Most inpatient units operate a general purpose approach, with diverse, individually planned treatments, in an institutional setting providing a therapeutic living experience. Attempts to simplify the situation, by adopting single-treatment approaches, e.g. the therapeutic community, or by limiting disorders treated, can have serious implications where one unit serves a large population. Sometimes, attention is directed at problems necessitating admission or one focal problem (Harper 1989). The short-term treatment model is employed increasingly.

Duration of stay is influenced by the severity and treatment resistance of disorders, non-clinical factors, e.g. deficiency of alternative placements, and by different ideological approaches to hospitalisation. If the objective is to make a diagnosis, control symptoms and review treatment, short admission is appropriate. Lengthy admission is inevitable, however, if substantial psychodynamic and personality changes are sought.

Adolescent inpatient care carries the added burden of promoting normal development, although this does not necessarily militate against hospitalisation designed primarily for symptom control. While brief hospitalisation is advocated, there is a group of highly resistant, disturbed adolescents requiring lengthy inpatient care. Despite disadvantages created by a small number of long-stay patients in a short-stay unit, this arrangement may be inevitable, in the absence of more appropriate accommodation.

There have been several outcome studies (Ainsworth 1984, Turner et al 1986, Rothery et al 1995) and consumer surveys (Wells et al 1978, Pyne et al 1986), although research and audit represent a lesser concern than the demands of clinical work, consultation and administration. This is of major significance in adolescent psychiatry, as evidence-based knowledge remains limited, causative models controversial and treatment largely empirical. Further, while scope for cost–benefit evaluation of mental health care is extensive, its application in adolescent psychiatry has been negligible (Knapp 1997).

REFERENCES

Achenbach T M 1991 Manual for the child behaviour checklist/4-18 and 1991 profile. University of Vermont Department of Psychiatry, Burlington

Ainsworth P 1984 The first 100 admissions to a regional general purpose adolescent unit. Journal of Adolescence 7: 337–348

Allsopp M, Verduyn C 1989 A follow-up of adolescents with obsessive–compulsive disorder. British Journal of Psychiatry 154: 829–834

Anders T F, Eiben L A 1996 Pediatric sleep disorders: a review of the last 10 years. Journal of the American Academy of Child and Adolescent Psychiatry 36: 9–20

Angold A 1989 Structured assessments of psychopathology in children and adolescents. In: Thompson C (ed) The instruments of psychiatric research. Wiley, Chichester, pp 271–304

Ashton C H 1990 Solvent abuse. British Medical Journal 300: 135–136

Bancroft J, Reinisch J M 1990 Adolescence and puberty. Oxford University Press, Oxford

Barker P 1986 Basic family therapy. Blackwell, Oxford

Barkley R A, Fisher M, Edelbrock C S, Smallish L 1990 The adolescent outcome of hyperactive children diagnosed by research criteria. I. An 8-year prospective follow-up study. Journal of the American Academy of Child and Adolescent Psychiatry 29: 546–557

Berg I 1985 The management of truancy. Journal of Child Psychology and Psychiatry 26: 325–331

Berg I 1991 School avoidance, school phobia, and truancy. In: Lewis M (ed) Child and adolescent psychiatry. A comprehensive text book. Williams & Wilkins, Baltimore, pp 1092–1098

Bernstein D P, Cohen P, Velez C N, Schwab-Stone M, Siever L J, Shinsato L 1993 Prevalence and stability of the DSM-IIIR personality disorders in a community-based survey of adolescents. American Journal of Psychiatry 30: 43–50

Bertagnoli M W, Borchardt C M 1990 A review of ECT for children and adolescents. Journal of the American Academy of Child and Adolescent Psychiatry 29: 302–307

Besag V 1989 Bullies and victims in schools. Open University Press, Milton Keynes

Biederman J 1988 Pharmacologic treatment of adolescents with affective disorders and attention deficit disorder. Pharmacological Bulletin 24: 81–87

Bogan A, Livingston M, Parry-Jones W Ll, Buston K, Wood S 1997 The experiential impact of head injury on adolescents: individual perspectives on long-term outcome. Brain Injury 11: 431–443

Bolton D, Collins S, Steinberg D 1983 The treatment of obsessive compulsive disorders in adolescence: a report of 15 cases. British Journal of Psychiatry 142: 456–466

Boyle M H, Offord D R, Racine Y et al 1993 Evaluation of the diagnostic interview for children and adolescents for use in general population samples. Journal of Abnormal Child Psychology 21: 663–681

Brandenburg N A, Friedman R M, Silver S E 1990 The epidemiology of childhood psychiatric disorders: prevalence findings from recent studies. Journal of the American Academy of Child and Adolescent Psychiatry 29: 76–83

Brent D A 1997 Practitioner review: The aftercare of adolescents with deliberate self-harm. Journal of Child Psychology and Psychiatry 38: 277–286

Brigham T A 1989 Self-management for adolescents: a skills training programme. Guilford Press, Hove

Brooksbank D 1984 Management of conversion reaction in five adolescent girls. Journal of Adolescence 7: 359–376

Campbell M, Green W H, Deutsch S I 1985 Child and adolescent psychopharmacology. Sage, London

Carlson G A 1990 Child and adolescent mania – diagnostic considerations. Journal of Child Psychology and Psychiatry 31: 331–341

Carlson G A, Cantwell D P 1980 Unmasking masked depression in children and adolescents. American Journal of Psychiatry 137: 445–449

Carlson G A, Kashani J H 1988 Manic symptoms in a non-referral adolescent population. Journal of Affective Disorders 15: 219–226

Carskadon M A, Dement W C 1987 Sleepiness in the normal adolescent. In: Guilleminault C (ed) Sleep and its disorders in children. Raven Press, New York, pp 53–66

Chadwick O, Anderson R, Bland M, Ramsay J 1989 Neuropsychological consequences of volatile substance abuse: a population based study of secondary school pupils. British Medical Journal 298: 1679–1684

Cohen D J, Brunn R D, Leckman J F (eds) 1988 Tourette's syndrome and tic disorders. Wiley, New York

Coleman J C, Hendry L 1990 The nature of adolescence, 2nd edn. Routledge, London

Conners C K, Barkley R A 1985 Rating scales and checklists for child psychopharmacology. Psychopharmacology Bulletin 21: 809–815

Costello E J 1989 Developments in child psychiatric epidemiology. Journal of the American Academy of Child and Adolescent Psychiatry 28: 836–841

Diamond G S, Serrano A C, Dickey M, Sonis W A 1996 Current status of family-based outcome and process research. Journal of the American Academy of Child and Adolescent Psychiatry 35: 6–16

DiGallo A, Barton J, Parry-Jones W Ll 1997 Road traffic accidents; early psychological consequences in children and adolescents. British Journal of Psychiatry 170: 358–362

Egan J 1986 Etiology and treatment of borderline personality disorder in adolescents. Hospital and Community Psychiatry 37: 613–618

Eminson M, Benjamin S, Shortall A, Woods T, Faragher B 1996 Physical symptoms and illness attitudes in adolescents: an epidemiological study. Journal of Child Psychology and Psychiatry 37: 519–528

Endicott J, Spitzer R L 1978 A diagnostic interview: the schedule for affective disorders and schizophrenia. Archives of General Psychiatry 35: 837–844

Eth S, Pynoos R (eds) 1985 Post-traumatic stress disorder in children. American Psychiatric Press, Washington, DC

Fairburn C G, Beglin S J 1990 Studies of the epidemiology of bulimia nervosa. American Journal of Psychiatry 147: 401–408

Farrington D P 1995 The development of offending and antisocial behaviour from childhood: key findings from Cambridge study in delinquent development. Journal of Child Psychology and Psychiatry

Flament M F, Whitaker A, Rapoport J et al 1988 Obsessive compulsive disorder in adolescence. Journal of the American Academy of Child and Adolescent Psychiatry 27: 764–771

Fosson A, Knibbs J, Bryant-Waugh R, Lask B 1987 Early onset anorexia nervosa. Archives of Disease in Childhood 62: 114–118

Freeman R D 1977 Psychiatric aspects of sensory disorders

and intervention. In: Graham P J (ed) Epidemiological approaches in child psychiatry. Academic Press, London, pp 275–304

Friedman A S, Glickman N W 1986 Program characteristics for successful treatment of adolescent drug abuse. Journal of Nervous and Mental Disorders 174: 669–679

Garralda M E 1985 Characteristics of the psychoses of late onset in children and adolescents (a comparative study of hallucinating children). Journal of Adolescence 8: 195–207

Gillies M, Parry-Jones W Ll 1992 Suitability of the paediatric setting for hospitalised adolescents. Archives of Disease in Childhood 67: 1506–1509

Goodyer I M (ed) 1995 The depressed child and adolescent: developmental and clinical perspectives. Cambridge University Press, Cambridge

Green R 1987 The 'sissy boy syndrome' and the development of homosexuality. Yale University Press, New Haven, CT

Gregory S, Bishop J, Sheldon L 1995 Deaf young people and their families. Cambridge University Press, Cambridge

Griffiths M D 1990 The acquisition, development and maintenance of fruit machine gambling in adolescents. Journal of Gambling Studies 6: 193–204

Gutterman E M, O'Brien J D, Young J G 1987 Structured diagnostic interviews for children and adolescents: current status and future directions. Journal of the American Academy of Child and Adolescent Psychiatry 26: 621–630

Hansen D J, Watson-Perczel M, Christopher J C 1989 Clinical issues in social-skills training with adolescents. Clinical Psychology Review 9: 363–391

Harper G 1989 Focal inpatient treatment planning. Journal of the American Academy of Child and Adolescent Psychiatry 28: 31–37

Hawker A 1978 Adolescents and alcohol. Edsall, London

Hawton K 1986 Suicide and attempted suicide among children and adolescents. Gaskell, London

Hawton K, O'Grady J, Osborn M, Cole D 1982 Adolescents who take overdoses: their characteristics, problems and contacts with helping agencies. British Journal of Psychiatry 140: 118–123

Hein K 1989 AIDS in adolescence: a response to the challenge. Journal of Adolescent Health Care 10: 510–536

Horowitz M J, Wilner N, Alvarez W 1979 Impact of event scale: a measure of subjective stress. Psychosomatic Medicine 41: 209–218

Jacobson R 1985a Child firesetters: a clinical investigation. Journal of Child Psychology and Psychiatry 26: 759–768

Jacobson R 1985b The subclassification of child firesetters. Journal of Child Psychology and Psychiatry 26: 769–775

Kafantaris V 1995 Treatment of bipolar disorder in children and adolescents. Journal of the American Academy of Child and Adolescent Psychiatry 34: 732–741

Kashani J H, Carlson G A, Beck N C 1987 Depression, depressive symptoms, and depressed mood among a community sample of adolescents. American Journal of Psychiatry 144: 931–934

Kazdin A E 1995 Conduct disorders in childhood and adolescence, 2nd edn. Sage, Beverley Hills

Kellerman J, Zeltzer L, Ellenberg L, Dash J, Rigler D 1980 Psychological effects of illness in adolescence. I. Anxiety, self-esteem, and perception of control. Journal of Pediatrics 97: 126–131

Kendall P C, Braswell L 1985 Cognitive-behavioral therapy for impulsive children. Guilford Press, New York

Knapp M 1997 Economic evaluations and interventions for children and adolescents with mental health problems. Journal of Child Psychology and Psychiatry 38: 3–25

Koocher G P, O'Malley J E, Gogan J L, Foster D J 1980 Psychological adjustment among pediatric cancer survivors. Journal of Child Psychology and Psychiatry 21: 163–173

Kovacs M, Paulanskas S, Gatsonis C, Richards C 1988 Depressive disorders in childhood III. A longitudinal study of comorbidity with and risk for conduct disorders. Journal of Affective Disorders 15: 205–217

Krener P G 1991 HIV-spectrum disease. In: Lewis M (ed) Child and adolescent psychiatry. A comprehensive textbook. Williams & Wilkins, Baltimore, pp 994–1004

Krener P G, Miller F B 1989 Psychiatric response to HIV spectrum disease in children and adolescents. Journal of the American Academy of Child and Adolescent Psychiatry 28: 596–605

Kumra S, Frazier J A, Jacobsen L K et al 1996 Childhood-onset schizophrenia. A double-blind clozapine–haloperidol comparison. Archives of General Psychiatry 53: 1090–1097

Kydd R R, Werry J S 1982 Schizophrenia in children under sixteen years. Journal of Autism and Developmental Disorders 12: 343–357

Leckman J F, Bradley S P, Anderson G M, Arnsten A F T, Pauls D L, Cohen D J 1997 Pathogenesis of Tourette's syndrome. Journal of Child Psychology and Psychiatry 38: 119–142

Leonard H, Swedo S, Rapoport J, Coltey M, Cheslow D 1988 Treatment of childhood obsessive-compulsive disorder with clomipramine and desmethylimipramine: a double-blind cross-over comparison. Psychopharmacological Bulletin 24: 93–95

Lewis M, Volkmar F R (eds) 1990 Clinical aspects of child and adolescent development, 3rd edn. Lea & Febiger, Philadelphia

Ludolph P S, Westen D, Misle B, Jackson A, Wixom J, Wiss F C 1990 The borderline diagnosis in adolescents: symptoms and developmental history. American Journal of Psychiatry 147:470–476

Lyons J A 1987 Post-traumatic stress disorder in children and adolescents. A review of the literature. Journal of Developmental and Behavioral Pediatrics 18: 349–356

McAdam E 1986 Cognitive behaviour therapy and its application with adolescents. Journal of Adolescence 9: 1–15

March J S 1995 Cognitive-behavioural psychotherapy for children and adolescents with OCD: a review and recommendations for treatment. Journal of the American Academy of Child and Adolescent Psychiatry 34: 7–18

Marsh A, Dobbs J, White A 1986 Adolescent drinking. HMSO, London

Masterton G 1979 The management of solvent abuse. Journal of Adolescence 2: 65–75

Merry J 1986 Art in the education of the disturbed adolescent. In: Steinberg D (ed) The adolescent unit. Wiley, Chichester, pp 43–51

NHS Health Advisory Service 1986 Bridges over troubled waters. HMSO, London

NHS Health Advisory Service 1995 Together we stand. The commissioning, role and management of child and adolescent mental health services. HMSO, London

Orvaschel H 1985 Psychiatric interviews suitable for research with children and adolescents. Psychopharmacology Bulletin 21: 737–746

Parry-Jones W Ll 1986 Multidisciplinary teamwork: help or hindrance? In: Steinberg D (ed) The adolescent unit. Wiley, Chichester, pp 193–200

Parry-Jones W Ll 1988 Obesity in children and adolescents. In: Burrows G D, Beumont P J V, Casper R C (eds)

Handbook of eating disorders, part 2. Obesity. Elsevier, Amsterdam, pp 207–219

Parry-Jones W Ll 1991 Target weight in children and adolescents with anorexia nervosa. Acta Paediatrica Scandinavica Supplementum 373: 82–90

Parry-Jones W Ll 1992 Adolescent psychoses: treatment and service provision. Archives of Disease in Childhood 66: 1459–1462

Parry-Jones W Ll 1994 History of child and adolescent psychiatry. In: Rutter M, Hersov L, Taylor E (eds) Child and adolescent psychiatry, modern approaches, 3rd edn. Blackwell, Oxford

Parry-Jones W Ll 1995 The future of adolescent psychiatry. British Journal of Psychiatry 166: 299–305

Parry-Jones W Ll 1996a Interventions and treatments In: Black D, Newman N, Mezey G, Harris Hendriks J (eds) Psychological trauma: a developmental approach. Gaskell, London, pp 230–234

Parry-Jones W Ll 1996b Adolescent psychiatric services: development and expansion. In: Hendriks J H, Black M (eds) Child and adolescent psychiatry: a new century. OP 33. Royal College of Psychiatrists, London, pp 86–93

Parry-Jones W Ll 1997 Adolescents. In: Detels R, Holland W W, McEwen J, Omenn G S (eds) Oxford Textbook of Public Health. Vol 3: The practice of public health. Oxford University Press, Oxford, pp 1397–1413

Parry-Jones W Ll 1998 Historical introduction. In: Green J, Jacobs B (eds) The inpatient child psychiatric treatment of children. Routledge, London

Petersen B S 1995 Neuroimaging in child and adolescent neuropsychiatric disorders. Journal of the American Academy of Child and Adolescent Psychiatry 34: 1560–1576

Puig-Antich J 1986 Psychobiological markers: effects of age and puberty. In: Rutter M, Izard C E, Read P B (eds) Depression in young people: developmental and clinical perspectives. Guilford Press, New York, pp 341–381

Pyne N, Morrison R, Ainsworth P 1986 A consumer survey of an adolescent unit. Journal of Adolescence 9: 63–72

Pynoos R S, Eth S 1986 Witness to violence: the child interview. Journal of the American Academy of Child Psychiatry 25: 306–319

Quay H C 1983 A dimensional approach to behaviour disorder: the revised behaviour problem checklist. School Psychology Review 12: 244–249

Ramsey J, Anderson H R, Bloor, K, Flanagan R J 1989 An introduction to the practice, prevalence and chemical toxicology of volatile substance abuse. Human Toxicology 8: 261–269

Rapoport J L 1989 Obsessive compulsive disorder in children and adolescents. American Psychiatric Press, New York

Remschmidt H E, Schulz E, 1995 Psychopharmacology of depressive dates in childhood and adolescence. In: Goodyer I M (ed) The depressed child and adolescent: developmental and clinical perspectives. Cambridge University Press, Cambridge, pp 253–279

Remschmidt H E, Schulz E, Martin M, Warnke A, Trott G-E 1994 Childhood-onset schizophrenia: history of the concept and recent studies. Schizophrenia Bulletin 20: 727–745

Reynolds C R, Richmond B O 1978 What I think and feel. A revised measure of children's manifest anxiety. Journal of Abnormal Child Psychology 6: 271–280

Riddle M A, Scahill L, King R A et al 1992 Double-blind, crossover trial of fluoxetine and placebo in children and adolescents with obsessive compulsive disorder. Journal of

the American Academy of Child and Adolescent Psychiatry 31: 1062–1069

Robins L N 1978 Sturdy childhood predictors of adult antisocial behaviour: replications from longitudinal studies. Psychological Medicine 8: 611–622

Robins L N 1991 Conduct disorder. Journal of Child Psychology and Psychiatry 32: 193–212

Rosenberg D R, Holttum J, Gershon S 1994 Textbook of pharmacotherapy for child and adolescent psychiatric disorders. Brunner Mazel, New York

Rothery D J, Wrate R M, McCabe R J R et al 1995 Treatment goal-planning: outcome findings of a British prospective multi-centre study of adolescent in-patient units. European Child and Adolescent Psychiatry 4: 209–221

Russell G F M, Szmukler G I, Dare C, Eisler I 1987 An evaluation of family therapy in anorexia nervosa and bulimia nervosa. Archives of General Psychiatry 44: 1047–1056

Rutter M 1986 The developmental psychopathology of depression: issues and perspectives. In: Rutter M, Izard C E, Read P B (eds) Depression in young people: developmental and clinical perspectives. Guilford Press, New York, pp 3–30

Rutter M 1987 Temperament, personality and personality disorder. British Journal of Psychiatry 150: 443–458

Rutter M 1989 Annotation: child psychiatric disorders in ICD-10. Journal of Child Psychology and Psychiatry 30: 499–513

Rutter M, Giller H 1983 Juvenile delinquency: trends and perspectives. Guilford Press, New York

Rutter M, Graham P, Chadwick O, Yule W 1976 Adolescent turmoil: fact or fiction. Journal of Child Psychology and Psychiatry 17: 35–56

Ryan N D 1990 Heterocyclic antidepressants in children and adolescents. Journal of Child and Adolescent Psychopharmacology 1: 21–31

Ryan N D, Puig-Antich J, Cooper T B et al 1986 Imipramine in adolescent major depression: plasma level and clinical response. Acta Psychiatrica Scandinavica 73: 275–288

Shaffer D, Pettigrew A, Wolkind S, Zajicek E 1978 Psychiatric aspects of pregnancy in schoolgirls: a review. Psychological Medicine 8: 119–130

Solomon Y, Farrand J 1996 'Why don't you do it properly?' Young women who self-injure. Journal of Adolescence 19: 111–119

Steinberg D 1982 Treatment, training, care or control? The functions of adolescent units. British Journal of Psychiatry 141: 306–309

Steinberg D (ed) 1986 The adolescent unit: work and teamwork in adolescent psychiatry. Wiley, Chichester

Steinberg D 1989 Management of crises and emergencies. In: Hsu L K G, Hersen M (eds) Recent developments in adolescent psychiatry. Wiley, New York, pp 87–114

Steinhausen H-C 1997 Annotation: Outcome of anorexia nervosa in the younger patient. Journal of Child Psychology and Psychiatry 38: 271–276.

Terr L 1991 Childhood traumas: an outline and overview. American Journal of Psychiatry 148: 10–20

Tomb D A 1991 The runaway adolescent. In: Lewis M (ed) Child and adolescent psychiatry. A comprehensive textbook. Williams & Wilkins, Baltimore, pp 1066–1071

Turner T H, Dessetor D R, Bates R E 1986 The early outcome of admission to an adolescent unit: a report on 100 cases. Journal of Adolescence 9: 367–382

Tyrer P J 1988 Personality disorders: diagnosis, management and course. Wright, Bristol

Watson J M 1986 Solvent abuse: the adolescent epidemic? Croom Helm, London

Wells P G, Morris A, Jones R M, Allen D J 1978 An adolescent unit assessed: a consumer survey. British Journal of Psychiatry 132: 300–308

Werry J S, Wollersheim J P 1989 Behaviour therapy with children and adolescents: a twenty-year overview. Journal of the American Academy of Child and Adolescent Psychiatry 28: 1–18

Will D, Wrate R M 1985 Integrated family therapy. A problem centred psychodynamic approach. Tavistock, London

Williams R A, Feibelman N D, Moulder C 1989 Events precipitating hospital treatment of adolescent drug abusers. Journal of the American Academy of Child and Adolescent Psychiatry 28: 70–73

Wolff S, Cull A 1986 'Schizoid' personality and antisocial conduct: a retrospective case note study. Psychological Medicine 16: 677–687

Wood A, Harrington R, Moore A 1996 Controlled trial of a brief cognitive-behavioural intervention in adolescent patients with depressive disorders. Journal of Child Psychology and Psychiatry 37: 737–746

Woodroffe C, Glickman M, Barker M, Power C 1993 Children, teenagers and health. The key data. Open University Press, Buckingham, pp 149–151

Wynn B 1986 Creative therapy. In: Steinberg D (ed) The adolescent unit. Wiley, Chichester, pp 73–82

Youngerman J, Canino I 1978 Lithium carbonate use in children and adolescents. Archives of General Psychiatry 35: 216–224

Yule W, Williams R M 1990 Post-traumatic stress reactions in children. Journal of Traumatic Stress 3: 279–295

Zanarini M C 1989 Childhood experiences of borderline patients. Comprehensive Psychiatry 30: 18–25

Zeltzer L, Kellerman J, Ellenberg L, Dash J, Rigler D 1980 Psychological effects of illness in adolescence. II. Impact of illness in adolescents – crucial issues and coping styles. Journal of Pediatrics 97: 132–138

Zeitlin H 1986 The natural history of psychiatric disorders in children. Oxford University Press, Oxford

Zucker K J 1990 Treatment of gender-identity disorders in children. In: Blanchard R, Steiner B W (eds) Clinical management of gender-identity disorders in children and adults. American Psychiatric Press, Washington, DC, pp 1–23

Zucker K J, Green R 1992 Psychosexual disorders in children and adolescents. Journal of Child Psychology and Psychiatry 33: 107–151

25
Old age psychiatry

A. Jacques   K. Woodburn

INTRODUCTION

In Britain 15.8% of the population was aged over 65 years in 1991. The male-to-female ratio falls steadily from 1:1.2 in the 65–69 year age band to 1:3.0 at over 85 years (patients will therefore generally be referred to as female). Table 25.1 shows how the elderly population has expanded during the 20th century. The very elderly group, the 'old-old', will continue to expand for several further decades, whilst the 'young-old' population has already peaked, though there will be a further rise when people born in the postwar 'baby boom' enter old age. In other developed countries the pattern is similar, and in developing countries an even more rapid population explosion will occur later (WHO 1986).

Only 5% of the total elderly population of Britain lives in any type of institutional care. Altogether, between 10 and 20% of the elderly have a major psychiatric problem, so psychiatric illness is a community problem. Nearly half the elderly female population and

a fifth of the elderly male population who live at home live alone, and the availability of potential carers is lessening with smaller family size, increased social mobility and changes in working practices, especially among women, so patients are often relatively isolated compared with their younger counterparts. On the other hand, about 65% of psychiatric hospital residents in Britain are aged over 65 years, and this figure may increase in the future.

Despite its growing importance, old age psychiatry is still in some areas an underdeveloped specialty. Some services are still plagued by bed blocking, inadequate staffing levels and poor morale. The pessimism and carelessness of 'ageism' or 'gerontophobia' can occasionally infect even the most enthusiastic services. Nevertheless, considerable success has been achieved in transforming a 'back-ward' non-specialty to a subject of major clinical, teaching and research interest.

HISTORY

The idea that elderly psychiatric patients might need separate attention first arose in the late 1940s. The gradual increase in older age groups (due to better housing, nutrition and social conditions during their childhood in the late 19th century) led to an increase in the elderly population of the long-stay wards of mental hospitals. Most of these patients were presumed to be suffering from 'senile dementia', but inevitably some had other, reversible conditions. Roth's (1955) simple demonstration that five diagnostic groups of elderly patients (senile dementia, arteriosclerotic dementia, delirium, depression and late paraphrenia) had different prognoses for discharge and survival showed the importance of accurate diagnosis. *Psychogeriatric assessment wards* for the elderly (Robinson 1975) began to be set up in the 1950s in a few hospitals and the idea gradually spread.

In the 1960s, problems of waiting lists for long-term care and assessment wards, and of 'misplacement' of

Table 25.1 Population trends and projections for the United Kingdom 1901–2011			
Year	Population (millions)		
	65–74 years	75–84 years	> 85 years
1901	1.29	0.47	0.06
1931	2.46	0.84	0.11
1951	3.69	1.55	0.22
1971	4.71	2.12	0.47
1991	5.03	3.12	0.89
2001	4.79	3.23	1.17
2011	5.18	3.15	1.32
% change 1901–2011	+300	+570	+2050
% change 1991–2001	−4.5	−3.6	+23

Adapted from the Central Statistical Office (1991).

dementing patients in medical wards (Kidd 1962), preoccupied psychiatrists. One solution was the development of *day hospitals* as an alternative to admission. Unfortunately it has not been proven that day hospitals either avoid or delay admission (Greene & Timbury 1979, Eagles & Gilleard 1984, Murphy 1994).

The 1970s was a decade of plans for coping with the population explosion of elderly people (Department of Health and Social Security 1972, Scottish Home and Health Department 1979). The concepts of *relief admission* (to relieve carers in a crisis) and *respite admission* (regular, preplanned breaks from caring) were introduced and, together with specialist *EMI (elderly mentally infirm) homes* for dementia sufferers in some areas (de Zoysa & Blessed 1984, Norman 1987), began to show that continued increases in long-stay hospital provision might not be necessary.

In the 1980s the burgeoning of private sector *nursing* and *residential homes*, some specialising in dementia, meant that in many areas unsatisfactory accommodation in old asylums was closed down. Increased interest in *community care* led to patchy development of sitter services, non-hospital day care and attempts at multi-agency care planning.

Paralleling this slow evolution of services was an equally slow growth of *old age psychiatry* as a specialty. The first consultants with a special interest in the field were appointed in the 1950s, a special section of the College of Psychiatrists was founded in the 1970s, academic posts were created in the 1980s, specialist journals such as the International Journal of Geriatric Psychiatry were founded and in 1989 Royal College subspecialty status was granted.

The 1990s has seen further extension of these developments. The shift away from provision of long-stay care by hospitals has focused the old age psychiatry team even more than in the past on diagnosis, assessment, acute treatment and rehabilitation, with outreach to the community and to those living in care homes. It is still unclear to what extent good community care as envisaged in legislation (Department of Health/Department of Social Security 1989) can replace institutional care for dementia (Challis & Davies 1986), as much of the effect of changes in the past 15 years has been to replace one type of long-stay institutional care (in hospital) with another (in residential and more especially nursing homes). Keeping people in their own homes, or providing alternative supported living in the community is still often a marginal exercise. The prospect of active *treatments* for Alzheimer's dementia is likely in the future to alter radically the style and practice of old age psychiatry. In the meantime the subspecialty's maturity has been marked by a huge growth in research publications and in text-

books (Copeland et al 1994, Jacoby & Oppenheimer 1997).

THE OLD AGE PSYCHIATRY SERVICE

Catchment area

Most old age psychiatrists believe that a defined catchment area for a service is not only desirable but essential. Care is provided locally for patients and relatives who may find travel difficult, 'boundary disputes' between services are unlikely and some attempt at planning the use of scarce resources is possible. There are inevitable inequalities between areas that are rich and poor in resources, or between active, optimistic teams and passive, pessimistic teams, though such differences may lessen with better education and audit. However, the catchment area principle has stood the test of time.

Age limit policy

Clear, carefully negotiated age policies on dementia and on 'functional' disorders are vital for good relationships between old age psychiatry and other specialties. Many old age services do not take referrals for diagnosis of early onset ('presenile') dementia, but provide day, respite or long-term care to selected cases. Very young dementia sufferers do not fit easily with their elderly counterparts, and the boundaries between primary dementia and head injury, Korsakov's syndrome and other disorders are vague, so it is wise to be selective. Many services have an older cut-off age, perhaps of 70 or 75 years, for 'functional' disorders, placing the emphasis on careful physical assessment as well as psychiatric treatment.

A comprehensive approach

In the few areas which offer pure dementia services, staff recruitment and morale may pose problems. Debates about *segregation or integration* of dementia sufferers have been prolonged. Old long-stay hospital wards were often examples of segregation at its worst, suffering from 'back-ward' mentality, distant from relatives and familiar territory, and rarely visited by outsiders. Meacher's broadside (1972) against some specialist EMI homes was an early plea for integration of dementia sufferers with the non-demented elderly. Rabins (1986) and Norman (1987) have emphasised the merits of 'segregated' dementia services, which can provide a separate environment where staff build up special skills and patients feel safe from the frequently stigmatising attitudes of their fit contemporaries. Wilkin et al (1985) concluded that there may be a 'right mix' for any integrated institution. Residential homes which had over about 30% of dementing residents appeared less successful than those with lower percentages.

In old age psychiatry services, similar conflicts of interest between 'organic' and 'functional' patients are found. About half of most services' referrals are for organic disorders, though they require much more than half of the resources.

Multidisciplinary teamwork

The multiple problems of elderly patients require multiple assessment and treatment skills. Psychiatric expertise should be backed up by readily available advice from geriatric medical colleagues and access to other specialist medical services. The multidisciplinary team of doctors, clinical psychologist, community psychiatric nurses (CPNs – in some areas based in primary care, but nevertheless most important members of the team), hospital nurses, occupational therapist, physiotherapist, social worker and pharmacist should regularly attend patient reviews in respite and long-stay care as well as in the day hospital and assessment wards. Good access to speech therapy and to dietetic, chiropody and dental services are essential.

The practice of inviting relevant outsiders to multidisciplinary discussions on particular patients is becoming more widespread encouraged by the development of the Care Programme Approach. Such 'network meetings' may involve the patient herself if she is able to participate, and any of – relatives, other friends or neighbours, home help, voluntary sector staff, area team social workers, housing agency representatives, general practitioner, primary care nurses, solicitor, police and clergy.

A range of services

Domiciliary assessment

Most referrals come from general practitioners, and consultants customarily see patients in their own homes. This not only provides better information on the social circumstances of the patient, her practical abilities and family relationships, but it avoids the disturbing or artificial effect of outpatient clinics, and usually starts the psychiatrist on a better footing with the patient. It often allows useful contact with relatives, though lack of privacy to interview the patient on sensitive topics, or the interference of a 'helpful' relative can lessen the value of the visit. Domiciliary assessment should help avoid hasty decisions and unnecessary admission. In some areas other members of the multi-disciplinary team contribute to domiciliary assessment and in a few areas the multiagency approach of the 'dementia team' is used.

Outpatient clinics

Only some services run outpatient clinics. These help to overcome the few limitations of domiciliary visiting. More privacy can be accorded to patient or informants. Physical examination and investigations can be carried out and a geriatric opinion obtained.

Open-access clinics, called *memory clinics* (Philpott & Levy 1987, Wright & Lindesay 1995) have become popular in the last 10 years. A multidisciplinary group involving perhaps the psychiatrist, physician, clinical psychologist, CPN and social worker can investigate complaints of memory problems from the general public, concerned families or professionals. Such a system may overcome the reluctance of general practitioners to refer patients with possible early dementia, allows differential diagnosis which would otherwise be neglected and gives some reassurance to the 'worried well'. Memory clinics do not fully meet the needs of patients if they do not offer information and continuing support after diagnosis.

Day hospital

Day hospitals now exist in most areas. In some, mainly rural, districts facilities are shared with geriatric medicine and other services, or 'mobile' day hospitals have been developed. The trend in day hospitals in recent years has been away from 'granny sitting' for patients with milder dementia. This role is being increasingly taken over by local day centres, run by social services, voluntary or private organisations, thus allowing day hospitals to concentrate on their diagnostic, assessment, treatment and rehabilitative functions, and to offer long-term intensive support to those who need nursing care with multidisciplinary back-up.

Flexibility in day care is essential if the actual needs of patients and carers are to be met. For carers in employment, for example, a 5-day day hospital may mean that they know where their relative is while they are working, but gives them no respite from caring when they are at home. In many areas, evening or weekend day care is now being offered, whilst 'night hospital' has been developed in one or two places.

Day hospital care can help effectively in the management of affective disorders and psychosis in the community. For dementia, it has been shown to be highly acceptable to carers (Gilleard et al 1984b) and it may be that, if sufficiently intensive and flexible, it can prevent admission to hospital.

Assessment beds

Dementing patients should be assessed in a separate ward from the 'functional' group, though there are of course some patients with both types of disorder and some who need considerable assessment before it is clear which category of bed is most suitable, so flexibility is required. Since domiciliary and day hospital assessment have become the norm, and as respite care has reduced the load of crisis admissions to short-stay wards, the need for assessment beds for dementia is lessening. Only a few patients need inpatient diagnosis. Some can benefit from inpatient treatment of specific behaviour problems. However, assessment beds are still often used for what are essentially 'relief' admissions, with no clear assessment purpose. If that function can be transferred to a respite facility, and if patients waiting for longer-term care do not wait for transfer for long periods, then the need for dementia assessment beds proper is perhaps as low as 0.3 per 1000 of the population over 65 years of age.

Respite beds

Respite for carers is of course an essential function of much domiciliary and day care. Residential respite care is most suited for dementing patients who live with their carers. A few patients are confused or develop minor infections as a result of the move, so respite care away from home is generally unsuitable for patients who live alone.

A choice of respite services is now available in most areas, including: holidays for groups of couples arranged by the Alzheimer Society; 'fostering' breaks with specially trained families; residential or nursing home care; and geriatric and psychiatric hospital care for those who need nursing. The system is most helpful if admissions come at regular intervals, planned with the relatives so that each break comes *before* the stress of caring becomes too great, rather than giving relief *after* a crisis. In severe cases this may mean that the patient spends half (or even more) of her time in hospital and half at home with day hospital support. If respite care is well planned very few patients fail to return home. A clear contract between the hospital and relatives avoids unplanned 'ditching' of patients.

Because hospital respite care developed rapidly without central planning it was of necessity fitted into available spaces. The beds may be in either assessment or long-stay wards, and neither is entirely satisfactory. Some respite admissions can be seen as short term or intermittent assessment admissions and there is a trend to redesignate respite beds accordingly. An alternative is to have specially designated and designed small wards for respite care. Whatever the title there is a need for a significant number of these beds for people with major nursing needs, perhaps up to 0.8 beds per 1000 of the population over 65 years of age. A recent idea is of a *dementia resource centre*, a small local unit providing support, day care and respite care in one place.

Continuing care

The need for long-term hospital care for those with functional disorders is very small. Residential homes or other supported accommodation are able to cater for most who cannot return home after admission, with the exception of the few psychotic or chronically depressed patients who make no response to drug treatments or have intractable side-effects. These sorry patients fit equally badly into a ward of young disturbed patients as into a ward of dementia sufferers.

There is still a place for continuing multidisciplinary hospital care for dementia associated with major behaviour disturbance. Nursing and residential homes are unlikely, unless highly specialised, to be able to tolerate such residents (Capewell et al 1986). Better training and greater numbers of staff, regular support by consultants, CPNs and other psychiatric team members, judicious drug treatments, and the promise of admission if a difficult situation does not improve, should enable such patients to survive longer in non-hospital care. Some services even offer 'respite care' for homes. A small number of hospital beds, and certainly less than the old norms of 3/1000 elderly for England and Wales (Department of Health and Social Security 1972, already reduced to around 2.5/1000 by the RCP/RCPsych report of 1989) or 5/1000 for Scotland (Scottish Home and Health Department 1979), should suffice, depending on local conditions. Here and elsewhere in service planning the 'balance of service' model is most important. If beds are provided in another service sector, even if their core function is slightly different, then the need for hospital beds will be less. Similarly, community provision, if sufficiently intensive, and regular respite services can lessen the need for long-stay hospital care. But if these alternatives are not available the burden of care will inevitably fall on hospital provision. The concept of NHS *nursing homes* or *'Domus' units* (Lindesay et al 1991) is one way forward in ensuring specialist dementia care for those who need it.

Liaison psychiatry

A third of referrals to most services are from geriatricians and general physicians. High rates of psychiatric disorder have been demonstrated in geriatric patients

(Bergmann & Eastham 1974, Copeland et al 1975). The value of a separate old age psychiatry liaison service has been shown by Scott et al (1988) and Swanwick et al (1994). The special diagnostic and treatment skills of the old age psychiatrist and special knowledge of local services allow patients to be more effectively treated in the medical wards, enable better discharge planning and help avoid unwise disposal or unnecessary long-term care. Organic disorders comprise 60% of referrals. In a good liaison service, which makes itself readily available, most referrals will be for diagnosis and advice, rather than for transfer.

Liaison geriatric medicine

The chances of finding physical illness among a psychogeriatric population are very high, and in many cases this illness will contribute to the psychiatric disorder, or interfere with treatment or rehabilitation. Readily available advice from a geriatric physician in the outpatient clinic, day hospital and wards can be very helpful, and can minimise the transfer of patients between the services.

Joint activities

To overcome the problems of overlap between psychiatric and geriatric services (Murdoch & Montgomery 1992), and to help each other with difficult patients, some centres have developed the concept of joint working (Arie & Dunn 1973, Pitt & Silver 1980). Part of the service is managed together by the two specialties, as in a joint assessment ward, joint day hospital or joint long-stay care. The patients involved will be both physically and mentally disabled, or require further assessment to determine which service should become responsible. The logical consequence is a 'department of care of the elderly' in which all facilities are shared.

Links with community services

Old age psychiatrists are very aware that their patients do not depend on the efforts of the psychiatric service alone if they are to be maintained in the community. A wide network of caring agencies and professions is also involved (Table 25.2). General practitioners are central to case finding, assessment and treatment of elderly people with mental disorders. CPNs provide continuing assessment and treatment services, and in some areas are introducing intensive home nursing care. Home care services and home helps are rightly said to be the backbone of community care. In their different ways primary care nurses also contribute greatly, though they have traditionally concentrated their efforts

Table 25.2   Community services for elderly people with psychiatric disorders

Service	Potential providers
Informal support and supervision	Family, friends, neighbours, shopkeepers, police, clubs, church groups, 'sitting' circles
Home help	Social services
Sitting services, day or night	Private agencies
	Voluntary agencies
	Private, including nursing agencies
	A few hospitals and social services departments
Meals on wheels	Social services
	Voluntary agencies
Aids, adaptations and safety	District nurses
	Occupational therapists (community or hospital based)
	Housing agencies
	Gas and electricity companies
Incontinence care	District nurses and health visitors, some specialist incontinence nurses
	Laundry services (social services or community health)
Day care	Social services
	Voluntary agencies
	Private agencies
Respite care	Informal carers
	Social services
	Voluntary agencies
	Private agencies
Long-term care at home	Informal carers
	All agencies
Planning and coordination of care – the 'key worker'	Informal carers
	Social workers
	Community psychiatric nurses
	Health visitors
	General practitioners

on the physically disabled. Care needs assessment and management in the community have been the particular responsibility of social workers since 1993. Social services departments may provide or purchase from others day care, respite care and other services. Workers in a growing number of voluntary organisations offer advice, support, counselling, and sitter, day care or other respite services. Some housing associations have recently been developing extra-care housing for dementia sufferers. A growing private sector is providing not only residential and nursing home care, but also home support services. This expansion has been greatly encouraged by community care legislation (Department of Health/Department of Social Security 1989) with its emphasis on a 'mixed economy of care'.

In the last 15 years great initiative has been shown in developing alternative forms of care for elderly people with psychiatric disorders. An effective old age service spends much of its efforts on liaising with agencies who share the care of patients living in the community, and on supporting them, whether in care planning, training and support of staff, project development, or just by paying them a regular visit. Two particular models of cooperation have been developed – the mental health liason meeting and the community dementia team.

The mental health liaison meeting

Representatives of the various agencies covering a particular community meet regularly, usually monthly, and discuss those patients with mental disorders who are of mutual interest to at least two of them. Such meetings help in care planning, avoid overlaps or gaps in care, and are mutually supportive and educative. Patients may be referred between the services. The meetings also develop a political role. Gaps in service provision become obvious and ideas about how to fill these gaps can be pursued. The liaison group is an efficient, effective and remarkably cheap method of organising care in the community, though it may challenge the rigid application of the social work lead role in care management. Such groups can provide the structure for developing the Care Programme Approach for those with specially complex care needs.

The community dementia team

A dementia team (Lodge & McReynolds 1985) is also a multiagency group, and is formed by representatives of the relevant bodies, usually by secondment or special appointment. After local consultation and advertisement, it provides an open-access point for people in the community who are worried about dementia in themselves, their relatives or those they care for professionally (cf. the 'memory clinic' concept, but here the emphasis is on care planning rather than diagnosis). Inevitably most referrals come from professionals, but informal referral of patients who would otherwise fail to come to the attention of mainstream services is encouraged. A particular member of the team, who may come from any of the agencies involved, is selected to make an initial assessment and may become the 'key worker' for that patient and family over the succeeding months

or years, introducing the patient to the services she needs, and providing continuing support. Such teams have not always succeeded. Referral rates may be low and, to be effective, they need to be able to have direct access to the necessary services.

Links with residential and nursing homes

Between 30 and 80% of residents in care homes are likely to suffer from dementia (Ineichin 1990) and perhaps 40% suffer from significant depressive symptoms (Mann et al 1984, Ames 1990). Links between the old age psychiatry service and residential or nursing homes may be informal or formal. The consultant may regularly visit homes within his catchment area to review the progress of known patients and give informal support to staff. CPNs or clinical psychologists may provide a regular advice and support service, particularly where hospital patients are discharged to the homes. Formal training sessions by doctor, CPN or clinical psychologist and formal liaison groups are found in a few areas.

Partnership with carers

Carers' groups have always been part of normal day hospital practice. Now Alzheimer Society, social work and other community-based carers' groups are commonplace. Carers form an essential part of the treatment team in dementia, having much information to provide about the patient, and wishing to be involved in decisions which are made throughout the illness. In day and respite care the psychiatric team is truly 'sharing care' with relatives and needs to recognise this.

Community bias

Attention in old age psychiatry is moving away from the problems of seemingly endless waiting lists for long-stay care to the opportunities of community care coupled with, if anything, brief contact with hospital. This trend is welcomed by almost all patients and most families. Indeed, long-term care of patients with dementia is more and more being seen as the responsibility of extra-care housing, residential and nursing homes, which may give patients a better living environment than hospital, and sometimes also better care. The financial implications of this shift in care arrangements for individuals, the statutory agencies and taxpayers, are the subject of continuing political debate in all developed countries. Psychiatric services which are less involved in providing long-stay care can concentrate their efforts on specialist advice and treatment.

INTERVIEW METHODS

Interviewing the patient

Interviewing elderly psychiatric patients requires special skills.

Normal changes of ageing

In response to the almost universal slowing of all mental processes the interviewer must slow his pace, and learn patience. Older people tend to be more cautious in their responses to questions, so the interviewer may need to be more encouraging than for a younger patient, and use more multiple-choice or forced-choice questions. A tendency to greater introspection makes some elderly people more reticent about personal problems than is the norm for younger generations. A 'transference' effect may add to this. Inevitably, the interviewer is considerably younger than the patient, and may be treated as an inexperienced person, who needs to be protected from unpleasant reality.

In addition, 'countertransference' attitudes may interfere with the interviewer's willingness to ask personal questions of someone who could be their grandparent. Some doctors seem to believe that elderly people have inevitably led sheltered lives. They therefore avoid important questions about alcohol or sexual behaviour. Even worse is the still prevalent tendency to infantilise elderly people. This can have strange effects on interviewers, who fail to explain the interview process, 'speak down' to the patient, assume that she lacks understanding, general knowledge or wisdom, ignore her right to make or be involved in decisions, or speak to her relatives as if they were her parents. Some elderly people prefer a formal approach to interviewing. On the other hand, many become less inhibited than younger adults are about touch, probably because it has less obvious sexual connotations. Not only a shake of the hand, but holding the hand and other reassuring bodily contact is often both acceptable and helpful.

Elderly people of the present generation sometimes have surprisingly fatalistic, ageist *attitudes towards illness*. This affects not only patients themselves but also their families and even professional carers, who may treat quite serious symptoms as evidence of 'just old age', fail to report them or underplay their significance. Persistence may be required to elicit the full clinical picture.

Difficulty with or *dislike of change* is also common. This may be a real biological aspect of ageing or may be culturally determined. Introducing new concepts or new activities can lead to considerable resistance, most obvious when the doctor is recommending a course of action or therapy. Considerable time and gradual persuasion may be necessary to get the patient to consider even quite simple changes. Major changes such as accepting a home help for the first time or leaving home may be met in the first instance by total resistance.

Disabilities

Disabilities, often unconnected with the patient's psychiatric disorder, may interfere with the interviewing process. *Impairment of hearing* is the most common, and, if not recognised, can easily lead to misdiagnosis of mental impairment. Access to a voice amplifier or communicator is essential. In severe cases it is necessary to write questions or use behavioural evidence of the mental state. *Visual impairment* brings difficulties with certain tests. Like deafness it may not be mentioned by a proud or self-conscious patient, and so is misconstrued. Patients who are physically ill, fatigued or in discomfort may not concentrate, so questioning will have to be simple, repetitive and carefully explained. *Parkinsonism* leads to mumbled speech which hinders interviewing, and can tempt the interviewer to diagnose depression or dementia.

Mental impairment

Impaired comprehension means that the interviewer has to explain carefully the rationale, content and duration of the interview. These explanations will have to be repeated several times for patients who show poor concentration, forgetfulness or suspiciousness. Difficulty with attention span, receptive dysphasia, poor vocabulary and grammar, impaired comprehension and abstract thinking all mean that questions or instructions should use simple words and simple one-clause sentences, dealing with only one item at a time, avoiding abstractions. It is not unusual for a patient to recall only the beginning (primacy effect) or the end (recency) of a long sentence. Retention of an instruction to be carried out in the future ('future memory') is likely to be impossible. Since attention and concentration are often impaired it is usually necessary to intersperse short periods of questioning with more informal talk. A patient whose impairment of simple mental tasks is being revealed will need the reassurance of a spell of interesting reminiscence before new embarrassment is caused. Patients with expressive dysphasia may need assistance from the interviewer who guesses what words she is trying to say, or with prompt cards. Considerable skill and inventiveness is required to interview a patient who has no idea that the interviewer is a doctor, has severe receptive dysphasia or has no insight into her condition. Skill is also required in dealing with the defensive patient who has developed the ability to side-track interviewers into repetitive reminiscence to cover amnesia.

Interviewing informants

In general psychiatry it is usual for the patient to be able to give enough information about the history to allow accurate diagnosis. This is much less true in old age psychiatry. In organic disorders, interviewing the patient can *never* give a reliable or comprehensive history. Even at very early stages of dementia, sufferers fail to time-code information properly, so that vital questions about the natural history of the illness cannot be answered. However, the patient's history should not be ignored. Her attitude to her illness is important in assessing insight, working out treatment strategy and predicting compliance. And she may have more knowledge of some details than even her close relatives have. Furthermore, some patients do not have any available informant, or their informants themselves may have dementia or other disabilities.

It is important, even in severe dementia, to ask the patient's permission before seeing the relative. Relatives (and professionals) often need to be reminded that they are not legally in charge of the patient, even though they may feel or act 'in loco parentis'. The doctor must also remind himself that he is the patient's *advocate* as well as trying to help the relatives. He may have to balance the distress of an exhausted relative who is demanding help against strong resistance from the patient who does not believe that any help is needed.

The relatives' history itself may be inaccurate, either because they wish to emphasise their need for help, or because they wish to carry on caring without outside intrusion. Clarifying questions are very important, to pin down the exact time when a symptom started, or how often it has been obvious. These details are most important in diagnosis and in assessing what action is needed.

A useful procedure with informants for a patient who may have dementia is:

- Explain the purpose, structure and timing of this interview, and of the interview with the patient.
- Details of relevant past history, personality, abilities and medical history will provide a baseline which is essential to diagnosis, and gives some currently relevant information.
- Obtain the general history of the mental decline and enough information to indicate that the impairment is *global*. Pin down timing as accurately as possible and clarify whether the process has been acute, gradual or irregular. Information from relatives may

be as important as mental testing of the patient and other investigations in suggesting a diagnosis of dementia. A standardised questionnaire such as the Information questionnaire on cognitive decline in the elderly (IQCODE, Jorm & Jacomb 1989) may be helpful.

- Using a *problem check-list*, such as Table 25.8 or that of Gilleard (1984), list the problems experienced by the relatives, patient and others. There may be as many as 15–20 dementia-related problems for one patient. Clarify the seriousness, circumstances, timing, frequency, consequences and variations of each problem separately and record any treatment or management strategies which have been tried. Review the problem list with the relative and ask them if any other significant problems have been missed out. This essential part of the interview enables the relative to feel that all their concerns have been covered, yet the whole process has been quick and effective. The extensive Present Behavioural Examination of Hope & Fairburn (1992) concentrates on the various 'non-cognitive' symptoms of dementia and is useful for research purposes.
- Ask about current supports, make a *timetable* of regular visitors or outings during the week and establish how long the patient can be left alone. This locates gaps and overlaps in care and support.

MENTAL STATE EXAMINATION

Much of the mental state examination is, as in younger patients, composed of information gathered during history taking, by observation of the patient's behaviour and from responses to questions. Organic mental testing (Hodges 1994) is central to much of the work of the old age psychiatrist. A few points are worth stressing:

- The principles of history taking from elderly people, particularly about explanation, pace, breaks from questions and simplicity of communication apply equally to mental testing.
- No individual item tests only one function. For example, to ask 'What day is it today?' can lead to information about receptive dysphasia, general comprehension, immediate memory, recent memory, motivation and affect, expressive ability, hearing and sight as well as telling how oriented the person is. The serial 7 test may reveal dyscalculia or dysphasia as well as poor concentration. Very non-specific tests such as clock drawing (Shulman et al 1986) can be invaluable.
- Impairments can interact. A patient who has

significant receptive dysphasia will be unable to participate in other mental tests which involve spoken questions or commands; this must not be taken to mean that she is impaired in these respects. Poor attention or low mood may interfere with all testing.

- Although some standard questions are useful, imagination and flexibility are also essential. For example, questions about general knowledge, remote memory and new learning must all be varied according to the individual's premorbid intelligence, education, interests and experience. And, as information emerges, the doctor may need to employ additional tests to explore, say, parietal lobe function or dysphasia.
- A patient's performance may vary from time to time. Mood, motivation, fatigue, time of day, and her attitude to the particular examiner may all make the difference between good and bad performance in tests. The doctor should never assume that what she has presented to him is how she always is. Mental state examination gives a tiny snapshot of her whole mental condition. Indeed, variations in presentation at different times provide useful information for both diagnosis and functional assessment.
- The mental state examination is carried out for diagnostic purposes or to monitor progress. It is not an assessment of the practical needs of the patient. That is a separate exercise.

FURTHER INVESTIGATIONS

Rating scales

Intellectual rating scales, such as the Mini-Mental State Examination (MMSE, Folstein et al 1975), the information–orientation section of the Clifton Assessment Procedure for the Elderly (CAPE, Pattie & Gilleard 1979) or Hodkinson's Abbreviated Mental Test (1973), provide a general rating of mental impairment which can be used to assess severity or chart progress or decline. They are widely used as screening tests but are not diagnostic. They do not substitute for a thorough mental state examination, for they do not provide enough evidence to demonstrate the global impairment and natural history of delirium or dementia. They are reasonably sensitive for mental impairment, but not very specific.

Ratings of behaviour using scales such as the Crichton Behaviour Rating Scale (Robinson 1975), the behaviour section of the CAPE, and the REPDS (Fleming & Bowles 1994) are in regular use. Again these are not in any way diagnostic, and many of the

items they test could relate to a variety of illnesses or disabilities. They do, however, give some estimate of severity of general impairment, after diagnosis has been carried out, and can be used to chart changes or to predict the level of care needed by the patient (Pattie & Gilleard 1976).

Standard depression rating scales are not very appropriate to old age psychiatry, as questions about biological symptoms will not clearly distinguish depressive from physical illness. The Geriatric Depression Scale (GDS, Yesavage et al 1983) and the Cornell Scale for depression in dementia (Alexopoulos et al 1988) have been specifically developed for use in elderly and dementing populations respectively.

Research interview schedules

Two major instruments were introduced in Britain in the 1980s, the Geriatric Mental State Schedule (GMS) of Copeland et al (1986), which links with the AGE-CAT computerised diagnostic programme, and the Cambridge Diagnostic Examination (CAMDEX) of Roth et al (1986), both covering the major diagnoses of old age psychiatry. These are making epidemiological surveys more reliable and valid, and providing a common language for researchers. They are not for routine use, but can be useful in examining difficult cases.

Psychological testing

The role of the clinical psychologist in mental state assessment in the elderly has expanded and contracted at different times over recent decades. Most claims that one particular psychological test can distinguish early dementia from normal ageing (e.g. Kendrick 1987), or distinguish pseudodementia from true dementia, have failed to convince, largely because they have been validated on pure samples of classical cases, rather than examining the grey areas. Nevertheless, psychological testing can be an extremely useful adjunct to examination, clarifying thinking, providing more detail about particular impairments, and adding weight for or against a particular diagnosis. The subject has been reviewed by Morris (1996).

Activities of daily living (ADL)

The psychological abilities examined in mental state or psychological testing represent only a sample of brain activity that may be affected by brain damage. Behaviour rating scales give some evidence of other impairments, but the most practically useful evidence comes from assessment of the 'activities of daily living'. This is the special province of the occupational therapist, and is best carried out on a visit to the patient's own home, rather than in an artificial 'ADL suite'. Improved performance under scrutiny, performance anxiety, variations with mood, motivation, time of day and the relationship with the therapist must be taken into consideration when interpreting the results. The Barthel index is widely used to summarise ADL information (Wade & Collin 1988).

Physical examination, blood tests and other investigations

Screening of the elderly in the community has generally brought little success in case finding, but screening of groups of elderly people at special risk of physical illness has been much more productive. Elderly patients with any major psychiatric diagnosis are such a group. Table 25.3 lists some possible tests and the rationale behind their use.

The *electroencephalogram (EEG)* still has some place in old age psychiatry, but mainly in the diagnosis of possible fits and Creutzfeldt–Jakob disease (CJD).

Table 25.3 Investigations and some differential diagnoses in old age psychiatry

Test	Diagnosis (examples)
Routine tests	
Full blood count	Infections, alcohol problems
ESR	Infections, tumours
Urea and electrolytes	Uraemia, metabolic disorders
Liver function	Alcohol problems, secondary tumours
Thyroid function	Hypothyroidism
Calcium and phosphorus	Parathyroid disorders
Mid-stream urine	Infections
Chest radiography	Secondary tumours
ECG	Cardiac arrhythmias
Other possible tests	
Vitamin B_{12} and folate (if MCV raised)	B_{12} and folate deficiency
Syphilis serology	Tertiary syphilis
HIV testing	AIDS dementia
EEG	Creutzfeldt–Jakob disease
CT	Normal pressure hydrocephalus
MRI	Vascular dementias, tumour
SPECT	Frontal lobe dementias

Computerised tomography (CT), *magnetic resonance imaging (MRI)*, *single photon emission CT (SPECT)* and *positron emission tomography (PET)* are variably available. They are lengthy procedures which can be distressing for confused or anxious people. Furthermore, they are not perfect diagnostic tools, and, being relatively expensive, and in the case of SPECT and PET invasive, are not in routine use. The sense of this practice is emphasised by the fact that probably 95% of dementias in old age are of the more common types. A scan should be ordered when there are unusual clinical features or course, specific reasons to suspect a space-occupying lesion, subdural haemorrhage or hydrocephalus, or a particularly difficult differential diagnosis. The value of MRI in showing white matter and vascular lesions, and the suggestions that SPECT could distinguish specific features of dementia of Alzheimer type (DAT) at early stages and frontal lobe dementia suggest that use of these tests will increase. As specific treatments for DAT or vascular dementias (VD) become more available, diagnosis at the earliest possible stage will become essential.

THERAPIES

Psychotherapy

Most older neurotic patients do not suit or show interest in explorative psychotherapy. Therapists tend to agree that brief, problem-solving therapy related to current life difficulties is more likely to be relevant and effective and a counselling approach is sometimes best. Possibly the biggest problem encountered is the resistance of some older people to change.

The psychodynamic issues that are relevant to older people differ from those which preoccupy young adults (Brink 1979, Knight 1996). Coming to terms with the losses of old age and with decreasing independence and increasing dependence is often central. This is particularly difficult for active, independent personalities who have never anticipated such changes. Coming to terms with the past is also likely to be relevant, typical issues being regrets, renunciation of hopes, forgiveness or lack of forgiveness of perceived wrongs, and putting past preoccupations into perspective (Butler 1963). Although for many people reminiscence is an entirely enjoyable experience, some achieve that enjoyment by idealisation and denial, and others fail to find happiness in their recollections or are entrenched in bitterness. Erikson's (1963) counterpoint of 'ego integrity' versus 'despair' is relevant here.

Changed relationships and power structures in the family and among friends may cause both external and internal conflicts, and family therapy is a growing interest. Previously held expectations of old age may cause a variety of problems. Many had expected that they would be surrounded by a family who have instead moved away physically or emotionally. Many looked forward to activities which they are kept from by disability or illness. Most are unprepared for the fact that old age can last for a very long time (average expectation of life at the age of 65 years is now 14 years for a man and 18 years for a woman). Personal and social attitudes to ageing may conflict. Older persons who wish to 'disengage' may find themselves at odds with those around them who think continuing activity and engagement are important. Conversely, those who wish to be working, physically energetic or sexually active may meet with disapproval from family and friends who expect them to 'retire'.

Psychological therapies

Clinical psychologists have recently begun to show a greater interest in treating elderly people (Stokes & Goudie 1990, Woods 1996) and have successfully applied cognitive and behaviour therapy techniques in treating anxiety, phobias, depression and sexual problems. Some fear that learning-based theories may have less value because older people tend to be more rigid psychologically and less inclined to change, but there is ample evidence that normal older people can continue to learn.

The same is not true of dementia sufferers. Nevertheless, psychology has contributed much to their treatment, from the use of memory management (Wilson & Moffat 1992) and specific examples of behaviour modification to evaluation of more general therapies (Woods 1996).

Reality orientation (RO)

This originated as a resocialisation technique in the back wards of American mental hospitals, but became metamorphosed into a treatment for dementia. It was enthusiastically embraced by staff in day care, residential homes and wards, partly because it was optimistic. But the optimism became excessive, RO was used as a universal 'therapy' whether it suited individual patients or not, and eventually got a bad name. Research (Brook et al 1975, Holden & Woods 1988) shows that the principle of encouraging orientation can help some patients in some aspects of their mental state, but perhaps only verbal orientation. Active involvement of the patient, and learning which makes use of procedural memory, are particularly effective. 'Classroom RO' has probably now had its day, but as a '24 hour' technique RO may

be useful in dealing with disorientation, mistaken ideas and distorted memories.

Reminiscence

This is less a specific therapy than a general principle (Butler 1963, Norris 1986, Thornton & Brotchie 1987) that elderly people often gain satisfaction, confidence and a sense of identity from reminiscing. Dementia sufferers may find reminiscence particularly satisfying. Lack of recent memory and helplessness in the present make them fall back on remote memories in a search for identity and security. Of course their stories may be fragmentary or repetitive, but good reminiscence therapy allows for this and helps the person expand from the merely stereotyped. Photographs, slides and films, old objects, old songs and dances, 'theatre' where the person 'performs' old work or domestic activities, handling old objects, and visits to the person's school, childhood home or other familiar scenes have all been effectively used. However, like reality orientation, reminiscence is not for all. For some, old memories evoke only sadness, regret or bitterness which they would rather avoid and may not be able to work through.

Validation therapy

This technique was introduced to escape from some of the impersonal excesses of 'classroom' style reality orientation (Feil 1993). It looks to the emotional state which underlies a patient's disoriented speech and behaviour. If she talks of wanting her mother, is it because she is feeling insecure, and would be helped by reassuring emotional or physical contact? If she wants to go off to work, is it because she is bored, and would benefit from exercise or activity? Although popular, there is no research evidence of its effectiveness.

Psychopharmacology

The changes in drug absorption, pharmacodynamics and activity with age are complicated. From the practical point of view certain principles are of day-to-day use:

- Most research in pharmacology and therapeutics has until recently been carried out on younger subjects. Check that any statements about a drug are relevant to elderly people.
- The body's ability to handle drugs changes in various ways with the process of ageing, but not in any absolute sense. Age is not in itself a contraindication to any drug.
- The normal interpersonal variation in drug handling and effects is greater in old age. One person may both need and tolerate large doses of a particular drug,

while another, apparently similar, person may obtain the same therapeutic effect with a lower dose, and even that low dose may cause harmful side-effects.

- Because of this great variability, it is important to start most drugs at a very small dose and build up gradually, particularly when using drugs with long half-lives or persistent metabolites.
- Gradual reduction in renal function and in some hepatic enzymes is the norm in old age so drugs which are cleared by these pathways need particular care.
- Side-effects of drugs may appear at much lower doses than in younger patients, and in some cases at well below the therapeutic dose for that patient. Patients with dementia of Lewy body type (DLBT) are at particular risk. There is also a small number of elderly schizophrenic patients who seem unable to tolerate therapeutic doses of any antipsychotic drug without major parkinsonian side-effects.
- Even simple or mild side-effects may have disastrous consequences. Mild postural hypotension from an antidepressant can lead to a fractured femur, and mild anticholinergic effects can cause severe urinary retention or constipation.
- Drug interactions are common, partly because of some doctors' penchant for polypharmacy. The assessment of any elderly patient should include a careful listing of all her medications. In many cases cutting or stopping drugs, simplifying schedules or changing to safer equivalents will lead to improvement in some or all of her symptoms (Findlay et al 1989).
- It may not be clear what drugs the patient is actually taking, and compliance can be a major problem. Again polypharmacy may be responsible. The patient may have a cupboard full of drugs whose purpose she does not understand, or which she has forgotten about. The drug list which the general practitioner has may not be the list of drugs that the patient is taking. Patients who are being treated both at home and in a day hospital or respite ward are in particular danger of mix-up and poor communication about changes. It is good practice, where possible, to provide clear instruction and counselling, and to monitor compliance carefully.

ORGANIC CONDITIONS

Delirium

Incidence

Delirium as a consequence of physical illness or toxic effects is more common in elderly people than in younger age groups (Lindesay et al 1990). It affects between 10 and 25% of patients aged over 65 years admitted to medical wards (Hodkinson 1973, Bergmann & Eastham 1974), and is particularly common after fractures. Unknown numbers suffer delirious states at home. The incidence may be high partly because elderly people are more prone to have one or more physical illnesses, and to be taking one or more drugs. In addition the ageing brain is more susceptible to insult, perhaps involving the cholinergic and noradrenergic systems which are important in cognition and the wake–sleep cycle. Dementing people are especially susceptible to superadded delirium (Hodkinson 1973).

Causes

The causes of delirium are no different in the elderly than in younger people, though some are relatively more important. Common infections and other general illnesses are potent causes and even quite simple conditions like constipation can lead to delirium in susceptible patients. Delirium is also a side-effect of a wide variety of drugs. Delirium tremens and benzodiazepine withdrawal should always be considered, and head injury, with the possibility of subsequent subdural haemorrhage, may not be reported. It is always sensible to consider these common conditions before subjecting the patient to more intensive investigation. Even a move ('translocation') can cause temporary delirium, though this is probably only true of those with an early or latent dementia.

Some patients suffer from more than one potential cause of the delirium. In some cases, particularly of possible stroke or transient ischaemic attack, the cause of the delirium may remain obscure even after scanning. Disentangling possible delirium in a dementia sufferer may be even more difficult. An acute change in mental state, or the emergence of one or more of the characteristic features (Table 25.4) should suggest possible delirium, but may be simply due to further progress in the illness, particularly in multi-infarct dementia or DLBT. On the other hand, many dementing people will suffer physical illnesses which do not cause delirium or worsening of their mental state. Lipowski (1983) reported no detectable cause for delirium in between 5 and 20% of cases.

Clinical features

The characteristic variability of delirium means that a doctor's assessment does not necessarily reflect the patient's mental state over the whole day. Family or nursing reports of delirious symptoms at other times of day or night must be taken seriously.

Table 25.4   Clinical features which tend to distinguish delirium from dementia. Global mental impairment is common to both conditions

Delirium	Dementia
Rapid onset	Slowly progressive
Acute medical cause	Slowly progressive cause
Clouding of consciousness	Clear consciousness
Sleep disturbance	Normal sleep pattern, but 'clock' may be wrong
Irregular variability	Tends to be worse towards evening but otherwise stable
Restlessness and unease	Usually settled apart from aimless wandering or searching
Affect laden visual perceptual disturbances	Hallucinations less common and not usually disturbing
Lability of affect and distress	Lability less common

Delirium is a serious condition and many delirious elderly medical ward patients die of the underlying cause. However, the rest have a good prognosis and only 5% or less go on to develop dementia. It is important to find the cause quickly and then to be relatively optimistic. The condition may last longer in old age; for example, delirium tremens or delirium after a stroke may last for many weeks. Patients who do not instantly recover after their physical state or investigations have apparently returned to normal should not be prematurely diagnosed as suffering from dementia. At the very least they should be physically well for 2 weeks before even medium-term decisions are made.

Differential diagnosis

Dementia   The classical distinction between delirium and dementia (Table 25.4) is an important but not absolute guide; features of delirium can appear during dementia, particularly if progress is rapid, and especially in DLBT. Many cases of delirium have few or none of the distinguishing features except for the acute course.

Affective disorders and psychosis   The lability of affect common in delirium sometimes becomes pervasive and patients may develop mood congruent ideas or delusions which suggest a diagnosis of primary affective disorder. In a somewhat similar way psychotic symptoms in delirium may suggest a primary psychosis. It is

in fact most unlikely that a primary affective disorder or primary psychosis would begin coincidentally with a physical illness.

Management

As at all ages the treatment of delirium is the treatment of the cause. Lindesay et al (1990) rightly emphasise psychological aspects of management, which should aim at:

- Reducing understimulation and maximising the clarity of perceptions, whilst avoiding overstimulation
- Minimising the unfamiliarity of the environment
- Minimising disorientation
- Reassurance that the illness is physical and temporary, and that any hallucinations are really being experienced by the patient, but will soon disappear
- An emotionally calm environment.

Drug treatment should be reserved for those who are severely disturbed, or whose sleep pattern is severely disrupted. Thioridazine should be avoided, since it not uncommonly increases disorientation or restlessness. Cautious use of promazine, haloperidol or droperidol, or a short course of a benzodiazepine or chlormethiazole, are among the therapeutic possibilities.

Hospital is not the best environment for an elderly delirious patient, and home treatment should always be considered, though the need for investigation and supervision may make admission necessary. As with dementia, no branch of medicine has sole responsibility for the treatment of delirium. Most patients quite rightly go to medical wards. Liaison psychiatric help is often needed for differential diagnosis and for advice on associated behaviour problems.

Dementia

Epidemiology

Henderson (1986) pointed to considerable difficulties in conducting community surveys of dementia:

- Defining the population: are residents in care included or not?
- Allowing for differing age structures of different populations
- Differential survival in different populations
- Using a valid diagnostic test: most simple tests measure impairment at the time of interview, only one of the steps in diagnosis; comprehensive tests are laborious to administer

- Estimating mild dementia: many surveys give estimates for moderate and severe cases only
- Differentiating between dementia of Alzheimer type (DAT) and other dementias.

Jorm et al (1987; Fig. 25.1) suggested from a meta-analysis of the many epidemiological studies of dementia that the *prevalence* rises exponentially with age, doubling with each successive period of 5.1 years, as shown by the classic Newcastle study (Kay et al 1964) and more recent studies (Bond 1987, Rocca et al 1991, Copeland et al 1992). The median age for suffering from dementia is about 82 years. Overall prevalence for populations over 65 range from 2 to 7% for moderate and severe dementia, with great variability in the figures for mild cases. In a chronic illness like dementia *incidence* is low compared with prevalence, with figures around 1.0–1.5% being typically reported from elderly community samples. Epidemiological studies now concentrate on finding *risk factors* for the individual illnesses which cause dementia, only old age being a general risk factor.

Because of the anticipated growth in older age bands the number of sufferers will rise (though there is growing evidence that prevalence does not continue its expo-nential rise beyond 90–95 years; Ritchie & Kildea 1995). Absolute numbers are uncertain, but the percentage rise in a particular community can be estimated, using Jorm's formula. In some areas of Britain there will be an increase of nearly 20% in the number of dementia sufferers in the next 10 years. The service needs of these extra sufferers and their carers are more important than absolute numbers or percentage increases, but there are few available estimates. The pool of available caring younger people is diminishing because of changes in population structure and social mobility, and because patients' children are increasingly likely to be either working or elderly and frail themselves.

About 70% of elderly dementia sufferers in Britain live in private houses, so the emphasis has always been on community care. About half of those living at home are living with close relatives, who may be coping with a severely disabled or disturbed individual. Slightly less than half are on their own and the focus of attention is on the risks of independent living.

Assessment

Identification O'Connor et al (1988) found that general practitioners knew of roughly 80% of severe dementia sufferers, but they were aware of only 30% of mild sufferers. Regular primary care visits to those aged over 75 years and the use of simple screening instruments such as the MMSE (Iliffe et al 1991b) may improve these figures. Memory clinics and the advent of drug therapies will encourage more to come forward early and more and more patients wish to know and discuss their diagnosis, but there is still a great deal of pessimism about help for dementia, which together with stigma, lack of insight, ignorance of services and isolation from potential identifiers of the problem conspires against early presentation. It is not yet clear how far early diagnosis helps prevent disability, or whether it helps institute community services which delay admission to costly and unpopular long-stay care. Early diagnosis may bring relatives the help they need to continue caring; or it may 'desensitise' them to outside help, and so speed admission.

Diagnosis of the syndrome The essential steps in diagnosis are:

1. Demonstrating a global mental impairment compared with that individual's normal performance
2. Showing that this impairment has been gradually progressive over a period of some months
3. Ruling out other causes of a similar clinical picture.

These steps require a clear history from the patient

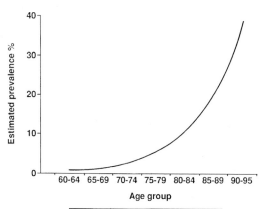

Age group	Estimated prevalence %
60-64	0.7
65-69	1.4
70-74	2.8
75-79	5.6
80-84	10.5
85-89	20.8
90-95	38.6

Fig. 25.1 Prevalence rates of dementia by 5 year age intervals for baseline population, pooled from selected studies (adapted from Jorm et al 1987). The graph can probably be extrapolated to younger age groups, but rates in the over-90s may level out, and almost certainly do not continue to rise exponentially.

and informants, a full mental state examination and at the very least some simple screening investigations. While these are usually carried out if the patient is referred to a psychiatrist, the same cannot be said for all general practitioners and physicians. The most common mistakes are to rely only on the mental state examination, to use only tests of orientation instead of demonstrating global impairment, and to fail to talk to another informant.

In old age neither CT nor MRI are sensitive or specific enough to use for syndrome diagnosis, though combinations of tests increase accuracy to acceptable levels, except in very mild cases (Jacoby & Levy 1980a). In the first few months of dementia a 'wait and see' approach is advisable, asking the patient to return for repeat assessment in 3–6 months.

Differential diagnosis The differential diagnosis of dementia in an elderly patient includes the following.

Normal old age A difficult problem for early cases (Henderson & Huppert 1984), and also in people with a lifelong mental impairment, those who are deaf and those with communication problems because of stroke. Attempts to find tests which differentiate very early dementia from normal old age have so far been largely unsuccessful and some argue that there is a continuum between normal old age and dementia. Bergmann (1977) found that roughly one-third of mild or doubtful cases proved not to have dementia 1 year later and that a further third were still in the doubtful category.

Age-associated memory impairment More recently concepts such as age-associated memory impairment (AAMI), age-consistent memory impairment (ACMI), late-life forgetfulness (LLF) and cognitive impairment–no dementia (CIND) have been developed, extending an original idea of Kral (1962), that there is a form of 'benign senescence' or impairment which does not progress to dementia. Attempts to follow up such cases have led to results not dissimilar to those found by Bergmann; some prove to have had early dementia, some may have non-progressive vascular or other pathology, and some have had temporary impairment, but some remain in diagnostic uncertainty.

Chronic brain damage which is not progressive This is often quite reasonably called dementia, but the non-progressive nature of the damage following head injury or other insults, and the possibility of some gradual improvement, makes care planning a very different matter in the two conditions, and it is important to differentiate them.

Delirium See above.

Korsakov's syndrome An alcohol history is essential in all cases. The restriction of impairment to recent memory, with relative sparing of immediate memory and other intellectual functions, should be suggestive

and MRI scanning may be helpful.

Pseudodementia of depression See section on affective disorders.

Pseudodementia of physical illness There is some overlap and realistic lack of clarity between this term and the term *reversible dementia*. Is, for example, secondary mental impairment in a hypothyroid patient a true dementia which is reversible or an artefact of the illness? In practice it does not matter, since treatment of the thyroid problems in either case will cure the 'dementia'. Unfortunately, it is more common for thyroid disorder and dementia to coexist as completely unconnected problems.

Diagnosis of the cause It is unclear what proportion of the elderly dementing population suffers from each of the many causes of dementia. Clinical and post-mortem studies alike are liable to bias, depending on whether they use community or hospital samples and their age structure. Clinical differentiation of DAT from vascular dementia (VD) and DLBT is not reliable, with many apparently mixed cases. Even at post mortem there are debates about definitions. It is probable, however, that over 95% of elderly patients suffer from the common forms of dementia – DAT, VD and DLBT – and that DAT is the most common cause, perhaps accounting for 60% of all sufferers.

● *Dementia of Alzheimer type (DAT)* Roth (1986) and others have noted differences between 'old-old' type 1 and 'young-old' type 2 DAT. Pathological and neurochemical evidence suggests that in older patients damage is more topographically restricted, and more limited to the acetylcholine system. There are less obvious differences between older DAT sufferers and normal people of the same age in their cholinergic systems, in psychological tests, and in their expectation of life (Christie & Train 1984). Some have suggested that in young cases there is a more malignant course (Naguib & Levy 1982, Loring & Largen 1985), but others disagree (Jorm 1985, O'Carroll et al 1991, Newens et al 1993). It is also possible to explain some apparent differences between older and younger sufferers using the concept of 'cerebral reserve'. If older people have less reserve then smaller amounts of cerebral damage will emerge earlier and have greater clinical effects.

Diagnosis is largely on clinical grounds. The NINCDS–ADRDA criteria provide good descriptions of definite, probable and possible DAT and have been widely used in research (McKhann et al 1984).

Genetic testing The identification of the apolipoprotein E (ApoE) ε4 allele as a 'dose-dependent' risk factor for late-onset DAT and of the ε2 allele as a protective factor have been well established (Corder et al 1993, Strittmatter et al 1993). However ApoE allele testing is not in routine use in current clinical practice.

Table 25.5   Genes implicated in familial and sporadic DAT

Chromosome product	Gene type	Age of onset (years) All	% age of Familial cases (Total c.120)	% of all cases	Protein
1 (3 mutations)	Autosomal dominant (var. penetrance)	40–90	c. 20	c. 2	Presenilin II (STM 2)
14 (28 mutations)	Autosomal dominant	30–55	70–80	5–10	Presenilin I (S182)
21 (4 mutations)	Autosomal dominant	40–65	2–3	<1	Amyloid precursor protein (APP)
19 (ε2,3,4 alleles)	Risk factor	40–very old		40–50	APOE

Modified from Barinaga (1995) and Eastwood (1996).

The absence of the ε4ε4 genotype does not preclude a diagnosis of DAT and its presence does not inevitably lead to DAT, so testing cannot be used predictively and for diagnostic purposes it should not be used as the sole test (Tanzi et al 1996). Table 25.5 summarises the current knowledge of genetic influences in familial DAT (covering all age groups). Other risk factors which have been implicated are summarised in Table 25.6.

Neuroimaging   Jobst et al (1992) have suggested that particular CT scan measurements indicating hippocampal atrophy may be of diagnostic significance. MRI studies (reviewed by O'Brien 1996) bring conflicting results but have indicated that periventricular white matter lesions are more common in DAT, though they are not specific to the illness and their relationship to neuropsychological dysfunction is not clear. Claims that particular patterns of lobar perfusion deficits in DAT can be shown on SPECT and PET scans (Herholz 1995) remain to be clarified.

Other tests   The search for a peripheral marker of the central cholinergic deficit continues. For example, Scinto et al (1994) claimed that the pupillary response to tropicamide application was significantly altered in DAT. This however has not been confirmed by others (Zerfass et al 1995). Kennard et al (1996) found the serum concentration of the iron-binding protein p97 to be elevated in DAT.

● *Vascular dementia (VD)*   After DAT, this group of disorders is probably the second most common cause of dementia in old age, although DLBT has also been suggested for this position. Amar & Wilcock (1996) report that histopathological studies show *multi-infarct dementia* to be the sole cause in 9–33% of cases, and that it contributes to dementia in a further 10–36%. In

Table 25.6   Risk and protective factors in late-onset non-familial DAT

Risk factors

Proven
    Age
    Down's syndrome
    ApoE ε4
Likely
    Female sex
    Head injury
    Postmenopausal oestrogen decline
Possible
    Vascular factors
    Family history of Down's syndrome
    Family history of Parkinson's disease
    Herpes simplex virus HSV-1

Protective factors

Proven
    ApoE ε2
Possible
    Oestrogen
    Premorbid intelligence and education
    Smoking
    Non-steroidal anti-inflammatory drugs

addition to the multi-infarct pattern of damage (which usually results from thromboembolic disease, but can also be caused by cerebral vasculitis or multiple lacunar infarcts), ischaemia leading to dementia may be caused by a *single infarct* in a crucial site or by white matter ischaemia (*Binswanger's disease*). Vascular dementia (not always progressive) may be due to hypoxia or haemorrhage (e.g. subdural haematoma, subarachnoid haemorrhage).

The borderland between vascular and Alzheimer-type dementia is complicated by the cerebral amyloid angiopathy characteristic of DAT which may perhaps lead to haemorrhage, by the existence of illnesses related to DAT where the damage is largely vascular (hereditary haemorrhagic cerebral angiopathy of Dutch type), and by findings such as those of Thomas et al (1996), that the β-amyloid protein may alter the endothelium of small cerebral β-blood vessels by stimulating the production of superoxide radicals. Alzheimer would perhaps not have been surprised, since his original patient had autopsy findings suggesting arteriosclerosis.

For many years the Hachinski score (Hachinski et al 1975) was used as a diagnostic test for multi-infarct dementia but it is probably insufficiently reliable or valid. History taking, examination and MRI scanning are currently the best diagnostic tools for diagnosis of the various types of VD. The NINDS–AIREN criteria provide a research diagnostic tool (Roman et al 1993).

• *Dementia of Lewy body type (DLBT)* Lewy bodies, which are eosinophilic inclusion bodies classically associated with Parkinson's disease, are in fact found in a spectrum of conditions now covered by the term Lewy body disease (McKeith 1995). Where there is predominant subcortical pathology the symptoms are largely neurological – perhaps as many as 30% of patients who are diagnosed as having idiopathic Parkinson's disease have evidence of dementia (Mayeux et al 1992). Where cortical pathology predominates there will be a combination of mental impairment, psychiatric symptoms and various extrapyramidal symptoms. Criteria for diagnosing DLBT have been proposed by McKeith et al (1992)

Table 25.7 Operational criteria for DBLT
Fluctuating cognitive impairment
At least one of:
Visual or auditory hallucinations
Mild spontaneous extrapyramidal features
Increased sensitivity to neuroleptics
Repeated unexplained falls or transient clouding
or loss of consciousness
Persistent and often rapidly progressive course
Exclusion of a physical cause of the syndrome
Exclusion of vascular pathology

Modified from McKeith et al (1992).

(Table 25.7) and others. Many cases may in the past have been diagnosed as of Alzheimer or vascular type, and many research findings may therefore have been based on impure samples.

• *Other causes* Among rarer causes it is worth noting that *Huntington's chorea* can begin in late life, though dementia is usually less prominent than in younger patients. *Syphilis* continues to contribute occasional cases of dementia, usually in a forme fruste of classical general paralysis. Secondary or primary *brain tumours* and non-metastatic effects present more often to neurologists than to psychiatrists. *Metabolic* and other 'medical' causes, often reversible, may be detected by simple screening tests (Table 25.3); but thyroid dysfunction and vitamin B_{12} and folate deficiencies are usually coincidental findings rather than causes of the dementia. *Alcoholic* brain damage must always be considered. *Normal pressure hydrocephalus* is worth searching for when early unexplained incontinence, abnormal gait or an atypical pattern of impairment are found. The future contribution in old age of *AIDS* dementia and of prion-related dementias is unpredictable, but these diagnoses must be kept in mind. So far, the cases of a new variety of *Creutzfeldt–Jakob disease* (Will et al 1996), which have raised the possibility of interspecies transmission of prion disease from cattle, have occurred in younger people.

Estimation of severity Although there have been many attempts to grade dementia into three or more categories (Hughes et al 1982, Reisberg et al 1982), they have been unsuccessful because of the complexity of the illness. Staging has anyway little practical significance for the sufferer or carers, who are more interested in practical problems. For example, wandering may be severe at mild stages, when the patient is physically fit and partially aware of her situation, and mild at severe stages, when she is frail and unmotivated. Severity is best rated using one of the simpler rating scales. In earlier stages neuro-cognitive rating scales are appropriate (reviewed by Morris & Kopelman 1992); later, behaviour and non-cognitive (affective, psychotic or neurological) assessments are more useful (Weiner 1990, Hope & Fairburn 1992, Hope & Patel 1993).

Listing problems The causes of symptoms in dementia are extremely complicated.

First, there are gradual losses of function. Some are simple and progressive losses of clearly localised brain functions such as recent memory impairment, agnosias and dyspraxias, the various dysphasias, and, later, more hard neurological signs. Others seem to be due to more generalised damage, such as the impairment of abstract thinking, remote memories and intelligence.

Second, there is the loss of standards, judgement, conscience, self-control and planning ability commonly found in frontal lobe disorder, and relating to the 'executive' and monitoring functions of the brain. Loss of inhibition on cognition, action and feeling can lead to disturbed behaviour, particularly at mild and moderate stages. Similar mechanisms explain loss of control of the bladder and, later, the bowel, emergence of primitive reflexes, some psychotic symptoms and fits.

Third are the reactions of the patient to her illness. There is a growing interest in exploring and understanding the experiences of people who suffer dementia (Goldsmith 1996). Insight and emotions decline only gradually and sufferers retain some ability to react into quite late stages, though these reactions become distorted by other impairments and by disinhibition. Estimates of the prevalence of depression range from 30 to 80% of cases (Sunderland et al 1988). Anxiety is common, and paranoid reactions and hoarding of possessions may occur. Covering up the embarrassment of the condition and social withdrawal are probably the most common reactions. Some sufferers may sense the frightening disintegration of personality. When insight is lost, the patient may react to what she sees as unnecessary intrusions into her life when she feels entirely competent. Later she is likely to become more passive and may end her days in a mildly disinhibited euphoria quite out of keeping with the seriousness of her condition.

Fourth, family interactions contribute to the problems of dementia. The family is aware of and remembers all the impairments and disturbances of the patient. They are likely to experience grief for the loss of her mind and personality and be more distressed than she is about her embarrassing behaviour, while simultaneously coping with the burden of her physical and psychological care and arranging services which can feel like an intrusion into family life. Worse still, they are likely to get no thanks from the increasingly withdrawn or egocentric patient. When other relatives and friends desert the patient out of embarrassment, it is no wonder if the now isolated remaining carer is very distressed on occasions, and that the relationship between carer and patient may become disturbed, with effects on the patient's behaviour.

Caring for a dementia sufferer is not usually a role taken on by choice. The research on stress among caring relatives has been well reviewed by Morris et al (1988). The majority of carers are either daughters in middle age or spouses. The burden of caring at home can be enormous. As many as 65% of close carers of day hospital attenders (Gilleard et al 1984a) experience distress at levels equivalent to a psychiatric case. Others, looking perhaps at more willing carers, have found lower levels of distress (Eagles et al 1987). Donaldson et al (1997) have emphasised the effect of

'non-cognitive' symptoms in the patient on the stress felt by carers.

Whether this strain is tolerable to the carer or not depends somewhat on the patient's symptoms, but more on the nature of the carer's previous relationship with the patient (Gilhooley 1984). Other important factors include the support that the carer feels she receives from her family and others, the services and financial assistance she receives and her methods of coping, some lifelong, some learnt during the experience of caring. Levin et al (1994) and others have shown that carers generally feel better when their relative finally moves into longer term care.

Other factors which may influence the presentation of dementia and which should be assessed are the environment and regimen in which the patient is living (Moos & Lemke 1980), which can make the difference between a dangerous symptom and a trivial complaint, the physical health of the patient and other disabilities that she may be suffering from.

Finally, it is important to assess the ability of the patient to understand and make decisions on matters such as finances, care and medical treatment.

If all these aspects are covered in discussions with the patient, the caring relatives and others who know her, it is likely that a comprehensive list of problem titles can be prepared (Table 25.8). Estimates of the frequency of individual problems in dementia (e.g. Sunderland et al (1988), Burns et al (1990b) and Ballard et al (1996) on *mood disorders*; Berrios & Brook (1985), Burns et al (1990a) and Ballard & Oyebode (1995) on *psychotic symptoms*) have not been entirely successful, as so much depends on which population of sufferers is studied. Other research usefully analyses the nature and causes of behaviour disturbances in detail (e.g. Morris et al (1989) and Keene & Hope (1996) on *eating disorders*; Hope et al (1994) on *wandering*; Stokes (1987), Ware et al (1990) and Patel & Hope (1993) on *aggression*; and Stokes (1986) on *screaming and shouting*).

Management

Treatment of the cause of dementia Ideally, treatment should address the cause of the neuronal damage in dementia. At present this is not possible except in the relatively few cases of reversible dementia. Even in the 'untreatable' cases of DAT and VD there are signs of hope.

Dementia of Alzheimer type Kelly & Hunter (1995) review current pharmacological strategies for DAT. Treatments which can boost cholinergic activity are becoming available. Among anticholinesterase drugs, tetrahydroaminoacridine has been extensively studied and donepezil has been licensed for use in the

Table 25.8   A short check-list of potential problems in dementia (Jacques 1992)

Problem	Examples
Memory impairment	Forgets appointments
	Forgets to change clothes, wash, go to toilet
	Forgets to eat, take tablets
	Loses possessions
Disorientation	Time, day or night
	Around house
	Recognising family or other visitors
Needs physical help	Dressing
	Washing, bathing
	Toileting
	Eating
	Housework
	Mobility
Risks in the home	Falls
	Fire from cigarettes, cooker, heating
	Flooding
	Letting strangers in
	Wandering out
Risks outside	Driving, road sense
	Gets lost
Apathy	Little conversation
	Lack of interest
	Poor self-care
Poor communication	Dysphasia
Repetitiveness	Questions or stories
	Actions
Uncontrolled emotion	Distress
	Anger or aggression
	Demands for attention
Uncontrolled behaviour	Restlessness, day or night
	Vulgar table or toilet habits
	Undressing
	Sexual disinhibition
	Shop lifting
Incontinence	Urine
	Faeces
	Inappropriate excretion
Emotional reactions	Depression
	Anxiety
	Frustration
	Embarrassment or withdrawal
Other reactions	Suspiciousness
	Hoarding
Mistaken beliefs	Still at work
	Parents or spouse still alive
Decision making	Indecisiveness
	Easily influenced
	Poor judgement
	Refuses help
Burden on family	Disruption of social and family life
	Distress, guilt, rejection
	Family discord

UK. These treatments have been shown to delay the decline in some patients with DAT, perhaps by 6–9 months. It has been suggested that ApoE genotype may help predict response to anticholinesterase treatment (Poirier et al 1995) and there have been hints that people with DLBT may respond better to the drugs (Harrison & McKeith 1995). Tang et al (1996) found evidence that oestrogen may protect against the development of DAT in postmenopausal women.

The advent of therapeutic possibilities for dementia in the current political climate of health services brings old age psychiatrists into difficult discussions on health care rationing and clinical criteria for the use of expensive treatments. Christie & Train's (1984) worry that longer survival times in dementia put a huge burden on services may prove to be prophetic.

Vascular dementia   Vascular dementias may be preventable to some extent by controlling vascular risk factors such as hypertension (Meyer et al 1987) and diabetes, and hypertension has been implicated in other impairments in old age including DAT (Skoog et al 1996). In multi-infarct dementia aspirin prophylaxis may prove to be helpful. Other specific treatments such as calcium-channel blockers are being evaluated.

Treatment of the symptoms of dementia   In practice, management of most cases of dementia consists of trying to find solutions to the problems on the individual's problem list.

Losses   The sufferer should be encouraged to use her remaining abilities to the full. Where there are gaps in her ability, the task is to fill those gaps so that she is not struggling helplessly. Gap fillers relate to all aspects of daily living, ranging from a phone call to remind her to get up in the morning to full nursing care. The carer's imagination and the experience of other carers are the most helpful guides. Sometimes a modest amount of retraining is possible. A patient who has recently forgotten how to use her cooker may be retrained after the device has been simplified, and so gain a few more months of independence. Patients who are repeatedly distressed by constantly rediscovering the death of their spouse may be helped by repeated but sensitive exposure to the facts of the death.

Behavioural and psychotic symptoms   Although disinhibited or poorly judged behaviour may have an organic basis, it is nevertheless influenced by environment and circumstances. For this reason encouraging normal behaviour can have dramatic effects on patients who otherwise seem to be uncontrollable. For similar reasons simple behaviour modification techniques, altering the reactions of others rather than trying to alter the patient's behaviour directly, can be effective. A labile aggressive man may be more placid with his wife if she realises that his anger is not intended and so learns to react in an unemotional way. However, relatives or staff often have to act as 'external conscience' for the patient, restraining her in a non-punishing way from unwise actions, like walking into the road or taking her clothes off in public. The fine balance between this reasonable care towards vulnerable brain-damaged people and unreasonable intervention in their lives should be debated in each case.

Traditionally, antipsychotic drugs have been used to control disturbed behaviour in dementia, but there is conflicting evidence about their efficacy (Schneider et al 1990) and they have sometimes been used more as sedatives. There has probably been overuse of these drugs, for example in nursing homes (McGrath & Jackson 1996), they may even worsen mental impairment (McShane et al 1997) and stopping the drugs may bring improvement (Findlay et al 1989). Sometimes small doses of antipsychotic drugs are both safe and effective, but often, for example in repetitive shouters, such large doses are required to quieten that major side-effects occur. When specific antipsychotic effects are required, say for hallucinations, the newer antipsychotic drugs, with potentially fewer side-effects, should probably be tried, but still have to be evaluated in dementia. Particular caution is necessary in DLBT, where neuroleptic sensitivity can lead to serious side-effects.

Less toxic tranquillisers such as chlormethiazole have some use. Possible 5-hydroxytryptamine mechanisms in repetitive behaviour have led to the use of antidepressants such as fluoxetine and trazodone. Carbamazepine is helpful in some cases. None of these drugs have been systematically evaluated in well-designed trials. The best practice is to avoid drug treatment where other measures or greater tolerance of the behaviour are possible.

Reactions   Patients' emotional reactions to early dementia should not be dismissed as part of the illness, but listened to with empathy. In some early cases, talking directly about the diagnosis will be both possible and reassuring. As public awareness of dementia grows and stigma disappears, more will wish to know their diagnosis and its consequences. Later, of course, there is a limit to the usefulness of repeated reassurance of any sort. Sometimes the best response to recurrent distress is to change the subject gently, or engage the patient in other activities. The outraged, insightless patient requires skillful and imaginative handling.

If emotional reactions are severe then drug treatment is appropriate, using therapeutic doses of specific drugs for specific problems such as depression, anxiety or paranoid reactions.

Carers   Support for families is of cardinal importance in the management of dementia. First, they need to be clearly informed of the diagnosis. This may bring enormous relief if they are blaming the sufferer for laziness or obstinacy, or themselves for impatience or lack of concern. Then they need to be educated fully about the problems which dementia may bring and the services and benefits which are available, using talks and literature (Mace et al 1985, Wilcock 1990, HEBS 1996). They need moral support, practical advice from others and the feeling that they are not alone in caring. Carers' groups are invaluable, though not for everybody. Stress management techniques may be useful, and counselling may help in coping with grief or with disturbances to family and social life. There is considerable scope to use family and individual therapies to help carers develop their coping skills (Richardson et al 1994). The particular needs of families from differing ethnic groups and of younger carers need to be catered for in any catchment area service. Most of all, all families will need regular, planned respite. Finally, when the patient dies the process of grief counselling should not end.

Environment   For patients who live at home it is often necessary to 'treat' the environment. This may mean providing reminders and aids around the house, or reducing risks from gas and electrical appliances. Similar principles apply to the design of homes and wards for dementing residents. Ideally, dementia sufferers should be in an environment which combines homeliness, privacy and individuality with compensation for lost abilities and a reasonable level of stimulation, while allowing freedom to wander under good observation (Norman 1987, Weisman et al 1991, Marshall 1997).

Physical care   Patients with dementia may forget physical symptoms, be unable to communicate them, or suffer anosagnosia or autotopagnosia. They must be treated in this respect (though not in others) rather like infants. The only outward evidence of illness may be restlessness, a deterioration in mental state or frank delirium. Poor medical care leads to both physical and psychiatric problems.

Decisions   Impairment of comprehension, insight, memory, reasoning, judgement, conscience, motivation and communication make it inevitable that dementing patients are less able to make either day-to-day or major decisions from early in the illness. At first the sufferer will be entirely competent, but gradually her competence to make some decisions or judgments will be more and more doubtful, until she becomes legally incapable (British Medical Association/The Law Society 1995).

In Britain the law on incapacity separates financial issues from issues of care and treatment. Most of the common and statute law regarding control of finances, testamentary capacity, guardianship or admission under the Mental Health Act, and consent to treatment was not developed with dementia sufferers in mind. The result is that it is both unwieldy and sometimes quite inappropriate. Law reform is urgently needed (Law Commission 1995, Scottish Law Commission 1995).

In all areas of decision making the choice for a dementia sufferer is:

- She takes her own decisions.
- She arranges to hand them over to others because she feels unable to handle them herself.
- Decisions are taken over from her through a legal process, because she is not only unable to manage them herself, but is also unable to direct other people to manage for her.

In addition she may be more or less suggestible as a result of her illness, and the motives of families and financial advisers may not always be entirely altruistic. Her ability to communicate her views will be impaired to some extent. It is nearly impossible to define exactly when the patient becomes unable to understand enough to decide for herself. And it is perfectly possible to be competent in one area, such as whether to accept help at home, and not another, such as whether to sell one's house.

A lot will depend on the patient's level of understanding of her current situation. It is very likely that at the beginning of the illness she will be able to understand the diagnosis. At later stages the clinician will need to judge how best to give the necessary information to help decision making.

Patient's expressed views are an amalgam of previously held views ('substitute judgement'), present views expressed in words or actions and passive 'behavioural' consent. Many cannot express their views even if they hold them. Many become excessively apathetic or suggestible. The consequence of all this is that there are decisions which theoretically only the patient herself can ever take but which she may become effectively incapable of taking. In such a circumstance the views of relatives may be assumed to be more important. Relatives have no legal right (unless through a court) to take decisions for incapable patients, although doctors and others sometimes informally give them such rights. Professionals, and to a lesser extent relatives, may be protected by the common law if their actions can be shown to benefit the patient and to do no harm ('best interests'), though this is gradually less so as the arguments for *personal autonomy* become increasingly powerful. The powers of a mental health guardian, the responsible medical officer, the Court of Protection (England and Wales), the Office of Care and Protection (Northern Ireland) or a curator bonis (Scotland) are limited by law.

Finances One of the great advantages of early diagnosis of dementia is that it gives the sufferer the chance to appoint an agent to collect benefits, grant *power of attorney* to someone she trusts, or to make or update her will. The old age psychiatrist may be called in to declare whether someone is competent to make such decisions, but all too often this occurs after the event. Where she has not given advance directions the patient has to depend on arrangements such as Department of Social Security appointeeship, special arrangements for hospitals to manage affairs, or court-appointed agents. There are considerable gaps in the current legal framework to protect dementia sufferers from potential financial abuse from unscrupulous relatives or others.

Restraint Conflict may arise between a patient's wish to move about autonomously and the fears of relatives or professionals about her safety. A variety of restraining practices have been developed. Restricting the right to drive a car is relatively uncontroversial (Bahro et al 1995), but physical and mechanical restraints, the use of drug treatment as a form of restraint, locking the doors of care facilities, surveillance cameras in care and living areas, electronic tagging and 'passive' alarms have all been subject to considerable criticism. The 'best interests' argument has often been used to justify such measures, but, in the unequal power relationship between dementia sufferers and their carers, this can be tantamount to justifying impersonal treatment or even frank neglect or abuse. Where a patient with dementia is actively and consistently objecting to advice from carers which would restrict her freedom the powers of the Mental Health Act, including admission and guardianship, should always be considered. If these powers are seen as too draconian in a particular case, those caring for the patient need to be very aware of the potential for abuse of their power over a vulnerable adult and the distress likely to be caused by restraint in her 'best interests'.

Medical treatment The Mental Health Act covers medical treatment only where it can be seen as treatment for mental disorder. Doctors and other professionals who prescribe or administer medical, surgical or other investigation or treatment do so 'in good faith', in accordance with professional expectations, and with the protection of the common law where its principles would suggest that it was neglectful if the treatment was necessary but was not given. This is all very well in life-saving treatment in early dementia and where everybody is agreed. If there are disagreements or uncertainties about the necessity of the treatment the patient's voice may be missing from the discussion, and a domineering relative or a strong doctor might override other views. Full consultation, a second opinion if necessary, clear recording of decisions and in difficult cases referral to a court procedure are the essentials of good practice in this area.

Terminal care   Terminal care of dementia sufferers is a particularly sensitive subject. At this stage the patient cannot contribute to discussions about how far investigation or treatment should proceed. It is normal practice to consider any previously expressed wishes of the patient, to consult with relatives and staff caring for her, but for the doctor to make the decision to treat or not on the basis of her present quality of life, expectation of recovery and level of distress. *Advance directives* (often misleadingly called 'living wills'), by which a person declares that they do not wish to be actively treated under certain conditions, are not yet legally binding in Britain, but should be carefully taken into consideration. Active *euthanasia* for dementing people is difficult even to conceive of, since the patient's request would, to be valid, necessarily have been made before the dementia began, probably several years before the event, and it is almost impossible for an individual to predict what their own experience of dementia would be. Consent by relatives could hardly be valid, and the suspicion might be that relatives and staff were motivated by impatience at caring, when a more appropriate response would be to try to improve the lot of the vulnerable sufferer.

Research   This is another controversial and difficult area (Brooke 1988, Berghmans & ter Meulen 1995). Here there is rarely the protection of necessity. Even in therapeutic research, it is hard to argue that the patient will necessarily be better off as a result, and the argument that fellow patients may benefit later is difficult to sustain. The discussions, explanations and consents which ethics committees rightly demand in all research on patients will be impracticable beyond the early stages. Some have got round this problem by concentrating their efforts on the earliest stages of the illness. Others have suggested an important role for ethics committees or emphasise the possible use of advance directives or proxy decision making. The subject deserves wide debate both by psychiatrists, lawyers and the public.

Genetic testing   It is now becoming possible to predict whether a member of a family with familial DAT is carrying the disease gene, and to predict whether an individual has an APOE status which carries a high or low risk of DAT. In general genetic testing is only of value where the test is highly accurate and where there is an available treatment (Lovestone 1996). The very simple test for apolipoprotein alleles in blood will tempt some, but people who contemplate this type of genetic testing need careful counselling about the

consequences, and need to know that the result could be used to their disadvantage, for example by insurance companies.

Advocacy   In response to some of the deficiencies of the law and to the risk that vulnerable dementing patients may be exploited or neglected, or not have their views represented, the concept of advocacy has been introduced. Family and professionals of course act as advocates in many cases but, where the patient is isolated or at particular risk, there is virtue in having someone whose sole function is to represent her in seeking help or benefits, in discussions about decisions, or in commenting on standards of care. The appointment of a lay advocate, perhaps through the Alzheimer Society, may be appropriate. Law reformers need to address the peculiar needs of insightless patients who desperately need advocacy but would reject it if offered.

Case conference   In the absence of an adequate legal framework or developed advocacy, the best practice, when there is debate about a dementing patient's competence and if she may be at risk in any way, is to hold a case conference involving all concerned. This helps avoid compulsory measures in most cases, while encouraging creative thinking about ways of reducing risks or helping her come to rational decisions. Case conferences must never, however, be used to bully vulnerable patients or reluctant carers.

Psychosis

'Old' psychosis – the 'graduate' population

The advent of antipsychotic drugs in the 1950s led to a progressive decrease in the long-stay schizophrenic population of psychiatric hospitals, the so-called 'graduates'. Elderly chronic schizophrenic patients are now more likely to be found in the community, often living alone or in hostel accommodation which cannot always offer the physical or psychiatric nursing care which they need, particularly since severe negative symptoms may be the predominant feature of illness (Soni & Mallik 1993). The result has been a slow increase in referrals from this group, often physically frail and living in poor conditions.

'New' psychosis – late life schizophrenia (late paraphrenia) and related disorders

Kraepelin (1919) used the term paraphrenia to describe an illness with delusions and hallucinations but without schizophrenic changes in affect, form of thought and personality. Roth & Morrissey (1952) noted that illnesses of this description were the most common form of psychosis in old age and called this 'late paraphrenia'. Since that time there has been considerable debate as to whether late paraphrenia is or is not schizophrenia of late onset (Reicher-Rossler et al 1995).

Epidemiology Old age psychotic disorder is not common. Only 10% of hospital admissions are for psychosis, and population studies, if they locate any cases at all, have shown prevalence rates of less than 1% (Eastwood & Corbin 1985, Castle & Murray 1993). The peak incidence of schizophrenia in males is between the ages of 15 and 30 years, and male hospital admission rates fall through old age, but for women a later peak has been found and admission rates rise in the eighth and ninth decades. If the figures for late life psychosis are added to those from younger people the lifetime risk is roughly equal between the sexes, but with more of the risk for females occurring in late life.

Aetiology Some aetiological factors support the link with schizophrenia but others suggest specific environmental factors.

Sex In Kay & Roth's series (1961) the sex ratio for old age schizophrenia was 9:1 for females to males, though others have found it as low as 4:1. Even allowing for the preponderance of elderly women in the community this is a very striking sex difference. Perhaps susceptible women are protected from psychosis in earlier life and need particular environmental stresses for it to emerge later (Castle & Murray 1993).

Genetics The risk of schizophrenia and paraphrenia in first-degree relatives of late paraphrenics is roughly half that found in first-degree relatives of younger schizophrenics.

Personality Kay & Roth (1961) found that 45% had lifelong paranoid or schizoid personality traits, and that this factor was independent of genetic and sensory causes.

Sensory deprivation Deafness has been shown to be associated with old age schizophrenia in between 25 and 40% of cases (Kay & Roth 1961, Post 1966, Cooper 1976). Visual impairment is less commonly relevant. Prager & Jeste (1993) have proposed that some of the association is due to suboptimal correction of the sensory deficits.

Social isolation All studies have found that the great majority of these patients are socially isolated. They are often unmarried, divorced or separated, or they married late and had few children. Their personality may have also led to isolation, and deafness increases this tendency.

Life events Some studies have shown a preponderance of life events preceding old age schizophrenia. However, in many cases the isolation and suspiciousness of the sufferer delay referral so that events before onset are unclear or modified by paranoid misinterpretation.

Organic factors Naguib & Levy (1987) showed that some patients with old age schizophrenia have CT evidence of organic brain changes. The relationship of these changes to the cognitive impairment which some patients exhibit, or to outcome, is unclear (Hymas et al 1989). Some evidence would suggest a spectrum of disorders, with at one end a pure delusional disorder with organic changes and at the other hallucinosis associated with sensory deprivation (Flint et al 1991 using CT, Howard et al 1994 using MRI).

Clinical features The onset is usually insidious, and in the past some cases of late-onset delusional disorder have been thought of as personality developments in schizoid or suspicious individuals rather than true psychosis. Resistance to help because of lack of insight may prevent diagnosis for years after the first psychotic experiences.

Paranoid symptoms may include any combination of persecutory, grandiose, erotic and jealous ideas or delusions. Hallucinations are most commonly auditory, but olfactory hallucinations, somatic hallucinations of electricity or rape and visual hallucinations, usually of flashes, also occur. In some patients, perhaps 10–20%, only delusions are present, as in Kraepelin's *paranoia* (1919), or *persistent delusional disorder* (see Ch. 15), though some of these may have had organic brain lesions (Flint et al 1991). Typical first-rank symptoms are found in about 30% of cases. These may include experiences of intrusion into the thoughts or body of the sufferer. Complaints of intrusions into her personal space in the sense of house or property are much more typical. An important consequence of this is that when the patient is admitted to hospital or moves house to escape from her persecutors, the symptoms may temporarily disappear (Post 1966). This can give the impression that the symptoms were exaggerated at home, or that the patient is now cured. However, a return visit home, or time to settle into a new personal space in hospital or a new house brings a resurgence of symptoms. Typical negative symptoms are uncommon, and indeed patients often preserve strong paranoid personality traits, making management difficult.

Various symptoms of neuropsychological impairment are found in a small proportion of patients, though estimates vary widely and their cause is unclear (Almeida et al 1995), depending largely on the exclusion criteria of individual studies. Many patients are proud of their continuing mental alertness and see this as protection against their persecutors. Possibly no more than expected develop dementia in the long run. If dementia does develop, the psychotic symptoms may 'dissolve' and antipsychotic treatment is no longer needed.

Depression secondary to the persecutions is not uncommon, and causes difficulties in differentiating old age schizophrenia from affective or schizoaffective disorders. The more usual reaction is of outrage and anger. The patient retaliates against her persecutors, who are likely to be unsuspecting neighbours. Calling in the police or a solicitor is as likely as calling in the doctor, and lack of insight usually leads the patient to suggest that the neighbours rather than she need treatment.

Treatment Antipsychotic drugs are effective in old age schizophrenia and delusional disorder (Post 1966, Hymas et al 1989, Jeste et al 1996), and long-term treatment is necessary. Christie (1982) has shown the quite dramatic effect on the need for hospital long-stay care by comparing 1970s figures with Roth's figures from the 1940s (Roth 1955). Compliance is a problem and the psychiatrist may have to resort to indirect means to persuade the patient to take drugs. Some patients have a trusted 'ally' who can persuade them. A CPN who gradually gets to know her can become such an ally. Suggestions that the drug will help her 'cope with the persecution better' or 'will put the problem into the background' may help. Few patients have enough insight to feel that treatment is fully justified. Compliance is not helped by the tendency of antipsychotic drugs to produce more side-effects the older the patient. Oral drugs which are relatively free of the common side-effects of antipsychotics, such as sulpiride, pimozide and risperidone and newer drugs, are more likely to be acceptable, and age is not a contraindication to clozapine treatment. Depot treatment is tolerated by some patients and is easier to monitor over a long period but occasionally leads to intractable side-effects. Relieving isolation and deafness have also been proposed as possible treatments.

Other conditions with paranoid or hallucinatory symptoms

The differential diagnosis of paranoid symptoms and of hallucinations in old age is complicated and there is considerable overlap between some of the conditions.

Secondary paranoid states A variety of organic cerebral conditions and treatment with steroids, antiparkinsonian or other drugs can sometimes produce psychotic phenomena without obvious mental impairment. History and investigation of the patient's physical state are important in all cases of paranoid psychosis.

Delirium The psychotic symptoms of delirium may be mistaken for symptoms of a primary paranoid psychosis. The acute time-course, relation to physical illness, evidence of cognitive impairment, and characteristic symptoms of delirium (Table 25.4) should help to distinguish between the disorders. In delirium, visual hallucinations are more common than auditory hallucinations, while the reverse is the case in schizophrenia.

Dementia Paranoid and other psychotic symptoms are common in dementia (Ballard & Oyebode 1995). Paranoid ideas may be a reaction to memory impairment in a sensitive individual, or may relate to the basic disease process. Agnosias, receptive dysphasia, impairment of comprehension and other related disorders may explain misinterpretations which lead on to more fixed paranoid ideas. Visual hallucinations have traditionally been ascribed to delirium occurring in the course of multi-infarct dementia, but are now more clearly linked to a diagnosis of DLBT (Table 25.7).

Paranoid ideas and hallucinatory experiences in dementia are usually relatively transient and ill formed. They respond, though often incompletely, to antipsychotic medication.

Affective disorders Psychotic symptoms are common in both severe depressive illness and in hypomania in old age. The admixture of symptoms helps to differentiate, as does the affective colouring of the experiences. A curious phenomenon is the persistence of psychotic symptoms between episodes in some patients with a long history of recurrent affective disorder.

Schizoaffective disorder Post (1971) described a number of cases who did not fit into either the description of paranoid psychotic illness or affective illness, but who were intermediate in clinical features, aetiology and outcome.

Hallucinations of sensory deprivation Berrios & Brook (1984) suggested that visual hallucinations without marked paranoid ideas might be a non-specific phenomenon in elderly patients, linked to visual impairment rather than to any particular diagnosis. The 'visions' are of people, animals or scenes and the patient has a degree of or even complete insight. If there is no other associated psychiatric disorder then the term *Charles–Bonnet syndrome* is appropriate (Damas-Mora et al 1982). Teunisse et al (1995) studied a large group of these patients and confirmed the association with visual sensory deprivation and old age. Some may prove to have DLBT. Small doses of antipsychotic drugs can be helpful, but some patients can use reassurance to help them pay less attention to the hallucinations.

The same is true of what is probably the auditory equivalent of this phenomenon, musical hallucinations (Berrios 1990) in those with a hearing impairment.

Affective disorders

Epidemiology

Longitudinal studies of the natural history of affective disorder show a general trend for episodes to occur more frequently and to last longer (Zis & Goodwin 1970, Cutter & Post 1982). The incidence of new cases of major affective disorder is at its peak in young adulthood, and probably declines steadily through the rest of life. Possibly less than 10% of new cases emerge in old age, and few of them are bipolar. Angst (1973) described a worse prognosis in later onset cases and Alexopoulos et al (1996) suggested that older-onset cases have a greater tendency to chronicity, but Winokur (1975) found no difference from early-onset cases.

A review of several community studies suggested a rate of between 1 and 2.5% for severe or psychotic depression (Eastwood & Corbin 1985) and Henderson et al 1993 found similar rates for DSM-IIIR major depressive disorder. However some (Copeland et al 1987, Lindesay et al 1989) give rates of 4–5%. Female rates are always higher than male rates, but may fall somewhat in later age groups. On the other hand, less severe depressions are common and may increase with ageing. Figures of 10–15% are regularly found, though of course the difficulties of defining mild disorders are notorious. Figures for all degrees of depression reach 22–33% and particularly high rates may be found in residential or nursing care homes (Ames 1990).

Aetiology

Genetic factors are much less important causally in affective disorder beginning in late life (Mendlewicz et al 1972, Young & Klerman 1992), while physical illness is significant in between 60 and 75% of cases. In a community study of major depression Murphy (1982) showed the importance of life events, physical illness and lack of a confiding relationship. The many losses to which elderly people are susceptible explain the relatively high prevalence of milder depressions, though sufferers may hesitate to complain because such losses are expected (Parkes 1964).

Cerebral pathology as an aetiological factor in late life severe depression is unlikely to be very important as the prevalence of the condition probably does not rise with increasing age. Jacoby & Levy (1980b) and others have shown CT abnormalities in some elderly depressives, and some have shown relationships between these changes and apparent cognitive impairment (Beats et al 1991). The nature and significance of the changes are disputed, and it is not proven that they have any effect on treatment or prognosis. MRI again brings conflicting results (O'Brien et al 1996), but deep white matter lesions are commonly described. Interpretation of these lesions is complicated because they have also been associated with normal ageing and with vascular disease.

Shulman & Post (1980), Stone (1989) and Broadhead & Jacoby (1990) have emphasised that new cases of mania are often related, perhaps causally, to brain disease, at least in men. And a link between onset of depressive illness in elderly men and a later diagnosis of abdominal cancer has been postulated, though not all are agreed.

Clinical features

Since the concept of involutional melancholia was abandoned, it has been clear that there are few significant differences between early- and late-onset depressions. There are cohort, period and age differences in, for example, the prevalence of religious delusions, and in the content of hypochondriacal ideas, including the very common fear of dementia.

Atypical presentations of depressive disorder are relatively common. The most debated is *pseudodementia*, or *cognitive change in depression*. Measurable intellectual impairment is often found during late-life depressions, but usually returns to normal after treatment. One possible explanation of pseudodementia is that it represents a crossing of the threshold of dementia in a person whose cerebral reserve is already compromised. If this were true then depressive illness with pseudodementia would predict the later development of dementia, as Kral & Emery (1989) and Devanand et al (1996) have suggested, though others have disputed this. The following list of clinical features (adapted from Wells 1979) distinguishing pseudodementia from dementia is helpful:

- past history of depressive illness
- depressed mood
- diurnal variation in mood
- other biological symptoms
- islands of normality
- exaggerated presentation of symptoms.

Agitation is described much more commonly in older depressives, as are *paranoid symptoms*. Hypochondriacal symptoms and other abnormal illness behaviour, pseudopersonality disorder and *mixed affective disorder* are also quite common, but it is possible that these descriptions are due to a sampling bias, as most studies have concentrated on inpatient populations.

Hypomania usually occurs in people with a past history of bipolar affective disorder. There is some evidence that male admission rates rise with age (Eagles & Whalley, 1985). Its first onset in old age should raise the suspicion of a physical illness or cerebral pathology (see Aetiology). It is particularly rare to have severe mania in old age, and the mental overactivity and elation of hypomania is not always matched by outward signs of overactivity. Indeed, the prevailing affect may be irritability. Delirium is an important and sometimes difficult differential diagnosis, as it can present with some of the features of hypomania, while more severe cases of hypomania tend to develop a pseudo- or real delirium.

Differential diagnosis

Dementia As well as the problem of pseudodementia, there are often difficulties in distinguishing the social withdrawal, lack of self-care and apathy of early dementia from depression. Depression during dementia causes particular difficulties (Ballard et al 1996). If there is doubt a trial of antidepressants is advisable.

Other organic depressive disorder The diagnosis of affective disturbance after a stroke is difficult, most of all in patients with communication problems. Robinson et al (1984) linked lesions in the left frontal cortex to depressive symptoms, but depression may also be due to emotional lability, reactive distress, organic apathy or lack of motivation and side-effects of drugs (House et al 1991). Lability is particularly common and may respond to small doses of antipsychotic drugs or, more specifically and sometimes dramatically, to antidepressants such as fluoxetine.

Differentiating depression and mild *parkinsonism* is sometimes difficult as retardation and a downcast expression occur in both conditions. Poor communication may impede examination. The picture is confused further because the side-effects of antiparkinsonian drugs include delirium, hallucinations, depression, elation and sexual disinhibition, paranoid states and even obsessional symptoms.

Depression is a feature of other physical illnesses common in old age, such as infections, hypothyroidism and tumours, and it is a side-effect of many drugs used in elderly patients. Every new case of depression requires a full medical history including alcohol and drugs, physical examination and screening investigations.

Treatment

Antidepressant drug treatment Age is not in itself a contraindication to any antidepressant, and some patients, particularly those with a long past history, can tolerate large doses of standard tricyclic drugs. However, the likelihood of anticholinergic and cardiovascular side-effects rises with age, and for many the classic drugs are unacceptable. Other tricyclics which may have fewer side-effects are still popular; these include doxepin, dothiepin and lofepramine. Careful supervision is essential when starting these drugs and adjusting doses, with daily lying and standing blood

pressure measurement if possible and education of the patient and her family about potential side-effects. Access to blood level monitoring may be helpful, but does not always predict side-effects or efficacy. Newer less toxic drugs are becoming more widely used, including trazodone, the selective serotonin reuptake inhibitors (SSRIs, reviewed by Newhouse 1996), venlafaxine and moclobemide. Some clinicians use traditional monoamine oxidase inhibitors as second-line drugs with good effect, even in major depression, though delayed postural hypotension may be a problem with these otherwise relatively safe drugs. With all antidepressants, small starting doses, gradual increases and prolonged trial periods of up to 2 months are required. Jacoby & Lunn (1993) propose that medication should continue for 2 years or more after recovery. Lithium augmentation (Flint 1995) and other combination treatments are worth trying in intractable cases.

Electroconvulsive therapy (ECT) Problems with antidepressant drugs have persuaded many clinicians that ECT has an important part to play in the treatment of late-life depression, as a first-line treatment in severe illness, and where drugs are contraindicated, fail or have undesirable side-effects. Benbow (1989) reviewed the literature and concluded that it is a safe and effective treatment for major depressions in old age, with a good response in 70–80% of cases. Unfortunately, the failure of a course of ECT to provide prophylaxis leaves a problem if drug treatment has been impossible. Benbow also concluded that, provided there is no evidence of a space-occupying lesion, dementia is not a contraindication to ECT if coexisting depression warrants its use.

Psychological treatment of depression Cognitive behaviour therapy for depression and anxiety-related symptoms in older people can be effective (Koder et al 1996) and appropriate referral should always be considered. In reactive depressions counselling, for example from the Cruse bereavement counselling service or other agencies, can be helpful.

Treatment of mania Neuroleptic drugs should be used in the same way as for younger patients, though in age-appropriate doses. Lithium can be used as first-line treatment or as a prophylactic mood stabiliser. Clearance of lithium declines steadily in later life. Equivalent doses lead to higher blood levels and relatively low blood levels can lead to toxic effects. For these reasons it must be administered with considerable care, and in lower doses than for younger patients. Blood levels of 0.4–0.7 mmol/l may be effective (Foster et al 1977). Regular thyroid and renal function checks are most important in this age group, and the lithium level should be retested if there is any intercurrent infection, or change in drug treatment, especially diuretics.

Prognosis There has been considerable controversy about the prognosis of depressive illness in elderly people. Post's classical study in 1962 suggested that with treatment most patients had a good outcome, though only 26% showed full recovery at follow-up and 12% were continually ill. Murphy (1983) was pessimistic, finding 35% well but 29% continually ill and 14% dead at 1 year follow-up of a mixed hospital and community group. Psychotic patients did particularly badly. Baldwin & Jolley (1986), however, found a much better prognosis, with 60% well and only 18% continually ill. Perhaps the samples from these and other studies come from rather different populations, but it is also possible that those who obtained better outcomes may have used more active treatments, particularly for severe cases. Cole (1990) carried out a meta-analysis of studies and showed that in the longer term (over 2 years) only a quarter of cases remained well, though 60% were in the well or well with relapse category, and only 10% were continuously ill. Alexopoulos et al (1996) emphasise the importance of continuing active treatment on prognosis. Murphy and others have found that poor physical health and adverse life events contribute to poor outcome. Many studies have found increased mortality among older people with depressive and manic illnesses, but estimates of death rates have varied greatly.

Suicide and parasuicide

Suicide

In Britain, around 20% of all suicides are elderly people, despite the fact that only 15% of the population is over 65 years in age. The rate declined in the 1960s due to detoxification of the gas supply and has remained fairly steady since (Shulman 1978, Lindesay 1991b). Rates for men are roughly twice those for women, and continue to increase with advancing age, while the female rate may gradually fall.

The main factors which predict late-life suicide include not only age and male sex, but physical illness (estimates range from 35 to 85% of cases), social isolation, widowed or separated status, alcohol abuse and, most especially, depressive illness and a past history of depression (Barraclough's (1971) series included 80% who had depressive illness). De Alarcon (1964) stressed the particular relevance of hypochondriacal ideas. Barraclough emphasised that around 80% of suicides had contacted their general practitioner in the 3 months before death, but Cattell & Jolley (1995) found somewhat lower rates of contact and low rates of onward referral to psychiatric services.

Parasuicide

In contrast, parasuicide is relatively uncommon in older age groups, contributing only about 5% to the total (Kreitman 1976, Hawton & Fagg 1990). The male:female ratio is much more even than in younger people. Elderly parasuicides are more likely to represent failed suicide rather than being gestures of distress, interpersonal difficulties or personality problems. Draper (1996) emphasised that the factors associated with parasuicide in old age were similar to those associated with completed suicide and relationship problems may be important in some cases. Pierce (1987) found that 90% of attempters had depressive illness (though not necessarily severe), and 50% were admitted to a psychiatric hospital. Over 60% were physically ill. Kreitman found that 8% of parasuicides (and 20 times the expected rate in men) went on to complete suicide within 3 years of the attempt.

All suicidal behaviour in the elderly should be taken seriously, and depressive illness should be suspected. Of course, there are also some personality-disordered individuals who have habitually harmed themselves over many years and continue to do so.

Neurosis

Prevalence

It is not always recognised that depression and anxiety problems are overall more prevalent in old age than dementia. Epidemiological studies of neurosis are beset with methodological difficulties. Differing case-finding methods, arguments about definition of syndromes, the issue of 'caseness', the boundary between personality and neurotic disorders, and the correct classification of 'depressive neurosis' are but some of the pitfalls. Kessell & Shepherd (1962) showed that whilst there was no great decline in community prevalence in neurosis in older people, and general practitioner attendances for neurotic disorders fell little, there was a marked fall in referrals to psychiatrists. Elderly people with neurotic disorders probably accept their complaints more readily, and general practitioners may be reluctant to refer on, perhaps considering such disorder to be 'just old age'. Estimates of prevalence range between 1 and 10% (Eastwood & Corbin 1985). Saunders et al (1993) found rates of clinical neurosis of 2.5% but there may also be a penumbra of 'subcases', perhaps a further 15%. Male prevalence rates are always lower and there have been suggestions that rates may decline in the very old age groups. Most studies find 'old' and 'new' cases to be roughly equal in frequency.

Clinical features

Bergmann (1978) examined a group of subjects with late-onset neurosis and found that most had symptoms of anxiety or depression. Anxiety symptoms may be generalised or may present as panic attacks or phobias (Lindesay 1991a). A particular phobia, uncommon in younger people but relatively common in the elderly, has been named *space phobia* by Marks (1981). Agoraphobics experience anxiety in crowded places, while space phobics become anxious in open spaces where they have no supports to hold on to. They usually have few background neurotic traits, and have had some physical illness or accident which has led them to fear falling or lack confidence in their mobility. They often become housebound. They respond relatively poorly to both physiotherapy and behaviour therapy.

Aetiology

By factor analysis of background variables Bergmann showed that physical illness, a feeling of loneliness (as distinct from actual isolation), impaired self-care and 'anxiety-prone' or 'rigid, insecure' personality traits contributed to the development of new cases of neurosis in old age. More recent studies come to similar conclusions, adding an emphasis on the role of life events.

Differential diagnosis

Obsessional disorders, eating disorders, hypochondriasis or abnormal illness behaviour rarely emerge for the first time in late life. New symptoms suggestive of any of these disorders should make the clinician think first of other diagnoses, using a hierarchical approach.

Physical illness   Patients who feel ill but cannot identify clear symptoms may present pseudoneurotic symptoms, or present their symptoms in an exaggerated fashion. An apparent eating disorder is much more likely to be caused by serious physical illness than by a late-onset neurosis, though rare cases of primary eating disorder do occur (Cosford & Arnold 1992). Kay & Bergmann (1966) found that one of the best predictors of mortality in elderly psychiatrically ill patients was a physical complaint.

Acute or chronic brain disease   Disinhibitory mechanisms can lead to the emergence or magnification of neurotic personality traits or symptoms.

Affective disorder   Depressive illness, hypomania or a mixed affective disorder can present in old age with pseudoneurotic symptoms and there is considerable comorbidity between depressive illness and anxiety (Flint 1994). In particular, the complaint of hypochondriasis, which only rarely begins as a neurotic disorder in later life, is much more likely to be caused by a depressive illness.

Treatment

Those with long-standing neurotic illness will be likely to require continuing treatment which has been effective. Given the likely causal factors in 'new' late-life neurosis, treatment of these cases should aim at resolving, or helping the patient come to terms with, problem issues such as physical ill health, losses or loneliness. Unfortunately, older people's tendency to dislike change can make even simple counselling or brief problem-solving psychotherapy hard work. Anxiolytic drugs should in general be avoided, though in severe or intractable cases sedative antidepressants are helpful, especially where there is evidence of a marked change from the person's normal self.

Alcohol problems

Prevalence

There are more elderly abstainers, and those who do drink take on average less than younger people (Dight 1976, Saunders et al 1989, Iliffe et al 1991a). Cohort effects play a large part in this and current cohorts may be gradually raising the levels of intake (Bennett et al 1995). However, many individual elderly people cut down their alcohol intake. As an individual ages, tolerance to alcohol is likely to decrease, because of reduction in important liver enzymes and changes in the response of the brain to alcohol. The same dose of alcohol produces higher blood levels, more intoxication and more adverse effects. Financial considerations also play a part; elderly people are often relatively poorer than they were when of working age. Furthermore, at present there are social pressures against drink among many, but not all, elderly groups, and many social activities for older people are not associated with drinking as they would be for younger people.

As might be expected the prevalence of heavy drinking is lower than in younger people (Saunders et al 1989). Defining the numbers who have alcohol problems is difficult, for there is probably considerable underreporting. Often the relevant questions are simply not asked, in the mistaken belief that older people, and especially older women, rarely drink. Fink et al (1996) have described a variety of possible screening interview questionnaires. In fact, although the female rate of problem drinking remains significantly below the male rate (Edwards et al 1973), it rises in old age, and the highest prevalence among women is in the 80s. Recent changes in the drinking habits of younger women will change this pattern in the future.

New and old cases of alcohol abuse tend to show some differences (Rosin & Glatt 1971, Atkinson 1994). In late-onset cases family history is not as great a factor as in younger cases. Risk factors in late-onset cases include female gender, higher socioeconomic class, precipitating life events (including not only losses but also sudden access to excess time and money at retirement) and physical ill health. These 'new' cases are more neurotic in type, with less evidence of a background personality disorder. The alcohol abuse tends to be milder, and may fluctuate more with greater chance of spontaneous remission.

Alcohol abuse may also be a symptom of or a reaction to psychiatric illness, though this is not the explanation for most 'new' cases. The elderly depressive or the mild dementia sufferer may begin drinking heavily for the first time in their lives, and here cause and effect can be difficult to disentangle. Alcohol-related dementia remains a controversial subject, but in all cases of dementia enquiry about past alcohol consumption is essential. *Korsakov's syndrome* is, of course, a common finding in 'old' cases, including the important subgroup of 'graduates' who were admitted with the Korsakov syndrome in middle age.

Treatment

The link between practical problems and recent onset allows greater optimism about treatment, which can focus on the person's circumstances and social milieu. Treatment is assisted by the availability of non-drinking social activities, by the absence of social stigma about abstinence and by a greater willingness among families to control an elderly person's finances in order to control her drinking. Effects of alcohol on the elderly person's physical state and mobility further encourage abstinence.

People who have abused alcohol over many years may also cut down their intake. But it is also quite common for their drinking to continue along the pattern of earlier years, and the associated physical or psychiatric problems continue or intensify. Those in lodgings and hostels may be particularly at risk.

Drug abuse

Drug abuse is not a major problem among elderly people except in relation to prescribed drugs such as benzodiazepines, opiates and other analgesics, occasionally barbiturates and other 'older' drugs, and less obvious drugs of abuse, particularly laxatives. Abuse of 'street' drugs by older people is likely to gradually increase as a problem over the next decades as a cohort effect.

It is sometimes felt that withdrawal of drugs of dependence from an elderly person is cruel, as they have 'not long to go'. However, the subtle personality and cognitive changes, which can lead to mistaken diagnoses of personality disorder, depression, dementia or a physical illness, are such that abstinence may greatly improve a person's quality of life. The greatest arguments arise over hypnotics in patients who show no obvious adverse effects, but are clearly psychologically dependent.

Sexual problems

It is commonly believed that older people, especially older women, have little sexual interest and limited sexual ability. Many couples continue to have active sex lives and sexual interest continues into advanced old age in most people, though social pressures and lack of opportunity inhibit many. Physiological changes can make intercourse more difficult, especially for women, and slower responses may work for or against a particular couple. Illness and drugs sometimes interfere with sexual activity, and, even though these may be temporary problems for one or other partner, reinstituting sexual relations after a break can be a major problem.

Some dementia sufferers begin to make sexual demands on their partners after years of lack of interest, or show disinhibited sexual interest in other adults or children (Haddad & Benbow 1993a, 1993b). Indiscriminate sexual behaviour by a resident in a care home or ward can cause considerable distress among staff and relatives.

Doctors and others may have to overcome a 'countertransference' difficulty in addressing sexual problems in people who could be their parents or grandparents. This may interfere with questioning and therapy, especially where subjects such as extramarital relationships, cross-generation relationships or homosexuality are concerned.

PERSONALITY

Normal changes of old age

In the past, social gerontology has been divided between those who believed that it was normal for older people to *disengage* from social life and activities, and become more introspective, a process sometimes seen as a preparation for death, and those who stressed the benefits of continued *engagement* in physical and mental activity. Both theories have been replaced by an emphasis on *continuity*, that is, that ageing individuals usually retain the attitudes, interests and styles of relating which have made up their personality throughout life. However, whether for biological, psychological or social reasons, it is commonly found that cautiousness, introversion and obsessionality do tend to increase with age, but there is great interpersonal variation. Those who had these characteristics as lifelong traits may adjust to old age relatively easily.

People who had disordered personalities in younger years rarely come to psychiatric attention, except as residents in homes and hostels, where their egocentricity, impulsiveness or lack of concern for the consequences of their actions make them less than ideal residents. 'Mellowing' is said to occur in some psychopaths in later life. Those with lesser degrees of personality disorder are only likely to see psychiatrists if they suffer another psychiatric disorder or in response to adverse life events.

During the decades of old age many planned or unplanned changes occur in family and other relationships, social circumstances and housing. It is unlikely that all will be entirely consonant with the individual's personality characteristics. At a time when change is becoming more difficult to cope with, major problems can arise. The independent-minded individual who develops parkinsonism or a stroke where outside help becomes essential may be a very 'bad' patient, resenting the dependent position, reacting violently against any hints of infantilisation and so responding poorly to attempts at rehabilitation. She may present to the liaison psychiatrist as depressed, but the depression hides an underlying resentment of her predicament.

Personality disorder and illness

Personality disorders are generally found in around 5–10% of older people in epidemiological studies (Abrams 1996). Some elderly people present with an exaggeration of previous personality traits, even to the point of caricature. It is frequently assumed that this is a part of the normal ageing process, but it may be a manifestation of psychiatric illness, including depressive illness, hypomania or paranoid psychosis; or of organic (especially frontal lobe) disorder, other brain damage, or early dementia without obvious global impairment. Personality disorder is lifelong by definition, and therefore personality *change* or *exaggeration* in old age demands an explanation. A careful history is essential, concentrating particularly on lifelong traits of personality, the time sequence of changes, their relationship to important life events and other possible

symptoms of illness. Neuroimaging is appropriate in cases of apparent personality change where organic disorder is a possibility.

'Senile squalor'

Clark et al (1975) and Macmillan & Shaw (1966) described elderly people who seemed to become by choice reclusive and eccentric in old age, and could end up living in squalor. Many seemed oblivious of the conditions they were living in and were very resistant to help. Many of Clark's group were physically ill and half died after admission to hospital. In Macmillan & Shaw's group there was a preponderance of psychiatrically ill people. A variety of names have been used to describe these patients, such as senile squalor syndrome and Diogenes syndrome. A related, probably obsessive problem of compulsive collecting, which can also lead to squalor, is called *syllogomania*. It is likely that elderly people may live in squalor for very varied reasons, including unrecognised physical illness, frontal lobe dysfunction due to early dementia or other organic disorder (Orrell et al 1989), other psychiatric illness, alcohol or drug misuse and lifelong eccentricity of personality. Old age is not in itself a cause of eccentricity. There is no need to define a syndrome of squalor, but squalor as a symptom merits further investigation.

THE ELDERLY WITH MENTAL HANDICAP

A growing number of people with mental handicap are entering old age. Some of these will suffer dementia, especially those with *Down's syndrome* (Lai & Williams 1989, Mann 1993), and some will have other psychiatric conditions (Cooper 1992). The expansion of community care for people with learning difficulties means that most will be living at home, perhaps with very elderly relatives, or in supported accommodation. The difficult decisions about who should take responsibility for this small but important group need further debate.

LEGAL CONSIDERATIONS

The elderly mentally disordered offender

Police and the courts can be unreasonably lenient to elderly law breakers, due either to an ageist belief that the elderly are inevitably less responsible for their actions or to a protective paternalism. Courts may feel that harrowing trials are not appropriate for relatively frail elderly people, and cautioning by the police is relatively common. An elderly person fits uncomfortably into a prison system geared to managing young offenders. This set of attitudes can act against elderly people. It removes their right to answer accusations made against them, and may brand them as sick or incapable when they are in fact perfectly well and responsible for their actions. It also leaves the victims of crime with no redress.

Crime is less common among the elderly than among younger groups, and it is important to emphasise the possible links between crime and psychiatric illness, particularly organic conditions, affective disorder and alcohol abuse (Taylor & Parrott 1988). Elderly people who have traffic accidents, shop-lift, are violent or make disinhibited sexual advances to others require careful assessment for early dementia and other disorders, though unfortunately they may not be referred for reports. The same is true of the elderly who are putting themselves at risk without necessarily committing any crime. Incautious drivers, wanderers, people who make repeated complaints about their neighbours can all come to the attention of police, but no further action is taken.

The same attitude can infect the legal system when the elderly person is the victim of crime. This can relate to violence in the home, bogus workmen or accusations of stealing by home helps. The older person's evidence is taken as less valid than that of a younger person, and investigations are not pursued as vigorously as they should be.

Abuse of and by elderly people

Elderly victims of abuse by family or other carers are the subject of increasing concern (Eastman 1984). Carers' groups often discuss angry and violent feelings once the group has become cohesive (Homer & Gilleard 1990). Figures are difficult to interpret, because definitions of abuse vary greatly, and underreporting is likely. At its broadest, abuse can include irritability and verbal abuse, physical neglect, financial exploitation, sexual abuse as well as direct physical assault. Objective evidence of physical abuse is difficult to assess in elderly people prone to falls, or those who bruise easily. The problem of whom to believe is particularly thorny when the possible victim is dementing. Vulnerable elderly people can also be victims of abuse by those whose job it is to care for them. Financial exploitation by solicitors, neglectful treatment by doctors, undue restraint in institutions, physical aggression and sexual abuse by nursing or other care staff all need considerably more attention than they get at present.

Psychiatrically ill elderly people may also become verbally abusive, or physically or sexually aggressive towards their informal and formal carers. In close relationships carers may find it difficult to discuss such problems openly. Once again, carers' groups are helpful.

Prevention is the best approach to problems of abuse. Better training and support of staff and informal carers is vitally important (Pritchard 1995). The value of regular visits by relatives, senior nursing staff, medical staff and students to long-stay wards and care homes should not be underestimated. Openness in discussing the mixed feelings that caring for elderly people induces should be encouraged. Respite from caring is most important of all.

THE FUTURE

Only effective treatments or preventative measures will be able to slow the increase in the number of cases of the common forms of dementia which is expected over the next three decades. Even massive programmes of hospital or nursing home building will not cope with this increase. The majority of sufferers will live in their own homes, without much support, unless the problem is solved of how to finance true home care for the increasing population of non-productive elderly people in a world of decreasing tolerance of high taxes. The public may anyway have little enthusiasm for community care of dementia sufferers, which has yet to prove its effectiveness. Nevertheless, that is generally what people with dementia want and what the future holds for hundreds of thousands of them. Research must concentrate on finding simple, valid and reliable procedures for early detection and diagnosis of dementia, assessment of these patients' needs and evaluation of community care programmes, alongside the search for cures.

The prevalence of other psychiatric disorders will not rise significantly with demographic changes. But changes in the attitudes of future cohorts of older people are likely to bring the full range of mental disorders increasingly to psychiatric attention. Future generations of elderly people are likely to be less passive, more educated in the facts of ageing, and more aware of their rights. They may expect that effective help, including good-quality institutional care where it is absolutely necessary, will be available, and will wish to participate in decisions about their care. Old age psychiatry will be a more varied but even more challenging field of work than it is at present. The challenge for professionals is not only to be well educated and enthusiastic, but to learn to work together and communicate effectively with those in other agencies who will inevitably be involved in care planning and provision for the individual older person who has a mental disorder.

REFERENCES

Abrams R 1996 Personality disorders in the elderly. International Journal of Geriatric Psychiatry 11: 759–763

Alexopoulos G S, Abrams R C, Young R C, Shamonian C A 1988 Cornell scale for depression in dementia. Biological Psychiatry 23: 271–284

Almeida O P, Howard R J, Levy R, David A S, Morris R G, Sahakian B J 1995 Cognitive features of psychotic states arising in late life (late paraphrenia). Psychological Medicine 25(4): 685–698

Amar A, Wilcock G 1996 Vascular dementia. British Medical Journal 312: 227–231

Ames D 1990 Depression among elderly residents of local-authority residential homes: its nature and the efficacy of intervention. British Journal of Psychiatry 156: 667–675

Angst J 1973 Classification and predicion of outcome of depression. Schatlauer, Stuttgart

Arie T, Dunn T 1973 A 'do-it-yourself' psychiatric–geriatric joint patient unit. Lancet ii: 1313–1316

Atkinson R 1994 Late onset problem drinking in older adults. International Journal of Geriatric Psychiatry 9: 321–326

Bahro M, Silber E, Box P, Sunderland T 1995 Giving up driving in Alzheimer's disease: an integrative therapeutic approach. International Journal of Geriatric Psychiatry: 871–874

Baldwin R C, Jolley D J 1986 The prognosis of depression in old age. British Journal of Psychiatry 149: 574–583

Ballard C, Oyebode F 1995 Psychotic symptoms in patients with dementia. International Journal of Geriatric Psychiatry 10: 743–752

Ballard C G, Bannister C, Oyebode F 1996 Depression in dementia sufferers. International Journal of Geriatric Psychiatry 11: 507–515

Barinaga M 1995 New Alzheimer's gene found. Science 268: 1845–1846

Barraclough B 1971 Suicide in the elderly. In: Kay D W K, Walk A (eds) Recent developments in psychogeriatrics. Headly, Ashford, pp 87–97

Beats B 1996 The biological origin of depression in later life. International Journal of Geriatric Psychiatry 11: 349–354

Benbow S M 1989 The role of electroconvulsive therapy in the treatment of depressive illness in old age. British Journal of Psychiatry 155: 147–152

Bennett N, Jarvis L, Rowlands D, Singleton N, Haselden L 1995 Living in Britain. HMSO, London.

Berghmans R I P, ter Meulen R H J 1995 Ethical issues in research with dementia patients. International Journal of Geriatric Psychiatry 10: 647–651

Bergmann K 1977 Prognosis in chronic brain failure. Age and Ageing 6(suppl): 61–66

Bergmann K 1978 Neurosis and personality disorder in old age. In: Isaacs A D, Post F (eds) Studies in geriatric psychiatry. Wiley, Chichester

Bergmann K, Eastham E J 1974 Psychogeriatric ascertainment and assessment for treatment in an acute medical setting. Age and Ageing 3: 174–188

Berrios G E 1990 Musical hallucinations: a historical and clinical study. British Journal of Psychiatry 156: 188–194

Berrios G E, Brook P 1984 Visual hallucinations and sensory delusions in the elderly. British Journal of Psychiatry 144: 652–664

Berrios G E, Brook P 1985 Delusions and the psychopathology of the elderly with dementia. Acta Psychiatrica Scandinavica 72: 296–301

Bond J 1987 Psychiatric illness in later life: a study of prevalence in a Scottish population. International Journal of Geriatric Psychiatry 2: 39–57

Brink T L 1979 Geriatric psychotherapy. Human Sciences Press, New York

British Medical Association/The Law Society 1995 Assessment of mental capacity: guidance for doctors and lawyers. BMA, London

Broadhead J, Jacoby R 1990 Mania in old age: a first prospective study. International Journal of Geriatric Psychiatry 5: 215–222

Brook P, Degun G, Mather M 1975 Reality orientation, a therapy for psychogeriatric patients: a controlled study. British Journal of Psychiatry 127: 42–45

Brooke H 1988 Consent to treatment and research. In: Hirsch S R, Harris J (eds) Consent and the incompetent patient. Gaskell/Royal College of Psychiatrists, London

Burns A, Jacoby R, Levy R 1990a Psychiatric phenomena in Alzheimer's disease: I: disorders of thought content. British Journal of Psychiatry 157: 72–75

Burns A, Jacoby R, Levy R 1990b Psychiatric phenomena in Alzheimer's disease: III: disorders of mood. British Journal of Psychiatry 157: 81–85

Butler R N 1963 The life review: an interpretation of reminiscence in the aged. Psychiatry 26: 65–76

Capewell A E, Primrose W R, MacIntyre C 1986 Nursing dependency in registered nursing homes and long term care geriatric wards in Edinburgh. British Medical Journal 291: 1719–1721

Castle D J, Murray R M 1993 The epidemiology of late-onset schizophrenia. Schizophrenia Bulletin 19: 691–700

Cattell H, Jolley D 1995 One hundred cases of suicide in elderly people. British Journal of Psychiatry 166: 451–457

Central Statistical Office 1991 CSO annual abstract of statistics, 1991. HMSO, London

Challis D, Davies B 1986 Case management in community care. Gower, Aldershot

Christie A B 1982 Changing patterns in mental illness in the elderly. British Journal of Psychiatry 140: 154–159

Christie A B, Train J D 1984 Changes in the pattern of care for the demented. British Journal of Psychiatry 144: 9–15

Clark A N G, Mankiker G D, Gray I 1975 Diogenes syndrome: a clinical study of gross neglect in old age. Lancet i: 366–373

Cooper A F 1976 Deafness and psychiatric illness. British Journal of Psychiatry 129: 216–226

Cooper S 1992 The psychiatry of elderly people with mental handicaps. International Journal of Geriatric Psychiatry 7: 865–874

Copeland J R M, Kelleher M J, Kellett J M, Barron G, Cowan D, Gourlay A J 1975 Evaluation of a psychogeriatric service: the distinction between psychogeriatric and geriatric patients. British Journal of Psychiatry 126: 21–29

Copeland J R M, Dewey M E, Griffiths-Jones H M 1986 Computerized psychiatric diagnostic system and case nomenclature for elderly subjects: GMS and AGECAT. Psychological Medicine 16: 89–99

Copeland J R M, Gurland B J, Dewey M E, Kelleher M J, Smith A M R, Davidson I A 1987 Is there more dementia, depression and neurosis in New York? A comparative study of the elderly in New York and London using the computer diagnosis AGECAT. British Journal of Psychiatry 151: 466–473

Copeland J R M, Dewey M E, Wood N et al 1992 Range of mental illness among the elderly in the community: prevalence in Liverpool using the GMS-AGECAT package. British Journal of Psychiatry 150: 815–823

Copeland J R M, Abou-Saleh M T, Blazer D G 1994 Principles and practice of geriatric psychiatry. Wiley, Chichester

Corder E H, Saunders A M, Strittmatter W J et al 1993 Gene dose of apolipoprotein E type 4 allele and the risk of Alzheimer's disease in late onset families. Science 261: 921–923

Cosford P, Arnold E 1992 Eating disorders in later life: a review. International Journal of Geriatric Psychiatry 7: 491–498

Cutter N R, Post R M 1982 Life course of illness in untreated manic–depressive illness. Comprehensive Psychiatry 23: 101–115

Damas-Mora J, Skelton-Robinson M, Jenner F A 1982 The Charles–Bonnet syndrome in perspective. Psychological Medicine 12: 251–261

de Alarcon R 1964 Hypochondriasis and depression in the aged. Gerontologica Clinica 6: 266–277

Department of Health 1989 Working for patients. HMSO, London

Department of Health and Social Security 1972 Services for mental illness related to old age. HMSO, London

Department of Health/Department of Social Security 1989 Caring for people: community care in the next decade and beyond. HMSO, London

Devanand D P, Sano M, Tang M-X et al 1996 Depressed mood and the incidence of Alzheimer's disease in the elderly living in the community. Archives of General Psychiatry 53: 175–182

de Zoysa A S R, Blessed G 1984 The place of the specialist home for the elderly mentally infirm in the care of mentally disturbed old people. Age and Ageing 13: 218–223

Dight S 1976 Scottish drinking habits: a survey of Scottish drinking habits and attitudes to alcohol. HMSO, London

Donaldson C, Tarrier N, Burns, A 1997 The impact of the symptoms of dementia on caregivers. British Journal of Psychiatry 170: 62–68

Draper B 1996 Attempted suicide in old age. International Journal of Geriatric Psychiatry 11: 577–587

Eagles J M, Gilleard C J 1984 The functions and effectiveness of a day hospital for the demented elderly. Health Bulletin (Edinburgh) 42: 87–91

Eagles J M, Whalley L J 1985 Ageing and affective disorder: the age of first onset of affective disorders in Scotland 1969–1978. British Journal of Psychiatry 147: 180–187

Eagles J M, Craig A, Robinson F, Restall D B, Beattie D A G, Besson J A 1987 The psychological well-being of supporters of the demented elderly. British Journal of Psychiatry 150: 293–298

Eastman M 1984 Old age abuse. Age Concern England, London

Eastwood R, Corbin S 1985 Epidemiology of mental disorders in old age. Recent Advances in Psychogeriatrics 1: 17–33

Eastwood R and Writing Committee, Lancet Conference 1996 The challenge of the dementias. Lancet 347: 1303–1307

Edwards G, Hawker A, Hensman C, Peto J, Williamson V 1973 Alcoholics known or unknown to agencies: epidemiological studies in a London suburb. British Journal of Psychiatry 123: 169–183

Erikson E 1963 Childhood and society. Triad Granada, London, pp 241–242

Feil N 1993 The validation breakthrough: simple techniques for communicating with people with 'Alzheimer's type dementia'. Health Profession's Press, Baltimore

Finch E J L, Catona C L E 1989 Lithium augmentation in the treatment of refractory depression in old age. International Journal of Geriatric Psychiatry 4: 41–46

Findlay D J, Shamara J, McEwen J, Ballinger B R, MacLennan W J, McHarg A M 1989 Double-blind controlled withdrawal of thioridazine treatment in elderly female inpatients with senile dementia. International Journal of Geriatric Psychiatry 4: 115–120

Fink A, Hays R, Moore A, Beck J 1996 Alcohol-related problems in older persons: determinants, consequences, and screening. Archives of Internal Medicine 156: 1150–1156

Fleming R W, Bowles J 1994 How, when and why to use the REPDS. University of Western Sydney: MacSearch

Flint A 1994 Epidemiology and comorbidity of anxiety disorders in the elderly. American Journal of Psychiatry 151: 640–649

Flint A 1995 Augmentation strategies in geriatric depression. International Journal of Geriatric Psychiatry 10: 137–146

Flint A J, Rifat S I, Eastwood M R 1991 Late-onset paranoia: distinct from paraphrenia? International Journal of Geriatric Psychiatry 6: 103–109

Folstein M F, Folstein S E, McHugh P R 1975 Mini-mental state. Journal of Psychiatric Research 12: 189–198

Foster J R, Gershell W J, Goldfarb A I 1977 Lithium treatment in the elderly. Journal of Gerontology 32: 299–302

Gibb W R G 1989 Dementia and Parkinson's disease. British Journal of Psychiatry 154: 596–614

Gilhooley M L M 1984 The impact of caregiving on caregivers: factors associated with the psychological wellbeing of people supporting a dementing relative in the community. British Journal of Psychological Medicine 57: 35–44

Gilleard C J 1984 Living with dementia: community care of the elderly mentally infirm. Croom Helm, London

Gilleard C J, Belford H, Gilleard E, Whittick J E, Gledhill K 1984a Emotional distress amongst the supporters of the elderly mentally infirm. British Journal of Psychiatry 145: 172–177

Gilleard C J, Gilleard E, Whittick J E 1984b Impact of psychogeriatric day hospital care on the patient's family. British Journal of Psychiatry 145: 487–492

Goldsmith M 1996 Hearing the voice of people with dementia. Kingsley, London

Greene J G, Timbury G C 1979 A geriatric psychiatry day service: a five year review. Age and Ageing 8: 49–53

Hachinski V C, Iliff L D, Zilhka E et al 1975 Cerebral blood flow in dementia. Archives of Neurology 32: 632–637

Haddad P, Benbow S 1993a Sexual problems associated with dementia: part I: problems and their consequences. International Journal of Geriatric Psychiatry 8: 547–551

Haddad P, Benbow S 1993b Sexual problems associated with dementia: part 2: aetiology, assessment and treatment. International Journal of Geriatric Psychiatry 8: 631–637

Harrison R W S, McKeith I G 1995 Senile dementia of Lewy body type: a review of clinical and pathological features:

implications for treatment. International Journal of Geriatric Psychiatry 10: 919–926

Hawton K, Fagg J 1990 Deliberate self-poisoning and self-injury in older people. International Journal of Geriatric Psychiatry 5: 367–373

HEBS 1996 Coping with dementia: a handbook for carers. Health Education Board for Scotland, Edinburgh

HEC 1986 Who cares: information and advice for those caring for a confused person. Health Education Council, London

Henderson A S 1986 The epidemiology of Alzheimer's disease. British Medical Bulletin 42: 3–10

Henderson A S, Huppert F A 1984 The problem of mild dementia. Psychological Medicine 14: 5–11

Henderson A, Jorm A F, Mackinnon A et al 1993 The prevalence of depressive dosorders and the distribution of depressive symptoms in later life: a survey using draft ICD-10 and DSM-III-R. Psychological Medicine 23: 719–729

Herholz K 1995 FDG PET and differential diagnosis of dementia. Alzheimer Disease and Associated Disorders 9: 6–16

Hodge J 1984 Towards a behavioural analysis of dementia. In: Psychological approaches to the care of the elderly. Croom Helm, London

Hodges J R 1994 Cognitive assessment for clinicians. Oxford University Press, Oxford

Hodkinson H M 1973 Mental impairment in the elderly. Journal of the Royal College of Physicians 7: 305–317

Holden U P, Woods R T 1988 Reality orientation: psychological approaches to the 'confused' elderly. Churchill Livingstone, Edinburgh

Homer A C, Gilleard C 1990 Abuse of elderly people by their carers. British Medical Journal 30: 1359–1362

Hope T, Fairburn C G 1992 The present behavioural examination (PBE): the development of an interview to measure current behavioural abnormalities. Psychological Medicine 22: 223–230

Hope T, Patel V 1993 The assessment of behavioural phenomena in dementia. In: Burns A (ed) Ageing and dementia: a methodological approach. Edward Arnold, London, pp 221–236

Hope T, Tilling K M, Gedling K, Keene J M, Cooper S D, Fairburn C G 1994 The structure of wandering in dementia. International Journal of Geriatric Psychiatry 9: 149–155

House A, Dennis M, Mogridge L, Warlow C, Hawton K, Jones L 1991 Mood disorders in the year after first stroke. British Journal of Psychiatry 158: 83–92

Howard R, Almeida O, Levy R, Graves P, Graves M 1994 Quantitative magnetic resonance imaging volumetry distinguishes delusional disorder from late onset schizophrenia. British Journal of Psychiatry 165: 474–480

Hughes C P, Berg L, Danziger W L, Coben L A, Martin R L 1982 A new clinical scale for the staging of dementia. British Journal of Psychiatry 140: 566–572

Hymas N, Naguib M, Levy R 1989 Late paraphrenia – a follow-up study. International Journal of Geriatric Psychiatry 4: 23–29

Iliffe S, Haines A, Booroff A, Goldenberg E, Morgan P, Gallivan S 1991a Alcohol consumption by elderly people: a general practice survey. Age and Ageing 20: 120–123

Iliffe S, Haines A, Gallivan S, Booroff A, Goldenberg E, Morgan P 1991b Assessment of elderly people in general practice: social circumstances and mental state. British Journal of General Practice 41: 9–12

Ineichin B 1990 The extent of dementia among old people in residential homes. International Journal of Geriatric Psychiatry 5: 327–335

Jacoby R, Levy R 1980a Computerized tomography of the elderly: 2: dementia: diagnosis and functional impairment. British Journal of Psychiatry 136: 256–259

Jacoby R, Levy R 1980b Computerized tomography of the elderly: 3: affective disorders. British Journal of Psychiatry 136: 270–275

Jacoby R, Lunn D 1993 How long should the elderly take antidepressants? A double-blind placebo-controlled study of continuation/prophylaxis therapy with dothiepin. Old Age Depression Interest Group. British Journal of Psychiatry 162: 175–182

Jacoby R, Oppenheimer C (eds) 1997 Psychiatry in the elderly. Oxford University Press, Oxford

Jacques A 1992 Understanding dementia. Churchill Livingstone, Edinburgh

Jeste D V, Eastham J H, Lacro J P, Gierz M, Field M G and Harris M J 1996 Management of late-life psychosis. Journal of Clinical Psychiatry 57(suppl 3): 39–45

Jobst K A, Smith A D, Szatmari M et al 1992 Detection in life of confirmed Alzheimer's disease using a simple measurement of medial temporal lobe atrophy by computed tomography. Lancet 340: 1179–1183

Jorm A F 1985 Subtypes of Alzheimer's dementia: a conceptual analysis and critical review. Psychological Medicine 15: 543–553

Jorm A F, Jacomb P A 1989 The information questionnaire on cognitive decline in the elderly (IQCODE): socio-demographic correlates, reliability, validity and some norms. Psychological Medicine 19: 1015–1022

Jorm A F, Korten A E, Henderson A S 1987 The prevalence of dementia: a quantitative survey of the literature. Acta Psychiatrica Scandinavica 76: 465–479

Kay D W K, Bergmann K 1966 Physical disability and mental health. Psychosomatic Research 10: 3–12

Kay D W K, Roth M 1961 Environmental and hereditary factors in the schizophrenias of old age (late paraphrenia) and their bearing on the general problem of causation in schizophrenia. Journal of Mental Science 107: 649–686

Kay D W K, Beamish P, Roth M 1964 Old age mental disorders in Newcastle upon Tyne. British Journal of Psychiatry 110: 146–158

Keene J M, Hope T 1996 The microstructure of eating in people with dementia who are hyperphagic. International Journal of Geriatric Psychiatry 11: 1041–1049

Kelly C, Hunter R 1995 Current pharmacological strategies in Alzheimer's disease. International Journal of Geriatric Psychiatry 10: 633–646

Kendrick D C 1987 Psychological assessment. In: Pitt B (ed) Dementia. Churchill Livingstone, Edinburgh

Kennard M L, Feldman H, Yamada T, Jefferies W A 1996 Serum levels of the iron binding protein p97 are elevated in Alzheimer's disease. Nature Medicine 2: 1230–1235

Kessell N, Shepherd M 1962 Neurosis in hospital and general practice. Journal of Mental Science 108: 159–166

Kidd C B 1962 Misplacement of the elderly in hospital. British Medical Journal 2: 1491–1495

Knight B R 1996 Psychotherapy of older adults. Sage, Thousand Oaks

Koder D-A, Brodaty H, Anstey K 1996 Cognitive therapy for depression in the elderly. International Journal of Geriatric Psychiatry 11: 97–107

Kraepelin E 1919 Dementia praecox and paraphrenia. Barclay R M (trans). Churchill Livingstone, Edinburgh

Kral V 1962 Senescent forgetfulness: benign and malignant. Journal de l'Association Medical Canadien 86: 257–260

Kral V, Emery O B 1989 Long-term follow-up of depressive pseudodementia of the aged. Canadian Journal of Psychiatry 34: 445–446

Kreitman N 1976 Age and parasuicide ('attempted suicide'). Psychological Medicine 6: 113–121

Lai F, Williams R S 1989 A prospective study of Alzheimer's disease in Down's syndrome. Archives of Neurology 46: 840–853

Law Commission 1995 No. 231. Mental incapacity. Law Commission, London

Levin E, Moriarty J, Gorbach P 1994 Better for the break. HMSO, London

Lindesay J 1991a Phobic disorders in the elderly. British Journal of Psychiatry 159: 531–541

Lindesay J 1991b Suicide in the elderly. International Journal of Geriatric Psychiatry 6: 355–361

Lindesay J, Briggs K, Murpy E 1989 The Guy's/Age Concern survey: prevalence rates of cognitive impairment, depression and anxiety in an urban community. British Journal of Psychiatry 155: 317–329

Lindesay J, MacDonald A, Starke I 1990 Delirium in the elderly. Oxford University Press, Oxford

Lindesay J, Briggs K, MacDonald A, Herzberg J 1991 The Domus philosophy: a comparative evaluation of a new approach to residential care for the demented elderly. International Journal of Geriatric Psychiatry 6: 727–736

Lipowski Z J 1983 Transient cognitive disorders in the elderly. American Journal of Psychiatry 140: 1426–1436

Lodge B, McReynolds S 1985 The use of multidisciplinary assessment by the community dementia team. Age Concern, Leicester

Loring D W, Largen J W 1985 Neuropsychological patterns of presenile and senile dementia of the Alzheimer's type. Neuropsychologia 23: 351–357

Lovestone S 1996 The genetics of Alzheimer's disease: new opportunities and new challenges. International Journal of Geriatric Psychiatry 11: 491–497

Mace N L, Rabins P V, Castleton B, Cloke C, McEwen E 1985 The 36-hour day: caring at home for confused elderly people. Hodder & Stoughton/Age Concern England, London

McGrath A M, Jackson G A 1996 Survey of neuroleptic prescribing in residents of nursing homes in Glasgow. British Medical Journal 312: 611–612

McKeith I G 1995 Lewy body disease. Current Opinion in Psychiatry 8: 252–257

McKeith I G, Perry R H, Fairbairn A F, Jabeen S, Perry E K 1992 Operational criteria for senile dementia of Lewy body type (SDLT). Psychological Medicine 22: 911–922

Macmillan D, Shaw P 1966 Senile breakdown in standards of personal and environmental cleanliness. British Medical Journal 2: 1032–1037

McShane R, Keene J, Gedling K, Fairburn C, Jacoby R, Hope T 1997 Do neuroleptic drugs hasten cognitive decline in dementia? Prospective study with necropsy follow up. British Medical Journal 314: 266–270

Mann A H, Graham N, Ashby D 1984 Psychiatric illness in residential homes for the elderly: a survey of one London borough. Age and Ageing 13: 257–265

Mann D M A 1993 Association between Alzheimer's disease and Down's syndrome: neuropathological observations. In: Berg J M, Karlinsky H, Holland A J (eds) Alzheimer's disease, Down's syndrome and their relationship. Oxford University Press, Oxford

Marks I 1981 Space phobia: syndrome or agoraphobic variant? Journal of Neurology, Neurosurgery and Psychiatry 44: 387–390

Marshall M 1997 Better quality environments for people with dementia. In: Jacoby R, Oppenheimer C (eds) Psychiatry in the elderly. Oxford University Press, Oxford

Mayeux R, Denaro J, Hemenegildo N et al 1992 A population-based investigation of Parkinson's disease with and without dementia. Archives of Neurology 49: 492–497

Meacher M 1972 Taken for a ride. Longman, London

Mendlewicz S, Fieve R, Rainer J 1972 Manic–depressive illness: a comparative study of patients with and without a family history. British Journal of Psychiatry 120: 523–530

Meyer J S, Rogers R L, Judd B W, Mortel K R, Sims P 1987 Cognition and cerebral blood flow fluctuate together in multi-infarct dementia. Stroke 19: 163–169

Moos R, Lemke S 1980 Assessing the physical and architectural features of sheltered care settings. Journal of Gerontology 35: 571–583

Morris C H, Hope R A, Fairburn C G 1989 Eating habits in dementia: a descriptive study. British Journal of Psychiatry 154: 801–806

Morris R G 1996 The neuropsychology of Alzheimer's disease and related dementias. In: Woods R T (ed) Handbook of clinical psychology and ageing. Wiley, Chichester, pp 219–242

Morris R G, Kopelman M D 1992 The neuropsychological assessment of dementia. In: Crawford J R (ed) A handbook of neuropsychological assessment. Parker, McKinlay Erlbaum, Hove, pp 295–321

Morris R G, Morris L W, Britton P G 1988 Factors affecting the emotional wellbeing of the caregivers of dementia sufferers: a review. British Journal of Psychiatry 153: 147–156

Murdoch P S, Montgomery E A 1992 Revised guidelines for collaboration between physicians in geriatric medicine and psychiatrists of old age. Psychiatric Bulletin 16: 583–584

Murphy E 1982 Social origins of depression in old age. British Journal of Psychiatry 141: 135–142

Murphy E 1983 The prognosis of depression in old age. British Journal of Psychiatry 142: 111–119

Murphy E 1994 The day hospital debate. International Journal of Geriatric Psychiatry 9: 517–518

Naguib M, Levy R 1982 Prediction of outcome in senile dementia: a computerized tomography study. British Journal of Psychiatry 140: 267–271

Naguib M, Levy R 1987 Late paraphrenia: neuropsychological impairment and structural brain abnormalities on computed tomography. International Journal of Geriatric Psychiatry 2: 83–90

Newens A J, Forster D P, Kay D W K, Kirkup W, Bates D, Edwardson J 1993 Clinically diagnosed presenile dementia of the Alzheimer type in the Northern Health Region: ascertainment, prevalence, incidence and survival. Psychological Medicine 23: 631–644

Newhouse P 1996 Use of serotonin selective reuptake inhibitors in geriatric depression. Journal of Clinical Psychiatry 57 (suppl 5): 12–22

Norman A 1987 Severe dementia: the provision of longstay care. Centre for Policy on Ageing, London

Norris A 1986 Reminiscence. Winslow Press, London

O'Brien J T, Ames D, Schwietzer I 1996 White matter changes in depression and Alzheimer's disease: a review of magnetic resonance imaging studies. International Journal of Geriatric Psychiatry 11: 681–694

O'Carroll R, Whittick J, Baikie E 1991 Parietal signs and sinister prognosis in dementia: a four year follow-up study. British Journal of Psychiatry 158: 358–361

O'Connor D W, Pollitt P A, Hyde J B, Brook C P B, Reiss B B, Roth M 1988 Do general practitioners miss dementia in elderly patients? British Medical Journal 297: 1107–1110

O'Connor D W, Pollitt P A, Roth M, Brook C P B, Reiss B B 1990 Problems reported by relatives in a community study of dementia. British Journal of Psychiatry 156: 835–841

Orrell M, Sahakian B J, Bergmann K 1989 Self-neglect and frontal lobe dysfunction. British Journal of Psychiatry 155: 101–105

Parkes C M 1964 The effects of bereavement on physical and mental health: a study of the case records of widows. British Medical Journal 2: 274–279

Patel V, Hope T 1993 Aggressive behaviour in elderly people with dementia: a review. International Journal of Geriatric Psychiatry 8: 457–472

Pattie A H, Gilleard C J 1976 The Clifton assessment schedule: further validation of a psychiatric assessment schedule. British Journal of Psychiatry 129: 68–72

Pattie A H, Gilleard C J 1979 Manual of the Clifton assessment procedures for the elderly (CAPE). Hodder & Stoughton, Sevenoaks

Perris C 1968 The course of depressive psychosis. Acta Psychiatrica Scandinavica 44: 238–248

Perry E K, Kerwin J, Perry R H, Irving D, Blessed G, Fairbairn A 1990 Cerebral cholinergic activity is related to the incidence of visual hallucinations in senile dementia of Lewy body type. Dementia 1: 2–4

Philpott M P, Levy R 1987 A memory clinic for the early diagnosis of dementia of Alzheimer type. International Journal of Geriatric Psychiatry 2: 195–200

Pierce D 1987 Deliberate self-harm in the elderly. International Journal of Geriatric Psychiatry 2: 105–110

Pitt B, Silver C P 1980 The combined approach to geriatrics and psychiatry: evaluation of a joint unit in a teaching hospital district. Age and Ageing 9: 33–37

Poirier J, Delisle M-C, Quirion R et al 1995 Apolipoprotein E4 allele as a predictor of cholinergic deficits and treatment outcome in Alzheimer's disease. Proceedings of the National Academy of Sciences of the USA. 92: 12260–12264

Post F 1962 The significance of affective illness in old age. Maudsley monograph 10. Oxford University Press, Oxford

Post F 1966 Persistent persecutory states of the elderly. Pergamon Press, Oxford

Post F 1971 Schizo-affective symptomatology in late life. British Journal of Psychiatry 118: 437–445

Prager S, Jeste D V 1993 Sensory impairment in late-life schizophrenia. Schizophrenia Bulletin 19: 755–772

Pritchard J 1995 The abuse of older people. Kingsley, London

Rabins P V 1986 Establishing Alzheimer's disease units in nursing homes: pros and cons. Hospital and Community Psychiatry 37: 120–121

Reicher-Rossler A, Rossler W, Forstl H, Meise U 1995 Late-onset schizophrenia and late paraphrenia. Schizophrenia Bulletin 21: 345–354

Reisberg B, Ferris S H, de Leon M J, Crook T 1982 The global deterioration scale for assessment of primary degenerative dementia. American Journal of Psychiatry 139: 1136–1139

Richardson C A, Gilleard C, Lieberman S, Peeler R 1994 Working with older adults and their families: a review. Journal of Family Therapy 16: 225–240

Ritchie K, Kildea D 1995 Is senile dementia 'age-related' or 'ageing-related'? Evidence from meta-analysis of dementia prevalence in the oldest old. Lancet 346: 931–934

Robinson R A 1975 The assessment center. In: Howells G (ed) Modern perspectives in the psychiatry of old age. Churchill Livingstone, Edinburgh

Robinson R G, Kubos K L, Starr L B, Krishna R, Price T R 1984 Mood disorders in stroke patients: importance of location of lesion. Brain 107: 81–94

Rocca W A, Hofman A, Brayne C et al 1991 Frequency and distribution of Alzheimer's disease in Europe: a collaborative study of 1980–1990 prevalence findings. Annals of Neurology 30: 81–90

Roman G C, Tatemichi T K, Erkinjuntti T, Cummings J L, Masdeu J C, Garcia J H 1993 Vascular dementia: diagnostic criteria for research studies. Neurology 43: 250–260

Rosin A J, Glatt M M 1971 Alcohol excess in the elderly. Quarterly Journal of Studies on Alcohol 32: 53–59

Roth M 1955 The natural history of mental disorder in old age. Journal of Mental Science 101: 281–301

Roth M 1986 The association of clinical and neurobiological findings and its bearing on the classification and aetiology of Alzheimer's disease. British Medical Bulletin 42: 42–50

Roth M, Morrissey J F 1952 Problems in the diagnosis of mental disorder in old age. Journal of Mental Science 98: 66–80

Roth M, Tym E, Mountjoy C Q et al 1986 CAMDEX: a standardised instrument for the diagnosis of mental disorders in the elderly with special reference to early detection of dementia. British Journal of Psychiatry 149: 698–709

Royal College of Physicians of London and Royal College of Psychiatrists 1989 Care of elderly people with mental illness. Royal College of Physicians, London

Saunders P A, Copeland J R M, Dewey M E et al 1989 Alcohol use and abuse in the elderly: findings from the Liverpool longitudinal study of continuing health in the community. International Journal of Geriatric Psychiatry 4: 103–108

Saunders P, Copeland J, Dewey M et al 1993 The prevalence of dementia, depression and neurosis in later life: the Liverpool MRC-ALPHA study. International Journal of Epidemiology 22: 838–847

Schneider L S, Pollock V E, Lyness S A 1990 A meta-analysis of controlled trials of neuroleptic treatment in dementia. Journal of the American Geriatrics Society 38: 553–563

Scinto L F M, Daffner K R, Dressler D et al 1994 A potential noninvasive neurobiological test for Alzheimer's disease. Science 266: 1051–1054

Scott J, Fairbairn A, Woodhouse K 1988 Referrals to a psychogeriatric consultation–liaison service. International Journal of Geriatric Psychiatry 3: 131–135

Scottish Home and Health Department 1979 Scottish health authorities priorities for the eighties. HMSO, Edinburgh

Scottish Home and Health Department 1989 Scottish health authorities review of priorities for the eighties and nineties. HMSO, Edinburgh

Scottish Law Commission 1995 No.151. Report on incapable adults. HMSO, Edinburgh.

Shulman K 1978 Suicide and parasuicide in old age. Age and Ageing 7: 201–209

Shulman K, Post F 1980 Bipolar affective disorder in old age. British Journal of Psychiatry 136: 26–32

Shulman K I, Shedletsky R, Silver I L 1986 The challenge of time: clock drawing and cognitive function in the elderly. International Journal of Geriatric Psychiatry 1: 135–140

Skoog I, Lernfelt B, Landahl S et al 1996 15-year longitudinal study of blood pressure and dementia. Lancet 347: 1141–1145

Soni S D, Mallik A 1993 The elderly chronic schizophrenic inpatient: a study of psychiatric morbidity in 'elderly graduates'. International Journal of Geriatric Psychiatry 8: 665–673

Stokes G 1986 Screaming and shouting. Winslow Press, London

Stokes G 1987 Aggression. Winslow Press, London

Stokes G, Goudie F 1990 Working with dementia. Winslow Press, London

Stone K 1989 Mania in the elderly. British Journal of Psychiatry 155: 220–224

Strittmatter W J, Saunders A M, Schmechel D et al 1993 Apolipoprotein E: high-avidity binding to β-amyloid and increased frequency of type 4 allele in late-onset familial Alzheimer's disease. Proceedings of the National Academy of Sciences of the USA 90: 1977–1981

Sunderland T, Alterman I, Yount D et al 1988 A new scale for the assessment of depressed mood in demented patients. American Journal of Psychiatry 145: 955–959

Swanwick G R J, Lee H, Clare A W, Lawlor B A 1994 Consultation–liaison psychiatry: comparison of two service models for geriatric patients. International Journal of Geriatric Psychiatry 9: 495–499

Tang M-X, Jacobs D, Stern Y et al 1996 Effect of oestrogen during menopause on risk and age at onset of Alzheimer's disease. Lancet 348: 429–432

Tanzi R, National Institute on Aging/Alzheimer's Association Working Group, I 1996 Apolipoprotein E genotyping in Alzheimer's disease. Lancet 347: 1091–1095

Taylor P J, Parrott J M 1988 Elderly offenders: a study of age-related factors among custodially remanded prisoners. British Journal of Psychiatry 152: 340–346

Teunisse R J, Cruysberg J R, Verbeek A, Zitman F G 1995 The Charles–Bonnet syndrome: a large prospevice study in the Netherlands. a study of the prevalence of the Charles–Bonnet syndrome and associated factors in 500 patients attending the University Department of Opthalmology at Nijmegen. British Journal of Psychiatry 166: 254–257

Thomas T, Thomas G, McLendon C, Sutton T, Mullan N 1996 β-amyloid-mediated vasoactivity and vascular endothelial change. Nature 380: 168–171

Thornton S, Brotchie J 1987 Reminiscence: a critical review of the empirical literature. British Journal of Clinical Psychology 26: 93–112

Wade D T, Collin C 1988 The Barthel ADL index: a standard measure of physical disability? International Disability Studies 10: 64–67

Ware G J G, Fairburn C G, Hope R A 1990 A community-based study of aggressive behaviour in dementia. International Journal of Geriatric Psychiatry 5: 337–342

Weiner M F, Koss E, Wild K V et al 1996 Measures of psychiatric symptoms in Alzheimer patients: a review. Alzheimer Disease and Associated Disorders 10: 20–30

Weisman G D, Cohen U, Ray K, Day K 1991 Architectural planning and design for dementia care units. In: Coons D H (ed) Specialized dementia care units 83–106. Johns Hopkins University Press, Baltimore

Wells C E 1979 Pseudodementia. American Journal of Psychiatry 136: 895–900

West P, Illsey R, Kelman H 1984 Public preferences for the care of dependency groups. Social Science and Medicine 18: 287–295

WHO 1986 Dementia in later life: research and action. World Health Organization Technical Report Series 730

Wilcock G K 1990 Living with Alzheimer's disease and similar conditions. Penguin, London

Wilkin D, Hughes B, Jolley D 1985 Quality of care in institutions. In: Arie T (ed) Recent advance in psychogeriatrics. Churchill Livingstone, Edinburgh

Will R G, Ironside J W, Zeidler M et al 1996 A new variant of Creutzfeldt–Jakob disease in the UK. Lancet 347: 921–925

Wilson B A, Moffat N 1992 Clinical management of memory problems. Chapman & Hall, London

Winokur G 1975 The Iowa 500: heterogeneity and course in manic – depressive illness. Comprehensive Psychiatry 16: 125–131

Woods R T 1996 Psychological 'therapies' in dementia. In: Woods R T (ed) Handbook of clinical psychology and ageing. Wiley, Chichester, pp 575–600

Wright N, Lindesay J 1995 A survey of memory clinics in the British Isles. International Journal of Geriatric Psychiatry 10: 379–385

Yesavage J A, Brink T L, Rose T L et al 1983 Development and validation of a geriatric depression screening scale: a preliminary report. Journal of Psychiatric Research 17: 37–49

Young R, Klerman G 1992 Mania in late life: focus on age at onset. American Journal of Psychiatry 149: 867–876

Zerfass R, Sattel H, Daniel S, Besthorn C, Forstl H 1995 Pupillary response to tropicamide: not a simple bedside test for Alzheimer's disease. International Journal of Geriatric Psychiatry 10: 993–994

Zis A P, Goodwin F K 1970 Major affective disorder as a recurrent illness. Archives of General Psychiatry 36: 835–839

26
Suicide and deliberate self-harm

J.T.O. Cavanagh   G. Masterton

SUICIDE

Definition

Suicide is not a diagnosis, rather it is a verdict or category of death which is broadly defined by the following requirements:

- the death was unnatural
- it was the result of the victim's own actions
- the victim intended to kill him/herself.

There can be doubts at all three stages of this process (Farmer 1988) particularly in regard to the motive of a person who cannot be interviewed.

Determination

Countries vary in how suicide is determined, which makes national comparisons of suicide statistics unreliable. In Britain, for instance, the English system relies on the coroner who investigates every case where violent or unnatural death is suspected. A verdict is reached at a public inquest when self-inflicted deaths are recorded as a suicide, an accident or, if undecided, an open verdict is reached. Variation occurs not only among courts, but between a coroner and his deputy (Barraclough 1978) and within the same court and jury with different coroners (O'Donnell & Farmer 1995). In Scotland, there is rarely a formal or public inquiry: the police investigate sudden, suspicious or unnatural deaths, and the procurator fiscal, on behalf of the Crown Office, determines whether a self-inflicted death is categorised as an accident, a suicide or it is undetermined whether the death was an accident or suicide.

The higher suicide rate recorded in Scotland compared with England is probably because the Scottish verdict is based on the evidence indicating that suicide was the most probable and reasonable explanation, whereas the coroner must apply a stricter test, that suicide has been proved by the evidence (Dolman 1994).

It is argued that the Scottish figures more accurately reflect the true suicide rate (Pounder 1991).

With a few exceptions such as hara-kiri, death by suicide has been disowned and despised by society. It was well into the 20th century before attempting suicide was decriminalised in Britain, and up to 200 years ago English law stated that individuals who committed suicide and their spouses should 'forfeit all chattels real and personal which he has in his own right', which resulted in penury for the victim's family.

From the 17th century, sympathetic coroners sought to avoid returning verdicts of suicide, and this humanitarian trend has continued to the present day with efforts being made to spare the feelings of relatives from the guilt and anguish that a suicide frequently generates. Since 1975, when Lord Chief Justice Widgery ruled on an appeal against a coroner's verdict of suicide, this has been reinforced by the legal requirement for conclusive proof before suicide is established (Dolman 1994). The consequence is that most research into suicide includes the victims of undetermined deaths, although the characteristics of these individuals lie midway between those of suicides and accidents in many respects (Holding & Barraclough 1978). When psychiatrists have investigated the Crown's decisions there is a consensus that between a third and a half of probable suicides are categorised as accidental or undetermined deaths.

Epidemiology

Basic statistics

Despite the vagaries of statistical interpretation, suicide remains a serious public and mental health problem worldwide. In many countries suicide is included among the top ten causes of death for all ages, and among the 15–34 age group it ranks second or third. What remains an international problem is the fragmentary nature of basic data on suicide. For example, only 39 of the 166 member states of the UN are listed as reporting data on suicide mortality. Along with this, there is great variety in the methods which exist to report and ascertain the cause of death.

The magnitude of suicide rates can be illustrated when they are compared with that other major cause of death in industrialised societies, road traffic accidents (RTAs). The number of people dying by their own hand is now significantly higher than those who die in RTAs. Indeed, the rates of these two causes of death have been going in opposite directions over the last two decades, with RTA mortality decreasing and suicide increasing (especially among adolescents and young adults).

Validity and reliability of statistics

Despite the increasingly prominent profile of suicide as a cause of death in many countries, there are major difficulties in comparing rates between nations as there are no global standardised criteria for the classification and reporting of suicide. However, within Europe this situation is improving. The 1982 WHO review indicated that differences in methods of determining whether deaths are suicide do not explain differences in suicide rates between populations. When the methods of ascertainment were controlled for, several authors found that differences in the rank order of suicides of countries or cultural groups were essentially the same (Sainsbury & Barraclough 1968, Whitlock 1971, Lester 1972, Barraclough 1973, Sainsbury et al 1981). Moreover, differences in rates between national, demographic and social groups have been recorded over significant time periods and have remained stable despite political upheaval which, in certain countries, has resulted in altered criteria and methods for determining suicide (Diekstra 1996).

Suicide is thus underreported for a variety of reasons and rates are subject to a number of errors but the random nature of these errors means that it is possible to compare rates between countries and over time.

Geographical patterns

Within the European region there is a pattern to the suicide rates. The lowest rates are seen in southern European countries followed by those in the north-west e.g. the UK and the Netherlands which show slightly higher rates. Higher still rates are prevalent in the Scandinavian countries and those counties which form the 'belt' of Europe, i.e. France and Belgium in the west through Switzerland, Austria and Hungary to Russia in the east. This position has remained virtually unchanged throughout the last century. The trend of suicide in the European region depends upon the countries studied. These differ but it can be said that the per period averaged rate has increased over the course of the century.

The evidence to date suggests that the prevalence of suicide continues to vary in accordance with international differences in traditions, customs, religious practice and other influences; but it also suggests that the strength of these differences is decreasing and that there is homogenisation among these countries. Although global rates of suicide are increasing, comparisons are compromised by differences in ascertainment and reporting, and by differences age and sex rates and urban:rural ratios (Table 26.1).

Suicide in the UK

Scotland   In Scotland there are 500–600 deaths per annum attributed to suicide and approximately 200 to undetermined causes (Registrar-general's Office (RGO) Scotland). There is estimated underreporting of about 30% (Ovenstone 1973) which is easily corrected by assuming all undetermined deaths to have been suicides, and adding undetermined deaths to suicides gives the probable maximum number of deaths (Pounder 1991). Over the last 15–20 years male deaths and male death rates from suicide have increased while those of females have remained static or fallen slightly. There has also been a disproportionate increase in the rates of suicide among the younger cohort of Scottish males (RGO Scotland 1988; Lowy et al 1990). Scotland is not especially unusual in this regard, particularly in the European context. The reversal of Scotland's position relative to England and Wales is a matter for concern. Until the 1950s the suicide rate in Scotland was lower than that in England and Wales for both sexes. Convergence of the rates occurred around the 1960s but by the 1970s rates in both sexes in Scotland were higher. Moreover, in England and Wales there was an overall decrease in female suicide between 1956 and 1976. Scottish rates are now higher by 30% in men and 20% in women and data analysis demonstrates that this is not an artefact of allocating deaths to the undetermined category (Crombie 1990).

Durkheim's statement in 1897 that international differences in suicide rates remained fairly constant over time has been borne out for most of the 20th century until this reversal of the rates in Scotland compared with England and Wales (Fig. 26.1).

England and Wales   For the first time since 1911 male suicide rates are increasing in England and Wales, while female rates are decreasing. There is also a change in the age distribution, with males under 45 now at greater risk of death by suicide than the older group (Charlton et al 1993).

Table 26.1	International patterns in suicide
Country	Pattern
Australia	Highest youth rate in industrialised world: 16.4 per 100 000 15–24 year group
Germany	Decline 1989–1991 from 18.4 to 17.5 per 100 000. Sex rate stable at 2.2:1 male:female. Higher rate in former East Germany
Denmark	Good records. One of Europe's highest rates. Majority males aged 30–59 years. Greatest increase females aged 40–54 years. In last 70 years, male rate risen by 3% to 33.5 per 100 000 and females by 58% to 17.2 per 100 000
Brazil	Poor records. Highest incidence in the 25–44 year group; increasing trend is in the 15–24 year group
Japan	Rate falling; no longer regarded as 'honourable'. Peak in 1986 of 21.2 per 100 000 now falling. Most cases in 55 and over group. Worrying trends – doubling of rate in 10–14 year group within a year
USA	Controversy over rates doubling in last 20 years; these figures relate especially to males
Netherlands	Fall of 10% overall since 1985. Most cases in elderly men, but rates in 30–39-year-old males have increased
France	Among the highest in Europe. Upward trend over last 10 years from 16 per 100 000 to 20.1 per 100 000. May reflect underestimation. Male:female = 3:1. Rates in males 30–34 years doubled and increased by 50% in 20–29-year-olds in <20 years. Higher in rural compared with urban centres

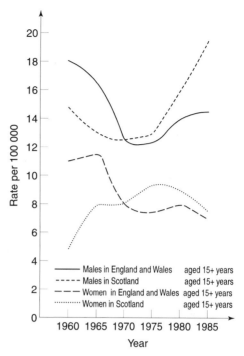

Fig. 26.1 Trends in suicide rates per 100 000 population (Crombie 1990).

Using trends of 5 year average death rates analysis showed that since the 1970s rates for men of 45 and over have fallen, while those for men under 45 have risen such that they now exceed the rates for the older age group, excepting those men aged 75 and over, who continue to have the highest rates. All age groups converged to similar rates by 1986–1990 with the exception of the 15–24 year group – despite their rising rates they are still lower than the older group. The female population saw a peak in all age groups in the period 1956–1965 and since then the rates in all age groups have fallen, apart from those under 25. Consistent with the pattern for men, there was convergence of the suicide rates for different age groups. In contrast to the male figures, however, women aged 45 and over continued to experience higher suicide rates by 1986–1990.

The trends in suicide and undetermined death rates became very similar for every age group under 75 by the 5 year period 1986–1990. The rates for men of 45 and over have fallen as the rates for those under 45 have increased. The rates for women of all age groups have fallen, with the most pronounced decreases in those of 45 and over; notwithstanding, the suicide rates for females under 45 still remained lower than those for older age groups.

Age and gender

Suicide increases as a function of age (Vaillant & Blumenthal 1990). It is rare in children under 12; it increases after puberty and the incidence continues to increase with each adolescent year (Moens 1990). A change in the picture can be seen in late adolescence and early adulthood onwards with a divergence in the age–mortality relationship. This can be seen in two parameters: between countries and between sexes within a country. There are two separate methods of analysing age–mortality relationships. The first method is age–suicide mortality correlation. Using this technique, the highest suicide rates are among older men in almost all European countries but the rate among females peaks at younger age (45–64) in a significant number of countries, especially Scandinavia. The majority of European countries, nevertheless, demonstrate a high correlation between age and suicide.

The other technique uses proportional mortality rates. If the rank order of suicide in the range of causes of death is related to age, then the ranking of suicide in that list decreases with increasing age. If all age groups are taken together, then suicide ranks as the 9th or 10th cause of death in most European countries. This translates to roughly 1% of all female deaths and 2% of all male deaths.

There are important changes in the epidemiology of suicide. There has been a real increase in youth suicide in the last 20 years. In industrialised nations there has been an increase in male rates within all age groups but most worryingly in the younger cohorts, which show mean changes of 70+% in the period 1970–1986. In women this youth suicide phenomenon is also evident, but to a lesser extent, with an increase of 40+% in the 15–29 group. However, in several countries, e.g. Canada and the US, there has been a decrease in the female rate while the male rate has increased.

Methods

By custom, methods of committing suicide are categorised as non-violent (drugs and poisons) and violent (all other methods). The most common methods vary among nations, cultures and age groups, between sexes and over time. In general, violent methods are more commonly employed by males and by the mentally ill. In Britain, suicides by hanging and by poisoning with vehicle exhaust fumes account for two in three male suicides but only one in three women; over half of female suicides are attributed to drug overdoses. Suicides involving firearms are associated with men, while suffocation using a plastic bag is more common among women. Two modes show an age rather than a sex bias – jumping from a high place among young adults and drowning among older victims.

Studies of cohorts of victims based on the violent method by which they ended their lives have revealed interesting features about suicidal behaviour and factors that determine the method employed. One example is self-immolation, where there are associations with a particular mental illness (schizophrenia), an independent cultural element (Asian-born women) and combined homicide–suicide (Soni Raleigh & Balarajan 1992, Prosser 1996).

A study of survivors of attempting suicide by deliberately throwing themselves in front of London Underground trains found most of these individuals suffered from severe mental illness and were currently in treatment; the method was determined not only by its perceived dangerousness but by its ready availability, and often there was little or no planning involved (O'Donnell et al 1996).

Methods are subject to fashion. There are well-known suicide 'hot spots' such as Beachy Head (Surtees 1982) and the Golden Gate Bridge (Seiden 1978), with victims sometimes travelling hundreds of miles to end their life at a special place. Suicides may follow the death of an idol, particularly if this has been by suicide, when the method may be copied. Mass suicides occasionally occur, often in the setting of an isolated and extreme religious sect, although forensic examination usually reveals a mixture of suicides and homicides among these victims. In suicide pacts, which account for 1 in 40 suicides, the couple invariably choose the same method, which is most often poisoning by car exhaust fumes (Brown et al 1995). Murder-suicides are not uncommon, with 20% of partner homicides being followed by the suicide of the perpetrator – and two-thirds of cases in which firearms are involved (Easteal 1994).

An important consideration is whether suicides can be prevented by reducing the availability of potentially more lethal methods. Between 1945–65 carbon monoxide poisoning by domestic gas accounted for around 40% of suicides in men and 60% in women. The detoxification of town gas during the 1960s prevented the 'head in the gas oven' suicide, and a corresponding fall in the total number of suicides by about one third occurred (Kreitman 1976) (Fig. 26.2).

In the USA, states with the strictest handgun control laws have the lowest rates of suicide involving firearms, and as there is almost no compensatory increase among other methods, these states also have the lowest suicide rates overall (Lester & Murrell 1982): the same relationship has been confirmed using the circulation of firearm magazines as an index of gun ownership (Lester 1989).

However, the fiercest debate in Britain about whether restricting a lethal method would result in an overall reduction in suicides or a compensatory increase by other methods has raged over antidepressant drugs, notwithstanding such deaths account for only 4% of suicides, 7% if undetermined deaths are included. The newer antidepressants are certainly less toxic in over-

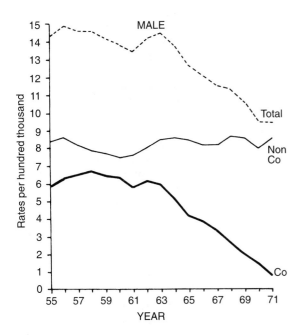

Fig. 26.2 Male suicide rates by mode of death for England and Wales. Co, deaths by carbon monoxide poisoning; non-co, deaths by other means.

(1858–1917). This involved three suicide types: anomic, egoistic and altruistic. Anomie occurs in social situations where the normative values of a social group lose their force and the usual standards which guide in times of stress are lost. The egoistic variety refers to individuals being separated from their social grouping and losing their sense of belonging to a community, the social norms of that society, therefore, having no significance for them. The altruistic form, as the term implies, refers to ending of one's own life for the greater good. A recent examination of Durkheim's concept of anomie investigated whether, as Durkheim proposed, factors which increase social cohesion or integration decrease suicide. Reviewing the birth and marriage rates of ten countries from 1900 till 1988, the birth rates were more strongly and consistently associated with suicide rates than were marriage rates (Lester 1996). This confirms the results of a Bavarian study (Wiedemann and Weyerer 1994) and provides some evidence in favour of Durkheim's hypothesis.

It is important to note that explicit distinction between the three varieties, especially between anomic and egoistic, is not always possible. Social isolation, subjective sense of loss of contact and loss of values remain prominent characteristics of those who die by their own hand.

The variables which recur consistently in studies of the social variables in suicide include: unemployment, social marginalisation and isolation, and economic variables such as recession and poverty (Table 26.2). A recent study addressing social factors operating in suicide found that several factors varied across age groups among completed suicides, with some age-related sex differences. In comparison with the general population, the suicides were more commonly never married (especially men aged 30–39), or were divorced or widowed (especially women 60–69). Suicides had more often lived on their own, although living with parents was more common among young male suicides (25–39). The latter group also had a greater incidence of psychiatric admission. Social isolation was a particularly

dose (Henry et al 1995) but whether lower fatal toxicity indices translate to a reduced suicide rate is debateable (Edwards 1995).

Proponents argue that not only are these drugs safer in overdose but compliance is improved because they have fewer side-effects, and patients may begin immediately at a therapeutic dose. It has been estimated that 300–450 lives per year may be saved by using SSRIs as first-line treatment but this did not take method substitution into account (Freemantle et al 1995). On the other hand, only one in seven suicide victims who were taking antidepressants employed the drug to end their life (Jick et al 1995), and this population-based study found no difference in the suicide rates by antidepressant compound after other variables were taken into account.

It is possible that some patients' lives will be saved by the use of the newer antidepressant compounds, whereas others taking these drugs will switch to another method if they are determined to kill themselves – where the balance lies is extremely difficult to establish because of the confounding variables.

Social variables

The earliest classification of sociological variables operating in suicide was proposed by Emil Durkheim

Table 26.2 Environmental variables associated with suicide

Social
Unemployment
Social marginalisation
Isolation
Economic
Recession
Poverty

common feature of those middle-aged males who had misused alcohol. While many of these features replicate sociological findings in suicide, the authors highlight the fact that some social variables might be related to the victim's psychopathology and excessive alcohol use. Gender-related psychopathology and alcohol misuse could be seen as confounders and future studies may reveal more if these are controlled for (Heikkinen et al 1995).

While there is strong evidence of a marked rise in male suicides, especially in the 15–24 age group, there appears to be no strong evidence that severe mental illness has increased among young adults in particular (Der et al 1990, Lehtinen et al 1991), which suggests the increase is attributable, at least in part, to environmental influences. Rises in the general male suicide rate are statistically associated with rises in unemployment in most of the EU.

Unemployment is often a significant variable (Platt 1984) and this is supported by a number of international studies (Pritchard 1988, Diekstra 1989, Dooley et al 1989). Although the causal mechanism is not fully understood it may be that the trigger is the demoralisation and depressive mood associated with being jobless (Warr 1987). In young men such pressure may be experienced more acutely as they seek to establish an adult identity.

The association between increased male suicide rates and unemployment is not unexpected in view of the known 'depressive' reaction and poorer health associated with being out of work, especially over a prolonged period (Platt 1984, Warr 1987, Whitehead 1987, Warr and Jackson 1987, Platt and Kreitman 1990).

The demands placed on men and women by a changing society, altered roles and changing social norms can be seen as a form of anomie. The loss of hope associated with prolonged unemployment creates a culture of hopelessness that may exacerbate the stresses upon those who are economically and psychologically vulnerable. Such individuals are often the first among the victims of socioeconomic recession (Pritchard 1992).

An association between age, socioeconomic grouping and suicide was found in a study of suicide and undetermined death in the UK. There was a concentration of suicide and undetermined deaths in the middle age groups of the lower socioeconomic category. Taking into account methodological considerations, these results could be explained in terms of the downward social drift associated, among other things, with long-term unemployment (Kreitman et al 1991).

The weight of evidence to date shows that suicide results from a complex interaction of biological, psychological, social and situational/personal factors.

Several sociodemographic factors characterise those who commit suicide, including the finding that suicide is more common in males and in those who are unmarried, separated, widowed or divorced (Buda & Tsuang 1990). Decreased social integration, increased social isolation and unemployment have also been shown to be significant interacting variables.

Biological variables in suicide and deliberate self-harm

The search for biological substrates of suicide and suicidal behaviour is a new and growing area of research endeavour. Dysfunction of monoaminergic neurotransmission has been implicated in suicidal behaviour (Roy 1994) based on postmortem studies of the serotonergic and, to a lesser extent, noradrenergic systems. It is difficult to control for the confounding variables associated with postmortem findings. They can only be a snapshot of brain function at the moment of death and are subject to genetic effects, developmental and early life processes, associated psychiatric disease and treatment for this, environmental stressors and artefacts of postmortem delay. Specific diagnostic categories, e.g. depression, mania and schizophrenia, may account for some of the reported biological changes, independently of suicidal behaviour. Research in this area is still dominated by studies with small sample sizes, multiple paradigm testing and retrospective designs. The search for biological substrates for deliberate self-harm (DSH) is likely to be just as difficult. Overall, results from biological studies in this area represent continuing research and experimentation and are not yet at the stage of providing clinical tools (Tables 26.3 and 26.4).

Clinical variables

One of the seminal studies attempting to determine the extent of mental illness among those who commit suicide was conducted by Barraclough (Barraclough et al 1974). Over 90% of the 100 cases could be diagnosed as having a mental disorder. Of these, 70% were depressed, 15% were alcohol dependent and 3% were schizophrenic. The findings of this study implied that suicide is rare among those with good mental and physical health and is more strongly associated with depression and alcoholism.

These results were mirrored by Cheng et al (1995) in a different cultural setting. In a case-controlled study in East Taiwan, 97–100% of the sample suffered from mental illness prior to suicide. Again the two most prevalent diseases were depression and alcoholism and the most common comorbid pattern was depression accompanied by substance abuse.

Table 26.3 Biological variables of suicide

Authors	Biological variables	Findings
Asberg et al 1976	5-HIAA	Depressed patients with low CSF 5-HIAA made more suicide attempts than other depressed patients
Mann et al 1989	5-HT/5-HIAA	No evidence for greater reduction in violent rather than non-violent suicides
Mann et al 1994	5-HT/5-HIAA	Postmortem brain tissue from suicide victims; modest reduction in brainstem 5-HT and 5-HIAA – independent of diagnosis
Arango et al 1996	Noradrenaline	Neuronal reduction in locus coeruleus in completed suicides versus controls? specific to suicide or also associated with depression
Arango et al 1990 Biegon & Israeli 1988 Mann et al 1986	β-receptors	Increased binding to β-adrenoceptors in cortex of suicides versus controls
De Paermentier et al 1990 Little et al 1993 Stockmeier & Meltzer 1991	β-receptors	Did not concur with β-receptor findings
Arango et al 1993 Meana & Garcia-Sevilla 1987	α-receptors	Increased binding in cortex of suicides
Gross-Isseroff et al 1990		Decreased α-receptor binding
Garcia-Sevilla et al 1996	Imidazoline receptors	Adrenergic receptors in brain and platelets. Platelet subtypes show upregulation in depression. Brain subtypes show downregulation in suicide victims
Arato et al 1989	CRF	Increased CRF concentration in CSF of suicide victims
Nemeroff et al 1988	CRF	Decreased receptor density in frontal cortex of suicide victims attributed to downregulation of CRF binding sites due to CRF hypersecretion by the hypothalamus
Banki et al 1987	CRF	No differences in CSF CRF concentrations between suicidal and non-suicidal depressed patients
Sundman et al 1997	GABA	No differences in the ligand binding of GABA receptors in frontal cortex of suicides and normal controls post mortem.
Linkowsky et al 1983 Linkowsky et al 1984	TSH	Lower TSH response to TRH in depressed patients who subsequently die by their own hand. Many inconsistencies and contradictions in the literature
Muldoon et al 1990	Cholesterol	Long-term follow-up of effect of cholesterol-lowering drugs – significant increase in suicide accidents and violence. Questions as to causal link. Hypotheses on biological plausibility, i.e. lower neuronal lipid viscosity and knock-on effect on 5-HT receptor availability

CRF, corticotrophin-releasing factor; CSF, cerebrospinal fluid; GABA, γ-aminobutyric acid; 5-HIAA, 5-hydroxyindole-acetic acid; 5-HT, 5-hydroxytryptamine; TRH, thyrotrophin-releasing hormone; TSH, thyroid-stimulating hormone.

Affective disorder

Psychotic depression Controversy surrounds the role of psychotic symptoms in depressed people who die by their own hand and whether they have a different suicide risk. Roose et al (1983) found delusions to be an important risk factor for suicide in depressed patients but both Coryell & Tsuang (1982) and Black et al (1988) found no such correlation. More recent studies found no major differences between psychotic and non-psychotic subgroups in sociodemographic features, comorbidity, clinical history or communication of suicidal intent.

One distinction noted by Isometsa et al (1994) was that those with psychotic features were more likely to use violent methods in the suicidal act (88% versus

Table 26.4	Biological variables in deliberate self-harm	
Authors	Biological variables	Findings
Mann et al 1992 Malone et al 1994	5-HT	Reduced 5-HT activity correlates with planned and medically serious attempts
Hildebrand et al 1990 Menachem et al 1989	5-HIAA	CSF 5-HIAA do not correlate with the recency of the DSH but remain stable on repeated testing. Implication that this is a trait-related variable
Nielsen et al 1994	Tryptophan	Tryptophan hydroxylase polymorphism found associated with history of DSH in violent offenders
Malone et al 1996	5-HT	Study using the prolactin response to fenfluramine – serotonergic dysfunction associated with more lethal forms of DSH
Agren et al 1980, 1982	MHPG	Report decreased urinary concentrations of MHPG
Roy et al 1994	HVA	Reports of reduced CSF HVA and reduced urinary HVA in DSH compared to controls. Reattempters over 5 years showed lower CSF and urinary HVA than those who did not reattempt
Sullivan et al 1994	Cholesterol	Suggestion of link between lower cholesterol and increased suicidality
Gallerani et al 1995		Noted low serum cholesterol following an act of DSH

CSF, cerebrospinal fluid; 5-HIAA, 5-hydroxyindoleacetic acid; 5-HT, 5-hydroxytryptamine; HVA, homovanillic acid; MPHG, 3-methoxy-4-hydroxyphenolglycol

59%). However, 'purity' of diagnosis is difficult to correlate directly as comorbidity is the rule rather than the exception.

Major depression It is generally accepted that major depression is one of the most important risk factors for suicide (Black et al 1990). The lifetime risk of suicide in major depression has been estimated at 19% or a suicide risk 30 times greater than the general population (Guze & Robins 1970). This puts the mortality risk of this illness in a league comparable with many severe physical illnesses (Goodwin & Jamison 1990).

Recent studies include that of Isometsa et al (1994), who found that 85% of a sample of suicides were complicated by comorbid diagnoses. This comorbidity varied with age and sex. Although 50% of the suicide victims with major depression were receiving psychiatric care at the time of death, only a minority were receiving adequate treatment . This is a problem identified in several studies, and the improvement of treatment and follow-up of patients with this potentially lethal illness needs to be addressed.

What clinical features are associated with depression? Barraclough et al (1974), Barraclough & Pallis (1975) and Modestin & Kopp (1988) found insomnia, impaired memory and self-neglect as well as greater overall severity of illness to be more common among depressed suicide victims (Table 26.5).

Table 26.5	Main correlates of suicide in major depression
Greater severity of illness
Self-neglect
Impaired concentration/memory
Hopelessness
Alcohol abuse
Mood cycling
History of suicidal behaviour

Fawcett and colleagues' (1990) prospective cohort study found that there were two main groups of predictors: short-term and long-term. The former comprised anhedonia, anxiety, impaired concentration and alcohol abuse. The latter consisted of hopelessness, mood cycling and a history of suicidal behaviour.

Comorbidity and its relationship to increased risk has been a feature in many study findings and suicide risk assessment must always account for this.

Non-major depression Non-major depressive disorder probably ranks among the most common psychiatric disorders (Angst 1992, Maier et al 1992). One secular trend noted among those who die by suicide has been the increase in the proportion of comorbid depression (Carlson et al 1991). Isometsa et al (1996) com-

Table 26.6 Main correlates of suicide in non-major depression
Male sex
Comorbid substance abuse
Younger age
Limited contract with health services

Table 26.7 Main correlates of suicide in bipolar affective disorder
Relatively early in course of illness
Current major depressive episode or mixed affective state
Recent adverse life events

pared depressive suicides who had unipolar depression which did not fulfil criteria for major depression with suicides who did have major depression. The vast majority (95%) of suicide victims with non-major depression were comorbid with, for example, alcoholism, personality disorder and/or physical illness. The characteristics of non-major depressives who died through suicide were: younger age; more men; more substance abusers; more 'secondary' depressives; less contact with health care services; less communication of suicidal intent despite contact with health care services; more recent life events reported in the final week (Table 26.6).

Bipolar affective disorder Despite having a lifetime risk of suicide comparable with that of unipolar depression (Fawcett et al 1987, Black et al 1988, Goldstein et al 1991), there has been little research specifically addressing the issue of suicide in those with bipolar affective disorder (Goodwin & Jamison 1990). Those studies which have been carried out suffer from selectivity or low numbers.

Reports indicate that bipolars tend to commit suicide early in the course of the disease (Guze & Robins 1970, Weeke 1979, Black et al 1985) and that there are no major differences between the sexes (Goodwin & Jamison 1990) (Table 26.7). However, a recent Finnish study found that early suicides appear to be more common among male than female bipolars (Isometsa et al 1994).

The majority (71%) of the bipolar suicides were complicated by comorbidity, in particular alcohol dependence – especially in males.

The majority (79%) of bipolars have a major depressive episode immediately before death. A minority have mixed states, which has been linked to high suicide risk (Goodwin & Jamison 1990, Dilsaver et al 1994, Strakowski et al 1996). Adverse life events constitute risk factors for both deliberate self-harm and suicide itself (Paykel & Dowlatshani 1988, Heikkinen et al 1993). In bipolar illness, life events not connected to the individual's own behaviour appear to be associated, in time, with the onset of the first episode of illness (Glassner & Haldipur 1983, Ambelas 1987, and a majority of controlled studies indicate a similar associa-

tion with subsequent episodes (Sclare & Creed 1990, Hunt et al 1992, McPherson et al 1993). As the illness progresses, the importance of adverse life events appears to decline (Post 1992). A recent study which compared recent life events and suicide in bipolar and unipolar patients found a majority of both bipolar and unipolar suicides to have suffered adverse life events during their last 3 months. In contrast, however, to unipolar cases, the stressors affecting bipolars appear to have been more dependent on the behaviour of bipolar patients than on extraneous events. There was also a sex difference, with more male bipolar suicide victims experiencing adversity than females.

Both the unipolar and the bipolar group appeared to have a clustering of life events in the week prior to the suicidal act, implying some form of trigger. Whatever the mechanism, there is the possibility that an adverse life event during an illness episode increases the risk of suicide in the patient (Isometsa et al 1995) and this has implications for treatment and suicide prevention in this patient group.

Along with many studies in the field of suicide research, a major confounding factor is the lack of living control populations with which to make valid comparisons.

Hopelessness

The relationship between extreme pessimism or hopelessness and suicidal intent has traditionally been regarded as a close one (Beck et al 1975, Cole 1980, Minkoff et al 1973, and Wetzel et al 1980) and clinical strategies for alleviating hopelessness have been found to be useful for countering the suicidal crisis (Beck et al 1979).

What is unclear is whether all suicidal thinking is related to hopelessness. One study which examined this issue concluded that factors other than hopelessness are relevant for understanding suicidal ideation (Mendonca and Holden, 1996). Self-reported 'unusual thinking' was found to be the most important predictor of various aspects of suicidal intent in their sample.

The definition of 'unusual thinking' is a cognitive distortion which involves feelings of loss of control over one's thoughts. The findings imply that this aspect of cognitive distortion may be an important predictor and thus its evaluation may be integral to the assessment of suicidal ideation and risk. However, unusual thinking is regarded as a *state* related to current risk rather than a *trait* variable such as pessimistic attitude, problem-solving rigidity or perfectionism all of which have been implicated in the long-term risk of suicide (Hewitt et al 1994, Beck et al 1990, Linehan 1987).

The preoccupation with a method of self-harm was significantly associated with hopelessness for depressed patients but not for subgroups of personality disorder, anxiety disorder or substance abuse. The question of the latter co-existing with depression needs to be addressed.

Schizophrenia

Bleuler (1950) described the suicidal drive or intent as 'the most serious of schizophrenic symptoms'. Follow-up studies over the last 50 years have confirmed that schizophrenia has an increased risk of suicide. Estimates of this risk are of the order of 10–15% (Niskanen et al 1975, Winokur & Tsuang 1975, Miles 1977, Tsuang 1978, Black et al 1985).

Several risk factors appear with regularity in the literature. These include: young age and male sex; previous deliberate self-harm; and comorbid depression – there is consistent evidence of association between depression and suicide in schizophrenia (Table 26.8).

Schizophrenic suicides have been shown to present with depressed mood, as well as other features of depression, during their index admission to hospital. However, they are not more likely to fulfil criteria for major depression. Schizophrenics tend to show the psychological features of depressive illness, e.g. hopelessness, but less of the somatic features (Drake & Cotton 1986).

Some researchers have suggested that patients with insight into their illness are at greater risk of suicidal behaviour (Faberow et al 1965, Warnes 1968, Drake et al 1984, Cotton et al 1985). These individuals develop a sense of hopelessness and demoralisation, leading to suicidal behaviour.

Improvement of awareness of illness should be tempered with caution with regard to the effects of such increased awareness on the patient's degree of demoralisation, self-concept and hopelessness about the future.

Neuroses

Panic disorder has been associated with suicidal ideation and suicide attempts, but whether there is a causal link is unclear (Weissman et al 1989, Beck et al 1991, Friedman et al 1992). Approximately 20% of deaths among those previously hospitalised with anxiety disorders are suicides, a figure comparable to the mortality in depressive disorders (Coryell 1988, Noyes 1991). One of the largest studies in this area examined suicide and mortality patterns in anxiety neurosis and depressive neurosis which had no comorbidity with other psychiatric diagnoses (Allgulander 1994). Standardised mortality ratios of suicide before age 45 among men and women with anxiety neurosis was 6.7 and 4.9 respectively; and for depressive neurosis was 12.6 and 15.7 respectively. The risk of completed suicide among former inpatients with primary anxiety neurosis was higher than in previous smaller studies. The risk was higher still in those with depressive neurosis.

Substance abuse

The San Diego Suicide Study investigated young suicides. It was set up partly because the predictive power of known variables in relation to suicide is poor. The identification of new risk factors or combinations of variables is necessary for the improvement of this situation. More than any other disorders, substance abuse and depression are associated with suicide.

As part of the San Diego Suicide Study, relationships between interpersonal and other stressors and diagnoses of substance abuse and depression were examined. It was demonstrated that interpersonal loss or conflict occurred more frequently near the time of death for substance abusers with/without depression than for those with affective disorder alone. These results are consistent with other results in this area and suggest that there may be differences in the manner in which suicidal individuals with substance abuse and those with affective illness alone respond to external stressors (Rich et al 1988). More specifically, suicide associated with alcoholism and substance abuse may be preceded more often by interpersonal loss and conflict 6 weeks before death.

Table 26.8   Main correlates of suicide in schizophrenia
Young and male
Relapsing pattern of illness
Past history of depression
Current depressive illness/comorbid with depression
Recent discharge from inpatient care to outpatient care
Social isolation in the community
Relatively good insight into illness

There is evidence that those dependent on alcohol or other substances are confronted with a broader range of stressors than those with mood or anxiety disorder who commit suicide. In the weeks before death, those with substance abuse disorders/alcoholism experience more in the way of conflicts/arguments and attachment disruptions (Duberstein et al 1993).

Alcohol Alcoholism is a disorder with an increased risk of suicide. Murphy & Wetzel (1990) reviewed the world literature and concluded that the lifetime risk varied according to the type of treatment received:

- 2.2% for alcoholics with a history of outpatient treatment
- 3.4% for those with a history of inpatient treatment.

This represents a lifetime risk twice that of the general population and 60–120 times that of the non-psychiatrically ill in the general population. Examination of the general population of suicides indicates that about 20% of them have alcohol problems.

Risk factors for suicide among those suffering from alcohol dependence include the following:

- *Sex* The sex ratio in alcohol dependence is male:female = 5:1 (Goodwin 1982, Robins et al 1984). Barraclough et al (1974) found the same sex ratio among their alcoholic suicide victims as was found in a survey of alcoholics, i.e. 4:1, and thus concluded that 'the sex of an alcoholic does not apparently predispose to suicide' of itself. However, both Berglund (1984) and Nicholls et al (1974) found that male alcoholics had a suicide rate twice that of female alcoholics.
- *Age* In five studies that recorded age, the mean age of alcoholics who killed themselves was 46.8 years. The consensus from most studies is that the longer the alcoholism persists the more likely the adverse nature of the personal and social consequences.
- *Marital status* Loss of spouse and divorced status are recognised as predisposing to suicide in the alcoholic dependent, as well to alcoholism itself.
- *Natural history of illness* Robins (1986) reported that alcoholic suicides are not usually abstinent but currently drinking at the time of the act.
- *Depression and alcohol dependence* Depression is common among alcoholics (Roy et al 1991) but the extent to which alcoholic suicide victims have developed an associated depression during which they commit suicide has been little studied. In four studies which did examine this (with a total of 111 suicide victims), 56.8% victims were assessed as having an associated depressive syndrome. There is evidence that the presence of depressive symptoms

has an additive effect with regard to the risk of suicide in patients suffering from alcoholism (Berglund 1984).

With regard to life events, a significant proportion experience loss of a close interpersonal relationship in the year before death, and a smaller, but significant proportion, in the last 6 months (Murphy et al 1979), replicating previous findings (Murphy & Robins 1967). The period after discharge from a psychiatric admission is a period of increased risk for suicide (Roy 1982, Berglund 1984). Moreover, approximately one-third of alcoholic suicides have made a previous attempt (Roy & Linnoila 1986). One study found that 1 in 5 had attempted suicide and that both male and female alcoholic suicide attempters were more likely to have had an episode of major depression or to have antisocial personality disorder. Males were also significantly more likely to have abused drugs, have panic disorder, phobias and generalised anxiety disorder. These and comparable data suggest that the alcoholic who attempts suicide manifests greater psychopathology than the alcoholic who never does so.

A problem with studies on the prediction of suicide is that of the prediction of too many false negatives and false positives to be clinically useful. Multiple risk factors predict suicide in alcohol dependence. One study (Murphy et al 1992) identified seven features that appear to be intimately linked to suicide: continued drinking, major depressive episode, suicidal communication, poor social support, serious medical illness, unemployment and living alone. All these factors were significantly more common among subsequent completed suicides than among controls (Murphy et al 1992). Comorbidity is important especially with regard to depression which may be related to recent interpersonal loss.

The identification of groups of risk factors (Table 26.9) means that alcohol-dependent patients can be, potentially, more easily monitored for increased risk, and treatment of any comorbid depression will reduce the risk of suicide. These steps, along with securing abstinence, remain the treatment goal.

Table 26.9   Main correlates of suicide in those with alcohol problems
Male sex Longer duration of problems Single/divorced/widowed Currently drinking Presence of depressive symptoms

Personality disorder

Some personality disorders are thought to be associated with greater suicidal mortality (Weissman 1993, Samuels et al 1994, Isometsa et al 1996). Comorbidity is, however, important here: one large study found that all suicide victims with a personality disorder received at least one DSM-IV Axis I diagnosis. In 95% of cases this included depressive syndrome, psychoactive drug abuse or both. Depression was present in most of the suicide victims and did not differentiate between those with or without a personality disorder. No evidence was found of impulsive suicides that would have occurred without the presence of an Axis I disorder (Isometsa et al 1996).

These findings are in keeping with those which have found comorbidity in affective disorder or with psychoactive substance abuse to be related to a particularly high risk in subjects with borderline personality disorder (Brent et al 1994, Lesage et al 1994, McGlashan 1987, Stone 1990). It therefore appears that suicides among those with personality disorder are almost always to be associated with a depressive syndrome, psychoactive drug abuse, or both. There is some differentiation between those suicide victims with Cluster B personality disorder (dramatic, emotional or erratic) (DSM-IIIR), who are more commonly associated with psychoactive drug abuse and non-fatal suicide attempts and less commonly with physical disorder, and those with Cluster C (anxious or fearful), who are unlikely to differ much from suicide victims who do not fulfil criteria for personality disorder.

Suicide in special groups

Psychiatric patients

Barraclough & Pallis (1975) asked which type of depressive commits suicide. They found significantly more of the suicides were unmarried, lived alone and had a history of DSH. These characteristics are similar to a case–control study of risk factors for suicide in psychiatric patients (Roy 1982). Paykel et al (1969) and Brown & Harris (1978) have shown that life events, especially those involving loss, are associated with the development of depression. Roy's 1982 study indicates that depression needs to be recognised and treated, especially in those with certain risk factors, for example: past suicide attempt; chronic psychiatric disorder; recent admission; living alone; unemployed; unmarried; and vulnerable to depression. The immediate period when changing from inpatient to outpatient care is one of increased risk for suicide. These findings are consistent with previous results in this area.

Table 26.10 Features which might increase the risk of suicide in psychiatric patients (Appleby, 1992)

Feature	Factors
Mental state	Psychosis, depressed mood, hopelessness suicidal ideas, suicidal content to psychotic phenomena, communication of intent
Past history	Previous parasuicide, history <4 years,? several admissions,? long history with recent change
Social/demographic features	Living alone, single/divorced/ widowed, unemployed male, young
Current episode features	Acute relapse, recent discharge, inpatient or recent outpatient, recent transition in care
Ward and staff	Staff hostility to patient, high staff or patient turnover, low morale, insufficient observation facilities, inadequate staff expertise

Risk factors for the psychiatric inpatient population have been the focus of recent attention (Table 26.10). In a recent case–control study, those psychiatric inpatients at particular risk had previously exhibited suicidal behaviour, suffered from schizophrenia, were admitted involuntarily and lived alone (Roy & Draper 1995). There is further evidence which contends that, once age, sex and diagnosis are controlled for in discharged psychiatric patients, the conventional risk factors of being unmarried, being unemployed, living alone, substance misuse and previous DSH, are common to cases and controls and may be characteristic of people with mental illness generally.

The suicide rate in patients discharged from hospital has been reported to be at its highest in the first month after discharge and this emphasises the need for targeted care after discharge, especially against a background trend of reduced inpatient beds and shorter inpatient stay in hospital (Geddes & Juszczak 1995).

The apparent reduction in male standardised mortality ratios in figures concerning psychiatric patients are likely to reflect the fact that young males, whose suicide rates in the general population are rising, are not in contact with health services at all prior to suicide (Vassilas & Morgan 1993).

A problem with most risk factors is that they are relatively common in all psychiatric patient groups. They correlate well with suicide but predict it badly. Taken together, however, they offer an opportunity to identify high-risk groups within an already high-risk population of psychiatric patients.

It appears that there are two major vulnerability points in an episode of illness: the initial acute phase when a patient may be treated at home; and the period of recovery when they may be discharged earlier than was once conventional clinical practice, perhaps at a time of incomplete recovery.

Pregnancy and the puerperium

Issues relating to pregnancy and the puerperium deserve special consideration. During pregnancy and in the first postnatal year women have a low risk of suicide despite having increased rates of psychiatric morbidity. Motherhood appears to act as a protective factor against suicide and concern for dependants in a general sense may provide an important focus for preventative measures in the clinical setting (Appleby 1991). The effects of pregnancy and childbirth on rates of suicide provides an important balance to the assumption that suicide risk is determined solely by the mental state and psychiatric history. Social factors must be taken account of, particularly from the viewpoint of preventative measures (Kendell 1991).

Physical health variables

An increased risk of suicide has been associated with many physical illnesses, particularly chronic neurological, gastrointestinal, cardiovascular and malignant disorders (Whitlock 1986), so, for example, the relative risk of committing suicide among patients with cancer of all types is 2.5 (Allebeck & Bolund 1991). Some well-known associations are indirect, for instance the link between suicide and peptic ulceration is almost entirely explained by coexisting alcohol dependence.

Thinking that particular diseases and drugs are associated with increased suicide risk produces a false dichotomy; it is more useful to think in general terms about features that are linked to increased risk (Table 26.11).

Physical ill health is a significant factor in 25–75% of suicides, the higher figures being reported in studies of suicide among older victims. Two recent studies illustrate this. Among all suicides in Scotland in 1988 and 1989, 40% of men and 50% of women suffered from a chronic physical illness (Milne et al 1994), while in a review of 100 cases of suicide among elderly people, 65% had significant physical illness and 23% had been medical inpatients within the preceding year (Cattell & Jolley 1995).

Table 26.11 Factors associated with a disease or drug side-effect that increase the likelihood of suicide

Mood disorder, especially depression, emotional lability

Motor overactivity, e.g. agitation, akathisia

Disinhibition, reduced impulse control

Severe chronic or recurrent pain that is inadequately controlled

Disfigurement, especially in women

Severe disability, especially loss of mobility

Extensive sick role limitations, e.g. loss of job, family role

Prospect of a degenerating disease without hope of recovery

There is a strong relationship between physical ill health and depression or subclinical distress (Mayou & Hawton 1986), and although these emotional disorders are usually mild, it is likely this factor largely mediates the association between physical ill health and suicide.

Management

All psychiatrists will encounter suicides among their patients and will have to manage the aftermath of the event, particularly if the death occurred in an inpatient. All unnatural deaths, whether definite suicides or not, must be reported to the statutory authorities – the procurator fiscal in Scotland and the coroner in England and Wales. The police will have to investigate the death on behalf of the Crown, so a death certificate cannot be issued and a postmortem examination will be required. In Scotland the Mental Welfare Commission should be informed of all suicides among psychiatric patients, irrespective of whether or not they are detained under mental health legislation. Psychiatrists should also provide details to the Royal College of Psychiatrists' Confidential Enquiry into Suicides and Homicides by Mentally Ill People (Royal College of Psychiatrists 1995, Appleby 1996).

Consideration must be given to the relatives who have to cope with the untimely death and the inevitable statutory procedures (and delays). Of course their emotional process is one of grief, but the nature and circumstances of the death predispose to extreme or atypical reactions, profound guilt or anger, and an increased risk of deliberate self-harm or suicide among the bereaved (Wertheimer 1991). Managing the survivors is a delicate process in which the help that is offered must be sensitive to the wishes of the individual – inappropriate help, or that which is pressed too vigorously, can be as distressing as providing no assistance at all.

The emotional impact on the individual who found the body or inadvertently caused the death must also be borne in mind, particularly if the death was gruesome. Post-traumatic stress disorder (PTSD) may develop in these circumstances.

Among train drivers involved in railway suicides PTSD occurred in 17% and other mental illnesses in a further 23% (Farmer et al 1992). Psychological debriefing is also necessary for ward staff when a suicide has occurred on the ward or been carried out by an inpatient. It is important to avoid scapegoating the staff on the one hand and sweeping the event under the carpet on the other.

Staff need to have an opportunity to talk through the event as quickly as possible in a safe, non-judgemental environment – a task that should be separated from the audit of such deaths that should become a routine part of clinical practice (NHS Health Advisory Service 1996).

Prevention

Despite all the uncertainties, confusion and controversy surrounding suicidal behaviour, suicide prevention is high on the health agenda. A reversal of the internationally rising trends in suicide and attempted suicide is one of the World Health Organization's targets for Europe as part of its Health For All strategy, whereas in England and Wales the Health of the Nation has set key targets of reducing the overall suicide rate by 15%, and the suicide rate among severely mentally ill people by at least 33%, by the year 2000 (Department of Health 1993). These aims were amplified in two documents (Department of Health 1994, NHS Health Advisory Service 1996) in which the emphasis was on implementation rather than feasibility – although it is by no means indisputable that the intervention of doctors may reduce the suicide rate (Wilkinson & Morgan 1994).

The main problem with preventing suicide is that it remains a rare and unpredictable event, even among patients who are identified as being at high risk. Suicidal intent is not constant, it waxes and wanes, often suddenly and unexpectedly. Further, the risk can be greater when the patient is becoming ill, or is recovering, or has recovered from illness rather than when the disorder is severe. The difficulty in predicting suicide even among likely victims is illustrated in an American study of 2000 patients with mood illness who were admitted to a psychiatric hospital. A statistical model determined risk based on established factors such as previous suicide attempts, suicidal ideation and outcome at discharge but this failed to pinpoint with 50% probability any of the 46 patients who committed suicide, and only one victim at 15% probability – i.e. at the same likelihood of suicide as for depressive illness (Goldstein et al 1991). Further, the changing epidemiology of suicide has reduced the potential opportunity for doctors to intervene, as young men who commit suicide are much less likely to have consulted their general practitioner in the weeks leading up to their death (Vassilas & Morgan 1993), or to have a psychiatric diagnosis other than substance abuse (Milne et al 1994).

These consistent findings have led to a call to focus therapeutic attention on the substance misuse of younger patients who present to hospital following DSH as the key clinical suicide prevention strategy in this group (Hawton et al 1993). Another doubt is whether medical intervention can prevent suicide even when high risk is identified. The debate centres on the Gotland study (Rutz et al 1989). The aim of this study had been to test the effect of increasing general practitioners' knowledge about the diagnosis and treatment of patients with affective disorders, and the suicide rate on the island had been monitored primarily to ensure the treatment strategies did not increase the risk for individual patients. The investigators discovered a reduction in suicides from an average 11 per year in 1982–1984 to four in the year of the study, a finding that was not mirrored by a reduction in Sweden as a whole. The suicide rate returned to normal in subsequent years (Rutz et al 1992). The Gotland study had major drawbacks, not least that the base population was only 56 000 and its effect was fleeting, but its significance has been considerable, and perhaps mainly symbolic – that if doctors learned to identify high-risk patients and treat depressive illnesses energetically an appreciable impact on the suicide rate will follow. Both sides of the argument have valid points: on the one hand, preaching that medical interventions will prevent suicide raises false hopes and expectations among the public, and encourages grieving relatives to blame health care professionals inappropriately, while on the other, scientific evidence cannot always determine medical practice, a leap of faith is sometimes necessary, and complacent or slipshod practice may make the difference between life and death, even if it cannot be proved. Irrespective of their position, all medical authorities agree that it is impossible to prevent all suicides and that medical considerations are but one element of the strategy.

Measures that could form part of a comprehensive suicide prevention strategy have been discussed (Gunnell & Frankel 1994). Broadly these interventions fall into three categories:

- Public health measures, which are subdivided into

method-targeted, person-targeted and general and have the potential to make the greatest impact

- Primary care measures, which focus on the identification and treatment of depression in particular
- Psychiatric practice measures.

None of these interventions has been demonstrated to be effective in well-conducted clinical trials: they reflect the opinions of respected authorities and the recommendations of expert committees, as well as the results of descriptive or methodologically inadequate studies.

Based on the assumption that one in three individuals who fail to commit suicide with one method will not switch to an alternative (Gunnell & Frankel 1994), the single intervention with the greatest impact on the suicide rate would be the fitting of catalytic converters and modification of car exhaust design which would reduce total suicides by 7%, almost entirely among men. Among women, the single most effective measure would be the addition of methionine to paracetamol, which would cut female suicides by around 5%.

The greatest challenge facing suicide prevention arises from the rapid increase among young men who abuse alcohol and drugs and are not in contact with health services (Hawton 1992). Until the reasons for this international 'epidemic' are understood, interventions which are acceptable to the at-risk individuals and likely to be effective cannot evolve.

DELIBERATE SELF-HARM

Terminology

There has been difficulty in finding a suitable term to define presentations of self-injury and self-poisoning that have not resulted in death. 'Attempted suicide' is widely used by the media and general public, although Kessel argued over 30 years ago that this term was not simply misleading, it was wrong and ought to be discarded, as the intent to die applied to less than half the patients (Kessel 1965). 'Parasuicide' is defined as an act of deliberate self-injury or self-poisoning which mimics the act of suicide but does not result in a fatal outcome; the term indicates a behavioural analogue of suicide but without conveying a psychological orientation towards death (Kreitman 1977). While dissociating the behaviour from a specific motive, the fact that 'suicide' remains in the term obfuscates the meaning to all bar the experts. The term (non-fatal) deliberate self-harm avoids all reference to suicide, and merely describes the common end-point of aberrant behaviour that is the basis for study. Deliberate self-harm (DSH) is the term used by the Royal College of Psychiatrists

(Royal College of Psychiatrists 1994) and government bodies (Department of Health and Social Security 1984) – and it is the preferred term for this chapter.

Features

The core features of DSH are:

- the behaviour is self-initiated
- harm is intended
- the act results, or may result, in injury and possibly death to the individual.

Therefore, self-harm where the intent is pleasure or experiment, or injury occurs accidentally, is excluded. Factitious disorders, in which deliberate self-injury often occurs, are distinguished from DSH by the elements of intentional deception and the simulation or induction of disease. Other forms of self-injurious behaviour which are not usually considered as forms of DSH are trichotillomania and bingeing and self-induced vomiting among psychiatric presentations, and medical presentations where injury results from intentional non-compliance, such as a patient who has diabetes refusing to take insulin or a patient with chronic renal failure refusing to continue on haemodialysis.

Basic statistics

The epidemiological study of DSH is dogged by the fact that no country anywhere in the world collects official data on DSH. Thus, it is not possible to correlate national trends with those in suicide. What can be done is to examine data from studies which looked at specific groups of cases of DSH in well-defined sample areas over several years (Kreitman 1977, Kreitman & Schreiber 1979, Diekstra 1982, Hawton & Goldacre 1982, WHO 1982). What these studies demonstrate is that hospital discharge rates for DSH by young people showed a marked increase in tandem with their suicide rates in the 15 year period 1965–1980 (Diekstra 1996). This pattern has been confirmed by data from British and Dutch hospital inpatient records (Diekstra 1982). On the basis of results from these studies and others, it is apparent that the trends of suicide and DSH rates are very similar. An important reason for examining epidemiological data on DSH is that one of the most consistent features of this phenomenon is as one of, if not the most, powerful predictors of suicide (Van Egmond & Diekstra 1989). Longitudinal follow-up studies of DSH indicate that 10–14% of those who harm themselves ultimately die by their own hand. In terms of risk, this translates to a risk of dying through suicide of 100 times that of the general population (Brent & Kolko 1990). How common DSH is can be ascertained using data from two epidemiological methods: the service utilisation study and the population sample survey. Two international studies using the former method (Diekstra 1982, Platt et al 1992) demonstrated higher female than male rates of DSH and a peak age for DSH in the first half of the life cycle (15–44 years).

Due to the differences in referral and data recording procedures, there is considerable variation in the groups with the highest rates, both between sexes and between countries. The information gathered from the other type of study method, i.e. the population sample survey, is at variance with that obtained from service utilisation studies. On the whole, they reveal higher rates of DSH and raise the issue of underreporting of cases of DSH (Diekstra 1985, Centers for Disease Control 1991).

With regard to prevalence rates of DSH, estimations vary from around 1% (Paykel et al 1974) to 20% (Rubinstein et al 1989) for those individuals aged 12/13 and above. A considerable proportion of studies only detail lifetime prevalence rates for adolescents and young adults, but those which examine rates in the general population indicate that lifetime prevalence rates for the general population do not overtake, and sometimes are below, those for the younger cohort. Therefore, it would seem that lifetime prevalence rates of DSH are not a function of age. These figures would bear the interpretation that the age at which people first deliberately harm themselves is decreasing. If this is the case, then the pre-eminence of DSH as a risk factor for subsequent suicide would indicate a lowering of the age at which people take their lives (Diekstra 1996).

Methods

In the UK, poisoning by drugs accounts for 90% of all hospital presentations of DSH. Of the remainder, two-thirds present with cutting of the wrist(s) or arm(s), while all other methods combined contribute the remaining 3–4%. These proportions have remained constant in Britain over the years and similar in Scotland (Edinburgh) and England (Oxford) (Platt et al 1988). In a comparison between England (Oxford) and Holland (Utrecht) the same 9:1 ratio between self-poisoning and other forms of DSH was found, but within the self-injury subgroup most of the English sample presented with wrist cutting, whereas the majority of the Dutch sample employed more dangerous methods such as jumping, hanging and attempting drowning (Grootenhuis et al 1994).

There are important temporal trends apparent in the drugs used for overdoses by patients seen at British hospitals, which are due to changes in prescribing practices. Hence barbiturate hypnotics and metha-

qualone accounted for 40% of admissions to Edinburgh's Regional Poisoning Treatment Centre during the late 1960s, but were superseded by the benzodiazepines during the 1970s (Proudfoot & Park 1978), and had virtually ceased to be a method of poisoning by the mid-1980s (Platt et al 1988). Likewise, benzodiazepine self-poisoning peaked at over 40% of referrals in the late 1970s, fell gradually during the early 1980s and then steeply, following curbs in prescribing, so that less than 20% of presentations now involve these compounds (Hawton & Fagg 1992, McLoone & Crombie 1996). Between 1981 and 1993, hospital presentations of paracetamol self-poisoning increased fourfold in Scotland (McLoone & Crombie 1996). The same trend was apparent in Oxford: in 1978–1979 paracetamol accounted for 17% of cases of self-poisoning, by 1983–1984 this had risen to 28% (Platt et al 1988) and in 1993 to 48% of all overdoses (Hawton et al 1996). Curiously, self-poisoning as a result of the other well-known 'over the counter' analgesic, aspirin, has remained constant throughout this period. The increasing popularity of paracetamol, particularly among younger patients, has also been reported in other European countries (Hawton et al 1996), and is of particular concern because of its serious medical complications. Indeed most patients admitted to liver transplant units because of fulminant hepatic failure have taken paracetamol overdoses (>80% of such presentations to the Scottish centre), and this poses major ethical dilemmas as transplantable organs are a scarce resource and adequate psychiatric assessment is often prevented by encephalopathy (O'Grady et al 1991). The reasons why patients choose paracetamol vary, although ready availability and knowledge that it is potentially fatal (without knowing how this would occur) appear to be the main factors (Hawton et al 1995). Deterring paracetamol self-poisoning, or reducing the harm it causes, would probably be best achieved by limiting the number of tablets available in all over-the-counter paracetamol preparations to 25 or fewer (Hawton et al 1996).

Social variables

The social variables which appear to operate most frequently around DSH include socioeconomic factors, unemployment and adverse life events. Situational crises have been accepted as important precursors to DSH (Kessel 1965, Lukianowicz 1972, Litman & Faberow 1961). For example, there have been reports which have found that those who deliberately harmed themselves had experienced the recent death of a parent more commonly than other psychiatric patients (Birtchnell 1970) or suffered a variety of separations

(Levi et al 1966). However, there has been a dearth of studies which have used controlled comparison of both healthy and psychiatrically unwell individuals. A notable exception to this (Paykel et al 1975) found that the events encountered by those who deliberately self-harm are different from controls in amount, type and temporal distribution. Generally, those who deliberately self-harm experience substantially more events than the general population and the attempts at suicide show a strong relationship to life events. The single event reported most often was interpersonal relationship difficulties – arguments with spouse. There is evidence that those who harm themselves deliberately report more life events than depressed controls, but of a specific sort. Those who attempted suicide reported more events of a threatening nature, for example: more undesirable but not more desirable events; more uncontrolled events but not more controlled ones; and more events major and intermediate in upset but not more minor in upset.

Paykel and colleagues concluded that these events of a threatening nature are more closely linked to DSH than to the onset of a depressive episode. Serious physical illness of self or of a close family member was also reported more often than by controls. The entrance or exit of someone from the social environment was more frequent before an episode of DSH than in the general population. As far as the timing of life events was concerned, Paykel et al found that there was a peak in the month before the episode of DSH. Overall, their findings indicate a strong and immediate relationship between episodes of DSH and life events.

Unemployment

Economic instability and recession and the relationship with suicidal behaviour has been the source of dispute over the last century and a half. On the relationship between DSH and unemployment, there has been a preponderance of studies using a cross-sectional design. They have shown that significantly more people who deliberately self-harm are unemployed than would be expected among the general population (Hawton et al 1982b) and DSH rates among the unemployed are always considered higher than among those in work (Kreitman 1973, Bancroft et al 1975, Kessel et al 1975). Caution must be exercised in ascribing causal links, as it is likely that DSH results from the complex interaction of many factors. Clinical experience, for example, suggests that many males who deliberately self-harm lead chronically marginalised existences with lives characterised by irregular employment, petty crime, excessive alcohol consumption and loneliness. In a sense, they are detached from the majority of society. The role of

Table 26.12   Environmental variables associated with deliberate self-harm
Adverse life events, especially interpersonal relationship difficulties
Unemployment
Socioeconomic adversity

unemployment as a major contributing factor to this situation must not be underestimated. Unemployment is a predisposing variable as it leads to increases in family and interpersonal strife, hopelessness and depression, social isolation, financial hardship, loss of self-esteem, and combinations thereof. Consequently, the likelihood of an adverse event, for example loss or argument with a partner, leading to an act of DSH is greater in the context of unemployment (Platt 1984). Hawton & Rose (1986) indicate that unemployment may worsen risk factors for DSH. In order to tease out the variables more research is needed in the context of evidence that the long-term unemployed are at a significantly higher risk of DSH (Table 26.12).

Motives

The reasons why a patient should self-harm are varied and sometimes complex or even mutually contradictory, but it is important to establish motives to form an appropriate management plan (Table 26.13). The motives patients report on assessment after DSH may not be what they would have said when they decided to harm themselves or during the act. Often the patient may genuinely not know what their motive was, particularly when the act was impulsive and in a setting of intoxication with alcohol or drugs (and alcohol is a factor in half the presentations). However, some acutely suicidal patients will set out to trivialise or deny the gravity of their act so that they have another opportunity to kill themselves if they manage to avoid detection. On the other hand, some patients may justify their act by infusing it with a degree of seriousness and life threat

Table 26.13   Motives underlying deliberate self-harm
Wish to die
Trial by ordeal
Time out
Cry for help
Communication with others
Unbearable symptoms

that are out of keeping with the circumstances surrounding their presentation.

Bearing these factors in mind, the main reasons patients offer for an act of DSH are as follows:

- *To die* The wish to die is cited as a motive by about 50% of patients who are hospitalised (Bancroft et al 1976) – but much less often by psychiatrists (Bancroft et al 1979) or by their spouse or other next of kin (James & Hawton 1985). The same findings apply to adolescents (Hawton et al 1982a). Ambivalence about death is reported more often than an unequivocal intent to die, and this is characteristically expressed as indifference about survival.
- *Trial by ordeal* Again reflecting ambivalence, patients may test the benevolence of fate by gambling with their life, usually by harming themselves in circumstances in which someone may or may not discover them. Survival is then interpreted as a sign of destiny or of divine intervention and the patient may then proceed to address the problems that precipitated the act.
- *Time out* Patients may harm themselves in a blind reaction to obtain respite from acute or chronic social difficulties, and the unpleasant thoughts and feelings these have engendered; this has been described as seeking an interruption to an unendurable state of tension (Shneidman 1964).
- *Cry for help/'cri du coeur'* The intent here is to enlist the assistance and sympathy of other people such as a disenchanted partner or family, or authorities such as the police or housing, usually after more acceptable methods have failed. In practice this motive is uncommon, its exaggerated importance arising from the fact it fits readily into the stereotype of DSH patients as inadequate and manipulative.
- *Communication with other people* This is a motive reported by about 30% of DSH patients admitted to hospital (Bancroft et al 1976). These interpersonal acts take two basic forms: either the expression of a powerful emotion, particularly anger but also guilt or love, to another person or people; or ascertaining how someone regards them through their reaction to the act.
- *Unbearable symptoms* Escape from intolerable symptoms, by death if necessary, is not uncommon and needs to be distinguished from accidental overmedication for symptom relief. The most common reasons are inadequately controlled pain and/or insomnia; panic, akathisia, constipation and fatigue are other symptoms which may lead to DSH.

Clinical variables

Deliberate self-harm is approximately 10 times more common than suicide (Diekstra 1993) and is a strong predictor of suicide. In completed suicide, depression and substance misuse disorders are the most prevalent mental disorders and the majority have comorbidity in which there may be important sex differences. Few studies of DSH have been based on well-defined operationalised criteria for mental disorders. One recent study (Suominen et al 1996) interviewed consecutive cases of DSH over 6 months and found that 98% had at least one Axis I diagnosis, with depressive syndromes more common in women than men and alcohol dependence more common in men. They concluded that a high proportion of DSH suffered from comorbid mental disorders and that comorbidity appears to play an important role in DSH, as is the case in completed suicide. A case–control study found that of those who made a serious attempt, 90.1% had a mental disorder at the time of the attempt and that there were high rates of mood disorders, substance abuse, conduct disorder or antisocial personality disorder, and non-affective psychosis. The relationship between psychiatric morbidity and suicide risk varied with age and gender. The incidence of comorbidity was high, with 56.6 % of those who made serious suicide attempts having two or more disorders. Also, the risk of a suicide attempt increased with increasing psychiatric morbidity, i.e. those with two or more disorders had odds of serious attempts that were 89.7 times the odds of those with no psychiatric disorder (Beautrais et al 1996). So, it can be concluded that those who make serious attempts have high rates of mental disorder and of comorbid disorders and that subjects with high levels of psychiatric comorbidity have higher risk of serious suicide attempts.

Affective illness

Major depression An examination of the risk of DSH in those inpatients with major depression found that the first 3 months after the onset of an episode of major depression and the first 5 years after the lifetime onset of major depression represented the highest risk period for attempted suicide, independent of the severity or duration of the depression. There is also some evidence which suggests that familial and genetic factors, early loss experiences and comorbid alcoholism may be causal factors (Malone et al 1995). Controversy surrounds whether there are clinically meaningful differences between depressed patients who deliberately harm themselves and those who do not. Large representative case-controlled studies are required to discover whether such differences exist. In 1898 Clouston wrote that 'the greatest danger of suicide is near the commencement of the attack'. There is contemporary data supporting this statement from a study which showed that most depressed patients who made a suicide attempt did so within the first 12 months of the depressive episode (Vieta et al 1992). The timing of suicidal behaviour in the course of major depression may indicate whether depression is a precipitant for 'latent' suicide attempters to cross the threshold to overt suicidal behaviour . If there is a biopsychological vulnerability for suicidal behaviour, then suicide attempters should manifest overt suicidal behaviour after exposure to the same or less duration and severity of depression as compared with non-attempters. Evidence indicates that, despite at least comparable levels of depression, non-attempters appear to tolerate severe depression without crossing the threshold into suicidal behaviour, whereas suicide attempters exceed the threshold during a similar depressive syndrome (Malone et al 1995). The extent to which age and duration of affective illness interact with the risk of DSH is another area under investigation. The view that the risk of DSH manifests itself in the early stages of the illness and decreases as the illness progresses has been challenged by results which indicate that the risk of DSH is unchanged in all age groups and throughout all stages of untreated illness (Ahrens et al 1995).

Bipolar illness   In a meta-analysis of the available literature, Lester (1993) highlighted two possible trends of suicidal behaviour in unipolar and bipolar illness: an excess of subsequent completed suicides in unipolar depression; and an excess of subsequent DSH in bipolar illness. Investigating suicidality in bipolar illness is beset by the major problem of which descriptive constructs are used, i.e. dimensional constructs based on symptom severity or categorical constructs which divide syndromes into discrete entities. While it is accepted that suicidality is more common in the depressive rather than the manic phase of bipolar illness, the risk in mixed states is less clear. In a study which analysed the relationship between suicidality and the affective state of bipolar patients, i.e. mixed or manic, the severity of concurrent depressive symptoms in mania, i.e. mixed state, rather than the presence of a depressive syndrome, was associated with suicidality in bipolar patients (Strakowski et al 1996). In rapid cycling bipolar illness there appears to be no significant difference in DSH compared with non-rapid cyclers (Wu & Dunner 1993).

Panic disorder

In panic disorder, the presence of comorbid illness appears to be intimately linked with the risk of DSH.

Retrospective studies found DSH to be associated with depression, substance abuse, eating disorders, PTSD and personality disorder, as well an early age of onset of the first episodes of anxiety or depression. Prospective data records all suicidal behaviour as occurring in those with comorbid depression and that the rate of DSH among those with panic disorder in the absence of depression is no greater than that found in the general population (Warshaw et al 1995). Whether the presence of panic disorder increases the risk of DSH in those with comorbid conditions like depression remains unclear, but it appears that suicidal behaviour in those with panic disorder is related more to other factors not peculiar to panic disorder itself, e.g. depression, substance abuse, PTSD, eating disorders, personality difficulties and factors related to quality of life. In common with all other syndromes, it is important to characterise coexisting disorders, Axis I and Axis II, when examining suicidal behaviour.

Personality disorder

One study which looked at suicidal behaviour in those with major depression and comorbid personality disorder concluded that those with borderline personality disorder symptoms are at risk for serious suicide attempts. The presence and severity of Axis II personality disorder has been positively related to indicators of suicidality (Corbitt et al 1996). This supports previous research findings that the presence of personality disorder may increase the risk of suicidal behaviour, especially in borderline personality disorder. Group differences also supported previous findings that major depression with comorbid borderline personality disorder carries a higher risk for attempted suicide than major depression alone. Therefore, it is important to consider the severity of comorbid Cluster B personality disorder characteristics when assessing suicide risk in those with major depression, even those who have not been categorised as having a personality disorder. This provides a salutary warning contradicting the clinical folklore that those with borderline personality disorder tend to make frequent, trivial suicidal gestures which are not highly life-threatening. Recent research findings suggest that if borderline personality disorder is comorbid with depressive disorder it can lead to serious suicide attempts. Research findings support the hypothesis that the higher levels of suicidality in borderline personality disorder are due to a vulnerability for suicidal behaviour in these patients. The threshold for such behaviour is lowered in the presence of comorbid stressors such as major depression (Malone et al 1993).

Subtance abuse

Aggression, impulsivity and comorbid Cluster B Axis II personality disorder are reproducible trait-related predictors of suicidal behaviour in adolescence (Brent et al 1994) and in adulthood (Brown et al 1982, Frances et al 1986) and those who have these trait-related features have greater risk of comorbid alcohol and substance abuse (Hawton et al 1993), which may also contribute to lowering the threshold for suicidal behaviour. Research comparing depressed alcoholics with non-depressed alcoholics and depressed non-alcoholics found that depression with alcoholism was associated with greater suicidality, implying that alcoholism can also lower the threshold for suicidality or is associated with other factors which underly a lower threshold (Cornelius et al 1996).

Alcohol Alcohol use has been found to increase the risk of suicidal behaviour in both alcoholic and non-alcoholic populations and is thought to be associated with approximately 50% of all suicides (Frances et al 1987). There is extensive use of alcohol in connection with DSH. The use of alcohol also adds to the potential danger of an overdose because alcohol increases the toxicity of psychotropic drugs and, clinically, it is not unusual for unconsciousness to be attributed to alcohol alone and thus delay medical treatment for the overdose.

The association of alcohol intoxication and suicidal risk has been extensively reported (Barraclough et al 1974, Goldney 1981). Among those receiving hospital treatment for the sequelae of DSH, 40–75% of males and 12–50% of females had taken alcohol at the time of the act or up to 6 hours before it (Patel et al 1972, Morgan et al 1975, Kreitman 1977, Adam et al 1978, Goldney 1981, Hawton et al 1989). In a study of DSH in which alcohol was involved in an accident and emergency setting, the consumption of alcohol just before or at the time of an episode of DSH was found to be more common among young or socially isolated men with a past history of DSH. This group were less often referred to a psychiatrist and their risk of suicide was judged to be less serious. At the end of a $5^{1}/_{2}$ year follow-up period, 3.3% had killed themselves and the suicide mortality in the year following the initial attempt represented a 51-fold risk compared with that of the local general population They are, therefore, a group at risk (Suokas & Lonnqvist 1995).

Psychosis

Generally, the clinical risk factors consistently associated with suicidal behaviour in patients with psychosis are: depression, hopelessness and severity of illness (Roy et al 1984, Drake & Cotton 1986, Roy 1986, Dassori et al 1990, Addington & Addington 1992). A high frequency of depressive symptoms has also been found among consecutive completed suicides with psychotic disorder (Rich 1988). Other clinical and demographic variables have less consistent significance, perhaps because samples have been composed of consecutive admissions and therefore vary in the distributions of illness stage and treatment experience. With regard to bipolar patients with psychotic symptoms, who have a high risk of completed suicide, a study of index admissions found they have a significantly reduced risk of DSH (Goldstein et al 1991). This finding is consistent with results in which psychotic patients with bipolar disorder had the highest rate of completed suicide but a relatively lower rate of attempts than the rest of the sample (Axelsson & Lagerkvist-Briggs 1992).

On comparing schizophrenics and depressed patients, one recent study compared positive and negative symptoms of psychosis and found that positive symptoms predicted later suicidal activity only for the schizophrenic group. Deficit or negative symptoms such as psychomotor retardation, concreteness, etc. predicted later suicidal activity only for the depressed group. The general adequacy of overall functioning predicted later suicidal activity for both diagnostic categories (Kaplan & Harrow 1996).

DSH specifically related to women

A variety of social risk factors relevant to women indicate that several factors, such as divorce, illegitimacy, unemployment, family factors, education, income and other factors affecting the status of women, play a major role in influencing the prevalence of DSH among females. There is also evidence of a special relationship between premenstrual syndrome and mood disorder (Rubinow & Schmidt 1987) in that women with premenstrual syndrome have a greater lifetime prevalence of affective disorder (Mackenzie et al 1986). A recent study examining the relationship between premenstrual syndrome and DSH found that those reporting suicidal ideas during the premenstrual phase were more commonly college students and working women rather than housewives. Depressive premenstrual syndrome symptoms were significantly more often reported by women who had suicidal ideas than those without (Chaturverdi 1995). The relationship between childhood sex abuse and DSH in women was examined in the specific group of women who met criteria for borderline personality disorder. The vast majority of those with a history of at least two DSH episodes reported a history of some form of childhood sexual abuse. Moreover, this group engaged in acts of DSH which were more lethal, more medically serious and with greater suicidal intent than those who reported no such abuse (Wagner & Linehan 1994). Asking about childhood trauma is important when examining any case of DSH, but it may have important predictive value in the case of women with borderline personality disorder. Similarly, sexual assault is associated with an increased lifetime rate of DSH (Davidson et al 1996).

Past abuse and suicidal ideation

Although caution should always be exercised when ascribing causal links, there are indications that a history of past physical and sexual abuse are predictive of suicidal ideation. One study found abuse victims to have been suicidal at a younger age and to have made multiple attempts. Among abuse victims, those who had made attempts were distinguished from non-attempters by higher levels of dissociation, depression and somatisation (Kaplan et al 1995).

Assessment

Current guidance remains 'the consultant who has charge of the patient whether in the Accident and Emergency Department or in a ward will be responsible for ensuring that a full physical assessment is made and that before patients are discharged from hospital, a psychosocial assessment is carried out by staff specifically trained for this task' (Department of Health and Social Security 1984). This requirement took into account research which demonstrated DSH patients who were assessed by non-psychiatrists did not appear to be at greater risk of subsequent repetition or suicide. However, the reality has been that patients are often not assessed by staff with adequate training and supervision in psychosocial assessment, and this includes junior psychiatrists (Owens & House 1995). Further, a national survey of practice discovered there had been little movement towards the guidelines recommended (Butterworth & O'Grady 1989), and it was widely accepted that these services were in a state of disarray.

This led to an important consensus statement on minimum standards for service provision in regard to the general hospital management of adult DSH (Royal College of Psychiatrists 1994). This document took into account that DSH patients might be assessed in the accident and emergency department or on an inpatient ward, and the assessment might be undertaken by specialist psychiatric staff or by general medical staff. The procedure was considered in terms of:

- The assessment of the immediate risk on arrival in the accident and emergency department or the ward, where a triage process probably undertaken by a trained nurse was advised
- The provision of suitable assessment facilities in 'a setting which accords with privacy, confidentiality and respect'
- The suitability of staff to undertake psychosocial assessment whatever their professional background, with emphasis on minimum standards of training and supervision
- Clinical assessment and management which covered further assessment procedures and the provision of appropriate facilities to maintain safety for the patient
- Communication, both among the clinical team and with those who were going to be involved in follow-up, and notably the general practitioner.

The fundamental recommendation was that each service should establish a self-harm services' planning group with a multidisciplinary membership. This would determine specifications, policies and minimum quality; it would supervise a designated self-harm specialist clinical team, organise training and monitor the service, by audit of the case notes and aftercare arrangements. While ambitious in their scope and perhaps unrealistic in their scale, these recommendations are undoubtedly valuable. In particular they establish an essential framework on which the assessment and management of individual patients can be based.

Patients

The purpose of the psychosocial assessment is to identify among DSH patients those who have a psychiatric illness, a high suicide risk, or potentially remediable coexisting problems such as substance misuse, interpersonal or social difficulties. The principles are those of any emergency psychiatric assessment, hence an exhaustive account of interview procedures is unnecessary. The element that is different, in terms of emphasis, is the evaluation of suicide risk, of which there are four components.

Recognised risk factors The sociodemographic and clinical factors associated with repetition of DSH and suicide are widely known. They are of limited clinical value: they represent a statistical stereotype of suicide and, with the exception of past episodes of DSH being a reasonable predictor of further episodes, they have proved uniformly poor predictors of outcome, especially in the short term. Further, these risk factors almost invariably do not enable the clinician to plan interventions that will reduce further risk. However, entirely disregarding established risk factors would be a mistake, mainly because their presence should act as a warning sign to the clinician that a more intensive assessment of suicide risk is warranted, particularly if the apparent risk seems low.

Suicidal intent An essential element in assessing suicide risk is to establish a factual account of the DSH, as well as the patient's expectations and motives. Scales of suicidal intent have been developed for use by clinical staff undertaking assessments, the most widely used being the Beck Suicide Intent Scale (Beck et al 1974). While suicidal intent is associated with medical lethality (Power et al 1985), its usefulness in predicting outcome is poor (Pallis et al 1984); it is most helpful among patients who make repeated high-intent attempts (Pierce 1981). It is also unclear how useful the dangerousness of the attempt is in predicting outcome (Hawton 1987). Plainly patients who opt for violent methods are more likely to die, but this outcome may reflect greater impulsivity, copycat activity, cultural factors and ready availability rather than greater intent.

Present psychiatric state Assessing the present psychiatric state adequately requires first and foremost a responsive and cooperative patient who is fit for interview, i.e. not drowsy, intoxicated or distressed by symptoms like pain or vomiting. Other requirements include sufficient time, a suitable milieu, the opportunity to reassess if necessary, and finally a good collateral informant who becomes essential when the patient is uncooperative or unfit.

The doctor's approach should be methodical, serious and sensitive. In general the topic of suicidal ideation should not be broached until rapport has been established. The precise wording and directness of the initial enquiry is a matter of opinion and style; however, this should be flexible, depending on the patient's age, culture and emotional state as well as the perceived threat of suicide. Although silences should be sanctioned, unanswered questions must be returned to later on, perhaps expressed in another way. Ambiguous comments must be clarified: remarks like 'I don't want to live' or 'There is no future for me' may or may not indicate suicidal ideation, it all depends on their context.

Where doubt exists or increased risk is established or suspected, asking more than once during the interview and repeating the enquiries at subsequent interviews become essential. Indicating willingness to listen to such thoughts, then or later facilitates this process. It is neither valid nor acceptable to regard suicidal risk as present or absent on the basis of a one-off enquiry like 'Do you feel suicidal?'

Plainly the presence of mental disorder is important to establish. Particular attention needs to be paid to indicators of depressive illness, and hopelessness has been established as an important predictor of eventual suicide in depressed patients (Beck et al 1985). Other depressive features which distinguished depressed patients who committed suicide from those who did not included insomnia, impaired memory, self-neglect and delusions; contrary to popular belief psychomotor retardation was not protective (Barraclough & Pallis 1975).

Among patients with schizophrenia, those who committed suicide were more likely to be depressed, and/or to report hopelessness or fear of mental disintegration. They also tended to have high non-delusional expectations of themselves and had struggled to adjust to their illness. Finally, the presence of akathisia and the abrupt discontinuation of medication may also increase the risk of suicide (Hawton 1987). These features probably explain why suicide among patients with schizophrenia occurs particularly in the early years of their illness and during what appears to be a quiescent phase. With alcoholism, the majority of patients who killed themselves were concurrently depressed (Barraclough et al 1974); the same applied for patients with neurotic conditions (Sims & Prior 1978). Particularly among younger patients, personality disorder characterised by impulsivity, aggressiveness and lability of mood were prominent. Of course such individuals often abuse alcohol or drugs, and indeed the best predictor of suicide after DSH in young people is substance misuse (Hawton et al 1993).

Social support Adverse social circumstances contribute to an increased risk of repetition or suicide, so it is essential to establish the circumstances from whence the patient came and, more often than not, to which they will return. Patients who live alone, particularly if this is not through choice such as following rejection by the family or the death of a partner, are at greater risk, partly because they have nobody to seek help on their behalf or to supervise any treatment they require. This group is particularly a problem with first presentations when the circumstances are not already known to the general practitioner or the mental health or social services.

Homicide risk

Finally, when assessing suicide risk it should become automatic practice to consider the potential risk to others as well – as indeed the risk of suicide or DSH should be considered in patients who are primarily regarded as at risk of harming other people (Royal College of Psychiatrists 1996). Classically, the risk to others is associated with the baby of a woman who has postnatal depression, but suicide following murder is not rare (Easteal 1994) and is certainly not confined to puerperal women. It is most important where children or other dependants are involved, and particularly when the breakup of a relationship is a prominent factor in the presentation.

Management

Management is determined by the outcome of the psychosocial assessment, the wishes of the patient and perhaps the family, and the availability of appropriate resources. For patients who are already known to services, communicating with the key worker and teeing up an appointment may be all that is required if the patient has not deteriorated to the extent that more intensive intervention is warranted.

DSH can be problem-solving rather than problem-indicating behaviour, so there is not always a need for further intervention. Self-harm may have a cathartic effect: for instance, the prevalence of mental disorder fell from 60 to 40% in a week in one study in which there had usually been no other treatment (Newson-Smith & Hirsch 1979). In one study 13% of the sample considered that DSH had led to a moderate improvement in their circumstances (Adam et al 1980), while in another, 15 of 88 patients were not followed up because the act had produced a positive change (Lawson 1988). However, others have found problem resolvers did improve on many psychological measures, yet their repetition rate was the same as those whose problems were not resolved (Sakinofsky et al 1990).

It has long been known that DSH patients have a very poor compliance rate with psychiatric follow-up, with non-attendance remaining likely even when the appointment was offered for 1–3 days later (Owens et al 1991), but a study of their consultation behaviour in primary care found DSH patients were, if anything, less likely to miss appointments than matched controls (Gorman & Masterton 1990). Hence the need for follow-up, and the acceptability and appropriateness of the arrangements are crucial considerations. 60% (Newson-Smith & Hirsch 1979) to 90% (Morgan et al 1975) of DHS patients have been found to have a mental disorder. The majority of these are borderline conditions reflecting distress and only about 30% have a significant mental illness, which is usually an adjustment reaction, anxiety state or depressive disorder (Newson-Smith & Hirsch 1979, Urwin & Gibbons 1979). The management of patients with severe mental illness and high suicide risk is usually straightforward, in that inpatient care, under a compulsory detention order if necessary, is often the only viable option. Paradoxically, less severe presentations can prove more difficult propositions, particularly given the tendency of suicidal ideation to fluctuate.

Patients in this category may still warrant a period of inpatient psychiatric assessment, given the limitations of a single interview at a point of crisis, but the widespread pressure on psychiatric admission beds and the understandable reluctance of patients to be admitted means that other options may have to be used. For many of these patients a day hospital assessment or early outpatient appointment with the psychiatric service is appropriate, although in some services specialist psychiatric nurses have been employed to followup selected patients (Evans et al 1992). The nurse's role has been extended to undertake cognitive behavioural problem solving with a reduction in depression, suicidal ideation and target problems – and possibly a reduction in repeat DSH (Salkovskis et al 1990).

If psychiatric follow-up is undertaken, the first appointment must take place within a few days of discharge; it should preferably be community based, with domiciliary visiting if necessary. Given that most of these patients' mood disorders are mild, and antidepressant medication confers little or no benefit in these circumstances, the prescription of antidepressant treatment should be restricted to those patients who have lasting, moderate or severe mood illness.

In these circumstances it is obviously sensible to take precautions that reduce the risk of the patient overdosing with their prescribed medication. The patient's compliance with past treatment, the toxicity of the drug and the prescribing arrangements should all be taken into account. Weekly prescriptions have been advocated, particularly when antidepressants with greater fatal toxicity are being used, but this arrangement is only worthwhile if there is somebody at home to supervise the taking of the drug, as the isolated individual can quickly stockpile a lethal quantity.

Specific psychological interventions to reduce the risk of repeat DSH and possible suicide are presented in Table 26.14. The samples in all studies were too small to show a statistically significant reduction in the repetition rate: for example, to reduce this rate from 15 to 10% would require about 1000 patients in a randomised control trial (House et al 1992). However, treatment consisting of brief, focused problem-solving therapy and cognitive-behavioural psychotherapy improved the patient's sense of well-being and reduced the level of psychiatric symptoms, whereas intensive follow-up conferred no additional benefit. Most of these studies also reported a reduction in social problems, together with an improvement in social adjustment.

There are two other elements the DSH service should offer: a contact arrangement in the event of crisis, and established links or referral routes to the social services and non-statutory agencies. Regarding a contact arrangement, the Bristol Green Card Scheme demonstrated in a controlled trial that, when patients were given a contact card which enabled them to have

Table 26.14 Controlled (randomised) treatment trials after deliberate self-harm (*n*>50)				
Authors	Sample size	Intervention	DSH repetition rate	
			Treatment (%)	Control (%)
Allard et al 1992	126	18 therapy sessions + home visits	35[*]	30[*]
Hawton et al 1987	80	Brief problem-oriented counselling (OP versus GP care)	7	15
Hawton et al 1981	96	Brief problem-oriented counselling (domicillary versus OP care)	10	15
Gibbons et al 1978	400	Task-centred social work	13.5	14.5
Welu 1977	120	Individual treatment programme versus routine psychiatric follow-up	5[**]	16[**]
Chowdhury et al 1973	197	General psychiatry	24[***]	23[***]

GP, general practitioner; OP, outpatient.

[*]2 years follow-up; [**]4 months follow-up; [***]6 months follow-up – subjects were established repeaters. All others 1 year follow-up.

immediate access to on-call junior psychiatric staff, the repeat DSH admission rate was halved (Morgan et al 1993), although only 15% of the group used the scheme. There is no reason why other staff cannot undertake this task, for example designated DSH nurses would be even more appropriate. If such systems are not available then the patient should be informed about the Samaritans: this is an organisation which has a vital role to play in helping the suicidal but is often disregarded by hospital services. Discussion and agreement with the patient on an arrangement for dealing with a recurrence of suicidal ideation or impulses should be a routine element of management.

Given that many DSH presentations are linked to interpersonal and social problems which lie outwith the scope of the hospital service, the satisfactory management of these patients often depends on establishing contact with community resources, where again the specialist DSH nurse can take a lead role. An exhaustive list of the possibilities would be tiresome – the service ought to be able to put patients in touch with reputable counsellors or counselling organisations, and should have recognised ways of dealing with common, serious problems such as homelessness, domestic violence, sexual abuse, substance misuse and bereavement.

While hospital staff tend to trivialise DSH, it should be remembered that for many patients this act is of great personal significance, a bridge between life and

death, and the doctor or nurse who undertakes their psychosocial assessment has a chance, which may be fleeting, to influence the outcome. It is not acceptable to expect these patients to find out for themselves what is available in the neighbourhood, nor to pass this task over to the general practitioner, by which time the opportunity may have passed.

Prognosis

The outcome following an act of DSH is traditionally considered in terms of repeat DSH and suicide, but other causes of death are also of interest.

Repeat deliberate self harm

British reports over the past 30 years have consistently given the proportion of first-evers among all DSH hospital admissions in the range 40–60%, which implies that about half the admissions involve repeaters (Kreitman & Casey 1988). Follow-up studies report 1–2 year follow-up rates of repeat admission in the range of 12–26%, with the larger cohorts clustering around a 15% 1 year rate (Table 26.15). Repetition is much more likely to occur in the first 3 months, for example Bancroft & Marsack (1977) found 10% of their sample had their first repeat within the first 3 months, 6% in the following 9 months and only another 2% during the second year. The authors postu-

Table 26.15   UK outcome studies for hospital admission following repeat deliberate self-harm (*n*>200)

Study	Follow-up period (years)	Sample size	Repeated admission (%)
Owens et al 1994	1	992	12
Wilkinson & Smeaton 1987	1–2	1376	19
Bancroft & Marsack 1977	1	690	16
Kreitman 1977	1	847	16
	1	910	17
	1	1052	17
Buglass & Horton 1974	1	2809	16
Greer & Bagley 1971	1–2	204	26

Table 26.16   Suicide following deliberate self-harm (*n*>200)

UK studies	Sample size	Follow-up (years)	Rate (%)
Hawton & Fagg 1988	1959	8	2.8
Pierce 1981	500	5	2.6
Buglass & Horton 1974	2809	1	0.8
Greer & Bagley 1971	204	1.5	2.0
Buglass & McCulloch 1970	511	3	3.3
Recent studies elsewhere			
De Moore & Robertson 1996	1223	18	6.7
Nordentoft et al 1993	974	10	10.6
Suokas & Lonnqvist 1991	1018	5	3.2
Ekeberg et al 1991	934	5	4.0
Nielsen et al 1990	207	5	11.6
Beck & Steer 1989	413	5–10	4.8
Rygnestad 1988	253	5	8.3

lated three patterns of repetition were occurring: chronic repetition arising because of recurrent crises; bursts of repetition during periods of stress; and one-off repetition in severe crisis. Kreitman & Casey (1988) subdivided repeaters into 'minor repeaters', who had a lifetime history of 2–4 episodes, and 'major/grand repeaters' who had a lifetime history of five or more episodes. They found in a sample of over 3000 admissions that repeaters were actually more common than first-episode patients among men and only marginally less frequent in women, while grand repeaters accounted for 1 in 6 men and 1 in 8 women. Hence the multiple repeater is no rarity. Much less common are patients who are admitted frequently within a short

space of time: patients with three or more admissions within a week accounted for less than 1% of the individuals admitted as a result of DSH over a 6 year period (Stocks & Scott 1991).

Suicide

The rate of death by suicide following an act of DSH is considerably increased. Studies vary in the proportion of patients who go on to commit suicide, with UK studies consistently reporting lower rates (Table 26.16). The UK results are certainly underestimates, given the constraints already described in reaching a verdict of suicide: in Hawton and Fagg's study the observed against expected rate of deaths was 23.7 for suicides, 40.2 for undetermined causes and 18.6 for accidents due to poisoning, which accords with these restrictions. A consistent finding is that the highest risk of suicide is in the first few years after DSH, and especially during the first year. However, these patients continue to be at greater risk of suicide compared with the general population for at least 20 years, and probably for the rest of their lives (De Moore & Robertson 1996).

Other causes of death

Hawton & Fagg (1988) also reported that deaths from natural causes were more than double the expected number, the excess being greater among females and associated with accidents (other than due to poisoning), endocrine disorders (especially diabetes), nervous disorders and respiratory disorders. Nordentoft et al (1993) also found deaths from natural causes were 2–3 times the expected rate in a cohort of 974 patients followed up for 10 years, with the excess being marked among younger men. Alcohol-related conditions, digestive disorders, sudden unexplained deaths and a ragbag of single cases of rare diseases were particularly associated.

REFERENCES

Adam K, Bianchi G, Hawker F, Nairn L, Sandford M, Scarr G 1978 Interpersonal factors in suicide attempts: a pilot study in Christchurch. Australian and New Zealand Journal of Psychiatry 12: 59–63

Adam K S, Bouckoms A, Scarr G 1980 Attempted suicide in Christchurch: a controlled study. Australian and New Zealand Journal of Psychiatry 14: 305–314

Addington D E, Addington J M 1992 Attempted suicide and depression in schizophrenia. Acta Psychiatrica Scandinavica 85: 288–291

Agren H 1980 Symptom patterns in unipolar and bipolar depression correlating with monoamine metabolites in the CSF. II. Suicide. Psychiatry Research 3: 225–236

Agren H 1982. Depressive symptom patterns and urinary MHPG excretion. Psychiatry Research 6: 185–196

Ahrens B, Berghofer A, Wolf T, Muller-Oerlinghausen B 1995 Suicide attempts, age and duration of illness in recurrent affective disorders. Journal of Affective Disorders 36: 43–49

Allard R, Marshall M, Plante M-C 1992 Intensive follow-up does not decrease the risk of repeat suicide attempts. Suicide and Life-Threatening Behaviour 22: 303–314

Allebeck P, Bolund C 1991 Suicides and suicide attempts in cancer patients. Psychological Medicine 21: 979–984

Allgulander C 1994 Suicide and mortality patterns in anxiety neurosis and depressive neurosis. Archives of General Psychiatry 51: 708–712

Amador X F, Friedman J H, Kasapis C, Yale S A, Flaum M, Gorman J M 1996 Suicidal behaviour in schizophrenia and its relationship to awareness of illness. American Journal of Psychiatry 153: 1185–1188

Ambelas A 1987 Life events and mania: a special relationship? British Journal of Psychiatry 150: 235–240

Angst J 1992 Epidemiology of depression. Psychopharmacology 106(suppl): 71–74

Appleby L 1991 Suicide during pregnancy and in the first postnatal year. British Medical Journal 302: 137–140

Appleby L 1992 Suicide risk in psychiatric patients: risk and prevention. British Journal of Psychiatry 161: 749–758

Appleby L 1996 New confidential inquiry established into homicides and suicides by mentally ill people. British Medical Journal 313: 234

Arango V, Ernsberger P, Marzuk P M et al 1990 Autoradiographic demonstration of increased serotonin 5-HT 2 and beta adrenergic receptor binding sites in the brain of suicide victims. Archives of General Psychiatry 47: 1038–1047

Arango V, Ernsberger P, Sved A F, Mann J J 1993 Quantitative autoradiography of alpha 1 and alpha 2 adrenergic receptors in the cerebral cortex of controls and suicide victims. Brain Research 630: 271–282

Arango V, Underwood M D, Mann J J 1996 Fewer pigmented locus coeruleus neurons in suicide victims: preliminary results. Biological Psychiatry 39: 112–120

Arato M, Banki C, Bissette G, Nemeroff C 1989 Elevated CSF CRF in suicide victims. Biological Psychiatry 35: 355–359

Asberg M, Traskman L, Sjostrand L 1976 Monoamine metabolites in CSF and suicidal behaviour. Archives of General Psychiatry 33: 1193–1197

Axelsson R, Lagerkvist-Briggs M 1992 Factors predicting suicide in psychotic patients. European Archives of Psychiatry and Clinical Neuroscience 241: 259–266

Bancroft J, Marsack P 1977 The repetitiveness of self-poisoning and self-injury. British Journal of Psychiatry 131: 394–399

Bancroft J, Skrimshire A, Reynolds F, Simkin S, Smith J 1975 Self-poisoning and self-injury in the Oxford area: epidemiological aspects 1969–1973. British Journal of Preventive and Social Medicine 29: 170–177

Bancroft J, Skrimshire A M, Simkins 1976 The reasons people give for taking overdoses. British Journal of Psychiatry 128: 538–548

Bancroft J, Hawton K, Simkin S, Kingston B, Cumming C, Whitwell D 1979 The reasons people give for taking overdoses: a further inquiry. British Journal of Medical Psychology 52: 353–365

Banki C, Bissette J, Arato M, O'Conner L, Nemeroff C 1987 CSF CRF-like immunoreactivity in depression and schizophrenia. American Journal of Psychiatry 144: 873–877

Barraclough B 1973 Differences between national suicide rates. British Journal of Psychiatry 122: 95–96

Barraclough B M 1978 Reliability of violent death certification in one coroner's district. British Journal of Psychiatry 132: 39–41

Barraclough B, Pallis D J 1975 Depression followed by suicide: a comparison of depressed suicides with living depressives. Psychological Medicine 5: 55–61

Barraclough B, Bunch J, Nelson B, Sainsbury P 1974 A hundred cases of suicide: clinical aspects. British Journal of Psychiatry 125: 355–373

Beautrais A L, Joyce P R, Mulder R T, Fergusson D M, Deavoll B J, Nightingale S K 1996 Prevalence and comorbidity of mental disorders in persons making serious suicide attempts: a case–control study. American Journal of Psychiatry 153: 1009–1014

Beck A T, Steer R A 1989 Clinical predictors of eventual suicide: a 5- to 10-year prospective study of suicide attempters. Journal of Affective Disorders 17: 203–209

Beck A T, Herman I, Schuyler D 1974 Development of suicidal intent scales. In: Beck A T, Resnik H L P, Lettieri D (eds) The prediction of suicide. Charles Press, Maryland, pp 45–56

Beck A T, Kovacs M, Weissman A 1975 Hopelessness and suicidal behaviour: an overview. Journal of the American Medical Association 234: 1146–1149

Beck A T, Rush A J, Shaw B F, Emergy G 1979 Cognitive therapy for depression; a treatment manual. Guilford Press, New York

Beck A T, Steer R, Kovacs M, Garrison B 1985 Hopelessness and eventual suicide: a 10 year prospective study of patients hospitalised with suicidal ideation. American Journal of Psychiatry 145: 559–563

Beck A T, Brown G, Berchik R J, Stewart B L, Steer R A 1990 Relationship between hopelessness and ultimate suicide: a replication with psychiatric outpatients. American Journal of Psychiatry 147: 190–195

Beck A T, Steer R A, Sanderson W C, Madland Skeie T 1991 Panic disorder and suicidal ideation and behaviour: discrepant findings in psychiatric outpatients. American Journal of Psychiatry 148: 1195–1199

Berglund M 1984a Mortality in alcoholics related to clinical state at first admission. Acta Psychiatrica Scandinavica 70: 407–416

Berglund M 1984b Suicide in alcoholism – a prospective study of 88 alcoholics. The multi-dimensional diagnosis at first admission. Archives of General Psychiatry 41: 888–891

Biegon A, Israeli M 1988 Regionally selective increases in beta adrenergic receptor density in the brains of suicide victims. Brain Research 442: 199–203

Birtchnell J 1970 The relationship between attempted suicide, depression and parent death. British Journal of Psychiatry 116: 307–313

Black D W, Warrak G, Winokur G 1985 The Iowa record linkage study I–III. Archives of General Psychiatry 42: 71–88

Black D W, Winokur G, Nasrallah A 1987 Suicide in subtypes of major affective disorder: a comparison with general population suicide mortality. Archives of General Psychiatry 44: 878–880

Black D W, Winokur G, Nasrallah A 1988 Effect of psychosis on suicide risk in 1593 patients with unipolar and bipolar affective disorders. American Journal of Psychiatry 145: 849–852

Black D W, Winokur G 1990 Suicide and psychiatric diagnosis. In: Blumenthal S J, Kupfer D J (eds) Suicide over the life cycle: risk factors, assessment and treatment of suicidal patients. American Psychiatric Press, Washington, DC

Bleuler E 1950 Dementia praecox or the group of schizophrenias. International Universities Press, New York, p 488

Brent D A, Kolko D J 1990 The assessment and treatment of children and adolescents at risk for suicide: In: Blumenthal S J, Kupfer D J (eds) Suicide over the life cycle. American Psychiatric Association Press, Washington, DC, pp 253–302

Brent D A, Johnson B A, Perper J et al 1994 Personality disorder, personality traits, impulsive violence and completed suicide in adolescents. Journal of the American Academy of Child and Adolescent Psychiatry 33: 1080–1086

Brown G, Harris T 1978 Social origins of depression. Tavistock, London

Brown G L, Ebert M H, Goyer P F et al 1982 Aggression, suicide and serotonin; relationships to CSF amine metabolites. American Journal of Psychiatry 139: 471–746

Brown M, King E, Barraclough B 1995 Nine suicide pacts: a clinical study of a consecutive series 1974–1993. British Journal of Psychiatry 167: 448–451

Buda M, Tsuang M T 1990 The epidemiology of suicide: implications for clinical practice. In: Blumenthal S J, Kupfer D J (eds) Suicide over the life cycle: risk factors, assessment and treatment of suicidal patients. American Psychiatric Association Press, Washington, DC, pp 17–38

Buglass D, Horton J 1974 The repetition of parasuicide: a comparison of three cohorts. British Journal of Psychiatry 125: 168–174

Buglass D, McCulloch J W 1970 Further suicidal behaviour: the development and validation of predictive scales. British Journal of Psychiatry 116: 483–491

Butterworth E, O'Grady T J 1989 Trends in the assessment of cases of deliberate self-harm. Health Trends 21: 61

Carlson G A, Rich C L, Grayson P, Fowler R C 1991 Secular trends in psychiatric diagnoses of suicide victims. Journal of Affective Disorders 21: 127–132

Cattell H, Jolley D J 1995 One hundred cases of suicide in elderly people. British Journal of Psychiatry 166: 451–457

Centers for Disease Control 1991 Attempted suicide among high school students – US; leads from the morbidity and mortality weekly report. Journal of the American Medical Association 266: 911

Charlton J, Kelly S, Dunnell K, Evans B, Jenkins R 1993 Suicide deaths in England and Wales: trends in factors associated with suicide deaths. Population Trends 71: 33–42

Chaturvedi S K, Chandra P S, Gururaj G, Dhanasekara Pandian R, Beena M B 1995 Suicidal ideas during the premenstrual phase. Journal of Affective Disorders 34: 193–199

Cheng A T A 1995 Mental illness and suicide. Archives of General Psychiatry 52: 594–603

Chowdhury N, Hicks R C, Kreitman N 1973 Evaluation of an after-care service for parasuicide (attempted suicide) patients. Social Psychiatry 8: 67–81

Cohen S, Lavelle J, Rich C L, Bromet E 1994 Rates and correlates of suicide attempts in first admission psychotic patients. Acta Psychiatrica Scandinavica 90: 167–171

Cole D A 1980 Hopelessness, social desirability, depression and parasuicide in two college samples. Journal of Consulting Clinical Psychology 56: 131–136

Corbitt E M, Malone K M, Haas G L, Mann J J 1996 Suicidal behaviour in patients with major depression and comorbid personality disorders. Journal of Affective Disorders 39: 61–72

Cornelius J R, Salloum I M, Day N L, Thase M E, Mann J J 1996 Patterns of suicidality and alcohol use in alcoholics with major depression. Journal of Alcoholism, Clinical and Experimental Research 20: 1451–1455

Coryell W 1988 Panic disorder and mortality. Psychiatric Clinics of North America 11: 433–440

Coryell W, Tsuang M T 1982 Primary unipolar depression and the prognostic importance of delusions. Archives of General Psychiatry 39: 1181–1184

Cotton P, Drake R, Gates C 1985 Critical treatment issues in suicide among schizophrenics. Hospital and Community Psychiatry 36: 534–536

Crombie I K 1990 Suicide in England and Wales and in Scotland. British Journal of Psychiatry 157: 529–532

Dassori A M, Mezzich J E, Deshavan M 1990 Suicidal indicators in schizophrenia. Acta Psychiatrica Scandinavica 81: 409–413

Davidson J R T, Hughes D C, George L K, Blazer D G 1996 The association of sexual assault and attempted suicide within the community. Archives of General Psychiatry 53: 550–555

De Moore G M, Robertson A R 1996 Suicide in the 18 years after deliberate self harm: a prospective study. British Journal of Psychiatry 169: 489–494

De Paermentier F, Cheetham S C, Crompton M R, Katona C L E, Horton R W 1990 Brain beta adrenoceptor binding sites in antidepressant-free depressed suicide victims. Brain Research 525: 71–77

Department of Health 1993 The health of the nation. Mental illness. HMSO, London

Department of Health 1994 The prevention of suicide. Jenkins R, Griffiths S, Wylie I et al (eds). HMSO, London

Department of Health and Social Security 1984 The management of deliberate self-harm. HN(84) 25 DHSS, London.

Der G, Gupta S, Murray R M 1990 Is schizophrenia disappearing? Lancet 335: 513–516

Diekstra R F W 1982 Epidemiology of attempted suicide in the EEC. In: Wilmotte J, Mendlewicz J (eds) New trends in suicide prevention. Bibliotheca Psychiatrica, Karger, Basel, pp 1–16

Diekstra R F W 1985 Suicide and suicide attempts in the EEC: an analysis of trends with special emphasis on trends among the young. Suicide and Life-Threatening Behaviour 15: 402–421

Diekstra R F W 1989 Suicide and attempted suicide: an international perspective. Acta Psychiatrica Scandinavica 80: 1–24

Diekstra R F W 1993 The epidemiology of suicide and parasuicide. Acta Psychiatrica Scandinavica Supplementum 371: 9–20

Diekstra R F W 1996 The epidemiology of suicide and parasuicide. Archives of Suicide Research 2: 1–29

Dilsaver S C, Chen Y W, Swann A C, Shoaib A M, Krajenski K J 1994 Suicidality in patients with pure and depressive mania. American Journal of Psychiatry 151: 1312–1315

Dolman W F G 1994 The coroner's response. In: Jenkins R, Griffiths S, Wylie I et al (eds) The prevention of suicide. HMSO, London, pp 135–139

Dooley D, Catalano R, Rook K et al 1989 Economic stress and suicide: multivariate analysis of economic stress and suicidal ideation. Part 2. Suicide and Life-Threatening Behaviour 19: 337–351

Drake R, Cotton P 1986 Depression, hopelessness and suicide in chronic schizophrenia. British Journal of Psychiatry 148: 554–559

Drake R, Gates C, Cotton P 1984 Suicide among schizophrenics: who is at risk? Journal of Nervous and Mental Disease 172: 613–617

Duberstein P R, Conwell Y, Caine E D 1993 Interpersonal stressors, substance abuse and suicide. Journal of Nervous and Mental Disorders 181: 80–85

Easteal P 1994 Homicide-suicides between adult sexual intimates: an Australian study. Suicide and Life-Threatening Behaviour 24: 140–151

Edwards J G 1995 Suicide and antidepressants (editorial). British Medical Journal 310: 205–206

Ekeberg O, Ellingsen O, Jacobsen D 1991 Suicide and other causes of death in a five-year follow-up of patients treated for self-poisoning in Oslo. Acta Psychiatrica Scandinavica 83: 432–437

Evans M, Cox C, Turnbull G 1992 Parasuicide response. Nursing Times 88: 34–36

Faberow N, Shneidman E, Leonard C 1965 Suicide among schizophrenic mental hospital patients. In: Faberow N, Shneidman E (eds) The cry for help. McGraw-Hill, New York, pp 78–109

Farmer R 1988 Assessing the epidemiology of suicide and parasuicide. British Journal of Psychiatry 153: 16–20

Farmer R, Tranah T, O'Donnell I, Catalan J 1992 Railway suicide: the psychological effects on drivers. Psychological Medicine 22: 407–414

Fawcett J, Scheftner W, Clark D, Hedeker D, Gibbons R, Coryell W 1987 Clinical predictors of suicide in patients with major affective disorders; a controlled prospective study. American Journal of Psychiatry 144: 35–40

Fawcett J, Scheftner W A, Fogg L et al 1990 Time-related precipitators of suicide in major affective disorders. American Journal of Psychiatry 147: 1189–1194

Frances A, Fyer M, Clarkin J 1986 Personality and suicide. In: Mann J J, Stanley M (eds) Annals of the New York Academy of Sciences 487: 281–293

Frances R, Franklin J, Flavin D 1987 Suicide and alcoholism. American Journal of Drug and Alcohol Abuse 13: 327–341

Freemantle N, House A, Song F, Mason J M, Sheldon T A 1994 Prescribing selective serotonin reuptake inhibitors as a strategy for prevention of suicide. British Medical Journal 309: 249–253

Freidman S, Jones J C, Chernen L, Barlow D H 1992 Suicidal ideation and suicide attempts among patients with panic disorder; a survey of two out-patient clinics. American Journal of Psychiatry 149: 680–685

Gallerani M, Manfredini R, Caracciolo S, Scapoli C, Molinari S, Fersini C 1995 Serum cholesterol concentrations in parasuicide. British Medical Journal 310: 1632–1636

Garcia-Sevilla J A, Escriba P V, Sastre M, Walzer C, Busquets X, Jaquet G, Reis D J, Guimon J 1996 Immunodetection and quantitation of Imidazoline receptor proteins in platelets of patients with major depression and in brains of suicide victims. Archives of General Psychiatry 53: 803–810

Geddes J R, Juszczak E 1995 Period trends in rate of suicide in first 28 days after discharge from psychiatric hospital in Scotland, 1968–1992. British Medical Journal 311: 357–360

Gibbons J S, Butler J, Urwin P, Gibbons J L 1978 Evaluation of a social work service for self-poisoning patients. British Journal of Psychiatry 133: 111–118

Glassner B, Haldipur C 1983 Life events and early and late onset bipolar disorder. American Journal of Psychiatry 140: 215–217

Goldney R 1981 Alcohol in association with suicide and attempted suicide in young women. Medical Journal of Australia 2: 195–197

Goldstein R B, Black D W, Nasrallah A, Winokur G 1991 The prediction of suicide. Sensitivity, specificity, and predictive value of a multivariate model applied to suicide among 1906 patients with affective disorders. Archives of General Psychiatry 48: 418–422

Goodwin D 1982 Alcoholism and suicide: associated factors. In: Pattison E M, Kaufman E (eds) Encyclopaedic handbook of alcoholism. Gardner Press, New York

Goodwin F K, Jamison K R 1990 Manic depressive illness. Oxford University Press, Oxford

Gorman D, Masterton G 1990 General practice consultation patterns before and after intentional overdose: a matched control study. British Journal of General Practice 40: 102–105

Greer S, Bagley C 1971 Effect of psychiatric intervention in a attempted suicide. British Medical Journal 1: 310–312

Grootenhuis M, Hawton K, Van Rooijen L, Fagg J 1994 Attempted suicide in Oxford and Utrecht. British Journal of Psychiatry 165: 73–78

Gross-Isseroff R, Dillon K A, Fieldust S J, Biegon A 1990 Autoradiographic analysis of alpha-1 noradrenergic receptors in the human brain postmortem. Archives of General Psychiatry 47: 1049–1053

Gunnell D, Frankel S 1994 Prevention of suicide: aspirations and evidence. British Medical Journal 308: 1227–1233

Guze S, Robins E 1970 Suicide and primary affective disorder. British Journal of Psychiatry 117: 437–483

Hawton K 1987 Assessment of suicide risk. British Journal of Psychiatry 150: 145–153

Hawton K 1992 By their own young hand (editorial). British Medical Journal 304: 1000

Hawton K, Fagg J 1988 Suicide, and other causes of death, following attempted suicide. British Journal of Psychiatry 152: 359–366

Hawton K, Fagg J 1992 Trends in deliberate self poisoning and self injury in Oxford, 1976–1990. British Medical Journal 304: 1409–1411

Hawton K, Goldacre M 1982 Hospital admission for adverse effects on medical agents (mainly self-poisoning) among adolescents in the Oxford region. British Journal of Psychiatry 141: 166–170

Hawton K, Rose N 1986 Unemployment and attempted suicide among men in Oxford. Health Trends 18: 29–32

Hawton K, Bancroft J, Catalan J, Kingston B, Stedeford A, Welch N 1981 Domiciliary and outpatient treatment of self-poisoning patients by medical and non-medical staff. Psychological Medicine 11: 169–177

Hawton K, Cole D, O'Grady J, Osborn M 1982a Motivational aspects of deliberate self poisoning in adolescents. British Journal of Psychiatry 141: 286–291

Hawton K et al 1982b Adolescents who take overdoses; their characteristics, problems and contact with helping agencies. British Journal of Psychiatry 140: 118–123

Hawton K, McKeown S, Day A, Martin P, O'Connor M, Yule J 1987 Evaluation of outpatient counselling compared with general practitioner care following overdoses. Psychological Medicine 17: 751–761

Hawton K Fagg J, McKeown S 1989 Alcoholism, alcohol and attempted suicide. Alcohol 24: 3–9

Hawton K, Fagg J, Platt S, Hawleins M 1993 Factors associated with suicide after parasuicide in young people. British Medical Journal 306: 1641–1644

Hawton K, Ware C, Mistry H et al 1995 Why patients choose paracetamol for self-poisoning and their knowledge of its dangers. British Medical Journal 310: 164

Hawton K, Ware C, Mistry H et al 1996 Paracetamol self-poisoning: characteristics, prevention and harm reduction. British Journal of Psychiatry 168: 43–48

Hawton K, Cole D, O'Grady V, Osborn M 1982a Motivational aspects of deliberate self-poisoning in adolescents. British Journal of Psychiatry 141: 286–291

Heikkinen M, Aro H, Lonnqvist J 1993 Life events and social support in suicide. Suicide and Life-Threatening Behaviour 23: 343–358

Heikkinen M E, Isometsa E T, Marttunen M H, Aro H M, Lonnqvist J K 1995 Social factors in suicide. British Journal of Psychiatry 167: 747–753

Henry J A, Alexander C A, Sener E K 1995 Relative mortality from overdose of antidepressants. British Medical Journal 310: 221–224

Hewitt P H, Flett G L, Weber C 1994 Dimensions of perfectionism and suicide ideation. Cognitive Therapy Research 18: 439–460

Hildebrand J, Bourgeois F, Buyse M, Przedborski S, Goldman S 1990 Reproducibility of monoamine metabolite measurements in human CSF. Acta Neurologica Scandinavica 81: 427–430

Holding T A, Barraclough B M 1978 Undetermined deaths – suicide or accident? British Journal of Psychiatry 133: 542–549

House A, Owens D, Storer D 1992 Psycho-social intervention following attempted suicide: is there a case for better services? International Review of Psychiatry 4: 15–22

Hunt N, Bruce-Jones W, Silverstone T 1992 Life events and relapse in bipolar affective disorder. Journal of Affective Disorder 25: 13–20

Isometsa E, Henriksson M, Aro H et al 1994a Suicide in psychotic major depression. Journal of Affective Disorders 31: 187–191

Isometsa E, Henriksson M, Aro H M, Lonnqvist J K 1994b Suicide in bipolar disorder in Finland. American Journal of Psychiatry 151: 1020–1024

Isometsa E, Henriksson M, Aro H M, Heikkinen M E, Kuoppasalmi K I, Lonnqvist J K 1994c Suicide in major depression. American Journal of Psychiatry 151: 530–536

Isometsa E K, Henriksson M M, Hillevi M A, Heikkinen M E, Kuoppasalmi K I, Lonnqvist J K 1994d Suicide and mental disorders: a case control study of young men. American Journal of Psychiatry 152: 1063–1068

Isometsa E, Heikkinen M, Henriksson M 1995 Recent life events and completed suicide in bipolar affective disorder. A comparison with major depressive suicides. Journal of Affective Disorder 33: 99–106

Isometsa E, Heikkinen M, Henriksson M et al 1996 Suicide in non-major depressions. Journal of Affective Disorders 36: 117–127

James D, Hawton K 1985 Overdoses: explanations and attitudes in self-poisoners and significant others. British Journal of Psychiatry 146: 481–485

Jick S S, Dean A D, Jick H 1995 Antidepressants and suicide. British Medical Journal 310: 215–218

Kaplan K J, Harrow M 1996 Positive and negative symptoms as risk factors for later suicidal activity in schizophrenics versus depressives. Suicide and Life-Threatening Behaviour 26: 105–121

Kaplan M L, Asnis G M, Lipschitz D X, Chorney P 1995 Suicidal behaviour and abuse in psychiatric out-patients. Comprehensive Psychiatry 36: 229–235

Kendell R E 1991 Suicide in pregnancy and the puerperium. British Medical Journal 302: 126–127

Kessel A, Nicholson A, Graves G, Krupinski J 1975 Suicidal attempts in an outer region of metropolitan Melbourne and in a provincial region of Victoria. Australian and New Zealand Journal of Psychiatry 9: 255–261

Kessel N 1965 Self-poisoning I. British Medical Journal 2: 1265–1270, 1336–1340

Kreitman N 1973 Social and clinical aspects of suicide and attempted suicide. In: Forrest A (ed) A companion to psychiatric studies. Churchill Livingstone, Edinburgh, vol 1, pp 38–63

Kreitman N 1976 The coal gas story. British Journal of Preventive and Social Medicine 30: 86–93

Kreitman N 1977 Parasuicide. Wiley, London

Kreitman N, Casey P 1988 Repetition of parasuicide: an epidemiological and clinical study. British Journal of Psychiatry 153: 792–800

Kreitman N, Schreiber M 1979 Parasuicide in young Edinburgh women, 1968–75. Psychological Medicine 9: 469–479

Kreitman N, Carstairs V, Duffy J 1991 Association of age and social class with suicide among men in Great Britain. Journal of Epidemiology and Community Health 45: 195–202

Lawson C W 1988 Deliberate self harm and outpatient attendance. British Journal of Psychiatry 152: 575

Lehtinen V, Lindholm T, Veijola J et al 1991 Stability of prevalence of mental disorders in a normal population cohort followed for 16 years. Social Psychiatry and Psychiatric Epidemiology 26: 40–46

Lesage A D, Boyer R, Grunberg F et al 1994 Suicide and mental disorders: a case-control study of young men. American Journal of Psychiatry 151: 1063–1068

Lester D 1972 Why people kill themselves; a summary of research findings on suicidal behaviour. Springfield, Thomas, pp 5–12

Lester D 1989 Gun ownership and suicide in the United States. Psychological Medicine 19: 519–521

Lester D 1993 Suicidal behaviour in bipolar and unipolar affective disorders: a meta-analysis. Journal of Affective Disorders 27: 117–121

Lester D 1996 Testing Durkheim's theory of suicide: a comment (letter.) European Archives of Psychiatry and Clinical Neuroscience 246: 112–113

Lester D, Murrell M E 1982 The preventive effect of strict gun control laws on suicide and homicide. Suicide and Life-Threatening Behaviour 12: 131–140

Levi L D, Fales C H, Stein M et al 1966 Separation and attempted suicide. Archives of General Psychiatry 15: 158–164

Linehan M M, Camper P, Chile J A, Strosahl K, Shearin E 1987 Interpersonal problem solving and parasuicide. Cognitive Therapy Research 11: 1–13

Linkowski P, Wettere J, van Kerkhofs M, Brauman H, Mendlewicz J 1983 Thyrotrophin response to thyrostimulin in affectively ill women: relationship to suicidal behaviour. British Journal of Psychiatry 143: 401–405

Linkowski P, Wettere J, van Kerkhofs M, Gregoire F, Brauman H 1984 Violent suicidal behaviour and the TRH-TSH test: a clinical outcome test. Neuropsychobiology 12: 19–22

Litman R E, Farberow N L 1961 Emergency evaluation of self-destructive potentiality. In: Farberow N L, Schneidman N S (eds) The cry for help. McGraw-Hill, New York, pp 48–59

Little K Y, Clark T B, Ranc J, Duncan G E 1993 Beta adrenergic receptor binding in frontal cortex from suicide victims. Biological Psychiatry 34: 596–605

Lowy A, Burton P, Briggs A 1990 Increasing suicide rates in young adults. British Medical Journal 30: 643

Lukianowicz N 1972 Suicidal behaviour; an attempt to modify the environment. British Journal of Psychiatry 121: 387–390

McGlashan T H 1987 Borderline personality disorder and unipolar affective disorder; long-term effects of comorbidity. Journal of Nervous and Mental Disorders 175: 467–473

Mackenzie T B, Wilcox K, Baron H 1986 Lifetime prevalence of psychiatric disorders in women with premenstrual difficulties. Journal of Affective Disorders 10: 15–19

McLoone P, Crombie I K 1996 Hospitalisation for deliberate self-poisoning in Scotland from 1981 to 1993: trends in rates and types of drugs used. British Journal of Psychiatry 169: 81–85

McPherson H, Herbison P, Romans S 1993 Life events and relapse in established bipolar disorder. British Journal of Psychiatry 163: 381–385

Maier W, Lichtermann D, Oerhlein A, Fickinger M 1992 Depression in the community: a comparison of treated and non-treated cases in two non-referred samples. Psychopharmacology 106 (suppl): 79–81

Malone K M 1994 Psychobiology of suicidal behaviour in major depression. MD Thesis. National University of Ireland

Malone K M, Haas G L, Sareney J A, Mann J J 1993 Familial effects on attempted suicide and depression. American Psychiatric Association annual meeting, San Francisco CA, NR 119

Malone K M, Haas G L, Sweeney J A, Mann J J 1995 Major depression and the risk of attempted suicide. Journal of Affective Disorders 34: 173–185

Malone K M, Corbitt E M, Li S, Mann J J 1996 Prolactin response to fenfluramine and suicide attempt lethality in major depression. British Journal of Psychiatry 168: 324–329

Mann J J, Arango V, Marzuk P M, Theccanat S, Reis D J 1989 Evidence for the 5-TH hypothesis of suicide. A review of post-mortem studies. British Journal of Psychiatry 155 (suppl.8) 7-14

Mann J J, McBride P A, Brown R A et al 1992 Relationship between central and peripheral serotonin indexes in depressed suicidal psychiatric inpatients. Archives of General Psychiatry 49: 442–446

Mann J J, Stanley M, McBride P A, McEwen B S 1986 Increased serotonin-2 and beta adrenergic receptor binding in the frontal cortices of suicide victims. Archives of General Psychiatry 43: 954–959

Mann J J, Underwood M D, Arango V 1994 Postmortem studies of suicide victims. In: Watson S J (ed.) Biology of schizophrenia and affective disease. Raven Press, New York

Mayou R, Hawton K 1986 Psychiatric disorder in the general hospital. British Journal of Psychiatry 149: 172–190

Meana J J, Garcia-Sevilla J A 1987 Increased alpha adrenoceptor density in the frontal cortex of depressed suicide victims. Journal of Neural Transmission 70: 377–381

Menachem B E, Persson L, Schechter P J, Haeggele K D, Huebert N, Hardenberg J 1989 CSF parameters in healthy volunteers during serial lumbar punctures. Journal of Neurochemistry 52: 632–635

Mendonca J D, Holden R R 1996 Are all suicidal ideas closely linked to hopelessness? Acta Psychiatrica Scandinavica 93: 246–251

Miles P 1977 Conditions predisposing to suicide: a review. Journal of Nervous and Mental Diseases 164: 231–246

Milne S, Matthews K, Ashcroft G W 1994 Suicide in Scotland 1988–1989. Psychiatric and physical morbidity according to primary care case notes. British Journal of Psychiatry 165: 541–544

Minkoff K, Bergman E, Beck A T, Beck R 1973 Hopelessness, depression and attempted suicide. American Journal of Psychiatry 130: 455–459

Modestin J, Kopp W 1988 Study on suicide in depressed in-patients. Journal of Affective Disorders 15: 157–162

Moens G F G 1990 Aspects of the epidemiology and prevention of suicide. Leuven University Press, Leuven

Morgan H G, Burns-Cox C J, Pocock H, Pottle S 1975 Deliberate self harm; clinical and socio-economic characteristics of 368 patients. British Journal of Psychiatry 127: 564–574

Morgan H G, Jones E M, Owen J H 1993 Secondary prevention of non-fatal deliberate self harm: the green card study. British Journal of Psychiatry 163: 111–112

Motto J A 1996 Clinical applications of biological aspects of suicide. Archives of Suicide Research 2: 55–74

Muldoon M, Manuck S, Mathews K 1990 Lowering cholesterol concentrations and mortality: a quantitative review of primary prevention trials. British Medical Journal 301: 309–314

Murphy G E, Robins E 1967 Social factors in suicide. Journal of the American Medical Association 199: 303–308

Murphy G E, Wetzel R D 1990 The lifetime risk of suicide in alcoholism. Archives of General Psyhiatry 47: 383–392

Murphy G E, Armstrong J W, Hermele S L, Fischer J R, Clendenin W W 1979 Suicide and alcoholism; interpersonal loss confirmed as a predictor. Archives of General Psychiatry 36: 65–69

Murphy G E, Wetzel R D, Robins E, McEvoy L 1992 Multiple risk factors predict suicide in alcoholism. Archives of General Psychiatry 49: 459–463

Nemeroff C, Owens M, Bissette G, Andorn A, Stanley M 1988 Reduced CRF binding sites in the frontal cortex of suicide victims. Archives of General Psychiatry 45: 577–579

Newson-Smith J G B, Hirsch S R 1979 Psychiatric symptoms in self-poisoning patients. Psychological Medicine 9: 493–500

NHS Health Advisory Service 1996 Suicide prevention: the challenge confronted. Williams R, Morgan H G (eds). HMSO, London

Nicholls P, Edwards G, Kyle E 1974 Alcoholics admitted to four hospitals in England, II; general and cause-specific mortality. Quarterly Journal of Studies in Alcohol 35: 841–855

Nielsen B, Wang A G, Bille-Brahe U 1990 Attempted suicide in Denmark. IV. A five-year follow-up. Acta Psychiatrica Scandinavica 81: 250–254

Nielsen D A, Goldman D, Virkkunen M, Tokola R, Rawlings R, Linnoila M 1994 Suicidality and 5-HIAA concentration associated with a tryptophan hydroxylase polymorphism. Archives of General Psychiatry 51: 34–38

Niskanen P, Lonnqvist J, Achte K, Rinta-Manty R 1975 Suicides in Helsinki psychiatric hospitals 1964–72. Psychiatrica Fennica 5: 275–280

Nordentoft M, Breum L, Munck L K, Nordestgaard A G, Hunding A, Bjaeldeger P A L 1993 High mortality by natural and unnatural causes: a 10 year follow up study of patients admitted to a poisoning treatment centre after suicide attempts. British Medical Journal 306: 1637–1641

Noyes Jr R 1991 Suicide and panic disorder; a review. Journal of Affective Disorders 22: 1–11

O'Donnell I, Farmer R 1995 The limitations of official suicide statistics. British Journal of Psychiatry 166: 458–461

O'Donnell I, Farmer R, Catalan J 1996 Explaining suicide: the views of survivors of serious suicide attempts. British Journal of Psychiatry 168: 780–786

O'Grady J G, Wendon J, Tan K C et al 1991 Liver transplantation after paracetamol overdose. British Medical Journal 303: 221–223

Ovenstone I M K 1973 Spectrum of suicidal behaviours in Edinburgh. British Journal of Preventive Social Medicine 27: 27–35

Owens D, House A 1995 Assessment of deliberate self-harm in adults. Advances in Psychiatric Treatment 1: 124–130

Owens D, Dennis M, Jones S, Dove A, Dave S 1991 Self-poisoning patients discharged from accident and emergency departments: risk factors and outcome. Journal of the Royal College of Physicians of London 25: 218–222

Owens D, Dennis M, Read S, Davis N 1994 Outcome of deliberate self-poisoning: an examination of risk factors for repetition. British Journal of Psychiatry 165: 797–801

Pallis D J, Gibbons S, Pierce D W 1984 Estimating suicide risk among attempted suicides: II Efficiency of predictive scales after the event. British Journal of Psychiatry 144: 139–148

Patel A, Roy M, Wilson G M 1972 Self-poisoning and alcohol. Lancet ii: 1099–1103

Paykel E S, Dowlatshani D 1988 Life events and mental disorder. In: Fisher S, Reason J (eds) Handbook of life stress, cognition and health. Wiley, Chichester, pp 241–263

Paykel E, Myers J, Dienelt M et al 1969 Life events and depression. Archives of General Psychiatry 21: 753–760

Paykel E S, Myers J K, Lindentall J J, Tanner J 1974 Suicidal feelings in the general population: a prevalence study. British Journal of Psychiatry 124: 460–469

Paykel E S, Prusoff B A, Myers J K 1975 Suicide attempts and recent life events. Archives of General Psychiatry 32: 327–333

Pierce D W 1981 The predictive validation of a suicide intent scale: a five year follow-up. British Journal of Psychiatry 139: 391–396

Platt S 1984 Unemployment and suicidal behaviour: a review of the literature. Social Science and Medicine 19: 93–115

Platt S, Kreitman N 1990 Long-term trends in parasuicide and unemployment in Edinburgh 1968–1987. Social Psychiatry and Psychiatric Epidemiology 25: 56–61

Platt S, Hawton K, Kreitman N, Fagg J, Foster J 1988 Recent clinical and epidemiological trends in parasuicide in Edinburgh and Oxford: a tale of two cities. Psychological Medicine 18: 405–418

Platt S, Bille-Brahe U, Kerhof A et al 1992 Parasuicide in Europe: the WHO/EURO multicentre study on parasuicide I; introduction and preliminary analysis for 1989. Acta Psychiatrica Scandinavica 85: 97–104

Post R M 1992 Transduction of psychosocial stress into the neurobiology of recurrent affective disorder. American Journal of Psychiatry 149: 999–1010

Pounder D J 1991 Changing patterns of male suicide in Scotland. Forensic Science International 51: 79–87

Power K G, Cooke D J, Brooks D N 1985 Life stress, medical lethality, and suicidal intent. British Journal of Psychiatry 147: 655–659

Pritchard C 1988 Suicide, gender and unemployment in the British Isles and the EEC 1974–85. Social Psychiatry and Psychiatric Epidemiology 23: 85–89

Pritchard C 1992 Is there a link between suicide in young men and unemployment. British Journal of Psychiatry 160: 750–756

Prosser D 1996 Suicides by burning in England and Wales. British Journal of Psychiatry 168: 175–182

Proudfoot A T, Park J 1978 Changing pattern of drugs used for self-poisoning. British Medical Journal 1: 90–93

Rich C L, Motooka M S, Fowler R C, Young D 1988 Suicide by psychotics. Biological Psychiatry 23: 595–601

Robins E 1986 Completed suicide. In: Roy A (ed) Suicide. Williams & Wilkins, Baltimore

Robins L N, Helzer J E, Weissman M M et al 1984 Lifetime prevalence of specific psychiatric disorders in three sites. Archives of General Psychiatry 41: 949–958

Roose S P, Glassman A H, Walsh B T, Wooring S, Vitar-Hekne J 1983 Depression, delusions and suicide. American Journal of Psychiatry 140: 1159–1162

Roy A 1982 Risk factors for suicide in psychiatric patients. Archives of General Psychiatry 39: 1089–1095

Roy A 1986 Depression, attempted suicide and suicide in patients with chronic schizophrenia. Psychiatric Clinics of North America 9: 193–207

Roy A 1994 Recent biological studies on suicide. Suicide and Life-Threatening Behaviour 24: 10–14

Roy A, Dejong J, Lamparski D, George T, Linnoila M 1991 Depression among alcoholics. Archives of General Psychiatry 48: 428–432

Roy A, Draper R 1995 Suicide among psychiatric hospital in-patients. Psychological Medicine 25: 199–202

Roy A, Linnoila M 1986 Alcoholism and suicide. Suicide and Life-Threatening Behaviour 16: 162–191

Roy A, Mazonson A, Pickar D 1984 Attempted suicide in chronic schizophrenia. British Journal of Psychiatry 144: 303–306

Roy A, Pollack S 1994 Are CSF or urinary monoamine metabolite measures stronger correlates of suicidal behaviour in depression? Neuropsychobiology 29: 164–167

Royal College of Psychiatrists 1994 The general hospital management of adult deliberate self-harm: a consensus statement on standards for service provision. CR 32 Royal College of Psychiatrists, London

Royal College of Psychiatrists 1995 Report of the confidential inquiry into homicides and suicides of mentally ill people. Royal College of Psychiatrists, London

Royal College of Psychiatrists 1996 Assessment and clinical management of risk of harm to other people. Royal College of Psychiatrists, London, CR53

Rubinow D R, Schmidt P J 1987 Mood disorders and the menstrual cycle. Journal of Reproductive Medicine 32: 389–374

Rubinstein J L, Heeren T, Housman D, Rubin C, Stechler G 1989 Suicidal behaviour in 'normal' adolescents: risk and protective factors. American Journal of Orthopsychiatry 59: 59–71

Rutz W, von Knorring L, Walinder J 1989 Frequency of suicide on Gotland after systematic postgraduate education of general practitioners. Acta Psychiatrica Scandinavica 80: 151–154

Rutz W, von Knorring L, Walinder J 1992 Long term effects of an educational programme for general practitioners given by the Swedish Committee for the Prevention and Treatment of Depression. Acta Psychiatrica Scandinavica 85: 83–88

Rygnestad T 1988 A prospective 5-year follow-up study of self-poisoned patients. Acta Psychiatrica Scandinavica 77: 328–331

Sainsbury P, Barraclough B M 1968 Differences between suicide rates. Nature 220: 1252

Sainsbury S, Jenkins J, Baert A E 1981 Suicide trends in Europe ICP/MNH 036. World Health Organization, Copenhagen

Sakinofsky I, Roberts R S, Brown Y, Cumming C, James P 1990 Problem resolution and repetition of parasuicide: a prospective study. British Journal of Psychiatry 156: 395–399

Salkovskis P M, Atha C, Storer D 1990 Cognitive behavioural problem solving in the treatment of patients who repeatedly attempt suicide: a controlled trial. British Journal of Psychiatry 157: 871–876

Samuels J F, Nestadt G, Romanoski A J, Folstein M F, McHugh P R 1994 DSM-III personality disorders in the community. American Journal of Psychiatry 151: 1055–1062

Sclare P, Creed F 1990 Life events and the onset of mania. British Journal of Psychiatry 156: 508–514

Seiden R J 1978 Where are they now? A follow-up study of suicide attempters from the Golden Gate Bridge. Suicide and Life-Threatening Behaviour 8: 203–216

Shneidman E 1964 Suicide, sleep and death. Journal of Consulting Psychology 28: 95–106

Sims A, Prior P 1978 The pattern of mortality in severe neuroses. British Journal of Psychiatry 133: 299–305

Soni Raleigh V, Balarajan R 1992 Suicide and self-burning among Indians and West Indians in England and Wales. British Journal of Psychiatry 161: 365–368

Stockmeier C A, Meltzer H Y 1991 Beta adrenergic receptor binding in frontal cortex of suicide victims. Biological Psychiatry 29: 183–191

Stocks R, Scott A I F 1991 What happens to patients who frequently harm themselves? A retrospective one-year outcome study. British Journal of Psychiatry 158: 375–378

Stone M H 1990 The fate of borderline patients: successful outcome and psychiatric practice. Guilford Press, New York

Strakowski S M, McElroy S L, Keck P E, West S A 1996 Suicidality among patients with mixed and manic bipolar disorder. American Journal of Psychiatry 153: 674–676

Sullivan P E, Joyce P R, Bulik C M, Mulder R T, Oakley-Browne M 1994 Total cholesterol and suicidality in depression. Biological Psychiatry 36: 472–477

Sundman I, Allard P, Eriksson A, Marcusson J 1997 GABA uptake sites in frontal cortex from suicide victims and in aging. Neuropsychobiology 35: 11–15

Suokas J, Lonnqvist J 1991 Outcome of attempted suicide and psychiatric consultation: risk factors and suicide mortality during a five-year follow-up. Acta Psychiatrica Scandinavica 84: 545–549

Suokas J, Lonnqvist J 1995 Suicide attempts in which alcohol is involved; a special group in general hospital emergency rooms. Acta Psychiatrica Scandinavica 91: 36–40

Suominen K, Henriksson M, Suokas J, Isometsa E, Ostamo A, Lunnqvist J 1996 Mental disorders and comorbidity in suicide. Acta Psychiatric Scandinavica 94: 234–240

Surtees S J 1982 Suicide and accidental death at Beachy Head. British Medical Journal 284: 321–324

Tsuang M T 1978 Suicide in schizophrenics, manics, depressives and surgical controls: a comparison with general population suicide mortality. Archives of General Psychiatry 35: 153–155

Urwin P, Gibbons J L 1979 Psychiatric diagnosis in self-poisoning patients. Psychological Medicine 9: 501–507

Vaillant G E, Blumenthal S J 1990 Introduction: suicide over the life cycle-riser factors and lifespan development. In: Blumenthal S J, Kupfer D J (eds) Suicide over the life cycle. American Psychiatric Press, Washington, DC pp 1–16

Van Egmond M, Diekstra R F W 1989 The predictability of suicidal behaviour: results of a meta-analysis of published studies. In: Diekstra R F W et al (eds) Suicide prevention; the role of attitude and imitation. Brill, Leiden

Vassilas C A, Morgan H G 1993 General practitioners' contact with victims of suicide. British Medical Journal 307: 300–301

Vieta E, Nieto E, Gasto C, Cirera E 1992 Serious suicide attempts in affective patients. Journal of Affective Disorders 24: 147–152

Wagner A W, Linehan M M 1994 Relationship between childhood sexual abuse and topography of parasuicide among women with borderline personality disorder. Journal of Personality Disorders 8: 1–9

Warnes H 1968 Suicide in schizophrenia. Diseases of the Nervous System 29: 35–40

Warr P 1987 Unemployment and mental health. Oxford University Press, Oxford

Warr P, Jackson P 1987 Adapting to the unemployed role: a longitudinal investigation. Social Science and Medicine 25: 1219–1224

Warshaw M G, Massion A O, Peterson L G, Pratt L A, Keller M B 1995 Suicidal behaviour in patients with panic disorder: retrospective and prospective data. Journal of Affective Disorders 34: 235–247

Weeke A 1979 Causes of death in manic–depressives. In: Schou M, Stromgren E (eds) Origin, prevention and treatment of affective disorders. Academic Press, London

Weissman M M 1993 The epidemiology of personality disorders: a 1990 update. Journal of Personality Disorders 7 (suppl 1): 44–62

Weissman M M, Klerman G L, Markowitz J S, Oullette R 1989 Suicidal ideation and suicide attempts in panic disorder and attacks. New England Journal of Medicine 321: 1209–1214

Welu T 1977 A follow-up programme for suicide attempters – evaluation of effectiveness. Suicide and Life-Threatening Behaviour 7: 17–30

Wertheimer A 1991 A special scar. The experiences of people bereaved by suicide. Routledge, London

Wetzel R D, Margulies T, Davis R, Karam E 1980 Hopelessness, depression and suicidal intent. Journal of Clinical Psychiatry 41: 159–160

Whitehead M 1987 (ed) The health divide: inequalities in health in the 1980s. Health Education Council, London

Whitlock F A 1971 Migration and suicide. Medical Journal of Australia 2: 840–848

Whitlock F A 1989 Suicide and physical illness. In: Roy A (ed) Suicide. Williams & Wilkins, Baltimore

WHO 1982 Changing patterns in suicide behaviour. WHO/Euro reports and studies 74. World Health Organization, Copenhagen

Wiedenmann A, Weyerer S 1994 Resting Durkheim's theory of suicide. European Archives of Psychiatry and Clinical Neuroscience 244: 284–286

Wilkinson G, Morgan H G 1994 Can suicide be prevented (controversies in management). British Medical Journal 309: 860–862

Wilkinson G, Smeeton N 1987 The repetition of parasuicide in Edinburgh 1980–1981. Social Psychiatry 22: 14–19

Winokur G, Tsuang M T 1975 The Iowa 500: suicide mania, depression and schizophrenia. American Journal of Psychiatry 132: 650–651

Wu L H, Dunner D L 1993 Suicide attempts in rapid cycling bipolar disorder patients. Journal of Affective Disorders 29: 57–61

27

Psychiatry in relation to other areas of medicine

Michael Sharpe

This chapter is devoted to a consideration of how our thinking about the psychiatric disorders considered elsewhere in this book has to be adapted if it is to be successfully applied to the presentation, aetiology and management of patients attending non-psychiatric medical services. It should be read in conjunction with others in this book, especially Chapter 26 on deliberate self-harm and Chapter 11 on organic disorders.

INTRODUCTION AND OVERVIEW

Conceptual issues

It is useful to begin our consideration of the application of psychiatric knowledge to patients attending medical services by considering what we mean by 'psychiatric disorder', how it differs from 'medical conditions' and what the implications of this distinction are.

Body and mind

Psychiatric disorders are, in a literal sense, simply those syndromes defined in the psychiatric diagnostic classifications of ICD-10 (WHO 1992) and DSM-IV (APA 1994). The designation of an illness as psychiatric (as opposed to medical or surgical) simply means that it has been traditionally regarded as lying within the scope of that subspeciality of medicine (see Ch. 1). Psychiatric disorders have also been assumed to be 'mental' in nature. This allocation to a 'mental' category of illness as opposed to 'physical' illness was based on an absence of known bodily pathology, a tendency to present with disturbed mental states, or both. The underlying assumption that mind can be meaningfully separated from body and that mental illnesses are fundamentally different from physical ones has been called mind–body dualism, an hypothesis commonly attributed to the writings of the philosopher Descartes (Kirmayer 1988). Cartesian dualism has exerted and

continues to exert a profound influence on Western medical thinking (Fabrega 1990), several aspects of which are illustrated below. It is especially important that the psychiatrist working in general medical settings is aware of these.

Conceptual dualism

Dualistic medical thinking encourages the view that the origin of psychological symptoms lies in mental pathology and that of somatic symptoms in physical pathology. By and large this simplistic view works in day-to-day practice. Difficulties arise however when clinical problems are encountered that do not readily fit into this dichotomous view. The two principal types of problem are shown in italics in Table 27.1.

The first problem is posed by patients who have somatic symptoms but no evidence of bodily pathology. It is unclear whether their illness should be categorised as mental or as physical, and whether they are psychiatric patients or medical patients. As a result they are often regarded as being *neither* and are banished to a medical 'no-man's land'. They can only be regarded as mentally ill by proposing the concept of 'somatisation' (Murphy 1989) in order to explain how mental pathology could lead to bodily symptoms. This manoeuvre leads to a disregard of the patient's somatic symptoms in favour of an exploration of psychopathology – an

Table 27.1 Traditional 'dualistic' categories of mental and physical illness		
	Mental symptoms	Physical symptoms
Bodily pathology	*Comorbidity*	Medical condition
No bodily pathology	Psychiatric condition	*Somatisation*

approach patients often resent. They can only be accepted as physically ill if they are regarded as having actual, albeit undetected, bodily pathology. Consequently they may either be diagnosed as having a 'functional' medical condition or be subjected to relentless medical investigation – a process that may lead to iatrogenic harm. These opposite and often opposing approaches to medically unexplained somatic symptoms have been particularly well illustrated by the confusion, controversy and conflict that has surrounded the chronic fatigue syndrome, sometimes called myalgic encephalomyelitis (ME) (Sharpe 1996a).

The second problem is posed by patients who have both prominent psychological symptoms and definite bodily pathology. They fall into *both* mental *and* physical categories. They are consequently regarded as being *both* physically *and* mentally ill, a situation referred to as comorbidity (Mayou & Sharpe 1995). While they may be accepted as both medical and as psychiatric patients, their needs may not be fully met by either speciality, a focus on one aspect of their illness leading to neglect of the other. Perhaps the most prominent example of this is the widespread neglect of depression in patients with medical disease (Freeling et al 1985).

Classificatory dualism

One consequence of conceptual dualism is classificatory dualism: separate classifications for psychiatric and medical conditions consequently poorly understood conditions may attract either no diagnosis or diagnoses from both medical and psychiatric classification, the choice depending only on the doctor's belief about the nature of the illness. For example, a patient with medically unexplained gastroenterological symptoms may be diagnosed as having either a 'medical' irritable bowel syndrome or a 'psychiatric' anxiety disorder, depending on the preference and theoretical orientation of the doctor (Tollefson et al 1991).

Patients who have symptoms of both a medical condition and a psychiatric disorder also give rise to diagnostic conundrums: for example, should a given symptom be attributed to the medical condition or to the psychiatric disorder (Cohen-Cole et al 1993); should the mental disorder be regarded as being caused by the physical disorder (and then be called an organic mental disorder) or as a separate entity?

Organisational dualism

Another result of the dualistic conceptualisation of illness is the division of medical services and specialities into medical/surgical and psychiatric. Medical and psychiatric services are not only professionally and organisationally distinct but often also geographically separate. Many of the practical difficulties encountered in the management of patients with psychiatric disorders in general medical settings arise from this split in medical thinking and separation of medical services.

Moral dualism

Finally, it is important to be aware of the different moral connotations placed on psychiatric and medical diagnoses both by the general public and by many medical colleagues. Medical disorders are by and large regarded as unfortunate failures of the body outside the person's control. Consequently they attract the sympathy of others. Psychiatric disorders on the other hand are regarded as illnesses of mind, that is as a failure of the faculties of reason and self-control. Consequently they carry the implication of failure of will and culpability, views that encourage fear and contempt in others, rather than eliciting care and comfort (Kirmayer 1988). Awareness of this stigmatising aspect of psychiatric diagnosis and treatment may influence how a patient presents, to whom they are referred and how they are managed. Stigma is a major issue for psychiatrists working in non-psychiatric settings (Bursztajn & Barsky 1985).

Beyond dualism

The dualism hypothesis is now under attack. New knowledge, such as the demonstration of a neural basis to psychiatric disorders, is rendering dualistic thinking increasingly untenable and recent evidence for the effect of psychiatric disorder on bodily illness (Frasure-Smith et al 1995) is making its application to medical thinking appear increasingly unhelpful. Consequently dualism is being replaced by the view that mind and brain are more appropriately regarded as two sides of the same coin – the mind/brain (Granville-Grossman 1993) – than as separate entities. An important implication of this modern view of medicine is that 'psychiatric disorders' are rendered no more distinct from 'medical conditions' than the brain is from the rest of the body. Consequently there have been calls to make psychiatry less 'brain-less' and medicine less 'mind-less' (Eisenberg 1986).

For the present however, the legacy of dualism continues to shape much everyday medical thinking and practice. It is important therefore that the psychiatrist working in it is aware of the resulting problems so that the clinical errors that may result are avoided. Perhaps the best way to do this is to ensure that biological, psychological and social aspects of aetiology and management are considered in each and every case – that is, always to apply the biopsychosocial approach to patient assessment and treatment (Engel 1977).

Characteristics of psychiatric disorder in medical settings

The patient with a psychiatric disorder in a medical setting is likely to differ from the patient seen in a specialist psychiatric service in several ways: differences are found in the presentation, the likelihood of coexisting medical conditions, and in the types of psychiatric illness encountered.

Presentation

In medical settings psychiatric disorder is more likely to present either with somatic symptoms or with a behavioural problem related to medical illness and its treatment. For example, the patient with depressive disorder may present with pain (Wilson et al 1994) or with poor compliance with medical treatment (Carney et al 1995), rather than as depressed mood and social withdrawal.

Coexistence with medical conditions

Patients with psychiatric disorder in medical settings, especially in general hospitals, often have coexisting medical conditions. Such *comorbidity* has important implications for the aetiology and management of the psychiatric disorder. For example, a stroke may cause both a depressive disorder (see below) and complicate its management by reducing the patient's tolerance of antidepressant medication.

Relative prevalence

The relative prevalence of specific psychiatric disorders encountered in medical settings is very different from that found in specialist psychiatric services. Adjustment disorders, neuroses, somatoform disorders and alcohol problems are the psychiatric disorders most commonly seen in primary care (Goldberg 1996) and in medical outpatient services (Van Hemert et al 1993b), while acute organic disorders are particularly common among medical and surgical inpatients (Taylor & Lewis 1993). The functional psychoses which form such a large part of specialist psychiatric work are uncommon in all these medical settings. The relative prevalence of specific psychiatric disorders in various medical settings is illustrated in Table 27.2.

Importance of psychiatric disorder in medical settings

Psychiatric disorder is not only a cause of suffering to medical patients but also has major implications for the prognosis and treatment of their medical condition. Psychiatric disorder magnifies the disability resulting from medical conditions (Wells et al 1989), complicates medical management (Sharpe et al 1994), leads to poorer outcome (Francis et al 1990; Frasure-Smith et al 1995) and increases the consumption of general medical resources (Levenson et al 1990). It is also a common reason why non-psychiatric doctors find their patients difficult to help with the application of standard medical approaches (Sharpe et al 1994).

Principles of psychiatric treatment in medical settings

The effective treatment of psychiatric disorder in medical settings requires that the differing presentation and type of disorder be taken into account. It also requires an appreciation of the medical context and a capacity to collaborate effectively with non-psychiatric physicians. These issues are now examined in more detail.

Table 27.2 Relative prevalence of psychiatric disorders in various medical settings				
	General practice	Casualty	Medical /surgical	
			Outpatients	Inpatients
Adjustment disorders	++	+++	++	+++
Depression/anxiety	++	++	+++	+++
Somatoform disorders	+	++	+++	++
Delirium	–	+	–	+++
Alcohol abuse	++	+++	++	+++
Psychosis	+	+	–	–

–, rare; +, uncommon; ++, common; +++, very common.

PRESENTATION OF PSYCHIATRIC DISORDER IN MEDICAL SETTINGS

As indicated above, the presentation of psychiatric disorder in patients attending medical services may differ from those more familiar to those working in specialist psychiatric services and may lead to the diagnosis of psychiatric disorder being missed.

Behavioural presentations

As in psychiatric settings, abnormal, disturbed or potentially self-destructive behaviour is a common presentation in medical settings. However, in the latter context it is more likely to indicate a diagnosis of delirium or adjustment disorder than psychosis. Often the presenting behavioural problem is more subtle and manifests as a medical problem. Common examples are the medical consequences of deliberate self-harm, abnormal or exaggerated illness behaviour and non-adherence to medical treatment.

Deliberate self-harm

Perhaps the most conspicuous example of self-destructive behaviour is deliberate self-harm, most commonly by overdose of drugs. Deliberate self-harm is one of the most common reasons for a patient to be admitted to a general hospital medical unit and for a general hospital inpatient to be referred to a psychiatrist (Hawton 1996). It is considered in more detail in Chapter 26.

Abnormal illness behaviour

Other forms of behavioural presentation include variations or exaggerations in the way in which a medically ill person behaves, that is in 'illness behaviour'. A patient may be regarded as manifesting *abnormal* illness behaviour if he or she behaves as if he is medically ill when not, or if he or she is ill, as more ill than he actually is (Pilowsky 1969). Examples are frequent attendance for medical care, excessive demands on family and friends, exaggerated claims for financial benefits and the unnecessary use of equipment such as wheelchairs. The term 'abnormal illness behaviour' may therefore be used to describe a clinical presentation. Its use requires caution, however, as the judgement of what illness behaviour should be regarded as abnormal is largely subjective. The most common diagnoses associated with abnormal illness behaviour are the somatoform disorders. Extreme forms of abnormal illness behaviour, in which patients deliberately manufacture somatic symptoms and physical signs, are best described as factitious disorder (see below).

Non-adherence to treatment

Non-adherence to the physician's recommended treatment is a common behaviour in all patients. It is less common for patients to actively refuse the treatment recommended by their physician. The most common reason for these behaviours is simply patient choice, although in both cases the patient's judgement may have been influenced by psychiatric disorder (Katon 1996a). For example, elderly patients with ischaemic heart disease who also have depression adhere less well to their recommended medication regimens (Carney et al 1995). The question of whether psychiatric disorder is influencing a patient's judgement is of even greater importance when life-saving treatment is refused or help to die is requested. A determination of competence and an assessment for depressive disorder is essential in all such cases (Sullivan & Youngner 1994).

Somatic presentations

Somatic symptoms that are unexplained by a medical condition are commonly encountered in all medical settings (Goldberg 1996). A large number of terms have been coined to describe this clinical problem:

- medically unexplained somatic symptoms
- medical symptoms not explained by organic disease
- functional somatic symptoms
- somatisation symptoms
- hysterical (conversion) symptoms
- hypochondriasis
- somatoform symptoms.

None of these terms is ideal. The more neutral descriptive terms, such as 'medically unexplained physical symptoms', and 'medical symptoms not explained by organic disease' are preferable to others such as 'hysteria' that carry conceptual baggage. From a medical perspective a case has also been made for a rehabilitation of the word 'functional', now often used to imply 'hysterical' but originally meaning a disturbance of bodily function, as opposed to structure (Trimble 1982). The modern ICD and DSM psychiatric classifications favour the term somatoform to describe the general problem, although some of the older terms such as hypochondriasis still appear as labels for specific disorders within this wider grouping.

Relative frequency

An American population survey found that between quarter and a third of the population had been severely troubled with symptoms such as pain and fatigue at some time in their lives and that in one-third of these cases the symptoms remained medically unexplained

(Kroenke & Price 1993). In primary care, as many as 1 in 5 new consultations are for somatic symptoms for which no specific cause is found (Goldberg & Bridges 1988). In hospital practice, medically unexplained somatic complaints are among the most common reasons for referral from primary care. Specific symptoms tend to cluster in medical specialities according to the organ system they appear to relate to: hence, abdominal and bowel symptoms predominate in gastroenterology clinics (Holmes et al 1987), headache in neurology clinics (Fitzpatrick & Hopkins 1981) and chest pain and palpitations in cardiac clinics (Mayou et al 1995). The somatic symptoms of fully one-third of all patients seen in neurology, cardiology and gastroenterological clinics remain medically unexplained at the time of discharge (Hamilton et al 1996).

Diagnoses

When making a diagnosis in a patient who has presented somatically there are three important pitfalls to be aware of: First, a presentation with somatic complaints does not necessarily imply a specific diagnosis, in particular somatic symptoms do not automatically mean a diagnosis of somatoform disorder (see below). In fact, a diagnosis of depressive and anxiety disorders (especially panic disorder) is more likely (Katon et al 1991). Second, a diagnosis of somatoform disorder does not exclude a medical condition. The patient's symptoms may be subsequently explained by a medical condition that was missed at initial assessment. Patients may also have a medical condition that explains some symptoms but not others: that is, they can have *both* a medical condition *and* a somatoform disorder. Third, it is important to be aware that a medical classificatory scheme of functional disorders exists for somatic complaints unexplained by conventionally defined disease. These functional medical diagnoses should not be regarded as alternatives to psychiatric diagnosis. They are simply alternative labels for the same phenomenon seen from different perspectives. The common functional medical disorders are:

- irritable bowel syndrome
- non-cardiac chest pain
- hyperventilation syndrome
- chronic fatigue syndrome
- fibromyalgia syndorme
- chronic pain
- tension headache.

In the absence of a satisfactory non-dualistic classification that is shared by medicine and psychiatry, the best working solution is for the clinician to note both medical and psychiatric diagnoses while being mindful that these are essentially descriptions of the same condition. Hence the patient may be given a diagnosis of irritable bowel syndrome/generalised anxiety disorder.

Importance

While in many cases medically unexplained somatic symptoms are mild and transient, in a significant minority of patients they are an important clinical problem: The associated disability may be severe (Smith et al 1986) and persistent (Kroenke & Mangelsdorff 1989). Presentation to disease-oriented medical services may lead to repeated investigation without benefit to the patient and at considerable cost (Larson et al 1980). A Danish study found that the small number of patients who, during an 8 year period, were admitted at least 10 times to general hospitals for physical symptoms for which no organic cause was found consumed 3% of the entire budget for admissions to non-psychiatric hospital departments (Fink 1992).

Neglect of psychiatric diagnosis and treatment

In a large proportion of cases of somatic presentation the psychiatric diagnosis is missed and no psychiatric treatment is given. Medical practitioners may not be aware that pain and fatigue are common symptoms of depression (Mathew et al 1981), and breathlessness, muscle pain, dizziness and palpitation of anxiety and panic (Katon et al 1996). Consequently depression and anxiety disorders are often not detected (Goldberg 1996). The effective recognition management of somatically presenting psychiatric disorder has the potential not only to reduce the patient's distress and disability but also to achieve significant savings in the overall cost of their medical care (Simon et al 1995).

COEXISTENCE OF PSYCHIATRIC DISORDER AND MEDICAL CONDITIONS

The other problem highlighted in the introduction was those cases in which the patient's illness is described in such a way that he is deemed to have both a medical and a psychiatric disorder.

Nature, terminology and classification

The psychiatric disorders most commonly comorbid with medical conditions are adjustment disorders, depressive disorders, anxiety disorders, substance misuse disorders and organic disorders. In order to examine the implications of comorbidity, depressive comorbidity will be used as an example.

The current classifications of psychiatric disorder offer two different ways of coding comorbidity. One is to code the medical condition separately from the psychiatric disorder. In DSM-IV, which is multiaxial, psychiatric disorder is recorded on Axis I and the comorbid medical condition on Axis III. The ICD-10 classification is not currently fully multiaxial but does require that comorbid medical conditions be recorded. The other way of coding comorbidity refers only to circumstances where the psychiatric disorder is judged to be a direct consequence of the medical condition. A different psychiatric diagnosis, referred to as 'mental disorder due to a general medical condition' in DSM-IV and organic mental disorders' in ICD-10, is then used. The use of these special diagnoses for comorbid depression and anxiety is however controversial. While it is likely that a medical condition such as a stroke *can* give rise to depression by a direct action on the nervous system (Robinson et al 1990), it is doubtful whether a reliable decision about the aetiology of the patient's depression can be made simply on the basis of a clinical assessment. Furthermore, a firm diagnosis of organic mood disorder has disadvantage for the patient if it leads to a neglect of psychological and social aspects of aetiology and management. While the above categories may be appropriate for delirium, in the case of depression it is probably wise to use the multiaxial method to record comorbidity and only to use the special diagnostic categories described above sparingly, if at all (see below).

Conceptual and research issues

The research literature devoted to the association between medical conditions and psychiatric disorders is a large one. Much of it describes the prevalence of psychiatric disorder in samples of hospitalised patients selected on the basis of a common medical diagnosis. Although this information is potentially important, the psychiatrist must be aware of its limitations. These result from problems in the definition of psychiatric disorder in the medically ill, biases in the way the sample of patients is selected and in the measurement of association between psychiatric disorder and the medical condition.

Defining psychiatric disorder

The criteria for defining psychiatric diagnoses were designed for use in psychiatric populations; they are not always readily applied to medical populations. A specific problem arises with somatic symptoms such as weight loss which form part of the criteria for depressive and anxiety disorders. Hence we have to ask, when a

patient with a medical condition such as cancer has weight loss, whether this symptom should be regarded as evidence of psychiatric disorder or as a symptom of the medical condition? Four main methodological approaches to the diagnosis of depression in the medically ill have been employed in order to address this problem (Kathol et al 1990):

- The psychiatric diagnostic criteria are simply applied unmodified; symptoms are counted whatever their cause is believed to be (the inclusive approach).
- The criteria are modified to exclude symptoms such as weight loss that might be a reflection of physical disease (the aetiological approach).
- The diagnostic criteria are applied unmodified but a judgement is made about the aetiology of individual symptoms; they are only counted if they are deemed not to be a direct manifestation of the physical disease (the exclusive approach).
- The criteria developed in psychiatric populations are redefined; new criteria are developed specifically for use in the medically ill (the substitution approach).

Each of these approaches has its merits but none is more obviously correct than another. In practice, the choice of approach may be less of a problem than appears from the above (Kathol et al 1990) and it is probably best to adopt the inclusive approach. This means applying psychiatric diagnostic criteria unmodified while being aware of the risk of overdiagnosis. A useful discussion of these problems is provided by House (1988).

Selection of sample

Another problem may arise from the way in which the patient sample is recruited; a sample of hospital patients may have a higher prevalence of psychiatric disorder than a primary care sample because patients with psychiatric disorder are more likely to be hospitalised, and treatment and because hospitalisation itself may cause emotional disturbance.

Measuring the association between psychiatric disorder and physical disease

Physical disease is generally defined in terms of objectively demonstrable abnormalities in the structure and/or function of bodily organs and systems. Patients selected solely on this basis, while admittedly sharing the same pathology (such as cancer or stroke), may be heterogeneous on many other variables potentially relevant to the aetiology of any associated psychiatric disorder. These variables include:

- Site(s) of body affected
- Duration and course of medical condition
- Meaning of the medical condition for the patient
- The effect on the patient's social and occupational context.

Consequently, determining the association between a psychiatric disorder and a medical condition simply by assessing the prevalence in patients who share a medical diagnosis is simplistic and may lead to misleading conclusions.

Prevalence of comorbidity

For the reasons described above the reader should be cautious when interpreting studies of comorbidity. None the less it is reasonable to conclude that persons who have a medical condition are also significantly more likely to have a psychiatric disorder (Weyerer 1990). Furthermore some medical conditions do appear to have a stronger association with psychiatric disorder than others. For example, the prevalence of depressive disorder is particularly high among patients with heart disease and neurological disorders (approximately 25%), but only just higher than the general population in patients with hypertension and diabetes (nearer 15%) (Wells et al 1988).

Aetiology

Why should persons with medical conditions be more likely to have psychiatric disorder? There are four main possible reasons:

- Coincidence
- Common causation
- Psychiatric disorder causes the medical condition
- Medical condition causes the psychiatric disorder.

Coincidence

Both physical disease and psychiatric disorder are common in persons in the general population. In clinical practice it is common to see patients whose psychiatric disorder appears to be unrelated to their medical condition. For example, in as many as a quarter of patients with comorbid depression the depression was present before the onset of the medical condition (Moffic & Paykel 1975).

Common causation

Both the psychiatric disorder and the medical condition may share a common cause. For example, stressful life events in a vulnerable person may precipitate both a stroke (House et al 1990) and a depressive illness (Emmerson et al 1989). Common causation seems unlikely however to be a major reason for the association of medical and psychiatric disorder.

Psychiatric disorder causes the medical condition

Psychiatric disorder can certainly cause a medical condition. The most clearly established examples are where the patient's behaviour has produced direct physical damage. Examples are deliberate self-harm and alcohol misuse (Sharpe & Peveler 1996). The question of whether psychiatric disorder and personality traits can cause medical conditions via non-behavioural mechanisms is much more controversial. A failure to establish the hypothesis proposed by psychosomatists in the 1930s and 1940s, that personality type was associated with specific medical conditions such as asthma (Alexander 1950), has led to considerable caution in subsequent aetiological speculation. Modern research has instead attempted to elucidate mechanisms whereby psychological factors could *influence* physical health. An example is the link between the nervous system and the immune system, an area of research called psychoneuroimmunology (Kiecolt-Glaser & Galser 1989). At present there is however little convincing evidence that depression and anxiety are major factors in the aetiology of medical conditions, but there is evidence that comorbid depression can influence the outcome of pre-existing medical conditions such as ischaemic heart disease (Frasure-Smith et al 1995) and stroke (Morris et al 1993).

Medical condition causes the psychiatric disorder

A medical condition may cause the predisposed individual to develop a psychiatric disorder. This may be a consequence of either a direct biological effect on the central nervous system or a psychological reaction.

Direct biological mechanism The following criteria are listed in DSM-IV (APA 1994) as being useful in deciding whether the psychiatric disorder in question can be regarded as being directly biologically caused by the medical condition:

- The presence of an organic cause (disease, drug)
- The organic cause was present before the psychiatric disorder
- Treatment of the organic cause results in relief of the psychiatric symptoms
- The psychiatric disorder is atypical in some way (e.g. lack of family history)

- There is evidence from the literature that the medical condition in question can cause psychiatric disorder by an established biological mechanism.

These requirements are easily met for clearly organic disorders such as delirium. Their value when applied to other disorders such as anxiety and depression is less clear (see above). In general, a medical condition may be considered more likely to cause psychiatric disorder by a biological mechanism if it affects the nervous system either structurally or chemically. Medical conditions that do affect the central nervous system and that can probably cause depression via a biological mechanism include:

- *Endocrine conditions*
  Cushing's syndrome (Kelly et al 1996)
  Hypothyroidism (Whybrow et al 1969)
- *Neurological conditions*
  Parkinson's disease (Cummings 1992)
  Stroke (Burvill et al 1995)
  Multiple sclerosis (Sadovnick et al 1996)
  Advanced cancer (Godding et al 1995).

Psychological reaction   It is easy to understand how a medical condition could give rise to a psychiatric disorder by acting as a psychosocial stressor. In such, the critical factor is the *meaning* of the condition to the patient. For example, it is not surprising that the person who finds that he or she has cancer becomes depressed, and that depression is more likely to occur in persons who believe their disease to be incurable (Alexander et al 1993). Similarly patients with skin disease are more likely to be depressed if they regard the skin disease as disfiguring (Wessely & Lewis 1989). In general, medical conditions are more likely to cause depression if they are perceived as disfiguring, disabling or potentially fatal.

Risk factors for the development of psychiatric disorder in the physically ill

In practice, rather than trying to decide whether an individual patient's psychiatric disorder is either biologically or psychologically caused, it is more useful to seek evidence for multiple aetiological factors. These factors are likely to include the medical treatment, the premorbid characteristics of the individual and aspects of his or her situation as well as the medical condition and its meaning for the patient.

Nature of the treatment

Medical consultation and hospital admission can be distressing, and major medical and surgical treatments can have considerable effects on a patient's mental state (Maguire 1990). Examples include major investigations and procedures such as genetic counselling, surgery, radiotherapy and drug therapy. Many drug treatments commonly used in medicine are known to cause depression. Important examples include:

- steroids (O'Carroll 1987)
- H_2-receptor antagonists, e.g. cimetidine (Billings & Stein 1986)
- antihypertensive drugs, e.g. beta blockers (Carney et al 1987).

Nature of the patient

For any given medical condition it is only a minority of patients who suffer from psychiatric disorder. Individual vulnerability is therefore an important additional factor. For affective and anxiety disorders it is probable that the constitutional factors predisposing to emotional disorders in the general population also apply to the medically ill. The most easily identifiable indicator of this vulnerability is a previous history of psychiatric disorder (Mayou & Sharpe 1995).

Context

In keeping with research on uncomplicated depression, the social context, and especially the degree of support the person enjoys, is of importance. Lack of social support has been repeatedly found to be an important risk factor for adverse emotional reactions to medical conditions such as cancer (Godding et al 1995).

Summary

A number of factors may be regarded as risk factors for the development of depression and these are listed below; personal vulnerability is especially important:

- The medical condition: involves the central nervous system; is perceived as threatening
- The treatment: affects the central nervous system; is disfiguring or disabling
- The person: has a previous history of psychiatric disorder
- The context: offers inadequate social support.

GENERAL PRINCIPLES OF MANAGEMENT

In this section the general principles of the management of psychiatric disorder in general medical settings are outlined. It is important to note that relatively few patients with psychiatric disorder seen in such settings receive any specific treatment for it and briefly to consider why this might be. Special features of the medical context relevant to psychiatric management are examined and the issues of detection, assessment and treatment reviewed.

Obstacles to effective management

Potential obstacles to effective psychiatric treatment include the following:

Failure of detection

The first obstacle to the effective management of patients with psychiatric disorder is a low rate of detection (Goldberg 1996). There are a number of reasons for this. As described, the patient may present with somatic complaints (Munk-Jorgensen et al 1997); the doctor may not ask the right questions (Freeling et al 1985); and the focus of the doctor on medical aspects of the patient's complaints may distract him from concern with the psychiatric disorder (Metcalfe et al 1988). While it is often appropriate for the needs of the medical condition to take priority, in some cases this may lead to ineffective treatment. For example, the complaint of pain may lead to a focus on medical causes while a coexisting and aetiologically important major depressive disorder, the treatment of which may reduce or even eliminate the pain, is ignored (Von Korff & Simon 1996). Any attempt to improve detection of psychiatric disorder must take these obstacles into account.

Failure to perform adequate assessment and treatment

Even if detected, psychiatric disorder may not be adequately assessed and treated. Two commonly held attitudes may prevent the physician from actively assessing and treating the psychiatric disorder. First, the psychiatric disorder may be regarded merely as an understandable result of the medical condition and consequently, but wrongly, be viewed as requiring no specific treatment. Second, the physician may believe wrongly that psychiatric treatment would be ineffective in any case, and is therefore pointless (Mayou & Smith 1986). The effect of these attitudes is compounded by a lack of psychiatric expertise, time and facilities in the non-psychiatric part of the health care system (Creed 1991).

Medical undergraduate training in psychiatry devotes relatively little attention to those aspects of psychiatry of importance to the non-psychiatric physician (Sharpe et al 1996) and only a minority of doctors receive relevant postgraduate training (Royal College of Physicians and Royal College of Psychiatrists, 1995). Furthermore, doctors working in general medical services often feel under pressure and consequently regard psychiatric assessment of the patient as too time consuming a task (Mayou & Smith 1986). Often there is a simple lack of basic facilities for psychiatric assessment such as a private interview room and a shortage of the resources needed for effective treatment such as the ready availability of adequately trained cognitive behaviour therapists (Royal College of Physicians and Royal College of Psychiatrists 1995). Finally, both patient (Wells et al 1994) and doctor (Mayou & Smith 1986) may wish to avoid the stigma that a psychiatric diagnosis and the acceptance of psychiatric treatment might imply. Strategies intended to improve psychiatric assessment and treatment in medical settings must address these problems.

Psychiatric management in the medical context

The first consideration for the effective detection, assessment and treatment of psychiatric disorder outside specialist psychiatric settings is an appreciation of the special characteristics of the medical context. As can be seen from the foregoing, the psychiatrist working in this setting cannot simply transplant the usual approach. Essential modifications include the following.

Addressing the medical patient's concerns

It is likely that patients seen in a medical setting will be more concerned about their medical state (whether an established medical condition or an unexplained somatic symptom) and its management than about their psychiatric state – a factor that the psychiatrist must be sensitive to if he or she is to obtain their cooperation. Not infrequently the patient will express reluctance about seeing a psychiatrist at all. Therefore, whatever the reason for the assessment, it is wise to begin the interview by taking time to explain the reason for the psychiatric consultation and to elicit the patient's own concerns about somatic complaints and medical treatment before going on to ask about psychological symptoms.

Other doctors and nurses

The medical patient is under the care of non-psychiatric physicians, nurses and other staff and their cooperation is essential. Their provision of a positive explanation of the reason for a psychiatric assessment is a necessary preliminary, and the collection of information about the patient from these important informants is a valuable contribution to the assessment process. Once assessment is completed, those concerned with the patient's ongoing management require detailed feedback and practical guidance about their role in the psychiatric management. A brief written note is rarely sufficient and frequently results in the psychiatrist's suggested treatment plan, however appropriate, not being carried out (Huyse et al 1990).

Facilities

Although the facilities for psychiatric assessment and treatment in non-psychiatric settings are often poor, the psychiatrist should persevere in finding an appropriately private and undisturbed place to interview the patient. Suggestions that the patient be given psychological therapy must take into account the extent to which skilled therapists are actually available, and may require that the psychiatrist takes responsibility for this aspect of the patient's treatment. If psychotropic drug treatment is recommended it is necessary to check that the drugs are readily available; frequently they are not and an unanticipated delay may result while the drugs are ordered from the pharmacy.

Follow-up

It is usually desirable carry out a follow-up consultation to check on the patient's progress. The psychiatrist should not rely on others, who may lack the necessary skill, to monitor the patient's mental state.

Detecting psychiatric disorder

As with all medical diagnoses the most important requirement is for the assessing doctor to have a high 'index of suspicion' based on an awareness of the prevalence of and risk factors for psychiatric disorder as described above. The practical task of detection may be aided by systematic screening procedures.

Questionnaires

One approach to screening is the use of questionnaires. These may be administered in pencil and paper form or by other means such as touch screen computer. Examples of aspects of illness screened for and associated questionnaires are:

- Depression and anxiety: Hospital depression and Anxiety Scale (HAD) (Zigmond & Snaith 1983)

- Alcohol misuse: Alcohol Use Disorder Identification Test (AUDIT) (Barbor et al 1992)
- Cognitive impairment: Mini-Mental State Examination (MMSE) (Folstein et al 1975)
- 'Quality of life': Medical Outcomes General Health Survey (SF-36) (Ware & Sherbourne 1992).

Interviews

An alternative to the questionnaire is simply to add a few questions to the routine medical and nursing assessment of every patient. For example, merely asking patients if they have suffered depressed mood may be as useful as giving them a questionnaire to measure depression (Van Hemert et al 1993a).

Assessment, diagnosis and formulation of psychiatric disorder

Once the presence of psychiatric disorder is suspected, it is necessary to make a diagnosis. Full diagnostic interviews are of course time consuming, but cut-down versions are now being developed specifically for use in medical settings. An example is the PRIME-MD interview that can be conducted in minutes (Spitzer et al 1994). Assessment requires more than diagnosis; and an assessment of the person, his concerns, his social context and of any comorbid medical condition is also necessary. The assessment may be usefully summarised as a diagnosis supplemented by a formulation covering biological, psychological and social aspects of the problem.

Treatment of psychiatric disorder

The usual principles of psychiatric management can be applied in the medical setting as long as attention is paid to the contextual issues outlined above.

Pharmacotherapy

There are several complications in the use of pharmacotherapy for psychiatric disorder in medical patients. Patients may not wish to take 'psychiatric drugs', they may be intolerant of them or the drugs may be contraindicated by a patient's medical condition or ongoing medical treatment. Therefore care must always be taken to check for potential contraindications and treatment interactions by using appropriate references such as the *British National Formulary* (British Medical Association & Royal Pharmaceutical Society of Great Britain, 1996). It is also desirable to begin treatment with a lower dose of the drug than is usual in general psychiatric practice.

Psychological therapy

Psychological treatments lack the potential of drug therapy to cause adverse effects and interaction; however, some patients and their physicians may be reluctant to accept an explicitly 'psychological therapy'. Time devoted to explaining the nature and relevance of this form of treatment to the patient is well spent. Simple psychological interventions such as information giving have been shown to be of value for alcohol problems (Chick 1991) and could be profitably extended to other conditions. More elaborate therapies, especially cognitive-behaviour therapy, have a proven role in the management of both comorbid emotional disorder and a wide range of somatoform disorders (Enright 1997).

Compulsory treatment

Patients may occasionally have to be given treatment for disturbed behaviour secondary to psychiatric disorder (such as an attempt to harm themselves) without their consent. In such cases the application of legal powers of compulsory treatment may be considered. It must be remembered that legislation such as the UK Mental Health Acts cannot be used to force a person to have medical treatment unless they have a mental disorder and the treatment is directed at the relief of that disorder.

Special problems

Specific additional issues arise in the management of the patient with a somatic presentation and the patient with a comorbid medical condition.

The patient with medically unexplained somatic complaints

Whatever the final diagnosis, certain strategies are needed in managing all patients who present with somatic complaints (Bass & Benjamin 1993).

- Accept the patient's experience of somatic complaints
- Ensure medical conditions have been excluded
- Widen the agenda to include psychological symptoms and stressors
- Make a psychiatric diagnosis and formulation
- Prevent further unnecessary medical investigation and treatment
- Explain and administer psychiatric treatment.

The patient with a comorbid medical condition

Management is similar to that of an uncomplicated psychiatric disorder but the comorbid medical condition must be taken into account: its course is likely to influence the outcome of psychiatric disorder and will limit the choice of treatment.

- Determine both the psychiatric and the medical diagnosis
- Ensure optimal treatment of the medical condition
- Take account of the medical condition when choosing treatment.

SPECIFIC PSYCHIATRIC DISORDERS AND THEIR MANAGEMENT

The psychiatric disorders most commonly encountered in medical settings are reviewed below. Specific aspects of management are also reviewed for each category of disorders as a supplement to general aspects of management outlined above.

Reactions to stressors

Reactions to stress can be broadly divided into acute, persistent and chronic forms. Transient but severe *acute stress reactions* are common in patients who have suffered acute stresses such as accidents (Koopman et al 1995). In medically ill patients the onset of, or exacerbation of disease, as well as hospitalisation and treatment are all potent stressors that can produce marked psychological reactions. The patient with an acute stress reaction to the sudden onset of severe illness such as myocardial infarction is likely to be aroused and anxious and may become disturbed in behaviour. He may also deny the reality or implications of what has happened to him for some time so that the adverse psychological reaction is delayed (Cassem & Hackett 1977).

More long-lasting *adjustment disorders* usually manifest as depressed or anxious mood and may also lead to disturbed behaviour and to poor compliance with medical treatment (Cassem & Hackett 1977, Oxman et al 1994). The symptoms of distress often wax and wane in severity in association with improvements and deteriorations in the course of the illness, and successes and failures in its treatment. For example, distress in patients having haemodialysis for renal failure fluctuates according to problems occurring in treatment (Reichsman & Levy 1973). Adjustment reactions are, by definition, usually transient but a proportion of patients who manifest them will go on to develop persistent psychiatric disorders, usually depression (Kovacs el al 1995). The precise boundary between adjustment disorder and established mood disorder can be hard to draw (Strain et al 1989).

A persistent emotional response to a past event that was perceived as life-threatening (e.g. serious road accident, invasive medical procedure) may be termed a *post-traumatic stress disorder*. The onset is usually weeks to months or more after the trauma. The key symptoms are the repeated reliving of the event in images ('flashbacks') and nightmares, as well as chronic anxiety and insomnia and tendency to avoid reminders of the trauma. This disorder has been described in a significant proportion of persons who have experienced severe accidents such as car crashes (Mayou et al 1993). It is also increasingly recognised to be a potential complication of acute medical illness and its treatment (Mayou & Smith 1997).

Management

Most emotional reactions to illness are transient and require no specific treatment other than ensuring that the patient has adequate and accurate information. More persistent or severe reactions are likely in persons who have a history of previous psychiatric disorder (Blanchard et al 1996). Such persons should therefore be regarded as being at risk. Attempts to prevent later problems with counselling or 'psychological debriefing' early after a trauma do not seem to be effective (Hobbs et al 1996). Established disorders should be treated with either antidepressant drugs or psychological therapy (Shalev 1996).

Mood disorders

Mood disorders are classified as either bipolar or unipolar; if unipolar, they are further subclassified on the basis of severity and persistence. ICD-10 subdivides unipolar depression into mild, moderate and severe forms and DSM-IV into major depression and a chronic milder form, termed dysthymia.

The prevalence of depressive disorder identified in surveys of medical populations depends on the threshold of severity used and the particular group of patients assessed. Differing practices for the differentiation of adjustment disorder from established mood disorder contribute to variations in quoted rates. None the less, general conclusions can be drawn; first the prevalence of more severe depressive disorder (usually defined as DSM *major depression*) is approximately 5% in primary care, 5–10% in medical outpatients, and 10–20% in medical inpatients. Second, when milder forms of depression are included the overall rate is 2–3 times higher than for major depression (Katon & Schulberg 1992). Third, chronic depressive states such as *dysthymia* are particularly common in patients with chronic medical conditions (Howland 1993). The depressive disorder of many hospitalised medical patients recovers on discharge without any specific psychiatric treatment

(Kathol & Wenzel 1992). However, continuing depression occurs in 10–20% and is associated with persistence of the medical condition and with ongoing social problems (Mayou et al 1991). Depressive disorder is particularly important in medical patients as it not only represents considerable distress but also amplifies disability (Wells et al 1989) and increases the cost of medical care (Simon et al 1995).

Management

The first stage of effective management of depression in the medically ill is detection and diagnosis. Once a depressive disorder has been diagnosed, management is based on pharmacological treatment with an antidepressant agent or with psychological treatment, usually cognitive behaviour therapy. Relatively few randomised trials have examined the effectiveness of such treatments specifically in medical populations. However, a review of the available trials shows that antidepressants are effective in treating depression in patients with significant coexisting medical conditions (Gill & Hatcher 1997) as well as in those who present with somatic complaints (Katon & Sullivan 1995). There is less evidence for the effectiveness of psychological treatments for patients with comorbid depression, although they have been shown to be effective for somatic presentations of depression (Guthrie 1996). A combination of antidepressant drugs and cognitive behaviour therapy has been shown to be particularly effective in relieving major depressive disorder in US primary care, including in patients with comorbid medical conditions (Katon et al 1996).

Anxiety disorders

Anxiety disorders are common in medical settings but, like depression, the precise prevalence reported from surveys depends on both the threshold of severity required and the sample of patients studied (Goldberg 1996). Furthermore, if a hierarchical approach to diagnosis which subsumes anxiety under depression is employed, anxiety will be under-reported (Sherbourne et al 1996). The main subtypes of anxiety disorders are paroxysmal anxiety or panic, generalised anxiety and phobic anxiety.

Panic disorder is a frequent cause of presentation to medical services. This is perhaps not surprising for a condition which has fear of dying and somatic symptoms as core features. Panic is a common cause of the somatic complaints of dizziness, paraesthesia, breathlessness, palpitations and chest pain and is a common accompaniment of hypochondriasis (Noyes et al 1994a). It also has an association with increased use of medical services (Katon 1996b). *Generalised anxiety disorder* is also common (Sherbourne et al 1996) but has been relatively neglected in liaison psychiatry research. Its contribution to multiple medically unexplained symptoms, disability and excessive use of medical services may have been underestimated (Roy-Byrne & Katon 1997). *Specific phobias* such as blood injury or needle phobias pose particular problems in medical and surgical care. This is particularly the case for conditions requiring frequent injections, such as insulin-dependent diabetes mellitus (Steel et al 1986).

Management

The information given to patients about their symptoms may be an important determinant of anxiety. For example, physicians who correctly address the illness concerns of patients with irritable bowel syndrome achieve a greater reduction in the patient's anxiety (Dulmen et al 1995). Treatment of established anxiety states is with psychological treatments and with antidepressant drugs, although, as with depression, there are few evaluations of therapy specifically in medical populations. Benzodiazepines may be useful for short periods, such as anxiety-provoking medical procedures, but their prolonged use may lead to dependence and should be avoided.

Somatoform disorders

The diagnostic category of somatoform disorders was defined to accommodate those patients who seek medical attention for somatic symptoms or concerns about health that are unexplained by, or disproportionate to, the medical findings. It is only applied if the patient does not meet criteria for an alternative psychiatric diagnosis, such as depressive disorder, and in this sense is a residual category. Somatoform disorders are also a 'mixed bag' and some of the subcategories may have a more comfortable home elsewhere. For example, it has been suggested that somatisation disorder is better regarded as a personality disorder (Bass & Murphy 1995) and hypochondriasis as an anxiety disorder (Warwick & Salkovskis 1990); however, there are simi-

larities in the presentation of somatoform disorders that make them worth considering together. Although the DSM and ICD classifications distinguish many discrete subtypes, somatoform disorders may be usefully and more simply conceptualised as a continuum, with one end typified by the patient who is principally concerned with their somatic *symptoms* – 'somatisation' – and the other by the patient who is preoccupied with the *fear or belief* that he has a serious disease – 'hypochondriasis' (Kirmayer & Robbins 1991). The majority of patients have both somatic symptoms and concerns about disease and therefore lie somewhere between these two extremes (Fig. 27.1).

Somatisation and associated disorders

Somatisation is a hypothetical process purporting to explain why patients develop somatic complaints in response to psychological stress. Somatisation disorder, or Briquet's syndrome, is the most chronic and severe form of somatisation. The predominantly somatising disorders include conversion disorder (where there is loss of function), pain disorder (where the main complaint is of pain) and undifferentiated somatoform disorder (a catch-all category for all other symptoms). Additional disorders described in ICD-10, but not DSM-IV, are neurasthenia (chronic fatigue syndrome) and somatoform autonomic dysfunction (which includes irritable bowel syndrome) (World Health Organization, 1992).

Briquet's syndrome (somatisation disorder)

This was defined to describe those patients, usually women, who present with long histories of multiple medically unexplained somatic complaints. They are sometimes referred to as 'fat file' patients. Definitions of the disorder require that the patient has a history of more than a certain number of medically unexplained complaints for which they have seen a physician. The frequency of medically unexplained complaints that patients report is continuously distributed in the general population; the setting of a specific number (various numbers between 4 and 13 have been used) serves merely to define a threshold for the purpose of case definition. The prevalence of somatisation disorder found in the general population lies between 1 and 4% (Escobar et al 1987), and in medical settings between 10 and 20%, depending on which case definition is used (Kirmayer & Robbins 1991).

There is a strong association between Briquet's syndrome and both personality disorder (Stern et al 1993) and affective disorder (Brown et al 1990). A tendency for somatisation disorder to run in families (Guze 1993) has been demonstrated, suggesting a genetic factor, and there is also an association with childhood

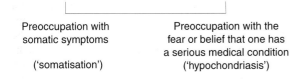

Fig. 27.1 The continuum of somatoform disorders

deprivation and abuse (Pribor et al 1993). Iatrogenic factors may also play a part in maintaining the disorder (Elks 1994). Without specific treatment the prognosis is very poor (Guze et al 1986).

Dissociative/conversion disorder (hysteria)

Conversion disorder is the modern equivalent of hysteria. The essential difference from other somatoform disorders is a clear 'alteration or loss of physical functioning' with deficits in motor or sensory function unexplained by a medical condition and not intentionally produced (as in factitious disorder). The prevalence of classical conversion symptoms, such as inability to move an arm or blindness, appears to be less common in modern medical practice than it was 100 years ago (Shorter 1992), but conversion disorders continue to be seen in modern specialist medical practice. There is some evidence for the general belief that hysteria is caused by stress in vulnerable persons (House & Andrews 1988). The actual form of the symptom is probably shaped by the patient's personal experience of medical illness as well as by cultural factors. It has been argued that the incidence of 'classical' hysteria has decreased in recent times because hysteria has changed its form and now manifests in more 'subtle' ways, such as the general weakness of chronic fatigue syndrome (Shorter 1992). Such a conjecture is intriguing but of course difficult to test.

The prognosis for acute conversion symptoms is good, but once established they can be enduring and patients may become chronically disabled and even wheelchair bound. A much quoted study suggesting that most patients diagnosed as having conversion disorder turned out to have neurological disease (Slater 1965) has been refuted by a more recent study (Mace & Trimble 1996).

Specific somatic symptoms (pain and fatigue)

Specific somatic symptoms may occur as a sole or predominant complaint as well as occurring together with many others, as is the case in patients with somatisation disorder. The current psychiatric classifications have singled out the symptom of pain and have dignified it with the diagnosis of *somatoform pain disorder*. Unexplained pain is extremely common in medical patients, common sites being the back, abdomen, pelvis and muscles (Kroenke et al 1993). Widespread pain complaints may also be diagnosed as the functional medical syndrome of fibromyalgia (Wolfe et al 1990).

Fatigue as a symptom is singled out in ICD-10 where, if it occurs in the absence of a depressive or other specific diagnosis, it is associated with a diagnosis of neurasthenia. In DSM-IV, however, chronic fatigue enjoys no special status and falls into the residual category of undifferentiated somatoform disorder. Chronic fatigue states may also be diagnosed as the functional medical syndrome of chronic fatigue syndrome (Fukuda et al 1994).

The causation of these specific somatoform disorders is uncertain but chronic pain and chronic fatigue have a strong association with previous and current depressive disorder (Hudson & Pope 1994). Both are frequently persistent and profoundly disabling.

Other somatoform disorders

Other subcategories of somatoform disorders are described in the psychiatric classifications. *Undifferentiated somatoform disorder* is designed as a residual category but is very common in community surveys (Escobar et al 1987). *Somatoform autonomic dysfunction* is an ICD-10 category describing patients who present with concerns about symptoms that are the result of autonomic arousal rather than disease and include 'cardiac neurosis, irritable bowel syndrome and hyperventilation'. Its utility is unclear.

Hypochondriasis and associated disorders

The other end of the 'somatoform continuum' (Fig. 27.1) is represented by hypochondriasis. The central feature of this syndrome is a preoccupation with the possibility that one has, or may have, a serious (usually fatal) disease, based on a misinterpretation of somatic symptoms that persists despite adequate medical evaluation and reassurance. Anxiety and depressive symptoms are common in such patients (Noyes et al 1994a) and it has been suggested that hypochondriasis should not be considered as a *diagnosis* but only as a symptom of depression (Kenyon 1964) or anxiety (Salkovskis & Warwick 1986); however, there are a sizable number of patients who meet criteria for hypochondriasis in the absence of these disorders (Appleby 1987). Clinically, a dimensional approach in which the degree of anxiety, depression and hypochondriacal concern are assessed and treated separately is often more useful than trying to determine which of these aspects of the patient's illness is primary and which secondary. Occasionally hypochondriacal concerns may be delusional and a diagnosis of psychotic disorder made (Scarone & Gambini 1991) is appropriate.

The prevalence of established hypochondriasis in medical outpatients is approximately 5%, although transient hypochondriacal states are more common (Barsky et al 1990). The aetiology is uncertain but is associated with both anxiety disorders and persistent fears about vulnerability to severe illness (Barsky & Wyshak 1989). Repeated reassurance from doctors and others may be a perpetuating factor (Warwick & Salkovskis 1985). The outcome is variable, with severe and untreated hypochondriacal states having a poor prognosis (Noyes et al 1994b).

Body dysmorphic disorder This disorder, which was previously known as dysmorphophobia, is regarded as a type of hypochondriasis in ICD-10 but classified separately in DSM-IV. The essential ingredient is a perceived defect in appearance for which there is inadequate objective evidence (Veale et al 1996). The disorder is relevant to medicine in so far as persons afflicted by it often attend doctors, especially plastic surgeons, in order to seek alteration of their appearance. While minor dissatisfaction with appearance is extremely common, severe morbid preoccupation (for example, with shape of nose or size of breasts) is relatively rare. As with hypochondriasis, these concerns may occasionally be delusional in intensity (de Leon et al 1989).

Management of somatoform disorders

The management of the somatoform disorders can be considered as having general and specific aspects. In addition to the points listed above, general aspects that are applicable to all somatoform diagnoses include:

- Provide information about the diagnosis to patient and physician
- Limit medical investigation and treatment
- Ensure treatment of associated depression and anxiety
- Coordinate the patient's overall management
- Encourage a return to normal behaviour.

Specific management may include both pharmacological and psychological treatment. Antidepressant drugs have been shown to have a role in reducing many unexplained complaints, including pain (Katon & Sullivan, 1995). Psychotherapy, especially cognitive-behaviour therapy is superior to conservative medical care for a range of unexplained somatic complaints (Speckens et al 1995). There are individual trials demonstrating its effectiveness in chronic pain, chronic fatigue, irritable bowel syndrome and hypochondriacal disorders (Sharpe 1995). Group therapy may also be helpful in the treatment of patients with somatisation disorder (Kashner et al 1995) and hypochondriasis (Stern & Fernandez 1991).

For chronic severe disability associated with somatoform disorder physical rehabilitation may have a role, especially for chronic pain and fatigue and for conversion disorders.

Factitious disorders and malingering

Factitious disorders and malingering are conditions in which the patient deliberately feigns or otherwise manufactures symptoms (such as abdominal pain) and signs (such as haematemesis by swallowing and regurgitating animal blood) with the aim of being regarded as sick and being given medical treatment (see below). Factitious disorder is differentiated from *malingering* on the basis that in the latter there is an obvious goal other than medical care (such as avoiding an exam) that the patient is trying to attain. Both are differentiated from somatoform disorders, which are conditions in which the patient is considered not to have deliberately produced the symptoms. In practice these distinctions are often not so clear-cut.

Patients presenting with factitious disorder may be dramatic, dishonest and have extensive medical knowledge. They may also use an actual bodily abnormality as evidence to support their story, for example, a scar to suggest an abdominal condition that has required previous emergency surgery. Severe cases who move from hospital to hospital have been described as having Munchausen's syndrome after Baron von Munchausen who told fantastic tales of his exploits (Asher 1951). Factitious disorder is relatively rare but memorable because of the degree of difficulty it creates.

Management of factitious disorders

Usual management is first to prevent iatrogenic harm by stopping investigation and treatment, and then to combine confrontation of the patient with the evidence that they are deliberately creating signs of illness (e.g. evidence of self-injection) with the offer of psychological help. Psychiatric help is rarely accepted however (Sutherland & Rodin 1990).

'Organic' mental disorder

These are disorders grouped on the basis that they result from demonstrable cerebral dysfunction. ICD-10 retains this grouping but it has been avoided in DSM-IV (in order to avoid the implication that other disorders are not organic). All organic disorders are more commonly encountered in medical than in psychiatric settings. The most important is delirium associated with medical conditions and their treatment and with substance misuse.

Delirium

This is the term for a general syndrome of transient impairment of consciousness and cognitive function. It is more common in elderly inpatients, in whom it may afflict as many as a quarter (Francis et al 1990). In most cases the delirium will be due to the effect on the central nervous system of a coexisting medical condition or its treatment. It is especially common in the elderly and in those with pre-existing cognitive impairment. It is important because it is associated with a poorer medical outcome and with a greater length of stay in hospital (Francis et al 1990).

Dementia

Dementia is a major problem in the population and consequently for general medical services. As elderly persons are increasingly represented among hospital patients, the prevalence of dementia found there increases. The most difficult task is often to differentiate dementia from delirium.

Other organic disorders

A variety of other organic disorders may occur, especially in those with cerebral disease. These include the effect of damage to specific parts of the brain such as the frontal lobes. The symptoms may result from damage or from seizure activity. Misdiagnosis of such medical conditions as functional psychosis may occur and results in a lost opportunity for effective medical treatment (such as in the case of an operable cerebral tumour). Mood syndromes or *organic mood disorders* may occur because of the direct effect of a medical condition on the brain (see comorbidity above).

Management

A prerequisite of management is detection. The diagnosis may be missed even if the patient is assessed. There are three common reasons for this. First, the cognitive impairment typically fluctuates (it is usually worse at night) and a 'snapshot' assessment may miss it. Second, the patient may present with mood changes, a focus on which may lead to a misdiagnosis of mood disorder. Third, cognitive impairment in an elderly patient may be diagnosed as dementia when in fact it is of recent onset. A careful history from an informant and, if necessary, repeated assessments will overcome these difficulties.

Once the diagnosis has been made the important management tasks are to limit potential damage to the patient (and to others) and to identify and if possible remove the cause. Close nursing observation and sedation may be required to prevent wandering and accidents. Nursing in a side room will minimise disruption to others (Taylor & Lewis 1993). It is particularly important to suspect alcohol withdrawal as this may explain the delirium. It also indicates a risk of seizures and of Wernicke–Korsakoff syndrome. Treatment for the latter (with thiamine) can prevent permanent memory impairment in many cases (Zubaran et al 1997).

Substance misuse disorders

A history of substance misuse is very common among patients in medical settings. The acute effects are a common cause of casualty attendance: the behavioural effects (such as accidents) and complications (such as liver damage) a cause of medical illness; and the physiological effects (such as gastrointestinal disturbance) a cause of unexplained somatic complaints (Sharpe & Peveler 1996).

Alcohol misuse

The most common substance misuse disorder encountered in medical settings is with alcohol. Alcohol problems are encountered particularly frequently in accident and emergency departments (Conigrave et al 1991). The problem is greater in males and as many as 20% of male medical admissions are problem drinkers (Orford et al 1992).

Other drugs commonly misused

The misuse of drugs other than alcohol is an increasing problem. It may present because of intoxication, withdrawal or associated disease. Drug misusers are most likely to be encountered in inner city casualty departments where they may represent 20% of attenders (Ghodse 1981).

Management

The physician is in a particularly good position to educate patients and to use their concern for their health as a motivating factor. The rate of detection without specific screening is low, but is improved by a systematic approach including specific questions, physical examination and appropriate investigations (Persson & Magnusson 1988). There is evidence that simple advice and education can have a worthwhile effect on alcohol intake (Chick 1991). Similarly, for patients who misuse other drugs it is useful to give information, help to those who wish to abstain and advice on harm limitation for those who do not.

Psychotic disorders

Other than presentations of persons with known psychotic disorders, these are encountered in general medical settings relatively rarely. Patients may present with bizarre complaints (such as 'my bowels are rotting'). Occasionally psychotic states arise during inpatient treatment, when they are often transient (Cutting 1980).

Management

Management may require the use of antipsychotic drugs and the application of compulsory powers to enable removal to a psychiatric ward.

Other disorders

Eating disorders (see Ch. 17) are occasionally encountered in medical settings. They may be a cause of unexplained symptoms, such as vomiting or weight loss, or may complicate the management of a medical condition, such as diabetes mellitus (Robin & Daneman 1992).

Sexual problems are also common in medical patients, where they may result either from the medical condition or its treatment (Hawton 1984) (see also Ch. 19).

PSYCHIATRIC SERVICES FOR GENERAL MEDICAL SETTINGS

In an effort to improve the management of psychiatric disorder in patients attending non-psychiatric settings, attempts have been made to improve the level of psychiatric expertise available. One approach is to educate the physicians working in these settings, another is to have psychiatrists or other mental health workers become directly involved in patient care.

Primary care

In primary care efforts have focused on improving the management of patients with depressive disorder. One approach has focused on improving recognition and the other on improving treatment. Recognition has been tackled by training physicians in interview methods, especially in the eliciting of depressive symptoms in patients who present somatically (Kaaya et al 1992). However, studies in the USA have found that this approach alone does not necessarily produce better patient outcome (Katon & Gonzales 1994). Improvement in the number of patients successfully treated for depression appears to require also the involvement of a professional trained in psychiatric treatment (Katon et al 1996).

Secondary and tertiary care

Similar approaches have been tried in hospital care. Progress has been made in training medical specialists to elicit and recognise depressive disorder in specific areas such as oncology (Parle et al 1997) but the biomedical focus of many hospital physicians is a potential obstacle to the widespread adoption of this approach.

In order to improve treatment of psychiatric illness in general hospitals, a number of small dedicated general hospital psychiatric departments have been established specifically for this purpose. These units have hitherto been devoted principally to the management of conspicuous psychiatric morbidity, especially deliberate self-harm (see Ch. 26), and obvious psychiatric emergencies on wards rather than to the systematic detection and management of the range of psychiatric disorder encountered in general hospital patients. Two principal ways of working have been described: *Liaison*, which involves meeting with medical staff and discussing both general management issues and the management of individual patients; and *Consultation* which is the management of individual referred patients. Most services now use a combination of both approaches – referred to as consultation–liaison or C-L services in the USA and simply as liaison psychiatry services in the UK. The staff of a liaison psychiatry service usually includes a consultant psychiatrist together with a clinical psychologist and specialist nursing staff. Are these services effective? The studies that have set out to demonstrate the overall effectiveness of such generic C-L services on the outcomes of medical inpatients have so far failed to do so (Goldberg 1992, Levenson et al 1992). However, evaluations of more targeted liaison psychiatric services have demonstrated substantial effects on both patient outcome (Sharpe 1996b) and on the cost of care (Strain et al 1991).

Medical–psychiatric units

A recent development in the USA has been the establishment of medical–psychiatric (or med-psych) units (Kathol 1994). These are general hospital inpatient units, staffed by physicians trained in both general medicine and in general psychiatry. Anyone who has been involved in the management of a patient with both a severe medical condition and a significant psychiatric disorder (such as severe debility in a woman with anorexia nervosa) will immediately see the need for such a facility. However, they require specially trained staff and are likely to have only a small number of beds so great care needs to be taken in selection of patients admitted to them. There are no such units in the UK.

Future developments

Future trends in the development of psychiatric liaison services are likely to include:

- a greater focus on outpatients
- the development of collaborative working, e.g. joint clinics

- the greater use of specialist nurses
- increased focus on reducing medical costs.

The role of primary care, the relationship between specialist hospital liaison psychiatry and general psychiatry services, and the question of who pays for the care of patients with unexplained somatic symptoms and with medical psychiatric comorbidity will no doubt continue to generate argument and controversy. However, the interface between psychiatry and medicine is likely to remain a clinically important one and to become increasingly central to the future of psychiatry as a medical speciality.

REFERENCES

Alexander F 1950 Psychosomatic medicine: its principles and applications. Norton, New York

Alexander P J, Dinesh N, Vidyasagar M S 1993 Psychiatric morbidity among cancer patients and its relationship with awarenecss of illness and expectations about treatment outcome. Acta Oncologica 32: 623–626

APA 1994 Diagnostic and statistical manual of mental disorders, 4th edn. American Psychiatric Association, Washington, DC

Appleby L 1987 Hypochondriasis: an acceptable diagnosis? British Medical Journal 294: 857

Asher R A J 1951 Munchausen's syndrome. Lancet i: 339–341

Barbor T F, de la Fuente J R, Saunders J, Grant M 1992 AUDIT: the alcohol use disorders identification test. World Health Organization, Geneva

Barsky A J, Wyshak G 1989 Hypochondriasis and related health attitudes. Psychosomatics 30: 412–420

Barsky A J, Wyshak G, Klerman G L, Latham K S 1990 The prevalence of hypochondriasis in medical outpatients. Social Psychiatry and Psychiatric Epidemiology 25: 89–94

Bass C, Benjamin S 1993 The management of chronic somatization. British Journal of Psychiatry 162: 472–480

Bass C, Murphy M 1995 Somatoform and personality disorders: syndromal comorbidity and overlapping developmental pathways. Journal of Psychosomatic Research 39: 403–427

Billings R F, Stein M B 1986 Depression associated with ranitidine. American Journal of Psychiatry 143: 915–916

Blanchard E B, Hickling E J, Taylor A E, Loos W R, Forneris C A, Jaccard J 1996 Who develops PTSD from motor vehicle accidents? Behaviour Research and Therapy 34: 1–10

British Medical Association, Royal Pharmaceutical Society of Great Britain 1996 British national formulary, 31th edn. BMA, London

Brown F W, Golding J M, Smith G R J 1990 Psychiatric comorbidity in primary care somatization disorder. Psychosomatic Medicine 52: 445–451

Bursztajn H, Barsky A J 1985 Facilitating patient acceptance of a psychiatric referral. Archives of Internal Medicine 145: 73–75

Burvill P W, Johnson G A, Jamrozik K D, Anderson C S, Stewart Wynne E G, Chakera T M 1995 Anxiety disorders after stroke: results from the Perth Community Stroke Study. British Journal of Psychiatry 166: 328–332

Carney R M, Rich M W, teVelde A, Saini J, Clark K,

Freedland K E 1987 Prevalence of major depressive disorder in patients receiving beta-blocker therapy versus other medications. American Journal of Medicine 83: 223–226

Carney R M, Freedland K E, Eisen S A, Rich M W, Jaffe A S 1995 Major depression and medication adherence in elderly patients with coronary artery disease. Health Psychology 14: 88–90

Cassem N H, Hackett T P 1977 Psychological aspects of myocardial infarction. Medical Clinics of North America 61: 711–721

Chick J 1991 Early intervention for hazardous drinking in the general hospital. Alcohol Alcohol Suppl 1: 4779: 477–479

Cohen-Cole S A, Brown F, McDaniel J S 1993 Diagnostic assessment of depression in the medically ill. In: Stoudemire A, Fogel B (eds) Psychiatric care of the medical patient. Oxford University Press, New York, pp 53–70

Conigrave K M, Burns F H, Reznik R B, Saunders J B 1991 Problem drinking in emergency department patients: the scope for early intervention. Medical Journal of Australia 154: 801–805

Creed F H 1991 Liaison psychiatry for the 21st century: a review. Journal of the Royal Society of Medicine 84: 414–417

Cummings J L 1992 Depression and Parkinson's disease: a review. American Journal of Psychiatry 149: 443–454

Cutting J 1980 Physical illness and psychosis. British Journal of Psychiatry 136: 109–119

de Leon J, Bott A, Simpson G M 1989 Dysmorphophobia: body dysmorphic disorder or delusional disorder, somatic subtype? Comprehensive Psychiatry 30: 457–472

Dulmen van A M, Fennis J F, Mokkink H G, Velden van der H G, Bleijenberg G 1995 Doctor-dependant changes in complaint related cognitions and anxiety during medical consultations in functional abdominal complaints. Psychological Medicine 25: 1011–1018

Eisenberg L 1986 Mindlessness and brainlessness in psychiatry. British Journal of Psychiatry 148: 497–508

Elks M L 1994 On the genesis of somatization disorder: the role of the medical profession. Medical Hypotheses 43: 151–154

Emmerson J P, Burvill P W, Finlay Jones R, Hall W 1989 Life events, life difficulties and confiding relationships in the depressed elderly. British Journal of Psychiatry 155: 787–792

Engel G L 1977 The need for a new medical model: a challenge for biomedicine. Science 196: 129–196

Enright S J 1997 Cognitive behaviour therapy – clinical applications. British Medical Journal 314: 1811–1816

Escobar J I, Burnam M A, Karno M, Forsythe A, Golding J M 1987 Somatization in the community. Archives of General Psychiatry 44: 713–718

Fabrega H J 1990 The concept of somatization as a cultural and historical product of Western medicine. Psychosomatic Medicine 52: 653–672

Fink P 1992 Surgery and medical treatment in persistent somatizing patients. Journal of Psychosomatic Research 36: 439–447

Fitzpatrick R M, Hopkins A 1981 Referral to neurologists for headaches not due to structural disease. Journal of Neurology. Neurosurgery and Psychiatry 44: 1061–1067

Folstein M F, Folstein S E, McHugh P R 1975 Mini-mental state. Journal of Psychiatric Research 12: 189–198

Francis J, Martin D, Kapoor W N 1990 A prospective study of delirium in hospitalized elderly. Journal of the American Medical Association 263: 1097–1101

Frasure-Smith N, Lesperance F, Talajic M 1995 Depression and 18-month prognosis after myocardial infarction. Circulation 91: 999–1005

Freeling P, Rao B M, Paykel E S, Sireling L I, Burton R H 1985 Unrecognised depression in general practice. British Medical Journal 290: 1880–1883

Fukuda K, Straus S E, Hickie I B, Sharpe M, Dobbins J G, Komaroff A L 1994 Chronic fatigue syndrome: a comprehensive approach to its definition and management. Annals of Internal Medicine 121: 953–959

Ghodse H 1981 Drug-related problems in London accident and emergency departments. A twelve month survey. Lancet ii: 859–862

Gill D, Hatcher S 1997 A systematic review of the treatment of depression with antidepressant drugs in patients who also have a physical illness. (submitted for publication)

Godding P R, McAnulty R D, Wittrock D A, Britt D M, Khansur T 1995 Predictors of depression among male cancer patients. Journal of Nervous and Mental Disease 183: 95–98

Goldberg D 1996 psychological disorders in general medical settings. Social Psychiatry and Psychiatric Epidemiology 31: 1–2

Goldberg D P 1992 The treatment of mental disorders in general medical settings. General Hospital Psychiatry 14: 83–85

Goldberg D P, Bridges K 1988 Somatic presentations of psychiatric illness in primary care setting. Journal of Psychosomatic Research 32: 137–144

Granville-Grossman K 1993. Mind and body In: Lader M (ed) Handbook of psychiatry. Cambridge University Press, Cambridge, vol 2

Guthrie E 1996 Emotional disorder in chronic illness: psychotherapeutic interventions. British Journal of Psychiatry 168: 265–273

Guze S B 1993 Genetics of Briquet's syndrome and somatization disorder. A review of family, adoption, and twin studies. Annals of Clinical Psychiatry 5: 225–230

Guze S B, Cloninger C R, Martin R L, Clayton P J 1986 A follow-up and family study of Briquet's syndrome. British Journal of Psychiatry 149: 17–23

Hamilton J, Campos R, Creed F 1996 Anxiety, depression and the management of medically unexplained symptoms in medical clinics. Journal of the Royal College of Physicians of London 30: 18–20

Hawton K E 1984 Sexual adjustment of men who have had strokes. Journal of Psychosomatic Research 28: 243–249

Hawton K E 1996 Self-poisoning and the general hospital. Quarterly Journal of Medicine 89: 879–880

Hobbs M, Mayou R, Harrison B, Worlock P 1996 A randomised controlled trial of psychological debriefing for victims of road traffic accidents. British Medical Journal 313: 1438–1439

Holmes K M, Salter R H, Cole T P 1987 A profile of district hospital gastroenterology. Journal of the Royal College of Physicans of London 21: 111–114

House A 1988 Mood disorders in the physically ill – problems of definition and measurement. Journal of Psychosomatic Research 32: 345–353

House A O, Andrews H B 1988 Life events and difficulties preceding the onset of functional dysphonia. Journal of Psychosomatic Research 32: 311–319

House A O, Dennis M, Mogridge L, Hawton K E, Warlow C 1990 Life events and difficulties preceeding stroke. Journal of Neurology, Neurosurgery and Psychiatry 53: 1024–1028

Howland R H 1993 General health, health care utilization, and medical comorbidity in dysthymia. International Journal of Psychiatry in Medicine 23: 211–238

Hudson J I, Pope H G 1994 The concept of affective spectrum disorder: relationship to fibromyalgia and other syndromes of chronic fatigue and chronic muscle pain. Baillère's Clinical Rheumatology 8: 839–856

Huyse F J, Strain J J, Hammer J S 1990 Interventions in consultation/liaison psychiatry. Part II: Concordance. General Hospital Psychiatry 12: 221–231

Kaaya S, Goldberg D, Gask L 1992 Management of somatic presentations of psychiatric illness in general medical settings: evaluation of a new training course for general practitioners. Medical Education 26: 138–144

Kashner T M, Rost K M, Cohen B S, Anderson M, Smith G R 1995 Enhancing the health of somatization disorder patients. Psychosomatics 36: 462–469

Kathol R G 1994 Medical psychiatry units: the wave of the future. General Hospital Psychiatry 16: 1–3

Kathol R G, Wenzel R P 1992 Natural history of symptoms of depression and anxiety during inpatient treatment on general medicine wards. Journal of General Internal Medicine 7: 287–293

Kathol R G, Mutgi A, Williams J, Clamond G, Noyes R 1990 Diagnosis of major depression in cancer patients according to four sets of criteria. American Journal of Psychiatry 147: 1021–1024

Katon W J 1996a The impact of major depression on chronic medical illness. General Hospital Psychiatry 18: 215–219

Katon W 1996b Panic disorder: relationship to high medical utilization, unexplained physical symptoms, and medical costs. Journal of Clinical Psychiatry 57 (suppl 10): 11–8; discussion 19–22

Katon W J, Gonzales J J 1994 A review of randomized trials of psychiatric consultation liaison studies in primary care. Psychosomatics 35: 268–278

Katon W J, Schulberg H 1992 Epidemiology of depression in primary care. General Hospital Psychiatry 14: 237–247

Katon W J, Sullivan M D 1995 Antidepressant treatment of functional somatic symptoms. In: Mayou R, Bass C, Sharpe M (eds) Treatment of functional somatic symptoms. Oxford University Press, Oxford, pp 89–102

Katon W J, Lin E H, Von Korff M, Russo J E, Lipscomb P, Bush T 1991 Somatization: a spectrum of severity. American Journal of Psychiatry 148: 34–40

Katon W J, Robinson P, Von Korff M et al 1996 A multifaceted intervention to improve treatment of depression in primary care. Archives of General Psychiatry 53: 924–932

Kelly W F, Kelly M J, Faragher B 1996 A prospective study of psychiatric and psychological aspects of Cushing's syndrome. Clinical Endocrinology 45: 715–720

Kenyon F 1964 Hypochondriasis: a clinical study. British Journal of Psychiatry 100: 478–488

Kiecolt-Glaser J K, Galser R 1989 Psychoneuroimmunology: past, present, and future. Health Psychology 8: 677–682

Kirmayer L J 1988 Mind and body as metaphors: hidden values in biomedicine. In: Lock M, Gordon D (eds) Biomedicine examined. Kluwer, Dordrecht, pp 57–92

Kirmayer L, Robbins J M 1991 Three forms of somatization in primary care: prevalence co-occurrence and sociodemographic characteristics. Journal of Nervous and Mental Disease 179: 647–655

Koopman C, Classen C, Cardena E, Spiegel D 1995 When disaster strikes, acute stress disorder may follow. Journal of Traumatic Stress 8: 29–46

Kovacs M, Ho V, Pollock M H 1995 Criterion and predictive validity of the diagnosis of adjustment disorder: a prospective study of youths with new-onset insulin-dependent diabetes mellitus. American Journal of Psychiatry 152: 523–528

Kroenke K, Mangelsdorff D 1989 Common symptoms in ambulatory care: incidence, evaluation, therapy and outcome. American Journal of Medicine 86: 262–266

Kroenke K, Price R K 1993 Symptoms in the community. Prevalence, classification, and psychiatric comorbidity. Archives of Internal Medicine 153: 2474–2480

Kroenke K, Lucas C A, Rosenberg M L, Scherokman B J 1993 Psychiatric disorders and functional impairment in patients with persistent dizziness. Journal of General Internal Medicine 8: 530–535

Larson E B, Omenn G S, Lewis H 1980 Diagnostic evaluation of headache. Impact of computerized tomography and cost-effectiveness. Journal of the American Medical Association 243: 359–362

Levenson J L, Hamer R M, Rossiter L F 1990 Relation of psychopathology in general medical inpatients to use and cost of services. American Journal of Psychiatry 147: 1498–1503

Levenson J L, Hamer R M, Rossiter L F 1992 A randomized controlled study of psychiatric consultation guided by screening in general medical inpatients. American Journal of Psychiatry 149: 631–637

Mace C J, Trimble M R 1996 Ten-year prognosis of conversion disorder. British Journal of Psychiatry 169: 282–288

Maguire P 1990 The psychological consequences of the surgical treatment of cancer of the breast. Surgery Annual 22: 77–91

Mathew R J, Weinman M L, Mirabi M 1981 Physical symptoms of depression. British Journal of Psychiatry 139: 293–296

Mayou R A, Sharpe M 1995 Psychiatric illness associated with physical disease. Baillière's Clinical Psychiatry 1: 201–224

Mayou R A, Smith E B O 1986 Hospital doctors' management of psychological problems. British Journal of Psychiatry 148: 194–197

Mayou R A, Smith K A 1997 Post traumatic symptoms following medical illness and treatment. Journal of Psychosomatic Research 43: 121–123

Mayou R A, Hawton K E, Feldman E, Ardern M 1991 Psychiatric problems among medical admissions. International Journal of Psychiatry in Medicine 21: 71–84

Mayou R A, Bryant B, Duthie R 1993 Psychiatric consequences of road traffic accidents. British Medical Journal 307: 657–651

Mayou R A, Bryant B, Forfar C, Clark D M 1995 Non-cardiac chest pain and benign palpitations in the cardiac clinic. British Heart Journal 72: 548–553

Metcalfe R, Firth D, Pollock S, Creed F H 1988 Psychiatric morbidity and illness behaviour in female neurological in-patients. Journal of Neurology, Neurosurgery and Psychiatry 51: 1387–1390

Moffic H S, Paykel E S 1975 Depression in medical in-patients. British Journal of Psychiatry 126: 346–353

Morris P L, Robinson R G, Samuels J F 1993 Depression, introversion and mortality following stroke. Australian and New Zealand Journal of Psychiatry 27: 443–449

Munk-Jorgensen P, Fink P, Brevik J I et al 1997 Psychiatric morbidity in primary public health care: a multicentre investigation. Part II. Hidden morbidity and choice of treatment. Acta Psychiatrica Scandinavica 95: 6–12

Murphy M R 1989 Somatisation: embodying the problem. British Medical Journal 298: 1331–1332

Noyes Jr R, Kathol R G, Fisher M M, Phillips B M, Suelzer M T, Woodman C L 1994a Psychiatric comorbidity among patients with hypochondriasis. General Hospital Psychiatry 16: 78–87

Noyes Jr R, Kathol R G, Fisher M M, Phillips B M, Suelzer M T, Woodman C L 1994b One-year follow-up of medical outpatients with hypochondriasis. Psychosomatics 35: 533–545

O'Carroll R 1987 Psychiatric effects of steroids. Lancet i: 1212

Orford J, Somers M, Daniels V, Kirby B 1992 Drinking amongst medical patients: levels of risk and models of change. British Journal of Addiction 87: 1691–1702

Oxman T E, Barrett J E, Freeman D H, Manheimer E 1994 Frequency and correlates of adjustment disorder related to cardiac surgery in older patients. Psychosomatics 35: 557–568

Parle M, Maguire P, Heavan C 1997 The development of a training model to improve health professionals' skills, self efficacy and outcome expectances when communicating with cancer patients. Social Science in Medicine 44: 231–240

Persson J, Magnusson P H 1988 Comparison between different methods of detecting patients with excessive consumption of alcohol. Acta Medica Scandinavica 223: 101–109

Pilowsky I 1969 Abnormal illness behaviour. Psychological Medicine 42: 347–351

Pribor E F, Yutzy S H, Dean J T, Wetzel R D 1993 Briquet's syndrome, dissociation, and abuse. American Journal of Psychiatry 150: 1507–1511

Reichsman F, Levy N 1973 Problems in adaptation to maintainance haemodialysis: a four year study of 25 patients. Archives of Internal Medicine 130: 859–865

Robinson R G, Morris P L, Fedoroff J P 1990 Depression and cerebrovascular disease. Journal of Clinical Psychiatry 51 (suppl): 26–31

Rodin G M, Daneman D 1992 Eating disorders and IDDM. A problematic association. Diabetes Care 15: 1402–1412

Roy-Byrne P P, Katon W 1997 Generalized anxiety disorder in primary care: the precursor/modifier pathway to increased health care utilization. Journal of Clinical Psychiatry 58 (suppl 3): 34–38; discussion 39–40

Royal College of Physicians, Royal College of Psychiatrists 1995 Joint working party report: the psychological care of medical patients; recognition of need and service provision. Royal College of Physicians, London

Sadovnick A D, Remick R A, Allen J et al 1996 Depression and multiple sclerosis. Neurology 46: 628–632

Salkovskis P M, Warwick H M 1986 Morbid preoccupations, health anxiety and reassurance: a cognitive–behavioural approach to hypochondriasis. Behaviour Research and Therapy 24: 597–602

Scarone S, Gambini O 1991 Delusional hypochondriasis: nosographic evaluation, clinical course and therapeutic outcome of 5 cases. Psychopathology 24: 179–184

Shalev A Y 1996 Treatment of posttraumatic stress disorder: a review. Psychosomatic Medicine 58: 165–182

Sharpe M 1995 Theories, concepts and terminology. In: Mayou R, Bass C, Sharpe M (eds) Treatment of functional somatic symptoms. Oxford University Press, Oxford, pp 89–102

Sharpe M 1996a Chronic fatigue syndrome. Psychiatric Clinics of North America 19: 549–574

Sharpe M 1996b Psychosomatic medicine and evidence based treatment. Journal of Psychosomatic Research 41: 101–107

Sharpe M, Peveler R 1996 Deliberate self-harm, substance misuse and eating disorders. In: Creed F, Guthrie E (eds) Seminars in liaison psychiatry. Royal College of Psychiatrists, London

Sharpe M, Mayou R A, Seagroatt V et al 1994 Why do doctors find some patients difficult to help? Quarterly Journal of Medicine 87: 187–193

Sharpe M, Guthrie E A, Peveler R, Feldman E 1996 The psychological care of medical patients: a challenge for undergraduate medical education. Journal of the Royal College of Physicians of London 30: 202–204

Sherbourne C D, Jackson C A, Meredith L S, Camp P, Wells K B 1996 Prevalence of comorbid anxiety disorders in primary care outpatients. Archives of Family Medicine 5: 27–34

Shorter E 1992 From paralysis to fatigue: a history of psychosomatic illness in the modern era. Free Press, New York

Simon G E, Ormel J, Von Korff M, Barlow W 1995 Health care costs associated with depressive and anxiety disorders in primary care. American Journal of Psychiatry 152: 352–357

Slater E O 1965 Diagnosis of hysteria. British Medical Journal 1: 1395–1399

Smith G R, Monson R A, Ray D C 1986 Patients with multiple unexplained symptoms. Archives of Internal Medicine 146: 69–72

Speckens A E, Van Hemert A M, Spinhoven P, Hawton K E, Bolk J H, Rooijmans H G 1995 Cognitive behavioural therapy for medically unexplained physical symptoms: a randomised controlled trial. British Medical Journal 311: 1328–1332

Spitzer R L, Williams J B, Kroenke K et al 1994 Utility of a new procedure for diagnosing mental disorders in primary care. The PRIME-MD 1000 study. Journal of the American Medical Association 272: 1749–1756

Steel J, Taylor R, Lloyd G 1986 Behaviour therapy for phobia of venepuncture. Diabetic Medicine 3: 481

Stern J, Murphy M, Bass C 1993 Personality disorders in patients with somatisation disorder. A controlled study. British Journal of Psychiatry 163: 785–789

Stern R, Fernandez M 1991 Group cognitive and behavioural treatment for hypochondriasis. British Medical Journal 303: 1229–1231

Strain J J, Stoudemire G A, Hales R E, Wolf D 1989 Critical issues in the review of diagnostic criteria for 'adjustment disorders' and 'psychological factors affecting physical conditon'. General Hospital Psychiatry 11: 153–155

Strain J, Lyons J S, Hammer J S et al 1991 Cost offset from a psychiatric consultation–liaison intervention with elderly hip fracture patients. American Journal of Psychiatry 148: 1044–1049

Sullivan M D, Youngner S J 1994 Depression, competence, and the right to refuse lifesaving medical treatment. American Journal of Psychiatry 151: 971–978

Sutherland A J, Rodin G M 1990 Factitious disorders in a general hospital setting: clinical features and a review of the literature. Psychosomatics 31: 392–399

Taylor D, Lewis S 1993 Delirium. Journal of Neurology, Neurosurgery and Psychiatry 56: 742–751

Tollefson G D, Tollefson S L, Pederson M, Luxenberg M 1991 Comorbid irritable bowel syndrome in patients with generalized anxiety and major depression. Annals of Clinical Psychiatry 3: 215–222

Trimble M R 1982 Functional diseases. British Medical Journal 285: 1768–1770

Van Hemert A M, Hawton K E, Bolk J H, Fagg J R 1993a Key symptoms in the detection of affective disorders in medical patients. Journal of Psychosomatic Research 37: 397–404

Van Hemert A M, Hengeveld M W, Bolk J H, Rooijmans H G, Vandenbroucke J P 1993b Psychiatric disorder in relation to medical illness among patients of a general medical outpatient clinic. Psychological Medicine 23: 167–173

Veale D, Boocock A, Gournay K et al 1996 Body dysmorphic disorder. A survey of fifty cases. British Journal of Psychiatry 169: 196–201

Von Korff M, Simon G 1996 The relationship between pain and depression. British Journal of Psychiatry 168 (suppl 30): 101–108

Ware J E, Sherbourne C D 1992 The MOS 36-item short-form health survey. Medical Care 30: 473–481

Warwick H M, Salkovskis P M 1985 Reassurance. British Medical Journal 290: 1028

Warwick H M, Salkovskis P M 1990 Hypochondriasis. Behaviour Research and Therapy 28: 105–117

Wells J E, Robins L N, Bushnell J A, Jarosz D, Oakley-Browne M A 1994 Perceived barriers to care in St Louis (USA) and Christchurch (NZ): reasons for not seeking professional help for psychological distress. Social Psychiatry and Psychiatric Epidemiology 29: 155–164

Wells K B, Golding J M, Burnam M A 1988 Psychiatric disorder in a sample of the general population with and without chronic medical conditions. American Journal of Psychiatry 145: 976–981

Wells K B, Stewart A, Hays R D 1989 The functioning and well-being of depressed patients. Journal of the American Medical Association 262: 914–919

Wessely S, Lewis G H 1989 The classification of psychiatric morbidity in attenders at a dermatology clinic. British Journal of Psychiatry 155: 686–691

Weyerer S 1990 Relationships between physical and psychological disorders. In: Sartoris N, Goldberg D, de Girolamo G, Costa e Silva J A, Lecrubier Y, Wittchen H U (eds) Psychological disorders in general medical settings. Hogrefe & Huber, Toronto, pp 34–46

WHO 1992 The ICD-10 classification of mental and behavioural disorders, 10th edn. World Health Organization, Geneva

Whybrow P C, Prange Jr A J, Treadway C R 1969 Mental changes accompanying thyroid gland dysfunction. A reappraisal using objective psychological measurement. Archives of General Psychiatry 20: 48–63

Wilson D R, Widmer R B, Cadoret R J, Judiesch K 1994 Somatic symptoms: a major feature of depression in a family practice. Journal of Affective Disorders 5: 199–207

Wolfe F, Smythe H A, Yunus M B et al 1990 The American College of Rheumatology 1990 criteria for the classification of fibromyalgia. Report of the Multicenter Criteria Committee. Arthritis and Rheumatism 33: 160–172

Zigmond A S, Snaith R P 1983 The hospital anxiety and depression scale. Acta Psychiatrica Scandinavica 67: 361–370

Zubaran C, Fernandes J G, Rodnight R 1997 Wernicke–Korsakoff syndrome. Postgraduate Medical Journal 73: 27–31

28

The relationship between crime and psychiatry

Derek Chiswick

INTRODUCTION

This chapter is about the relationship between crime and mental disorder, the forensic aspects of certain psychiatric disorders, risk assessment, the clinical aspects of certain crimes, and the mentally disordered offender in the criminal justice system.

Biological basis for crime

In 1995 police in England and Wales recorded over 5 million crimes, an increase of 31% since 1987. Increases, not quite as high, have been reported over the same period elsewhere in the Western world. Crime is therefore common. A third of men, and 8% of women, born in 1953 were convicted of an offence by the age of 40, though one-fifth of the men (7% of the male population) accounted for more than 60% of the crimes (Home Office 1996). Crime is an activity of teenagers and young adults; the rates peak at 15–17 years for males and decline after the age of 18. Females account for about 1 in 5 offenders and their peak age for offending is 2–3 years earlier than for males. Theft in its various forms, car crimes and criminal damage account for over 90% of notifiable crimes.

Before considering the association between individual psychiatric disorders and crime, we will briefly consider the biological basis for criminal behaviour generally. For an activity as common, and yet diverse, as crime most observers agree that explanations must be multifactorial in type, and that postulating a single mental condition as the 'cause' of criminal behaviour would be absurd. None the less researchers continue to seek evidence of a criminal trait and to explore whether biological factors make a contribution to criminal behaviour. Farrington (1993) has provided an excellent review of the psychosocial factors associated with criminal behaviour, and Smith (1995) in the distinguished report of the *Academia Europaea* (Rutter & Smith 1995) describes how the complex correlates of the recent increase in juvenile crime might act together.

Farrington points out that few studies in this area meet optimal criteria of prospectively studying a large general population sample, over a long period, recording a wide range of variables, and using both self-report and criminal records for measures of offending. Many of the factors identified by Farrington as contributory to criminal behaviour are beyond the scope of this chapter but they are included below to emphasise that crime is multifactorial:

- genetic factors
- personality and impulsivity
- intelligence
- the natural history of offending behaviour
- family influences
- peer influence
- schools
- socioeconomic deprivation
- community influences
- ethnicity.

It is probably unwise to consider criminal behaviour in youngsters as though it were a unitary phenomenon. Offending behaviour that begins and ends in adolescence may be a separate phenomenon from preadolescent-onset offending which often continues throughout adolescence into adult life (Moffitt 1993a). The former is probably less pathological than the latter, which is more likely to be associated with hyperactivity in childhood and neuropsychological deficits (Rutter 1996).

Genetics, personality and intelligence factors

The bedrock of genetic evidence for criminality is in the classical twin and adoption studies of heritability reviewed by McGuffin & Thapar (1992), Carey (1994) and Rutter (1996). Concordance for criminality is up to six times greater in monozygotic than in dizygotic twins (Dalgaard & Kringlen 1976, Christiansen 1977). Adoption studies show much greater correlations of criminal behaviour of adopted children with their biological than with their adoptive parents (Cloninger et al 1982, Mednick et al 1984).

These findings are not universally accepted. A meta-analysis of the genetic literature found only a 'low-moderate correlation' between heredity and crime, and the role of inheritance in violent crime (as distinct from property crime) has not been demonstrated (Walters 1992, Carey 1994, Alper 1995). Even if genetic transmission plays a part in the endowment (or potential endowment) of a personal characteristic that is conducive to offending, the nature of that characteristic, how it is modified by other factors, and how its expression leads to offending remain unknown. These conclusions are far removed from popular notions of a 'gene for crime' which were fuelled in the 1960s by the hypothesis that people with an extra Y chromosome were predisposed to criminal behaviour. Later research failed to support the original hypothesis (Borgaonkar & Shah 1974).

The genetic element, if present, may have its effect on the constellation of hyperactivity/inattention/impulsivity; certainly attention deficit hyperactivity disorder (ADHD) in childhood is associated with later offending (Sandberg 1996) and is also a disorder of adults (Toone & van der Linden 1997). The genetic risk may be mediated through abnormal neuropsychological or cognitive functioning (Moffitt 1993b). There is evidence of neuropsychological impairment in some offenders (Taylor 1993a).

Findings from studies of neuroanatomical pathways thought to be associated with violence in animal models may have applicability in man (Garza-Trevino 1994). The possibility of genetically-determined abnormal neurotransmission in the central nervous system of offenders has been explored, principally by Virkkunen in Finland. He reported low turnover of brain serotonin in alcoholic violent offenders, together with an abnormality in the gene thought to control serotonin breakdown (Virkkunen et al 1996). There is also some evidence of low cholesterol levels in American army veterans with antisocial personality disorder, but a Scottish study showed no association between serum cholesterol and aggressive personality traits (Fowkes et al 1992, Freedman et al 1995). The significance of these biochemical findings in relation to criminal behaviour is uncertain.

Any gene expression is likely to act in concert with environmental factors such as violent or incompetent parents, or inadequate role models. In a Danish study of 397 males followed from birth to early adult life, a subgroup with both early neuromotor deficits and unstable families showed more than twice the adolescent disturbance and adult criminal behaviour than subgroups with either neuromotor deficits or family

instability alone (Raine et al 1996). This psychosocially damaged subgroup (44% of the cohort) accounted for 70% of the total crime committed by the cohort.

There is a long established link between low intelligence and delinquency (Rutter & Giller 1983). The inference that this results from an increased likelihood of duller offenders being caught is not borne out by research. The finding holds for self-reported, as well as recorded, offending even though offending by less intelligent youngsters is more likely to be 'missed' in self-report research. Low intelligence is probably related to general neuropsychological deficits, particularly the ability to manipulate abstract concepts. Conversely high intelligence may be protective for high-risk children, giving them the opportunity to escape from a ghetto background.

The interaction of biological and social disadvantage is encapsulated in a disturbing study of 14 juveniles on death row in America (Lewis et al 1988). The youths showed serious central nervous system deficits, low intelligence and multiple psychotic symptoms. Five had been sodomised by a relative and nearly all came from violent families.

Finally, evidence of a genetic basis for criminal behaviour has obvious social and legal implications. So far, the admissibility of such evidence in cases coming before the courts in America and elsewhere has met with varying success. The XYY syndrome has been introduced but failed as a defence in five major American cases; in Australia, France and Germany it may have been a factor affecting sentence in some cases (Denno 1996). Of more interest is the case of Stephen Mobley, who in 1991 shot and killed a pizza store manager in Georgia during an armed robbery. On the basis of his personal, criminal and family history, his lawyer requested the court that he undergo testing for a possible genetic absence of isoenzyme monoamine oxidase A to establish whether he suffered from a syndrome reported in a Dutch family by Brunner et al (1993). The court refused the testing and Mobley now has an appeal pending while he awaits execution on death row.

CRIME AND MENTAL DISORDER

Some people with a psychiatric disorder may behave in a criminal manner, and some offenders have psychiatric disorders. Crime and psychiatric disorder is therefore a legitimate area for psychiatric study but attempts to understand what, if any, is the relationship between crime and psychiatric disorder are fraught with problems. These arise for five principal reasons:

- Crime is a man-made concept; it is whatever a

society chooses at any particular time to decree as unlawful. The classifications of crime change within the same country over time (e.g. in the UK in relation to abortion, homosexual acts and prostitution), and they vary from country to country.

- The use of a person's criminal record as a measure of his offending is unreliable: most crime is unreported and undetected. It is also impossible to glean the nature and gravity of an offence simply from its statutory description. Indecent assault, for example, may be the merest contact between perpetrator and victim or a sexual attack of homicidal intensity. Classification of the degree of violence in an assault is an inexact science.

- Most research is based on captive populations of offenders (and patients) because this is more easily conducted. There are no systems for the routine psychiatric examination of court-based samples. Thus criminals in prison are more likely to be studied than either criminals in the community or criminals who are never caught. Extrapolating findings from such samples may be misleading. Self-report studies and criminal surveys of community samples are of greater value and are beginning to be reported. Similarly, psychiatric research cohorts in this field tend to be on inpatient rather than community-based samples. It may not be possible to generalise findings from these restricted samples. Recently research has been on cohorts which include undetected sufferers of psychiatric disorder.

- Great care must be taken before extrapolating findings from one population to another. The relation between crime and mental disorder is affected by overall rates of crime, the operation of the criminal justice system, social policy in respect of offenders and the nature and the provision of health and social care for mentally disordered people. These factors differ between countries and in different areas of the same country; they also vary over time within individual countries. Conclusions must therefore be considered in the context of prevailing circumstances.

- Use of standardised diagnostic criteria in research on offender populations is relatively recent. Older studies tend to group together all diagnostic categories, often including personality disorders and substance misuse disorders.

While bearing in mind the limitations imposed by these factors it is convenient to consider the relationship between crime and mental disorder by examining:

- the extent of mental disorder among offenders
- the criminality of psychiatric populations

- the manner in which specific psychiatric disorders might sometimes be associated with criminal acts.

Mental disorder in offenders

Prison studies

There are no published reports in Britain on the psychiatric condition of all offenders either arrested or passing through the criminal courts on a particular day or at a particular time. Studies of people arrested by the police are referred to later in this chapter. There have been many studies of imprisoned offenders. These may tell us a little about the psychiatry of offending but the findings are affected by the selective processes of criminal prosecution and of imprisonment.

Prisons contain two distinct populations. Untried or remanded prisoners are those awaiting trial or sentence. Sentenced prisoners are those who have been convicted and are serving a sentence. The remanded population is an unsifted population, whereas the sentenced population has gone through various filtering processes in which psychiatric assessment may have led to the removal of mentally disordered prisoners. There have been three large psychiatric studies of remanded prison populations in Britain (Davidson et al 1995, Birmingham et al 1996, Brooke et al 1996). There has also been a comprehensive survey of sentenced prisoners in England (Gunn et al 1991) (Table 28.1).

The findings for psychotic disorders in remanded prisoners (2–5%) are in keeping with the previous studies comprehensively reviewed by Coid (1984) but markedly less than the 9% reported by Taylor & Gunn (1984) in their study of all receptions at Brixton Prison, London. Prevalence figures of psychiatric disorder, particularly in the remand populations, are largely dependent on the availability of local alternatives to prosecution and remand in custody. The impact of alcohol- and drug-related conditions in both remanded and sentenced prisoners is clear. Comorbidity of substance misuse and psychotic disorders is common, and there is evidence that subgroups of schizophrenia such as delusional disorder and 'not otherwise specified' are more common in prison than in hospital populations (Cote et al 1997).

Female prisoners Women in prison show higher rates of neurotic conditions, personality disorder and substance abuse than men (Maden et al 1990). Prison has become a receptacle for some very disturbed women. They are less likely than male prisoners to be serving a sentence for violence or burglary but are more likely to have committed a drug offence, theft, fraud or deception (Player & Jenkins 1994). High levels of psychiatric morbidity have been reported elsewhere. A

Table 28.1 British studies of psychiatric disorder in male prisoners					
Study	No. of subjects	Psychosis (%)	Neurosis (%)	Personality disorder (%)	Substance abuse (%)
Sentenced: England (Gunn et al 1991)	1769	2	6	10	23
Remand: Scotland (Davidson et al 1995)	371	2.3	NR	NR	73
Remand: England (Birmingham et al 1996)	569	5	9	7	36
Remand: England (Brooke et al 1996)	750	5	26	11	38

NR not recorded.

study of 1272 remanded women in Chicago found that 80% had a lifetime prevalence of at least one psychiatric disorder and 70 were symptomatic within the 6 months prior to the research interview. Substance abuse and post-traumatic stress disorder were the most common diagnoses (Teplin et al 1996).

Criminality in psychiatric populations

The traditional view

Criminal behaviour, particularly violence, by the mentally ill has become a major public issue in the Western world. In the context of an increasing crime rate the public has identified the mentally ill as a significant contributory factor (Appleby & Wessely 1988, Levey & Howells 1995), and politicians have responded with various initiatives (see below). The question 'How criminal are people with psychiatric disorder?' can never be answered with certainty and any answer requires qualification. In the context of all psychiatric admissions, the number of patients admitted compulsorily as a consequence of an offence is tiny; less than 1% of the 300 000 admissions in 1995 were under Part III (the criminal provisions) of the Mental Health Act 1983. During a 2 year period between 1992 and 1995 a confidential inquiry into suicides and homicides identified 39 homicides committed by current or recent psychiatric patients (Steering Committee of the Confidential Inquiry 1996). During that period there were approximately 1000 homicides in England and Wales.

This sanguine view of the relation between mental illness and violent offending prevailed for some years. It was held that the well-established factors associated with offending, such as poverty, criminality in the family, poor parenting, school failure, and hyperactivity and antisocial behaviour in childhood, were powerful fac-

tors that overshadowed any effect due to metal illness (Walker & McCabe 1973, Gibbens & Robertson 1983).

Early research in this area concentrated on arrest rates in former psychiatric patients. These were shown to be equal to, or marginally higher than, those of the general population, or only higher for certain offences (Zitrin et al 1976, Cocozza et al 1978, Sosowsky 1978). However, when arrest rates of former mental hospital patients were compared with samples matched for demographic variables, the differences disappeared (Monahan & Steadman 1983).

A reappraisal

More recently these conclusions have been reappraised by Wessely & Taylor (1991), Monahan (1993), Monahan & Steadman (1994) and Wessely (1997), driven by the fact that other research continued to show associations between violence and certain diagnostic groups. These included high rates of serious mental illness, particularly schizophrenia, in prisoners remanded in custody (see above), high rates of violence by mentally ill people before admission to hospital (MacMillan & Johnson 1987, Humphreys et al 1992) and during admission (McNiel et al 1988, Noble & Rodger 1989).

The limitations previously described apply to many of these studies. Some have been addressed, to varying degrees, in recent epidemiological surveys of community populations and in studies of birth cohorts. These have the advantages of unbiased population cohorts, inclusion of never-treated cases, robust diagnostic interviewing schedules, and self-report in addition to formal hospital and criminal records for information. The latest Danish birth cohort study (Hodgins et al 1996) has a truly huge sample (see below).

Two American population studies showed that violence was six times more common in people with a diagnosis of schizophrenia (Swanson et al 1990), and that violence was more likely in those with current psychotic symptoms irrespective of whether or not they had ever been hospital patients (Link et al 1992). Two Swedish studies of birth cohorts also found an association between schizophrenia and violence. Lindqvist & Allebeck (1990) found crimes of violence (usually minor) were four times higher among a 39 year birth cohort treated for schizophrenia than among controls. Hodgins (1992) conducted a 30 year follow-up of 15 117 people born in Stockholm in 1953. Men with a major mental disorder were 2.5 times more likely to have a criminal record than men without, and four times more likely to have been convicted of violence. For women the increased likelihood was five and 27 times respectively.

A study of all 0.36 million people born in Denmark between 1944 and 1947 and followed up until aged 43 was able to utilise the high-quality information available in the Danish psychiatric and criminal registers (Hodgins et al 1996). Those who had been hospitalised had higher rates of offending. Although this was an 'ever-hospitalised' cohort, and therefore did not include less disordered cases, these patients will have spent most of their lives in the community rather than in hospital. In this respect the patients are typical of those currently seen by psychiatric services. The rates for commission of a violent crime in various diagnostic categories, which were hierarchical, are shown in Table 28.2.

The likelihood of a person with a major mental disorder committing a violent crime was increased nearly 4.5 times in men and 8.5 times in women compared with controls. These relative risk rates were substantially lower than in those with admissions for mental retardation, antisocial personality disorder and substance misuse disorders. This lower risk rate of schizophrenia compared with other mental disorders was not found in a study of a much smaller cohort and matched controls

based on the Camberwell case register (Wessely et al 1994). In schizophrenic men the rate of overall offending was the same as that in men with other disorders, but for crimes of violence the rate was increased 3.8 times. However, the fraction of higher risk attributable to schizophrenia (assessed by survival analysis techniques) was less than that attributable to gender, substance abuse, ethnicity and early onset of the illness. For women with schizophrenia the increased rate applies to all types of offending.

Other studies and reviews point to the extremely high risk rates in those with dual diagnoses of mental illness and substance misuse (Smith & Hucker 1994). In a Finnish study, schizophrenia with secondary alcohol misuse increased the risk of homicide by 17 times in men and 80 times in women (Eronen et al 1996a).

In summary, we can conclude that the presence of any psychiatric disorder increases the chance of having a criminal conviction. Major metal illness increases the likelihood of acquiring a conviction for violence by up to five times in men and 30 times in women. Substance misuse in combination with mental illness greatly increases these risks and singly carries a higher risk than mental illness. These conclusions must be treated with caution. The strongest predictors of crime in those with schizophrenia are still the same as those that predict crime in people who do not have the disorder. Schizophrenia seems to multiply the power of these predictors. Finally, it should be emphasised that people with a mental illness make a tiny contribution to the overall amount of violent crime.

Specific psychiatric disorders and criminal acts

Schizophrenia The phenomena of schizophrenia and their association with offending have attracted relatively little research. Most investigations are of acting on delusions. Of 20 people who had pushed strangers on to New York's subway tracks, 10 were influenced by delusions or hallucinations (Martell & Dietz 1992). Taylor (1985) found that 47% of a cohort of psychotic prisoners described psychotic motivation, usually delusions, for their offences; passivity, religious and paranormal delusions were particularly noted (Taylor 1993b).

In a study that supplemented the patient's account with that of an informant, Buchanan et al (1993) found that 50% of their sample reported acting on delusions in the previous week, though rarely with violence. Patients who reported acting on delusions were more likely to have sought further evidence for their beliefs, reduced the conviction of their belief when challenged and registered accompanying affective symptoms.

Almost all types of delusions have in various studies

Table 28.2 Danish 1944–1947 birth cohort study (Hodgins et al 1996): relative risk estimates of at least one violent crime between 1978 and 1990		
Psychiatric disorder	Females (*n*=158 799)	Males (*n*=165 602)
Major mental disorder	8.66	4.48
Mental retardation	11.81	7.65
Antisocial personality disorder	12.15	7.20
Drug use disorder	15.08	8.67
Alcohol use disorder	14.87	6.68
Other mental disorder	3.97	3.15

been said to indicate a potential for violence; there are major methodological problems relating chiefly to accurate identification of phenomena. The presence of acute symptoms may be more important than their nature (Humphreys et al 1992, McNiel et al 1988); the early years of the illness seem to produce more violence than the later years (Hafner & Boker 1982). Junginger (1996) has produced a theoretical model of the way other factors in the illness, and the presence of absence of psychiatric treatment, might act as modifiers of psychiatric phenomena. A fully independent life is rarely compatible with having schizophrenia. Reliance on family, carers, health and social care staff, and housing and welfare agencies is likely to impinge significantly on daily life. Shelter, warmth and nourishment may not be easily obtained. Crime and violence even when attributable to psychotic symptoms need to be considered in the wider context. All types of offence may be committed by people with schizophrenia, including the random killing of a stranger. However, all the studies previously described report that the majority of crimes are not serious.

Affective disorders In clinical practice major affective disorder in association with crime is less commonly encountered than is schizophrenia. Grandiosity of mood and disinhibition in mania and hypomania commonly leads to public disorder and driving offences or fraud from failure to pay for restaurant and hotel bills. Less commonly there may be a serious sexual or violent crime.

The role of depressive disorders in offending behaviour is controversial and probably rare (Guze 1976). The literature on shoplifting and depression is largely historical; a recent study of 1649 shoplifters in Montreal found 1% who were suffering from depression or bipolar disorder (Lamontagne et al 1994). Of greater significance is the rare but well-recognised phenomenon of extended or altruistic homicide in which a depressed person (usually a parent) kills one or more family members (usually including a child) and then commits or attempts suicide. Given the frequency of depression and the rarity of altruistic homicide it seems an impossible task to identify these cases in advance. The epidemiology of this rare phenomenon is difficult to study but may show some similarities with that of depressive disorder (Marzuk et al 1992).

Personality disorder Surveys of offender populations always find high rates of personality disorder; this is expected as offending will often be a component in reaching the diagnosis. In practice, 'pure forms' of antisocial personality disorder are uncommon; there is often overlap with other categories of personality disorder (Coid 1992), together with other Axis I diagnoses and multiple psychiatric symptoms.

The situation is further complicated by the confusing clinical and legal terminology in relation to psychopathic disorder. The term that appears in the Mental Health Act 1983 has a legal definition and refers to a disorder that results in abnormal aggression or serious irresponsibility. It became a legal entity in the 1950s, replacing its predecessor, the moral imbecile (Home Office & Department of Health and Social Security 1975). It is therefore incorrect to assume that the disorder defined in law 50 years ago is the equivalent of any particular category of psychiatric disorder in current use. A Government working party has recommended review of the law in this area (Department of Health & Home Office 1994).

Only 35 offenders in the category psychopathic disorder were sent to hospitals by courts in 1995 (Department of Health 1996) and even this level of practice is contentious (Coid & Cordess 1992, Criminal Behaviour & Mental Health 1992). The most serious clinical difficulties are in measuring change in personality-disordered patients while they are detained in secure settings, and in making decisions about discharge (Norton & Dolan 1995). Follow-up studies show that psychopathic disorder patients discharged from secure hospitals reoffend at twice the rate of those with mental illness (Bailey & MacCulloch 1992).

Neuroses Neurotic symptoms are common in offenders but it is unusual to find a causal relationship between an offence and a disorder that satisfies ICD-10 diagnostic criteria for a neurotic, stress-related or somatoform disorder. Whether an offence is attributed to the effects of post-traumatic stress disorder or to an underlying personality disorder may depend on whether a transverse or longitudinal view of the offender's psychopathology is taken. Neurotic conflicts, as distinct from disorder, may play a speculative role in any offending behaviour, e.g. shoplifting, fire-setting or sexual offending. West (1988) has given a perceptive account of the role of individual psychopathology in crime.

Learning disability Only 76 offenders with a learning disability were admitted to hospital from courts in 1994–1995 (Department of Health 1996). Over the last 30 years there has been a major reduction in such court disposals (Langton et al 1993), though an unknown number may have dual diagnoses and be detained in the category of mental illness. Early literature contained grossly exaggerated prevalence figures for 'feeble-mindedness' among offenders (Walker & McCabe 1973). Offending by the learning disabled does not occur in a vacuum; it is subject to all the influences which typically affect offending, i.e. unstable families, poor parenting, socioeconomic disadvantage, educational underachievement and substance misuse.

Property offending predominates but the range of offences committed is wide. There is some evidence to support increased arrest rates among the learning disabled (Robertson 1988). Crimes of serious violence may be less common but arson and sexual offences were overrepresented in studies of hospital-based cohorts (Day 1990, 1994).

Substance abuse The relationship between substance abuse and crime is complex and not necessarily causal, even though problems of substance abuse are almost endemic among offender populations (Davidson et al 1995, Brooke et al 1996) and offending is common in those with alcohol and drug problems (Gordon 1990). Hore (1990) has pointed out that even intoxication at the time of the offence, which is commonly described, does not exclude other contributory factors, e.g. the social setting in which perpetrator and victim meet and consume alcohol, or the crime may be conditional upon, for example, an argument. These issues reinforce the fact that any crime rarely has unitary causation.

Alcohol consumption has been implicated in family violence (Gayford 1975), child abuse, rape and other sex offences (Rada 1975, Lindqvist 1991). In a Scottish sample of 400 individuals charged with murder, Gillies (1976) reported that 58% of the males accused and 30% of the females accused were intoxicated at the time of the offence. Over a third of the victims had also been abusing alcohol. Similar findings were reported recently from Finland, where 39% of men and 32% of women convicted of homicide had diagnoses of alcoholism (Eronen et al 1996b). Occasionally offending may be associated with the neuropsychiatric sequelae of alcoholism, such as delirium tremens or alcoholic hallucinosis. Chronic drinkers with multiple social handicaps form a large proportion of the short-sentence populations in most prisons. Many receive their only medical care when in prison.

One in 10 men and 1 in 4 women in prison have been regular users of opiates or stimulants before imprisonment (Maden et al 1990, 1991). More than a third of prisoners in Scotland have injected drugs, and the majority of these have injected in prison (Dye & Isaacs 1991). An outbreak of human immunodeficiency virus (HIV) infection has occurred in a Scottish prison (Gore & Bird 1993). The management of drug misuse in prison and measures to control HIV infection are huge tasks for prison services.

Organic conditions In theory disinhibition and impaired judgment, characteristic of organic brain disease, may lead to minor crimes of dishonesty or sexual offences. In practice elderly sexual offenders rarely have psychiatric or organic disorders (Clark & Mezey 1997). Elderly offenders convicted of other crimes have high

rates of alcohol misuse. In younger men offending may be associated with any cause of organic brain disease such as head injury or Huntington's chorea.

Epilepsy Epilepsy is a rare contributory factor to offending. Twenty years ago Gunn (1977) reported an increased prevalence of epilepsy in prisoners compared with the general population but not with a population showing the same socioeconomic disadvantage from which the prison population is typically drawn. Gunn's sample of epileptic prisoners showed no excess rates for crimes of violence. The most likely explanation for any excess, if present, is that the socioeconomic and psychosocial correlates of epilepsy are similar to those for crime in general. Serious violence as an ictal phenomenon is exceedingly rare. Even violence in temporal lobe epilepsy is not simply the result of an electrical discharge in the brain (Herzberg & Fenwick 1988).

Pathological jealousy and other disorders of passion Delusional syndromes characterised by pathological feelings of jealousy, love or entitlement are commonly associated with criminal behaviour. Pathological (or morbid) jealousy is the most common. Normal jealousy can generate criminal behaviour and the distinction between normal and pathological jealousy cannot be defined in scientific terms. The syndrome is seen in a variety of disorders. A consecutive study of over 8000 inpatients treated in Munich gave a prevalence for delusional jealousy of 1.1%, slightly more than half of whom were female (Soyka et al 1991). Organic and paranoid disorders, alcohol psychosis and schizophrenia were the most common underlying conditions, while affective disorders were rare.

The syndrome classically described by Shepherd (1961) is that of a symptomatic manifestation of one of the disorders mentioned above. The behaviour involves repeated, often violent, questioning, checking and following of the partner. There are attempts to force a 'confession'. Elaborate delusional beliefs lead to searches for 'evidence' of infidelity by the partner. The treatment is that of the underlying condition.

More difficult to assess are the remaining jealousies which Mullen (1990, 1993) refers to as normally or pathologically reactive. These have no clear boundary between them. Mullen emphasises that pathological reactive jealousy may occur in response to real or imagined infidelity: the latter is not the issue. A pathological reaction is manifested by exaggerated responses which come to dominate personal functioning and relationships. It is commonly related to problems in personality development. What then remains are 'the jealous reactions experienced by most of us at some time in our lives' (Mullen 1993).

As for offending behaviour, this is seen in all types of

jealousy, including normal reactive jealousy. Careful assessment is crucial and requires appraisals of premorbid personality, the relationship with the partner and the nature of the provoking incident or behaviour. The couple are often disparate in terms of social skills, educational attainment or occupational status. The syndrome has a high association with violence and homicide. Both partners need to be made aware of the risks, and often separation is required; this clearly does not eliminate the risk of further violence.

The delusional conviction of being loved by someone who is identified but unattainable, usually by reason of their social class or importance, is the basis of erotomania or de Clerambault's syndrome. Pursuing the object of the delusion and repeatedly pestering them by telephone, by letter and with gifts is typical. Some erotomanics 'arrange' holidays or weddings with their victims. The condition is rare but surfaces in forensic populations as a result of criminal acts secondary to the delusion (Taylor et al 1983). Menzies et al (1995) found that multiple delusional objects and a history of other antisocial behaviour were predictive of future violence. The syndrome has various aetiologies (schizophrenic and affective), though it can present as a single delusional disorder (Segal 1989). It is only one of a number of behaviours that may be associated with stalking (Mullen & Pathe 1994), a behaviour that has recently been recognised as an offence in the Protection from Harassment Act 1997.

The conviction of having been wronged by others (e.g. a doctor or lawyer or employer) and of consequent entitlement to redress is the basis of morbid querulousness. The convictions dominate, usually in fluctuating outbursts, the lives of sufferers, who hound their victims with letters, distribute leaflets, daub walls and write to newspapers and members of parliament. Often they are declared 'vexatious litigants' and become banned from using the courts. There is a high likelihood of assaults on the perceived 'wrongdoer' or damage to his or her property. As with other disorders of passion, there are various aetiologies (Rowlands 1988).

Factitious illness by proxy   This term (also known as Munchausen syndrome by proxy), correctly describes a situation rather than a psychiatric disorder (Meadow 1989, Bools 1996). The behaviour is the fabrication of symptoms in, or the injury of, a child by its carer (usually mother) who then presents the child to a doctor or other agency for treatment. Bools describes a wide range of injurious behaviours from verbal fabrications and tampering with specimens and charts to poisoning, smothering and withholding of nutrients. The condition may be a factor in child abuse and has been implicated in acts of serial killings by health care workers. Underlying psychiatric conditions include person-

ality disorders (particularly antisocial and borderline types), somatisation, affective and eating disorders and substance misuse.

Young offenders   Offending among under 16-year-olds is increasing at a higher rate than it is for older teenagers (Home Office 1996). Nearly half the youngsters serving custodial detention in excess of 12 months have committed murder, manslaughter, arson, rape and wounding. The remainder have committed robbery and burglary, nearly always having previous similar convictions. Bailey (1995) has emphasised that young offenders convicted of serious crimes have high rates of previous psychiatric contact, substance misuse, previous criminality, mental illness within the family and parental marital conflict.

Elderly offenders   Elderly offenders constitute a very small proportion of the offending population but they have high rates of psychiatric disorder. In a sample of over 1000 men remanded in prison, half the men aged over 55 had active psychiatric symptoms on admission, mostly the result of alcohol abuse (Taylor & Parrott 1988). Needham-Bennett et al (1996) studied 50 consecutive police referrals of offenders aged over 60 to a community service. Shoplifting accounted for 63% of offences and 28% of the sample scored as 'cases' on a computerised diagnostic screening device for the elderly.

Risk assessment and dangerousness

Dangerousness is not a scientific concept and has no satisfactory clinical definition (Chiswick 1995). It refers to the perception by others that a person who has behaved in a violent manner will do so again. Consideration of this aspect of a patient forms part of daily decision making. In relation to mentally disordered offenders it has particular relevance when considering:

- the appropriate security environment for treatment
- discharge to a community setting
- the application of a restriction order under section 41 of the Mental Health Act 1983.

Research findings

Research has concentrated on the relationship between psychiatric disorder and reoffending, the fate in the community of discharged 'dangerous' patients and the reliability of predictions of dangerousness.

The most dangerous psychiatric patients may be expected to be those who have been detained under restriction orders and/or are discharged from high security hospitals. Special hospital follow-up studies in the last decade show that up to 50% reoffended and 10% did so seriously (Chiswick 1995). Restricted patients conditionally discharged to the community between 1972 and 1990 had a reconviction rate within 5 years of 27%, of which 5% were for a grave offence; reconviction rates since 1987 have lessened compared with earlier years (Kershaw et al 1997). These rates are much lower than for prisoners released from custody: 50% of men released from prison between 1983 and 1992 reoffended within 2 years (Kershaw et al 1997). Factors known to be associated with reoffending on discharge from high security care are (Murray 1989):

- previous criminal record, particularly extensive property offending
- younger age
- admission offence (property offender more likely to reoffend, homicidal offender less likely to reoffend than other violent offenders)
- shorter length of stay
- absolute discharge rather than conditional discharge
- discharge by a mental health review tribunal
- legal category of psychopathic disorder.

The reliability of predictions of dangerousness have been criticised for their inaccuracy. For example, Monahan (1984) famously concluded that for every one person detained in hospital due to dangerousness, a further two are detained unnecessarily, and that the best predictor of future offending is the previous criminal record irrespective of any mental disorder. These observations are based, in part, on outdated literature with methodological problems. Accuracy in prediction studies is affected by:

- the nature of the cohort, e.g. whether hospital or community based and whether community-based patients received any treatment
- whether allowance is made for unreported crime
- whether allowance is made for the institutional suppression of violence, i.e. violence that may occur is prevented in hospital settings
- whether data has been collected in a standardised manner.

Risk assessment in practice

The notion that certain psychiatric patients possess an innate makeup that marks them out from other patients as dangerous has outlived its usefulness. Research and practical experience have shown that, even if this were true, the ability of psychiatrists to identify dangerous patients from among others with similar conditions has not been good. Furthermore, the contextual element for violence by psychiatric patients is so important that the once-and-for-all categorisation of a patient as 'dangerous' or 'not dangerous' is of no clinical value.

The approach in psychiatry is therefore shifting from the prediction of dangerousness to:

- systematic consideration of what factors in the patient, his treatment and personal and social circumstances increase the chances of harm to others and to himself (risk assessment)
- systematic procedures to ensure that the risk assessment is made and reviewed, and that measures have been adopted to deal with the identified risks (risk management).

Risk assessment and management have become the 'new money' of dangerousness. They are not psychiatric discoveries but rather the combination of psychiatric knowledge with systematic methods sufficiently robust to withstand scrutiny. Added impetus to the importance of these issues has come from three sources:

- public perception of psychiatric patients as dangers to the community has forced a political response manifested by mandatory independent inquiries into homicides by psychiatric patients (Peay 1996), supervision registers (Baker 1997), and new legislation such as the supervised discharge order (Eastman 1997) and hybrid hospital order (see below)
- increased litigation by victims in respect of acts of violence by psychiatric patients
- business-orientated provision of health care has led to the adoption of business methods to promote 'quality'.

Risk assessment and management Risk assessment is part of daily clinical care in all psychiatric settings and with all psychiatric patients. Here we are concerned with offender patients when discharge to the community, or transfer from higher to lower level of security, is under consideration. The findings of the Kim Kirkman inquiry (West Midlands Regional Health Authority 1991) refer to the application of clinical judgement in risk assessment and Chiswick (1995) has described the factors on which this should be based. Risk assessment requires questions to be asked about:

- The individual patient
  - What is the psychiatric disorder and its relationship to previous violence?
  - Has it been modified by treatment?
  - Is clinical change a matter of observation or speculation?
  - Does clinical improvement lessen the likelihood of further offending?
  - What is the relevance of premorbid personality,

substance misuse or inappropriate sexual behaviour?
- What is the patient's understanding of his offending behaviour?
- Is his 'inner world' accessible to staff?
- Do his actions match his words?
- Does he appreciate the need for continuing treatment?
- Are your clinical views similar to those of colleagues?
- The circumstances of his previous violent behaviour
  - Did situational factors contribute to violence?
  - Can they be identified and modified?
- Potential victims
  - Why was the original victim involved?
  - Can potential victims be identified, and if so warned?
  - Do potential victims know of the patient's disorder?
- The condition(s) from which he suffers
  - What is known, from the literature, about the disorder and special risk factors for offending?
- Aftercare
  - Will the patient cooperate with aftercare?
  - Will those at greatest risk be involved in aftercare planning?
  - Do potential victims have access to appropriate professional advice?

Clinical risk management requires, at the very least, that a risk assessment is conducted, documented in an assimilable form and is available to those involved in the patient's care. It should identify how early deterioration may be manifested and indicate what action is to be taken.

It is impossible to separate clinical risk assessment from the fear of culpability if 'things go wrong'. This has been reflected in increased, perhaps defensive, use of the Mental Health Act in recent years (Department of Health 1996). Fears have been accentuated at a time when patients seem to be more violent, resources are stretched and expectations of what can reasonably be guaranteed have become unrealistic (Coid 1996). A series of independent inquiries into homicides have revealed common failures (Sheppard 1996):

- risk assessment not carried out
- risks denied or minimised
- information not transmitted
- vague identification of clinical responsibility
- lack of community support
- carer ignorant about services and how to access them
- inadequate resources
- incompetent management of the service
- inadequately trained staff.

All these factors require correction if clinical risk is to be properly assessed and managed. This is a multiprofessional task in which clinicians and managers have equal responsibilities. It cannot be done quickly or cheaply.

Offences and offenders

Every crime is a unique event in which offender, victim and circumstances interact in a manner that is 'special' for that particular episode. The notion that evidence about the crime and other behaviour of an unidentified criminal can be used to infer the motivation and personality of the perpetrator lies at the heart of offender profiling or criminal investigative analysis. Enthusiasts claim it provides a 'psychological signature' of the criminal. Evidence based on offender profiling was firmly rejected by the court in a notorious case where speculation based on profiling was used to try and entrap a man suspected of the brutal murder in 1992 of a young mother on Wimbledon Common, London. In essence, the prosecution case appeared to consist of the offender profile, and when this was disallowed by the trial judge, the prosecution dropped its case against the defendant (Ormerod 1996). Proponents of profiling point to one or two 'successes' but rarely has the exercise resulted in an arrest that would not have been made on other grounds. The process has a place but only in conjunction with other routine and scientific methods of police inquiry (Canter & Heritage 1990, Grubin 1995).

Homicide

The homicide rate has increased annually in England and Wales over the last 40 years and in 1995 there were 699 killings, which included the crimes of murder, manslaughter and infanticide (Home Office 1996). All defendants charged with murder are examined for the purpose of a psychiatric report. The legal definition of murder is 'the unlawful killing of any reasonable creature under the Queen's peace, with malice aforethought, death occurring within a year and a day of the act'.

Over half the male, and nearly 75% of female, victims are usually known to their killers. Half of the women killed in 1995 were killed by a current or former partner or lover. Death other than by means of a sharp or blunt instrument, brute force or strangulation is unusual. Quarrels, revenge or a loss of temper account for 50% of killings.

For statistical purposes homicide is normal where the outcome is conviction for murder, or for manslaughter other than by reason of diminished responsibility (see below). 'Abnormal' murder comprises convictions for manslaughter due to diminished responsibility (the majority of abnormal homicides), infanticide, homicide in a failed suicide pact and legal findings of insanity. On this basis, in England, abnormal homicides account for less than 1 in 5 killings (Home Office 1996). Findings of diminished responsibility are falling as the homicide rate rises; in recent years diminished responsibility has applied in less than 15% of homicides.

Legal verdicts (e.g. of diminished responsibility) do not depend on research-based diagnostic criteria. Studies using such criteria in countries with low rates of homicide confirm an association between some psychiatric disorders (antisocial personallity disorder, alcohol misuse and schizophrenia, but not affective disorders or learning disability) and homicide (Eronen et al 1996b). The association with mental disorder is even stronger in women who commit homicide (Eronen 1995). Suicide of the suspect before coming to trial occurs in less than 10% of cases. A study of homicide–suicide in the north of England found these were mostly men who had killed wives, children or both. The most common factors were ending of relationships, depression and jealousy; in nearly a third of cases alcohol abuse contributed (Milroy 1995).

In practice, psychiatric findings in abnormal homicide usually relate to a domestic or family killing with a background of any one or more of the following: interpersonal strife, jealousy, substance misuse, chronic ill health in victim or suspect and, where mental illness is present, either psychotic or depressive disorder. Even in homicides by the mentally ill there is usually a large contextual component; the nature of the relationship between victim and killer, the victim's behaviour and situational factors may all have contributory roles in the homicide. Sometimes the homicide is the mercy-killing of a chronically disabled parent, child or spouse.

Infants under the age of 1 year are at the greatest risk of death by homicide and 60% are killed by their mothers. Some of these are the victim of a mentally ill parent (d'Orban 1979, McGrath 1992) but others have their origins in situational, relationship and personality problems (Resnick 1969, Scott 1973). Many of these, together with younger child victims, are killed in circumstances associated with chronic ill treatment, battering or neglect (Cordess 1995).

The killing of parents or siblings is the rarest form of family homicide. Patricide is more common than matricide (though both are rare), and was associated in a Scottish study with alcohol intoxication (Gillies 1976). An association between matricide and schizophrenia has been frequently described (Green 1981, Clark 1993) but may owe as much to opportunity as it does to the psychopathology of the disorder. Many adult schizophrenic sons live with, or are dependent on, their mothers; in the setting of these, often strained, relationships mothers can easily become the target of any aggression (Chiswick 1981).

Where the victim is a stranger, it is unusual to find any evidence of mental illness in the accused. An exception is the rare instance when a schizophrenic selects a stranger as a victim on the basis of psychotic phenomena. Sexual or sadistic murder of a random victim is rare, though such cases attract wide publicity, particularly when the killings are of a serial type. Grubin (1994a) compared a group of sexual murderers with non-homicidal rapists. The murderers were isolated men with few, if any, intimate relationships in their lives. They did not otherwise greatly differ from the rapists and did not meet the stereotypical picture of the sadistic killer described by Brittain (1970).

Sexual offences

Sexual offences account for less than 1% of all notifiable offences; since 1985 the rate of increase in sexual offences has been equal to that of recorded crime in general – about 4% per year. Sex offenders are almost exclusively men among whom mental illness is not prevalent. There is no absolute relationship between any particular type of sexual offence and any particular type of sexual disorder: none should ever be assumed or implied. A man who sexually assaults a child may or may not be a paedophile; while a person convicted of the offence of indecent exposure may or may not be an exhibitionist.

Sexual offences and sexual offenders are widely heterogeneous. Sexual offences have precise legal definitions but the same offence (e.g. indecent assault) may conceal a wide range of behaviours. This heterogeneity makes it impossible to arrive at a useful classification of sexual offenders. Indeed Grubin & Kennedy (1991) have argued that until we have such a classification, it is pointless to talk of the 'psychiatry' of sex offending. Such classifications as we have are usually based on one particular facet of the offence or the offender. Most reflect the personal bias of their creator. Few have been tested for validity, reliability or practicability. They are usually based on a confusing mishmash of offence behaviour, imputed motivation, type of victim, personality traits and psychological or psychodynamic theory. Legal categories of sexual offending undergo frequent change but a report by the Howard League for Penal Reform (1985) provides a useful guide. West (1994) has edited a broadly based account of sexual offending. The reader is also referred to Chapter 19. The following is a brief account of some of the more common sexual offences, with particular reference to any psychiatric aspects.

Rape Approximately 500 men are convicted of rape each year, while 5000 offences are recorded by the police; in the last decade there has been a 10% increase per year in recorded rapes, more than double that of the increase in sexual crimes generally (Home Office 1996). The Criminal and Public Order Act 1994 introduced the specific crime of male rape; 150 such offences were recorded in 1995 by police.

Rape is a sexual crime not a psychiatric disorder: therefore there can be no satisfactory clinical classification of rapists. Traditional classifications based on categories such as violent, sadistic or sexual rape depend largely on the perspective of the researcher and have not been shown to have inter-rater reliability (Knight & Prentky 1989). Robust definition and focused application is required if these types of behavioural classsifications are to have any value (Gibbens et al 1977). Studies of convicted (and usually imprisoned) rapists find they are predominantly young men with poor social backgrounds and education. There is usually an overrepresentation of people from black ethnic minorities (Amir 1971, Dietz 1978). Most rapists have criminal records, often for violence and up to a third for sex offences (Gibbens et al 1977). However, in all these respects they are not greatly different from other prisoners (Lloyd & Walmsley 1989, West 1993).

While some rapists describe sadistic fantasies and 'try-outs' prior to offending, the significance of these phenomena is uncertain (Grubin 1994b). Sadistic fantasy is common in men but it is probably the combination with social isolation and an impaired capacity for empathy that distinguish those who put sadistic fantasy into practice.

Incest and other sexual behaviour with children

For legal purposes incest is sexual intercourse (vaginal) within a forbidden relationship. Between 200 and 500 offences, mostly father–daughter incest, have been notified annually in recent years but there is gross underreporting compared with the frequency of the behaviour. Legally incest requires proof of penetration: much intrafamilial sexual abuse falls short of penetration. In England (though not in Scotland) step relationships do not come within the legal definition of incest. Therefore prosecution for stepfather–daughter sexual intercourse will be for a different crime. Sexual abuse by mothers of their sons is increasingly recognised. Family factors in incest have been emphasised, particularly findings of a dysfunctional family with generational blurring. Wives are often absent, incapacitated or unavailable or they commonly have a passive or dependent role in the family. Family pathology often coexists with pathology in the father (Finkelhor 1984).

Up to 30% of incest perpetrators have a sexual preference for children, nearly half having offended outside the family (Abel et al 1988). Other psychiatric features may be alcohol abuse and antisocial personality disorder. There are no consistent findings suggestive of low intelligence. A proportion of incest perpetrators have been victims of child sexual abuse. This appears to be more common in those with paedophilia, backgrounds of other crimes and in adolescent perpetrators (Hilton & Mezey 1996).

Other sexual offences against children vary from minor indecency to violent sexual activity. Among adolescent boys the criminal behaviour is associated with poor social skills, physical unattractiveness and peer group isolation. Adult offenders are more likely to show features of paedophilia. Such men become skilled in targeting vulnerable children, grooming them with behaviour designed to increase their trust and then gradually increasing the degree of intimacy in the relationship. Emotional bribery is employed to maintain secrecy; they commonly refer to their behaviour as a 'secret game'.

Indecent exposure

In the last 2 years there have been fewer than 900 convictions each year for indecent exposure (Home Office 1996) and the annual rate of offending seems to be falling. Only a minority of episodes are reported and an even smaller proportion result in conviction. Traditionally offenders have been divided into those who are exhibitionists, with the features classically described in the 19th century by Lasègue (1877), and those whose exposing occurs in the context of drunkenness or a disinhibiting psychiatric disorder such as schizophrenia, hypomania, organic brain disorder or a learning disability.

Typically exhibitionists (almost invariably men) expose their genitals to a female victim in a public but quiet location, or on public transport, or from their own home or car. They are sexually excited, often later masturbating to the image of the exposure. Few make any attempt to speak to or touch their victims. They are usually unable to explain their behaviour. It is known that a small proportion of exposers progress to more serious sexual crimes. Sugarman et al (1994) reviewed 210 cases and found subsequent more serious offending was associated with childhood conduct disorder, other criminal offences, and pursuing or touching the victim.

Psychiatric assessment of sexual offenders

Assessment of a person charged with, or convicted of, a sexual offence should be approached without preconceptions and with information from sources other than solely the accused. Establishing the presence or absence of a psychiatric disorder is a prerequisite, together with a detailed psychosexual history. In addition, assessment requires a consideration of the victim's behaviour and relationship (when present) to the accused, and situational factors such as the relevance of substance misuse by assailant and victim.

Psychotic illness in sexual offenders is unusual, though occasionally disinhibition due to a manic illness or to residual schizophrenia may be a factor. Rarely is the offence a response to delusional or hallucinatory symptoms. Abnormalities and disorders of personality and associated alcohol misuse are common.

In practice few sex offenders are seen at times other than when they face criminal charges or are being considered for release from prison. The appropriateness of offering treatment, and the conditions under which it may be provided, must be balanced with the requirements of the criminal justice system. Those few patients with an underlying mental illness usually require treatment for that illness. For sex offenders who do not consider that they have any problem, who minimise their offending and who present to psychiatrists for statutory purposes, there is little prospect of treatment being either feasible or beneficial.

Reoffending and community treatment There is a public perception that sex offenders always reoffend, and the political sensitivity of the issue is reflected in recent legislation. The Criminal Justice Act 1991 introduced mandatory supervision for certain sex offenders after release from prison. The Sex Offenders Act 1997 requires sex offenders discharged from prison or hospital to notify themselves to the police within 14 days of discharge. They must give the police their name, date of birth and home address and keep them notified of any changes in name or address. Studies of reoffending have been reviewed by Grubin & Wingate (1996) and do not generally support the public's impression. Sexual reoffending occurred in 7–19% of released offenders (Hanson et al 1993, Kaul 1993, Marshall 1994). Grubin and Wingate point out the limitations of reoffending studies based on criminal records and the fact that longer periods of follow-up reveal higher rates of reoffending. Nevertheless, reoffending rates of under 20% for sex offenders compare with rates of up to 80% for other offenders.

Can the 20% be identified and treated? Attempts to identify high-risk offenders have depended on gathering data of a demographic and historical type and seeking correlations with reoffending. The common variables with high correlations are childhood conduct disorder, parental instability, previous sex offending, early first conviction and a diagnosis of personality disorder (Grubin & Wingate 1996). These have predictive value for groups but not for the individual. As for their relevance for treatment, they are facts of history unamenable to change. In contrast, the factors that interest those who treat sex offenders are anger, self-esteem, social skills and victim empathy at the time when reoffending may take place (Hanson et al 1993). Thus the practical value of 'predictors' is limited.

Treatment for sex offenders in the community is in its infancy in Britain. Allam et al (1997) have described a programme for offenders undergoing community service; it is therefore targeted at less serious offenders. The programme attempts to address cognitive distortions, self-esteem and assertiveness, sexuality, the role of fantasy, victim empathy and relapse prevention techniques. The work is unevaluated but the treatment themes are familiar in other approaches to sex offender therapy.

In Denmark until 1970 surgical castration was carried out on selected sex offenders. Since 1989 aggressive medical castration using antigonadotrophin in combination with antiandrogen preparations has been used (Hansen & Lykke-Olsen 1997). Of 24 prisoners undergoing treatment, 12 have been released on probation still undergoing treatment and none has committed a further sex offence.

Offences against property

Arson Arson is among the leading causes of fires throughout the world (Geller 1992). It is a grave crime for which a sentence of life imprisonment can be imposed: the lawful form of the activity is a mark of public celebration. There were 30 000 episodes of arson reported to the police in 1995 and the clear-up rate of 16% was among the lowest for any crime (Home Office 1996). Studies based on captive populations of arsonists therefore exclude approximately 90% of people who commit the crime. As with other crimes, arson is multifactorial in origin and arsonists are a widely heterogeneous group (Geller 1992, Barker 1994, Prins 1994a, Rix 1994).

Most attempts to classify fire-setters have been based on assessment, or speculation, of their motivation; such classifications are bound to contain overlap between categories. Clare et al (1992) identified problems in classifications based on:

- arsonists' personal and social characteristics, e.g. classically by Lewis & Yarnell (1951)
- typologies of motives (Barnett & Spitzer 1994, Prins 1994a)
- functional analysis of the behaviour (Jackson et al 1987).

All methods have deficiencies. Few studies have used adequate control groups, motivation is often complex and multifactorial, while behavioural analysis does not help identify the weight of particular contributory factors in any given case. An historical association between fire-setting and sexual psychopathology (Freud 1929) is not borne out in current practice or literature. The following are examples of fire-raising and should not be seen as mutually exclusive categories within an all-embracing classification.

- *Motivated fire-setting* This is a deliberate act with the aim of a fraudulent insurance claim, engineering a change of housing, taking revenge in a broken relationship or failed business venture or concealing another crime, e.g. murder or burglary.
- *Political fire-setting* This is a group activity common at times of social unrest. Not all the perpetrators may be politically motivated.
- *Suicide by fire* An epidemic of self-immolation, as an apparent political gesture, occurred in the late 1960s. It is possible that some of the subjects were mentally disturbed. This method of suicide is sometimes employed by prisoners.
- *Psychiatric disorder or organic brain disease* Fire may be set by schizophrenics in response to psychotic phenomena, by people with a learning disability for reasons of excitement and by substance abusers in states of intoxication, delirium tremens, alcoholic hallucinosis or drug-related psychosis.
- *No psychiatric disorder* Fires may be set out of boredom or as a vague form of 'protest'.
- *Those with no motive* Some fire-setters gain satisfaction from watching the fire and the subsequent emergency. They may act heroically, often being early on the scene and appearing to help the fire brigade. Such men sometimes gain employment as firemen or security guards. For some of these offenders the condition defined as pyromania in ICD-10 may be relevant.
- *Female fire-setters* A comparison of imprisoned female fire-setters with other women in prison failed to show significant psychiatric or social differences between the two groups (Stewart 1993). Both had highly disturbed backgrounds, histories of abuse and unstable lives as adults.

Current classifications of fire-setters have not reached such sophistication that they provide a practical guide to treatment and prognosis. Individual assessment based on standard psychiatric examination together with full details of the fire-setting behaviour is necessary. Only a tiny proportion of fire-setters receive a psychiatric disposal in court; in the highly selected samples examined by psychiatrists, a mental illness may be present in 10–30% of cases (Molnar et al 1984, Puri et al 1995). Alcohol or other substance abuse is common, while mental illness, if present, is likely to be schizophrenia or an associated paranoid psychosis. Among the population of people with a learning disability in secure hospital settings, arson is a common index offence.

Studies of prognosis give widely different reoffending rates for arson from 4 to 30% (Lewis & Yarnell 1951, Soothill & Pope 1973, O'Sullivan & Kelleher 1987). In a Finnish follow-up study of 304 fire-setters who had pretrial psychiatric assessments, 40 had died within 2–15 years of the offence, 17 by suicide (Repo & Virkkunen 1997).

Shoplifting Shoplifting is a form of theft which is perpetrated on a massive scale with huge losses to the retail trade. Most shoplifting has nothing to do with any mental disorder. Gibbens et al (1971), in an early follow-up study of 532 women who had shoplifted 10 years earlier, found rates of subsequent psychiatric hospitalisation three times greater than expected. Depressive disorders were the most common but a unitary causal model for the offence is often inadequate (Gudjonsson 1990).

The disorder of kleptomania has a place in ICD-10 and DSM-IV. It refers to the repeated failure to control an impulse to steal objects that are not required and are then often discarded, given away or hoarded. The condition is exceedingly rarely encountered in clinical practice. A study of 20 patients who met diagnostic criteria for kleptomania were all found to have lifetime diagnoses of major mood disorders; 16 had additional diagnoses of anxiety disorders and 12 of eating disorders (McElroy et al 1991). Depressed shoplifters typically make little effort to conceal their actions or to escape arrest. Shoplifting is often seen in association with substance abuse and residual schizophrenia. It may also occur in organic states or in states of absent-mindedness.

Child abduction

Abduction or stealing of a child is notified to police with increasing frequency; there were 355 reported incidents in 1995 but annual convictions are less than 70. The great majority are carried out by men in custody disputes with their partners. The abduction of a child by a stranger for sexual purposes is rare (d'Orban & Haydn-Smith 1985) but understandably cases receive wide publicity.

Baby stealing is almost invariably carried out by women. Most stolen babies are found fairly quickly and have usually been well cared for by their abductors. The classification by d'Orban (1976) based on 24 cases remains useful. He described three types of offence:

- Comforting offences by deprived women with backgrounds of immaturity, and often having had their own child taken into care.
- A manipulative offence by an older woman with personality difficulties but with a better social

adjustment. Such women seek to manipulate a relationship by presenting the baby as their own.

- Mentally ill women who steal a baby impulsively with little or no planning during a psychotic illness.

The risk of repetition is a real issue, particularly in the third group in whom delusions concerning babies are often systematised.

Victims of crime

Current growth in crime rates brings a parallel growth in the numbers of victims. There is good evidence that being a victim is associated with psychiatric morbidity. This applies not only to victims of sexual abuse and sexual crimes but also to victims of violent and other offences (Taylor 1993c). Nearly 5% of men and 2% of women were victims of violent crimes, excluding domestic and sexual assaults, in 1991 (Mayhew et al 1993). Community surveys in America have reported even higher figures (Helzer et al 1987). Acute and longer-term psychiatric sequelae occur, including symptoms of fear, anger, guilt and irritability as well as recognised disorders such as adjustment reactions and post-traumatic stress disorder (Bisson & Shepherd 1995). Taylor (1993c) emphasises that variables such as the threat of extinction, extent of physical injury, duration of exposure to crime, victim isolation, knowledge of the assailant and specificity of the event all have implications for outcome.

The effects of child sexual abuse are well recognised, though up to one-third of adult survivors report no long-term effects (Hilton & Mezey 1996). Psychiatric morbidity is associated with abuse by a father or stepfather, violent sexual behaviour, penetrative sex and bizarre or repugnant sexual acts. Adult survivors of abuse show high rates of depression, guilt, low self-esteem, alcoholism, sexual problems, eating disorders, self-harm and further victimisation. Male survivors show similar psychiatric sequelae.

MENTALLY DISORDERED OFFENDERS AND THE CRIMINAL JUSTICE SYSTEM

Arrest, prosecution and diversion

The mentally disordered person who comes to the attention of the police faces a bewildering range of potential outcomes. These depend less on his offence and psychiatric condition than on the organisation of local psychiatric services to the police and courts, and on the quality of cooperation between health and criminal justice systems. Poor communication, misunderstandings and lack of accurate shared information

between the two systems have been recurring features reported by a series of inquiries into psychiatric homicides (Sheppard 1996).

An unknown number of mentally disordered people are referred directly by the police to mental health services. The use of section 136 of the Mental Health Act 1983 to arrest a mentally disordered person found in a public place and detain him at a designated place of safety fluctuates and is probably inaccurately recorded. The Mental Health Act Commission (1997) recommends that the place of safety should be in mental health premises but frequently police stations are used for this purpose. In London in 1995 1500 people were detained under section 136 by Metropolitan police; 20% of police divisions in the capital have no suitable 'place of safety' provision (Cherrett 1996). Section 136 is disproportionately applied to patients from black ethnic minorities (Dunn & Fahey 1990).

An observational study (Robertson et al 1996) of procedure at seven Metropolitan police stations over 18 weeks found that 37 of 2721 detainees (less than 2%) were definitely or probably suffering from acute mental illness and nearly all were speedily diverted to treating agencies. The most significant factor associated with a failure to divert at the arrest stage was black ethnicity. An American study refers to the police as the 'streetcorner psychiatrist' and describes their 'pivotal' role as a mental health resource (Teplin & Pruett 1992).

Government initiatives in the last decade have encouraged early removal of mentally disordered offenders from the criminal justice system and avoidance of remands to prison solely for the purpose of obtaining a psychiatric report (Home Office 1990, Department of Health & Home Office 1992). Court liaison and court diversion schemes have developed widely but vary in their operation. Some depend on attendance of a psychiatrist at court at fixed times (James & Hamilton 1991, Joseph & Potter 1993), while others involve the sifting of cases held in custody by a community psychiatric nurse (Rowlands et al 1996). Medium-term outcome is more favourable in patients diverted to inpatient rather than outpatient care (Holloway & Shaw 1993).

The importance of linking a central London court diversion scheme with appropriate inpatient beds has been emphasised by James et al (1997). Unfortunately the promotion of these schemes occurs at a time of reconfiguration of mental health services and a drastic reduction in psychiatric hospital beds. A significant proportion of patients with enduring illness, often complicated by substance misuse, are recycled through courts and court diversion schemes, with little evidence of long-term gain (Prins 1994b).

Police interviews and false confessions

A mentally disordered suspect who is interviewed by police may unwittingly provide information which is unreliable, misleading or self-incriminating. Unreliable or false confessions have been at the heart of many of the notorious miscarriages of justice that resulted in the Royal Commission on Criminal Justice (Gudjonsson 1993, Runciman 1993, Editorial 1994). False confessions may be of three types:

- *Voluntary false confessions* The individual goes voluntarily to the police and confesses to a crime he knows he has not committed, usually to satisfy a pathological need for notoriety. Some cases may involve a psychiatric disorder such as depression, schizophrenia or a personality disorder.
- *Coerced compliant false confessions* These are elicited during persuasive interrogation, are known to be false by the suspect but are offered for an immediate gain, e.g. a promise of release.
- *Coerced internalised false confessions* These occur in two situations. Firstly, where a suspect with amnesia (e.g. alcohol-related) comes to believe he committed a crime he did not do. Secondly, where subtle manipulation by a questioner convinces an innocent suspect that he committed the crime. This type of false confession is often associated with psychiatric factors in the suspect, such as a learning disability or states of anxiety, confusion, guilt or bereavement.

The codes of practice under the Police and Criminal Evidence Act (PACE) 1984, require that mentally disordered suspects (including those with a learning disability) should be interviewed in the presence of an appropriate adult. The role of the appropriate adult is regarded by many as unclear and unsatisfactory (Pearse & Gudjonsson 1996). Psychiatrists may occasionally be required to give an opinion on the fitness of a detainee to be interviewed (Norfolk 1997, Rix 1997).

Remand to prison

The mentally disordered offender remanded in custody joins the population of other remanded prisoners awaiting trial or sentence. This is a population with high psychiatric, physical and social morbidity in an environment the function of which is penal custody rather than the provision of welfare. Remand of mentally ill offenders to prison as a means of obtaining psychiatric treatment has been shown to be completely ineffective (Dell et al 1993, Robertson et al 1994). Remanded prisoners figure significantly in prison suicides (Backett 1987, Dooley 1990, Bogue & Power 1995). Female remanded prisoners have high rates of previous self-mutilation

(Wilkins & Coid 1991). For a general review of psychiatric practice in prisons, see Chiswick & Dooley (1995).

Mental disorder and court proceedings

The great majority of mentally disordered offenders who receive a psychiatric disposal in the criminal courts do so after conviction, i.e. they have pled, or been found, guilty and the judge imposes a disposal from the menu of psychiatric alternatives to punishment (see below). For a small minority of mentally disordered offenders, their psychiatric condition may affect their capacity to be tried or their responsibility for their crimes. These two situations are considered in turn before considering the psychiatric options available at the sentencing stage.

Fitness to plead

It would be unjust to try a person who, by reason of mental disorder, lacks the capacity to defend himself in court. Such a person is said to be unfit to plead or under disability such that he cannot be tried (section 2, Criminal Procedure (Insanity and Unfitness to Plead) Act 1991. Whether a person is unfit to plead is a matter for determination by a jury in a crown court after hearing psychiatric evidence. A defendant is fit to plead if he has the capacity to:

- understand the charge and its implications
- distinguish between a plea of guilty and one of not guilty
- challenge a juror to whom he might object
- follow the evidence in court
- instruct counsel on his behalf.

Psychiatric assessment is of the accused's ability, at the time of his trial, to comprehend his situation and adequately communicate instructions to his counsel. His mental condition at the time of the offence is irrelevant. Amnesia does not, of itself, render a person unfit to plead. The mental state of a defendant may fluctuate from day to day so a brief re-examination on the day of the court appearance is advisable. Schizophrenia, other psychoses and learning disability accounted for 87% of 286 unfit to plead cases reported by Grubin (1996); the sample was almost all unfit to plead cases in England and Wales between 1976 and 1988; 46% recovered from their unfitness to plead but only 26% returned to court for trial.

A defendant who makes no reply when asked to plead to the charges is said to be mute on arraignment. Here the jury is asked to decide if the mutism is the result of an unwillingness or an inability to speak. If mutism is the result of an inability to speak, then the jury proceeds to decide the issue of fitness to plead in the normal manner. The most likely example is that of a deaf mute, though some method of communication is usually possible, e.g. sign language, writing or even grunts and nods. Failure in communication compounded by lack of comprehension, as it might be in severe learning disability, renders a meaningful trial impossible. Grubin's sample contained seven deaf defendants, two of whom had a learning disability.

Prior to 1991 a finding of unfitness resulted in mandatory committal to hospital with no trial or opportunity to test the case against the accused. The 1991 Act introduced major changes including:

- a trial of the facts
- complete acquittal if the facts are not found
- flexible disposal by the judge if the facts are found, except for murder where there remains mandatory committal to hospital.

Criminal responsibility

A finding of guilt requires, for most crimes, not only that the defendant committed the unlawful act (the actus reus) but also that he had the necessary state of mind or mens rea for that particular crime. There are four factors of psychiatric relevance which might, but in practice rarely do, affect mens rea:

- age
- mental disorder
- the effects of alcohol or drugs
- automatism.

Age Children under the age of 10 in England and Wales (under 8 in Scotland) are not criminally responsible for their acts; it is assumed that they are incapable of forming a criminal intent. They may however be made the subject of a care order. Between the ages of 10 and 14 a child may be convicted of a crime if, in addition to proof of mens rea, there is evidence that the child knew, either in the legal or moral sense, that what he was doing was wrong. Psychiatric evidence may be led by the prosecution to help establish this fact; it requires a global consideration of the child's social, intellectual, moral and conative development.

Mental disorder The defence which rests upon an absence of mens rea due to insanity is known as the insanity defence and, if successful, it results in a special verdict of not guilty by reason of insanity (section 2, Trial of Lunatics Act 1883). This is a rare finding, almost confined to cases of murder. There are usually fewer than 10 cases per year but the introduction of the Criminal Procedure (Insanity and Unfitness to Plead) Act 1991 may increase its utilisation. It results in

acquittal and, prior to the 1991 Act, mandatory committal to hospital. Now, flexible disposal options are possible, except where the charge is one of murder.

The verdict continues to be governed by the McNaughton Rules, laid down in 1843 by the judges at the request of the House of Lords. Daniel McNaughton was acquitted of the murder of William Drummond, private secretary to Sir Robert Peel, then Prime Minister. McNaughton is said to have acted in response to paranoid delusions (West & Walk 1977). His crime caused public uproar; homicides by the mentally ill were no less a source of public concern then than they are now. The Rules established there was an initial assumption of sanity and legal responsibility in all cases. A successful insanity defence depends upon the following.

To establish a defence on the ground of insanity, it must be clearly proved that at the time of the committing of the act, the party accused was labouring under such a defect of reason, from disease of the mind, as not to know the nature and quality of the act he was doing, or if he did know it, that he did not know he was doing wrong.

Thus the defendant must prove three matters:

- that he was suffering from a disease of the mind at the time of the crime
- that this caused a defect of reason
- that the defect of reason robbed him of the capacity to either know what he was doing or know that it was wrong.

The Rules pose problems for the examining psychiatrist. Apart from the difficulties of establishing a retrospective diagnosis, the requirement to speak with authority on what the accused did, or did not, know when he committed the crime is an unfamiliar clinical task. Most cases are accounted for by schizophrenia, depression, epilepsy and the complications of substance misuse – see below (Mackay 1990). The results of positron emission tomography are regularly heard in evidence in criminal trials in America and increasingly in Britain. Abnormalities without clinical evidence of psychiatric disorder are not accepted as a disease of the mind, though Fenwick (1993) has provocatively argued that recent developments in neuroimaging would render much of the criminal law obsolete. Buchanan (1994) provides an alternative view.

Effects of alcohol or drugs Intoxication by drink or drugs does not in itself constitute a defence to a criminal charge; courts are understandably reluctant to broaden the opportunities for alcohol or drugs to be used as 'excuses' by defendants. However, there are three situations where the effects of substance misuse might affect an accused person's criminal responsibility.

- Evidence of intoxication may be used to demonstrate an inability to form the specific intent that is necessary for certain crimes (e.g. murder). Such a defence could not apply in crimes requiring only basic intent (e.g. manslaughter).
- If alcohol or drugs have caused a disease of the mind, an insanity plea under the McNaughton Rules may be possible.
- If alcohol or drugs have caused an abnormality of mind, a plea of diminished responsibility (in murder only) may be possible – see below. Griew (1991) reported a case where the compulsion to drink in an alcoholic was accepted as the abnormality of mind necessary to support diminished responsibility.

Automatism   An act performed by a person's body independently of that person's mind is for legal purposes an automatic act or automatism. It is a legal concept not to be confused with the clinical phenomenon of automatic behaviour. Because the act is regarded as involuntary, automatism is an accepted legal defence. The court is concerned with public protection. For this reason it distinguishes automatisms due to a disease of the mind (known as insane automatism) from those where there is no disease of the mind (non-insane automatism). Defendants whose crime was due to an insane automatism are dealt with under the flexible disposals introduced in 1991 for other insanity acquitees. Those with non-insane automatism walk free from court.

There is no logical thread by which the courts have determined which automatisms are due to diseases of the mind. Arteriosclerosis, epilepsy and sleep-walking have been declared diseases of the mind, but not organic states associated with a brain tumour and with hypoglycaemia (Dempster 1990, 1991, Fenwick 1991). Absent-mindedness. even in association with depression, was accepted in support of non-insane automatism in a case of shoplifting.

Diminished responsibility

Unfitness to plead and the insanity defence have important places in the development of the criminal law as it applies to the mentally ill. In practice, but only for murder, the arcane wrangles associated with insanity can be side-stepped by use of the plea of diminished responsibility, a Scottish invention in 1867 which did not become part of English law until the Homicide Act of 1957. Today nearly all offenders who escape conviction for murder on psychiatric grounds do so on the basis of diminished responsibility. There are approximately 70 cases per year in England and Wales.

Section 2 of the Homicide Act introduced a halfway stage between full and absent responsibility. Diminished responsibility is a legal concept and therefore it cannot be defined in clinical terms. It has the effect of reducing a charge of murder, which carries a mandatory sentence of life imprisonment, to the less serious charge of manslaughter, for which there is flexible sentencing. When it was introduced the mandatory sentence for murder was the death penalty; diminished responsibility was introduced to provide an escape route from hanging for cases seen as deserving. The relevant section states:

Where a person kills or is party to the killing of another, he shall not be convicted of murder if he was suffering from such abnormality of mind (whether arising from a condition of arrested or retarded development of mind or any inherent causes or induced by disease or injury) as substantially impaired his acts and omissions in doing or being a party to the killing.

To sustain the defence, proof is required on a balance of probabilities of three matters:

- that the accused was at the time of the crime suffering from an abnormality of mind
- that the abnormality of mind resulted from one of the causes specified in section 2 of the 1957 Act
- that the abnormality of mind substantially impaired mental responsibility.

Although psychiatrists seem willing to testify that an abnormality of mind exists, the phrase cannot be defined in medical terms. The authoritative judgement of the then Lord Chief Justice in *Byrne* in 1960 has given scope for some creative psychiatric court reports. He said an abnormality of mind was 'a state of mind so different from that of an ordinary human being's that the reasonable man would term it abnormal'.

Practical aspects   Resting as it does on such slender theory, it is not surprising that nearly all psychiatric diagnoses have, on occasions, been accepted as the basis for diminished responsibility. In a consecutive sample of 101 murder cases seen for psychiatric assessment, Mitchell (1997) found diagnoses of depression and psychotic conditions accounted for 73% and personality disorders 13% of diminished responsibility cases. Other diagnoses such as emotional immaturity, dissociative states and the premenstrual syndrome have also been successfully argued to support the plea. Depending on the circumstances, probation and even an absolute discharge are not unusual disposals (Dell 1984).

The finding is a more likely outcome in women than in men. Contested cases have a high failure rate and usually attract heavy media coverage. Psychotic cases are likely to go to hospital but the verdict is not always the key to leniency in sentencing. In Mitchell's sample 23 of the 36 depressed manslaughter cases were sent to prison, including five who received life sentences.

Infanticide

In the early part of this century mothers who killed an infant child of their own were sentenced to death for murder and then reprieved by the Home Secretary. The Infanticide Act 1938 provided an alternative. It states that if a woman causes the death of her child, who must be aged less than 12 months, and the court is satisfied that the balance of her mind was disturbed by reason of her not fully having recovered from the effect of giving birth to the child, or by reason of the effect of lactation consequent upon the birth, she is guilty of infanticide. The disposals are exactly as for manslaughter. Psychiatrists are required to put their evidence within the framework of the Infanticide Act 1938. The consequent need to 'drive a square peg into a round hole' can cause problems, similar to those described for diminished responsibility.

In recent years there have been fewer than five infanticides per year. Infant killing today has little to do with outdated notions of 'milk fever' but shows similar psychosocial antecedents to child battering and neglect (Home Office & Department of Health and Social Security 1975; Payne 1995).

Psychiatric disposals

Courts have the power to deal with accused and convicted defendants by a range of options, most of which are contained in Part III of the Mental Health Act 1983 (Table 28.3). Indeed the great majority of court disposals take place after conviction. These depend on opinions from psychiatrists concerning the presence of a mental disorder and the appropriateness of compulsory admission to hospital for its treatment. The direct transfer of prisoners from prison to hospital under sections 47, 48 and 49 is not a matter for the court but the Home Office.

Remands to hospital: sections 35 and 36
Assessment of an accused person in prison for a psychiatric report is often unsatisfactory. The psychiatrist does not have the benefit of clinical observation over a period of time and there may be a need to carry out investigations or seek other information, both of which may be more easily effected if the prisoner is in hospital. Remand to hospital under section 35 is only possible for an untried or unsentenced prisoner deemed unsuitable for bail. One medical report is necessary stating that there is reason to suspect that the defendant may be suffering from a mental disorder. In hospital, treatment, except in an emergency, can only be given with the patient's consent. If compulsory treatment is required, consideration must be given to detention under section 3. Section 36 provides for treatment, compulsory if necessary, of remanded patients in hospital. It can only be ordered by a crown court and cannot be applied if the charge is murder. Two medical recommendations are required; the mental disorder must be either mental illness or severe mental impairment.

Hospital order: section 37   The ordering of a convicted offender to hospital, as an alternative to prison, under the terms of a hospital order is the most common route of admission of offender patients to hospital. There are approximately 1000 made each year, and over 90% are in the category of mental illness (Department of Health 1996). The grounds are similar

Table 28.3	Compulsory admission for offenders under Part III of the Mental Health Act 1983		
Section	Purpose	Maximum duration	Authority
35	Remand for report	12 weeks	M,C
36	Remand for treatment	12 weeks	C
37	Hospital or guardianship order	6 months, renewable	M,C
38	Interim hospital order	12 months	M,C
41	Restriction on discharge	Without limit of time	C
47	Transfer of convicted prisoner	Unlimited	Home Secretary
48	Transfer of untried and other prisoners	Until further action by a court	Home Secretary
49	Restriction on discharge	Lapses on normal date of release from prison	Home Secretary

M, magistrates' court; C, crown court.
A hospital direction under section 46 of the Crime (Sentences) Act 1997 will be implemented in 1998.

to those for detention under section 3, except that the appropriateness of, rather than the necessity for, hospital treatment is specified. Courts must be satisfied on evidence that a bed is available for the patient. In hospital a patient detained under section 37 has almost identical rights to those of patients detained under civil powers. The responsible medical officer can send the patient on leave of absence or discharge him whenever he sees fit, irrespective of the length of sentence the court might have imposed for that crime.

Restriction order: section 41 Crown courts (but not magistrates' courts) have power to impose an order under section 41 restricting discharge. This removes authority of the responsible medical officer to discharge the patient and transfers it to the Home Secretary. In 1995 30% of hospital orders carried restriction orders and the absolute number of such orders has risen in recent years. The rise may reflect the fact that the conditional discharge of restricted patients provides a more effective legal framework for aftercare than other measures. The grounds for a restriction order are that the offender may commit further offences if at liberty and that it is necessary to protect the public from serious harm.

Public protection is the major issue in the Home Secretary's consideration of the discharge of restricted patients. In cases of particular concern he is advised by the Advisory Board on Restricted Patients, established in the wake of the Graham Young case (Egglestone 1990). This is an independent Board which gives advice on the likelihood of dangerousness upon release.

Interim hospital order: section 38 Where a patient detained under a hospital order subsequently proves unsuitable for treatment, the case cannot be returned to court for consideration of a penal sentence. A mechanism for assessing suitability for a hospital order is provided by the interim hospital order (section 38); approximately 100 are imposed each year. The offender must be suffering from a category of mental disorder for which admission under a hospital order may be appropriate.

Hospital direction ('the hybrid order'): section 46 Crime (Sentences) Act 1997 The principle whereby a court orders either imprisonment or hospital treatment was eroded with the introduction of the hospital direction, commonly known as a 'hybrid order', in the Crime (Sentences) Act 1997. For serious crimes (except that of murder) a crown court may impose a prison sentence which begins with treatment in hospital, followed by either transfer to prison or continued detention in hospital until the sentence is completed. At present it only applies to psychopathic disorder but its scope can be extended by the Home Secretary. The hybrid order has been criticised as a flawed attempt to combine punishment of mentally disordered offenders with protection for the public (Chiswick 1996, Eastman 1966).

Transfer of prisoners to hospital: sections 47, 48 and 49 Prisoners, whether untried or convicted, who become mentally disordered can only receive treatment in prison if they give consent. Untried and convicted prisoners may be transferred to hospital by direction of the Home Secretary. In hospital, the provisions of Part IV (consent to treatment) of the Mental Health Act apply to transferred prisoners. Prisoners awaiting trial may be transferred to hospital for urgent treatment under section 48. The mental disorder must be either mental illness or severe mental impairment. Transfers under section 48 have risen steeply since government policy was clarified in a 1990 circular; they now number approximately 500 per year (Robertson et al 1996). For convicted prisoners the requirements for a transfer direction (section 47) are similar to those for a hospital order. In most cases the Home Secretary also applies a restriction direction (section 49) so that in hospital these patients' situation is similar to that of any other restricted patient. The Home Secretary may direct transfer of the patient back to prison if he is satisfied that treatment in hospital is no longer required or appropriate.

Preparation of psychiatric reports for the court

Psychiatric reports are requested in only a small proportion of cases coming before the criminal courts. However they are of great importance to the accused and the court and demonstrate one aspect of what has been called 'the public face of psychiatry' (Bluglass 1995). Psychiatric recommendations may influence decisions about guilt, responsibility and sentence. The purpose of the report is to provide expert advice on one or all of these matters. The report is advice to the court which is the decision-making body. In practice recommendations for treatment, particularly where these are for inpatient care, are rarely disregarded.

Requests for reports may come from the Crown, the defendant's solicitor or from the court at the instigation of the sentencer (magistrate or judge). The defendant may be detained in prison, in hospital or on bail in the community. The psychiatrist should always satisfy himself that he understands the reason why a report has been requested and should not hesitate to clarify doubts with the referring agency. It will be necessary first to read all the background information, including statements of the accused and witnesses; second, to examine the accused; third, to seek additional information from relatives or staff where appropriate; and fourth, to reflect on the answers to the questions that have been asked before writing the report.

Examination of the accused is unusual in that it does not take place within the setting of the normal doctor–patient relationship (Chiswick 1985). The purpose of the interview and the fact that information will not remain confidential should be explained to the defendant and his agreement to it sought. History taking and mental state examination follow usual lines, but it is important to obtain an account from the accused of the offence in his own words, which should be noted.

The report should address the particular questions that have been asked; advice on disposal is usually the chief issue but sometimes fitness to plead or responsibility may be in doubt. In homicides it is essential to comment on the question of diminished responsibility. The report will be read by a non-psychiatric audience; it should therefore be clear, concise and free of jargon and technical terms (Bluglass 1995). It should be impartial and balanced and demonstrate sensitivity to the court's needs. It may be read out in court and should be free of moral judgements, sarcasm, humour or pompous language. Any recommendations should be unambiguous and practicable and be based on clinical findings contained in the report. Only treatment recommendations that are of a psychiatric nature should be made. The report should state the name of the accused and the charge; it is easier to read if arranged in sections:

- A note of when, where and for how long the accused was examined, together with a statement of the sources of information.
- A brief sentence giving his age, employment and social circumstances.
- A brief chronological account of his educational, occupational and social history, emphasising any factors of psychiatric relevance.
- Family history with any points of psychiatric importance.
- Previous medical and psychiatric history.
- A note of previous criminal convictions.
- A note of the circumstances of the offence as narrated by the accused with emphasis on any relevant psychiatric points. (Where the defendant pleads not guilty, the court must ensure that previously undisclosed material is not heard before guilt has been determined.)
- Features found on psychiatric examination.
- The psychiatrist's opinion, together with relevant discussion, on the particular questions that have been asked.
- A clear summary of conclusions or recommendations. The report should conclude with the name, designation and qualifications of the psychiatrist.

If called to give expert evidence in court, the psychiatrist should be properly prepared. He should answer the questions put to him clearly, avoid straying beyond his sphere of expertise and be able to support his statements with evidence. Grounds (1985) and Bluglass (1995) provide sensible advice for the prospective psychiatric witness.

Services for mentally disordered offenders

Any psychiatric service dealing with a defined geographical area will see patients whose contact is precipitated by an offence. Such patients may be referred at any stage of the criminal justice process through police, courts, lawyers, prisons, or from a secure psychiatric hospital. The needs of these patients are usually met by a combination of general and specialist forensic psychiatric services, the balance of which will be determined by local factors. A comprehensive service should contain the following elements:

- An effective emergency service to deal with police referrals
- An effective service to local courts, including provision for early diversion
- Accessible outpatient clinics for 'cold' referrals from courts, probation service, lawyers and other sources
- Liaison with probation and other community based services for offenders
- Liaison with the health care service for prisoners
- Access to a range of inpatient facilities, including open ward, intensive psychiatric care, and medium security for the assessment and treatment of patients before trial and after conviction
- Liaison with high security hospitals for patients returning from, or requiring treatment under, conditions of special security
- Access to accommodation in the community providing varying levels of support.

Mentally disordered offenders may receive treatment in a variety of settings or they may fail to receive treatment at all. A comprehensive government review of health and social services for mentally disordered offenders (Department of Health & Home Office 1992), known as the Reed report, made a careful analysis and produced 276 recommendations (Chiswick 1992). They rested on principles that mentally disordered offenders should receive care of high quality from health and social services. This should be appropriate to their need, at no greater level of security than is justified, with an emphasis on care near to their home area. Further reviews have considered the role of the special hospitals and the treatment of people with psychopathic disorder.

There remain severe problems with an underprovision of inpatient facilities providing intensive psychiatric care, medium secure care and long-term care with low security (Mental Health Act Commission 1997). The independent sector is filling some of the gaps in provision and now provides over a third of the medium secure beds in England and Wales. The provision of high secure care (formerly maximum security) is undergoing change, with contraction in the number of beds in the three existing special hospitals. At the time of writing a judicial inquiry into the treatment of psychopathic patients at Ashworth Hospital on Merseyside is in progress.

REFERENCES

Abel G G, Becker J V, Cunningham-Rathner J, Mittleman M, Rouleau J L 1988 Multiple paraphilic diagnoses among sex offenders. Bulletin of the American Academy of Psychiatry and Law 16: 153–68

Allam J, Middleton D, Browne K 1997 Different clients, different needs? Practical issues in community-based treatment for sex offenders. Criminal Behaviour and Mental Health 7: 69–84

Alper J 1995 Biological influences on criminal behaviour: how good is the evidence? British Medical Journal 310: 272–273

Amir M 1971 Patterns in forcible rape. University of Chicago Press, Chicago

Appleby L, Wessely S 1988 The influence of the Hungerford massacre on the public opinion of mental illness. Medicine, Science and the Law 28: 291–295

Backett S A 1987 Suicide in Scottish prisons. British Journal of Psychiatry 151: 218–221

Bailey J, MacCulloch M 1992 Characteristics of 112 cases discharged directly to the community from a new special hospital and some comparisons of performance. Journal of Forensic Psychiatry 3: 91–112

Bailey S 1995 Young offenders, serious crimes. British Journal of Psychiatry 167: 5–7

Baker E 1997 The introduction of supervision registers in England and Wales: a risk communications analysis. Journal of Forensic Psychiatry 8: 15–35

Barker A 1994 Arson. A review of the psychiatric literature. Oxford University Press, Oxford

Barnett W, Spitzer M 1994 Pathological fire-setting 1951–1991: a review. Medicine, Science and the Law 34: 4–20

Birmingham L, Mason D, Grubin D 1996 Prevalence of mental disorder in remand prisoners: consecutive case study. British Medical Journal 313: 1521–1524

Bisson J I, Shepherd J P 1995 Psychological reactions of victims of violent crime. British Journal of Psychiatry 167: 718–720

Bluglass R 1995 Writing reports and giving evidence. In: Chiswick D, Cope R (eds) Seminars in practical forensic psychiatry. Gaskell, London, pp 134–163

Bogue J, Power K 1995 Suicide in Scottish prisons, 1976–93. Journal of Forensic Psychiatry 6: 527–540

Bools C 1996 Factitious illness by proxy (Munchausen syndrome by proxy). British Journal of Psychiatry 169: 268–275

Borgaonkar D S, Shah S A 1974 The XYY chromosome – male or syndrome? Progress in Medical Genetics 10: 135–222

Brittain R P 1970 The sadistic murderer. Medicine, Science and the Law 10: 198–207

Brooke D, Taylor C, Gunn J, Maden A 1996 Point prevalence of mental disorder in unconvicted male prisoners in England and Wales. British Medical Journal 313: 1524–1527

Brunner H G, Nelen M, Breakfield X O, Ropers H H, van Oost B A 1993 Abnormal behaviour associated with a point mutation in the structural gene for monoamine oxidase A. Science 262: 578–580

Buchanan A 1994 Brain, mind and behaviour revisited. Journal of Forensic Psychiatry 5: 232–236

Buchanan A, Reed A, Wessely S et al 1993 Acting on delusions II: the phenomenological correlates of acting on delusions. British Journal of Psychiatry 163: 77–81

Canter D, Heritage R 1990 A multivariate model of sexual offence behaviour: developments in 'offender profiling'. I. Journal of Forensic Psychiatry 1: 185–212

Carey G 1994 Genetics and violence. In: Reiss A J, Miczek K A, Roth J A (eds) Understanding and preventing violence: biobehavioral influences. National Academy, Washington, vol 2, pp 21–58

Cherrett M 1996 Mentally disordered offenders and the police. Mental health review. Pavilion, London

Chiswick D 1981 Matricide. British Medical Journal 238: 1279–1280

Chiswick D 1985 Use and abuse of psychiatric testimony. British Medical Journal 290: 975–977

Chiswick D 1992 Reed report on mentally disordered offenders. British Medical Journal 305:1448–1449

Chiswick D 1995 Dangerousness. In: Chiswick D, Cope R (eds) Seminars in practical forensic psychiatry. Gaskell, London, pp 210–242

Chiswick D 1996 Sentencing mentally disordered offenders. British Medical Journal 313: 1497–1498

Chiswick D, Dooley E 1995 Psychiatry in prisons. In: Chiswick D, Cope R (eds) Seminars in practical forensic psychiatry. Gaskell, London, pp 243–271

Christiansen K O 1977 A preliminary study of criminality among twins. In: Mednick S A, Christiansen K O (eds) Biosocial bases of criminal behaviour. Gardner, New York, pp 89–108

Clare I C, Murphy G H, Cox D, Chaplin E H 1992 Assessment and treatment of fire-setting: a single-case investigation using a cognitive-behavioural model. Criminal Behaviour and Mental Health 2: 253–268

Clark C, Mezey G 1997 Elderly sex offenders against children: a descriptive study of child sex abusers over the age of 65. Journal of Forensic Psychiatry 8: 357–369

Clark S A 1993 Matricide: the schizophrenic crime? Medicine, Science and the Law 33: 325–328

Cloninger C R, Sigvardsson S, Bohman M, von Knorring A 1982 Predisposition to petty criminality in Swedish adoptees. II Cross-fostering analysis of gene–environment interaction. Archives of General Psychiatry 39: 1242–1247

Cocozza J J, Melick M E, Steadman H J 1978 Trends in violent crime among ex-mental patients. Criminology 216: 317–334

Coid J W 1984 How many psychiatric patients in prison? British Journal of Psychiatry 145: 78–86

Coid J W 1992 DSM-III diagnosis in criminal psychopaths: a way forward. Criminal Behaviour and Mental Health 2: 78–94

Coid J W 1996 Dangerous patients with mental illness: increased risks warrant new policies, adequate resources, and appropriate legislation. British Medical Journal 312: 965–969

Coid J W, Cordess C 1992 Compulsory admission of dangerous psychopaths. British Medical Journal 304: 1581–1582

Cordess C 1995 Crime and mental disorder 1. Criminal behaviour. In: Chiswick D, Cope R (eds) Seminars in practical forensic psychiatry. Gaskell, London, pp 14–51

Cote G, Lesage A, Chawky N, Loyer M 1997 Clinical specificity of prison inmates with severe mental disorders: a case control study. British Journal of Psychiatry 170: 571–577

Criminal Behaviour & Mental Health 1992 Psychopathic disorder. 2: 66–244

Dalgaard O C, Kringlen E 1976 A Norwegian study of criminality. British Journal of Criminology 16: 213–232

Davidson M, Humphreys M S, Johnstone E C, Owens D G C 1995 Prevalence of psychiatric morbidity among remand prisoners in Scotland. British Journal of Psychiatry 167: 545–548

Day K 1990 Mental retardation: clinical aspects and management. In: Bluglass R, Bowden P (eds) Principles and practice of forensic psychiatry. Churchill Livingstone, Edinburgh, pp 399–418

Day K 1994 Male mentally handicapped sex offenders. British Journal of Psychiatry 165: 630–639

Dell S 1984 Murder into manslaughter: the diminished responsibility defence in practice. Maudsley monograph 27. Oxford University Press, Oxford

Dell S, Robertson G, James K, Grounds A 1993 Remands and psychiatric assessments in Holloway Prison 1: The psychotic population. British Journal of Psychiatry 163: 634–640

Dempster T 1990 Defence of insanity. Journal of Forensic Psychiatry 1: 355–359

Dempster T 1991 Sleepwalking and insanity. Journal of Forensic Psychiatry 2: 327–330

Denno D W 1996 Legal implications of genetics and crime research. Ciba Foundation Symposium 194: 248–264

Department of Health 1996 Statistical bulletin 1996/10 In-patients formally detained in hospitals under the Mental Health Act 1983 and other legislation, England: 1989–90 to 1994–95. Government Statistical Service, London

Department of Health, Home Office 1992 Review of health and social services for mentally disordered offenders and others requiring similar services. Final summary report. CM 2088. HMSO, London

Department of Health, Home Office 1994 Working group on psychopathic disorder, report. Department of Health, Home Office, London

Dietz P E 1978 Social factors in rapist behaviour. In: Rada R T (ed) Clinical aspects of the rapist. Grune & Stratton, New York

Dooley E 1990 Prison suicide in England and Wales. British Journal of Psychiatry 156: 40–45

d'Orban P T 1976 Child stealing: a typology of female offenders. British Journal of Criminology 16: 275–281

d'Orban P T 1979 Women who kill their children. British Journal of Psychiatry 134: 560–571 McGrath 1992

d'Orban P T, Haydn-Smith P 1985 Men who steal children. British Medical Journal 290: 1784

Dunn J, Fahy T A 1990 Police admissions to a psychiatric hospital; demographic and clinical differences between ethnic groups. British Journal of Psychiatry 156: 373–378

Dye S, Isaacs C 1991 Intravenous drug misuse among prison inmates: implications for spread of HIV. British Medical Journal 302: 1506

Eastman N 1996 Hybrid orders: an analysis of their likely effects on sentencing practice and on forensic psychiatric practice and services. Journal of Forensic Psychiatry 7: 481–494

Eastman N 1997 The Mental Health (Patients in the Community) Act 1995. A clinical analysis. British Journal of Psychiatry 170: 492–496

Editorial 1994 Guilty innocents: the road to false confessions. Lancet 344: 1447–1450

Egglestone F 1990 The advisory board on restricted patients. In: Bluglass R, Bowden P (eds) Principles and practice of forensic psychiatry. Churchill Livingstone, Edinburgh, pp 1253–1257

Eronen M 1995 Mental disorders and homicidal behaviour in female subjects. American Journal of Psychiatry 152: 1216–1218

Eronen M, Tiihonen J, Hakola P 1996a Schizophrenia and homicidal behaviour. Schizophrenia Bulletin 22: 83–89

Eronen M, Hakola P, Tiihonen J 1996b Mental disorders and homicidal behaviour in Finland. Archives of General Psychiatry 53: 497–501

Farrington D P 1993 The psychosocial milieu of the offender. In: Gunn J, Taylor P J (eds) Forensic psychiatry, clinical legal and ethical issues. Butterworth-Heinemann, Oxford, pp 252–285

Fenwick P B C 1991 Brain, mind, insanity and the law. British Medical Journal 302: 979–980

Fenwick P 1993 Brain, mind and behaviour. Some medico-legal aspects. British Journal of Psychiatry 163: 565–573

Finkelhor D (ed) 1984 Child sexual abuse: new theory and research. Free Press, New York

Fowkes F G, Leng G C, Donnan P T, Deary I J, Riemersma R A, Housley E 1992 Serum cholesterol, triglycerides and aggression in the general population. Lancet 340: 995–998

Freedman D S, Byers T, Barrett D H, Stroup N E, Eaker E, Monroe-Blum H 1995 Plasma lipid levels and psychologic characteristics in man. American Journal of Epidemiology 141: 507–517

Freud S 1929 Civilisation and its discontents. In the standard edition of the complete works of Sigmund Freud, volume XXI, 1961. Hogarth, London, p 90

Garza-Trevino E S 1994 Neurobiological factors in aggressive behaviour. Hospital and Community Psychiatry 45: 690–699

Gayford J 1975 Wife-battering: a preliminary survey of 100 cases. British Medical Journal 1: 194–197

Geller J L 1992 Arson in review: from profit to pathology. Psychiatric Clinics of North America 15: 623–645

Gibbens T C N, Robertson G 1983 A survey of the criminal careers of hospital order patients. British Journal of Psychiatry 143: 362–369

Gibbens T C N, Palmer C, Prince J 1971 Mental health aspects of shoplifting. British Medical Journal 3: 612–615

Gibbens T C N, Way C, Soothill K L 1977 Behavioural types of rape. British Journal of Psychiatry 130: 32–42

Gillies H 1976 Homicide in the west of Scotland. British Journal of Psychiatry 128: 105–127

Gordon A 1990 Drugs and criminal behaviour. In: Bluglass R, Bowden P (eds) Principles and practice of forensic psychiatry. Churchill Livingstone, Edinburgh, pp 897–901

Gore S M, Bird A G 1993 No escape: HIV transmission in jail. British Medical Journal 307: 147–148

Green C M 1981 Matricide by sons. Medicine, Science and the Law 21: 207–214

Griew E 1991 Alcoholism and diminished responsibility. Journal of Forensic Psychiatry 2: 79–84

Grounds A 1985 The psychiatrist in court. British Journal of Hospital Medicine 34: 55–58

Grubin D 1994a Sexual sadism. Criminal Behaviour and Mental Health 4: 3–9

Grubin D 1994b Sexual murder. British Journal of Psychiatry 165: 624–629

Grubin D 1995 Offender profiling. Journal of Forensic Psychiatry 6: 259–263

Grubin D 1996 Fitness to plead in England and Wales. Maudsley monograph 38. Psychology Press, Hove

Grubin D H, Kennedy H G 1991 The classification of sexual offenders. Criminal Behaviour and Mental Health 1: 123–129

Grubin D, Wingate S 1996 Sexual offence recidivism: prediction versus understanding. Criminal Behaviour and Mental Health 6: 349–359

Gudjonsson G H 1990 Psychological and psychiatric aspects of shoplifting. Medicine, Science and the Law 30: 45–51

Gudjonsson G H 1993 The psychology of interrogations, confessions and testimony. Wiley, Chichester

Gunn J 1977 Epileptics in prison. Academic Press, London

Gunn J, Maden A, Swinton M 1991 Treatment needs of prisoners with psychiatric disorders. British Medical Journal 303: 338–341

Guze S B 1976 Criminality and psychiatric disorders. Oxford University Press, New York

Hafner H, Boker W 1982 Crimes of violence by mentally abnormal offenders. Oxford University Press, London

Hansen H, Lykke-Olsen L 1997 Treatment of dangerous sexual offenders in Denmark. Journal of Forensic Psychiatry 8: 195–199

Hanson R K, Steffy R A, Gauthier R 1993 Long-term recidivism of child molesters. Journal of Consulting and Clinical Psychology 6: 646–652

Helzer J E, Robins L N, McEvoy L 1987 Post-traumatic stress disorders in the general population. New England Journal of Medicine 318: 1630–1634

Herzberg J L, Fenwick P B C 1988 The aetiology of aggression in temporal lobe epilepsy. British Journal of Psychiatry 153: 50–55

Hilton M R, Mezey G C 1996 Victims and perpetrators of child sexual abuse. British Journal of Psychiatry 169: 408–415

Hodgins S 1992 Mental disorder, intellectual deficiency, and crime: evidence from a birth cohort. Archives of General Psychiatry 49: 476–483

Hodgins S, Mednick S A, Brennan P A, Schulsinger F, Engberg M 1996 Mental disorder and crime: evidence from a Danish birth cohort. Archives of General Psychiatry 53: 489–496

Holloway J, Shaw J 1993 Providing a forensic psychiatry service to a magistrates' court: a follow-up study. Journal of Forensic Psychiatry 4: 575–581

Home Office 1990 Provision for mentally disordered offenders. Circular no. 66/90. Home Office, London

Home Office 1996 Criminal statistics England and Wales 1995. Cm 3421. Stationery Office, London

Home Office, Department of Health and Social Security 1975 Report of the committee on mentally abnormal offenders. Command paper 6244. HMSO, London

Hore B 1990 Alcohol and crime. In: Bluglass R, Bowden P (eds) Principles and practice of forensic psychiatry. Churchill Livingstone, Edinburgh, pp 873–880

Howard League for Penal Reform 1985 Unlawful sex: report of a Howard League working party. Waterlow, London

Humphreys M S, Johnstone E C, MacMillan J F, Taylor P J 1992 Dangerous behaviour preceding first admission for schizophrenia. British Journal of Psychiatry 161: 501–505

Jackson H F, Glass C, Hope S 1987 A functional analysis of recidivist arson. British Journal of Clinical Psychology 26: 175–185

James D V, Hamilton L W 1991 The Clerkenwell scheme: assessing efficiency and cost of a psychiatric liaison service to a magistrates' court. British Medical Journal 303: 282–285

James D, Cripps J, Gilluley P, Harlow P 1997 A court-focused model of forensic psychiatry provision to central London: abolishing remands to prison? Journal of Forensic Psychiatry 8: 390–405

Joseph P L, Potter M 1993 Diversion from custody. 1: Psychiatric assessment at the magistrates' court. British Journal of Psychiatry 162: 325–330

Junginger J 1996 Psychosis and violence: the case for a content analysis of psychotic experience. Schizophrenia Bulletin 22: 91–103

Kaul A 1993 Sex offenders – cure or management? Medicine, Science and the Law 33: 207–212

Kershaw C, Dowdeswell P, Goodman J 1997 Restricted patients – reconvictions and recalls by the end of 1995: England and Wales. Home Office statistical bulletin 1/97. Home Office, London

Knight R A, Prentky R A 1989 Classifying sexual offenders: the development and corroboration of taxonomic models. In: Marsh W, Laws R, Barbaree H (eds) Handbook of sexual assaults. Plenum Press, New York

Lamontagne Y, Carpentier N, Hetu C, Lacerte-Lamontagne C 1994 Shoplifting and mental illness. Canadian Journal of Psychiatry 39: 300–302

Langton J, Krishnan V, Cumella S, Clarke D, Corbett J 1993 Detentions in a mental handicap hospital: a ten-year retrospective study. Journal of Forensic Psychiatry 4: 85–95

Lasegue C 1877 Les exhibitionnistes. L'Union Médicale Troisième Série 23: 709

Levey S, Howells K 1995 Dangerousness, unpredictability and the fear of people with schizophrenia. Journal of Forensic Psychiatry 6: 19–39

Lewis D O, Pincus J H, Bard B et al 1988 Neuropsychiatric, pseudoeducational and family characteristics of 14 juveniles condemned to death in the United States. American Journal of Psychiatry 145: 584–589

Lewis N D C, Yarnell H 1951 Pathological firesetting (pyromania). Nervous and mental disease monograph 82. Coolidge Foundation, New York

Lindqvist P 1991 Homicides committed by abusers of alcohol and illicit drugs. British Journal of Addiction 86: 321–326

Lindqvist P, Allebeck P 1990 Schizophrenia and crime: a longitudinal follow up of 644 schizophrenics in Stockholm. British Journal of Psychiatry 157: 345–350

Link B G, Andrews H, Cullen F T 1992 The violent and illegal behaviour of mental patients reconsidered. American Sociological Review 57: 275–292

Lloyd C, Walmsley R 1989 Changes in rape offences and sentencing. Home Office research study 105. HMSO, London

McElroy S L, Pope H G, Hudson J I, Keck P E, White K L

1991 Kleptomania: a report of 20 cases. American Journal of Psychiatry 148: 652–657

McGrath P 1992 Maternal filicide in Broadmoor Hospital 1919–69. Journal of Forensic Psychiatry 3: 271–297

McGuffin P, Thapar A 1992 The genetics of personality disorder. British Journal of Psychiatry 160: 12–23

Mackay R 1990 Insanity and fitness to stand trial. Journal of Forensic Psychiatry 1: 277–304

MacMillan J F, Johnson A L 1987 Contact with the police in early schizophrenia: its nature, frequency and relevance to outcome of treatment. Medicine, Science and the Law 27: 191–200

McNiel D F, Binder R L, Greenfield T K 1988 Predictors of violence in civilly committed acute psychiatric patients. American Journal of Psychiatry 145: 965–970

Maden A, Swinton M, Gunn J 1990 Women in prisons and the use of illicit drugs before arrest. British Medical Journal 301: 1133

Maden A, Swinton M, Gunn J 1991 Drug dependence in prisoners. British Medical Journal 302: 880

Marshall P 1994 Reconviction of imprisoned sexual offenders. Home Office research and statistics department. Research Bulletin 36: 23–29

Martell D A, Dietz P E 1992 Mentally disordered offenders who push or attempt to push victims onto subway tracks in New York City. Archives of General Psychiatry 49: 472–475

Marzuk P M, Tardiff K, Hirsch C S 1992 The epidemiology of murder–suicide. Journal of the American Medical Association 267: 3179–3183

Mayhew P, Elliott D, Dowds L 1993 The 1988 British crime survey. Home Office research study 111. HMSO, London

Meadow R 1989 Munchausen syndrome by proxy. British Medical Journal 299: 248–250

Mednick S A, Gabrielli W F, Hutchings B 1984 Genetic influences in criminal convictions: evidence from an adoption cohort. Science 224: 891–894

Mental Health Act Commission 1997 Seventh biennial report 1995–1997. Stationery Office, London

Menzies R P, Federoff J P, Green C M, Isaacson K 1995 Prediction of dangerous behaviour in male erotomania. British Journal of Psychiatry 166: 529–536

Milroy C M 1995 Reasons for homicide and suicide in episodes of dyadic death in Yorkshire and Humberside. Medicine, Science and the Law 35: 213–217

Mitchell B 1997 Diminished responsibility manslaughter. Journal of Forensic Psychiatry 8: 101–117

Moffitt T E 1993a Adolescence-limited and life course-persistent antisocial behaviour: a developmental taxonomy. Psychological Review 100: 674–701

Moffitt T E 1993b The neuropsychology of conduct disorder. Developmental Psychopathology 5: 135–151

Molnar G, Keitner L, Harwood B T 1984 A comparison of partner and solo arsonists. Journal of Forensic Science 29: 574–583

Monahan J 1984 The prediction of violent behaviour: toward a second generation of theory and policy. American Journal of Psychiatry 141: 10–15

Monahan J 1993 Mental disorder and violence: another look. In: Hodgins S (ed) Mental disorder and crime. Sage, London

Monahan J, Steadman H J 1983 Crime and mental disorder: an epidemiological approach. In: Tonry M, Morris N (eds) Crime and justice: an annual review of research. University of Chicago Press, Chicago

Monahan J, Steadman H J 1994 Violence and mental disorder. Developments in risk assessment. University of Chicago Press, Chicago

Mullen P 1990 Morbid jealousy and the delusion of infidelity. In: Bluglass R, Bowden P (eds) Principles and practice of forensic psychiatry. Churchill Livingstone. Edinburgh, pp 823–834

Mullen P E 1993 The crime of passion and the changing cultural construction of jealousy. Criminal Behaviour and Mental Health 3: 1–11

Mullen P, Pathe M 1994 Stalking and pathologies of love. Australian and New Zealand Journal of Psychiatry 28: 469–477

Murray D J 1989 Review of research on re-offending of mentally disordered offenders. Research and planning unit paper 55. Home Office, London

Needham-Bennett H, Parrott J, Macdonald A J D 1996 Psychiatric disorder and policing the elderly offender. Criminal Behaviour and Mental Health 6: 241–252

Noble P, Rodger S, 1989 Violence by psychiatric in-patients. British Journal of Psychiatry 155: 384–390

Norfolk G A 1997 'Fitness to be interviewed' – a proposed definition and scheme of examination. Medicine, Science and the Law 37: 228–234

Norton K, Dolan B 1995 Assessing change in personality disorder. Current Opinion in Psychiatry 8: 371–375

Ormerod D 1996 Psychological profiling. Journal of Forensic Psychiatry 7: 341–352

O'Sullivan G H, Kelleher M J 1987 A study of fire-setters in the south west of Ireland. British Journal of Psychiatry 151: 818–823

Payne A 1995 Infanticide and child abuse. Journal of Forensic Psychiatry 6: 472–476

Pearse J, Gudjonsson G 1996 How appropriate are appropriate adults? Journal of Forensic Psychiatry 7: 570–580

Peay J 1996 Inquiries after homicide. Duckworth, London

Player E, Jenkins M 1994 Prisons after Woolf: reform through riot. Routledge, London

Prins H 1994a Fire-raising: its motivation and management. Routledge, London

Prins H 1994b Is diversion just a diversion? Medicine, Science and the Law 34: 137–147

Puri B K, Baxter R, Cordess C C 1995 Characteristics of fire-setters. British Journal of Psychiatry 166: 393–396

Rada R T 1975 Alcoholism and forcible rape. American Journal of Psychiatry 132: 444–446

Raine A, Brennan P, Mednick B, Mednick S A 1996 High rates of violence, crime, academic problems, and behavioural problems in males with both early neuromotor deficits and unstable family environments. Archives of General Psychiatry 53: 544–549

Repo E, Virkkunen M 1997 Outcome in a sample of Finnish fire-setters. Journal of Forensic Psychiatry 8: 127–137

Resnick P J 1969 Child murder by parents. American Journal of Psychiatry 126: 325–334

Rix K J B 1994 A psychiatric study of adult arsonists. Medicine, Science and the Law 34: 21–34

Rix K J B 1997 Fitness to be interviewed by the police? Advances in Psychiatric Treatment 3: 33–40

Robertson G 1988 Arrest patterns among mentally disordered offenders. British Journal of Psychiatry 153: 313–316

Robertson G, Dell S, James K, Grounds A 1994 Psychotic men remanded in custody to Brixton Prison. British Journal of Psychiatry 164: 55–61

Robertson G, Pearson R, Gibb R 1996 The entry of mentally

disordered people to the criminal justice system. British Journal of Psychiatry 169: 172–180

Rowlands M W D 1988 Psychiatric and legal aspects of persistent litigation. British Journal of Psychiatry 153: 317–323

Rowlands R, lnch H, Rodger W, Soliman A 1996 Diverted to where? What happens to the diverted mentally disordered offender. Journal of Forensic Psychiatry 7: 284–296

Runciman, Viscount 1993 The Royal Commission on Criminal Justice Report. Cmnd 2263. HMSO, London

Rutter M 1995 Causal concepts and their testing. In: Rutter M, Smith D J (eds) Psychosocial disorders in young people. Wiley, Chichester, pp 7–34

Rutter M 1996 Concepts of antisocial behaviour, of cause, and of genetic influences. In: Bock G R, Goode J A (eds) Genetics of criminal and antisocial behaviour. Ciba Foundation Symposium 194: 1–20

Rutter M, Giller H 1983 Juvenile delinquency: trends and perspectives. Penguin, Harmondsworth

Rutter M, Smith D J 1995 (eds) Psychosocial disorders in young people. Wiley, Chichester

Sandberg S 1996 Hyperkinetic or attention deficit disorder. British Journal of Psychiatry 169: 10–17

Scott P 1973 Parents who kill their children. Medicine, Science and the Law 13: 120–126

Segal J H 1989 Erotomania revisited: from Kraepelin to DSM-III-R. American Journal of Psychiatry 146: 1261–1266

Shepherd M 1961 Morbid jealousy: some clinical and social aspects of a psychiatric symptom. Journal of Mental Science 107: 687–753

Sheppard D 1996 Learning the lessons, 2nd edn. Zito Trust, London

Smith D J 1995 Youth crime and conduct disorders: trends, patterns and causal explanations. In: Rutter M, Smith D J (eds) Psychosocial disorders in young people. Wiley, Chichester, pp 389–489

Smith J, Hucker S 1994 Schizophrenia and substance abuse. British Journal of Psychiatry 165: 13–21

Soothill K L, Pope P J 1973 Arson: a twenty year cohort study Medicine, Science and the Law 13: 127–138

Sosowsky L 1978 Crime and violence among mental patients reconsidered in view of the new legal relationship between the state and the mentally ill. American Journal of Psychiatry 135: 33–42

Soyka M, Naber G, Volcker A 1991 Prevalence of delusional jealousy in different psychiatric disorders. An analysis of 93 cases. British Journal of Psychiatry 158: 549–553

Steering Committee of the Confidential Inquiry 1996 Report of the confidential inquiry into homicides and suicides by mentally ill people. Royal College of Psychiatrists, London

Stewart L A 1993 Profile of female firesetters. Implications for treatment. British Journal of Psychiatry 163: 248–256

Sugarman P, Dumughn C, Saad K, Hinder S, Bluglass R 1994 Dangerousness in exhibitionists. Journal of Forensic Psychiatry 5: 287–296

Swanson J W, Holzer C E, Ganju V K, Jono R T 1990 Violence and psychiatric disorder in the community: evidence from the epidemiological catchment area surveys. Hospital and Community Psychiatry 41: 761–770

Taylor P 1985 Motives for offending among violent and psychotic men. British Journal of Psychiatry 147: 491–498

Taylor P J 1993a Organic disorders, mental handicap and offending. In: Gunn J, Taylor P J (eds) Forensic psychiatry, clinical legal and ethical issues. Butterworth-Heinemann, Oxford, pp 286–328

Taylor P J 1993b Psychosis, violence and crime. In: Gunn J, Taylor P J (eds) Forensic psychiatry, clinical legal and ethical issues. Butterworth-Heinemann, Oxford, pp 329–372

Taylor P J 1993c Victims and survivors. In: Gunn J, Taylor P J (eds) Forensic psychiatry, clinical legal and ethical issues. Butterworth-Heinemann, Oxford, pp 885–944

Taylor P J, Gunn J 1984 Violence and psychosis I – risk of violence among psychotic men. British Medical Journal 288: 1945–1949

Taylor P J, Parrott J 1988 Elderly offenders: a study of age-related factors among custodially remanded prisoners. British Journal of Psychiatry 152: 340–346

Taylor P, Mahendra B, Gunn J 1983 Erotomania in males. Psychological Medicine 13 :645–650

Teplin L A, Pruett N S 1992 Police as streetcorner psychiatrist: managing the mentally ill. International Journal of Law and Psychiatry 15: 139–156

Teplin L A, Abram K M, McClelland G M 1996 Prevalence of psychiatric disorders among incarcerated women I. Pretrial jail detainees. Archives of General Psychiatry 53: 497–501

Toone B K, van der Linden 1997 Attention deficit hyperactivity disorder or hyperkinetic disorder in adults. British Journal of Psychiatry 170: 489–491

Virkkunen M, Goldman D, Linnoila M 1996 Serotonin in alcoholic violent offenders. In: Bock G R, Goode J A (eds) Genetics of criminal and antisocial behaviour. Ciba Foundation Symposium 194: 168–182

Walker N, McCabe S 1973 Crime and Insanity in England. Vol 2: New solutions and new problems. University of Edinburgh Press, Edinburgh

Walters G D 1992 A meta-analysis of the gene-crime relationship. Criminology 30: 595–613

Wessely S 1997 The epidemiology of crime, violence and schizophrenia. British Journal of Psychiatry 170 (suppl 32): 8–11

Wessely S, Taylor P J 1991 Madness and crime: criminology versus psychiatry. Criminal Behaviour and Mental Health 1: 193–228

Wessely S C, Castle D, Douglas A J, Taylor P J 1994 The criminal careers of incident cases of schizophrenia. Psychological Medicine 24: 483–502

West D J 1988 Psychological contributions to criminology. British Journal of Criminology 28: 77–92

West D J 1993 Disordered and offensive sexual behaviour. In: Gunn J, Taylor P J (eds) Forensic psychiatry, clinical legal and ethical issues. Butterworth-Heinemann, Oxford, p 543

West D 1994 Sex crimes. Dartmouth, Aldershot

West D J, Walk A (eds) 1977 Daniel McNaughton: his trial and the aftermath. Healy, Ashford, Kent

West Midlands Regional Health Authority 1991 Report of the panel of inquiry appointed by the West Midlands Regional Health Authority, South Birmingham Health Authority and the Special Hospitals Service Authority to investigate the case of Kim Kirkman. West Midlands Regional Health Authority, Birmingham

Wilkins J, Coid J 1991 Self-mutilation in female remanded prisoners: 1. An indication of severe psychopathology. Criminal Behaviour and Mental Health 1: 247–267

Zitrin A, Hardesty A S, Burdock E M, Drossman A K 1976 Crime and violence among mental patients. American Journal of Psychiatry 133: 142–149

29
Legal and ethical aspects of psychiatry

S. G. Potts

Psychiatric practice is as much a moral as a medical endeavour.

(Mechanic 1989)

INTRODUCTION

After at most 20 hours devoted to ethics in a decade or more of training, would-be psychiatrists might take issue with Mechanic. This is because ethical issues, while ever-present, remain implicit in most psychiatric encounters, only becoming explicit when brought to the surface by conflict.

Contrast two cases. Ms Smith is referred by her general practitioner to a local psychiatrist who runs a private practice in behavioural psychotherapy. She has an uncomplicated spider phobia which causes her distress and interferes with her everyday life. She understands the principles of graded exposure, complies with the programme she is set, and after the six sessions she initially contracted for, is happy to report a substantial improvement. Mr Jones, on the other hand, is arrested after behaving bizarrely in busy traffic, endangering himself and others. Social services have already been alerted by neighbours about the apparent neglect of his two young children. Examination shows him to be floridly psychotic, and he is transferred under the Mental Health Act to a local psychiatric hospital against his will. There he becomes increasingly agitated and requires forcible medication, to which he develops an acute dystonic reaction. It becomes clear that he has schizophrenia, which responds to drug treatment, but is aggravated by continuing use of cannabis. His psychiatrist regrets that there are insufficient resources to offer him, in addition to drugs, the psychological treatment which is known to improve compliance with medication and reduce the risk of relapse.

Both types of case are common in psychiatric practice. While the ethical issues in the second case are multiple and manifest, at first glance there appear to be none raised by the first. This is because the ethical principles which govern all medical transactions, including both of these, are implicit, or embedded, but no less present, in the dealings between Ms Smith and her doctor. It is only when clinicians and commentators struggle to resolve conflicts, such as those raised in Mr Jones' case, that the principles involved are exposed, delineated and made explicit. Where there is no conflict between principles, they remain so hidden it is easy to suppose them absent.

While these ethical principles underlie the whole of medicine, they lie closer to the surface in psychiatry than many other disciplines. This means that some ethical issues, such as resource allocation, are no different in psychiatry than other medical specialities, while others, though shared with medicine generally, are highlighted in psychiatry because of its nature – an example being the potential for sexual abuse of the doctor–patient relationship. Finally, there is an important set of issues, such as involuntary commitment to hospital, which arise exclusively in psychiatry, although the principles which apply remain those in operation elsewhere. While all psychiatry takes place in a legal framework, the law, very properly, has more to say about this third group of issues, via mental health legislation and the common law.

In what follows I hope to set out the nature of these principles, their origins, in terms of history and philosophy, and their application within psychiatry. I will also discuss, in outline, the relevant legal issues, although the specifics will vary between jurisdictions.

HISTORICAL AND PHILOSOPHICAL BACKGROUND

Recent years have seen a dramatic expansion in the number and range of ethical controversies in medicine and psychiatry, with loudly voiced argument assailing the bewildered practitioner from all sides. Yet until the 1970s medical ethics meant little more in Britain than, firstly, the medical etiquette governing transactions between practitioners – for example, 'Any undisclosed division of professional fees is *unethical*' (British Medical Association 1981, italics added); and, secondly, exhortations to avoid alcohol (at least when on duty), adultery (at least with one's patients) and above all, advertising. The lay public, and many practitioners, took the view that any more specifically *ethical* questions could be resolved by reference to the Hippocratic Oath. This short and ancient text contains absolute but unargued prohibitions against euthanasia, abortion, sexual relationships with patients and breach of confidentiality. The model of medicine it advances is that of an art whose secrets are passed from one generation of adepts to the next, via a kind of masonic apprenticeship, and in which the overriding principle is one of benevolent devotion to the sick. The oath cannot possibly guide psychiatrists struggling with today's issues, partly because they were unanticipatable by Hippocrates and his peers, but mainly because the oath is a blunt list of dos and don'ts without an argued basis which could be extended to modern practice. The hippocratic tradition lives on in the modern equivalent of the oath, the Declaration of Geneva (World Medical Association 1948), which jettisons the archaic language, but which is still so generally phrased as to be of liittle value in guiding particular decisions. British medical schools have recognised this, if belatedly, in that none now requires its medical graduates to declare the oath, and the Declaration of Geneva has not generally been adopted as a replacement.

The best known specifically psychiatric codes are the Declaration of Hawaii (World Psychiatric Association 1977), a two-page list of 10 guidelines, and the rather more detailed *Principles of Medical Ethics with Annotations Especially Applicable to Psychiatry* (APA 1973). Even this last document is not specific enough to answer many questions, and its principles are again set forth as an unargued list, like the 10 commandments but without their vigour of expression. ('A physi-

cian shall recognise a responsibility to participate in activities contributing to an improved community'.) The problem, of course, with such unargued lists, is that they give no guidance on how to act when principles are in conflict: and it is in just such cases that guidance is most needed. Oaths and declarations are clearly not sufficient, but the psychiatrist who goes beyond them to the philosophy from which they emerge soon risks confusion. Moral philosophy is a huge and venerable discipline, as old as medicine itself. It is also an important living academic subject, represented on the campus of any self-respecting university, with all that implies for continuing disagreement. It is possible, however, to identify, at the risk of brutal oversimplification, two broadly competing camps within the subject as a whole: the deontological and the teleological traditions, whose main features and major problems are summarised in Table 29.1.

Deontology versus teleology

Deontology

Of the two, deontology is by far the older, taking its roots in a combination of Judeo-Christian theology and Ancient Greek philosophy, which were first fully synthesised 700 years ago in St Thomas Aquinas' *Summa Theologica* (Shapcote 1912–1936). Aquinas claimed that secular reason could arrive at the same moral laws as were handed down in religious precepts, and, particularly since Immanuel Kant in the late 18th century, the philosophy has been divorced from the theology to stand or fall independently. The term deontology derives from the Greek *deon* for duty, indicating the centrality of rules. Initially these were expressed primarily as *obligations*, akin to commandments, but, since the great revolutions of the 18th century, the more legalistic language of *rights* has taken precedence. By virtue of their status as human beings, people have

Table 29.1 Features and problems of contrasting moral theories		
	Deontology (absolutism)	Teleology (consequentialism, utilitarianism)
Main features	Rule based	Outcome based
	Rights and duties determine action	Greatest good of greatest number determines action
	Consequences irrelevant	Consequences all-important
Major problems	No procedure to resolve conflicts of rights	No common scale of measurement
	What kinds of things have rights, and why?	Individual interests easily overridden for greater good

rights, such as the rights to life, liberty and the pursuit of happiness enshrined in the American Declaration of Independence. It is generally (but not universally) acknowledged that rights and duties are correlate, so that granting someone a right confers a duty elsewhere, whether it falls on specific individuals, people in general, or institutions, including hospitals and the state. If I have a right to confidentiality, my doctor has a duty to observe it; if I have a right to life, everyone has a duty not to kill me; and if I have a right to medical treatment, the government has a duty to ensure its provision. There is no such thing as half a right or a partial duty: rights and duties act like trump cards (Dworkin 1977) and hold absolutely (hence *absolutism* as an alternative term for this philosophy). This is so whatever the consequences: 'though the heavens fall' in Anscombe's phrase (1981).

There are many difficulties in this outlook. Where do rights come from? What sort of entities possess them, and why? By virtue of what are they granted? When are they acquired: at conception, viability, birth, or later? Can they be lost, temporarily, as perhaps in delirium, or permanently, in dementia? On what grounds are they granted to the severely mentally handicapped but withheld from higher primates? More pressingly, what happens in situations where they appear to conflict, as in therapeutic abortion to save a woman's life? And how can it be right to ignore consequences so blithely?

Teleology

Teleology derives its name from the Greek *teleon*, purpose, and was elaborated by the 19th century English philosophers Jeremy Bentham and John Stuart Mill, each of whom owed much to their Scottish forebear, David Hume. Teleological morality is also called consequentialism or utilitarianism. The central concept is, that rather than rights, people have *interests*, whether these be concerns, desires or needs. Fulfilment or frustrations of these interests is the ultimate source of value, good or bad. Teleology relies heavily on the assumption that it is possible to measure the various possible outcomes of moral choices in terms of pleasure or pain, happiness lost or gained, for all those affected; and that, via some unspecified kind of moral calculus, a decision can be arrived at by applying the much-abused slogan 'the greatest good of the greatest number' as the determining principle.

Although teleological views have become very powerful in recent moral philosophy, and by extension, in medical ethics, there are again major problems. The system depends vitally on the claim that it is possible to measure, on the same scale of value, such widely varying outcomes as an examination passed, a cup final won, or a healthy baby born to a healthy mother. No such measuring system has been developed, and it strains credulity to accept without demur that it ever could be. Furthermore, such a system carries with it the inescapable risk that the interests of individuals or minorities could too readily be sacrificed to the common good, if the stakes were high enough. As the philosopher Bernard Williams (Smart & Williams 1973) has put it, in such a system the individual matters no more than do individual petrol tanks in the statistics on national petrol consumption.

Derivative principles

The psychiatrist who seeks guidance by taking a course in moral philosophy will thus probably emerge asking more questions than he started with; but it is neither necessary nor possible to resolve age-old questions of moral theory in order to arrive at a measure of consensus on general, but not fundamental, ethical principles at a lower level. John Stuart Mill, for example, famously argued that the greatest good of the greatest number can best be served by giving people as much liberty (or autonomy, as we would now put it) as possible to decide for themselves how to order their lives, limited only by the effects of their choices on others (Mill 1859).

It is possible, therefore, to arrive at a general principle of respect for autonomy both within a rights-based, deontological, moral outlook (people have a right to privacy and self-determination, and others have correlative duties), and from a teleological perspective, via Mill's argument (people's interests are most likely to be fulfilled if their freedom to choose is maximised).

The philosopher R.M. Hare (1981) has argued that the basic dispute between deontology and teleology can be resolved by making the latter primary, and deriving from it, by arguments like Mill's, a basic set of rules. These then acquire a secondary, derivative, deontological force, which can be used to guide practical decision-making. Where conflicts between these rules arise, they are resolved by resort to primary teleological reasoning.

While they do not explicitly adopt this approach, Beauchamp and Childress, in their widely influential work (1994), argue for a brief set of four prima facie principles: respect for autonomy, beneficence, non-maleficence and justice. While important, they are not necessarily fundamental, and can be supported by a variety of different moral theories, which are likely to take different approaches to the resolution of any conflict between them. Nor is the list immutable: Gillon (1994), for example, has added the further requirement of concern for the principles' scope of application. Figure 29.1 shows how these principles

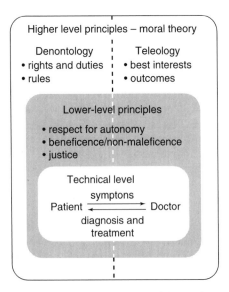

Fig. 29.1 Relationship between moral theory, lower-level principles and the clinical encounter.

might act as intermediary levels of ethical reasoning between individual doctor–patient encounters and abstract moral theory. The principles and their applications will be examined further below. First, however, it is necessary to explore further the reasons for the dramatically increased interest in ethical issues in the last 30 years.

Recent history 1: Abuses of psychiatry and the limits of paternalism

This change cannot be explained by moral theory or derived principles: rather it reflects powerful social forces that impinge upon doctors, patients, and the settings in which they meet. These forces need clarification.

Authors commonly cite new developments in medical technology as the primary driving force in generating interest in ethics. Although psychiatry lags behind other specialities in this respect, developments such as psychosurgery, electroconvulsive therapy (ECT), an ever-widening range of psychotropic drugs, brain imaging techniques, and the identification of genetic tests for such conditions as Huntington's chorea have made it possible for psychiatrists to *do* a great deal more than hitherto, raising the inevitable question of whether they *should*. While undoubtedly relevant, technological development is not the only, or even the foremost, factor behind ethics' expansion. Much more important has been the attack, from several directions, on the benevolent paternalism implicit in the hippocratic model.

Recent history has shown, all too shockingly, how easily such paternalism turns malevolent. Lifton (1976) has described how psychiatrists were at the forefront of the Nazi euthanasia campaign, from its beginnings well before the Second World War. Those patients they deemed *Lebensunwertes leben* – lives unworthy of life – were taken aside and murdered in their thousands. Even worse, this selective culling of schizophrenics, epileptics and the mentally handicapped served as the testing ground for methods, such as poison gas, which were later applied on a much wider scale in the wholesale slaughter of the Holocaust (Muller-Hill 1991). The motivation for this grotesque abuse of psychiatry appears to have been predominantly eugenic: the wish to preserve the purity of the race. No clearer illustration of the ease with which consequentialist reasoning can sacrifice the interests of individuals or minorities to a supposed higher good can be provided.

Although the abuses of the Nazi era are by far the worst, unchecked paternalism has an inbuilt tendency to overreach itself and turn malevolent. In the decades since, it has given rise to other abuses, all very different in their time, place and underlying motivation. From the 1950s to the 1980s, for example, the Soviet Union systematically abused psychiatry for political ends (Bloch & Reddaway 1977). A diagnosis not recognised elsewhere, sluggish schizophrenia, was defined so as to medicalise politically unacceptable dissident or reformist behaviour. Dissidents so labelled were detained in psychiatric hospitals and medicated against their will.

Although there were brave exceptions, many Soviet psychiatrists colluded with this practice. Some, no doubt, were well intentioned, and acted out of a belief in the validity of 'sluggish schizophrenia'. Others, more aware of the true nature of the diagnosis, turned a blind eye to its use, out of a mixture of political conformism, personal ambition, and fear of being labelled dissident themselves. It was only after a long campaign of criticism by Western psychiatrists, and the coming of glasnost and perestroika, that the practice ended.

Although the Nazi and Soviet abuses show that psychiatry is readily distorted in a totalitarian state, we should not complacently assume that it cannot also happen in a liberal democracy. Continuing concern about psychiatry in Japan (Harding 1991), the outrage that greeted the dumping of psychiatric patients in barbaric conditions on the Greek island of Leros (Ramsay 1990) and sporadic enquiries into conditions inside some British hospitals all attest to the need for continued vigilance. Nor should we forget the results of excessive therapeutic zeal. Between the end of the war and the development of effective psychotropic drugs in the 1950s, unmodified ECT, psychosurgery and insulin coma were the only effective physical treatments for serious mental illness. In the USA and Europe, well-intentioned but overenthusiastic use of these treatments became institutionalised, with the consequence that thousands of patients underwent inappropriate, unnecessary and dangerous physical procedures. The backlash against these excesses is still felt today in the profoundly negative public attitude to ECT, and the legislative barriers against its use in some American states. The initial overuse of a new intervention, followed by a rejecting overreaction, and then by due recognition of its proper place in treatment, is a pattern well recognized throughout medicine, but it seems to have been greatly exaggerated in the case of ECT and psychosurgery. No doubt this partly arose from the intense frustration engendered in psychiatrists responsible for large asylums with many disturbed patients and no effective treatment, but it was made more possible by the paternalistic attitude that the psychiatrists knew best, and that patient's views were irrelevant.

The dawning recognition of the defects of paternalism grew from the civil liberties campaigns and the counterculture movement of the 1960s and subsequently. These movements, their aims embodied in the slogan 'Question authority', challenged the assumption that authority figures, including doctors and psychiatrists, could be trusted to act benevolently, replacing it with the contrary view that patients, like citizens in general, needed protection from the inherently (if unconsciously) malevolent tendencies of unrestrained authority, echoing Shaw's dictum that all professions are conspiracies against the laity. In other words they rejected the very notion of paternalism as a valid basis for civil society, and therefore for medicine and psychiatry.

Paternalism is thus now largely (but not completely) replaced by a contractarian model of the relationship between doctor and patient in which the participants are contracting equals, much as car owners and garage mechanics might be. There is an asymmetry of knowledge between mechanic and carowner, just as there is between doctor and patient, but there is no asymmetry of power. The mechanic is contractually obliged to undertake an accurate assessment of the presenting problem, to explain it to the owner to the owner's satisfaction, to propose the appropriate repair work, and then to abide by the owner's decision. In return the owner is obliged to provide payment, but he is free to accept or reject the mechanic's advice. The expertise might lie on one side of the transaction, but the choice, and more importantly the money, lies on the other, thus balancing the power relationship. Of course a great deal of medicine, and especially psychiatry, cannot be fitted to this model, and it distorts practice to assume that it

can be. None the less the model is now predominant, although paternalism retains a place where the patient's ability to choose for himself is impaired, as is often the case in psychiatry; it is paternalism that justifies the detention and treatment against his will of Mr Jones and others like him.

Recent history 2: Antipsychiatry

A disconnected group of psychiatrists and others, influential beyond its size, and collectively known as the antipsychiatrists, went beyond the rejection of paternalism to deny altogether the validity of psychiatric diagnoses and therefore of treatment. Thomas Szasz is the first, foremost and longest-enduring. His central argument, stated in the title of his early work, *The Myth of Mental Illness* (1961), and reframed repeatedly since, is that mental illness, as a concept, has no validity. It is simply wrong, in his view, to medicalise mental distress and abnormal behaviour with a diagnostic label, and then to treat it: those who profess to do so are little more than frauds, acting as unwitting agents of social control. R. D. Laing's rather different argument – that schizophrenia is not so much a diagnosis as a sane response to an insane society, which psychiatrists protect via the labelling and segregation of dissenting victims – is expressed no less vigorously (Laing 1965). While these views still have their advocates, they are now less influential than when first promulgated, and have little influence on the day-to-day running of most psychiatric services.

Fulford (1989) has mounted a spirited defence against the antipsychiatrists' charge that psychiatric diagnosis is inherently value-laden and therefore oppressive, intolerant of deviance and scientifically invalid. His argument has a much stronger philosophical (as opposed to polemical) grounding, and therefore a greater strength, than those of Szasz or Laing, whose positions he essentially turns on their heads. Szasz and Laing argue from analogy, claiming that since medical diagnoses are rooted in purely factual descriptions of organic pathology and its consequences, and since such descriptions are generally lacking in psychiatry, then psychiatric diagnoses cannot lay claim to the validity accorded their medical counterparts. Fulford shows, to my mind convincingly, that medical diagnoses are no less value-laden than the psychiatric equivalents, and that it is simply false to claim that they rely universally on accounts of organic dysfunction: he thus rescues psychiatric diagnosis from the charge of scientific invalidity.

None the less it is vitally important that psychiatry remains aware of the very real abuses committed in its name in the past, when psychiatrists clearly *did* act as agents of social control, in order to guard against this ever-present risk in the present and the future. It could be argued that one function of mental health legislation, beyond protecting the rights of patients, is to protect psychiatry against well-intentioned, but damaging, excursions beyond its legitimate boundaries. In this respect psychiatry clearly differs from other medical specialities.

THE FOUR-PRINCIPLES APPROACH

Respect for autonomy

Respect for a patient's autonomy always heads the various shortlists of prima facie ethical principles, reflecting the primacy of the contractarian model. According to this principle, patients should be treated as rational autonomous agents, making their own decisions about their lives. From it flow further lower-level requirements, including confidentiality and informed consent (see below). Respecting a patient's autonomy assumes that the patient's capacity to make rational choices is not impaired, temporarily or permanently, by mental or physical disorder (or, in the case of children, by immaturity). Many ethical problems in medicine generally, and especially in psychiatry, turn on this issue of competence. Two sets of questions arise: those with a relatively narrow technical focus (What kinds of condition can limit a patient's competence? How is competence assessed? Is it a global matter, or can it be broken down to specific competences for specific issues?); and those with a broader, more ethical dimension (Where competence is limited, what principles then take over to guide action? The contractarian advance directive, the paternalism implied in a best interests standard, or the intermediate position afforded by a proxy judgement?).

Non-maleficence and beneficence

The Latin epithet *primum non-nocere*, meaning first (or above all) do no harm, has an obscure but ancient origin. It lives on in the clumsily labelled principle of non-maleficence, the requirement that doctors strive to avoid harming those in their care and their kin. Philosophers argue about the extent to which this principle can be separated from its correlate, the principle of beneficence (the requirement to do good or promote wellbeing), but it is clear that the primacy implied by the phrase 'above all' does not apply. If it did, no surgeon could ever operate because of the pain he might cause, and no psychiatrist could ever prescribe for fear of side-effects. In almost all therapeutic decisions, a judgement about the *balance* of burdens and benefits is

made, non-maleficence and beneficence being as inseparable as the opposing sides of a coin. However, differing philosophical models of the interaction between doctor and patient lead to different views about how this balancing is to be done, and who does it.

In the contractarian/deontological model, there is an agreement, explicit or implicit, between doctor and patient. Acting benevolently and avoiding harm is what the doctor offers and the patient wants. They make a contract, which derives its binding power from the general duty to tell the truth and to keep promises, both of which originate in the the principle of respect for autonomy. Furthermore, the judgement about what constitutes benefit and harm, and how they are to be balanced, is the patient's. The doctor's role is to provide the patient with sufficient information to enable the patient to make a considered judgement according to his own view of the possible outcomes, and then to abide by the patient's choice. In the teleological model, acting benevolently and avoiding harm is fundamental, for it is the very root of *all* morality, medical decisions forming a particular subset. In principle at least, benefits and burdens can be assigned values on some common scale, and moral mathematics then determines the right action. However, given the lack of consensus on any such scale, heavy emphasis is placed on the patient's own valuations as those offering most accuracy. Again, therefore, the doctor is required to provide sufficient information to enable the patient to choose between the options before him according to his own ranking of burdens and benefits. Maximum benefit and minimum harm is most assured when patient autonomy, or, in Mill's term, liberty, is greatest.

The two models therefore yield similar lower-level views of the doctor–patient interaction, but in the contractarian model autonomy is paramount and beneficence/non-maleficence derivative, while in the teleological model the reverse is the case.

Justice

The justice referred to in this principle is not retributive, concerned with the punishment of wrongdoing, but distributive, concerned with the sharing out of losses and gains between individuals.

In the hippocratic tradition, represented in the Smith case above, the relationship between doctor and patient is dyadic and exclusive, and questions of justice do not arise. But medical encounters do not take place in a vacuum. The patient will often have a family, and he will always be a citizen: no man is an island. The doctor, a citizen too, will have other patients, and usually limited access to expensive tests and treatments. Doctor and patient are thus both located in a moral web of rights and responsibilities owed to other parties, and the strands of duty which link them to each other can be distorted and sometimes broken by the weight of moral burdens falling elsewhere in the web.

Sometimes these tensions are specfic and therefore stark, as when a nephrologist has two patients needing dialysis, but only the resources to treat one. Whom should he choose: the patient who is more likely to benefit, who is the more 'deserving', who has more dependents, who has more to offer society, who is younger, or whose condition is not self-inflicted? Psychiatry does not readily offer such dramatic dilemmas, although in truth they are rare in medicine generally. Usually the choices are less clear-cut, and lie not between specific individuals with competing claims on the same scarce resource, but between unidentified future patients with potential claims on different resources. For example, a psychiatric hospital may choose to delay resettling long-stay patients in community housing in order to liberate funds for an urgently needed alcohol detoxification project; or a Health Authority may limit the number of patients started on clozapine in order to pay for new anti-HIV (human immunodeficiency virus) drugs.

Questions of justice are not confined to matters of resource allocation. They also arise whenever a clinical decision confers potential burdens and benefits on people other than the patient, even when access to treatment is not limited. In Jones' case above, part of the justification for detaining him in hospital comes from the risks he poses to other (unidentified) members of the public who might be endangered by his bizarre behaviour in traffic; and part of the justification for medicating him against his will is the risk his disturbed behaviour poses to other (identified) patients and staff. The principle of justice requires attention to the means by which the benefits and burdens for the patient of detention and enforced medication are balanced against the benefits and burdens accruing to other people, whether they be his children, fellow patients or the public in general.

Consideration of the principles underpinning such choices and issues leads directly into unresolved debates about the best structure for a health care system, and, beyond this, to questions of *political* as well as moral philosophy. Deontological and teleological views are probably more at variance in this area than elsewhere in medical ethics. Deontology would imply, for example, that when patients compete for a scarce treatment, the only way to respect their rights is to choose between them at random. If one patient is elderly, unskilled, free of dependents, and unlikely to benefit much from treatment, while another is young, with a dependent family, a valuable talent, and a good prospect of cure, teleolo-

gists would decry the inefficiency and waste that follows from tossing a coin to choose between them.

In practice such decisions are usually made via a muddled mixture of teleological and deontological thinking, superimposed on long-standing but never justified custom and practice. The British NHS was founded on the principle of equal access to treatment, free at the point of need, but decisions about the relative budgets for cardiology and orthopaedics turn more on matters of local history and practical politics than they do on philosophy, however much cost-effectiveness data and teleological argument might be cited to choose between hearts and hips.

Scope

As Gillon has argued, even full consensus about the above four principles might not guarantee agreement about their application, because of differing views about their scope. Whose rights, whose interests are to figure in ethical deliberation: where and how are the limits to be set? The widely debated Oregon experiment is a case in point. After a long consultation period, the state of Oregon proposed a rank ordering of a long list of medical treatments and surgical procedures, in an attempt to determine which would, and which would not, be funded by public money. Unfortunately the orderings produced by various groups differed, sometimes considerably, raising the question: whose views count? Current patients, who know what it is like to suffer the condition in question? The general population, as potential patients, trying to imagine what it might be like? Medical staff who know what it is like to treat such conditions, and who are more illness averse than the general population? Or the taxpayer, who pays for it all? Questions abound, but answers are few: a position familiar elsewhere in philosophy, but one on which, in this context, practical, real-world, decisions are based, sometimes with life and death consequences.

It is a common criticism of the four-principles approach that it gives no guidance about how to proceed when principles conflict. This reflects the principles' status as pragmatic, prima facie, lower-order rules of thumb, derived ultimately from more abstract moral theory about which there is much less agreement. The four principles provide a common ground for moral debate between people of very different philosophical or religious outlooks, just as the same pitch can be used to play rugby or football. Those hoping for a set of universal binding rules governing all situations requiring moral choices will face inevitable disappointment, but they should not be surprised, given that we live in a pluralist democracy.

In what follows, I hope to show how these principles

might bear upon a range of more specific areas of ethical concern in psychiatry.

CONFIDENTIALITY

What I may see or hear in the course of the treatment, or even outside of the treatment, in regard to the life of men, which on no account must spread abroad, I will keep to myself, holding such things shameful to be spoken about.

Hippocratic Oath

The hippocratic adherence to confidentiality is absolute but unargued, with a complete lack of guidance to its scope of application. What are these things which must not be spread abroad? And is it really the case that on no account may confidentiality be breached? (Indeed it is possible to demonstrate the weakness of the oath by paraphrasing it: 'whatever should be kept secret, I will keep secret, because it should be kept secret.') While priests and lawyers still enjoy relationships with their clients which preserve this hermetically sealed notion of confidentiality, doctors do not. Questions of what clinical information doctors may (or may be obliged to) divulge, and under what circumstances, grow ever more complex, and require doctors to make judgements balancing patient autonomy against the interests of the patient himself, other individuals, or society in general.

The complexity of medical practice already means that large numbers of staff have access to potentially sensitive information held in a patient's casenotes. Add up the number of nurses, doctors, social workers, psychologists, occupational therapists, medical secretaries and administrative staff employed on a typical psychiatric ward: the total is unlikely to be less than 20. Add in the primary care staff to whom the discharge letter is sent, not to mention the general medical team who referred the patient, and the total rises further. It is not surprising that patients sometimes feel they lose control over sensitive information about their own lives when they enter psychiatric services: yet all these professionals have a legitimate need for access, if treatment is to be effective. Problems arise when patients seek to restrict the range of dissemination within this circle (refusing permission, for example, for the psychiatrist to communicate with the general practitioner, or divulging something on the condition that the nurses not be told), or when others outside this circle seek access to such information. Of course many disclosures of information occur with the patient's full knowledge and permission. Codes of practice have developed to guide this process, whereby any information passed on

is the minimum necessary for the purpose at hand (such as ensuring payment by a health insurance company), and then only after the patient has given explicit written permission. Giving permission is not the same as conferring an obligation, however: there are circumstances in which the clinician may decline to pass on information at the patient's behest, if he feels it is detrimental enough to the patient's best interests.

More ethically interesting, however, are those cases in which confidentiality is breached in the face of opposition (or incompetence) on the part of the patient. It would be hard to construct a case where a competent patient's wish for confidentiality is overridden in the patient's own interest. If the patient is competent, then his autonomy is paramount, and he, not his psychiatrist, is the best judge of his own best interests. Where the patient is incompetent (see below), then breaches of confidentiality may be justifiable in his best interest. A surgeon may need to be told, for example, that the semiconscious and uncooperative patient he is operating on for injuries sustained in a road traffic accident is heavily alcohol dependent, and likely to develop delirium tremens without appropriate postoperative treatment. The principle of beneficence/non-maleficence thus overrides the principle of respect for autonomy in circumstances such as these, at least until such time as the patient's competence is restored. The same reasoning applies when divulging to others a depressed patient's suicidal ideation, in order to ensure his care in conditions of safety. In these cases the harm (breach of confidentiality) and the benefit (prevention of delirium tremens or suicide) accrue to the same person, the patient, and the temporary overriding of autonomy is generally readily justifiable. More troubling are those cases where the benefits involved accrue to someone else, raising the general issue of justice. Perhaps the most famous such case is that of Tarasoff (1976). Although the case was heard by California's Supreme Court, and is therefore not a precedent in other jurisdictions, it has influenced professional and legal attitudes in other US States and in Britain. Prosenjit Poddar, a student at the University of California who was receiving psychotherapy, divulged to his therapist murderous feelings towards a young woman, Tatiana Tarasoff, who had spurned his advances. Poddar's therapist informed his supervisor, and the police, but, crucially, not Tarasoff herself. Poddar later murdered her, and her parents sued. Rulings of the court made it clear that clinicians in such cases had a *duty* to warn and otherwise protect third parties potentially at risk from their patients. Subsequent rulings in various jurisdictions might have modified the expression of that duty, but Tarasoff remains a landmark case for affirming that such a duty exists, and the duty to observe confidentiality must be balanced against it. An unwelcome consequence of the ruling is to extend the psychiatrist's role as an agent of social control, and to impute to clinicians powers of predicting dangerousness they simply do not possess. It is significant that, after they were informed of Poddar's threats, the police arrested him, only to release him uncharged because he had committed no offence; no-one sued them.

Harm to third parties can come about in a variety of ways which fall short of direct threats to kill, raising the question of how severe the harm and what the level of risk must be before confidentiality is breached. In some areas the law imposes a statutory duty, and in others codes of practice apply. Examples include the provisions of child protection legislation obliging professionals to report continuing abuse or neglect; the (much-ignored) duty to report drug-dependent patients to the Home Office; and the requirement to report to the Driver and Vehicle Licensing Agency (DVLA) patients who are unfit to drive but ignore advice to stop. In general, in such cases, the clinician's duty is not so much to warn and protect potential victims (who are sometimes identifiable, sometimes not) but to inform the relevant regulatory agencies, and the limits of the clinician's duty are well marked. Where there is no statutory provision, matters are much less clear-cut. The developing law relating to HIV and the acquired immune deficiency syndrome (AIDS) is a case in point. In some jurisdictions HIV infection is a notifiable disease, and a body of case law is slowly building up around HIV transmission. The question of whether knowingly infecting another with HIV is an offence, and if so what, is one that courts in Britain, Cyprus and elsewhere have recently grappled with: not far behind it will come the question of whether a therapist who becomes aware that her HIV-positive patient is continuing to have unprotected sex has a duty to warn his unsuspecting spouse.

In other cases it is not so much the patient's private behaviour that might pose risks, but his ability to function in a job which confers responsibility for the welfare and safety of others. A clinician's threshold for breaching confidentiality about a depressed airline pilot or a paranoid air traffic controller will clearly be lower than for a librarian or a shopkeeper, for example. Teleological reasoning readily accommodates such variations, even in the absence of an agreed scale of risk, but a deontologist will struggle to justify such a willingness to vary the threshold at which a duty is breached.

The duty to warn and protect third parties placed at risk by a patient's action confers on the clinician a kind of vicarious responsibility, which is at times burdensome. The burden has been increased further by the General Medical Council's recent clarification that doctors may also owe a duty of care to the patients of colleagues whose competence is threatened by illness. A surgeon who becomes aware that a colleague has developed a drink problem, and is operating while intoxicated, for example, is held to owe a duty to the colleague's patients, as well as his own, which requires him to report the situation in such a way as to bring it to an end.

Examples such as these show that we have come a long way from the view of confidentiality enshrined in the Hippocratic Oath as absolute and total. It is now seen as important but relative, contingent and overridable. Respecting confidentiality is only one among an ever-growing list of duties which the clinician must balance against one another.

CONSENT

The law regarding consent to medical treatment makes it clear that any unconsented touching of a patient by a doctor may be both a civil wrong (a tort) and a criminal act (a battery). Doctors avoid action on these grounds in three ways: by reference to any relevant legislation, such as the Mental Health Act; by invoking common law rights and duties; or by showing the patient has consented to the treatment in question.

For some medical and psychiatric treatments (surgery, invasive procedures, ECT, entry into research projects), practice dictates that the patient must make explicit his consent by signing the requisite form. Elsewhere – that is, for nearly all psychiatric treatment – consent is implicit in the patient's attendance. Ms Smith, for example, is unlikely ever to be asked 'Do you consent to this programme of graded exposure for your spider phobia?' The boundary separating treatments in need of explicit consent is erratically drawn, however. In British practice, a signed consent form would always be required before a biopsy of a brain tumour, sometimes before a lumbar puncture, but only rarely before magnetic resonance imaging. As a result of social pressures in the mid-1980s, blood tests for HIV status now require explicit consent, but other blood tests (including those for hepatitis B, which raise many of the same issues) do not.

Whether implicit or explicit, a patient's consent will not be valid unless he is informed, competent and free of duress. Given the asymmetry of knowledge and expertise described above, there is a requirement on the doctor to impart sufficient understandable and relevant information to the patient to enable a choice based on the patient's own judgement of the alternatives. Only then is the patient fully capable of acting autonomously. But what counts as relevant? And how much is sufficient? Various tests apply, including, in order of increasing rigour, that which would generally be divulged by a reasonable body of medical opinion; that which any reasonable patient would need and wish to know; and that which the particular patient in question would need and wish to know. British practice favours the former, after the Sidaway case (1983) of a woman who suffered paralysis after cervical spine surgery. She claimed damages on the grounds that if she had been informed beforehand of the small but definite risk of this complication (approximately 1%), she would not have consented: but her claim was dismissed, it being argued that there was no requirement upon doctors to divulge risks of this magnitude, and most generally did not.

Freedom from duress is an obvious element of valid consent but duress can range widely in degree, from the blatant, which is easily identified as such and therefore excluded, to the very subtle, which may never be thought of by patient or doctor as duress at all: for where lies the boundary between duress and persuasion?

Particularly frequent and problematic in psychiatry is the kind of duress applied by the doctor who tells her patient: 'We want you to stay on the ward and take this medication, Mr Roberts; and I'm afraid that if you don't we'll have to consider sectioning you.'

Of the three elements of consent, that raising most ethical issues, especially in psychiatry, is, however, competence, a complicated medical and legal concept, which finds itself at the heart of many other ethical questions.

COMPETENCE

The primacy of autonomy discussed above relies heavily, but usually invisibly, on the assumption that the patient is competent to make choices about her treatment. Ethical debate tends to focus more on the issues raised if the patient is not competent, and her autonomy therefore impaired, than on what constitutes competence. This implies that competence is a dichotomous either/or phenomenon, and that there is consensus on how to assess it. Unfortunately this is not the case. Various definitions of competence (and its constituent elements) can be offered, the common thread being capacity to make a personal, reasoned choice between alternatives. As such, it requires several subcapacities, including the ability to acquire, retain and understand information, and then to use it, together with personal preferences or valuations, to deliberate, make a reasoned choice, and then to communicate that choice, together with, where necessary, the reasoning behind it.

All these abilities are dimensional, not categorical, so competence itself, being composed of them, cannot be otherwise: yet it is often discussed as if it were, and psychiatrists are regularly called in as the arbiters, especially in general hospitals. ('Is or is not Mr Johnson competent to refuse transfusion/discontinue dialysis/decline chemotherapy?') This is partly because, in medicine as in law, patients are *deemed* competent until proven otherwise, and the burden of proof falls upon the clinician (or the courts) to demonstrate sufficient impairment of competence for the matter at hand. Competence may be eroded in a gradual way, as in a dementing illness, without ever being called into question, until a situation requiring a significant choice arises. If the patient is then declared incompetent, it does not mean that he has just become so. Competence is often erroneously thought of as being global, as well as dichotomous, so that a patient considered incompetent in one area of his life is thereby so deemed in all other areas too. The psychiatrist who argues that, by virtue of his depression, Mr Johnson is indeed incompetent to discontinue his dialysis, should not assume he also becomes incompetent to make a will, manage his finances, or choose between steak and fish at dinner. The degree of evidence required to discharge the burden of proof varies between applications, as does the consequence of a judgement of incompetence. Competence is thus *task-specific*: of course Mr Johnson can choose between steak and fish, and even if he cannot manage his finances, he may well be competent to appoint a proxy to do it for him.

Legal aspects

The above example illustrates how competence has both legal and medical aspects. Legal applications embrace both the criminal and the civil law, and Chapter 28 has dealt with the former, under such heads as fitness to plead, diminished responsibility, and the McNaughton Rules. The large literature on mentally disordered offenders which that chapter reviews tends to consider the concept of *responsibility* more central than competence, although the two are closely related: the same factors which might lead to a defence of diminished responsibility may also call into question the defendant's competence to stand trial at all (i.e. his fitness to plead) or to be punished. In this last context British psychiatrists are thankfully spared a particularly painful ethical dilemma imposed on some of our American colleagues: namely, the requirement that an offender who becomes mentally ill after being sentenced to death should receive psychiatric treatment to render him competent for execution.

As far as the civil law is concerned, competence is

most commonly questioned in regard to money: specifically the ability to make a will (testamentary capacity) and the management of one's assets while still alive. In order to be 'of sound disposing mind' the testator must understand what a will is, and must know the nature and extent of his property and the identities of those who might have a claim on it. He must be free of undue influence, and of mental disorder which might distort those of his judgements which are relevant to the making of the will. He need not be free of mental disorder entirely, however. An encapsulated delusional system, such as the belief that he is spied upon by police-appointed pigeons, need not intrude at all upon large areas of a patient's life, and indeed may be apparent only on direct questioning by a trained interviewer. Such a patient would be psychotic, and yet, at the same time 'of sound disposing mind'.

Where a patient develops a mental illness, especially one which is chronic or irreversible, but may be expected to live for some time yet, the question of his competence to manage his affairs naturally arises, particularly if those affairs are complex or he is wealthy. The test of competence which applies is similar to that determing testamentary capacity, and is, once again, task-specific. For patients found incompetent, a proxy, such as a family member or lawyer, may be appointed to act on his behalf. Power of attorney is a legal instrument used to formalise the long-standing principle that whatever a person can legitimately do, he can appoint another to do on his behalf. Originally, however, power of attorney lapsed when capacity was lost. The recently developed durable power of attorney works differently: a proxy is appointed at a time when the patient retains competence, but anticipates that his illness will erode it. The proxy's powers are not enacted at this stage, but spring into effect when the patient loses capacity, and remain in effect until the patient dies (or, less commonly, since the illness in question is usually dementia, recovers).

Where there is no suitable proxy, or where conflicts of interests might arise, more formal procedures are available, the details of which vary between jurisdictions. In Britain, for example, application may be made to the Court of Protection, who can provide a disinterested third party to manage the patient's affairs on a best interests standard.

Medical applications

For most of this century, and especially in recent decades, campaigners have called for the legalisation of euthanasia, and are ever closer to success, particularly in Holland, the Northern Territory of Australia, and the west coast of the USA. The debate originally centred around core cases, real or rhetorical, in which incurable

physical illness was expected to cause death in the near future, and unrelievable pain and suffering, without diminution of awareness, until then. Euthanasia's advocates argue that to deny a person so afflicted a quick, painless, dignified death at the hands of a doctor is cruel and wrong.

While psychological or psychiatric factors do not figure large in this central case, the debate has expanded rapidly in the last 20 years, each expansion introducing more questions with a psychological content. Some of these now impinge directly upon clinical practice, even though euthanasia remains illegal. Public anxiety about facing incurable pain in a terminal illness has been matched, and perhaps surpassed, by the widespread (and demographically justified) fear of a long twilight of decline, via dementia, to a life stripped to bare existence and maintained by medical interventions the patient is now incapable of refusing. In an attempt to reassert control over this much feared indignity, the concept of a living will was first proposed in the late 1960s. Perhaps better known as an advance directive, this is a document drawn up by someone who is now competent and wishes to retain control over treatment decisions which might become necessary at some time in the future, when he might no longer be so. Different formats are available, the common feature being a list of interventions that prospective patients would accept or decline in variously specified circumstances (e.g. 'If I should develop a dementia or other incurable brain disease, then I would/would not – *delete as appropriate* – wish to have dialysis if it becomes necessary').

These documents are still much more widely used in the USA than Britain, where argument rages about whether they should be legally binding, or whether they merely provide guidance to the doctor. The Voluntary Euthanasia Society recently proposed that a doctor who flouts the terms of a patient's living will should be made criminally liable and punishable with up to 2 years' imprisonment. The legislation that finally emerged did not go this far: and the extent to which British doctors *must* abide by a living will probably requires a test case for clarification; as does the appropriate action where a patient now demented and incompetent expresses a wish to continue living, in direct contradiction to the terms of a previously enacted living will.

Given their inflexibility, and the impossibility of ever drafting living wills sufficiently specific to cover all possible future medical scenarios, the alternative (or additional) use of health care proxies has much to recommend it. The medical counterpart of the durable power of attorney for financial matters, a proxy decision maker for health care is a friend or family member nominated by a potential patient at a time when competent, who is empowered to take treatment decisions on the patient's behalf if, at some future time, he becomes incompetent to do so himself.

Ideally the proxy should apply a *substituted judgement* test to the decision at hand, and use her prior knowledge of the patient to determine what he would have wanted in the circumstances now prevailing.

The use of proxies is not without its difficulties, however. There is no reason to believe that the alternative *best interests* test is necessarily any better applied by a proxy than by the doctors involved, and it may be difficult for the proxy to distinguish between substituted judgement, best interests, and the further question of what *she* would want for the patient. Furthermore, in cases where the proxy stands to benefit from any legacy, there is a potential conflict of interest which may complicate matters; and, where the proxy is of an age with the patient, and therefore vulnerable to the same risks of dementia, the question of the proxy's *own* competence may arise.

Perhaps the best way to minimise these complications is to adopt an instrument which combines the function of an advance directive and the nomination of a proxy, whose function it is to apply the terms of the advance directive in the light of her knowledge of the patient's preference and values.

Euthanasia: other issues

The competence of those requesting treatment withdrawal (or, in Holland, where it has a quasi-legal status, euthanasia) can be called into question in another way, with a specifically psychiatric dimension. It is well known that depression is prevalent in the physically ill, often going unrecognised, and that physical illness, especially in the elderly, is a risk factor for suicide. The possibility therefore arises that requests for euthanasia, or an end to life-sustaining treatment, might represent suicide equivalents in patients whose judgement is distorted by depressive illness (Potts 1991). The recently enacted legislation in Australia's Northern Territory (Right of the Terminally Ill Act 1996, overturned by the Australian Senate in 1997) recognised this, and specifically required a psychiatric assessment to exclude the possibility. Oregon's 1994 Death with Dignity Act, which legalised physician-assisted suicide, but which has been held up by legal challenges, also made provision for 'counselling' where a psychological disorder is suspected. The Dutch provisions for euthanasia mandate no such psychiatric assessment, and, following a much-publicised 1991 case, the Dutch Supreme Court took the view that a treatment-resistant depression, in itself, and in the absence of any physical illness, might be a valid condition in which to honour a request for euthanasia (Ogilvie & Potts 1994).

COMPULSION

As long as euthanasia remains illegal, these ethically-debated medical decisions at the end of life will have a mainly passive character, restricted to choices to withdraw or withhold life-sustaining treatment. Elsewhere, and specifically in psychiatry, ethical questions have long reverberated around the very different issue of active treatments which patients might be *compelled* to undergo.

The occurrence of mental illness in its members has always demanded a response from society, especially when that illness leads sufferers into acts (or omissions) which put themselves or others at risk.

Western society's response, over the centuries, has three principal strands running through it: namely, the punitive, the segregating, and the therapeutic. Each has dominated in different eras, but all persist today. The punitive response implies that, notwithstanding any mental illness, people who offend retain autonomy and therefore responsibility for their actions, and are punishable for them. Repeated findings of high rates of mental illness in custodial settings (see Ch. 28) imply that this response is with us still. The segregating response grew out of discomfort with this purely punitive approach, and has a long history, going back at least as far as the founding of London's Bethlem Royal Hospital in 1247. Implicit in it is the view that the mentally ill may need to be separated from the public to minimise the risk to others, and separated under supervision, to minimise the risk to themselves. This response reached its peak in the Victorian asylum building era, but lives on, as do many of those very buildings.

The therapeutic response has a history too, rooted as it is in the efforts of Pinel and the Tukes to ensure that those segregated in this way are treated as humanely as possible. However, as became clear in the 1950s and 1960s, large institutions which act as warehouses for those declared deviant, can all too readily become punitive, however high-minded the intent. This recognition coincided with the development of increasingly effective physical treatments, which held out the promise, not only of a return to health, but to society. Maintaining mental health, for some people, requires continuing psychosocial support and long-term medication, and where these are either not forthcoming, or refused by the patient, there is an increased chance of relapse, with all that implies about re-emerging risk. The public are increasingly aware of these risks, and anxiety about them is both reflected in, and generated by, the publicity accorded to a series of cases in recent years, particularly those of Ben Silcock and Christopher Clunis.

Mental health legislation reflects this history, so that

the 1959 Mental Health Act (1960 in Scotland), concentrated on *admission to* hospital, while its 1983 successor (1984 in Scotland) had more to say about compulsory *treatment in* hospital. The Mental Health (Patients in the Community) Act 1995 is an attempt to provide greater powers for supervision and compulsory treatment *outside* hospital, but has met much criticism (Eastman 1997).

The Jones case set out in the Introduction above is typical of those for which compulsory admission and treatment might be mooted. Jones has an acute florid psychotic illness, manifested by behaviour which poses direct and indirect risks to himself and to others, and by impaired insight, which calls into question his competence to refuse offers of help. In these circumstances beneficence (acting in what others, particularly psychiatrists, judge to be his best interests) and justice (acting out of concern for the rights and interests of others) together lead to the overriding of his autonomy, which would otherwise be paramount, and an order for compulsory admission to hospital.

This compulsion can be justified in either teleological or deontological terms. A teleologist would say that ordinarily a person is the best judge of his own interests, and for these reasons his autonomy should be respected, but, where his judgement is impaired by illness, others have to judge his interests on his behalf, at least temporarily. A deontologist would argue that autonomy is paramount, but can only be properly exercised by a competent moral agent: in circumstances where illness limits competence, then respect for autonomy requires the minimal necessary intervention in order to restore it. It can be argued, indeed, that Mr Jones has a *right* to be detained and treated against his will.

Set against this paternalistic approach, however, must be the recognition that deprivation of liberty is a harm, that supposedly benevolent institutions such as hospitals can be damaging, and that physical treatments such as drugs and ECT carry risks, including the risk of death. The principle of non-maleficence therefore requires that the procedures for compulsory detention and treatment have built-in safeguards, such as second opinions, rights of appeal and review, and specific time limits.

Legislation varies between jurisdictions, but in general, the greater the potential harms, the more protection the patient is offered. Thus, in Scotland, the signature of a single doctor, who need not be a psychiatrist, can be sufficient to detain someone for up to 72 hours (in circumstances where a family member or mental health officer is not available), while a 6 month detention order requires the agreement of a mental health officer and two doctors, one of whom must be a trained psychiatrist while the other is usually the patient's general practitioner. The application is heard by a Sheriff

Court, where the patient is entitled to present his case and to be legally represented. The spirit behind the Mental Health (Scotland) Act 1984 and its 1983 English counterpart had intended to use these more formal provisions wherever possible, in order to maximise the protection they offer patients. It is no surprise to practising psychiatrists, who are familiar with the tendency for these problems to emerge at a crisis, requiring immediate action, that emergency detention is the rule rather than the exception.

British mental health legislation tends to separate provisions for admission and for treatment, with only the longer term detention orders specifically so labelled. Elaborate provisions are built in regarding consent to treatment, requiring, after 3 months of a 6 month order, that the Responsible Medical Officer either confirm the patient consents to the treatment plan then in place, or that he obtain a second opinion from an independent psychiatrist approving the plan. 'Treatment', in this context, almost always means the use of drugs, and specifically antipsychotics, whether by mouth or in depot form. Additional procedures apply to ECT and to other, much less frequently used physical treatments, such as psychosurgery or the use of hormones.

Complying with these procedures protects psychiatrists against unconsenting patients' subsequent civil or criminal claims (see Consent, above). In an emergency situation, however, such as that of an aggressive, agitated psychotic patient brought by police to the accident and emergency department after self-harm, it is the common law concept of necessity and not mental health legislation that is called upon to justify emergency restraint and sedation, even though a short-term detention order may be applied at the same time. Non-psychiatrists do not always appreciate this distinction. Several potential errors ensue, among them the mistaken assumptions that a disturbed patient has to be detained in order for sedation to be legal; and that detention can be used to justify urgent (or non-urgent) compulsory treatment for physical complaints. If such treatment is necessary, as say for a diabetic prone to hypoglycaemic attacks in which he aggressively refuses glucose or glucagon, then once again it is the common law that justifies the minimal necessary restraint and sedation, as well as the physical measures intended to raise his blood sugar level. In such a case it may not be necessary, appropriate or possible to invoke the Mental Health Act.

Compulsory treatment in order to prevent relapse, rather than to bring about remission, is more problematic, both practically and ethically. Psychiatrists everywhere will be familiar with patients who have recurrent psychotic episodes in which they risk harm to themselves and others, and who require compulsory admission and treatment, to which they respond well, but who repeatedly withdraw from follow-up and discontinue medication once outside hospital, thereby repeating the whole cycle. There are repeated calls for a power to compel these patients to continue taking medication outside hospital (Royal College of Psychiatrists 1993), which, in Britain at least, have so far been resisted. It might at first seem odd that so much could depend on where a patient is, so that compulsion is justified within but not without the hospital setting: but the crucial issue is competence, not geography. Patients now subject to compulsory treatment are, by definition, those whose competence and autonomy are impaired by *current* episodes of illness: that is why they are in hospital. Any proposed community treatment order would seek to impose treatment on people who are not currently ill, but who might become so: that is why they are out of hospital. Their competence would not be questioned, and their autonomy to decline medication not so much seen as impaired, as simply overruled, usually by appeal to the interests of others. This attitude to autonomy is much harder to justify, either teleologically or deontologically, and it is no accident that political pressures for greater control over the mentally ill have not yet led to the introduction of such powers; though that is not to say that they may not yet come.

CONCLUSION

Psychiatry, more than any other branch of medicine, throws up a host of ethical issues, some of which intersect with the law as well as with clinical practice. The practising psychiatrist has always needed a familiarity with the relevant civil law and mental health legislation, though not, of course, to the level of a lawyer. Now, given the ever-increasing complexity of modern practice, the psychiatrist also needs a working knowledge of basic ethical principles, and an ability to reason ethically in areas where there is disagreement, though not, of course, at the level of the moral philosopher.

REFERENCES

Anscombe GEM 1981 The collected philosophical papers of GEM Anscombe. Vol 3: Ethics, Religion and Politics. Basil Blackwell, Oxford

APA 1973 (revised 1988) Principles of medical ethics with annotations especially applicable to psychiatry. American Psychiatric Association, Washington, DC

Beauchamp T L, Childress J F 1994 Principles of biomedical ethics, 4th edn. Oxford University Press, New York

Bloch S, Reddaway P 1977 Russia's political hospitals: the abuse of psychiatry in the Soviet Union. Gollancz, London

British Medical Association 1981 The handbook of medical ethics. BMA, London

Dworkin R M 1977 Taking rights seriously. Harvard University Press, Cambridge, MA

Eastman N 1997 The Mental Health (Patients in the Community) Act 1995: a clinical analysis. British Journal of Psychiatry 170: 492–496

Fulford K W M 1989 Moral theory and medical practice. Cambridge University Press, Cambridge

Gillon R 1994 British Medical Journal 309: 184–188

Harding T 1991 Mental health service delivery abuses in Japan. In: Bloch S, Chodoff P (eds) Psychiatric ethics, 2nd edn. Oxford University Press, Oxford

Hare R M 1981 Moral thinking: its levels, method and point. Oxford University Press, Oxford

Laing R D 1965 The divided self. Penguin, Harmondsworth

Lifton R J 1986 The Nazi doctors: medical killing and the psychology of genocide. Basic Books, New York

Mechanic D 1989 Mental health and social policy, 3rd edn. Prentice-Hall, Englewood Cliffs

Mill J S 1859 On Liberty, London. (Rapaport E (ed) 1978 Hackett Publishing, Indianapolis)

Muller-Hill B 1991 Psychiatry in the Nazi era. In: Bloch S, Chodoff P (eds) Psychiatric ethics, 2nd edn. Oxford University Press, Oxford

Ogilvie A D, Potts S G 1994 Assisted suicide for depression: the slippery slope in action. British Medical Journal 309: 492–493

Potts S G 1991 Euthanasia and other medical decisions about the end of life. Lancet 338: 952–953

Ramsay R 1990 The scandal of Leros. British Medical Journal 300: 688

Royal College of Psychiatrists 1993 Community supervision orders. Royal College of Psychiatrists, London

Shapcote L 1912–1936 The summa theologica (English translation). Burns, Oates, London, 22 vols

Sidaway 1983 Reported as (1985) 1 All ER 643

Smart J J C, Williams B A O 1973 Utilitarianism: for and against. Cambridge University Press, New York

Szasz T S 1961 The myth of mental illness. Harper & Row, New York

Tarasoff v Regents of The University of California 1976. Supreme Court of California Suppl 131 Report 14

World Medical Association 1948 General Assembly, Geneva. (Amended 1968, Sydney and 1983, Venice)

World Psychiatric Association 1977 (revised 1983) General Assembly, Hawaii

30

Psychological therapies

C. P. L. Freeman

INTRODUCTION

In the last edition of this textbook there were four separate brief chapters on counselling and crisis intervention, interpretative psychotherapies, therapy with family and couples and behavioural and cognitive psychotherapies. In this edition we have reduced these to a single chapter. This is not because we think psychotherapy is unimportant but because: we felt it important to concentrate on evidence-based psychotherapy; there is increasing evidence that common factors in psychotherapy are important and that successful outcome in psychotherapy is largely independent of the school to which the psychotherapist belongs; we felt that the four previous chapters were so brief as not to do justice to any of the schools of psychotherapy described and that reference to key texts might be more helpful to the trainee.

Types of psychotherapy

There are many different classifications of the types of psychotherapy; examples are given in Tables 30.1–30.3. This chapter will review various schools of psychotherapy. I have given more space to those where there is a definite evidence-base and only briefly mentioned others because the roots of modern psychotherapy lie in psychodynamic theory. A more detailed historical description of psychodynamic psychotherapies and psychoanalysis is justified.

Table 30.1   Classification of psychotherapies (Roth, & Fonagy 1996)

Psychodynamic psychotherapy
Behavioural and cognitive psychotherapy
Interpersonal psychotherapy
Strategic or systemic psychotherapies
Supportive and experimental psychotherapies
Group therapies

Table 30.2   Types of psychotherapy

Supportive	Re-educative	Reconstructive
Guidance	Behaviour	Freudian analysis
Milieu therapy	Cognitive therapy	Kleinian analysis
Occupational therapy	Interpersonal therapy	Ego analysis
Music therapy	Client-centred therapy	Neo-Freudian therapy
Reassurance	Gestalt therapy	Adlerian therapy
Ventilation	Emotive release	Reichian analysis
	Psychodrama	Brief dynamic therapy
	Transactional analysis	

After Welberg (1977).

PSYCHOANALYTIC PSYCHOTHERAPY AND PSYCHOANALYSIS

In 1895, Freud with Joseph Breuer published studies on hysteria (Freud & Breuer 1895/1955). Together they had developed hypnosis to uncover hidden or forgotten memories. When these memories were brought into consciousness, the physical symptoms the patients were suffering from tended to disappear. They postulated that 'hysterical' symptoms were the result of traumatic experiences being 'converted' into physical, mainly neurological, symptoms, the process of conversion relieving the psychological pain. Freud had previously noted, while observing the work of Bernhein and Charcot, that where hypnosis was used only in a suggestive sense to implore the patient that he would, for instance, be able to walk or see, symptoms did disappear, but after a time another physical symptom appeared. He called this 'symptom substitution'.

Freud and Breuer then separated, mainly because of Freud's increasing use of 'free association', but partly because the patients began to talk about their sexual feelings towards Breuer, which Breuer found difficult to

Table 30.3   Types of psychotherapy
• *Psychotherapy 1* describes the basic relationship between any good doctor or other professional and his/her patient/client. It requires an ability to communicate and empathise • *Psychotherapy 2* is a deeper level of communication and understanding, involving recognition that the individual's present state is influenced by past experience. It recognises transference but does not explore it • *Psychotherapy 3* is the level of psychodynamic psychotherapy, focusing on the therapist–patient relationship and working on the transference occurring • *Psychotherapy 4* is behavioural psychotherapy. It uses techniques of behaviour modification based on learning theory and focuses on the patient's manifest behaviour

Levels of psychotherapy (Cawley 1977)

1. **Outer** *(support and counselling)*	(1) unburdening of problems to sympathetic listener
	(2) ventilation of feelings within supportive relationship
	(3) discussion of current problems with helper
2. **Intermediate**	(4) Clarification of problems, their nature and origins
	(5) confrontation of defences
	(6) interpretation of unconscious motives and transference
3. **Deeper** *(exploration and analysis)*	(7) repetition, remembering and reconstruction of past
	(8) regression to less adult and less rational
	(9) resolution of conflicts by working through

tolerate. The technique of free association, where the patient talks about anything that comes into his mind as completely as possible, however trivial or however irrelevant it may appear, is a key technique in psychoanalytic psychotherapy. The therapist listens without interrupting. Freud's view was that Breuer was not so charming or physically attractive that patients would naturally express their love for him and this led to his discovery of the process of 'transference'.

Basic principles of psychoanalysis

Freud defines psychoanalysis as 'the psychology of the unconscious'. Thoughts can be conscious, preconscious (not in the conscious at present but can be called

into it) and unconscious (existing outside conscious awareness) and not being able to be recalled. Freud believed that only thoughts and feelings that were conscious could be changed so that one of the main processes of therapy is to make what is unconscious conscious. Slips of the tongue and slips of the pen are said to be evidence of unconscious or preconscious thoughts (freudian slips).

Defence mechanisms

One of the greatest debts we owe to psychoanalysis, and to Freud in particular, is the description of a set of mental mechanisms which have helped to make some aspects of human behaviour more readily understandable. The use of such mechanisms seems to be universal and is not limited to sufferers from neurotic illness. Nor is it true to say they are necessarily signs of disturbance or underlying unhappiness, or that they indicate some preneurotic state. They are demonstrated most clearly and dramatically in certain types of neurotic illness but may in fact be indicative of health rather than disease. For instance, there is recent evidence that women who are diagnosed as having breast carcinoma and are told of that fact but who then deny it have a better long-term outcome than those who fail to use denial. In a fascinating study, Valliant et al (1986) studied the defence mechanisms of 307 healthy middle-aged men followed up for 40 years and described the defence styles associated with coping and success. Defence mechanisms, then, are universal phenomena which all of us use at times to limit and constrict awareness so that threatening cues, either from the inner or outer environment, can be excluded. They appear to be invoked automatically and not under conscious control and are psychological measures which allow stressful situations to be coped with by distorting reality.

Psychoanalytic theory maintains that excessive use of defence mechanisms leads to eventual neurotic breakdown. However, there is no objective evidence for this and the theory could easily be turned around to suggest that inadequate or inappropriate use of defence mechanisms leads to overt anxiety and neurotic breakdown. These concepts can be usefully invoked to help in the understanding of certain patients. They are certainly extremely useful when trying to help medical students understand psychological problems and it may sometimes be useful for the patient to understand his behaviour in such terms. However, as used to be said about masturbation, their excessive use may lead to blindness, and they should not be regarded as an all-embracing or comprehensive explanation of neurotic behaviour. Behavioural and learning theory approaches have as much, if not more, to offer in this regard and have certainly led to more effective forms of treatment. What follows is a brief description of the more common defence mechanisms which have been described.

Repression Freud considered this to be the central and basic defence mechanism and that other defence mechanisms only come into operation when repression starts to fail. Thoughts or feelings which the conscious mind finds unacceptable are repressed from consciousness; thus repression is a way of dealing with unbearable aspects of inner life, so that aggressive or sexual feelings, fantasies or desires are thrust out of consciousness. Freud saw repression as a mental process arising from conflict between the 'pleasure principle' and the 'reality principle', indicating that when impulses and desires are in conflict with enforced standards of conduct, painful emotions arise and the conflict is resolved by repression. It has been suggested that the term suppression should be used for this automatic process and that repression should be employed in its ordinary sense of 'actively thrusting out of the mind', but generally repression is still used to mean an unconscious process.

Denial Repression and denial are sometimes confused but, whereas the former refers to internal feelings, denial is the involuntary and automatic distortion of an obvious aspect of outer reality. Thus, when a patient is told by a doctor that he has cancer this fact may be denied at subsequent interviews, even though a clear and concise explanation was given which the patient obviously understood. Denial is not the same as lying, which is also a common human habit.

Projection This occurs when an individual unconsciously disowns an attitude or attribute of his own and ascribes it to somebody else. Children when they are angry or afraid commonly ascribe such feelings to inanimate objects or pets so that 'Be careful, the dog will bite you' or 'The table is very cross with you, mummy' are used instead of 'I would like to bite you' or 'I am cross with you' A husband who is unfaithful, or wishes to be, may project such attributes on to his wife and then become intensely jealous of her, constantly suspecting her infidelity. A person with latent homosexual tendencies may be quick to notice homosexual traits in others.

Reaction formation This term describes the process of developing the opposite attitude to the one being defended against. The obsessional traits of orderliness, neatness and punctuality can be seen as a reaction formation against inner feelings of squalor, dirt and chaos. Similarly, some very needy individuals who really desire to be cared for and cosseted cope with these feelings by caring for and cosseting others, sometimes very successfully.

Displacement This is the transfer of affect, usually fear or anger, from one person, situation or object to another to which it does not really belong. In psychoanalytic terms phobias are explained in this way, the phobia representing an unconscious fear of some other situation or person. Freud's case of Little Hans, who developed a phobia of horses, which in fact represented a fear of his father, is well known. Freud's explanation of phobias is almost certainly wrong and, as has been discussed earlier, a simple learning model is more appropriate. A more everyday example of displacement might be the wife who, furious and irritated with her husband for always coming home late or giving her no support with the children, vents her anger not on her husband but on the children instead. Actions such as kicking the cat or smashing plates when angry are not displacements in the analytic sense as these are usually quite conscious and deliberate actions.

Rationalisation This is the process of justifying reasoning after the event. An individual tries to provide logical and believable explanations for his behaviour to persuade himself and others that his irrational behaviour is justified and therefore should not be criticised. A patient who consistently and repeatedly arrives late for outpatient appointments but always has a plausible excuse, and assures you that he always tries to get to your sessions on time, may really be expressing his resentment at your failure to cure him, or devote more time to him, but he tries to conceal this from himself, and you, with talk of slow watches and missed buses.

Undoing This applies to unconsciously motivated acts, which magically or symbolically counteract, cancel out or otherwise reverse a previous act or thought motivated by an unacceptable, unconscious impulse. This is the main mechanism that operates in obsessional thoughts and compulsive rituals.

Regression This refers to reversion to modes of psychological functioning, characteristic of earlier life stages, especially childhood phases. It occurs when the individual is faced by some serious conflict in the present. A simple example is when an elder sibling becomes more infantile in his behaviour at the time of the birth of a younger sibling. Regressive behaviour occurs frequently in the context of psychiatric treatment and some treatment regimens encourage the development of such behaviours.

Turning against the self This is the process through which the subject deflects hostile aggressiveness and directs it on to himself, perhaps injuring himself physically or deliberately putting himself at a social or financial disadvantage. Examples are the destruction of one's valued possessions when one is distressed or depressed and self-damaging behaviour, such as hair pulling, self-mutilation, etc.

Sublimation This is one of the least harmful of the defensive formations. Urges particularly harmful to the person are given socially acceptable expression; for example, an extremely aggressive person may select the occupation of a butcher, or a latent homosexual can put his tendencies to social use by becoming a scoutmaster. Thus, sexual or aggressive impulses instead of being given free expression are sublimated to other activities, which are carried out with great vigour and often great success. Sometimes the term is used loosely to indicate any substitution of what appears to be a higher satisfaction for a more basic or instinctual one. Sublimation is the most effective of the defence mechanisms in that no symptoms or odd behaviour are produced and the impulse or fears in question find unconscious expression in activities which fulfil the subject and benefit others.

Compensation This is the development of abilities to an unusual degree, to conceal or make up for a defect. The childhood stammerer who eventually becomes a great orator is a classical example.

Resistance

This global concept refers to the sum of the defence mechanisms that an individual uses and a way in which they thwart the therapist's attempt to help him gain access to unconscious processes.

Transference

Transference in its most basic form is where an individual relives a past relationship in the context of a present one. Freud originally conceptualised transference as only occurring within psychotherapy so that patients who had experienced such feelings as love, anger or a profound sense of gratitude towards their therapist may be expressing feelings which originated from relationships in early childhood, particularly with their parents. Freud broadened his view to accept that transference reactions occur throughout ordinary life and are part of most, if not all, relationships.

Countertransference refers to the fact that therapists can have transference feelings towards patients. Analysis and interpretation of the transference is said to be one of the most powerful therapeutic agents in psychodynamic psychoanalytic psychotherapy.

Freud's structural theory of mind

The terms 'id', 'ego' and 'super-ego' are not Freud's. They were inserted by the translator of Freud's German into English. Even when they became widely accepted in the English language Freud refused to use them. He divided the mind into the 'it' (id) the 'I' (ego) and

Table 30.4	Freud's structural theory of mind

The It (id)
- experienced as if it were an external force
- entirely unconscious
- locus of unconscious motives and repressed memories

The I (ego)
- almost entirely conscious
- except that defence mechanisms may act unconsciously in the I
- represents conscious sense of self

The Over-me (super-ego)
- partly conscious and partly unconscious
- contains values and moral rules
- conflicts with the it
- may dictate behaviour either consciously or unconsciously

the 'over me' (super-ego) (Karon & Widener 1995) (Table 30.4).

Drives

Another important freudian concept is that of basic drives. Again, Freud never used the word instinct, which is another mistranslation. It is an important one because the term instinct implies something that is immutable. Initially Freud postulated two basic drives: the sexual and the self-preservation ('libido' and 'ego' drives). Later he introduced the 'death drive' (thanatos) but this never gained widespread acceptance. Conflict between these drives may result in symptoms.

Psychosexual stages

These are summarised in Table 30.5. The term 'fixation' refers to an individual becoming arrested at a certain point of development because particularly unpleasant or pleasurable events happened at that particular stage of development. When regression occurs this is often to a particular point of fixation.

The genital stage of development led to the development of the 'Oedipus complex'. This refers to the male child's wish to have an exclusive relationship with the mother and exclude or destroy the father. The fear of retaliation by father leads to the concept of 'castration anxiety'.

Freud and dreams

Freud saw the remembered dream as a distorted but relevant access to preconscious and unconscious thoughts. He saw the phenomena of reliving the day's

Table 30.5	Stages of development	
Freud	Abrahams	Erickson
Oral (1st year)	Oral receptive (sucking) Oral sadistic (biting)	Basic trust versus mistrust
Anal (2nd year)	Anal sadistic (expelling) Anal retentive (holding in)	Autonomy versus shame
Genital (3–5 years) Oedipus complex		Initiative versus guilt
Latency period (approx 7+ years)		Industry versus inferiority Adolescence – identity versus confusion Early adulthood – infancy and solidarity versus isolation Adulthood – generativity versus stagnation Maturity – ego integrity versus despair

Psychoanalysis as a treatment

Psychoanalytic psychotherapy involves 2 or more years of therapy, 5 days per week for 1 hour a day sessions. This is a completely inappropriate treatment for contemporary health care systems, however they are funded, and tends to treat only those individuals with the appropriate time and money to engage in it. Nevertheless the theoretical underpinning of much brief dynamic therapy relates directly to core analytic theory.

Post-Freudian developments

Jungian therapy emphasises the value of patients pursuing the products of unconscious fantasy through dreams, reveries and artistic creativity. In the course of analysis, patients encounter various typical primordial images or 'archetypes', which are familiar in myth, fable and fairy stories. In order to obtain balance and integration, the individual must recognise and differentiate himself from the immensely powerful influence of such archetypal images which are, in many instances, projected upon actual people in the external world. Jungian therapy facilitates this process of individuation.

Adlerian psychology reflects its founder's view that aggression, the drive to self-assertion and the will to power take precedence over sex as the prime mover of human behaviour. Adler conceived the infant and child as feeling weak and inferior and driven to achieve in order to overcome such feelings. Adler popularised the concept of striving and modified it into something akin to self-actualising, a goal of completion, aspired to but never attained. His view of 'organ inferiority', whereby infantile weaknesses could be expressed through deficiencies and dysfunctions in particular organs of the body, provided a psychological foundation for the development of psychosomatic medicine.

Harry Stack-Sullivan and Fromm-Reichmann moved away from Freud's emphasis on the structural and drive-related theory of mind and focused more on cultural and interpersonal influences. They developed the concept of the self and saw the self as an internal system which was constructed of a 'good me', 'bad me' and 'not me'. They felt that the basic drives were towards acquiring security and satisfaction rather than sex and self-preservation. They emphasised the interpersonal nature of the pre-adolescent period when same-sex friendships were important. It was a much less deterministic theory than that of Freud, in that difficulties at an earlier stage could be corrected by good experiences later.

Ego psychology has become a much more dominant school in the USA, whereas object relations theory has dominated in the UK. The former is a direct development of Freud's work and Anna Freud fits into this

experience as simply the elements from which a dream was then constructed. The dreams were seen as a type of wish fulfilment. For example, an unacceptable wish could be expressed openly in a dream while being repressed from conscious thought.

Sexual seduction

This is perhaps the most controversial area of Freud's theory and the one that has been most attacked (Masson 1984). Freud initially found it extremely difficult to believe that so many of his patients had been sexually abused in childhood but he became increasingly convinced that these sexual experiences had occurred. He then retracted this when he realised that in at least some of his patients these childhood memories were fantasy rather than fact. Masson attacks Freud for this retraction, making it appear that Freud believed that all his patients' experiences were fantasy, although it is clear that Freud was never this emphatic.

school with her description of normal development in psychoanalytic terms, defence mechanisms and the analysis of children. An important development in ego psychology was the work of Erik Erikson (1950) who reconceptualised these theories to include an important social perspective so that the anal stage became the stage of autonomy versus shame and self-doubt. The oedipal stage was characterised by initiative versus guilt, and the latency period by industry versus inferiority (Table 30.5).

The object relation schools

In psychoanalytic theory, the term 'object' refers to that which is used to gratify a need. Usually the object is a person. Freud described the original object for the child being the mother's breast. Later in development the whole mother becomes the object. This has been the dominant school in British analytic thinking and particularly in Scotland.

Melanie Kline placed most emphasis on the development that happened in the first year of life. At this time the infant is terrified of being devoured by the mother or the mother's breast. This is the 'paranoid position'. Towards the end of the first year of life, Kline said that the characteristic stage was that of the 'depressive position'. This is where the infant discovers that he or she both loves and hates the same individual (the mother). The concept of the good mother (good breast) and bad mother (bad breast) is initially perceived as being two different individuals. As they merge, so the depressive position may emerge because, if you reject the bad mother, you lose the good as well. 'Splitting' is a defence mechanism where good and bad object images cannot be integrated.

Ronald Fairbairn (1954) was the leader of the Scottish school of object relations. Parallel and equally influential work was carried out by Harry Guntrip (1969) in Leeds. The central theme is the drive towards forming a good object relationship. They described 'depressive anxiety' (the fear that your anger will destroy the object or drive it away) and 'schizoid anxiety' (that your love will destroy the object). They also emphasised the role of separation anxiety.

Otto Kernberg (1980) is the main exponent of object relations in the American literature. He emphasised the defence mechanisms of projection and splitting, particularly in borderline patients.

Brief or time-limited psychodynamic psychotherapy

Freud did very little in the way of long-term psychotherapy. Many of his cases he saw for only two or

three sessions and typically he saw people for 3–4 months. The very long term, high frequency treatment that characterises psychoanalysis slowly emerged during the 1920s and 1930s.

BEHAVIOURAL METHODS

In many early descriptions of behavioural approaches, emphasis was placed on the role of learning in the aetiology, maintenance and treatment of psychiatric problems. It was generally held that learning was a crucial concept in three main ways. First, some disorders were associated with lack of learning, e.g. enuresis, or psychopathic behaviour. Second, some disorders were associated with overlearning, e.g. obsessional rituals and phobias. Third, some disorders were associated with loss of previous learning, by neurological dysfunction, e.g. aphasia, or through insufficient or inappropriate reinforcement as in institutionalisation. These notions provided the rationale for the application of learning theory to the amelioration of psychiatric problems. The links between behavioural approaches and learning theory have gradually become less direct, and methods of behaviour change have been sought from wider experimental psychology and other areas.

Systematic desensitisation (SD) (general exposure)

The original technique developed by Wolpe (1958) involved three stages:

1. Training the patient to relax (see next section).
2. Constructing with the patient a hierarchy of anxiety-arousing situations.
3. Presenting phobic items for the hierarchy in a graded way, while the patient inhibits the anxiety by relaxation.

In this way, the patient, while never experiencing intolerable anxiety, proceeded from mildly frightening situations to previously terrifying ones.

Progress up the hierarchy can be made in imagination, in real life (in vivo) or by a combination of both, depending on such factors as the availability of the feared object or situation and how easily the graded steps can be reproduced in real life. Films, slides and recordings can also be used. The balance of evidence suggests that in vivo SD is more effective, possibly because the treatment setting is more like the real-life situation, thus facilitating generalisation.

When SD is being conducted in imagination, the length of the session is generally about 40 minutes, depending on how long it takes to get the patient relaxed; moving steps in the hierarchy rarely extends beyond 30 minutes. The number of sessions required varies (anything from 10 to 100 being possible), depending on the complexity of the problem and on the number of hierarchies to be worked through, for it is seldom that a patient presents with a single well-defined phobia. Patients are expected to practise at home what they have learned in the clinical session.

The following illustrates a section of a typical hierarchy for a patient with a phobia of shopping:

1. Entering a quiet shop to purchase one article, e.g. a newspaper, with the exact purchase money in hand
2. Waiting behind one person, otherwise as in (1)
3. Purchasing more than one article, as (1)
4. As (3), but having to wait for change
5. Asking to see an article before purchasing
6. As (4), but waiting in a queue of several people.

When SD is carried out in vivo, the patient is instructed how to relax and how and when to use relaxation in the clinic; but the actual desensitisation is done in the real situation. Often this 'homework' can be done while the patient is accompanied by a relative, and the presence of such a companion can act as an extra way of breaking down the hierarchy into smaller steps.

SD is one of the most intensively investigated of all kinds of psychological therapy, with over 100 studies looking simply at the relative importance of the various elements involved. There is little doubt about its effectiveness, and as a treatment for phobic anxiety it is extensively used.

Relaxation

Behaviour therapists are not the only practitioners of relaxation, other therapists having used it extensively. Nevertheless, since Wolpe (1958) advocated Jacobson's (1938) technique for SD it has earned a firm place in the behavioural armamentarium. Its role has also gradually extended. Formerly, when used alone, it was regarded as a control procedure, lacking the essential conditioning elements of SD; but gradually evidence accumulated showing that it was often at least as effective as the treatment with which it was compared. This was particularly striking when it was being used as a control procedure with which to compare biofeedback (see below). It has now earned a place in its own right as an effective treatment for anxiety management, headaches, chronic pain, hypertension and other problems. A useful review of relaxation procedures has been provided by Lichstein (1988).

Flooding (rapid exposure)

Flooding involves exposing patients to a phobic object in a non-graded manner with no attempt to reduce anxiety beforehand. As with SD, flooding can be conducted in vivo or in imagination. In the latter case it is often referred to as implosive therapy, and as such was originally put forward as a psychoanalytic technique, with some similarity to abreaction. A recent application of imaginal flooding is to post-traumatic stress disorder (Cooper & Clum, 1989).

Typically the patient is placed alone in a room with the phobic object, say a cat, and is required to stay there until the fear has diminished. It is argued that fear is maintained by the patient's avoidance of the phobic object or situation, and that if avoidance is not allowed the fear will diminish. The flooding session must be of long duration, normally an hour or more, to be effective. In general, the patient should stay in contact until there are clear indications of marked fear reduction; some reduction is normally seen after 15 minutes. Ending before this may represent another avoidance and could exacerbate the problem. This brings out a resemblance to SD which may not be obvious at first sight. In the initial stages of flooding, the anxiety is very high but, due to emotional exhaustion or habituation, after a time it starts to decline so that each recurrence of the frightening stimulus, e.g. a movement of the cat towards the patient, no longer leads to increased anxiety and the stimulus–response link between the cat and the fear has weakened. Another likely reason for success is the subject's 'reality testing' of the situation, whereby he discovers that he is less afraid of the phobic object than he had expected to be.

Several studies have compared flooding with SD in the treatment of phobias. Most have shown that there are no major differences in outcome. Flooding seems to be more effective with obsessive–compulsive patients when combined with response prevention (see below).

The decision whether to use flooding or not is by mutual agreement of patient and therapist. Most patients find it less frightening than they had imagined and it is usually much quicker acting than SD.

COGNITIVE THERAPY

Cognitive or cognitive-behavioural therapy refers to a method of therapy based on a theory of the emotional disorders (Ellis 1962, Beck 1967), a body of experimental and clinical studies (Blackburn 1988) and well-defined therapy techniques (Beck et al 1979, Beck & Emery 1985, Hawton et al 1989, Blackburn & Davidson 1990). Theoretically, the emphasis is on information processing; that is, individuals react, feel and behave according to how they process the information contained in their environment (Fig. 30.1).

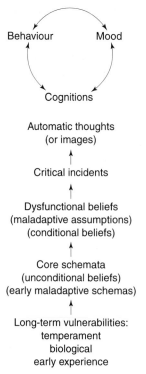

Automatic thoughts
(or images)

↑

Critical incidents

↑

Dysfunctional beliefs
(maladaptive assumptions)
(conditional beliefs)

↑

Core schemata
(unconditional beliefs)
(early maladaptive schemas)

↑

Long-term vulnerabilities:
temperament
biological
early experience

Fig. 30.1 The cognitive model.

Cognitive approaches to treatment were first developed for the management of depressive illness and labelled as cognitive therapy (Beck 1964) or as rational-emotive therapy (RET) (Ellis 1962). The theoretical underpinning and experimental studies were criticised (e.g. see Ledwidge 1978, Coyne & Gottlib 1983), but generally there has been a positive reaction which has resulted in a mushrooming of basic research and of therapeutic applications to disorders other than depression. The general principles of cognitive therapy will be described, followed by its specific applications. The main characteristics of cognitive therapy are described in Table 30.6.

General principles

Cognitive therapy, like behaviour therapy, is problem oriented. It is aimed at correcting psychological problems (emotional, cognitive and behavioural) and at improving coping skills (dealing with problem situations) to alleviate patients' distress. The main characteristics of cognitive therapy are that it is time limited, structured and problem oriented; it follows an explicit agenda, deals with the 'here-and-now', and adopts a learning rather than psychodynamic model. It is a scientific method, involving the setting up and testing of

Table 30.6	Main characteristics of standard cognitive therapy	
Time limited	15–22 sessions over 3–4 months
Structure	Each session lasts 1 hour
Agenda	Each session is structured by the use of an agenda to optimise the use of time
Problem-oriented	Therapist and patient focus on defining and solving presenting problems
A-historical	It deals with the here-and-now without recourse to the distant past history of the patient
Learning model	It does not use pychodynamic hypothetical constructs to explain the patient's behaviour. Rather dysfunctional behaviour is attributed to maladaptive learning. Relearning more functional behaviour is the goal
Scientific method	An experimental method is adopted; therapy involving collecting data (problems, thoughts, attitudes), formulating hypotheses, setting up experiments and evaluating results
Homework	The patient is given assignments for data collecting, verification of hypotheses and practice of cognitive skills
Collaboration	Patient and therapist work together to solve problems
Active	The therapist adopts an active and directive role throughout treatment. He can be didactic sometimes but his main role is to facilitate the definition and resolution of problems
Socratic questioning	The principal therapeutic method is socratic questioning, which is to ask a series of questions aimed at bringing the patient to identify his underlying thought, to perceive alternative solutions or to modify his opinions
Openness	The therapeutic process is not clouded in mystiques rather, it is explicit and open, therapist and patient sharing a common understanding of what is going on in therapy

hypotheses. Patients are given regular homework assignments and a collaborative relationship between therapist and patient is developed.

Table 30.7 How does cognitive-behavioural therapy differ from other psychotherapies?
Open, explicit, collaborative
Structured, e.g. agenda
Sets behavioural tasks
Therapist more active
Mainly uses here- and-now rather than past
Doesn't use symbolism
Uses specific cognitive technique

Patients are provided with a rationale for understanding their problems, a vocabulary for expressing themselves, and a training in techniques for overcoming distressing affects and for solving problems. In addition to cognitive methods, cognitive therapy uses the whole gamut of behavioural techniques described earlier in the chapter. This is done not only to change behaviour but also to change interpretations, expectations and self-concept. These changes are not taken for granted, but put forward as hypotheses, and discussed after the behavioural experiments, which are replicated until both the therapist and patient are satisfied that cognitive changes have taken place. The main differences between cognitive-behavioural therapy and other therapies are listed in Table 30.7.

Cognitive therapy is more than the routine application of a series of techniques. In addition to mastering the basic therapeutic skills (Truax & Carkhuff 1967), the therapist must conceptualise each case within a cognitive therapy framework following a functional analysis which is similar to that described earlier in this chapter. The focus is on the cognitive factors which maintain dysphoric mood and maladaptive behaviour. Blackburn & Davidson (1990) described the main areas of enquiry to reach a formulation in cognitive therapy. These are:

- Definition of the problem: what are the major complaints? Which particular functions are affected?
- Objective factors: what are the current stresses, main past traumatic events and current living situation?
- Internal vulnerability factors: what are the main attitudes and beliefs which the patient holds about himself and his world? What types of events does he appear to be sensitive to?
- Mediational cognitive factors: what are the typical automatic thoughts which are expressed and which processing errors do they contain? (See next section for a definition.)
- Current themes: the recurring theme, for example, failure, loss of control, loss of love or low self-image, will indicate particular vulnerabilities and help the therapist to hypothesise about basic schemata.

- Coping skills: what are the typical methods of dealing with problems? In what way are these helpful or unhelpful?
- Emotions: what are the predominant emotions and what situations trigger them?

Specific techniques

The techniques first described for the treatment of depression (Beck et al 1979) are applicable, with some modifications and additions, to many different disorders (Hawton et al 1989); for example, anxiety, obsessional–compulsive disorder, eating disorders, phobic disorders, somatic problems, sexual dysfunction and chronic psychiatric handicaps. Beck (1987) has described the cognitive dysfunctions which maintain depression. These are seen at three levels of thinking, and cognitive therapy techniques are aimed at modifying each of these levels. An example is given in Figure 30.2.

The general aims of cognitive therapy are:

- To monitor negative automatic thoughts
- To recognise connections between cognitions, affect and behaviour
- To examine evidence for and against distorted automatic thoughts
- To substitute more reality-oriented interpretations
- To learn to identify and alter dysfunctional schemata.

The automatic thoughts (so called because they are the habitual and reflexive commentaries that we make to ourselves and of which we are not necessarily fully conscious) are the basic data of cognitive therapy. Several techniques have been described to help the therapist elicit and modify these thoughts, which maintain low or anxious or angry moods and dysfunctional behaviour (e.g. inactivity, ruminating, checking, bingeing, avoiding, etc.). The patient can be helped to access these thoughts through direct questioning, inductive questioning (a series of questions which guide the patient to discover the related automatic thought), using moments of strong emotion, re-enacting situations in role-plays, using mental imagery to recreate situations or using behavioural tasks to trigger the thoughts. The patient is asked to keep a diary (the 'daily record of dysfunctional thoughts'), using changes in emotions as cues to monitor thinking. These records are also used to practise challenging the automatic interpretations and substituting alternative interpretations which may lead to less distressing emotions. A variety of other techniques can also be used to modify automatic thoughts; for example, examining the evidence for and against, listing probabilities and collecting information which may invalidate the original interpretation. The basic principle in all these techniques is that the patient

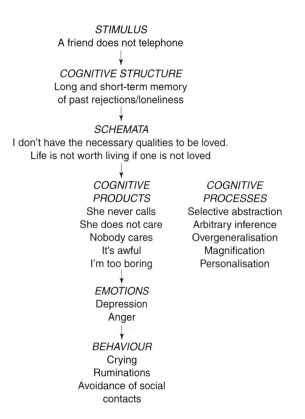

STIMULUS
A friend does not telephone

↓

COGNITIVE STRUCTURE
Long and short-term memory
of past rejections/loneliness

↓

SCHEMATA
I don't have the necessary qualities to be loved.
Life is not worth living if one is not loved

↓

COGNITIVE PRODUCTS	COGNITIVE PROCESSES
She never calls	Selective abstraction
She does not care	Arbitrary inference
Nobody cares	Overgeneralisation
It's awful	Magnification
I'm too boring	Personalisation

↓

EMOTIONS
Depression
Anger

↓

BEHAVIOUR
Crying
Ruminations
Avoidance of social
contacts

Fig. 30.2 Cognitive processes.

is taught to consider his thoughts not as facts but as interpretations which may be more or less accurate and which may be more or less functional in terms of the feelings and the behaviour that they trigger.

Identifying the basic schemata or beliefs which lead the patient to process information in idiosyncratic ways typically occurs later on in therapy and is, generally, more difficult and abstract than identifying automatic thoughts. It is also more difficult to modify the schemata, particularly in the personality disorders described in Axis II of DSM-IV (Beck et al 1990).

The schemata are inferred from the implicit or explicit rules which are exemplified in the automatic thoughts. The therapist and the patient, in collaboration, must look for common themes, for the 'shoulds' which are applied to the self and to others, and for the logical implications of automatic thoughts, by, for example, the 'downward arrow technique', of which an example (from Blackburn & Davidson 1990) is given in Figure 30.3.

As with the automatic thoughts, modifying the schemata is done through collaborative discussion and the use of behavioural tasks. Thus, the patient may be asked to weigh up the advantages and disadvantages of holding the belief, to examine the evidence for and

against the belief, to question the validity of the personal contract, to consider the short-term and long-term utility of the personal rule, to disobey the rule in a behavioural assignment and test the consequences. The latter technique is similar to response prevention in behaviour therapy.

Rational-emotive therapy (RET)

RET, developed by Ellis (1962), holds that 'neurotic' behaviour derives from about 12 irrational beliefs which put impossible demands on people, for example:

- The idea that it is mandatory for an adult to be loved by everyone for everything he does, instead of his concentrating on his own self-respect, on winning approval for practical purposes, and on loving rather than being loved.
- The idea that certain acts are awful or wicked, and that people who perform such acts should be severely punished, instead of the idea that certain acts are inappropriate or antisocial, and that people who perform such acts are behaving stupidly, ignorantly or neurotically and should be helped to change.
- The idea that it is horrible when things are not the way one would like them to be, instead of the idea that, if it is too bad, one ought to try to change or control conditions so they become more satisfactory and, if that is not possible, one had better temporarily accept their existence.

INTERPERSONAL PSYCHOTHERAPY

Interpersonal psychotherapy (IPT) is a structured, individual, time-limited (8–12 sessions) psychotherapy which has been shown to be effective in clinical trials of major depressive disorder and bulimia nervosa.

There are many different types of interpersonal psychotherapy but IPT refers specifically to the model of treatment proposed by Klerman & Weissman (1984). It is of particular interest because it was devised by a biological psychiatrist and an epidemiologist.

IPT is based on the work of Harry Stack-Sullivan (1953). Sullivan taught that psychiatry includes the scientific study of people and the processes between people rather than focusing exclusively on the mind, society or the brain, hence the unit of clinical study is the patient's interpersonal relations at any one particular time.

IPT has two focuses: to reduce depressive symptoms and to deal with the social and interpersonal problems associated with the onset of the symptoms. The initial sessions are devoted to establishing the treatment contract, dealing with the depressive symptoms, and identi-

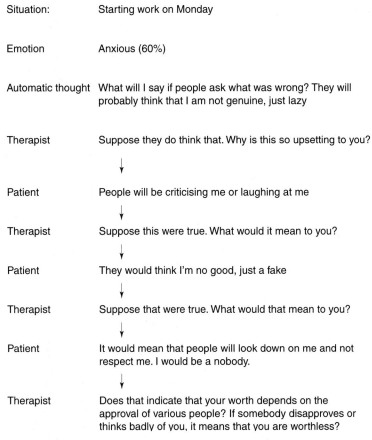

Situation:	Starting work on Monday
Emotion	Anxious (60%)
Automatic thought	What will I say if people ask what was wrong? They will probably think that I am not genuine, just lazy
Therapist	Suppose they do think that. Why is this so upsetting to you?
Patient	People will be criticising me or laughing at me
Therapist	Suppose this were true. What would it mean to you?
Patient	They would think I'm no good, just a fake
Therapist	Suppose that were true. What would that mean to you?
Patient	It would mean that people will look down on me and not respect me. I would be a nobody.
Therapist	Does that indicate that your worth depends on the approval of various people? If somebody disapproves or thinks badly of you, it means that you are worthless?

Fig. 30.3   Downward arrow technique.

fying the problem areas. During the initial sessions, both the depression and the interpersonal problems are diagnosed and assessed. In these sessions, the therapist should accomplish six tasks:

- Begin dealing with the depression
- Complete an interpersonal inventory and relate the depression to the interpersonal context
- Identify the principal problem areas
- Explain the rationale and intent of interpersonal therapy
- Set a treatment contract with the patient
- Explain the patient's expected role in the treatment.

Relating depression to the interpersonal context in the initial sessions

The interpersonal inventory

Once the review of the depression has been completed,

the therapist should direct the patient's attention to the onset of symptoms and to the reason for seeking treatment: what has been going on in the patient's social and interpersonal life that is associated with the onset of symptoms? The review of key persons and issues often follows easily. If not, it is useful to begin an inventory of current and past relationships to get a full picture of what the important current social interactions are in the patient's life.

The systematic review of current and past interpersonal relationships involves an exploration of the patient's important relationships with others, beginning with the present. This may all be done during the sessions or the psychotherapist may ask the patient to write an autobiographical statement containing interpersonal information.

In this inventory, the following should be gathered about each person who is important in the patient's life:

- Interactions with the patient, including frequency of contact, activity shares, and so on

- The expectations of each party in the relationship, including some assessment of whether these expectations were or are fulfilled
- A review of the satisfactory and unsatisfactory aspects of the relationship, with specific, detailed examples of both kinds of interactions
- The ways the patient would like to change the relationship, whether through changing his or her own behaviour or bringing about changes in the other person.

Although the inventory is concentrated in the first two sessions, it may be added to less systematically as treatment progresses.

Problem areas

It is important to define the problem areas because they can help the psychotherapist formulate a treatment strategy with the patient. Since IPT is short-term, it is usually concentrated on one or two of the four problem areas that depressed patients commonly encounter. The main problem areas are usually:

- Grief
- Interpersonal disputes with spouse, lover, children, or other family members, friends, coworkers
- Role transitions – a new job, leaving one's family, going away to school, relocation in a new home or area, divorce, economic or other family changes
- Interpersonal deficits – loneliness and social isolation.

Diagnosis of interpersonal disputes

For the therapist to choose role disputes as the focus of IPT, the patient must give evidence of current overt or covert conflicts with a significant other. Such disputes are usually revealed in the patient's initial complaints or in the course of the interpersonal inventory. In some IPT research, role disputes with the spouse have been the most common problem area. In practice, however, recognition of important interpersonal disputes in the lives of depressed patients may be difficult.

In developing a treatment plan, the therapist first determines the stage of the role dispute:

- *Renegotiation* implies that the patient and the significant other are openly aware of differences and are actively trying, even if unsuccessfully, to bring about changes.
- *Impasse* implies that discussion between the patient and the significant other has stopped and that the smouldering, low-level resentment typical of 'cold marriages' exists.

- *Dissolution* implies that the relationship is irretrievably disrupted.

Role transitions

Depression frequently results when a person recognises the need to make a normative role transition but has difficulty with the necessary changes required or when a person correctly recognises failure in a particular role but is unable to change the behaviour or to change roles. In depressions associated with role transitions, the patient feels helpless to cope with the change in role. The transition may be experienced as threatening to one's self-esteem and sense of identity, or as a challenge one is unable to meet.

In general, difficulties in coping with role transitions are associated with the following issues:

- Loss of familiar social supports and attachments
- Management of accompanying emotions, such as anger or fear
- Demands for a new repertoire of social skills
- Diminished self-esteem.

Training

Didactic seminar

In a 2–5 day seminar, an attempt is made to help the therapists identify what they are already doing that is like IPT, what they are doing that is not IPT, and the special skills needed for the IPT approach. This takes the form of an exegesis of the written material with extensive clinical illustration using videotaped case material.

Supervised casework

After the didactic seminar, therapists are assigned between two and four training cases each, on which they receive weekly supervision on a session-by-session basis. This is done on the telephone or in person after the supervisor has reviewed the videotape of the session. Both trainee and supervisor have videotape equipment and tapes available, so that they can watch specific segments as they discuss the session. The primary purpose of the supervision is boundary marking or helping the therapist learn which techniques are included and which are excluded in IPT. It is also helpful if the supervisor reviews the ratings made by the patient during the session as well as the observer ratings. The main differences between IPT and other therapies are shown in Table 30.8.

Klerman & Weissman (1993) is a text which reports new developments in IPT and describes IPT-M (maintenance treatment) as used by Kupfer et al (1992).

COGNITIVE ANALYTIC THERAPY (CAT)

This relatively new psychotherapy has a definite following in the UK but is little known elsewhere. It has been developed by Anthony Ryle and the key text is his 1990 book *Cognitive Analytic Therapy: Active Participation and Change,* a new integration in brief psychotherapy. Ryle describes how he recognises three essential patterns of what he calls neurotic repetition. These are:

- Traps – negative assumptions generate acts which produce consequences which reinforce the assumptions
- Dilemmas – the person acts as though available action or possible roles were limited to polarise alternatives (false dichotomies) usually without being aware that this is the case
- Snags – appropriate goals or roles are abandoned either because the individual makes an assumption that others would oppose them or because they are perceived as forbidden or dangerous. Ryle states that the central model underlying CAT is that of the procedural sequence model (PSM).

Several features differentiate CAT. The Psychotherapy file (produced in full in the above book) combines instructions for self-monitoring with descriptions of a range of traps, dilemmas and snags. It is normally given to patients at the end of their first interview. Ryle points out that the therapeutic relationship is clearly altered by a therapist who emphasises trying to work, offers concepts, prescribes reading, and suggests homework assignments but these techniques do not make working with the transference impossible. One of the key theoretical concepts underlying the basis of CAT is the procedural sequence model (PSM). This gives an account of the sequence of mental and behavioural processes involved in carrying out an aimed directed activity. Ryle believes that these procedures are hierarchally structured. Describing them and helping alter them is one of the main features of the treatment.

At the end of the assessment period, a re-formulation is produced. This is given to the patient in written form at the end of treatment. It is usually 10–12 sessions. A goodbye letter is written, training is more comprehensive than for IPT or CBT and normally takes two years of individual or group supervision. A number of trials evaluating CAT are under way but as yet no randomised control trials have been published.

SUPPORTIVE PSYCHOTHERAPY

This form of psychotherapy is as variously defined as it is widely used. Bloch (1979) describes it as a form of psychological treatment given to patients with chronic and disabling psychiatric conditions 'for whom basic change is not seen as a realistic goal'. This definition emphasises the notion of therapy as a prop or crutch and envisages the objectives of such an approach as the promotion of the patient's best possible psychological and social functioning, the bolstering of his self-esteem and self-confidence, the cultivation of his sense of and contact with reality, the prevention of relapse, and, in certain instances, the transfer of the source of support from professional to family or friends.

Table 30.8 Comparison of IPT with other psychotherapies	
IPT	Non-IPT psychotherapies
What has contributed to this patient's depression right now?	Why did the patient become what he is and/or where is the patient going?
What are the current stresses?	What was the patient's childhood like?
Who are the key persons involved in the current stress? What are the current disputes and disappointments?	What is the patient's character?
Is the patient learning how to cope with the problem?	Is the patient cured?
What are the patient's assets?	What are the patient's defences?
How can I help the patient ventilate painful emotions – talk about situations that evoke guilt, shame, resentment?	How can I find out why this patient feels guilty, ashamed or resentful?
How can I help the patient clarify his wishes and have more satisfying relationships with others?	How can I understand the patient's fantasy life and help him get insight into the origins of present behaviour?
How can I correct misinformation and suggest alternatives?	How can I help the patient discover false or incorrect ideas?

However, other definitions of supportive psychotherapy stress its role in enabling individuals to cope with and overcome psychological difficulties presenting more acutely. For example, a Royal College of General Practitioners' report (1981) on prevention of psychiatric disorders in general practice emphasised the importance of supportive intervention in enabling the individuals to negotiate 'psychosocial transitions' – particular life events and challenges which produce psychological reactions, symptoms and disorders commonly seen in patients presenting to general practitioners, health visitors and social workers. The objectives of such supportive psychotherapy include the minimising of the impact of the threatening event, the provision of protection and relief from responsibilities during the crisis or transition, the encouragement of the expression of emotions and talking through the difficulties, and support for the individual in his attempts to seek out new directions in life.

Supportive psychotherapy is also conceived of as the use of psychological means to build individuals up to a point where they can devote themselves to more profound, time-consuming and complex reconstructive psychotherapeutic interventions and as a temporary expedient to contain individuals who are acutely ill and who are awaiting the therapeutic impact of other forms of psychiatric treatment, most notably pharmacological.

There is much more general agreement as to what constitutes the key elements of the supportive forms of psychotherapy (Table 30.9). It is now recognised that the interview itself can exercise a psychotherapeutic effect – that the mere act of a doctor listening carefully to what the patient is saying, picking up verbal and non-verbal cues and enabling the patient to give a full account of his situation and problems can result in a significant improvement. This realisation has led in turn to attempts to dissect out those characteristics of the interview which may exercise particularly beneficial effect. To date, the bulk of the effort has been directed at identifying interview techniques which facilitate case detection but the implications for the facilitation of therapy seem clear. Among the interview techniques which appear important are the therapist's ability to note verbal and non-verbal cues, to ask questions in a sequence from open to closed, to avoid using too many direct questions and to emphasise the importance of

understanding the here-and-now situation (Marks et al 1979).

Reassurance provided by a therapist equipped to use the therapeutic relationship constructively, able to be both detached and compassionate, and skilled in listening and providing information simply and comprehensively is one of the basic elements of the supportive form of psychotherapy. Reassurance can be used to good effect to relieve fears, boost self-confidence and promote hope. But it is not without its problems. To promote a patient's hopes unreasonably by providing false reassurance, or to intervene prematurely before the patient has explained his situation fully, may be effective initially but will eventually prove useless. However, as Kessel has pointed out in a thoughtful essay on the subject, such a view reflects the perspective of the specialist psychotherapist concerned with the exploration rather than the alleviation of worry (Kessel 1979). The harmful effect of absolving a patient from his responsibilities and of getting between a patient and his recognition of underlying causes can be avoided once it is recognised.

Explanation is likewise an important element in psychotherapeutic support. Whereas reconstructive forms of psychotherapy emphasise non-directiveness, a degree of therapeutic passivity and active therapeutic interventions limited to the provision of interpretation, the supportive forms encourage the provision of explanations by the therapist of such diverse matters as the nature of the patient's symptoms, the choice of treatment, and the likely outcome. Explaining to a patient quite why certain symptoms are being experienced and the extent to which they are common can itself be reassuring and therapeutically effective. The goal is not so much depending on self-understanding as enhancement of the patient's ability to cope by clarifying the nature of the problem faced, the symptoms experienced and / or the treatment recommended.

Guidance and suggestion involve the provision of direct and indirect advice. In general, therapists are encouraged to refrain from advising patients, yet in supportive therapy teaching a patient how and when to ask for help is often a crucial component. Advice may be necessary with regard to particular problems, such as optimal ways of relating to a particularly difficult relative or handling a job interview, or to general issues, such as making contact with members of the opposite sex. Occasionally advice is ineffective, and persuasion, involving the therapist in a more direct, controlling posture, is required. Suggestion involves the therapist using such techniques as the showing or withholding of approval in attempts to modify a patient's situation. Suggestion operates in all forms of psychotherapy and it has even been postulated that the suitability of an individual for treatment is dependent on his potential openness to the suggestive

Table 30.9 Elements of supportive psychotherapy
The interview
Reassurance
Explanation
Guidance and suggestion
Ventilation

influence (Strupp 1978). Variables which appear to regulate the forcefulness of suggestion include the significance of the therapist to the patient, the degree to which the patient is or can become dependent and the depth of the patient's anxiety or depression. Individuals whose coping strategies have been overwhelmed are believed to be particularly prone to cling with desperation to any potential helping resource and to respond dramatically to proffered advice, reassurance and guidance.

In recent years, the value of *ventilation* of feelings within the psychotherapeutic setting has received support, and interest has been stimulated in the old notion of catharsis by the rise of the so-called 'emotive release (body) therapies'. It does seem useful for patients to be able to express emotions such as anger, frustration and despair openly. Unfortunately, the amount and quality of emotional expression has rarely been assessed independently and related to outcome, so its value has received little direct experimental verification.

Supportive psychotherapy is widely used in psychiatric settings, in general practice and in settings in which

patients with short-lived yet intense emotional crises are seen.

EFFECTIVENESS OF PSYCHOLOGICAL INTERVENTIONS

In the following section I will present a brief but structured introduction to the evidence for efficacy of psychological treatment. I have used major depressive disorder as an example and I have not covered alcohol and drug problems, sexual problems or eating disorders because these are covered in their respective chapters.

Meta-analyses have been conducted of the efficacy of psychotherapies in depressive illness and other neurotic disorders (Table 30.10). There are a number of areas of caution to be considered when interpreting such work. All the studies described look at efficacy from research trials rather than effectiveness in clinical settings. There is much less work in the latter area but one meta-analytic study by Weisz et al in 1995 showed no effect of psy-

Table 30.10 Comparisons of no treatment, placebo control and psychotherapy

Study	n^a	Psychotherapy versus no treatment ES(n^b, °ES$_c$)	Placebo versus no treatment ES(n^b, °ES$_c$)	Psychotherapy versus placebo ES(n^b, °ES$_c$)
Andrews & Harvey (1981)	81	0.72 (292, 0.003)*	—	0.55 (28,0.06)
Barker et al (1988)	17	1.06 (20, 0.136)*	0.47 (20, 0.071)	0.55 31, 0.11)
Bowers & Clum (1988)	69	0.76 (n=40)	0.55 (n=69)	—
Dush et al (1983)	31	—	0.21 (219,.03)	—
Dush et al (1989)	48	0.51 (n=60)	—	0.41 (n=142)
Eppley et al (1989)	70	0.43 (100, 0.076)*	0.23 (14, 0.14)	—
Hill (1987)	15	0.99 (39, 0.123)*	0.56 (60, 0.062)	—
Hyman et al (1989)	48/8^e	0.58 (55, 0.115)	—	0.66 (14, 0.142)
Jorm (1989)	63	0.53 (100, 0.048)	—	0.46 (10, 0.146)
Laesle et al (1987)	23	1.12^d (n=37)	—	0.10^d (n=8)
Landman & Dawes (1982)	42	0.80 (5, 0.30)	0.58 (4, 0.31)	0.51 (5, 0.32)
Miller & Berman (1983)	48	0.78	0.38	—
Prioleau et al (1983)	32	—	0.32	—
Quality Assurance Project (1983)	10	1.72^d	0.65^d (10, 0.17)	1.07^d
Smith et al (1980)	475	0.85(1761, 0.03)*	0.56 (200, 0.05)	—
Total^f	1,080	0.82 (n=2,309)	0.42 (n=596)	0.48 (n=250)

ES, effect size.
^{a} Number of studies.
^{b} Number of effects.
^{c} Standard error of the mean.
^{d} Effect sizes based on pre/post changes rather than control/treatment comparison.
^{e} Two separate meta-analyses were done.
^{f} Totals do not represent independent information because some reviews include studies also reviewed by other researchers.
*$P < 0.005$.
Reprinted with permission from Lambert et al (1993).

chotherapy in ordinary clinical settings but a large effect when delivered in carefully controlled trials with trained therapists in standardised conditions. Few studies have medium-term or long-term follow-up periods and many of the efficacy values reported represent only short-term outcomes. Given the chronic and relapsing nature of most of the psychological conditions in which psychotherapy is used, this is a serious deficiency. The concepts of recovery, relapse and recurrence and remission which have been now quite carefully defined in many drug studies are rarely applied to psychotherapy trials.

I will not discuss the limitations of meta-analysis except to say that most meta-analyses of psychotherapy combine different patient groups, different treatments, different outcome measures, though there are a few studies, particularly in cognitive-behavioural psychotherapy, which meet the homogeneity that the meta-analytic method requires (for example all using the BDI, Beck depression inventory) as an outcome measure. Figure 30.4 shows the concept of effect size (ES) in graphic form. This shows the average effect size for psychotherapy from all the studies in Table 30.10. as 0.82. This means that the average patient undergoing psychotherapy is better off than approximately 80% of those undergoing minimal or placebo treatment but that those undergoing placebo treatment are still 66% better off than no-treatment controls. Effect sizes are measured in standard deviation units.

Major depressive disorder (MDD): key review

Many of the large reviews of the efficacy of psychotherapy in major depression are now quite old and don't include many studies using modern psychotherapy techniques. Nevertheless, three studies have focused on the efficacy of psychotherapy contrasted with pharma-

Table 30.11 Meta-analyses of psychotherapy trials (Depression Guidelines Panel 1993)

Therapy	Overall efficacy (%)	No. trials analysed
Behaviour therapy alone	55.3	10
Brief dynamic therapy		
alone	34.8	6
Cognitive therapy		
alone	46.6	12
Interpersonal therapy		
alone	52.3	1
All therapies	50.0	29

cotherapy: the Quality Assurance Project (1983), Steinbruek et al (1993) and Conte et al (1986). The most influential of these, the Quality Assurance Project, showed an effect size for psychotherapy of 0.69, for tricyclic medication of 0.55 and for monoamine oxidase inhibitors of 0.39. The best, more recent review is the meta-analysis described by the Depression Guidelines Panel (1993). The results are reported somewhat differently from most meta-analyses in that effect size is not given but there is an expected response rate for each therapy. Details are given in Table 30.11. There are a relatively small number of studies on brief dynamic psychotherapy and only one on interpersonal psychotherapy in this review. In addition to considering meta-analysis I have thought it appropriate to mention two key studies.

Key studies

- Elkin 1994
- Hollon et al 1992

Specific/simple phobia: Key review

Emmelkamp (1994): This paper reviews behaviour treatments for specific phobias. Overall improvement rates appear to be achieved in approximately 75% of cases. The general conclusion is that exposure is more effective than systematic de-sensitisation and that in vivo exposure is the most effective. Treatments for circumscribed specific phobias can be brief, being carried out in a single prolonged session of two hours or over two to four sessions at weekly intervals.

Key studies

- Liddell et al 1994
- Ost 1989

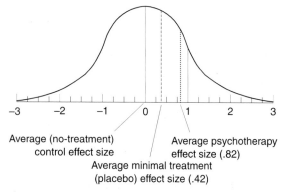

Fig. 30.4 Comparison of placebo and psychotherapy effects in relation to no-treatment control. (Reprinted by permission from Lambert et al 1993.)

Generalised anxiety disorder: Key review

Durham and Allan's review (1993) is important because they reviewed studies that had used the Hamilton Anxiety Scale and the state trait anxiety inventory as outcome measures. Their results show that CBT produces best results but there are some important qualifications. The rates of improvement varied markedly from study to study, CBT was not always the best treatment and outcome and rates of improvement were modest, though significantly better than placebo drugs or anti-anxiety medication. Not all studies had reasonable follow-up periods. Approximately 55% of those who had received cognitive therapy were in the normal range on the two above measures at the end of treatment, and this compared with 22% who had received behaviour therapy without cognitive intervention.

Key studies

- Butler et al 1991
- Durham et al 1994
- Power et al 1990

Panic disorder: Key review

Mattick et al (1990) reviewed studies on vivo exposure, medication and other less specific psychological techniques. The results are reported in effect sizes rather than percentage improvements. The authors comment on the low mean effect sizes for waiting list control or placebo treatments of around 0.3. Effect sizes for Alprazolam were 1.04, for Diazepam 0.56, Imipramine 1.01, Cognitive Therapy 1.43 and in vivo exposure 1.7.

Key studies

- Marks et al 1993
- Clark et al 1994

Social phobia: Key review

There is one good meta-analysis of 10 trials of behavioural and cognitive therapy: Chambless & Gillis, 1993, Evaluated controlled trials. There were significant effects both on the positive symptoms of social phobia and the fears of negative evaluation that social phobics exhibit. Given the chronicity of this disorder follow-ups were relatively brief being between 1 and 6 months.

Key study

- Heimberg et al 1990

Post-traumatic stress disorder: Key review

The most comprehensive review is that by Edna Foa (1995). She points out that most studies have either been on Vietnam veterans or on female rape victims. Effective techniques appear to be anxiety management, stress inoculation, training and cognitive restructuring. The role of exposure-based treatments remains controversial. The evidence-based psychodynamic psychotherapy is unclear largely because of the poor quality of the studies. Although not part of Foa's review it is perhaps worth emphasising that as yet there is little evidence base for post disaster counselling or post disaster psychological debriefing.

Key study

- Foa et al 1991

REFERENCES

Beck A T 1964 Thinking and depression: II. Theory and therapy. Archives of General Psychiatry 10: 561–571

Beck A T 1967 Depression: clinical, experimental and theoretical aspects. Harper & Row, New York

Beck A T 1987 Cognitive models of depression. Journal of Cognitive Psychotherapy I: 5–37

Beck A T, Emery G 1985 Anxiety disorders and phobias: a cognitive perspective. Basic Books, New York

Beck A T, Freeman A 1990 Cognitive therapy of personality disorders. Basic Books, New York

Beck A T, Rush A J, Shaw B F, Emery G 1979 Cognitive therapy of depression. Guilford Press, New York

Blackburn I M 1988 An appraisal of comparative trials of cognitive therapy. In: Peris G, Blackburn I M (eds) Cognitive psychotherapy: theory and practice. Springer Verlag, Heidelberg

Blackburn I M, Davidson K M 1990 Cognitive therapy for depression and anxiety. A practitioner's guide. Blackwell Scientific, Oxford

Bloch S (ed) 1979 Supportive psychotherapy. In: An introduction to the psychotherapies. Oxford University Press, London

Butler G, Fennell M, Robson P, Gelder M 1991 Comparison of behavior therapy and cognitive therapy in the treatment of generalised anxiety disorder. Journal of consulting and clinical psychology 59: 167–175

Cawley R H 1977 The teaching of psychotherapy. Association of University Teachers of Psychiatry Newsletter Jan 19:36

Chambless D L, Gillis M M 1993 Cognitive therapy of anxiety disorders. Journal of Consulting and Clinical Psychology 61: 248–260

Clark D M, Salkovskis P M, Hackmann A, Middleton H, Anastosiades P, Gelder M 1994 A comparison of cognitive therapy, applied relaxation and imipramine in the treatment of panic disorder. British journal of psychiatry 164: 759–769

Conte H R, Plutchik R, Wild, K V, Karasu T B 1986 Combined psychotherapy and pharmacotherapy for depression. Archives of General Psychiatry 43: 471–479

Cooper N A, Clum G A 1989 Imaginal flooding as a supplementary treatment for PTSD in combat veterans: a controlled study. Behavior Therapy 20: 381–391

Coyne J, Gottlib I 1983 The role of cognition in depression: a critical appraisal. Psychological Bulletin 94: 472–505

Depression Guidelines Panel 1993 Depression in primary care: detection, diagnosis and treatment: quick reference guide for clinicians. Clinical Practice Guideline No 5, AHCPR publication No 93-0552. US Department of Health and Human Services, Public Health Service, Agency for Health Care Policy and Research, Rockville, MD

Durham R C, Allan T 1993 Psychological treatment of generalized anxiety disorder: A review of the clinical significance of outcome studies since 1980. British journal of psychiatry 163: 19–23

Durham R C, Murphy T, Allan T, Brehard K, Treliving L R, Fenton G W 1994 Cognitive therapy, analytic psychotherapy and anxiety management training for generalised anxiety disorder. British journal of psychiatry 115: 315–323

Elkin I 1994 The NIMH treatment of depression collaboration research program: where we began and where we are. In: Bergin A E, Garfield S L (eds) Handbook of psychotherapy and behaviour change, 4th edn. Wiley, New York

Ellis A 1962 Reason and emotion in psychotherapy. Citadel Press, Secaucus, NJ

Emmalkamp P M G 1994 Behavior therapy with adults. In: Bergin A E, Garfield S L (eds) Handbook of psychotherapy and behavior change, 4th edn, Wiley, New York

Erikson E H 1950 Identity and the life cycle. International Universities Press, New York

Fairbairn W R D 1954 An object-relations theory of personality: psychoanalytic studies of the personality. Basic Books, New York

Freud S, Breuer J 1895/1955 Studies on hysteria. In: Strachey J (ed) The standard edition of the complete psychological works of Sigmund Freud. Hogarth Press, London

Foa E B, Davidson J, Rothbaum B O 1995 Treatment of post-traumatic stress disorders. In: Gabbard G O (ed) Treatment of psychiatric disorders: The DSM-IV version. American Psychiatric Press, Washington DC

Foa E B, Rothbaum B O, Riggs D S, Murdoch T B 1991 Treatment of PTSD in rape victims: A comparison between cognitive-behavioral procedures and counselling. Journal of consulting and clinical psychology 59: 715–723

Guntrip H 1969 Schizoid phenomena, object relations, and the self. International Universities Press, New York

Hawton K, Salkovskis P M, Kirk J, Clark D M 1989 Cognitive behaviour therapy for psychiatric problems: a practical guide. Oxford University Press, Oxford

Heimberg R G, Dodge C S, Hope D A 1990 Cognitive behavioral treatment of social phobia: Comparative to a credible placebo control. Cognitive therapy and research 14: 1–23

Hollon S D, Du Rubeis R J, Evans M D et al 1992 Cognitive therapy and pharmacotherapy for depression: singly or in combination. Archives of General Psychiatry, 49: 774–781

Jacobson E 1938 Progressive relaxation. University of Chicago Press, Chicago

Karon B P, Widener A J 1995 Psychodynamic therapies in historical perspective. In: Bonyar B, Beutler L E (eds). Oxford University Press, New York, pp. 24–27

Kernberg O 1980 Internal world and external reality: object relations theory applied. Aronson, New York

Kessel N 1979 Reassurance. Lancet i: 1128

Klerman G L, Weissman M M, Rounsaville B J, Chevron E S 1984 Interpersonal psychotherapy of depression. Basic Books, New York

Klerman G L, Weissman M M 1993 New applications of interpersonal psychotherapy. American Psychiatric Press, Washington, DC

Kupfer D J, Frank E, Perel J M et al 1992 Five year outcome for maintenance therapies in recurrent depression. Archives of General Psychiatry 49: 769–773

Ledwidge B 1978 Cognitive behaviour modification: a step in the wrong direction. Psychological Bulletin 85: 353–375

Lichstein K L 1988 Clinical relaxation strategies. Wiley, New York

Liddell A, di Fazio L, Blackwood J, Ackerman C 1994 Long-term follow-up of treated dental phobics. Behaviour research therapy 32: 604–610

Marks I M, Swinson R P, Basoglu M, Kuch K, Noshirvani H, O'Sullivan G, Lelliot P T, Kirby M, McNamee G, Sengun S, Wickwire K 1993 Alprazolam and exposure alone and combined in panic disorder with agoraphobia. Journal of psychiatry 162: 776–787

Marks J, Goldberg D P, Hillier V F 1979 Determinants of the ability of general practitioners to detect psychiatric illness. Psychological Medicine 9: 263–267

Masson J M 1984 The assault on truth: Freud's suppression of the seduction theory. Farrar, Straus & Giroux, New York

Mattick R P, Andrews G, Hadzi-Pavlovic D, Christensen H 1990 Treatment of panic and agoraphobia: An integrative review. Journal of nervous and mental disease 178: 567–576

Ost L G 1989 One session treatment for specific phobias. Behaviour research and therapy 25: 397–409

Power K G, Simpson R J, Swanson V, Wallace C A 1990 A controlled comparison of cognitive behaviour therapy, diazepam, and placebo alone and in combination, for the treatment of generalised anxiety disorder. Journal of anxiety disorders 4: 267–292

Quality Assurance Project 1983 A treatment outline for depressive disorders. Australian and New Zealand Journal of Psychiatry 17: 129–146

Roth A, Fonagy P 1996 What works and for whom. A critical review of psychotherapy research. Guilford Press, New York

Royal College of General Practitioners 1981 Prevention of psychiatric disorders in general practice. RCGP, London

Ryle A 1990 Cognitive-analytic therapy: active participation in change. Wiley, Chichester

Steinbruek S M, Maxwell S E, Howard G S 1983 A meta-analysis of psychotherapy and drug therapy in the treatment of unipolar depression with adults. Journal of Consulting and Clinical Psychology 51: 856–863

Strupp H M 1978 Psychotherapy research and practice – an overview. In: Bergin A E, Garfield S L (eds) Handbook of psychotherapy and behaviour change, 2nd edn. Wiley, New York

Sullivan H S 1953 Interpersonal theory of psychiatry. Norton, New York

Truax C B, Carkhuff R R 1967 Toward effective counselling and psychotherapy: training and practice. Aldine, Chicago

Valliant G E, Bond M, Valliant O 1986 An empirically validated hierarchy of defense mechanisms. Archives of General Psychiatry 43: 786

Weisz J R, Donenberg E R, Man S S, Weiss B 1995 Bridging the gap between laboratories and clinic in child and adolescent psychotherapy. Journal of Consulting and Clinical Psychology 63: 688–701

Welberg L R 1977 The technique of psychotherapy. Grune & Stratton, New York

Wolpe J 1958 Psychotherapy by reciprocal inhibition. Stanford University Press, Stanford

31

Evidence-based medicine and psychiatry

Stephen M. Lawrie   John R. Geddes

INTRODUCTION

Evidence-based medicine (EBM) can be simply defined as the identification (reliably and efficiently), critical appraisal (in terms of validity and usefulness) and implementation of the best available evidence (from research and experience) for a particular intervention or manoeuvre in a given clinical situation (Sackett et al 1997). The process of EBM depends crucially on a precise formulation of an answerable clinical question. The final stage of EBM is a constant evaluation of one's performance at each stage.

The strategies of EBM facilitate a career-long, problem-based, self-directed learning process with the fundamental aim of improving patient care. EBM was developed to assist the decision making of the individual clinician helping a particular patient; however, the same process is also increasingly being used by policy-makers and purchasers of services.

In this chapter we will briefly describe the main historical developments leading to EBM and then critically examine its potential clinical importance. We will then discuss in detail, with examples, how each of the components of EBM described above can be applied to the contemporary practice of psychiatry.

Although EBM promises benefits for practitioners (and their patients) throughout their career, we appreciate that most readers are studying for postgraduate exams and will therefore emphasise the processes of critical appraisal (Critical Review Paper Working Party 1997). This will be followed by an estimate of how much of current psychiatric practice is evidence based, and how it compares to other medical disciplines. Finally, we will discuss the main problems facing EBM in general and evidence-based mental health (EBMH) in particular.

Before we go any further, however, it is necessary to clarify what EBM is *not* (Sackett et al 1996). EBM is not 'old hat', as a few examples in the 'why we need it' section below will clearly demonstrate; nor is it impossible, as everyone can learn how to do it. It is most certainly not a purely academic pursuit – its whole theory and practice is targeted directly at the needs of clinicians and their patients. EBM does not simply consist of using results from randomised controlled trials (RCTs) or meta-analyses of RCTs, as it also applies to the rational use of diagnostic tests and making valid prognostic statements. EBM does not intend to tyrannise clinical practice with some form of 'cook-book' medicine as it explicitly seeks to integrate evidence from *both* research and clinical expertise. Lastly, it does not play into the hands of those who wish to cut the costs of health care, as the best available treatment is often not the cheapest (although it may have something to say about balancing optimal practice within resource constraints).

HISTORICAL DEVELOPMENT

Sackett & colleagues (1996) like to trace the philosophical origins of EBM to the spirit of enquiry and call for external evidence in 19th century Paris. More specifically, the development of the RCT as the clinical equivalent of a controlled scientific experiment – first described by Daniels & Hill (1952) – has probably done more than anything else to place medical practice on secure scientific foundations. The development and refinement of techniques of meta-analysis (Smith & Glass 1977; Mann 1990) has allowed the results of two or more studies to be summarised quantitatively.

EBM first became possible with developments in information technology which allowed rapid bibliographic searching and retrieval, coupled with the application of biostatistical principles derived from population-based epidemiology to the care of individual patients (Sackett et al 1991). At the same time, the increasing demand from consumers of health care and others for more explicit use of treatments of proven benefit increased the pressure on doctors to keep up to date and to ensure that their practice was based on the best available evidence (Cochrane 1972).

WHY EBM?

The central issue addressed by EBM is that keeping abreast of new medical developments is difficult. There are ever increasing quantities of medical journals containing an ever increasing literature to be sifted through. Relevant studies need to be read and assimilated and – when appropriate – new findings incorporated into clinical practice. Similarly, old practices need to be discarded as evidence emerges of lack of effectiveness or actual harm. For the average psychiatrist, as with most doctors, there are perhaps a handful of general medical journals and a similar number of specialist journals to be read, but time is limited and the journals are (clinically) disorganised. Moreover, there is evidence that the further physicians are from graduation, the more out of date they become (Ramsey et al 1991). Not only are we likely to need more time to study, but we are less likely to do so (and less able to assimilate new information due to age-related cognitive decline).

This is not merely an academic issue. Studies suggest that the average physician, when asked, could usefully seek clinically relevant information in two out of every three patients they see, and that such information would change their clinical decisions in one of every four (Covell et al 1985, Smith 1996). It has long been recognised that the mass of potentially relevant information needs to be reliably reviewed and formatted for easy access in everyday clinical situations. The problem is that traditional updating methods – books, review articles and even continuing medical education – are unreliable and don't change clinical practice.

Textbooks are almost inevitably out of date by the time they are published. Most 'expert' review articles are unsystematic (in the selection and interpretation of studies for review) and often outdated. For example, conventional narrative review methods delayed the use of thrombolysis for myocardial infarction by about 10 years after a systematic review/meta-analysis would have shown convincing benefit (Antman et al 1992); while the dangerous, sometimes lethal, use of lignocaine prophylaxis for ventricular fibrillation was extended by about the same length of time after it had been shown to be counterproductive. In psychiatry, it has been known since the early 1990s that illness education and social skills training improve outcome in schizophrenia, but these are still far from routinely provided (Benton & Schroder 1990, Mari & Streiner 1996). By contrast, systematic reviews require a comprehensive search for relevant studies using an explicit strategy, bias-free citations, accurate judgement of scientific quality of cited articles, and appropriate synthesis of the articles' conclusions. Unfortunately, but perhaps predictably, there is a strong inverse relationship ($r = -0.52$) between adherence to these standards and self-professed expertise of the reviewer (Oxman & Guyatt 1993).

Lastly, continuing medical education (CME), the relatively recent attempt to deal with these problems, doesn't work. As with reading, those motivated to attend CME courses are least likely to need to. Furthermore, it has been shown that many commonly used methods of CME do not change doctors' clinical behaviour and so are unlikely to bring about improvements in the quality of patient care (Davis et al 1995). The strategies of EBM offer a feasible alternative to haphazard reading and being at the mercy of pharmaceutical company representatives for keeping up to date. Although EBM itself is still in need of rigorous evaluation, there is some evidence that medical students at McMaster and Harvard University, where the teaching has been problem- rather than knowledge-based for several years, find their undergraduate teaching more stimulating and satisfying and are better able to keep up to date with medical advances as postgraduates than students taught in more traditional curricula (Sackett et al 1997).

The Cochrane collaboration

The recognition of the need for systematic reviews of RCTs and the development of the scientific methodology of review articles has been one of the most striking developments in health services research over the past decade. The first specialty to rise to Archie Cochrane's challenge was perinatology. Following the pioneering efforts of Iain Chalmers, the Oxford Database of Perinatal Trials, containing over 6000 RCTs, was published in 1992. To widen the scope of the reviews to include other fields of medicine, the Cochrane Collaboration was formed to 'prepare and maintain systematic reviews of randomised controlled trials of the effects of health care, and of other evidence when appropriate, and to make this information readily available to decision-makers at all levels of health care systems' (Cochrane Collaboration 1995). The first UK Cochrane Centre was established in Oxford in 1992 as part of the NHS Research and Development (R&D) Programme and centres have since been established in several other countries. The Cochrane Collaboration facilitates systematic reviews of RCTs of all aspects of health care, maintains a register of RCTs, organises training for reviewers and establishes systems to update and efficiently disseminate the findings. Within this network, there are collaborative review groups, which coordinate reviews in a specific area of medical practice – for example, the Cochrane Schizophrenia Review

Group. Thus far, there are four other groups in psychiatry – covering dementia, depression and anxiety, alcohol and drugs, and developmental disorders.

The Cochrane Library, containing all this information, is continually updated and published four times a year on compact and floppy disk and on the internet. As well as the Cochrane Database of Systematic Reviews (CDSR), the library contains the Database of Abstracts of Reviews of Effectiveness (DARE), the Cochrane Controlled Trials Register (of 160 000 controlled trials) and the Cochrane Review Methodology Database for those undertaking research synthesis (Cochrane Collaboration 1998).

By facilitating access to summaries of research evidence, the gradual evolution of the CDSR will greatly enhance the feasibility of evidence-based medical practice. Even now, the Cochrane Library is probably the best available source of systematic reviews of the effectiveness of health care interventions. Its main strengths are in the continual updating of information and the dramatic advances in the methodology of systematic reviews that has accompanied the development of the Cochrane Collaboration (NHS Centre for Reviews and Dissemination (CRD) 1996). Despite this impressive progress to date, it is likely to be several years before the CDSR comprehensively covers the majority of health care interventions. The Cochrane Collaboration builds upon contributors' existing interests, which no doubt ensures the commitment to continual updating but means that reviews of very specialist interventions may be undertaken before reviews of more common and important treatments.

Despite the limited number of completed reviews the Cochrane Library is surprisingly comprehensive because of the inclusion of the DARE maintained by the NHS CRD. The DARE contains abstracts of systematic reviews published since 1994 which have passed explicit quality criteria. Included are the abstracts of the Effective Health Care bulletins produced by the CRD, which cover topics in particular need of review (Sheldon 1996). The CRD approach is therefore complementary to that of the Cochrane Library in meeting the information needs of the NHS.

Improving current awareness

Although these initiatives fulfil an essential role in producing regularly updated systematic reviews of evidence of clinical effectiveness, an inevitable delay exists between the publication of important evidence and its incorporation into a review. Secondary publications are designed to bridge this gap – the first two being the *ACP Journal Club* (a supplement to the *Annals of Internal Medicine*) and *Evidence-Based Medicine*. The latter is aimed at primary care physicians and covers most of the main medical specialties, including psychiatry. The aim of these journals is to locate and summarise the small number of clinical research articles that are clinically important and to publish them as structured abstracts, with commentaries provided by experienced clinicians. Both journals have recently been published as a combined cumulative database on CD-ROM entitled *Best Evidence* (BMJ Publications, London) which will be updated annually.

Of particular relevance to psychiatrists, are the recent launch of a journal *Evidence-Based Mental Health* (*EBMH*) in early 1998 and the establishment of a Centre for Evidence-Based Mental Health (CEBMH) in Oxford, UK. All these developments, which have thus far concentrated on research synthesis, seek to help bring about a greater use of evidence in everyday clinical practice.

HOW TO PRACTISE EBM

Learning the principles of EBM and beginning to employ them to improve patient care can be relatively quick, but acquiring detailed knowledge and experience demands regular and continuing reading and practise. What follows is enough to begin this hopefully lifelong process. Readers who want to further satisfy their curiosity and/or to take things further should consider: learning EBM by attending EBM and critical appraisal skills workshops, subscribing to the journals and disks described above, and/or setting up channels for regular communication with EBM teachers. (Indeed, a case can be made for at least one person in each service, perhaps the audit or R&D coordinator, doing all of these with a view to staff development and service evaluation.)

The five components of the EBM process are:

1. framing answerable questions
2. searching for evidence
3. appraising the evidence
4. implementing the findings
5. evaluation.

These five principles will be introduced, illustrated with an example of a treatment study, and described in two further examples below that cover meta-analysis and prognosis. It should be noted, however, that EBM also covers issues of aetiology, diagnosis, clinical decision analysis, economics, quality improvement and clinical guidelines which are beyond the scope of this brief chapter. Those who are particularly interested or assiduous in preparing for exams are referred to Sackett et al (1991, 1997).

1. Framing questions

To be useful, such questions will be brief summaries of the clinical scenario and what information is required that are constructed in a way that makes searching for evidence likely to succeed. Specific questions will of course vary according to the situation, but productive questions tend to be composed of four parts ('the four-part clinical question'): the patient problem, the type of clinical issue or intervention being considered (e.g. diagnostic, prognostic or therapeutic), the comparison intervention (if appropriate) and the clinical outcome(s) of interest.

> *Treatment example: You are referred a 22-year-old female outpatient with a five year history of bulimia nervosa. She is not clinically depressed, but regularly abuses alcohol, and wishes some sort of talking rather than drug treatment. As a general adult psychiatrist, you are not sure what the best sort of treatment would be. You ask her to begin to record a diary of her eating and bingeing and arrange to do a literature search before you see her again in 2 weeks time.*

> *Question: In bulimia nervosa (problem), which psychotherapy (intervention) is most effective in securing recovery (outcome)?*

There are of course several questions that one could ask in this and any clinical situation – for example, how does drug treatment compare with psychotherapy? are there alternative treatments? The question will, of course, depend on what is most useful to you and your patient, what evidence you can actually find, and what might be of greatest benefit to know for similar common situations in the future. Of course, the number of possible questions will always be greater than the time available to answer them, but once one question is answered (and ideally recorded somewhere for easy access), others can be dealt with as and when the need and opportunity arises. Not only can several questions be asked within a domain (e.g. treatment) but several domains (such as clinical findings, aetiology, differential diagnosis, prognosis, therapy, prevention and even self-improvement) may be pertinent in any one consultation. However, as stated, we will limit ourselves to considering evidence about treatment (from single RCTs and systematic review) and prognosis in this chapter.

2. Searching for evidence

A really well-framed clinical question will make the literature search parameters obvious, but this may sometimes require further thought (and perhaps slight modification of the question). In obtaining evidence, one must next consider where and how to get it.

Electronic media for literature searching have several advantages, in terms of time taken and completeness, over hand searching journals. The quickest and easiest way of identifying reliable information is to use evidence-based medical summaries generated by others – as available from the Cochrane Collaboration or *Best Evidence* CDs mentioned above. However, the former may not, as yet, include a completed systematic review or meta-analysis in a relevant area, and the latter will only include recently published papers. A search on one of the computerised literature databases is therefore often required.

MEDLINE, BIDS (Bath Information Database Service) and PsychLit are all useful resources, but have different databases stretching back to 1975, 1981 and 1990, respectively. It is important to appreciate that even a well-conducted search on one of these databases will probably only detect 30–50% of the relevant studies and that each will identify a different set of publications, but in clinical practice MEDLINE has the advantage of being widely available.

A MEDLINE search demands search terms, as textwords or subject headings, to be typed in and allows certain operations to be performed to identify publications of a particular type. Ideally, when considering a treatment issue as in the brief example above, one would be able to identify one or more systematic reviews (indexed in MEDLINE under the heading 'meta-analysis') of RCTs which monitored and compared relapse rates on drug and placebo. However, it is more likely that no meta-analyses are available and one or more potentially relevant RCTs must be identified and then evaluated. *Evidence-Based Medicine* (EBM) suggests search terms to identify RCTs according to the year of publication – a 'high-quality yield search' with one item would use 'clinical trial (publication type [pt])' for 1990 and after, as well as 'random (textword [tw])' before 1990, although using more than one term will increase the number of studies identified (see inside back cover of *EBM* volume 1, part 7). If the clinical question is of a prognostic nature then the best evidence is likely to come from cohort (search 'cohort') studies (see below).

If you cannot find any relevant studies, a number of possible strategies are available. MESH search terms can be 'expanded' into a broader category, alternative words could be used, or another database may be worth consulting. However, it is more common to get too much rather than too little information from such a search. It is often useful to get help in searching, or learning how to search, from a trained librarian. Once the study or studies have been identified, they must be evaluated both in terms of their validity and usefulness.

Literature search example: You remember seeing a structured review of a paper on psychotherapy for bulimia in a recent edition of Evidence-Based Medicine *(on disk or in print). Searching the disk/journal you find the one-page summary, although it was published longer ago than you thought (EBM Jan/Feb 1996). You note that the summary contains some of the EBM summary data you require.*

3. Appraising the evidence

The evidence needs to be critically appraised for its scientific validity and clinical importance. Validity criteria are essentially the same as the questions to be answered in critical appraisal (Table 31.1)(Crombie 1996); while clinical importance can be determined by some of the summary measures EBM practitioners find useful (particularly for treatment studies).

Appraisal example: Although you know that Evidence-Based Medicine *only selects for inclusion treatment trials with random allocation, clinically important outcome measures and consistent data*

Table 31.1 Critical appraisal for single treatment studies	
Questions	**Answers**
• *Is the research valid?* **Was the assignment of patients to treatments randomised?** Was the randomisation list concealed? Were all subjects who entered the trial accounted for at its conclusion? Were they analysed in the groups to which they were randomised? Were subjects and clinicians blind to which treatment was being received? Apart from the experimental treatment, were the groups treated equally? Were the groups similar at the start of the trial?	
• *Is the research important?* Absolute risk reduction (ARR, i.e. CER−EER) Number need to treat (NNT, i.e. 1/ARR)	ARR = NNT =
• *Can I apply it to my patient?* Is this patient so different from those in the trial that the results don't apply? How great would the benefit be for this particular patient? What is the Patient Expected Event Rate (PEER) in my practice for patients like this one? (PEER−CER=F, or estimate) What is the NNT for this patient ?	 NNT/F =
• *Is it consistent with my patient's values and preferences?* Do I have a clear assessment of the patient's values and preferences? Are they met by this intervention and its potential consequences?	
• *Clinical 'bottom-line' comments:*	

Source: Sackett et al 1997

analysis, no system is infallible and therefore you evaluate the paper for yourself (Fairburn et al 1995), following the checklist for treatment studies (Table 31.1).

The paper compares the outcome after cognitive-behavioral therapy (CBT), interpersonal therapy (IPT) and behaviour therapy. Treatment allocation was random (although the paper doesn't mention whether or not the randomisation list was concealed); 90% of the patients were interviewed at follow-up and the groups were analysed as randomised; the treatment was not blind (but outcome assessment was), the groups were treated equally other than with the interventions of interest and did not differ significantly at the start of the trial. You decide therefore that the study is valid.

At this point, it is worth introducing some of the measures of clinical effectiveness and how to calculate them for treatment studies. We are primarily interested in comparing the proportion of patients treated with a new treatment who get the outcome of interest – or the experimental event rate (EER) – with the proportion of patients treated with an alternative (standard) treatment who get the outcome of interest – or control event rate (CER). The difference between these two outcome rates is the absolute risk reduction (ARR), i.e. CER −EER expressed as a percentage. This tells us the difference in the number of patients with a specific outcome for every 100 patients treated in either way. The next term to introduce transforms this ARR into a more clinically useful number – the number needed to treat (NNT) – which is simply the reciprocal of the ARR and tells us how many such patients we would need to treat in a particular way so as to avoid one outcome event. As a rough rule of thumb, NNTs of less than 10 usually denote a powerful and important treatment effect.

The results given in the paper are rates of still satisfying diagnostic criteria for bulimia at the end of the study – 37% for CBT, 28% for IPT and 86% for simple behavioural therapy. The ARR and NNT are therefore 49% (86−37%) and 2 (95% confidence interval 1 to 4) for CBT, and 58% (86−28%) and 2 (95% CI 1 to 3) for IPT. There seems little to choose between CBT and IPT, but the summary states that patients receiving CBT were less likely to have any symptoms than those receiving either IPT or behavioural therapy, and that CBT complete remission rates were highest.

4. Implementation

We are here concerned with whether the results of valid,

important studies can be applied to our particular patient or group of patients. In essence, this depends on the similarity and differences between the subjects in a paper and our own clinical population. Certain questions can be routinely asked for prognostic and therapeutic studies, as shown in Tables 31.1–31.3. In practice, it is often quickest to answer these applicability questions first, as this avoids the unnecessary evaluation of irrelevant papers, as long as the other stages of critical appraisal are not forgotten.

One further term needs to be introduced here. This is simply an estimate of your own patients' susceptibility to the outcome of interest as compared with the average patient in the trial – on the basis of age, sex, comorbidity, etc. This estimate is called F (for fraction), as many patients will be less susceptible than those in the RCT, although any patient may be more susceptible and the F will be greater than 1. The NNT for any particular patient can be simply calculated by dividing the NNT by F.

Implementation example: Your patient is clearly similar in age and sex to those described in the study and would have been eligible for inclusion in the study. Interpersonal psychotherapy is not available locally – but cognitive-therapy is (and it produces the best remission rates). In your team, the clinical psychologist provides the cognitive-behaviour therapy and so you refer her. You tell the patient that there is a good chance of successful outcome.

5. Evaluation

The final stage of EBM is the continual evaluation and improvement of the specific skills involved at each stage of the process. It is useful to review periodically the clinical questions you have asked and your success in answering them. How well can you critically appraise the scientific literature and is there any way that you can improve your skills (for example, by using critical appraisal checklists prepared by others)? Are you providing clinically useful summaries of the evidence – and keeping them up to date? It is useful to share any problems identified – by discussing with other local practitioners or clinical epidemiologists. You may benefit from attendance at an EBM or critical appraisal skills workshop.

One useful way of implementing EBM is to encourage a critical, but supportive, culture. Clinical colleagues should be asking each other for the evidence in support of some of their statements. Audit of how 'evidence-based' your practice is and what changes we should aim for, preferably with individualised feedback, will then be feasible. Similarly, it may be possible to begin to teach EBM principles to medical students or members of other disciplines. Existing structures, such as a journal club, can be reorganised along EBM lines (Sackett et al 1997).

Evaluation example: You ask the psychologist to inform you of the treatment outcome and decide to audit the treatments (and their outcome) you have offered to patients with bulimia you have seen over the past year. You discuss with your colleagues the possibility of a larger audit and ensuring that all such patients are treated with CBT in the future (for which resources will need to be identified).

FURTHER EXAMPLES OF CRITICAL APPRAISAL AND IMPLEMENTATION

Prognosis

Example: A 25-year-old male patient currently hospitalised for his first episode of schizophrenia is nearing discharge. His ageing parents ask to see you to discuss the likely outcome for their son. At the meeting they are particularly interested in whether he will be able to live independently and obtain paid employment in the future. You tell them that the conventional wisdom is that about half of all patients with schizophrenia will return to their premorbid social situation but that the other half are likely to deteriorate progressively. They thank you for your time, but you are dissatisfied with the information you gave and sense that the parents were too. You resolve to search the literature for a recent prognosis study.

1. Question

What percentage of patients in their first episode of schizophrenia will be living independently and in paid employment at 5–10 years?

2. Literature search

Using the MESH headings 'schizophrenia', 'cohort' and 'first episode' on MEDLINE (1993–1997) you identify several studies. However, one catches your eye as it describes the results of a 13 year follow-up in Nottingham and mentions disability and residence in the structured abstract (Mason et al 1995).

3. Appraisal

Using the critical appraisal checklist for prognosis studies (Table 31.2), you decide that the Mason et al (1995) study meets the validity criteria because it studied all first-episode psychosis patients in a defined catchment area, obtained follow-up information in 94%, objective outcomes were determined with good reliability and no subgroups with different prognoses were identified (making adjustment unnecessary), even though there was no independent 'test-set' group of patients. The results also look important – 57 of the 59 subjects (97%) had been living independently in the community for most of the past 2 years, 16 (28%) alone, and 22 (37%) had been employed for the past 2 years.

You then calculate *95% confidence intervals* for these outcomes to ensure that the results given in the paper are sufficiently precise to be useful in practice. The 95% confidence interval (CI) is the range of values in which you can be 95% sure that the true value lies. The approximate 95% CI for a proportion (expressed as a decimal) is the proportion plus or minus 1.96 times the square root of $\{[(\text{the proportion}) \times (1 - \text{proportion})] / \text{sample size}\}$. For living independently, this is 0.97 ± 1.96 times the square root of $(0.97 \times 0.03)/59$, or 0.97 ± 0.04, or 93 to 100%. The other confidence intervals are 17 to 39% for living alone and 26 to 48% for employment (check them yourself for practise). The 95% CI gives an estimate of the uncertainty of the proportion.

4. Implementation

Again using the checklist (Table 31.2), you decide that the results can be applied to your patient because the study was of an unbiased inception (first-episode) cohort and your patient is just recovering from his first episode. The study was in a UK secondary care setting similar to your own service. You also think that the information will be useful for you, your patient and his parents. You arrange to see them again briefly to discuss the results of your endeavours.

5. Evaluation

You note that the paper identified also gives information on symptoms and treatment outcomes and file your critically appraised summary of the paper under schizophrenia – prognosis. The summary will need to be updated as new evidence becomes available.

Systematic reviews and meta-analysis

Example: You want to improve the local implementation of care management for the severely mentally ill. You are aware that there has been considerable uncertainty about the effectiveness of care management and for which patients it is most useful.

Table 31.2   Critical appraisal for prognosis studies

Questions	Answers
● *Is the research valid?* Was the sample of patients unbiased and representative? Is it a study of a cohort of patients who are at a common (usually early) point in the course of their disease? Was the follow-up of the patients sufficiently long and complete? Were objective outcome criteria applied in a 'blind' fashion? If subgroups with different prognoses were identified, was there adjustment for important prognostic factors? Was there validation in an independent ('test-set') group of patients?	
● *Is the research important?* Outcome 1 Outcome 2 Outcome *n*	Rate (95% CI)
● *Can I apply it to my patient?* Were the study patients similar to my own? Will this evidence make a clinically important impact on my conclusions about what to offer or tell my patient?	
● *Clinical 'bottom-line' comments:*	

Source: Sackett et al 1997

1. Question

For patients with severe mental illness, what are the effects of care management on the clinical state and service utilisation?

2. Searching for evidence

You search for a relevant systematic review of RCTs in the CDSR on the Cochrane Library. You find a systematic review of case management for people with severe mental disorders which seems to address the issue (Marshall et al 1996).

3. Appraisal

Although the review has been conducted under the auspices of the Cochrane Collaboration, it is still important to critically appraise it for validity and usefulness (Table 31.3). The review includes nine RCTs of case management versus standard care. The reviewers clear-

ly describe the search strategy for identifying the primary studies, as well as the inclusion and exclusion criteria for including them in the review. All the studies investigated a form of case management which was broadly comparable; standard care was defined as the usual level of psychiatric care provided in the area where each study was conducted. The studies examined a range of clinical and health service utilisation outcomes. Although there was some variation between the studies, the reviewers investigated the reasons for this and concluded that it was mainly quantitative rather than qualitative. You decide that the results of the overview are probably valid. As the primary studies were performed in the UK and USA, and included patients with severe mental illness (however defined), you also think that the review can be applied to your own clinical situation.

4. Implementation

The main findings of the review are that case manage-

Table 31.3 Critical appraisal for a systematic review	
Questions	Answers
• *Is the research valid?*	
Did the review address a clearly focused issue? (i.e. did the review describe: the population studied? the intervention given? the outcome considered?)	
Did the authors select the right sort of studies for review? (i.e. addressing the review question, with adequate study design)	
Were the important, relevant studies included? (Look for which bibliographic databases were used, personal contact with experts, search for unpublished as well as published studies, search for non-English language studies)	
Did the reviewers do enough to assess the quality of the included studies?	
Did they use description of randomisation and/or a rating scale?	
• *What are the results?*	
Were the results similar from study to study?	
Are the results of all studies clearly displayed?	
If the results are not similar, are the reasons for the variations discussed?	
What is the overall result of the review?	
Is there a clinical bottom line?	
What is the numerical result?	ARR =
	NNT=
How precise are the results?	
Is there a confidence interval?	
• *Can I apply the results to my patient(s)?*	
Is my patient so different from those in the trial that the results may not apply?	
Should I apply the results to my patient(s)?	
How great would the benefit be?	
Is the intervention consistent with my patient's values and preferences?	
Were all the clinically important outcomes considered?	
Are the benefits worth the harm and costs?	

Source: Sackett et al 1997

ment assists community psychiatric teams to maintain contact with patients. However, it also increases the rate of admission to hospital. There was no significant effect on other outcome variables (such as possible improvements in symptom severity or quality of life). Of 600 case managed subjects, 151 were lost to follow-up (EER = 25.2%), as compared with 200 of 611 standard care subjects (CER = 32.7%). The absolute risk reduction is 7.5% and the NNT is 13 (95% CI 8 to 40). This means that 13 patients have to be treated with case management to prevent one less patient being lost to follow-up than would occur with standard care.

The ratio of the odds of being lost to follow-up in the case management group to the odds of the same in the standard care group was 0.68 (95% CI 0.53 to 0.88). You know from an audit of your own service, carried out before the implementation of the care programme approach, that only 10% of your own patients were lost to follow-up each year. This is the patient expected event rate (PEER) and is about 30% (0.100/0.327 = 0.306) of the CER in the review. Assuming that case management has a fairly constant effect in all patient groups, you can therefore adjust the NNT to apply the loss of follow-up rate of your service by dividing it by this proportion, which is called the F value (Cook & Sackett 1995). This revised NNT is approximately 42 (13/0.306). However, among patients with a previous history of loss of contact, your drop-out rate was 80%. Adjustment in a similar way produces a second revised NNT of about 5 for this 'high risk of drop-out' patient group.

5. Evaluation

You therefore decide not to use your scarce resources on routine case management (NNT 42), but to concentrate on those you have previously lost contact with (NNT 5). You audit the loss to follow-up in both groups over the next 6 months, both to ensure that your pre-case management audit figures are still applicable and to examine the effects of your decision to focus your care programming.

HOW EVIDENCE-BASED ARE WE?

An obvious place to begin to evaluate our individual and collective practice is to ask how much of contemporary medical and specifically psychiatric treatment is evidence-based? We tend to assume that, because we are *trying* to do good, we *are* doing good. However, few of our treatments are evidence-based in the sense that they are supported by high-quality studies that would meet strict critical appraisal guidelines. Indeed, it has been estimated that perhaps 'only 15% of medical interventions are supported by solid scientific evidence' (Smith 1991).

This debate raises the question: how can we deem a treatment to be 'evidence-based'? One way of answering this is to identify how well the intervention is supported by evidence – using a hierarchy to rate the evidence according to the likelihood of it giving an unbiased estimate of the true effect. Most reliable are findings from systematic reviews of good quality RCTs, followed by individual good quality RCTs. However, there are certain clinical situations where benefits could be said to be obvious, or where RCTs would be difficult and, arguably, even unethical (e.g. admission and observation for suicidal ideation). None the less, it might still be possible to conduct standard care versus alternative treatment RCTs in these areas. Alternatively, some useful information about treatments may be available from naturalistic follow-up studies, although the information gained from cohort studies and case–control studies is most reliable for prognosis and diagnosis, respectively. Lastly, uncontrolled studies, case series and individual case reports are too susceptible to bias to have general value, although they may sometimes identify a treatment effect or therapeutic hazard that would merit further study.

Using these criteria – where treatment is considered evidence-based if it is based on results from randomised evidence – either from systematic reviews or RCTs, or where benefit is obvious – how evidence-based is contemporary medicine and psychiatry? The answer crucially depends on whether we talk about treatments or diseases. Chalmers examined the evidence for 226 obstetric procedures: only 50% had been evaluated in RCTs, with only 20% of procedures having been shown to be beneficial; the other 30% were of dubious benefit or dangerous (Chalmers et al 1989). On the other hand, taking patients as the denominator, Ellis et al (1995) reviewed the evidence for the main treatment of 121 consecutive admissions to a medical ward in Oxford over 1 month. One hundred and nine patients had an identified primary diagnosis, 58 (53%) of whom received evidence-based interventions (e.g. heparin and warfarin for deep venous thrombosis), a further 32 (29%) received treatments supported by convincing non-experimental evidence (e.g. antibiotics for infections, resuscitation for cardiac arrest), and the remain-

Table 31.4 Primary diagnoses and evidence-based treatments for 40 psychiatry patients	
Primary diagnosis (No. patients)	Primary treatment
Alcohol withdrawal (1)	Individualised chlordiazepoxide regimen
Acute schizophrenia (12)	Antipsychotic medication
Chronic schizophrenia (4)	Oral/i.m. antipsychotic medication
Acute mania (3)	Lithium
Bipolar affective disorder prophylaxis (2)	Lithium
Depressive disorder (4)	Antidepressants
Treatment-resistant depression (3)	Lithium augmentation

ing 19 (18%) patients were given treatments without any substantial supporting evidence (e.g. support for stroke or overdoses, treatment of pain). Overall, therefore, 82% of the medical interventions were evidence-based, taking patients rather than procedures as the focus of interest. This apparent discrepancy between procedures or patients can be explained by the simple fact that there are many procedures which have never been evaluated, whereas patients tend to have common diseases which are easier to study and therefore more likely to have been subject to treatment trials. We can take issue with the Ellis and colleagues' approach, or some of the deficiencies of the study – such as potential problems with generalisability, the accuracy of diagnosis, the fact that few patients only have one problem in clinical practice, and that self-evident treatments are not necessarily effective – but the conclusion remains that most medical patients receive treatments backed up by evidence from RCTs. How does psychiatry compare?

Using a similar design, Geddes and colleagues (1996) evaluated the treatments received by 40 consecutive admissions to a general psychiatry ward in Oxford. The main diagnoses and treatments received are shown in Table 31.4. As can be seen from the table, 29 (65%) of these acute admissions received interventions supported by evidence from RCTs or meta-analysis. The other 14 (35%) acute admissions received treatments (usually combinations of medication) for which there was no good evidence of efficacy. This is a small study and subject to the same criticisms as apply to the study of Ellis et al (1995). Moreover, many of the primary trials were small and the study only considered medical interventions: many other interventions are used in multidisciplinary inpatient (and particularly outpatient) settings.

Summers & Kehoe (1996) addressed some of these issues by examining 160 treatment decisions in 158 patients (56 inpatients, 29 daypatients and 75 outpatients). They reported that there was RCT evidence for 85 (53%) of the patient interventions (especially drug treatments), that 16 (10%) of the interventions could not be ethically subject to RCT evaluation (e.g. observation levels in suicide), and that the remaining 59 (37%) patients received supportive practical measures and psychotherapy. Thus, inpatient psychiatric treatment may be more evidence based than outpatient services, but, overall, psychiatry compares reasonably well with acute medicine. There is still a need, however, for further and more all-encompassing assessments of these questions in psychiatry as in other specialties.

PROBLEMS FOR EBM AND EBMH

These studies highlight some of the problems facing EBM, although none are insurmountable. Most of the research done on treatments is conducted on patients with a particular diagnosis and no other comorbid or complicating conditions. This does not reflect the complexities of medical practice and raises questions about whether the results from RCTs apply to all patients. The adjustment of the results obtained from a trial using the PEER and F (see above) are attempts to deal with this, but there is also an increasing recognition of the need for clinical trials which more closely resemble real-life clinical practice. These large-scale *pragmatic* trials aim to include a representative sample of patients rather than highly selected 'super-patients', the standards of interventions are similar to those achievable in (good) clinical practice and outcomes are chosen which are meaningful to patients and clinicians. The science of research synthesis and statistical meta-analysis is complex and sometimes produces results which are inconsistent with subsequent large trials, but it is still in its infancy and methodological advances are occurring rapidly.

EBMH, in particular, probably has a number of other problems to solve (Geddes & Harrison 1997). Clinical diagnoses in psychiatry are reliable if diagnostic criteria are followed but this is probably rare in clinical practice. We need to continue to improve the quality of diagnostic decision making in clinical psychiatric practice (Zarin & Earls 1993). In psychiatry we have very few external validating criteria for diagnosis, so our diagnostic gold standard is the psychiatric interview – and yet symptom elicitation has low reliability unless a structured interview is employed (Mojtabai & Nicholson 1995). RCTs in psychiatry have tended to be small and from single centres. Treatment compliance is more of a problem in psychiatry than medicine, which demands more studies of attempts to increase compliance. We are alone in medicine in facing the problems of trying to treat detained patients against their will and need to find ethically satisfactory ways of including such patients in treatment trials. The RCTs that have been done have used a host of incomparable outcome measures, usually of symptom severity rather than hard, practically relevant, dichotomous outcomes (e.g. recovered or not, employed or not). At the same time, we should not forget that hard end-points used in medical studies (usually death) ignore morbidity and quality of life. Finally, although various talking treatments are supported by RCT evidence, there are likely to be considerable variations in how these are practised clinically and this requires some form of clinical quality control.

THE FUTURE

What can be and needs to be done to promote EBM in

general and EBMH in particular? The agenda could encompass virtually all aspects of medical care from research through to service provision and purchasing, but a few points merit particular mention.

Firstly, EBM itself requires better evidence of its effectiveness. There are clear *a priori* reasons to believe that EBM should lead to optimal patient outcomes, simply because it provides a coherent and consistent approach to helping clinicians ensure that patient care is based on the best available evidence. However, EBM itself has shown that such apparently convincing reasoning may be misguided, and that empirical, randomised evidence of efficacy is required. Moreover, is the time and effort required to practice EBM justified – that is, is EBM cost-effective?

There is some evidence for the effectiveness of specific components of EBM. Medical graduates of universities which offer courses in critical appraisal are more likely to keep up to date than their counterparts in traditional universities, but more work is required on the effects of evidence-based teaching on clinicians and any benefits for their patients.

Second, the numbers of people directly involved should hopefully steadily increase. EBM is most certainly not an elitist pursuit – it depends on the endeavours of too many and requires the help of still more. There is plenty of room, for example, for more contributors to the systematic reviews supervised by the Cochrane Collaboration, for ever-increasing numbers of EBM teachers, and local coordinators at a Trust or Directorate level.

Third, EBM readily identifies critical clinical areas that require further evaluation. As research becomes more responsive to the needs of patients and clinicians, and as clinicians become more skilled at basing their practice on high-quality evidence, it should become easier to coordinate the large-scale, pragmatic trials which are required. Equally as important, however, is the evaluation of the most effective methods of implementation, that is, changing clinical practice according to the evidence. Without this, even the highest quality research becomes irrelevant. Each stage of the process need to be carefully linked – EBM is a form of knowledge management in which high-quality knowledge is produced, disseminated and effectively implemented.

SUMMARY AND CONCLUSIONS

EBM attempts to help doctors to stay abreast of developments in medical research by integrating clinical epidemiology, biostatistics, pathophysiological knowledge and clinical experience. Its underlying rationale is that health care decisions should be based on the best available evidence. For each kind of clinical question it is usually possible to identify the study design most likely to provide the most valid and useful information. Evidence is identified using the most efficient available methods, critically appraised using empirically derived criteria and integrated with clinical practice using meaningful measures and indices.

There are at least four specific advantages of EBM over previous attempts to keep doctors up to date, such as traditional methods of continuing medical education, audit and clinical guidelines:

- It facilitates the incorporation of the best available treatments into clinical practice as soon as there is sufficient evidence for their efficacy.
- It can identify which time and resource consuming medical procedures are required and which are not (and which require further evidence).
- It provides a common language and rules for communicating about effectiveness.
- It shows promise in improving undergraduate education and postgraduate training.

Archie Cochrane criticised psychiatry in 1972 for 'using a large number of therapies whose effectiveness has not been proven', stated 'it is basically inefficient', and suggested increasing 'grants for well-designed evaluatory research'. Some progress has been made in the past 25 years and EBMH could deliver more. EBM offers a way of steadily improving patient care and job satisfaction throughout the average clinical career by replacing the tyranny of haphazard medical informatics with the rigour of a systematically gathered evidence base. Clinical freedom is dead (Hampton 1983) – long live clinical freedom!

REFERENCES

Antman E M, Lau J, Kupelnick B, Mosteller F, Chalmers T C 1992 A comparison of results of meta-analyses of randomized control trials and recommendations of clinical experts. Treatments for myocardial infarction. Journal of the American Medical Association 268: 240–248

Benton M K, Schroder H E 1990 Social skills training with schizophrenics: a meta-analytic evaluation. Journal of Consulting and Clinical Psychology 58: 741–747

Chalmers I, Enkin M, Keirse M J N C 1989 Effective care in pregnancy and childbirth. Oxford University Press, Oxford

Cochrane A 1972 Effectiveness and efficiency: random reflections on health services. Cambridge University Press, Cambridge, (reprinted 1989 by BMJ, London)

Cochrane Collaboration 1995 Cochrane collaboration handbook. Cochrane Collaboration, Oxford

Cochrane Collaboration 1998 The Cochrane library. Update Software, Oxford

Cook R J, Sackett D L 1995 The number needed to treat: a clinically useful measure of treatment effect. British Medical Journal 310: 452–454

Covell D G, Uman G C, Manning P R 1985 Information needs in office practice: are they being met? Annals of Internal Medicine 103: 596–599

Critical Review Paper Working Party 1997 MRCPsych part II examination: proposed critical review paper. Psychiatric Bulletin 21: 381–382

Crombie I K 1996 The pocket guide to critical appraisal. BMJ, London

Daniels M, Hill A B 1952 Chemotherapy of pulmonary tuberculosis in young adults. An analysis of the combined results of three Medical Research Council trials. British Medical Journal 1: 1162

Davis D A, Thomson M A, Oxman A D, Haynes R B 1995 Changing physician performance. A systematic review of the effect of continuing medical education strategies. Journal of the American Medical Association 274: 700–705

Ellis J, Mulligan I, Rowe J, Sackett D L 1995. Inpatient general medicine is evidence-based. Lancet 346: 407–410.

Fairburn C G, Norman P A, Welch S L, O'Connor M E, Doll H A, Peveler R C 1995 A prospective study of outcome in bulimia nervosa and the long-term effects of three psychological treatments. Archives of General Psychiatry 52: 304–312 (summarised in Evidence-Based Medicine 1: 48)

Geddes J R, Harrison P J 1997 Closing the gap between research and practice. British Journal of Psychiatry 171: 220–225

Geddes J R, Game D, Jenkins N E et al 1996 What proportion of primary psychiatric interventions are based on randomised evidence. Quality in Health Care 5: 215–217

Hampton J R 1983 The end of clinical freedom. British Medical Journal 287: 1237–1238

Mann C 1990 Meta-analysis in the breech. Science 249: 476–480

Mari J J, Streiner D 1996 Family intervention for those with schizophrenia. In: Adams C, De Jesus Mari J, White P (eds) Schizophrenia module of *the Cochrane database of systematic reviews* (updated 02 December 1996). Available in *the Cochrane library* (database on disk and CD-ROM). The Cochrane Collaboration, issue 3. Update Software, Oxford, 1996 (see also Psychological Medicine 24: 565–578; Evidence-Based Medicine 1: 121)

Marshall M, Gray A, Lockwood A, Green R 1996. Case management for people with severe mental disorders. In: Adams C, De Jesus Mari J, White P (eds) *module of the Cochrane database of systematic reviews* (updated 02 December 1996). Available in *the Cochrane library* (database on disk and CD-ROM). The Cochrane Collaboration, issue 1. Update Software, Oxford 1997. Updated quarterly. (See also Evidence-Based Medicine 1: 30)

Mason P, Harrison G, Glazebrook C, Medley I, Dalkin T, Croudace T 1995 Characteristics of outcome in schizophrenia at 13 years. British Journal of Psychiatry 167: 596–603

Mojtabai R, Nicholson R A 1995 Interrater reliability of ratings of delusions and bizarre delusions. American Journal of Psychiatry 152: 1804–1806

NHS Centre for Reviews and Dissemination 1996 Undertaking systematic reviews of research on effectiveness. Centre for Reviews and Dissemination, University of York

Oxman A, Guyatt G H 1993 The science of reviewing research. Annals of the New York Academy of Sciences 703: 125–134

Ramsey P G, Carline J D, Inui T S et al 1991 Changes over time in the knowledge base of practicing internists. Journal of the American Medical Association 266: 1103–1107

Sackett D L, Haynes R B, Guyatt G H, Tugwell P 1991 Clinical epidemiology: a basic science for clinical medicine. Little Brown, Boston

Sackett D L, Rosenberg W M, Gray J A, Haynes R B, Richardson W S 1996. Evidence-based medicine: what it is and what it isn't. British Medical Journal 312: 71–72

Sackett D L, Richardson S, Rosenberg W, Haynes R B 1997 Evidence-based medicine: how to practise and teach EBM. Churchill Livingstone, London

Sheldon T A 1996 Research intelligence for policy and practice: the role of the National Health Service Centre for Reviews and Dissemination (EBM note). Evidence-Based Medicine 1: 167–168

Smith M L, Glass G V 1977 Meta-analysis of psychotherapy outcome studies. American Psychologist September: 752–760

Smith R 1991 Where is the wisdom…? British Medical Journal 303: 798–799

Smith R 1996 What clinical information do doctors need? British Medical Journal 313: 1062–1068

Summers A, Kehoe R F 1996 Is psychiatric treatment evidence-based? Lancet 347: 409–410

Zarin D A, Earls F 1993 Diagnostic decision making in psychiatry. American Journal of Psychiatry 150: 197–206

32

Current controversies in psychiatry

Eve C. Johnstone   C. P. L. Freeman

SERVICE DELIVERY Eve C. Johnstone

There is currently much controversy about mental health issues, both among those responsible for psychiatric services and in the public domain. A good deal of this controversy relates to approaches to service provision. It should be no surprise that these issues provoke the interest that they do. Mental health services impose a large burden and they have been subject to more change than virtually any type of health service over the past four decades, both in the UK and in the USA (Rattery 1992). The UK is now in its fifth decade of moving towards a community orientated mental health service, although at the time of writing, the Minister of Health, the Right Honourable Paul Boateng, has just announced a stoppage of closures of mental hospitals. This is understood to be a pause rather than a reversal of the policy, now almost 40 years old, of moving the locus of patient care from large mental hospitals.

The policy of caring for the mentally ill in the UK in large mental hospitals lasted for 150 years. It began with the passage of the Asylum Act in 1808. Numbers of asylums expanded throughout the 19th century and it was not until after the end of the First World War that significant developments took place in the provision of outpatient services and in the later development of treatment facilities for psychiatric patients in general hospitals, made possible by the legislative changes of the Mental Treatment Act of 1930. The Mental Health Act (HMSO, 1959) emphasised the hospital's role as a place for treatment and not merely custody. It placed a duty upon local authorities to provide residential and other services for the mentally ill. In the 1960s and 1970s there had been a number of well-publicised scandals relating to standards of care in mental hospitals. The work of social psychiatrists such as Barton (1959) and Wing & Brown (1961, 1970) had indicated that the circumstances of institutional care could intensify the abnormalities of the patients living in mental hospitals, and the social climate of the 1960s, emphasising personal freedoms and rights, was very much against the imposition of such care.

The 'golden decade' (Ch. 4) from the 1950s to the 1960s, when effective psychotropics of various kinds were introduced, was associated with great therapeutic optimism, and against this background ideas were put forward to the effect that most patients could be discharged from mental hospitals and that no particular provision outside would be required for them (Tooth & Brooke 1961, Taylor 1962). It was made clear that these ideas had been crystallised into government policy when, in 1961, the then Minister of Health, the Right Honourable Enoch Powell, made his famous 'water tower' speech, in which he said there was to be 'nothing less than the total elimination of by far the greater part of the country's mental hospitals ... great isolated institutions which stood ... isolated, majestic, imperious, brooded over by the gigantic water tower and chimney combined'. Instead, patients were to be cared for in wards or wings of general hospitals.

In the almost four decades since then there have been a number of key changes in mental health policy and guidance to accompany the extensive changes in service which have taken place over the years. These have reached a crescendo in the 1990s. Thus the Ministry of Health's *Hospital Plan for England & Wales* (Ministry of Health 1962), predicting that by the 1970s bed requirements would have fallen by 50%, was followed in 1970 by the Local Authority Social Services Bill, which made local authority social services departments responsible for providing personal social services for the mentally ill. The 1975 white paper *Better Services for the Mentally Ill* set out the government's broad objectives of enabling multiprofessional assessment and relocating specialist services to local areas. The Mental Health Act 1983 and the Mental Health (Scotland) Act 1984 brought the legislation relating to the mentally ill closer to the principles of care in the community and reinforced the rights of mentally ill people.

In 1985, the Social Services Committee (DHSS, 1985) restated the elements of a comprehensive district mental health service and referred to poor provision for new long-stay patients, failure to provide new facilities before old ones were closed, and the difficulty of releasing money from hospital closures. These are, of course, themes that have recurred frequently in discussions of the mental health service. After this, the publication of new policy and guidance proceeded apace. The white paper *Caring for People: Community Care in the Next Decade and Beyond* (Department of Health 1989) and the NHS and Community Care Act (HMSO 1990), which was implemented in 1993 and made local authorities the key community care agency, both emphasised that the prime aim was to promote services which supported people in their own homes wherever feasible.

In 1990 NHS guidance in the Care Programme Approach (Department of Health 1990) stated that before patients were discharged from psychiatric hospitals it should be ensured that proper arrangements were made for their return home and for any continuing care. In 1991 the Reed report (Department of Health & Home Office 1991) emphasised that mentally disordered offenders should, if appropriate, receive care and treatment from Health and Social Services rather than in custodial care. The white paper (Department of Health 1992) *The Health of the Nation: A Strategy for Health in England* included among its objectives the reduction of ill-health and death from mental illness, and two of its main targets were to significantly improve the health and social functioning of mentally people and to reduce the suicide rate of severely mentally ill people by at least 33% by the year 2000. The well-meant objectives of these various papers and guidelines had provoked some concern amongst psychiatrists before this, but their confidence in the wisdom of those formulating policy was further weakened by this specific aim, which all might agree was worthy but the means of achievement of which was very much a matter for speculation, even by the best informed.

In 1993 a 10 point plan for developing successful and safe community care for discharged psychiatric patients (Department of Health Press Release H93/908) was announced by the Secretary of State. In 1994 supervision registers for mentally ill people (NHS Executive 1994) were implemented in England and Wales. These required all health authorities to ensure that provider units identify, and give priority to, patients at significant risk of suicide, of doing serious harm to others, or of serious self-neglect. Again, many psychiatrists held the view that while these were aims they might wish to achieve, they did not know how they might set about this successfully. Some of the legislation and guidance was, of course, the result of public concern about the fact that violent incidents involving such behaviour seemed greatly to have increased following the intro-

duction of the policy of community care. Between 1974 and 1988 there was only one independent inquiry in the UK into a homicide by someone with a mental illness. Between 1988 and 1996 there were 26 inquiry reports on homicides and other serious untoward incidents involving people with serious mental illness in England and Wales (11 of them in London) (King's Fund London Commission 1997).

The Ritchie report (Ritchie et al 1994) was highly critical of the case of Christopher Clunis, a man with paranoid schizophrenia who stabbed to death a total stranger on a platform of the London underground railway. Following upon this, the Department of Health issued further guidance on the discharge from hospital of mentally disordered people, emphasising the need to ensure safety and appropriate supervision (NHS Executive 1994). Thereafter, in 1996, the Mental Health Act (Patients in the Community) and the Mental Health Patients' Charter were both published. It will be clear that, as the 1990s progressed, the policy of transferring the locus of care of mentally ill people to the community, preferably to their own homes within that community, was pursued, while at the same time alarm bells were ringing about the major difficulties that could be associated with this policy. As a result of these concerns, numerous directives and notes for guidance were produced exhorting the general aims of achieving high standards of care and ensuring safety, but without practical suggestions as to how these aims could be achieved in the circumstances pertaining and following the general lines of government policy. This situation has been associated with much concern about the running of the psychiatric services and with declining morale in those who work in them.

This general concern has been expressed in several ways. Problems have perhaps been most acute in London and there have been a number of studies of London's health services. In 1992 both the Tomlinson report (1992) and the King's Fund Commission (1992) reported on London's health services in general, although the King's Fund report did not specifically address mental health services. The Tomlinson report emphasised the need to develop fully resourced community teams if community care policies were to work successfully. Following the publication of the Ritchie report (1994) into the case of Christopher Clunis, which was highly critical of the services, a Mental Health Task Force was set up by ministers to report upon London's mental health services (Department of Health 1994, Moore, 1996). This emphasised the need to address pressures on beds, further development of community-based support and better organisation of plans for closure of long-stay hospitals to ensure that timetables were realistic and that beds were not closed before effective alternative facilities were developed.

In 1995 the King's Fund London Commission was set up to further study London's health services, and on this occasion mental health services were included (King's Fund London Commission 1997). Many areas of concern were raised. These included substantial staff shortages in most relevant disciplines and the increasing difficulties of engaging with the services individuals of working age with severe and enduring mental health problems – this applied especially to young men. In the conclusion to this report it was stated that London's mental health services were operating in a manner which could not be allowed to continue without exposing service users, their families and carers to unnecessary risks and placing excessive strain upon staff. While this study concerned London as a whole, major inequalities in the service were found and the worst problems related to deprived city areas. It was considered that similar problems are likely to be found in the deprived parts of other metropolitan areas such as Birmingham, Manchester and Liverpool.

At the same time as these various governmental and other official bodies were reporting upon the mental health services, much attention was also being given to these matters in the mass media. Studies conducted in North America (Day & Page 1986, Matas et al 1986) have shown that in the newspapers the mentally ill are usually portrayed in a negative light, with few positive images. Scott (1994) reviewed the articles on psychiatry in six British national daily papers and their associated Sunday papers over a period of 3 months and found that the average number of articles per newspaper per month was 19. Forensic issues and the association between dangerousness and mental illness were emphasised, and in general mentally ill people and those who care for them were described in a negative way. Barnes & Earnshaw (1993) examined all reports relating to mental illness in the tabloid *Mirror* and the broadsheet *Independent* between October and December 1992. There were 55 in the *Mirror* and 46 in the *Independent*. A reasonable proportion of the articles in the *Independent* were informative accounts about mental illness or reviews of work published in psychiatric journals. By contrast, 71% of the tabloid articles were reports of individual cases. These concerned reports of suicides in noteworthy circumstances or reports of psychotic illness involving violent crime or murder. Those concerning non-psychotic illness linked the disorders to unusual and generally humorous presentations, e.g. 'Bizarre bagpipe phobia baffles doctors'. A majority of the articles relating to doctors in the psychiatric field suggested negligent practice. In these reports, therefore, the mentally ill were portrayed in a consistently negative light, with no positive images, in the tabloid press.

It can scarcely be denied, therefore, that psychiatry has had a bad press, but not all of the blame can be placed upon the media. The reader of, for example, the Ritchie report (1994) on the case of Christopher Clunis is not likely to be able to think of a way to describe the events recounted there in a positive light. None the less, these difficult issues feed upon one another, so that in part the staff shortages (many services in London are said to have levels of agency and non-permanent staff of 20% in all grades, Johnson et al 1997) are thought to relate to the staff feeling poorly supported in a service which is under intense public scrutiny (Johnson et al 1997).

At the time of writing, solutions to these difficulties have not been found, in spite of the extensive guidance that has been offered and the many reports that have been written. The situation is not, of course, entirely new. A number of different approaches to service provision have found favour over the past 300 years and the history of service delivery during that time has been one of circular change. There are few ideas which have not been round at least once before (Allderidge 1979) but, sadly, as each approach has fallen into disrepute (for this is what has happened) there has been a tendency to assume that any change will be for the better (Bennett & Freeman 1991), and little interest has been shown in clarifying the reasons behind the problems that have arisen. Certainly there has been ample scrutiny of the problems on this occasion and perhaps this time lessons will be learned.

The care of psychiatric illness is not easy. The problems associated with the mentally disordered are very distressing ones and there are no easy answers. The medical profession and society in general are, however, having to face these problems rather more directly at present than has been the case for many decades.

ISSUES OF COMORBIDITY Eve C. Johnstone

A very different issue which has had much recent discussion in psychiatric circles is that of comorbidity. As noted in Chapter 10, diagnostic classifications have been intended to divide the generality of patients into discrete groups to offer a guide to rational treatment and accurate prognosis, and to aid research and the advancement of knowledge. The introduction of a multiaxial system in DSM-III in 1980, so that the clinical disorder such as depression or dementia suffered by a patient could be considered at the same time as the question of personality disorder, mental retardation and other medical disorders, encouraged the consideration of comorbidity of clinical disorders such as depression and personality disorders of any kind. As noted in Chapter 27, there has of late been increasing interest in the comorbidity of physical illnesses such as cancer and stroke and clinical psychiatric disorders such as depression. Comorbidity of different clinical psychiatric disorders is increasingly recognised as an important issue. The occurrence of depression in patients with other psychiatric disorders such as schizophrenia (Ch. 13) has already been mentioned, but an issue of particular concern is comorbidity of schizophrenia or other major psychiatric disorder and substance abuse.

The role of some substances of abuse, especially amphetamine, LSD, cocaine and MDMA (Ecstasy), in producing psychotic symptomatology has long been known (e.g. Horowitz 1969, Angrist & Gershon 1970). Although the role of cannabis in this regard is less clear, the idea that there is a 'cannabis psychosis' separate from affective psychoses and schizophrenia has been promoted (Imade & Ebie 1991) and the diagnosis quite widely made. The thinking behind the making of such a diagnosis seemed, at least in part, to relate to the idea that the psychosis might be less serious and the prognosis less pessimistic than if the psychosis occurred in the absence of substance misuse. There is now evidence that the reverse is the case. The use of cannabis among schizophrenic patients is associated with worse psychotic symptoms and earlier and more frequent relapses (Martinez-Arevalo et al 1994). Comorbidity of substance misuse (in this context including alcohol as well as drugs) and schizophrenia – so-called 'dual diagnosis' – has received increasing attention in recent years (Regier et al 1990; Menezes et al 1996). It is clear that both drug misuse and alcohol misuse in schizophrenic patients are associated with a particularly malignant course and worse prognosis (Cantwell & Harrison 1996). The difficulties of engaging schizophrenic young men with comorbid substance abuse and chaotic lifestyles in orthodox psychiatric services are difficult to overestimate, and ensuring compliance with maintenance treatment programmes has proved very difficult indeed. There is an association with homelessness and dual diagnosis of this kind, and even keeping in touch with those affected is far from easy. These individuals are also prone to offending behaviour and have a complexity of needs extending across health, social services, housing benefits and criminal justice systems (King's Fund London Commission 1997). The organisation of such complex programmes of care is a formidable task but one that may need to be undertaken if the current, all too frequent, cycle of psychotic relapse $\longrightarrow$ situational crises + judicial involvement $\longrightarrow$ admission under the Mental Health Act $\longrightarrow$ discharge and loss to follow-up $\longrightarrow$ non-compliance + further substance abuse $\longrightarrow$ psychotic relapse/situational crisis,

is ever to be broken. The mismatch of expectations between these patients and the service, whereby some traditional services find these patients difficult to manage and are reluctant to accept them (Cantwell & Harrison 1996) and some dual diagnosis patients reject the help that they are offered, perceiving it as rigid, inflexible and inappropriate (King's Fund London Commission 1997), is a matter that will require to be addressed.

'RECOVERED MEMORIES' AND 'FALSE MEMORY SYNDROME' C.P. L. Freeman

The explosion of reports about childhood abuse has raised many questions about the nature of memory for traumatic events. The false memory debate has been heated and often abusive and centres on the validity and accuracy of recovered memories. For the purposes of this discussion I will use the definitions quoted in the Royal College of Psychiatrists report (1997).

A 'recovered memory' is one in which traumatic events have been totally forgotten until 'released' or recovered in therapy or as a result of some other trigger or experience. A 'false memory' is one which is not based on events which have occurred. The 'false memory' position is that many, if not all, of the memories that are recovered in the context of therapy are false and are the products of inappropriate therapeutic suggestions. There are two main organisations that promote this view: the False Memory Syndrome Foundation in the USA and the British False Memory Society. The issues for therapists working in this area include the following:

- Can traumatic childhood experiences be completely repressed from memory for very prolonged periods and then be recalled in intricate detail with associated sounds, smells, feelings and images 20, 30 or even 40 years later?
- If such memories appear, are they an accurate recall of early experience or are they subject to the same rules of distortion, forgetting and confabulation that occur with less emotional non-traumatic memory?
- Can grown-up children from apparently well-adjusted families who, for whatever reason, enter therapy have such memories 'implanted' in them by poorly trained, misguided or overenthusiastic therapists?
- How can therapists who work in this area proceed in a way that is safe for them and appropriately therapeutic for their patients?

Some high profile cases have reached the courts. Probably the most well known is that of Gary Ramona, who sued his daughter's psychiatrist, Richard Rose, her counsellor, Marche Isabella, and the hospital where they worked, The Medical Centre, Anaheim, California, USA, for $8m. He charged that they had implanted false memories of sexual abuse in his daughter Holly. Ramona's account was that his previously happy and well-adjusted family had been totally destroyed by his daughter Holly's treatment. She had gone to Isabella for counselling, while at university, for treatment of depression and bulimia. He contended that Isabella had suggested a link between bulimia and sexual abuse and that gradually during treatment false memories of incest were seeded, then amplified and finally became a certainty. He was then confronted by his daughter, his wife and the therapist and accused of sexually molesting his daughter. His wife divorced him, his three teenage daughters refused to speak to him and he later lost his job. Ramona won his case. The jury voted 10 to 2 in his favour and ruled that Holly's memories were probably false, that the therapists may not have implanted the memories but they had clearly reinforced them. They awarded Ramona $475 000 of the $8 m for which he had sued. The case was extensively reported by the False Memory Syndrome Foundation in the USA and hailed as a complete justification of their view. The detailed background to the case is somewhat different (*Guardian* 1994): Holly's memories certainly had been gradually revealed during the early stages of therapy but they had also been shared by her mother. Her mother remembered that as a child Holly had frequently complained that her 'bottom hurts' and that later she had repeated urinary tract infections. She remembered hearing her daughter cry out at night and going into the bedroom and finding her husband standing or lying next to Holly wearing only his underpants, saying that Holly had been having a nightmare. There were other memories like this which did not occur in the context of therapy. Behaviourally, Holly had always shown a terror of men, she always slept with her knees tightly against her chest, and she was stated to have nightmares at school of snakes entering her vagina. She had a terror of gynaecological examinations and even when watching movies avoided any scenes of intimate contact. She also had a sense of doom about the future and a conviction that she would never marry.

The therapists in this case did make some mistakes. They overestimated the prevalence of sexual abuse in patients with eating disorders, which is more like 25% than 75%, and late in the treatment they did use a sodium amytal interview in an attempt to confirm the accounts of abuse that had emerged.

Other court cases have had quite different outcomes. In 1990 a former fireman, George Franklin, was convicted of the murder of an 8-year-old, 20 years previously. This was largely based on the testament of his daughter, Eileen. She told the American court that she had been in her father's van when he had raped her friend and crushed her skull with a rock. She had forgotten this completely for 20 years until the memory was triggered by a particular look from her own daughter. The jury believed her and brought in a murder conviction. A recent documentary highlighted the case of Marilyn Van Derbur Atler, who was Miss America 1958. This was at a time when the Miss America Pageant had such a high profile that its winners became national celebrities, as well known as major film stars. Marilyn appeared to come from the 'perfect' middle-America family and was accompanied by her loving, kind father at all her engagements. At the age of 24 she remembered that she had been systematically abused by her father from the age of 5 until approximately 17. She had lost all memory of this. She disclosed the abuse in her 50s after her father had died. Her account was completely corroborated by her sister who had also been abused but who had never forgotten it.

The nature of memory

There is ample evidence that memory is malleable and prone to distortion. When we think we are remembering something clearly, our remembering is often a combination of memory traces, the context and the setting in which we are remembering, and our current and past experience. Memories for ordinary autobiographical events are not hard-wired. They are flexible, alter with time and alter with subsequent experience. Loftus and colleagues (1989) showed subjects slides of an automobile accident. They demonstrated that it was possible by verbal suggestion to implant things in the image which were not there and that these elements were then clearly remembered and described by subjects. Studies of the explosion of the space shuttle *Challenger*, which was watched live by thousands of individuals, showed many incorrect recollections of events (Neisser & Harsch 1992). Participants' certainty that they were accurate in their recall was not related to actual accuracy. Nevertheless, despite the distortions and inaccuracies, the central features of the memory were accurately retained.

Piaget (1962), the Swiss psychologist, recounted a personal pseudomemory. He had a clear visual memory of someone trying to kidnap him from his pram when he was 2 years old. The memory involved his nanny chasing the potential kidnapper and then coming home and telling Piaget's parents what had happened. Years later, when Piaget was 15, the nanny confessed that the incident had never occurred. She had been deliberately trying to enhance her status as a protector with the family, and yet Piaget had had a clear visual memory of the events.

Hyman and colleagues (1995) demonstrated that they could implant false memories of childhood events in college students. Participants were asked to describe both real and false events, the real events having been supplied by information from parents. Over a series of three interviews, 6% of participants developed vivid pseudomemories of false events. In a later experiment, the same group showed that if participants were asked to imagine these false events in detail, then the rate of vivid pseudomemories increased to 25%. These studies support the view that false memories can be induced, particularly with repeated suggestion, with rehearsal, and with the use of imagery, but that only a small proportion of subjects are vulnerable. In contrast, there is much work showing that traumatic memories may be laid down and remembered quite differently. They appear to be primarily imprinted in sensory and emotional modes and these sensory experiences remain stable over time and are altered by other life experiences (van der Kolk & van der Hart 1991). They may return, triggered by reminders, at any time during a person's life as vividly as if the subject were having the experience all over again. Support for this view comes not just from studying childhood sexual abuse but from repeated studies on other traumas. Psychiatrists studying 'shell shock' during the First World War (Rivers 1918) were struck by this. Sargant & Slater (1941) observed amnesia for trauma of the Dunkirk evacuation in 144 out of 1000 consecutive admissions to a field hospital and described how memories of personal experience relating to extremely traumatic or stressful events could not be retrieved in verbal form.

Semantic memory is primarily symbolic in nature and the usual symbolism used is language. This is the kind of memory that is examined in most day-to-day memory tests. Episodic memory refers to particular autobiographic experiences which involve elements of location, colour, smell, mood and the context of personal experiences. Typically, these memories are of emotionally-laden personal events. In contrast, procedural memory refers to acquired skills and habits, emotional responses, and reflex actions which have no verbal content. These vary from the highly tuned memories that make up a golfer's swing or a tennis player's serve, to traumatic memories that may be encoded in non-verbal form. The most widely quoted minor example of this is that of the French neurologist, Claparede (Claparede (Rapaport) 1951). In 1911, he reported his observations of a woman with Korsakoff's syndrome who consistently had no memory of him, even when he introduced himself repeatedly after short periods of time. Finally, on one introduction, he shook her hand with a drawing pin hidden in the palm of his own hand and pricked her. On the next occasion they met she still had no memory of him but refused to shake his hand. Although she had no conscious memory of Claparede she had some form of memory of the pain caused by the pin-handshake.

Clinical studies of traumatic memories have to some extent confirmed the view that childhood trauma can occur but it can be forgotten and remembered later. Herman & Schatzow (1987) examined 53 women who had sought treatment in an incest survivors' group. The majority of these women reported that at some point in the past they had experienced complete or partial amnesia for their sexual abuse. The amnesia appeared to be related to early onset of the abuse, chronic abuse and the severity of the abuse as characterised by violence or sadism. In an important study, Williams (1994) examined a non-clinical population. These were a group of women who had been treated for sexual abuse 17 years earlier. Of the 129 women in the study, whose age of abuse ranged from infancy to 12 years old, 38% of the adult subjects reported they were amnesiac and had no memory of any childhood abuse or they chose not to report it. Williams concluded that the majority of this 38% did have amnesia for the abuse because they were willing to disclose other intimate details of their lives. They found that greater amnesia was associated with the perpetrators being family members but that it was not correlated with any particular type or severity of abuse. They found that amnesia was greatest for those who had been abused between ages 4 and 6.

Conclusions

Where then do these single case studies, anecdotes, laboratory and clinical studies lead us and what guidance can they give us in the 'false memory debate'? Many of the studies seem contradictory but I think it is possible to arrive at some tentative conclusions.

- Semantic and autobiographical memories are liable to omission, distortion and confabulation and the certainty with which something is 'remembered' is not a good guide to whether it actually happened.
- Highly traumatic memories, whether they occur in childhood or adulthood, may be encoded differently without a clear verbal representation. They may be 'remembered' as bodily sensations, emotional states, smells or sounds and may be difficult to access through verbal means.
- Highly traumatic memories which are continuously remembered and never forgotten may be more resistant to the distortions and omissions described in the first point above.
- Highly traumatic memories which common sense would lead one to think are completely unforgettable

can be completely forgotten and remembered many years later. This process does not just apply to sexual childhood memories.

- How frequently this occurs is not yet clear. It may occur in approximately 25% of cases. Interestingly, this is about the same proportion of individuals who in an acute traumatic situation behave in a chaotic disorganised dissociative way and report acute episodes of amnesia.
- Much of the work on the distortion and fallibility of memory has been carried out on non-emotionally charged or moderately stressful experiences and not on the highly stressful experience of childhood physical or sexual abuse.
- False memories can be created. This does not only occur during the course of therapy but there may be particular therapeutic interventions which make this more likely. It is not known how commonly this occurs or what proportion of individuals are susceptible to it. Experimental work outwith the therapy setting suggests it occurs in only a small minority of individuals.

Guidelines for therapists

Several sets of guidelines have been produced (British Psychological Society 1996, Mollon 1996, Royal College of Psychiatrists 1997). Of these, that of the British Psychological Society is the most useful discussion document. The most disappointing is that produced by the Royal College of Psychiatrists. It consists of a list of defensive procedures which, if adhered to, would make sensible therapy with many patients completely impossible. Its impact has to some extent been mitigated by a helpful review article in the *British Journal of Psychiatry* (Brewin 1996). The assumption in many of these guidelines is that the danger lies in direct questioning, suggestion, and the use of imagery, etc. by the therapist. This, of course, completely misses the point that the very nature of non-directive analytically orientated psychotherapy is designed to produce a 'blank screen' which can be filled by fantasy, speculation and early memory.

It is clear that particular techniques such as sodium amytal interviewing and the use of hypnosis to recover memory should be used with extreme caution, if at all, and that the suggestion that certain diagnoses, such as eating disorders, are strongly associated with childhood abuse is wrong. It is also clear that the assertions of many therapists from Freud onwards have been misguided, overemphatic and probably done much more harm than good in dealing with a very difficult and delicate clinical area. As with most controversies in psychiatry, the most important thing is that we should keep an open mind and not be didactic. This is an area where our knowledge and understanding do need to be extended.

One hundred and three years separates the two quotes below showing that, so far, progress has been rather slow.

Before they come for analysis, the patients know nothing about these scenes. They are indignant as a rule if I warn them that such scenes are going to emerge. Only the strongest compulsion of the treatment can induce them to embark on a reproduction of them (Freud 1896).

I didn't remember anything about the abuse until I was 48 years old. That's when I remembered the incest. Seven or eight years after that, the ritual abuse started breaking through (Annette: Bass & Davis 1989).

REFERENCES

Alldridge P 1979 Hospitals, madhouses and asylums: a history of the York retreat. Cambridge University Press, Cambridge

Angrist B, Gershon S 1970 The phenomenology of experimentally induced amphetamine psychosis – preliminary observations. Biological Psychiatry 2: 95–107

Barnes R C, Earnshaw S 1993 Mental illness in British newspapers. Psychiatric Bulletin 17: 673–674

Barton R 1959 Institutional neurosis. John Wright, Bristol

Bass E, Davis L 1988 The courage to heal: a guide for women survivors of child sexual abuse. Harper Row, New York

Bennett D H, Freeman H L 1991 Community psychiatry. Churchill Livingstone, London

Brewin C R 1996 Scientific status of recovered memories. British Journal of Psychiatry 169: 131–34

British Psychological Society 1996 Symposium on recovered memories. PS Special Publication, Leicester, pp 1–44

Cantwell R, Harrison G 1996 Substance misuse in the severely mentally ill. Advances in Psychiatric Treatment 2: 117–124

Claparede E (Rapaport E) 1951 Recognition and 'me-ness'. In: Rapaport D (ed and trans) Organization and pathology of thought. Columbia University Press, New York. (Original Work published in 1911)

Day D M, Page S 1986 Portrayal of mental illness in Canadian newspapers. Canadian Journal of Psychiatry 31: 813–817

Department of Health 1989 Caring for people: community care in the next decade and beyond. HMSO, London

Department of Health 1990 The care programme approach for people with mental illness referred to specialist psychiatric services. HMSO, London

Department of Health 1992 The health of the nation: a strategy for health in England. HMSO, London

Department of Health 1994 Priorities for action: a report by the mental health task force London project. HMSO, London

Department of Health, Home Office 1991 Review of health and social services for mentally disordered offenders and others requiring similar services. Department of Health, London

Department of Health and Social Security 1985. Government response to the second report from the Social Services Committee 1984–1985 Session, HMSO, London

Freud S 1896 The aetiology of hysteria, Standard edition of the Complete Psychiatric Works of Sigmund Freud edited by J. Strachan in collaboration with Anna Freud, vol III, 1893–1899. Early Psychoaralytic Publications, Hogarth Press, London

Guardian 1994 You must remember this. July 23rd

Herman J L, Schatzow E 1987 Recovery and verification of memories of childhood sexual trauma. Psychoanalytic Psychology 4: 1–4

Horowitz M J 1969 Flashbacks: recurrent intrusive images after the use of LSD. American Journal of Psychiatry 126: 565–569

Hyman I E, Troy T H, Billings F J 1995 False memories of childhood experiences. Applied Cognitive Psychology 9: 181–197

Imade A G T, Ebie J C 1991 A retrospective study of symptom patterns of cannabis induces psychosis. Acta Psychiatrica Scandinavica 83: 134–136

Johnson S, Ramsay R, Thornicroft G (eds) 1997 London's mental health. King's Fund, London

King's Fund 1992 London's health care 2010: changing the future of services in the capital. King's Fund, London

King's Fund London Commission 1997 Transforming health in London. King's Fund, London

Loftus E F, Korf, N L, Schooler J W 1989 Misguided memories: sincere distortions of reality. In: Yuille J C (ed) Credibility assessment. Kluwer, Norwell, MA pp 155–173

Martinez-Arevalo M J, Calcedo-Ordonez A, Varo-Prieto J R 1994 Cannabis consumption as a prognostic factor in schizophrenia. British Journal of Psychiatry 164: 679–681

Matas M, El-Guebaly N, Harper D, Green M, Peterkin A 1986 Mental illness and the media. Canadian Journal of Psychiatry 31: 431–433

Menezes P, Johnson S, Thornicroft G et al 1996 Drug and alcohol problems among individuals with severe mental illness in South London. British Journal of Psychiatry 168: 612–619

Ministry of Health 1962 A hospital plan for England and Wales. Cmnd 1604. HMSO, London

Mollon P 1996 The memory debate: a consideration of clinical complexities and some suggested guidelines for psychoanalytic therapists. British Journal of Psychotherapy 13: 193–203

Moore R 1996 Lessons from the mental health task force London project. In: Thornicroft G, Strathdee G (eds) Commissioning mental health services. HMSO, London

Neisser U, Harsch N 1992 Phantom flashbulb: false recollections of hearing news about the Challenger. In Winograd E, Neisser U (eds) Affect and accuracy in recall. Cambridge University Press, New York, pp 9–31

NHS Executive 1994 Guidance on the discharge of mentally disordered people and their continuing care in the community. HSG (94) 27. HMSO, London

Piaget I 1962 Plays, dreams and imitation in childhood. Norton, New York

Rattery J 1992 Mental health services in transition: the United States and the United Kingdom. British Journal of Psychiatry 161: 589–593

Regier D A, Farmer ME, Rae D S et al 1990 Comorbidity of mental disorders with alcohol and other drug abuse: results from the epidemiological catchment area (ECA) study. Journal of the American Medical Association 264: 2511–2518

Ritchie J H, Dick D, Lingham R 1994 The report of the inquiry into the care and treatment of Christopher Clunis. HMSO, London

Rivers W H R 1918 The repression of war experience. Lancet Feb 2: 173–177

Royal College of Psychiatrists 1997 Reported recurred memories of childhood sexual abuse. Psychiatric Bulletin 21: 663–665

Sargant W, Slater E 1941 Amnesic syndromes in war. Proceedings of the Royal Society of Medicine 34: 757–764

Scott J 1994 What the papers say. Psychiatric Bulletin 18: 489–491

Taylor the Lord 1962 The public, parliament and mental health. In: Richter D, Tanner J M, Taylor the Lord, Zangwill P L (eds) Aspects of psychiatric research. Oxford University Press, Oxford

Terr L C 1991 Childhood traumas: an outline and overview. American Journal of Psychiatry 148: 10–20

Tomlinson B 1992 Report of the inquiry into London's health services, medical education and research. HMSO, London

Tooth G C, Brooke E M 1961 Trends in the mental health population and their effect on future planning. Lancet i: 710–713

van der Kolk B A, van der Hart O 1991 The intrusive past: the flexibility of memory and the engraving of trauma. American Imago 48: 425–454

Williams L M 1994 Recall of childhood trauma: a prospective study of women's memories of child sexual abuse. Journal of Consulting and Clinical Psychology 62: 1167–1176

Wing J K, Brown G W 1961 Social treatment of chronic schizophrenia: a comparative survey of three mental hospitals. Journal of Mental Science 107: 847–861

Wing J K, Brown G W 1970 Institutionalism in schizophrenia. Cambridge University Press, Cambridge

Appendix 1
Mental health legislation and definitions

Lindsay D. G. Thomson

Legislation	Mental Health Act 1983	Mental Health (NI) Order 1986	Mental Health (Scotland) Act 1984	Mental Treatment Act 1945
Definition	England & Wales	Northern Ireland	Scotland	Republic of Ireland
Mental disorder	Mental disorder means mental illness, arrested or incomplete development of mind, psychopathic disorder, and any other disorder or disability of mind	Mental disorder means mental illness, mental handicap and any other disorder or disability of mind	Mental disorder means mental illness or mental handicap however caused or manifested	
Mental illness	—	Mental illness means a state of mind which affects a person's thinking, perceiving, emotion or judgement to the extent that he requires care or medical treatment in his own interests or the interests of other persons.	—	—
Mental impairment	Mental impairment means a state of arrested or incomplete development of mind (not amounting to severe mental impairment) which includes significant impairment of intelligence and social functioning and is associated with abnormally aggressive or seriously irresponsible conduct on the part of the person concerned	—	Mental impairment means a state of arrested or incomplete development of mind, not amounting to severe mental impairment, which includes significant impairment of intelligence and social functioning and is associated with abnormally aggressive or seriously irresponsible conduct on the part of the person concerned	—

Legislation	Mental Health Act 1983	Mental Health (NI) Order 1986	Mental Health (Scotland) Act 1984	Mental Treatment Act 1945
Definition	England & Wales	Northern Ireland	Scotland	Republic of Ireland
Severe mental impairment	Severe mental impairment means a state of arrested or incomplete development of mind which includes severe impairment of intelligence and social functioning and is associated with abnormally aggressive or seriously irresponsible conduct on the part of the person concerned	Severe mental impairment means a state of arrested or incomplete development of mind which includes severe impairment of intelligence and social functioning and is associated with abnormally aggressive or seriously irresponsible conduct on the part of the person concerned	Severe mental impairment means a state of arrested or incomplete development of mind which includes severe impairment of intelligence and social functioning and is associated with abnormally aggressive or seriously irresponsible conduct on the part of the person concerned	—
Psychopathic disorder	Psychopathic disorder means a persistent disorder or disability of mind (whether or not including significant impairment of intelligence) which results in abnormally aggressive or seriously irresponsible conduct on the part of the person concerned	—	— N.B. Mental disorder includes a persistent disorder manifested only by abnormally aggressive or seriously irresponsible conduct	—
Mental handicap	—	Mental handicap means a state of arrested or incomplete development of mind which includes significant impairment of intelligence and social functioning	—	—
Severe mental handicap	—	Severe mental handicap means a state of arrested or incomplete development of mind which includes severe impairment of intelligence and social functioning	—	—
Exclusions from detention	Persons suffering from mental disorder by reason only of promiscuity or other immoral conduct, sexual deviancy, or dependence on alcohol or drugs	Persons suffering from mental disorder by reason only of personality disorder, promiscuity, or other immoral conduct, sexual deviancy or dependence on alcohol or drugs	Persons suffering from mental disorder by reason only of promiscuity or other immoral conduct, sexual deviancy, or dependence on alcohol or drugs	—

Legislation	Mental Health Act 1983	Mental Health (NI) Order 1986	Mental Health (Scotland) Act 1984	Mental Treatment Act 1945
Definition	England & Wales	Northern Ireland	Scotland	Republic of Ireland
Persons of unsound mind	—	—	—	Undefined
Addict	—	—	—	Addict is a person who: (a) by reason of his addiction to drugs or intoxicants is either dangerous to himself or others, or incapable of managing himself or his affairs, or of ordinary proper conduct; or (b) by reason of his addiction to drugs, intoxicants or perverted conduct is in serious danger of mental disorder

— Term not in Act/Order or undefined

Mental Health Act 1983: Part II Compulsory Admission to Hospital (England and Wales)

Purpose	Section	Grounds for detention	Duration	Signatories/ applicant	Appeal
Admission for assessment	2	• Mental disorder • Patient's health or safety/ protection of others • Requires hospitalisation for assessment	28 days	Two doctors (one approved) /nearest relative or approved social worker	Mental Health Review Tribunal • application by patient
Admission for treatment	3	• Mental illness, (severe) mental impairment & psychopathic disorder makes hospital treatment appropriate • If psychopathic disorder or mental impairment, such treatment is likely to alleviate or prevent deterioration of the condition • Necessary for patient's health or safety or for protection of others and it cannot be provided unless detained	6 months, renewable for a further 6 months and subsequently yearly	Two doctors (one approved)/ nearest relative or approved social worker	Mental Health Review Tribunal • application by patient, nearest relative or by hospital managers as prescribed in the Act
Emergency admission	4	• Mental disorder • Patient's health or safety, protection of others • Requires urgent hospitalisation for assessment	72 hours	One doctor/ nearest relative or approved social worker	None
Emergency detention of patient in hospital	5(2)	• It appears that an application for admission to a hospital should be made	72 hours	Doctor in charge or nominated deputy/none	None
Nurse's holding power	5(4)	• Mental disorder • Patient's health or safety/ protection of others • Requires to be immediately restrained from leaving hospital • Not practicable to obtain doctor immediately for Section 5(2)	6 hours	Nurse of the prescribed class/ none	None

Detention can proceed from S.4/S.5(2)→S.2→S.3 or commence with S.2 or S.3.
Detention can be terminated at any stage by the Responsible Medical Officer (RMO), hospital managers, nearest relative (if not opposed by the RMO); or following appeal, by the Mental Health Review Tribunal.

Mental Health (Scotland) Act 1984: Part V Compulsory Admission to Hospital

Purpose	Section	Grounds for detention	Duration	Signatories/consent	Appeal
Emergency admission	24	• Mental disorder • Patient's health or safety/or protection of others • Requires hospitalisation urgently	72 hours	One fully registered doctor/relative or Mental Health Officer if practicable	None
Emergency detention of patient in hospital	25(1)	• Mental disorder • Patient's health or safety/or protection of others • Requires ongoing hospitalisation urgently	72 hours	One fully registered doctor/relative or Mental Health Officer if practicable	None
Emergency detention of patient in hospital	25(2)	• Mental disorder • Patient's health or safety /or protection of others • Requires to be immediately restrained from leaving hospital • Not practicable to secure immediate attendance of a doctor for the purpose of making an emergency recommendation	2 hours or until arrival of doctor with power to make an emergency recommendation	Nurse of the prescribed class	None
Short term detention	26	• Mental disorder of a nature or degree to make hospital detention appropriate • Patient's health or safety/or protection of others	28 days (further to S.24 or S.25(1))	Approved doctor/nearest relative or Mental Health Officer	To Sheriff or Mental Welfare Commission
To extend S.26 if S.18 not applied for and patient suddenly deteriorates	26A	• Mental disorder • Detained under S.26 • Intention to lodge application for S.18	3 working days	Approved doctor/nearest relative or Mental Health Officer	To Sheriff or Mental Welfare Commission
Non-urgent admission or ongoing detention	18	• Mental disorder of a nature and degree which makes it appropriate to receive medical treatment in hospital; (1) in the case where the mental disorder is a persistent one manifested only by abnormally aggressive or seriously irresponsible conduct, such treatment is likely to alleviate or prevent a deterioration of his condition; or (2) in the case where the mental disorder from which he suffers is a mental handicap, the handicap comprises mental impairment (where such treatment is likely to alleviate or prevent a deterioration of his condition) or severe mental impairment; and • it is necessary for the patient's health or safety or for the protection of other people that he should receive such treatment and it cannot be provided unless he is detained	6 months, renewable for a further 6 months and subsequently yearly	Two doctors (one approved); application by nearest relative or Mental Health Officer; Sheriff's approval	To Mental Welfare Commission; to Sheriff if detention extended after 6 months

Detention can proceed from S.24/S.25 → S.26 (→ S.26A) → S.18 but a S.24/S.25 or S.26 cannot be reapplied during this process. In a non-urgent situation a direct application is made to the sheriff court for an S.18. Detention can be terminated at any stage by the Responsible Medical Officer (RMO), hospital managers or nearest relative (if not opposed by the RMO); or following appeal, by a Sheriff or the Mental Welfare Commission.

Mental Health (Northern Ireland) Order 1986: Part II Compulsory Admission to Hospital

Purpose	Article	Grounds for detention	Duration	Signatories/applicant	Appeal
Admission for assessment	4	• Mental disorder • Substantial likelihood of serious physical harm to self or others • Requires hospitalisation	7 days with possible extension to 14 days	One doctor in community, one hospital doctor on admission and RMO (if RMO not admitting doctor)/nearest relative or approved social worker	Mental Health Review Tribunal
Assessment of patients already in hospital	7(2)	• It appears that an application for assessment ought to be made	48 hours	One hospital doctor/none	None
Nurse's holding power	7(3)	• Mental disorder • Requires an application for assessment • Not practicable to secure immediate attendance of doctor	6 hours	Nurse of the prescribed class/none	None
Detention for treatment	12	• Mental illness or severe mental impairment • Substantial likelihood of serious physical harm to self or others • Requires hospitalisation	6 months, renewable for a further 6 months and subsequently yearly	RMO or if the patient is detained for more than one year, RMO and one doctor approved by the Commission/nearest relative or approved social worker	Mental Health Review Tribunal – automatic if patient detained for >2 years

Detention can proceed from Article 7(3) if required→A.7(2) if required→A.4→A.12.
Detention can be terminated at any stage by the Responsible Medical Officer (RMO), the Responsible Board or nearest relative (if not opposed by the RMO); or following appeal, by the Mental Health Review Tribunal.

Mental Treatment Act 1945 Republic of Ireland: Compulsory Admission to Hospital

Purpose	Section	Grounds for detention	Duration	Signatories/applicant	Appeal
Admission for treatment	184	• Mental illness, addiction • Unfit to be treated as a voluntary patient • Requires hospitalisation	6 months, renewable every 6 months up to a maximum of 2 years	Two doctors, one being the receiving consultant/nearest relative or involved social worker	The High Court (habeas corpus) The Minister for Health

Detention is terminated when the patient is discharged; or following a successful appeal.

Appendix 2
Electroconvulsive therapy

C. P. L. Freeman

EVIDENCE FOR THE EFFICACY OF ECT IN VARIOUS DISORDERS

Depressive illness

There is overwhelming evidence that ECT is an effective treatment for severe depressive illness, particularly psychotic depressions for which it is the most effective and rapidly acting treatment available. In the 1960s there were several large studies which compared ECT with different antidepressant drugs and with placebo tablets. These studies were double blind as far as the drug treatments were concerned but not for the comparison between ECT and drug. Wechsler et al (1965) reviewed 153 studies on a total of nearly 6000 patients where drugs and ECT had been compared. Percentage figures for overall improvement with different treatments were as follows: ECT 72%; tricyclics 65%; monoamine oxidase inhibitors 50%; and placebo tablets 23%. Two large multicentre trials were published in the mid-1960s. In the USA Greenblatt et al (1964) reported a trial on depressed patients admitted to three state hospitals in Greater Boston. Assessment was made at the end of 8 weeks and ECT was significantly more effective than all other treatments. In the UK the Medical Research Council trial (Medical Research Council Clinical Psychiatry Committee 1965) of the treatment of depressive illness compared ECT with imipramine, phenelzine and placebo. Percentages of patients with no or only slight symptoms were as follows: ECT 71%, imipramine 52%; phenelzine 30%; and placebo 39%. An interesting finding in this study was the sex difference between treatments. ECT was clearly more effective than all drug treatments in women, but in men ECT and imipramine were equally effective and both superior to phenelzine and placebo. When the patients were followed up for a further 6 months it was found that about half the imipramine non-responders recovered completely when given a course of ECT.

There have been six such studies in the last 15 years, all carried out in the UK. The results are summarised in Table Appendix 2.1. Five of these studies showed a clearly positive result in favour of real ECT, thus refuting the argument that ECT works because it is a powerful placebo. The one study that showed no difference was on a small number of patients and a unilateral brief pulse stimulus was used.

What is also clear from these studies is that improvement does occur with 'sham' or simulated ECT, at least in the short term. Unfortunately, none of the studies have included a rigorously controlled follow-up period and subjects have gone on to have further ECT and/or antidepressant drugs so that comparisons of the relative efficacy of real versus sham ECT several weeks after the end of treatment cannot be drawn.

Predictors of response to ECT in depression

Although a number of trials were carried out in the 1960s looking for clinical features which might be associated with a good response to ECT, it is not possible to say with any certainty that there are particular symptoms that predict good response and others that predict poor response. As a general rule, the more symptoms of classical 'endogenous' depression the depressed patient has, the more likely he is to respond; so that a cluster of symptoms such as severe depression, diurnal variation of mood, early morning wakening, loss of weight, loss of appetite and libido would indicate a likely good response. Two particular symptoms, retardation and depressive delusions, respond well to ECT and there is good evidence that patients with depressive delusions are more likely to fail to respond to tricyclic drugs. In the Northwick Park trial (Johnstone et al 1980), delusions were the most consistent predictor of response and, in those patients who had both delusions and retardation, retardation by itself did not predict response when this overlap was allowed for. Those features of illness which are said to predict poor response to the treatment such as hypochondriacal symptoms, ill-adjusted personality, neurotic traits and a fluctuating course to the illness may be associated with a poor response to all physical methods of treatment rather

Table Appendix 2.1   Recent trials of real versus simulated ECT

Reference	Number of patients	Groups compared	Stimulus	Rate of ECT	Outcome
Freeman et al (1978)	20 + 20	Bilateral temporal versus simulated for first two treatments then real for both groups	Sine wave	6 (2/week)	Significantly more rapid onset of response noted in simulated group, who also needed more treatments
Lambourn & Gill (1978)	16 + 16	Unilateral temporal versus simulated	Brief pulse	6 (3/week)	No difference between groups, both improved
West (1981)	11 + 11	Bilateral temporal versus simulated	Sine wave	6 (2/week)	Clear differences in favour of real ECT
Johnstone et al (1980)	35 + 35	Bilateral frontal versus simulated	Sine wave	8 (2/week)	Both groups showed steady improvement. Real group significantly greater improvement but accounted for mainly by deluded depressives. No difference between groups at I month follow-up
Brandon et al (1984)	42 + 53	Bilateral temporal versus simulated	Sine wave	8 (2/week)	Clear superiority of real ECT
Gregory et al (1985)	23 + 23 + 23	Bilateral temporal (Lancaster) versus simulated	Sine wave	Varied (2/week)	Bilateral superior to unilateral. Both superior to simulated

than to ECT in particular. Abrams & Vedak (1991) reported on 47 men given ECT for melancholia. No clinical predictors were found, suggesting that once patients with non-melancholic depression are excluded the ability to predict response from clinical features is lost. There was still sufficient variability in outcome to allow predictors to emerge but none of the core features of melancholia either alone or in clusters did so.

Effects of ECT on memory

Does ECT cause brain damage?   This topic has been extensively reviewed, Weiner (1984). There is no evidence from animal work in monkeys, cats or rats that ECT even though given in an unmodified form and at a

frequency and number greater than customary in clinical practice causes any neuropathological changes.

Selective brain damage including actual neuronal loss and gliosis can occur in the hippocampus but only following sustained generalised seizure activity lasting more than 90 minutes, multiple brief recurrent seizures (more than 26 in 8 hours) or sustained continuous limbic seizures (lasting longer than 3–5 hours). None of these conditions is likely to occur in clinically given ECT. Some early studies did show petechial haemorrhages but these were a consequence of the increase in arterial and central venous pressure associated with unmodified seizures. A recent description of the normal post mortem findings of a patient who had had 1250 treatments underlines these conclusions. There is, however, an important distinction between gross structural damage as revealed by routine neuropathology, computerised tomography (CT) or MRI and functional change of a more subtle kind. It is certainly not possible at this time to say that neurochemical and/or neurophysiological changes such as alteration in protein synthesis do not occur. Such changes might well form the basis of the enduring cognitive impairment that some patients experience.

Memory impairment is by far the most important undesirable effect of ECT. The interaction between depression, which also causes cognitive impairment, and ECT is complex and it is convenient to consider impairment of memory in four areas separately:

1. Short-term retrograde amnesia (0–3 months)
2. Retrograde amnesia for remote events
3. Short-term anterograde amnesia (0–3 months)
4. Long-term or permanent anterograde amnesia.

Short-term retrograde amnesia Some patients experience a retrograde amnesia for events leading up to and during a course of ECT. There may be complete amnesia for a few minutes or hours before each treatment, though many patients can remember events right up until the anaesthetic quite clearly. Patchy amnesia may stretch back in time for several weeks, but it should be remembered that such forgetfulness is also very common in severely depressed patients who do not receive ECT.

Such retrograde impairment is not usually distressing and may be welcomed by the patient for helping him to forget the painful experience of his illness.

Retrograde amnesia for remote events Testing personal remote memories is extremely difficult as each individual's experience is unique and standardised tests are impossible to construct. Some patients certainly do complain of gaps or holes in their memory stretching back several years. Squire & Chase (1981) have shown that B/ECT in particular may effect memory over the previous decade and that patchy loss of memory for some personal events, television programmes or major news items may occur.

Weiner (1986) has shown that B/ECT can produce long-term impairment of personal memories irrespective of whether a sine wave or pulsed stimulus is used, but that the combination of bilateral electrode placement with high-energy sine wave stimuli produced the greatest impairment.

Short-term anterograde amnesia There is usually some degree of anterograde amnesia, especially if the patient is confused after treatment. More importantly, some patients show difficulty in retaining new learning for a few days or even a few weeks after the course of ECT finishes. Clinicians should be aware of this and

appreciate that some patients may find it hard to remember phone numbers, messages, shopping lists, etc., for a few weeks after a course of ETC. There have been two large studies, by Weeks et al (1980) and Johnstone et al (1980), which have studied the magnitude and duration of cognitive impairment. Both are in agreement that such impairment is common but short lived. After 3 months of ECT treatment there is no impairment whatsoever. It must be remembered that depressive illness itself has a profound effect on cognitive function. Thus, patients' subjective complaints may be related as much to the memory impairment caused by depression as to that caused by ECT. Secondly, studies which show that patients do as well on cognitive tests after ECT as they did before do not necessarily show that ECT does not cause impairment. It may be that, as treatment progresses and depression lifts, cognitive impairment due to depression is replaced by cognitive impairment due to ECT. Both studies quoted above had control groups of either non-ECT treated depressives or depressives treated by simulated ECT to control for this factor.

There is overwhelming evidence that U/ECT given to the non-dominant hemisphere causes fewer side-effects, particularly less memory impairment and less post-ECT confusion. It is also clear that U/ECT must be given to the non-dominant hemisphere. When Halliday et al (1968) gave dominant-hemisphere ECT they found greater impairment on tests of verbal learning than occurred with B/ECT.

Long-term permanent anterograde amnesia The studies discussed so far compare groups of patients and show no permanent changes in memory and cognitive function due to ECT when treated and untreated groups are compared. It is more difficult to demonstrate that ECT does not cause impairment in an occasional individual. It is almost impossible to know in an individual patient who complains of permanent memory impairment after ECT whether the treatment really was responsible. It may be that because ECT affects memory in the short term it sensitises patients to further lapses in memory which would otherwise go unnoticed. Freeman et al (1980) examined a group of self-selected patients who were convinced their memories had been impaired by ECT. Some impairment was indeed found and there was no evidence of faking. Much of this impairment could be accounted for by continuing psychiatric symptomatology, drug and alcohol use. However, there remained some residual impairment which may have been due to ECT. All patients had had B/ECT, some of them many years previously. The degree of impairment was not related to the number of ECT treatments.

The question of long-term memory impairment must

for the time being remain an open one. If it does occur it appears to be mild and infrequent. The sort of complaints that patients have are of holes in their memory going back several years before ECT and/or a decreased ability to retain new learning over a period of several years after ECT. There is no evidence at present to implicate U/ECT in such a way.

The work of Ottosson (1960) suggests that when memory impairment does occur it is mainly due to the amount of electrical energy delivered to the patient's brain rather than to the magnitude or duration of the epileptic fit. Hamilton et al (1979) claimed that the degree of memory impairment following ECT is positively correlated with the magnitude of the associated rise in blood pressure and postulate that it may be the increased permeability of the blood–brain barrier which mediates this effect.

Other side-effects

The most common other side-effects are headache, post-ECT confusion and muscle aches and pains (Table Appendix 2.3). Although headache is quite common it is rarely troublesome and is well tolerated by patients.

The electrical stimulus

Most older ECT machines deliver a biphasic sinusoidal wave form with a frequency of 50 or 60 Hz, which is very little different from alternating current mains. This is not a particularly physiological stimulus and all the more recent machines deliver a string of high-voltage very brief direct current pulses, each pulse lasting between 1 and 2 ms, with 60–70 pulses being given per second. With this technique much less electrical energy is passed across the brain and Valentine et al (1968)

and Weaver et al (1977) have shown that fits can be as reliably induced as with conventional sine wave stimuli. All Royal College of Psychiatrists approved ECT machines give brief pulse stimuli and have a wide range of treatment settings.

The amount of electrical energy delivered to the brain varies considerably with different wave forms. The ranges given by manufacturers are only approximate as the interelectrode resistance (mainly the resistance of the patient's head) varies considerably.

Most of the electrical energy is dissipated in a series of shunts through skin, connective tissue and blood vessels and only a fraction passes through grey and white matter.

Seizure threshold determination The seizure threshold varies from patient to patient over a 40-fold range and stimulus dosing is a recently introduced technique to try and determine this threshold. This is important because stimuli marginally above the seizure threshold may be less effective than those at a higher intensity, particularly if brief-pulse U/ECT is used. The technique involves starting with what will almost certainly be a subthreshold stimulus and then at the same session increasing the stimulus intensity in stages until a seizure occurs. The technique does not appear to cause greater cognitive impairment or a higher rate of abortive or inadequate seizures. Seizure threshold determination is usually only required at the first treatment. If missed seizures occur during a course, restimulation is applied as described below.

How to tell if a fit has occurred

The most reliable way is to use EEG monitor, and most of the currently produced American machines have this facility. These machines have a simple one- or two-channel electroencephalograph which is automatically disconnected when the treatment stimulus is applied and can accurately measure the number of seconds of fitting that the treatment induces. There is some doubt that such single-channel recording is adequate, especially when electrodes are placed frontally, as there is much interference from frontalis muscle activity. Simple observation of the patient is probably unreliable in some cases though several studies have shown high correlations between careful clinical observation and EEG measures. The former tend to give fit length about 10 seconds shorter. The American Psychiatric Association has recommended that EEG monitoring should be routine. The facility for monitoring should be available for occasional patients. Unfortunately, no European-made machines have this facility. The muscle twitching that occurs with suxamethonium depolarisation can be mistaken for the clonic phase of a fit and

Table Appendix 2.3 Side-effects related to ECT (subjective complaints of patients)[a]			
Symptom	Total reported symptoms (%)	Severe	Mild
Memory impairment	64	27	37
Headache	48	19	29
Confusion	27	9	18
Clumsiness	9	4	5
Nausea/vomiting	5	3	2
Other side-effects	12		

From Freeman et al (1980).
[a]Only 20% reported no side-effects at all.

occasionally the patient is completely paralysed so that no external evidence of fitting can be seen. A simple technique can be used to overcome this problem. This involves isolating one forearm by inflating a blood pressure cuff to above systolic pressure before the muscle relaxant is given. The isolated forearm does not become paralysed and fitting can easily be observed in that limb. This has the advantage that, in the elderly or frail, the dose of muscle relaxant becomes less critical and patients can be completely paralysed yet fitting can still be observed. When U/ECT is given, the cuff should be applied to the ipsilateral forearm. It is thus possible to check that bilateral fitting has occurred.

What to do if no fitting ensues

Occasionally during the course of administering ECT a stimulus is applied but no fit is observed. The psychiatrist then has just a few seconds to decide whether to give a further stimulus before the patient comes round from the anaesthetic. The following routine should be employed:

1. Check with all members of the ECT team that no signs of a fit occurred. If a unilateral or localised fit was induced you may have missed it but it may have been seen by other observers. Because the fit threshold rises after a fit, there is no point in trying to induce a maximal seizure with a second stimulus.
2. Ask the anaesthetist to ventilate the patient with pure oxygen. This lowers the fit threshold. This should be for at least 20–30 inhalations.
3. Check that the electrode sites are well prepared, especially if the patient's hair is covered in insulating hair lacquer.
4. Check that the interelectrode space is dry and that the electrodes were spaced sufficiently far apart.
5. Increase the machine's settings by 25%.
6. Apply a second stimulus using very firm pressure on the electrodes.
7. If there is still no fit, do not repeat the stimulus; make a clear note in the ECT record that no fit has occurred.
8. Ask the doctor in charge to check the patient's medication. Although many psychiatric drugs are epileptogenic, some such as chlordiazepoxide, diazepam and the rest of the benzodiazepines are antiepileptic. Stop all such medication before the next ECT session.
9. At the next session make sure that the patient is well oxygenated, use a higher setting if available on the ECT machine and use the tourniquet technique to check if a fit has occurred.

10. Premedication with caffeine may be suitable for some patients or switch to different anaesthetic agent such as ketamine or etomidate.

A very small proportion of patients will not fit during ECT unless a very large or prolonged stimulus is given. If this is the case it is worth checking the thickness of the skull table with lateral skull radiography and placing the electrodes over the thinnest area. It may also be worth prescribing a small dose of a phenothiazine several hours before ECT in an attempt to lower the fit threshold.

What is an adequate fit?

The figure of 25 seconds is often quoted as the minimum length for an effective seizure. There is little or no evidence for this. In general, seizure length is not correlated with outcome but it may be that a fit of 25 seconds or greater is some rough guide that sufficient current has been passed or that deep structures have been stimulated. In routine clinical practice it seems reasonable to restimulate if a short fit occurs. If a fit lasts longer than 120 seconds, preparation should be made to terminate it before it goes over 180 seconds using either a further dose of barbiturate anaesthesia or intravenous diazepam. Long fits may be associated with cerebral hypoxia and marked cognitive impairment.

Number and frequency of treatments

A set number of treatments should not be prescribed. The patient should be assessed after each treatment to see if further ECT is necessary. A few patients respond dramatically to one or two applications of ECT and further treatments are unnecessary; some patients need as many as 10–12, though most respond to a course between four and eight. There is some evidence that older patients require more treatments and that response to the initial two treatments is highly correlated with overall change at the end of the course. Barton et al (1973) showed there was no prophylactic value in giving extra ECT after symptomatic improvement in the hope of preventing relapse. He also showed that if relapses do occur they tend to occur early, 69% developing within 2 weeks. Clinically then it is important to monitor a patient's condition carefully for 2 or 3 weeks, but only to give additional treatments if symptoms recur. The most difficult clinical decision is what stage to abandon ECT if it is not relieving symptoms. If there has been no change at all in the patient's depressive symptoms after six to eight treatments, the course should be stopped. Some patients appear to show a brief response early in a course but relapse quickly.

In such patients it is worth giving a course of up to 10 ECT treatments.

Treatment should be given two or three times a week. At present there is no convincing evidence that giving daily ECT produces more rapid recovery, and memory impairment is more severe. Once-weekly ECT may be indicated for elderly patients with marked post-treatment confusion or for patients who have brief hypomanic episodes during treatment. If a sustained hypomanic mood change is induced, the course should be stopped. Stromgren (1975) has reported that giving four unilateral treatments per week as compared with two unilateral treatments per week reduced the total treatment time by a mean of 11 days, though one or two more treatment applications were required. Memory impairment and other side-effects were not increased.

Maintenance (continuation ECT)

The term continuation refers to the use of ECT on a regular basis after the acute course. For example, after a course of say eight, twice-weekly ECT, the patient is moved to once-weekly and then once-fortnightly ECT for the next three months with no gap between the acute course and the continuation treatment. The main purpose of the continuation ECT is the prevention of early relapse after successful treatment with an acute course. It is not simply a very prolonged series of treatments. It should not be used unless there has been a definite and clinically relevant anti-depressant response.

The term maintenance ECT refers to the use of ECT in the longer term as a prophylactic treatment to prevent recurrence. Maintenance ECT is usually given every two, three or four weeks. It would appear that providing maintenance ECT is given bi-weekly or less frequently there is no progressive rise in seizure threshold, nor any cumulative effect on cognitive function.

Continuation ECT should be considered when:

1. The index episode of illness responded well to ECT
2. There is early relapse despite adequate continuation drug treatment or an inability to tolerate continuation drug treatment.
3. The patient's attitude and circumstances are conducive to safe administration.

Continuation ECT can be given safely to out-patients as long as the guidelines for out-patient ECT in the ECT Handbook are observed.

There has been renewed interest in main/ECT in the last few years. There have still been no controlled trials but there are numerous descriptive reports. Several studies have compared main/ECT with main/ECT refusers and all show marked reduction in relapse rates with main/ECT. A number of studies have shown that relapse rates after acute treatment with ECT are high even when adequate antidepressant medication is maintained. Godber et al (1987) followed up 163 elderly depressed patients (mean age 76 years) treated with ECT. Follow-up was up to 3 years and in that time 73% of patients experienced one or more relapses. Main/ECT may be indicated particularly in depressed elderly patients in whom other types of prophylactic treatment have failed or when drug treatment cannot be used because of adverse effects. All 12 of the reports that the author has found in the literature, ranging from 1949 to 1990, have shown advantages for main/ECT in terms of fewer episodes of depression, greater improvement and fewer relapses. There would now appear to be sufficient evidence for a properly controlled clinical trial.

REFERENCES

Abrams R, Vedak C 1991 Prediction of ECT response in melancholia. Convulsive Therapy 7(2): 81

Barton J L, Mehta S, Snaith R P 1973 The prophylactic value of ECT in depressive illness. Acta Psychiatrica Scandinavica 49: 386–392

Brandon S, Cowley P, McDonald C, Neville P, Palmer R, Wellstood-Eason S 1984 Electroconvulsive therapy: results in depressive illness from the Leicestershire trial. British Medical Journal 288: 23–25

Devanard D P, Dwork A T, Hutchison E R et al 1994 Does ECT alter brain structure? American Journal of Psychiatry 151: 957–970

Freeman C P L 1995 The ECT handbook. The Second Report of the Royal College of Psychiatrists' Special Committee on ECT. Royal College of Surgeon's Council Report 39, Jan 1995, London

Freeman C P L, Weeks D, Kendell R E 1980 ECT: patients who complain. British Journal of Psychiatry 137: 17–25

Godber C, Rosenvinge H, Wilkinson D et al 1987 Depression in old age: prognosis after ECT. Geriatric Psychiatry 2: 19

Gregory S, Shawcross C R, Gill D 1985 The Nottingham ECT study: a double blind comparison of bilateral, unilateral and simulated ECT in depressive illness. British Journal of Psychiatry 146: 520–524

Greenblatt M, Grosser G H, Wechsler H 1964 Differential response of hospitalised depressed patients to somatic therapy. American Journal of Psychiatry 120: 935–943

Halliday A M, Davison K, Browne M W, Kreeger L C 1968 A comparison of the effects on depression and memory of bilateral ECT and unilateral ECT to the dominant and non-dominant hemispheres. British Journal of Psychiatry 114: 997–1012

Hamilton M, Stocker M J, Spencer C M 1979 Post ECT cognitive defect and elevation of blood pressure. British Journal of Psychiatry 135: 77–78

Johnstone E C, Deakin J F W, Lawlor P, Frith C D, Stevens M, McPherson K, Crow T J 1980 The Northwick Park ECT trial. Lancet ii: 1317–1320

Lambourn J, Gill D 1978 A controlled comparison of

simulated and real ECT. British Journal of Psychiatry 133: 514–519

Medical Research Council Clinical Psychiatry Committee 1965 Clinical trial of the treatment of depressive illness. British Medical Journal i: 881–886

Ottosson J O 1960 Experimental studies of the mode of action of electroconvulsive therapy. Acta Psychiatrica et Neurologica Scandinavica suppl 145

Squire L R, Miller P L 1981 Retrograde amnesia and bilateral electroconvulsive therapy. Archives of General Psychiatry 38: 89–95

Stromgren L S 1975 Therapeutic results in brief interval unilateral ECT. Acta Psychiatrica Scandinavica 52: 246

Valentine M, Keddie K M G, Dunne D 1968 A comparison of techniques in electroconvulsive therapy. British Journal of Psychiatry 114: 989–996

Weaver L A, Ives J D, Williams R, Nies A 1977 A comparison of standard alternating current and low energy brief pulse electrotherapy. Biological Psychiatry 12: 525–543

Wechsler H, Grosser G H, Greenblatt M 1965 Research evaluating antidepressant medications on hospitalised mental patients: a survey of published reports during a five year period. Journal of Nervous and Mental Disease 141: 231–239

Weiner R D 1984 Does electroconvulsive therapy cause brain damage? Behaviour and Brain Science 7: 1–54

Weiner R D, Rodgers H J, Davidson J R T, Squire L R 1986 Effects of stimulus parameters on cognitive side effects. Annals of the New York Academy of Sciences 462

West E 1981 Electro-convulsion therapy in depression: a double-blind controlled trial. British Medical Journal 282: 355–357

Index